THE
UNBORN
PATIENT

THE UNBORN PATIENT

The Art and Science of Fetal Therapy

THIRD EDITION

MICHAEL R. HARRISON, M.D., F.A.C.S., F.A.A.P.
Professor of Surgery and Pediatrics
Director, The Fetal Treatment Center
Chief, Division of Pediatric Surgery
University of California, San Francisco
San Francisco, California

MARK I. EVANS, M.D.
Professor and Chairman of
Obstetrics and Gynecology
Professor of Human Genetics
Director, Center for Fetal Therapy
MCP/Hahnemann University
Philadelphia, Pennsylvania

N. SCOTT ADZICK, M.D.
C. Everett Koop Professor
of Pediatric Surgery
University of Pennsylvania
School of Medicine
Surgeon-in-Chief and
Director, The Center for Fetal Diagnosis
and Treatment
Children's Hospital of Philadelphia
Philadelphia, Pennsylvania

WOLFGANG HOLZGREVE, M.D.
Professor of Medicine
Head and Senior Consultant
Department of Obstetrics
and Gynecology
University of Basel
Basel, Switzerland

W.B. SAUNDERS COMPANY
A Harcourt Health Sciences Company

Philadelphia • London • New York • St. Louis • Sydney • Toronto

W.B. SAUNDERS COMPANY
A Harcourt Health Sciences Company

The Curtis Center
Independence Square West
Philadelphia, Pennsylvania 19106

Library of Congress Cataloging-in-Publication Data

The unborn patient : the art and science of fetal therapy / Michael R. Harrison—[et al.].—3rd ed.
     p. ; cm.
  Includes bibliographical references and index.
  ISBN 0-7216-8446-7
  1. Fetus—Abnormalities—Diagnosis. 2. Fetus—Diseases—Treatment. 3. Fetus—Surgery.
4. Surgery, Experimental. I. Harrison, Michael R. (Michael Richard),
  [DNLM: 1. Abnormalities—diagnosis. 2. Abnormalities—therapy. 3. Fetal
Diseases—diagnosis. 4. Fetal Diseases—therapy. 5. Prenatal Diagnosis. WQ 211 U54 2001]
RG626.H38 2001

618.3′2—dc21   00-058853

THE UNBORN PATIENT   ISBN 0-7216-8446-7

Printed in the United States of America

Last digit is the print number: 9   8   7   6   5   4   3   2   1

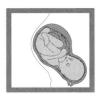

Contributors

N. SCOTT ADZICK, M.D.
C. Everett Koop Professor of Pediatric Surgery, University of Pennsylvania School of Medicine; Surgeon-in-Chief and Director, The Center for Fetal Diagnosis and Treatment, Children's Hospital of Philadelphia, Philadelphia, Pennsylvania
Open Fetal Surgical Techniques; The Fetus with a Lung Mass

CRAIG T. ALBANESE, M.D.
Associate Professor of Surgery and Pediatrics, and Co-Director, The Fetal Treatment Center, University of California, San Francisco, San Francisco, California
Operative Fetoscopy: FETENDO; The Fetus with Airway Obstruction; Fetal Hydrothorax; Ontogeny of the Fetal Immune System: Implications for Fetal Tolerance Induction and Postnatal Transplantation

W. FRENCH ANDERSON, M.D.
Professor of Biochemistry and Pediatrics, University of Southern California School of Medicine; Director, Gene Therapy Laboratories, Norris Cancer Center, Los Angeles, California
The Fetus with a Genetic Defect Correctable by Gene Therapy

ALICIA BÁRCENA, Ph.D.
Assistant Research Biologist, The Fetal Treatment Center, University of California, San Francisco, San Francisco, California
Ontogeny of the Fetal Immune System; Implications for Fetal Tolerance Induction and Postnatal Transplantation

HOWARD R. BELKIN, M.D., D.D.S., J.D.
Resident Physician in Psychiatry, Department of Psychiatry and Behavioral Neurosciences, Wayne State University School of Medicine, Detroit; Attorney-at-Law, Farmington Hills, Michigan
Legal Considerations in Fetal Treatment

PHILLIP R. BENNETT, M.D., B.Sc., M.B.B.S., Ph.D., M.R.C.O.G.
Professor, Institute of Obstetrics and Gynaecology, Imperial College School of Medicine, Queen Charlotte's and Chelsea Hospital, London, United Kingdom
Preterm Labor: The Achilles Heel of Fetal Intervention

RICHARD L. BERKOWITZ, M.D.
Professor and Chairman, and Director, Maternal-Fetal Medicine, Mount Sinai School of Medicine, New York, New York
The Fetus at Risk for Thrombocytopenia

OMAR S. BHOLAT, M.D.
Assistant Professor of Surgery, Department of Surgery, MCP-Hahnemann University School of Medicine, Philadelphia, Pennsylvania
Advanced Technologies for Future Fetal Treatment: Surgical Robotics

JOSEPH P. BRUNER, M.D.
Associate Professor, Departments of Obstetrics and Gynecology, and Radiology, Vanderbilt University Medical Center, Nashville, Tennessee
Intrauterine Myelomeningocele Repair

JAMES B. BUSSEL, M.D.
Associate Professor of Pediatrics, Weill Medical College, Cornell University; Associate Professor, New York Presbyterian Hospital, New York, New York
The Fetus at Risk for Thrombocytopenia

CHARLES B. CAULDWELL, M.D., Ph.D.
Clinical Professor of Anesthesia and Perioperative Care, University of California, San Francisco, San Francisco, California
Anesthesia and Monitoring for Fetal Intervention

FRANK A. CHERVENAK, M.D.
Professor and Acting Chairman, Department of Obstetrics and Gynecology, Cornell University Medical College, New York, New York
Ethical Considerations

FERGUS V. COAKLEY, M.B., B.Ch.
Associate Clinical Professor, Department of
Radiology, University of California, San Francisco,
San Francisco, California
*Magnetic Resonance Imaging and Computed
Tomography of the Fetus*

JOSHUA A. COPEL, M.D.
Professor of Perinatology, Departments of Diagnostic
Imaging, and Obstetrics and Gynecology, The Yale
Fetal Cardiovascular Center, Yale-New Haven
Medical Center, Yale University School of Medicine,
New Haven, Connecticut
The Fetus with Cardiac Arrhythmia

TIMOTHY M. CROMBLEHOLME, M.D.
Assistant Professor of Pediatric Surgery and
Obstetrics and Gynecology, The University of
Pennsylvania School of Medicine; Pediatric Surgeon,
The Center for Fetal Diagnosis and Treatment, The
Children's Hospital of Philadelphia, Philadelphia,
Pennsylvania
*The Fetus with Airway Obstruction; The Fetus with
Amniotic Band Syndrome*

WILLIAM J.B. DENNES, M.B.
Research Fellow, Institute of Obstetrics and
Gynaecology, Imperial College School of Medicine,
Queen Charlotte's and Chelsea Hospital; Specialist
Registrar, Department of Obstetrics and Gynaecology,
Chelsea and Westminster Hospital, London, United
Kingdom
Preterm Labor: The Achilles Heel of Fetal Intervention

JAN A.M. DEPREST, M.D., Ph.D.
Associate Professor, Department of Obstetrics and
Gynaecology, University Hospitals Leuven, Leuven,
Belgium
Obstetric Endoscopy

YASSER Y. EL-SAYED, M.D.
Assistant Professor of Gynecology and Obstetrics,
Stanford University School of Medicine; Division of
Maternal-Fetal Medicine, Lucile Packard Children's
Hospital at Stanford, Stanford, California
*New Tocolytic Strategies for Fetal Surgery: Efficacy and
Fetomaternal Safety of Nitroglycerin*

MARK I. EVANS, M.D.
Professor and Chairman of Obstetrics and
Gynecology, Professor of Human Genetics; Director,
Center for Fetal Therapy, MCP/Hahnemann
University, Philadelphia, Pennsylvania
The Fetus with a Biochemical Disorder

DIANA LEE FARMER, M.D.
Associate Professor of Surgery and Pediatrics,
Division of Pediatric Surgery, The Fetal Treatment
Center, University of California, San Francisco;
Associate Professor of Clinical Surgery, University of
California, San Francisco, San Francisco, California
Fetal Hydrothorax

JODY A. FARRELL, M.S.N., P.N.P.
Clinical Nurse Coordinator, University of California,
San Francisco, San Francisco, California
Postnatal Follow-up and Outcomes

DARIO O. FAUZA, M.D.
Instructor in Surgery, Harvard Medical School;
Surgical Associate, Fetal Medicine Program,
Children's Hospital, Boston, Massachusetts
Fetal Tissue Engineering

VICKIE A. FELDSTEIN, M.D.
Associate Professor, Department of Radiology,
University of California, San Francisco, San Francisco,
California
*Magnetic Resonance Imaging and Computed
Tomography of the Fetus*

ROY A. FILLY, M.D., F.A.I.U.M.
Professor of Radiology, Obstetrics and Gynecology,
and Reproductive Sciences, and Chief, Section of
Diagnostic Sonography, Department of Radiology,
University of California, San Francisco, San Francisco;
Clinical Professor of Radiology and Nuclear Medicine,
Stanford University, Standord, California
*Sonographic Anatomy of the Normal Fetus; Sonography
for Fetal Thoracic Intervention*

NICHOLAS M. FISK, M.B.B.S., Ph.D., F.R.C.O.G.,
F.R.A.N.Z.C.O.G., D.D.U.
Professor of Obstetrics and Gynaecology, Imperial
College School of Medicine; Honorary Consultant,
Queen Charlotte's and Chelsea Hospital, London,
United Kingdom
The Fetus with Twin-Twin Transfusion Syndrome

ALAN W. FLAKE, M.D.
Associate Professor of Surgery, and Obstetrics and
Gynecology, University of Pennsylvania; Director,
Children's Institute for Surgical Science, Children's
Hospital of Philadelphia, Philadelphia, Pennsylvania
*The Fetus with Sacrococcygeal Teratoma; The Fetus with
a Hematopoietic Stem Cell Defect*

ULRICH GEMBRUCH, M.D.
Professor of Obstetrics and Gynecology, Department
of Obstetrics and Gynecology, Medical University of
Lübeck, Germany
The Fetus with Nonimmune Hydrops Fetalis

JAMES D. GOLDBERG, M.D.
Co-Director, Prenatal Diagnosis Center, California
Pacific Medical Center, San Francisco, California
Prenatal Diagnostic Techniques

FRANÇOIS GOLFIER, M.D.
Attending Obstetrician and Gynecologist, Department
of Obstetrics and Gynecology, Hotel-Dieu, Lyon cedex
02, France
Fetal Hematopoietic Stem Cell Transplantation

RICHARD W. GRADY, M.D.
Assistant Professor of Urology, Children's Hospital and Regional Medical Center, The University of Washington Medical Center, Seattle, Washington
The Fetus with Complex Genitourinary Anomalies

BRYAN J. GUSHIKEN, M.D.
Assistant Clinical Professor, San Francisco General Hospital, University of California, San Francisco, San Francisco, California
Sonography for Fetal Thoracic Intervention

FRANK L. HANLEY, M.D.
Professor of Surgery and Pediatrics, Chief, Division of Cardiothoracic Surgery, University of California, San Francisco
The Fetus with Congenital Heart Disease

MICHAEL R. HARRISON, M.D., F.A.C.S., F.A.A.P.
Professor of Surgery and Pediatrics, and Director, The Fetal Treatment Center, Chief, Division of Pediatric Surgery, University of California, San Francisco, San Francisco, California
Professional Considerations in Fetal Treatment; Historical Perspective; The Rationale for Fetal Treatment: Selection, Feasibility, and Risk; Operative Fetoscopoy: FETENDO; Open Fetal Surgical Techniques; The Fetus with a Diaphragmatic Hernia

WOLFGANG HOLZGREVE, M.D.
Professor of Medicine, Head and Senior Consultant, Department of Obstetrics and Gynecology, University of Basel, Basel, Switzerland
The Fetus with Nonimmune Hydrops Fetalis

RUSSELL W. JENNINGS, M.D.
Assistant Professor of Surgery and Pediatrics, University of California, San Francisco, San Francisco, California
Anesthesia and Monitoring for Fetal Intervention

MARK PAUL JOHNSON, M.D.
Associate Professor, Departments of Obstetrics and Gynecology, and Surgery, University of Pennsylvania School of Medicine; Director of Obstetrical Services, Center for Fetal Diagnosis and Treatment, Children's Hospital of Philadelphia, Philadelphia, Pennsylvania
Fetal Obstructive Uropathy

CHARLES S. KLEINMAN, M.D.
Professor of Perinatology, Department of Pediatrics; Director, Pediatric Cardiology, Nemors Cardiac Center, Orlando, Florida; formerly, Professor of Pediatrics, Yale University School of Medicine, New Haven, Connecticut
The Fetus with Cardiac Arrhythmia

THOMAS M. KRUMMEL, M.D.
Chairman, Department of Surgery, Stanford University; Emile Holman Professor and Chair, Department of Surgery, Stanford University School of Medicine, Stanford, California
Advanced Technologies for Future Fetal Treatment: Surgical Robotics

JACOB C. LANGER, M.D., F.R.C.S.C.
Professor of Surgery, and Chief, Division of Pediatric General Surgery, University of Toronto; Chief, Division of General Surgery, Hospital for Sick Children, Toronto, Ontario, Canada
The Fetus with an Abdominal Wall Defect

COREY LARGMAN, Ph.D.
Adjunct Professor, Division of Metabolism, Department of Medicine, University of California, San Francisco Veterans Affairs Medical Center, San Francisco, California
Fetal Wound Healing: The Role of Homeobox Genes

MICHAEL T. LONGAKER, M.D.
John Marquis Converse Professor, Director of Surgical Research, New York University School of Medicine, New York, New York
The Fetus with Cleft Lip/Palate and Craniofacial Anomalies

LAWRENCE B. McCULLOUGH, Ph.D.
Professor of Medicine and Medical Ethics, Center for Medical Ethics and Health Policy, Baylor College of Medicine, Houston, Texas
Ethical Considerations

MARTIN MEULI, M.D., P.D.
Attending Pediatric Surgeon, Department of Surgery, University Children's Hospital, Univeristy of Zurich Medical School, Zurich, Switzerland
The Fetus with a Myelomeningocele

MICHAEL E. MITCHELL, M.D.
Professor of Urology, Children's Hospital and Regional Medical Center, The University of Washington Medical Center, Seattle, Washington
The Fetus with Complex Genitourinary Anomalies

KENNETH J. MOISE, JR., M.D.
Professor of Obstetrics and Gynecology, and Director, Divison of Maternal Fetal Medicine, University of North Carolina at Chapel Hill School of Medicine, Chapel Hill, North Carolina
The Fetus with Immune Hydrops

WALTER J. MORALES, M.D.
Florida Institute for Fetal Diagnosis and Therapy, St. Joseph's Women's Hospital, Tampa, Florida
Percutaneous Fetoscopically Guided Intervention

MARCUS O. MUENCH, Ph.D.
Assistant Research Cellular Biologist, University of California, San Francisco, San Francisco, California
Fetal Hematopoietic Stem Cell Transplantation

RODRIGO NEHGME, M.D.
Department of Pediatrics, The Yale Fetal
Cardiovascular Center, Yale-New Haven Medical
Center, Yale University School of Medicine, New
Haven, Connecticut
The Fetus with Cardiac Arrhythmia

MARY E. NORTON, M.D.
Assistant Professor, University of California, San
Francisco, San Francisco, California
Prenatal Diagnostic Techniques

PRANAV P. PANDYA, M.R.C.O.G.
Associate Professor of Obstetrics and Gynaecology,
Department of Obstetrics and Gynaecology,
University College London, London, United Kingdom
*Percutaneous Sonographically Guided Interventions:
Catheters and Shunts*

ROBERT PIECUCH, M.D.
Clinical Professor or Pediatrics, University of
California, San Francisco, San Francisco, California
Postnatal Follow-up and Outcomes

RUBÉN A. QUINTERO, M.D.
Medical Director, Florida Institute for Fetal Diagnosis
and Therapy, St. Joseph's Women's Hospital, Tampa,
Florida
Percutaneous Fetoscopically Guided Intervention

CHARLES H. RODECK, D.Sc., F.R.C.O.G., F.R.C.Path.
Professor and Chairman of Obstetrics and
Gynaecology, Department of Obstetrics and
Gynaecology, University College London, London,
United Kingdom
*Percutaneous Sonographically Guided Interventions:
Catheters and Shunts*

MARK A. ROSEN, M.D.
Professor of Anesthesia and Perioperative Care, and
Obstetrics and Gynecology, and Reproductive
Sciences; Director, Obstetrical Anesthesia, University
of California, San Francisco, San Francisco, California
Anesthesia and Monitoring for Fetal Intervention

NORMAN H, SILVERMAN, M.D., D.Sc. (Med)
Professor of Pediatrics and Radiology (Cardiology);
Director, Pediatric Echocardiography Laboratory,
University of California, San Francisco, San Francisco,
California
The Fetus with Congenital Heart Disease

ERIK D. SKARSGARD, M.D.
Assistant Professor of Surgery and Pediatrics,
Stanford University School of Medicine; Division of

Pediatric Surgery, Lucile Packard Children's Hospital
at Stanford, Stanford, California
*New Tocolytic Strategies for Fetal Surgery: Efficacy and
Fetomaternal Safety of Nitroglycerin*

ERIC J. STELNICKI, M.D.
Postdoctoral Research Fellow, The Fetal Treatment
Center, University of California, San Francisco, San
Francisco, California
Fetal Wound Healing: The Role of Homeobox Genes

PETER P. SUN. M.D.
Assistant Professor, University of Pennsylvania School
of Medicine; Attending Neurosurgeon, Children's
Hospital of Philadelphia, Philadelphia, Pennsylvania
The Fetus with Hydrocephalus

LESLIE N. SUTTON, M.D.
Professor of Neurosurgery, University of
Pennsylvania School of Medicine; Chief
Neurosurgeon, Children's Hospital of Philadelphia,
Philadelphia, Pennsylvania
The Fetus with Hydrocephalus

MYLES J.O. TAYLOR, B.M., B.Ch., M.R.C.G.P., M.R.C.O.G.
Research Fellow, Imperial College School of Medicine;
Horonary Senior Registrar, Queen Charlotte's and
Chelsea Hospital, London, United Kingdom
The Fetus with Twin-Twin Transfusion Sydnrome

NOEL B. TULIPAN, M.D.
Professor, Department of Neurosurgery, Vanderbilt
University; Neurosurgery Attending, Vanderbilt
University Medical Center, Nashville, Tennessee
Intrauterine Myelomeningocele Repair

JOSEPH P. VACANTI, M.D.
John Homans Professor of Surgery, Harvard Medical
School; Director of Pediatric Transplantation and
Director of the Laboratory of Tissue Engineering and
Organ Fabrication, Massachusetts General Hospital,
Boston, Massachusetts
Fetal Tissue Engineering

YVES VILLE, M.D.
Professor of Obstetrics and Gynecology, University
Paris Owest, and Head of Department, Chi
Poissy—St. Germain, Poissy, France
Obstetric Endoscopy

ESMAIL D. ZANJANI, Ph.D.
Professor of Medicine and Physiology, University of
Nevada School of Medicine; Professor of Medicine,
Veterans Affairs Medical Center, Reno, Nevada
*The Fetus with a Genetic Defect Correctable by Gene
Therapy*

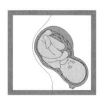

Preface

The third edition is late in arriving. That's not because the gestation was long, but rather the conception delayed. The second edition of *The Unborn Patient: Prenatal Diagnosis and Treatment* was so well received that the publisher expected a third edition many years ago. But both the playing field and the players had shifted so dramatically since the first edition in 1984 and the second edition in 1991 that a third edition seemed unlikely. The field was advancing exponentially, many textbooks on maternal-fetal medicine, prenatal diagnosis, and perinatology were available, and the enterprise of fetal diagnosis and treatment had spread from a few academic centers around the world to a much broader enterprise. Most important, only one of the original three editors could contemplate a replay of the exhausting task ahead.

The second edition was an exhausting labor of love which brought together international experts from widely diverse fields to synthesize a relatively new enterprise. If there were to be a third edition, it would have to be much more than a replay of the same approach, an internationally authored comprehensive textbook on fetology. It was the right time for a book focused sharply on fetal therapy. Much of the background of a more general nature would be eliminated and the concentration would be on the art and craft as well as the science of fetal treatment. Three new editors representing the breath and scope of modern fetal therapy joined the effort to produce a definitive reference for colleagues,

practitioners, and patients. The leading world authority in each of 45 areas was recruited to write a single- or double-authored chapter (without the usual complement of junior co-authors). The text was to be distinguished by its rich illustration.

There is a geography to this publishing adventure. It was conceived and launched at the International Fetal Medicine and Surgery Society meeting in Alaska, refined at the subsequent IFMSS meeting on Heron Island, and cemented when the four editors convened for four days of intensive work in the redwood forests of Tree Top Ranch (Timber Cove) on the wild Sonoma coast. It was here that artist Susan Quan converted the often fanciful imaginings of the editors into whimsical line drawings that illustrate each chapter of this book and tie together the many aspects of fetal intervention.

Now that we've gone from three editors from a single institution in San Francisco to four editors in four diverse international medical centers, we can no longer acknowledge by name all of our many wonderful professional colleagues who have contributed to the advancement of this field and the production of this book. We would be remiss not to mention our wonderful fetal fixers club, The International Fetal Medicine and Surgery Society, which has been the one cohesive forum and source of inspiration for most of the advances in fetal diagnosis and treatment in the last two decades. Finally we would like to acknowledge the creative and organizational talent of Vilma Zarate whose tireless efforts made this work come together.

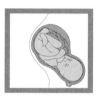

Preface to the First Edition

As originally conceived, this book was to be a small project of short gestation. A few years ago, this seemed appropriate because there was little information about fetal management and the field was changing so rapidly that a monograph would have to be frequently updated. But in the last two years, the field has exploded and information has accumulated so rapidly that our little mouse has become an elephant with correspondingly longer gestation. We have reluctantly conceded that our original plan to write a short monograph about our personal experience in developing the Fetal Treatment Program at the University of California, San Francisco (UCSF), would not do justice to the field. At the same time, we believed that this rapidly changing and exciting field was not ready for a "textbook" with the usual drawbacks of large, multiauthored works. With the help of a few carefully selected contributors in special fields, we have written a cohesive book based on our own experience, and we have incorporated the growing experience of other investigators around the world. We have tried to deal with all of the questions (e.g., medical, physiologic, social, ethical, legal) that may arise when a family seeks help with an abnormal fetus. We recognize that this is a very young book in a very new and rapidly growing field.

As is often the case, the conception of this book was an accident. In this case, three individuals with highly different backgrounds—a pediatric surgeon, an obstetrician geneticist, and a sonographer—shared an interest in fetal defects. Five years of constant discussion, speculation, experimentation, and interaction in caring for fetuses and their families led to the development of the Fetal Treatment Program at UCSF and eventually to the gestation of this monograph. The first trimester was taken up with clinical speculation and intense experimental investigation. In the second trimester, the first therapeutic maneuvers were attempted and then refined in human fetuses. With the initial flurry of interest and excitement surrounding the first human fetal cases, the Kroc Foundation agreed to sponsor a meeting that brought together pioneering investigators from around the world and produced the consensus statement on fetal treatment that was published in the New England Journal of Medicine. The Kroc Foundation also kindly agreed to underwrite the cost of color plates for this book. The third trimester, involving the actual writing, rewriting, and editing, has proved somewhat painful but has yielded, we hope, a healthy and vigorous issue.

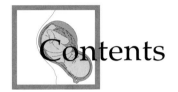

Contents

Color Plate follows page xvi

PLATE 1

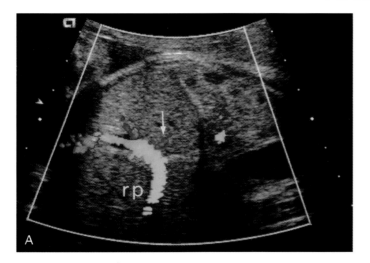

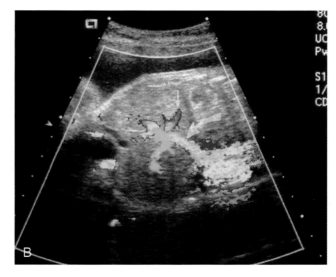

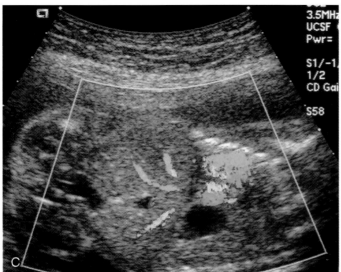

FIGURE 7–4. *A,* Left CDH without liver in the thorax. Color Doppler image in the coronal plane through the fetal thorax and abdomen shows normal hepatic vasculature: right portal vein (rp) and left portal venous branch (*arrow*) remaining below the expected region of the diaphragm. *B,* Color Doppler image in the coronal plane through the fetal thorax and abdomen shows normal hepatic vasculature: ductus venosus (*curved arrow*) and left lateral segment portal branches (*straight arrow*) remaining below the expected region of the diaphragm. *C,* Color Doppler image in the coronal plane through the fetal thorax and abdomen shows normal hepatic veins coursing toward but not above the diaphragm.

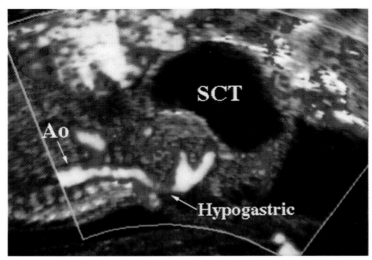

FIGURE 21–4. Power Doppler examination of fetal SCT demonstrating vascular supply arising from the internal iliac artery.

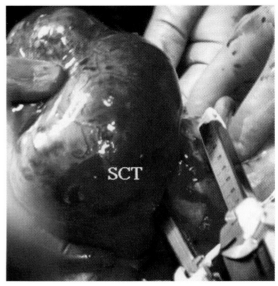

FIGURE 21–5. Photograph of open fetal surgical procedure for SCT. The GIA stapler is being applied across the pedicle of the tumor.

PLATE 2

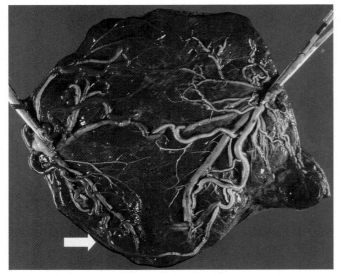

FIGURE 23–2. An injection study of a monochorionic placenta. Arteries from the left and right twins' placental cord insertions are shown in red and yellow with veins in blue and green, respectively. An AA anastomosis is seen (*arrow*).

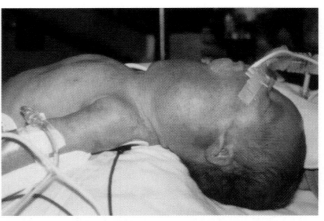

FIGURE 24–4. A complex cervical mass resulting in hyperextension of the neck due to a cervical teratoma. This has been referred to as the "flying fetus" sign, as the head extension is similar to that observed in ski jumpers. The appearance of the patient postnatally.

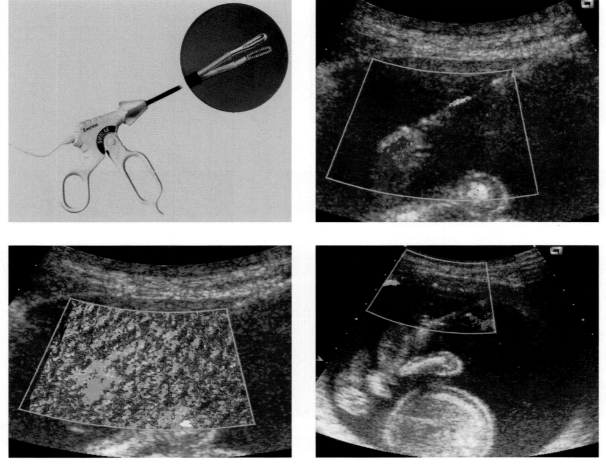

FIGURE 23–7. Cord occlusion with 3-mm bipolar diathermy forceps (*upper left*; Everst Medical Minneapolis, MN). The cord is identified (*upper right*), diathermied (*lower left*), and cessation of flow achieved in the umbilical cord (*lower right*).

PLATE 3

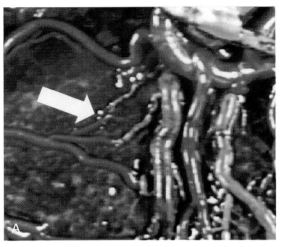

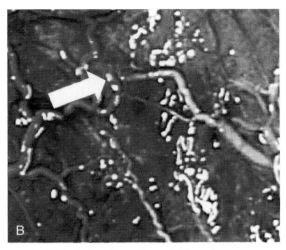

FIGURE 23–10. Placental injection study demonstrating variation in AV configurations. *A,* The vein emerges at approximately 180 degrees to the entering artery. *B,* In contrast, the angle between the artery and vein is only approximately 90 degrees.

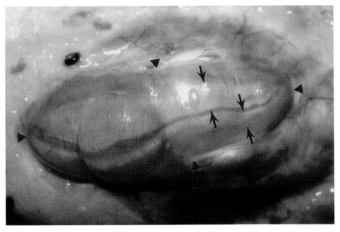

FIGURE 28–2. Experimental MMC lesion at birth. The spinal cord remnants rest on the dorsal aspect of a fluid-filled cystic sac (*markers*) and appear as two separated and extremely flattened parts ("hemicords") (*paired arrows*).

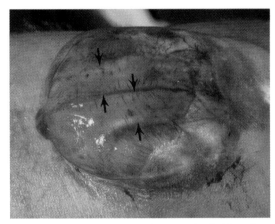

FIGURE 28–3. Human MMC lesion at birth. Note the striking similarities between the experimental and the naturally occurring phenotypes. The severely altered spinal cord tissue also appears split into two separate parts (*paired arrows*).

FIGURE 28–4. Transverse histologic section through the center of the experimental lesion shown in Figure 28–2. The spinal cord remnants are exposed on the surface and show massive alterations and complete loss of the characteristic cytoarchitecture. Each arrow points at one "hemicord." (V = vertebral body.) For comparison with an analogous human lesion, see Figure 28–12.

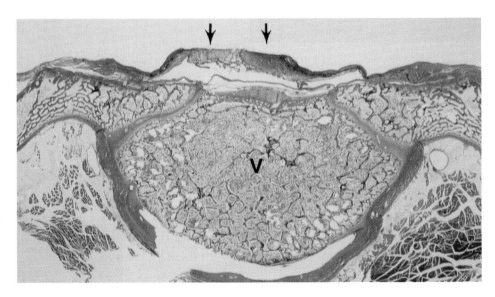

PLATE 4

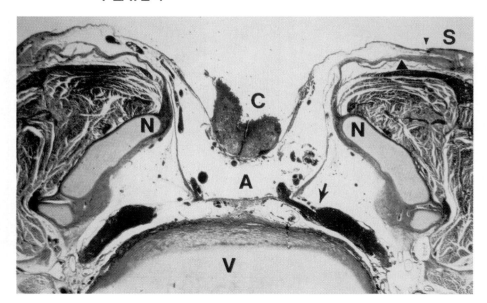

FIGURE 28–12. Classic morphology of human fetal MMC (23 gestational weeks) (histologic cross section). The exposed spinal cord tissue (C) appears grossly normal ventrally, while the dorsal part is lost (avulsion injury). The open pia fuses laterally to the epidermis (*small marker*), the open dura to the dermis (*large marker*) of the skin (S), thereby enclosing the enlarged and abnormally configured arachnoid space (A). Spinal nerve and dorsal root ganglia look normal (*arrow*). (N = open neural arch, V = vertebral body.)

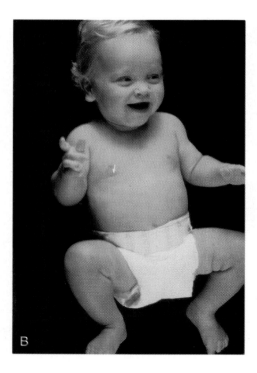

FIGURE 35–13. *B,* After in utero placement of a pleuroamniotic shunt, the healthy infant showed only a small scar below his right nipple where the catheter was located, marked by the *arrow.*

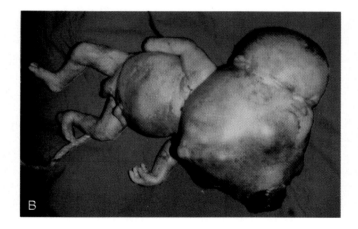

FIGURE 35–18. *B.* After a premature rupture of membranes and birth at 29 weeks' gestation, the intubation and ventilation of this newborn with neck teratoma were impossible.

PLATE 5

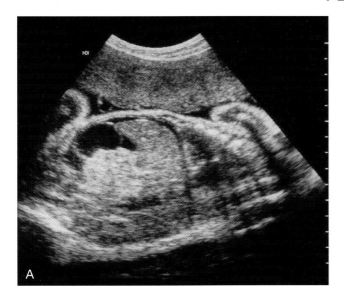

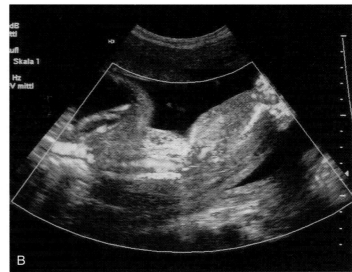

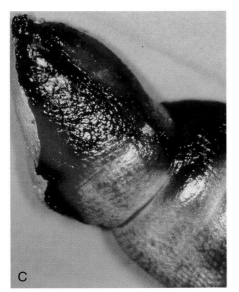

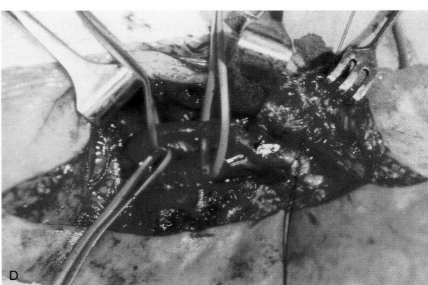

FIGURE 35–20. *A,* This fetus with Klippel-Trenaunay syndrome shows ascites, skin edema, and polyhydramnios at 29 weeks' gestation. *B,* B-mode ultrasound and power Doppler showed edematous left leg that seems to show an increased blood flow to the proximal part of the leg. *C* and *D,* Postpartum examination confirmed the prenatal diagnosis of Klippel-Trenaunay syndrome showing unilateral hypertrophy of the whole left leg, cutaneous "portwine" hemangiomas; furthermore, arteriovenous fistula was diagnosed and successfully operated.

PLATE 6

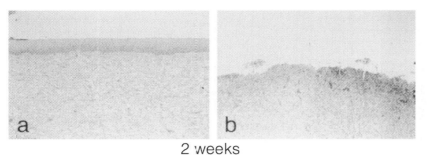

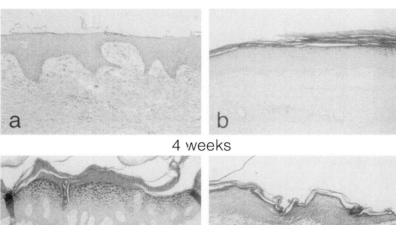

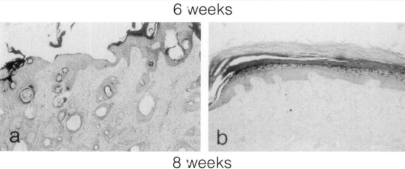

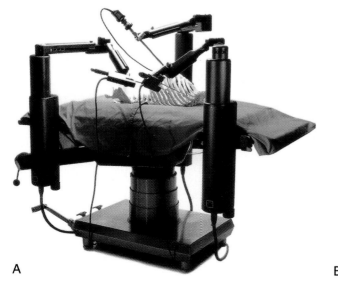

2 weeks

4 weeks

6 weeks

8 weeks

FIGURE 43–8. Comparative neoskin histologies from engineered (*A*) and acellular (*B*) sites at different times following implantation, in weeks. Notice the faster epithelization time and higher level of organization of the engineered specimens. (H&E, original magnification × 100.) (From Fauza DO, Fishman S, Mehegan K, et al: Videofetoscopically assisted fetal tissue engineering: Skin replacement. J Pediatr Surg 33:357–361, 1998, with permission.)

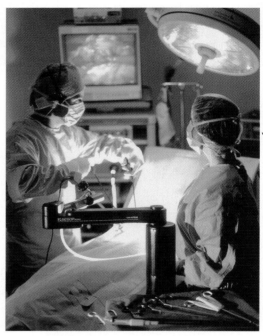

FIGURE 45–1. The Aesop robotic arm can serve as an assistant during laparoscopic surgery and eliminates the need for a human assistant. (Photograph by Bobbi Bennett for Computer Motion Inc., Santa Barbara, CA, copyright 1999.)

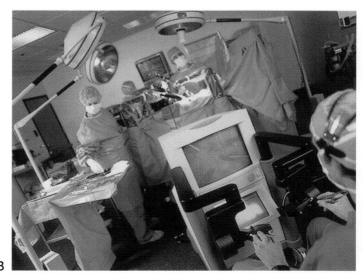

FIGURE 45–5. The Zeus™ Robotic Surgical System (*A*) is comprised of three slave-type robotic arms. During surgery (*B*), the surgeon sits at the workstation and performs delicate procedures using familiar instrumentation. (Courtesy of Computer Motion Inc., Santa Barbara, CA, copyright 1999.)

The Fetus as a Patient: A Womb with a View

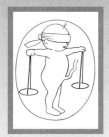

CHAPTER *1*

Professional Considerations in Fetal Treatment

MICHAEL R. HARRISON

Powerful new imaging and sampling techniques have stripped the veil of mystery from the once secretive fetus. Although most prenatally diagnosed malformations are best managed by appropriate medical and surgical therapy after maternal transport and planned delivery near term, a few simple anatomic abnormalities with predictable devastating developmental consequences may require correction before birth. In the 1980s, the developmental pathophysiology of several potentially correctable lesions was worked out in animal models; the natural history was determined by serial observation of human fetuses; selection criteria for intervention were developed; and anesthetic, tocolytic, and surgical techniques for hysterotomy and fetal surgery were refined.[1-3] In the 1990s, this investment in basic and clinical research has benefited an increasing number of fetal patients.

As we enter the 21st century, the enterprise of fetal treatment is solidly positioned for continued expansion. Our newfound ability to treat the fetus as a patient raises puzzling new problems and dilemmas for fetal caregivers and society. These go beyond the traditional "medical" problems, such as how to diagnose a condition, when and if to treat, and when a new therapy is ready to be tried. The newer problems raised by prenatal diagnosis and the availability of therapy include ethical, legal, and economic issues as well as logistic and professional issues. If the fetus is a patient: Who is the fetus' physician? How should care of the fetus be organized and delivered?

The Fetus' Physician(s)

It is clear from the historical development of fetal treatment that the fetus with an anomaly requires the attention of a team of specialists working together. Management of the defective fetus does not easily divide according to the sometimes artificial (and negotiable) time of delivery. Whether the patient is inside or outside the womb, its care is a continuum that requires the expertise of physicians trained in the care of mothers and babies. It is hard to imagine how one specialist, no matter how broadly trained, could take sole responsibility for the treatment of a fetus with a complex malformation.

The obstetrician will manage the pregnancy. The obstetric specialist (e.g., perinatologist, geneticist) who is an expert in prenatal diagnosis, amniocentesis, chorionic villus sampling, percutaneous umbilical blood sampling, and so forth, is indispensable in fetal diagnosis, family counseling, and management of the pregnancy and its complications. But he or she is not familiar enough with management of the neonate's disease process after birth to make decisions about exactly how it should be managed before birth. By the same token, the neonatologists or pediatric surgical specialist familiar with the disease process, its pathophysiology, and its treatment after birth, although indispensable in formulating treatment, and in some cases, performing the surgery, is not qualified to manage the pregnancy or the obstetric problems associated with intervention. In addition to physicians trained in the clinical care of the pregnant woman and the newborn with a defect, the expertise of other specialists is required. An obstetric sonologist who has expertise in prenatal diagnosis is indispensable in finding and defining the fetal defect, in excluding other associated fetal anomalies, and in performing sonographically guided diagnostic and therapeutic maneuvers, such as needle and catheter placement. Many other specialists from both the pediatric and the obstetric fields will be required to contribute in special circumstances. For example, a pediatric cardiologist will help with fetal arrhythmias, a neurologist or neurosurgeon will assist with hydrocephalus, and an endocrinologist will assist with endocrine disorders. There should be access to bioethical and psychosocial support and open communication with colleagues in the medical community, including people who may be critical of such an undertaking.

Fetal Procedures: Teams, Specialists, and Responsibility

A special problem arises with interventional fetal procedures, especially those that require the expertise of spe-

3

cialists from very different fields. For example, who should place vesicoamniotic shunts: the obstetrician expert in percutaneous sonographically guided fetal sampling and manipulation, or the pediatric surgical specialist expert in catheter drainage of obstructed urinary tracts in infants? Who should perform open fetal surgical procedures: the obstetrician experienced in uterine surgery, or the pediatric surgeon experienced in repair of complex anomalies in very small children? Because no single specialty training provides the total spectrum of skills and experience, this is an area in which "turf" battles between medical specialties and "ego" battles among team members may sabotage the fetal treatment enterprise. It is also an area in which cooperative efforts and teamwork can be productive.

Although there is no simple solution to this problem, some general principles have evolved during the last decade in centers in which obstetricians, sonologists, surgeons, and many other specialists have been working closely together to improve fetal treatment. The first principle is that fetal therapy is a team effort requiring varying amounts of input from all team members. The team must include an obstetrician, perinatologist, geneticist, sonologist, surgeon, neonatologist, anesthesiologist, and many other support personnel. This range of expertise can usually be provided by three or four individuals, depending on what roles are combined; that is, an obstetrician, a sonologist, a surgeon, and an anesthesiologist.

The second principle is that although all members of the team can contribute to any particular procedure, there must be a team leader who takes responsibility for the conduct of that particular procedure. Which member of the team becomes the leader depends on the nature of the procedure itself.

The third principle is that the procedure is done by the team member who is most likely to produce the best outcome. For example, if fetal outcome depends on skill and expertise in performing sonographically guided percutaneous procedures, the obstetrician/sonologist is usually in charge of the team and performs the procedure. In our center, we have found that percutaneous procedures are best performed by the obstetrician/geneticist working closely with the sonologist. The surgeon assists with technical details, such as catheter preparation, when his expertise in placing drainage catheters in babies will enhance the fetal effort. The anesthesiologist manages the sedation for local anesthesia or more commonly general anesthesia. An experienced operating room nurse and an obstetric nurse are always present. It is clear that an obstetrician who is experienced in fetal blood sampling, fetoscopy, and intrauterine transfusion is the best person to perform this procedure. For open surgical procedures, the roles are reversed because the outcome is related directly to the skill, judgment, and experience of the surgeon. The risks are higher than are those for closed procedures, and success depends on the ability of the surgeon to expose the fetus by hysterotomy, correct the defect, return the fetus, and close the still-pregnant uterus securely. The chance of success is highest when one physician takes responsibility for the procedure from the beginning to the end.

The Special Problem of Open Fetal Surgery

Although open fetal surgical procedures constitute a small minority of the procedures performed in this exciting field, the problem of who should lead the team and who (or how many) should perform the procedure deserves thoughtful consideration. The simplest solution is to ask each surgical specialist to do his or her part of the procedure; that is, the obstetrician opens the uterus, the pediatric surgical specialist (e.g., pediatric surgeon for hydronephrosis, pediatric neurosurgeon for hydrocephalus) operates on the fetus, and the obstetrician closes the uterus. Although this politically expedient solution is the easiest way to approach fetal surgery and is likely to keep team members comfortable in their accustomed roles, it is not likely to yield the best outcome for several reasons. This approach assumes that traditional skills will suffice; that is, the obstetricians can close the still-pregnant uterus as they do in the case of an empty uterus and that the pediatric surgeon can do with a fetus what he has learned in a neonate. Neither is true. Second, tag-team surgery is never ideal. Exposure of the fetus by hysterotomy and subsequent closure are too intimately intertwined with the procedure on the fetus itself to be divided up by specialty. The limiting factor in the development of fetal surgery is the ability to expose the fetus by hysterotomy without causing abortion, in the same way that the limiting factor in the development of cardiac surgery was the ability to stop the heart without killing the patient. Hysterotomy and closure without abortion is the same "enabling" step for fetal surgery as cardiopulmonary bypass was for cardiac surgery. Fetal surgery cannot develop and will not succeed unless a few surgeons are willing to devote considerable time and effort to developing, practicing, and perfecting all aspects of this new procedure: hysterotomy, fetal exposure, and correction; closure of the pregnant uterus; and control of labor.

The fetal surgeon and his or her team must deal with a broad spectrum of new unsolved surgical problems and questions. What is the optimal anesthetic agent for the mother and the fetus? How can the need for uterine relaxation for fetal exposure be balanced against the need for uterine tone to prevent bleeding? How can massive low-pressure venous bleeding from the incised myometrium be controlled during the time of fetal exposure before sutures can be placed for closure? How can uterine retraction be maintained and the fetus exposed without inciting umbilical vessel spasm and disturbing the umbilical circulation? How can fetal vital functions be monitored during surgery? How can the fetus be resuscitated with fluid if necessary? How can amniotic fluid volume be maintained during and after surgery? What fetal incisions are possible? What fetal exposure is necessary to correct that particular defect? Will abdominal fetal exposure compromise umbilical vein flow? Will thoracic exposure compromise venous return? Will manipulation of the umbilical cord endanger the placental circulation? How can intrauterine volume be maintained so that the fetus can be easily replaced when the procedure is complete? How can the membranes be sealed and closed to prevent a leak of amniotic fluid and its disastrous sequelae? How is the thick myometrial muscle best closed to allow optimal healing and to prevent thinning of the scar and liability to rupture of the uterus later on? How can uterine integrity be maintained during the immediate postoperative period when the uterine muscle may contract before healing is adequate? It is worth pointing out that whereas obstetricians feel competent and confident in closing the empty uterus, none has faced the formidable problems of closing a still-gravid uterus. Although surgeons usually feel confident in managing surgical bleeding and anatomic closure, none has dealt with the problems of water-tight closure of a membrane lining a thick muscle with a tendency to vigorous and sometimes uncontrollable contraction in the postoperative period. (The only contracting muscle that the surgeon repairs is the diaphragm.) Thus, the formidable list of problems facing the fetal surgery team covers broad areas of many different surgical specialties.

Cross-Training of Fetal Surgeons

Because the fetal surgeon requires broad new skills that can be developed only in extensive experimental work, his or her background can be in one of several specialties, none of which provides adequate training for all aspects of a fetal surgical procedure (Fig. 1–1). An individual with obstetric training must develop the necessary surgical skill to perform the corrective surgery on the fetus and to open and close the gravid uterus, an undertaking very different compared with doing a cesarean section. An individual with surgical training must practice and become skillful not only at surgical manipulation of the pregnant uterus but also at tocolytic management of preterm labor. Because the fetal surgeon will, by neces-

sity, be performing procedures that are traditionally part of another specialty, he or she will have to work with team members from all the subspecialties to learn and practice the procedures that are not part of their traditional training. It is obvious that the surgeon and the team members will have to practice the procedure together in a sufficiently rigorous model (the nonhuman primate is the only appropriate one) to work out the physiologic problems as well as the procedural details before attempting fetal surgery in humans. In fact, experimental surgery provides an invaluable opportunity to work out not only the procedures but also the professional relationships that will enable the team to function smoothly. The lines of responsibility must be drawn clearly among team members before the choice of doing a procedure is offered to a patient. If agreement cannot be reached, it is unlikely that the team will function properly. The necessity to demonstrate competence in fetal surgery on animals (preferably the primate) will undoubtedly be the limiting step in the development of fetal surgery programs, because few individuals from any specialty will be willing to devote enough time, effort, and money to develop a proper fetal surgical team.

Logistics of Fetal Care and the Development of Fetal Treatment Centers

Beyond the many individual specialists and their clinical expertise, the institutional setting and organization of this joint venture will prove to be crucial to its success. A close working relationship among perinatal specialists is mandatory. This is best achieved in a clinical setting that includes a high-risk obstetric unit familiar with maternal transport, in utero transfusion, management of preterm labor, and so forth, and a neonatal intensive care nursery equipped to manage the respiratory and metabolic problems of premature infants. The setting should be one in which research is intermingled with clinical care. Because most fetal treatment is "unproven," all clinical experience must be reviewed, analyzed, and reported to improve understanding of the diseases involved. Ideally, this commitment to clinical research will be bolstered by the more difficult, expensive, and time-consuming basic research in which the pathophysiology is explored and techniques for intervention are developed in experimental fetal models. The blend of skills and expertise required in a fetal treatment center is shown in Figure 1–2. At present, this combination is usually available only in large referral centers associated with university teaching programs.

The activity of a fetal treatment program should be reviewed by the uninvolved colleagues. There will not always be unanimity of opinion about difficult clinical decisions taken by many different specialists with many different backgrounds and motivations. For the safety of the patient-subject and the physician-investigator, innovative treatment must be addressed with the Committee on Human Research; protocols should be reviewed; and consent procedures should be approved. Only in

---

FETAL SURGERY TRAINING

MINIMALLY INVASIVE (Sono guided, Fetoscopy)

OB = Ped Surg = Interventional Radiology

OPEN SURGERY (Hysterotomy, FETENDO)

Fetal Exposure: OB = Surg = Laparoscopist

Fetal Repair: Surg Subspecialist (Ped , Neuro, Uro, etc)

FIGURE 1–1. Fetal therapy requires a broad range of skills and backgrounds. Minimally invasive procedures performed under sonographic or fetoscopic guidance can be performed by obstetricians, surgeons, and other interventionists. In open fetal surgery which requires hysterotomy or operative video-fetoscopy (FETENDO), obstetricians may provide fetal exposure, but surgical repair requires a surgical specialist with experience in small babies.

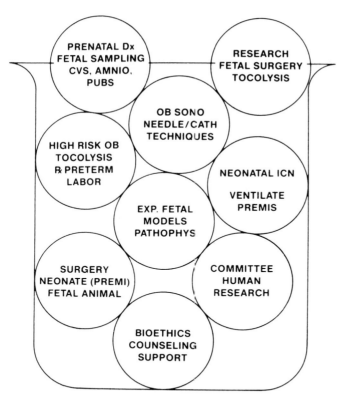

FIGURE 1–2. The fetal treatment program is a melting pot requiring the expertise of many different specialists and specialties in an institutional setting that promotes high-level primary care, clinical investigation, and experimental work on fetuses.

this setting can the difficult and unsolved problem of deciding whether a given intervention should be called innovative treatment or research can be resolved. In innovative therapy, the relationship is that of a physician with his or her patient and, in research, the relationship is that of an investigator with his or her subject. As fetal intervention develops further, elements of both must be balanced for the best interests of the fetus, the mother, the involved physicians, and society (Fig. 1–3).

It is also in this broader forum that issues of medical judgment can be openly debated and resolved. These issues include when a particular intervention is ready to be tried and how to weigh the risks and benefits for all the parties involved. Beyond these questions of medical judgment, the physician-investigator who contemplates innovative fetal treatment assumes an unshakable obligation to provide an open forum and to report all results, good or bad, so that the procedures can be evaluated fairly. The danger of overenthusiastic or ill-advised interventions would be minimized if everyone contemplating intervention realized that the decision to "try" was a commitment to report the results to the medical profession (not the media) and to accept the criticism of their colleagues. At this stage, "trying" a new procedure and not reporting the results is reprehensible.

Fetal Referral Process

Referrals to the Fetal Treatment Center (FTC) come from a referring physician or the patients themselves. More recently, many families confronted with a new fetal diagnosis find information, answers, support, and resources through the Internet. Many come well-informed about choices in treatment through information obtained on-line. Patients who self-refer are encouraged to contact their physician prior to the team's review of their case. Upon receiving the initial medical information from the referring physician, the nurse coordinator determines whether the patient condition is emergent, necessitating an immediate evaluation, or is nonemergent and is appropriate for presentation at the weekly FTC meeting. The FTC requests a detailed obstetric and medical history via fax and a copy of the sonogram by overnight mail prior to team review of each case. The referring physician and/or the patient are sent by mail or fax current publications regarding the fetal diagnosis, clinical course, and possible interventions for specific anomalies. They are encouraged to seek information on the Web and from other centers.

The records and sonograms are reviewed by the multidisciplinary FTC team and the referring physician is contacted regarding potential treatment options. If the patient diagnosis meets selection criteria for possible fetal surgical intervention, the patient is offered the opportunity to come to the FTC for consultation, but never with a commitment to specific treatment or intervention. That can be decided only after full evaluation on site, formal consultation, and full counseling about all alternatives. If the patient does not meet criteria for fetal intervention, recommendations for prenatal surveillance are given to the referring physician. Questions are addressed during follow-up telephone conversations.

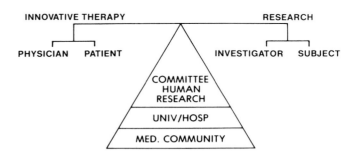

FIGURE 1–3. The institutional setting is important for a fetal treatment program. At this stage, fetal treatment involves elements of both innovative treatment (a physician–patient relationship) and research (an investigator–subject relationship). Decisions pertaining to treatment must have the support of the Committee on Human Research, the hospital, the university and, in the long term, society. Although a decision to attempt treatment may be a matter of medical judgment, it implies an inflexible obligation to report all results, whether good or bad, so that the benefits and liabilities of the treatment can be established as soon as possible.

If the family elects to travel to the FTC, a letter is sent to the parents prior to consultation that includes the scheduled studies, an evaluation schedule, travel directions, and suggestions for lodging. Reserving air flights and procuring lodging on short notice is difficult and costly. Fortunately, most of these families are eligible for free travel through programs like the United Airlines "Friendly Skies Program" and the American Airlines "Miles for Kids" travel program. If the patient's evaluation process involves an overnight stay, families will need to reserve a room at a guesthouse close to the hospital. Many centers have complimentary or low-cost housing for needy families like the "Kids 'n Moms House" or the "Ronald McDonald House."

Appointments for tests and consultations are scheduled and coordinated in such a manner that the family will have a smooth course throughout their evaluation process. Because the FTC is usually a busy tertiary facility, it can be difficult to obtain the necessary specialists at a time convenient for all. In our experience, evaluations and operations are best performed in the evening or early morning hours to accommodate hectic schedules.

The Indispensable Weekly Meeting

To facilitate communication amongst the team members, all new and active cases are reviewed at the weekly multidisciplinary FTC meeting. This forum provides an opportunity for all members of the multidisciplinary team to address specific patient care needs. Sonograms performed at the University of California at San Francisco (UCSF) and those received from referring centers that week are reviewed and discussed. The nurse coordinator maintains a status list of patients that is updated weekly and presented at the FTC meeting. This document assists in communicating the patient care management plan and aids in ensuring that patient follow-up data are maintained. Management issues are openly discussed and implemented, thus avoiding misunderstandings among team members. This time is also used to discuss clinical outcomes and the findings of fetuses who have delivered, and presents an opportunity to review recent maternal-fetal laboratory research. Management algorithms for the more common fetal anatomic anomalies have also been developed during these multidisciplinary sessions.

The weekly FTC conference is the heart of the FTC enterprise because it allows everyone involved—perinatologists, surgical subspecialists, sonographers, neonatologists, nurses, social workers, and the like—to come together and discuss the care of every patient. It is the one time every week when everyone's opinion can be heard and debated. It is the one time when all the activity of the previous week must be reported and criticized. It is the one time when special expertise can be summoned for individual cases (e.g., cardiologists and cardiac surgeons for complex heart disease, neurologists and neurosurgeons for hydrocephalus or myelomeningocele, etc.). It is the one time when visiting physicians, scientists, and scholars of all types can get a feel for the enterprise and share in the excitement and frustration of dealing with real problems of real patients. It is the one time when differences and misunderstandings, which are inevitable in such a multidisciplinary venture, can be expressed and resolved. The weekly meeting is indispensable for patient care.

Patient Evaluation, Counseling, and Informed Consent

Once the family arrives at the FTC, the mother and fetus undergo 1 or 2 days of outpatient evaluation. A detailed fetal sonographic survey is performed to confirm the diagnosis and detect any other anatomic abnormalities. With some diagnoses, a fetal echocardiogram is required. Karyotyping at the referring institution is preferable but, if not completed, percutaneous blood sampling can be performed here. Lastly, an informed consent conference is held with the family, pediatric surgeon, perinatologist, anesthesiologist, social worker, and nurse coordinator.

The informed consent conference provides an in-depth description of the fetal diagnosis, treatment options including the fetal surgery procedure if applicable, results, maternal risks, potential benefits, and alternatives of therapy. If the fetal malformation is best managed by planned delivery and postnatal surgery, the neonatologist and pediatric surgeon counsel the parents regarding the type of defect, the surgical repair, and the anticipated neonatal hospital course. Arrangements are then made for scheduled delivery at the referring institution or, if necessary, at the FTC. If the fetus has a fatal defect not amenable to fetal or postnatal surgery, the perinatologists or reproductive geneticist will provide the parents with options regarding either continuing or terminating the pregnancy. The family, with the aid of the social worker, are encouraged to ask questions. Follow-up telephone and written contact summarizing the conference is made immediately with the referring physician.

After the informed consent conference the patient and family are given the opportunity to consider all treatment options. In emergent situations, if the mother is considered a good candidate for fetal intervention, admission is planned for the following day. These parents undergo further preoperative teaching and preparation with the obstetric nurse specialist. A tour of the obstetric floor, the adult intensive care unit (ICU), and the intensive care nursery (ICN) is included. The mother has a preoperative medical history and physical examination by the perinatologist and anesthesiologist. In nonemergent circumstances, families are encouraged to take the information from the evaluation and return home to decide which option would be best for them. Families are encouraged to seek the advice of their referring physician, family, and friends and to notify the FTC coordinator with their decision. If fetal intervention is their choice, a date for the surgery is chosen and arrangements are made for them to return to the FTC at a mutually agreed upon time.

The Obstetric Unit and Operating Room

The obstetric unit provides complex antepartum, intrapartum, and postpartum care for the fetal surgical patient including nursing staff trained in the management of high-risk obstetric patients. If the patient has been admitted for postnatal management of the newborn, the delivery occurs on the obstetric unit. A neonatal resuscitation room, adjacent to the obstetric operating room, is available for immediate neonatal management by neonatologists, surgeons, intensive care nurses, and respiratory therapists. All deliveries take place in the obstetric unit. Vaginal delivery is appropriate for most fetal lesions, even abdominal wall defects. Planned cesarean is necessary for patients who underwent open fetal surgery. The more specialized EXIT procedure (ex utero intrapartum treatment) is necessary for all fetuses with threatened airway obstruction.

Fetal interventions requiring general anesthesia may be performed in the obstetric operating room or the pediatric surgical operating room depending on the complexity and requirements of the case. In addition to the pediatric surgeons and perinatologists, the fetal surgery operating room is staffed by a highly skilled team of surgical nurses as well as anesthesiologists with training in maternal-fetal anesthesia. Numerous items have required miniaturization and sterilization including special surgical instruments, fetal and uterine radiotelemetric monitors, specially devised uterine staplers and atraumatic retractors, the level I intrauterine warming unit, fetal medication, and fetal intravenous access equipment. Equipment for fetoscopic procedures is even more complex and crucial to success.

Fetal Intensive Care Unit

The patient undergoing open fetal surgery is extubated in the operating room and is then transported to the fetal intensive care unit (FICU), where intensive monitoring is provided for 48 hours. Those undergoing fetoscopic surgery (FETENDO) do not require such intensive monitoring and are recovered in a specially equipped room on the obstetric ward. During the postoperative recovery, intensive care is provided under the direction of the fetal surgery team including central venous and arterial access, tocolysis, vasoactive drugs, hemodynamic monitoring, and specialized fetal monitoring. Preprinted orders, standards of care, and a clinical pathway for fetal surgery patients are implemented in the care of these patients.

Once preterm labor is controlled, the monitoring lines are removed, tocolysis is weaned to oral medication, and the care of the mother is returned to the obstetric service where management is continued under the direction of the perinatologist.

Discharge Planning and Follow-up

After fetal surgery, plans are made by the social worker for patient discharge to the nearby facility such as a "Ronald McDonald House." In the majority of cases, the family will remain nearby the FTC for the duration of the pregnancy undergoing frequent sonography and obstetric care. Occasionally, the family is allowed to return home with monitoring done by the referring perinatologist and frequent contact with the FTC team.

For patients who do not undergo fetal intervention, close follow-up is crucial. The family and perinatologist are contacted to discuss how the pregnancy is progressing as well as to discuss perinatal management issues that may arise. If the patient is returning to San Francisco for delivery, we assist in the travel, the planning and timing of the delivery, and the coordination of services.

Short- and long-term follow-up is provided by the FTC including long-term follow-up of neurodevelopmental outcome. This follow-up enables the FTC to provide the most reliable information related to patient outcome and also provides reassurance to the family.

Financial Considerations

Extremely specialized interventions have been shown to be most cost effective if provided at a few centers. Morbidity and mortality have also been demonstrated to decrease as the number of procedures performed increases. The FTC is a regionalized approach to providing specialized care and as such requires funding and recognition of medical necessity from state and federal agencies as well as third-party payors. Third-party payors now recognize that these highly specialized interventions are not necessarily "experimental" and thus excluded from coverage and, in fact, often prove "preventative" and cost effective. But it is only recently that third-party payors in the United States, including Medicaid, and in other developed countries have approved reimbursement for prenatal treatment at our center. Coverage for each family has to be negotiated and confirmed prior to treatment. Sometimes coverage is denied and must be appealed.

The experience in San Francisco is instructive. We have been fortunate to have had a very strong institutional commitment to fetal therapy, which was absolutely necessary in the early years of little or no reimbursement. Hospital costs for the first series of patients were absorbed by the UCSF Medical Center. When coverage cannot be obtained, our medical center has generously agreed to heavily discounted or no charges in many cases. We feel strongly that the family should not take on a potentially heavy financial burden for fetal care. The present uncertainty about insurance coverage places the parents in an uneasy position, not knowing the outcome for their child, and not knowing how they will pay for medical treatment.

While coverage for individual families is improving, funding for the enterprise of fetal treatment and for the infrastructure of a fetal treatment center is always difficult. In the age of managed care, medical centers and medical schools balk at funding even those positions indispensable to good patient care and success of the program (e.g., nurse coordinator, long-term care coordinator, research fellows, etc.). Needless to say, outside funding for research and training is crucial to the enterprise but remains difficult to secure. Fundraising through grants and gifts is exhausting but necessary. For example, the UCSF FTC has raised and expended over $10 million on research and development.

It is important to point out that a successful fetal treatment program more than pays for itself not through reimbursement for the procedures but through obstetric and neonatal activity attracted to the medical center. In our enterprise, for every patient requiring fetal intervention, nine others not requiring fetal intervention require delivery and prolonged neonatal care at our center. A detailed financial analysis of the FTC clinical activity over 1 year revealed a more than $1 million contribution to the margin for the hospital, and a considerable contribution to the revenue of perinatologists, neonatologists, and surgical subspecialists.

Outreach and Communication

The FTC provides community outreach with the most current information concerning diagnosis and treatment of fetal abnormalities, as well as immediate phone consultation and review of sonographic material submitted by referring physicians. A Web page that can be accessed over the Internet is an excellent way to educate families and referring physicians. A newsletter is helpful, particularly for families who have been cared for and remain committed to the enterprise. For example, in San Francisco, we have established a toll-free telephone number so families and physicians can reach us (1-800-RX-FETUS), published a newsletter for 10 years, and more recently created a Web page (www.fetus.ucsf.edu). In the future, the use of telemedicine capabilities will expedite diagnostic assessment and assist providers and families with information and management of the fetus with anomalies.

"Spinoff" From the Fetal Treatment Enterprise

While only a few fetal defects are amenable to treatment at present, the enterprise of fetal treatment has produced some unexpected "spinoffs" that have significance beyond this narrow therapeutic field. For pediatricians, neonatologists, and dysmorphologists, the natural history and pathophysiology of many previously mysterious newborn conditions have been clarified by following the development of the disease in utero. For obstetricians, perinatologists, and fetologists, techniques developed in experimental work in lambs and monkeys will prove useful in caring for other high-risk pregnancies (e.g., an absorbable stapling device developed for fetal surgery has been applied to cesarean sections,[4] radiotelemetric monitoring has applications outside fetal surgery,[5] and videoendoscopic techniques, which allow fetal manipulation without hysterotomy, will greatly extend the indications for fetal intervention[6, 7]). Finally, the intensive effort to solve the vexing problem of preterm labor after hysterotomy for fetal surgery[8] has yielded new insight into the role of nitric oxide in myometrial contractions, and has spawned interest in treating spontaneous preterm labor with nitric oxide donors.[9]

Fetal treatment research has yielded advances in fetal biology with implications beyond fetal therapy. The serendipitous observation that the fetus heals incisions without scar has provided new insights into the biology of wound healing and stimulated efforts to mimic the fetal process postnatally. Fetal tissue appears biologically and immunologically superior for transplantation and for gene therapy, and fetal immunologic tolerance may allow a wide variety of inherited nonsurgical diseases to be cured by fetal hematopoietic stem cell transplantation.

The great promise of fetal therapy is that for some diseases the earliest possible intervention (i.e., before birth) will produce the best possible outcome (i.e., the best quality of life for the resources expended). However, the promise of cost-effective, preventative fetal therapy can be subverted by misguided clinical applications (e.g., a complex in utero procedure that "half-saves" an otherwise doomed fetus for a life of intensive [and expensive] care). Enthusiasm for fetal intervention must be tempered by reverence for the interests of the mother and her family, by careful study of the disease in experimental fetal animals and untreated human fetuses, and by a willingness to abandon therapy that does not prove effective and cost-effective in properly controlled trials.

REFERENCES

1. Harrison MR, Golbus MS, Filly RA (eds): The Unborn Patient: Prenatal Diagnosis and Treatment, 2nd ed. Philadelphia: WB Saunders Company, 1990.
2. Harrison MR, Adzick NS: The fetus as a patient: Surgical considerations. Ann Surg 213:279–291, 1990.
3. Harrison MR: Fetal surgery. West J Med 159:341–349, 1993.
4. Bond SJ, Harrison MR, Slotnick RN, et al: Cesarean delivery and hysterotomy using an absorbable stapling device. Obstet Gynecol 74:25–28, 1989.
5. Jennings RW, Adzick NS, Longaker MT, Harrison MR: Radiotelemetric fetal monitoring during and after open fetal surgery. Surg Obstet Gynecol 176:59–64, 1993.
6. De Lia JE, Cruikshank DP, Keye WR: Fetoscopic neodymium: YAG laser occlusion of placental vessels in severe twin-twin fusion syndrome. Obstet Gynecol 75:1046–1053, 1990.
7. Estes JM, MacGillivray TE, Hedrick MH, et al: Fetoscopic surgery for the treatment of congenital anomalies. J Pediatr Surg 27:950–954, 1992.
8. Sabik JF, Assad RS, Hanley FL: Halothane as an anesthetic for fetal surgery. J Pediatr Surg 28:542–546, 1993.
9. Lees C, Campbell S, Jauniaux E, et al: Arrest of preterm labor and prolongation of gestation with glyceryl trinitrate, a nitric oxide donor. Lancet 343:1325–1326, 1994.

CHAPTER 2

Historical Perspective

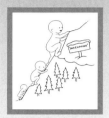

MICHAEL R. HARRISON

The concept that the fetus is a patient, an individual whose maladies are a proper subject for medical treatment as well as scientific observation, is alarmingly modern. It was not until the last half of the 20th century that the prying eye of the ultrasonographer rendered the once opaque womb transparent, letting the light of scientific observation fall on the shy and secretive fetus.

Historically, we approached the fetus with a wonder bordering on mysticism. Enid Bagnold's description in *The Door of Life* captures the awe engendered by a scene that no one had actually witnessed.

Hanging head downwards between cliffs of bone was the baby, its arms all but clasped about its neck, its face aslant upon its arms, hair painted upon its skull, closed, secret eyes, a diver poised in albumen, ancient and epic, shot with delicate spasms, as old as a Pharaoh in its tomb.

Whether this reverence is a reflection of our profound wonder at the "miracle" of differentiation of a fertilized egg into a human infant or a clandestine darwinian mechanism to ensure the survival of the species, it has certainly hindered investigation of fetal physiology and precluded any consideration of fetal therapy. Only in the last few decades have techniques for visualizing, monitoring, measuring, and prodding the fetus begun to alter our perceptions of the living human fetus. Only now are we beginning to consider the fetus seriously—medically, legally, and ethically. Now that our perspective is undergoing radical change, it is instructive to trace the medical history of our approach to this, our most reticent patient.[1]

The Ancients' View of the Fetus as Seed and Homunculus

Animal husbandry is quite complicated, although few view it in this fashion. In biblical times, it was enough to describe the phenomenon: someone begat someone who begat someone who, etc. The intricacies of the begetting—the conception and growth of the individual—were matters assigned to the realm of Solomon's wisdom: "And in my mother's womb was fashioned to be flesh in the time of ten months, being compacted in blood, of the seed of man, and the pleasure that came with sleep" (Wisdom of Solomon, 7:2). There was general recognition that physical characteristics passed from parent to offspring, and this idea was conceptualized as a seed passed from the father to the mother where it grew and later blossomed as a child. Even into the 2nd century, Marcus Aurelius could say: "A man passes seed into the womb and goes away, and anon another cause takes it in hand and works upon it and perfects a babe—what a consummation from what a beginning!" (Meditations, X:26) (Fig. 2–1).

In attempting to explain how the fetus was related to the child, the Greek and Roman thinkers conceived the idea of the homunculus—a miniature person living and growing within the mother before birth. This concept undoubtedly evolved from practical experience in animal husbandry and from observation of aborted human and animal fetuses. The fetus was seen to grow in resemblance to the child as gestation progressed. In the absence of "modern" biologic information, the homunculus provided a very good explanation for at least the older fetus.

The homunculus, a purely descriptive explanation, was sometimes carried to a wonderfully whimsical extreme. Lawrence Sterne, in *The Life and Opinion of Tristram Shandy, Gentleman* (Book 1, Chapter 2), had his hero soliloquize:

The homunculus, sir, in however low and ludicrous a light he may appear, in this age of levity, to the eye of folly or prejudice;—to the eye of reason in scientific research, he stands confessed—a being guarded and circumscribed with rights. The minutest philosophers who, by the by, have the most enlarged understandings (their souls being inversely as their inquiries), show us incontestably, that the homunculus is created by the same hand,—engendered in the same course of nature,—endowed with the same locomotive powers and faculties with us; that he consists, as we do, of skin, hair, fat, flesh, veins, arteries, ligaments, nerves, cartilages, bones, marrow, brains, glands, genitals, humors, and articulations,—is a being of as much activity,—and in all senses of the word, as much and as truly our fellow creature as my Lord Chancellor of England. He may be benefitted, he may be injured, he may obtain redress; in a word, he has all the claims and rights of humanity. . . .

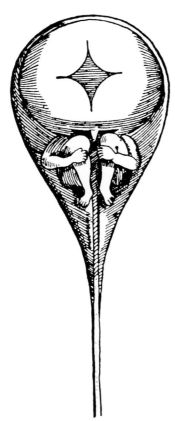

FIGURE 2–1. A human spermatozoon is shown containing a homunculus. (From Hartsoeker: Essai de Dioptrique, Sect. 88, Parks, 1694. In Meyer AW: The Rise of Embryology. Stanford: Stanford University Press, 1939.)

Attempts to Describe the Fetus

Prior to the 20th century, the development of both obstetrics and pediatrics contributed surprisingly little to our knowledge of the fetus. Although physicians were beginning to take an interest in children as early as 1472, when Paulus Bagellardus published *The Little Book of Diseases of Children*, it was not until 1748 that a scientific treatise on the care and feeding of infants appeared. William Cadogan of London, in his monograph *An Essay upon Nursing,* denounced the common practice of feeding the infant artificially until the mother's milk came down and noted that the infant "requires some intermediate time of abstinence and rest to compose and recover the struggle of the birth and the change of circulation (the blood running into new channels)," thus contributing the first significant observation about perinatal circulatory physiology.

The work of Charles Darwin had an indirect but significant impact on our scientific and philosophical attitude toward the fetus. His ideas about the evolution of species provided a macroscopic view of reproduction that posited a progression from seed to infant, as well as from generation to generation. Before his view of procreation and speciation became generally known, the relation between the seed and the infant was a religious matter, a continuum accepted on faith. This may account

for the derivation of the current religious doctrine that links copulation directly with procreation and, thus, ascribes the sacredness of life to the conceptus or homunculus from its very beginning. Darwin's ideas demystified the role of reproduction. In *The Descent of Man*, he wrote: "Man is developed from an ovule, about 125th of an inch in diameter, which differs in no respect from the ovules of any animal."

At the dawn of the 20th century, the fetus was shedding its metaphysical trappings in favor of biologic description. Still, the concepts of inheritance and evolution did little to explain exactly how the seed became an infant, and work on the development of the human fetus remained entirely descriptive during the first part of the 20th century. In the 1920s, Minkowski examined human fetuses obtained at cesarean operations by placing the recently delivered fetus in warm saline solution. Hertig and Rock studied aborted fetuses at various stages of gestation and were able to piece together the morphology of embryonic and fetal development. This descriptive information was supplemented by the study of animal fetuses in various species, an undertaking that also blossomed and bore fruit in the 20th century (Fig. 2–2).

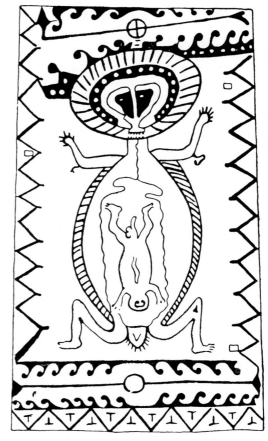

FIGURE 2–2. A fetus is displayed on a painted and carved door from Dutch New Guinea. (From deClercq FSA, Schmelz JDE: Ethnographische Beschrijving van de West-en Noordkust van Nederlansch, New Guinea. In Needham J: A History of Embryology. New York: Abelard-Schuman, 1959, p 19.)

Experimental Fetal Observation

Since early observations of the human fetus were limited to an occasional aborted "homunculus," fetal developmental anatomy and physiology had to be derived almost exclusively from observations made on animals. This is undoubtedly how Hippocrates arrived at the brilliantly intuitive proposal that the fetus urinated in utero and that amniotic fluid consists of fetal urine, an observation confirmed only during the 19th century. Andreas Vesalius must be credited with the first truly analytic observations on the living mammalian fetus. At the time when Galen's dogmatism reigned and before the circulation of blood was discovered, Vesalius described in *De Humani Corporis Fabrica* (1543) the anatomy of the fetoplacental unit and the experimental preparation on which observations were based:

> Quite pleasing is it, in the management of the fetus, to see how, when the fetus touches the surrounding air, it tries to breathe. And this dissection is performed opportunely in a dog or pig when the sow will soon be ready to drop her young . . . the naked fetus attempts and struggles for respiration and thereupon, when the coverings are punctured and broken, thou shalt see that when the fetus breathes that pulsations of the arteries of the fetal membranes and of the umbilicus stop. Up to this moment, the arteries of the uterus are beating in unison with the rest of the arteries outside of itself.

This remarkable description, based on direct observation of a dissected living fetus, marked the beginning of scientific fetal observation.

It was not until the 19th century that experimental animal preparations were used to make physiologic observations on the living mammalian fetus. Bichat in 1803 was the first to study fetal movements. Zuntz (1877) and later Preyer (1885) studied intact fetal guinea pigs suspended in warm saline. They noted that the fetus must be kept in warm physiologic salt solution and that a fetus, once allowed to breathe, could not be returned to its mother and survive.

Experimental fetal observation blossomed in the 20th century, at first reluctantly, and then with a crescendo of enthusiasm. By 1920, the first successful fetal operations had been performed: Mayer removed guinea pig fetuses from the uterus and placed them in the maternal abdominal cavity—a few guinea pigs survived for several days. Fetal movements had been studied by Graham Brown in the cat and also by Lane in the rat. In the 1920s, the first experimental in utero manipulation was demonstrated by Swenson, and the possibility of normal delivery after in utero surgery was established by Nicholas. In the 1930s and 1940s, experimental fetal observation gained momentum. Barcroft introduced the most productive fetal experimental model when he described operations on the lamb fetus using spinal anesthesia. Surgery was performed through a small uterine incision, without removing the fetus. Hall's work on development of the nervous system in the fetal rat and Barron's work on neurologic development in the fetal lamb extended the techniques for fetal surgery, including the use of pursestring sutures to avoid the loss of amniotic fluid.[2]

Experimental Fetal Intervention to Study Fetal Malformations

The first major dividend from experimental fetal manipulation came when Jost demonstrated that removal of the fetal rabbit testes had a profound influence on subsequent sexual development.[3] In the 1950s, Louw and Barnard produced intestinal atresia, similar to that seen in human neonates, by interrupting the mesenteric blood supply in fetal puppies.[4] This contribution was important, although it was less glamorous than was Barnard's later work with cardiac transplantation, because it not only established the ischemic pathogenesis of neonatal intestinal atresia but also demonstrated the feasibility of simulating human birth defects by appropriate fetal manipulation.

In the 1960s and 1970s, experimental fetal surgery was used to simulate a variety of human congenital anomalies: coarctation of the aorta in the puppy,[5] intestinal atresia in the rabbit,[6] congenital diaphragmatic hernia in the lamb,[7] congenital hydronephrosis in the rabbit[8] and lamb,[9] and congenital heart disease in the lamb.[10] Perhaps more important, the development of a chronically catheterized fetal lamb preparation led to intensive investigation of fetal cardiovascular, pulmonary, and renal physiology.[10, 11] Experimental fetal surgery proved to be more difficult in the primate, where uterine contractility and preterm labor were more difficult to control. However, in the last two decades, advances in surgical and anesthetic techniques and in the pharmacologic control of labor have made experimental manipulation of even the primate fetus feasible (Fig. 2–3).[12]

By the late 1970s, a variety of experimental fetal models were used widely to study both normal developmental physiology and the pathophysiology of several congenital defects. These models proved to be both descriptive and predictive; for example, removal of a piece of diaphragm not only produced a lesion that mimicked the human analogue (congenital diaphragmatic hernia) but also produced the associated developmental consequence (i.e., pulmonary hypoplasia).

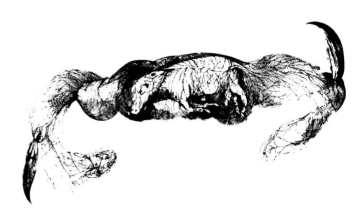

FIGURE 2–3. Dissection of the living mammalian fetus marks the beginning of scientific fetal observation. (From Adelmann HB [trans.]: The Embryological Treatises of Hieronymus Fabricius of Aquapendente. 2: The Formed Fetus. Copyright © 1942 by Cornell University. Used by permission of the publisher. Cornell University Press.)

Once the pathophysiology of certain congenital anomalies has been clarified, these models may be used to explore treatment. For instance, babies born with congenital diaphragmatic hernia die because their lungs are hypoplastic. It has been demonstrated experimentally that simulated correction of experimental diaphragmatic hernia in utero may prevent the development of fatal pulmonary hypoplasia.[13] Now that fetal malformations like diaphragmatic hernia can be detected prenatally, fetal experiments designed to explore the pathophysiology of correctable congenital anomalies will assume some practical clinical significance. In the natural evolution of thought, our ability to detect malformations clinically and our ability to study them experimentally raises the questions: What medical treatments can be applied to ameliorate these abnormalities? Must we await birth to apply our knowledge of treatment of congenital abnormalities?

The Fetus Demystified

The fetus could not be considered a patient until it was demystified; until the origin and development of the fetus from embryo to neonate could be explained scientifically. It is only with the development of molecular biology in the last century that we have been able to bridge the conceptual gap between the seed and the fully developed and marvelously complex human infant, between subcellular events like DNA-directed enzyme synthesis and subsequent complex biologic functions like the digestion of food. Modern molecular biology provided the conceptual framework for linking the seed to the infant: The seed contains a microscopic blueprint encoded in DNA for the future individual. We can now be confident that there is an explicable order in the differentiation of the seed into the individual, even if we do not know exactly how the microscopic blueprint is acted out in the orchestrated ballet of fetal development.

Although molecular biology provided a conceptual framework that demystified fetal development, the fetus could not be a patient until his or her ailments could be diagnosed. The ability to diagnose fetal disorders evolved slowly. Fetal activity felt by the mother or palpated by her physician was the first crude measure of fetal well-being. Then the fetal heartbeat, detected at first by auscultation and later by sophisticated electronic monitors, was found to reflect fetal stress and distress. Later, minute amounts of gestational hormones were detected in maternal blood and urine. These levels correlated with the condition of the fetus. Then came amniocentesis: Analysis of the constituents of amniotic fluid made possible the prenatal diagnosis of many inherited metabolic and chromosomal disorders and permitted assessment of fetal pulmonary maturity and the severity of fetal hemolytic reactions.

But the development that had the most profound effect on our approach to the fetus was the introduction of a safe, noninvasive imaging technique that permitted direct visualization of the living fetus. X-rays were recognized as being potentially harmful to the developing organism: Plain x-rays yielded little information, and introduction of radiopaque materials into the amniotic fluid (amniogram) increased the risk of premature rupture of the membranes or preterm labor without yielding much more diagnostic information. Sonography was then developed. This method enabled accurate delineation of normal and abnormal fetal anatomy with considerable detail and later on "live" moving pictures. Unlike previous techniques, ultrasonic imaging appears to have no harmful effect on the mother or on the fetus.

The sonographic voyeur, spying on the unwary fetus, finds that he or she is surprisingly active and does not at all resemble the passive parasite that we had imagined. The sonographer sees the fetus kicking and rolling, breathing in peculiar cyclical bursts, swallowing enormous quantities of amniotic fluid, and emptying its bladder. The sonographer can even see the rhythmic motion of the heart and its valves. Fetal parts can be measured to assess fetal growth, and an increasing number of anatomic malformations can be accurately delineated. Sonography can be used to guide needle puncture of the amniotic cavity for amniocentesis, or needle aspiration of fetal urine, ascites, and cerebrospinal fluid.

Real-time sonography can guide the safe acquisition of fetal blood and other fetal tissues (e.g., skin, liver, muscle). Such samples enable the diagnosis of fetal hematologic disorders and enzymatic defects that cannot be detected by amniocentesis alone. In addition, the newest noninvasive imaging technique, nuclear magnetic resonance, promises not only definition of fetal anatomy but actual chemical definition of fetal tissue without invasive sampling.

Most of the early techniques for prenatal diagnosis evolved to detect serious inherited diseases and malformations that were incompatible with normal postnatal life. The diagnosis of such diseases usually led to abortion. An indirect but more positive benefit of prenatal testing for potentially fatal lesions is, of course, reassurance when the test is negative. Nevertheless, through this early concentration on detecting uncorrectable fetal disorders, prenatal diagnosis has acquired, for some, an unsavory connotation: that the only way to prevent birth defects is to eliminate the defective fetus. In the past, the possibility of preventing certain birth defects by correcting the defect, rather than by eliminating the fetus, had not been seriously considered. Consequently, the diagnosis of potentially correctable disorders has attracted less attention than has the diagnosis of more lethal lesions.

Early Attempts to Treat Fetal Disease

Although we are only now beginning to attempt fetal treatment, the idea is not new. Hydrops fetalis, associated with maternal Rh sensitization, was the first fetal disorder to be treated successfully. In the early 1960s, treatment of the neonate with severe hydrops fetalis was so discouraging that Liley attempted to transfuse the fetus in utero. He demonstrated that intra-abdominal infusion of blood ameliorated severe hydrops, thus inaugurating fetal intervention.[14]

A little-known side to this story marked a rather inauspicious start for more invasive fetal treatment. A logical refinement in the treatment of the erythroblastotic fetus was complete exchange transfusion. This required direct access to the fetal circulation, which prompted the first in utero fetal operations. In the early 1960s, obstetricians in New York and Puerto Rico exposed several fetuses though uterine incisions to cannulate femoral and jugular vessels for exchange transfusion. The overall experience was apparently discouraging. Reports were sketchy, and this approach was quickly abandoned and laid dormant for the next decade. Surgical exposure of the living fetus would have to await development of better anesthetic agents and surgical techniques, but this initial experience at least raised the possibility of fetal surgery.[15]

The next fetal disease to be approached therapeutically was the devastating respiratory distress syndrome of prematurity. Through a combination of clinical experience with severely premature infants and laboratory experiments using fetal lamb and rabbit preparations, surfactant deficiency was established as being the physiologic basis for the respiratory distress syndrome. Effective treatment could then be devised. Glucocorticoids administered to the fetus via the mother increase fetal surfactant production, hasten fetal lung maturation, and ameliorate the respiratory distress syndrome. Glucocorticoid therapy to induce fetal lung maturation, combined with improved methods of respiratory support for tiny premature infants, has greatly reduced the mortality caused by this condition.

It is now apparent that there are other fetal disorders that not only can be diagnosed in utero but also can be treated by prenatal administration of appropriate medications or hormones. The severe developmental consequences of congenital hypothyroidism, for example, might be prevented by giving thyroid hormone to the fetus. Furthermore, certain other fetal deficiencies can be treated by providing blood cells, hormones, or medications.

By the 1980s, we were ready to take the next step, which is the correction of fetal anatomic defects. Although many fetal anatomic malformations can be detected by sonography, only selected cases warrant consideration for intrauterine therapy because only a few have a compelling physiologic rationale for prenatal correction. Congenital hydronephrosis, diaphragmatic hernia, and obstructive hydrocephalus are examples of malformations in which a simple anatomic lesion interferes with organ development and, if the anatomic defect is corrected, fetal development may proceed normally. The physiologic rationale for in utero correction of these lesions was defined, and the feasibility of in utero correction was established.[16, 17]

How the Fetus Became a Patient In Our Lifetime

It is important to recognize that it is only during our professional lifetime, and really only in the last decades of the 20th century, that the fetus has become a patient.

We now know that the fetus has disorders that can be diagnosed and treated, and society can now accept the fetus as an unborn patient. How did such a remarkable shift in attitude toward the fetus occur in such a short time?

The impetus for fetal treatment came from two fields of endeavor that developed rapidly during the last two decades. Neonatologists and surgeons traced the pathogenesis of the problems they treated after birth back to the fetus, and obstetricians, geneticists, and sonologists developed the ability to accurately diagnose human fetal disease (Fig. 2–4).

Clinical frustration provided the impetus for unraveling the pathophysiology on neonatal malformations, such as congenital diaphragmatic hernia, hydronephrosis, and hydrocephalus. Pediatric surgeons and neonatologists were frustrated by caring for newborn babies with problems that were discovered "too late to correct." This is the same frustration that all physicians feel when they discover a disease process that has already gone too far, whether it is a cancer that has already metastasized or the ulcer that has perforated; the same frustration that makes all healers say: "If only we had been here a little earlier—we might have changed the course of that disease." When physicians responsible for neonates who died with a diaphragmatic hernia or hydronephrosis realized that the disease process was already at the final stage at birth, they began to ask whether the course of the disease might be changed if something could be done earlier. Both diagnosis and treatment would have to be before birth. The questions then became: Can the lesion be diagnosed before birth? Will intervention have the desired effect? and Can it be done? Thus, clinical frustration in dealing with uncorrectable neonatal diseases led to the experimental stud-

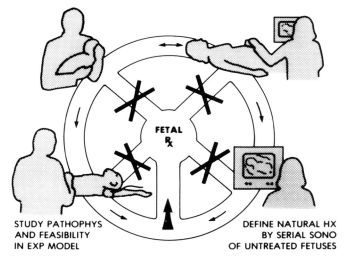

STUDY PATHOPHYS AND FEASIBILITY IN EXP MODEL

DEFINE NATURAL HX BY SERIAL SONO OF UNTREATED FETUSES

FIGURE 2–4. The impetus for fetal treatment came from pediatricians and surgeons who were frustrated by diseases that were already uncorrectable at birth and from obstetricians and sonographers who were seeing fetuses with potentially correctable defects before birth. However, before fetal treatment could be implemented, the pathophysiology of the disorder and the feasibility of repair had to be established experimentally, and the natural history of the disease in the untreated human fetus had to be defined by serial sonography.

ies in which a model of the human disease was created in fetal animals to study the pathophysiology of the process, to test whether the damage seen at birth was reversible if corrected before birth, and to establish the feasibility and safety of in utero intervention.

While researchers were exploring certain life-threatening neonatal problems that might lend themselves to correction before birth, obstetricians, geneticists, and sonographers were developing the techniques of prenatal diagnosis and were finding fetuses with similar defects. Although prenatal diagnosis by amniocentesis was aimed initially at potentially fatal fetal diseases, the development of sophisticated new imaging techniques allowed accurate delineation of other anomalies that were often found serendipitously during ultrasonography performed for obstetric indications. Thus, physicians primarily concerned with management of the mother and fetus through pregnancy (e.g., perinatologists, geneticists, obstetric sonologists) could detect fetal lesions, such as hydronephrosis and hydrocephalus, and they could begin to wonder what they could do for this fetus and how they could best manage this pregnancy. Physicians interested in all phases of fetoneonatal development began sharing information and ideas about how the fetal condition might determine the place, timing, and mode of delivery. Detection of fetal defects also led to serial sonographic studies that defined the natural history and pathophysiology of an increasing number of human fetal diseases, including hydronephrosis, diaphragmatic hernia, hydrocephalus, and nonimmune hydrops. Fetal medicine was established.

Thus, the impetus provided by the neonate who had an uncorrectable disorder at birth and the fetus who had a birth defect detected before birth led to the realization that many fetal diseases may require medical management before birth. Although neither impetus was sufficient in itself to justify fetal intervention, together they spurred the necessary clinical and experimental studies that would lead to successful fetal treatment. When the baby's physician and the mother's physician together began to define the natural history of the disease by serial sonographic examination of untreated human fetuses and to study the pathophysiology and feasibility of fetal intervention in experimental animal models, the stage was set for a full consideration of the fetus as a patient. Thus, fetal treatment is the flowering of more than a decade of clinical and experimental work in prenatal diagnosis and fetoneonatal physiology by physicians of diverse specialties and backgrounds.

A very brief summary of milestones in the development of fetal surgery are presented in Table 2–1. The advances in treating various fetal diseases are discussed in the relevant chapters of this book.

Fetal Physicians Found a Field

During the critical early stage in the development of promising but unproven fetal therapy, one of the most difficult issues was deciding when a new procedure could be offered to a patient. The diagnostic and therapeutic maneuvers discussed in the 1970s and 1980s in-

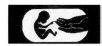

TABLE 2–1. MILESTONES IN THE DEVELOPMENT OF FETAL SURGERY

Hysterotomy → Vascular access (1960s)
Hysterotomy refined: Absorbable staples, retractor, fibrin glue (1982)
Maternal safety: Monkey model (1983)
First successful open fetal surgery (1983)
First edition of *The Unborn Patient* (1984)
Fetal monitoring: Radiotelemeter (1988)
First successful open CDH repair (1989)
Experimental fetoscopic techniques (1989)
Nitric oxide role in uterine relaxation (1991)
Fetoscopic techniques refined [FETENDO] (1995)
First successful FETENDO clip (1997)
Myelomeningocele repaired (1997)

volved risks not only to the fetus but also to the mother. This raised difficult ethical problems concerning the rights of the fetus and the mother, the assessment of risk versus benefit, and the responsibilities of those involved in innovative therapy and research.

Because work in this area was new, controversial, and liable to misinterpretation, some general guidelines were developed by leaders in the field and adopted by almost all the early practitioners of innovative fetal treatment. For example, in the early stages of development of the Fetal Treatment Program (FTP) at the University of California at San Francisco (UCSF) in the early 1980s, we established guidelines for intervention. We agreed that intervention should not be considered until the following criteria were met: (1) the natural history of the disease was defined by serial sonography in untreated cases, (2) the pathophysiology of the disease was studied in an appropriate animal model, (3) the feasibility and safety of intervention must be discussed with noninvolved physicians and opposing viewpoints presented to the patient, (4) informed consent procedures must be approved by the Committee on Human Research, and finally, (5) every case of attempted fetal treatment must be reported to the medical profession regardless of outcome.

More specific criteria for individual cases emerged as experience with fetal treatment grew at centers around the world. In 1982, we asked the Kroc Foundation to host a conference called "Unborn: Management of the Fetus with a Correctable Defect." This conference brought together 24 obstetricians, surgeons, sonologists, pediatricians, bioethicists, and physiologists from centers active in fetal treatment around the world. Experimental and clinical experience with fetal treatment was reviewed intensively to assess the potential benefits and liabilities of various interventions, the directions that should be pursued, and the problems that should be avoided. The participants agreed to pursue a cooperative exchange of information, to establish a registry of treated cases, and to formulate some tentative guidelines for use in selecting patients and procedures.

This informative exchange of information, which all agreed should be carried on at annual meetings (the founding of the "International Fetal Medicine and Surgery Society"), produced the following general consensus about fetal treatment, which is still generally applicable today:

1. The fetus should be a singleton in whom a detailed sonographic examination and genetic studies reveal no concomitant abnormalities.
2. The family should be fully counseled about risks and benefits and should agree to treatment, including long-term follow-up to determine efficacy.
3. A multidisciplinary team that includes a perinatologist experienced in fetal diagnosis and fetal sampling or intrauterine transfusion, a geneticist, a sonologist experienced in the diagnosis of fetal anomalies, and the pediatric surgeon and neonatologist who will manage the infant after birth should concur in the plan for innovative treatment; and the approval of an institutional review board should be obtained.
4. There should be access to a level III high-risk obstetric unit and intensive care nursery and also to bioethical and psychosocial consultation.

By coming to agreement on some principles that would guide the few teams involved in fetal treatment during the early years (1980s), the enterprise of fetal therapy avoided the treacherous and potentially ruinous debacle of teams rushing to attempt "spectacular" fetal interventions for media attention, as happened with cardiac transplantation in the 1970s.

The early practitioners of fetal treatment realized that they could find and define many birth defects in utero. They anticipated that as diagnostic abilities improved, so also would their ability to select for treatment only those fetuses who would benefit from intervention. They then set about refining their ability to measure fetal organ function so that they would no longer have to make important clinical decisions based on morphologic criteria alone. Treatment of several fetal disorders proved feasible, but a great deal of clinical and laboratory expertise was required to determine which procedures were safe and effective. The teams involved understood that treatment of more complicated congenital anomalies would expand as techniques for fetal intervention improved, and that this progress would require a great deal of work, both clinical and experimental.

The evolution of fetal therapy over the last two decades parallels the founding and evolution of the International Fetal Medicine and Surgery Society from the first meeting in Santa Barbara, California, in 1982 to the most recent meeting at Carlisle, England, in 1999.

The Maturation of Fetal Therapy: From Registries to Trials

New technologies usually start in a single, highly committed center, and initially remain confined to a relatively small number of centers with the interest, expertise, and resources to achieve reasonable results. This was fetal therapy in the 1980s. In this phase, registries are often useful. Such was the case for the initial registries sponsored by the International Fetal Medicine and Surgery Society for cases of hydronephrosis and hydrocephalus treated with shunts. But as technologies like fetal treatment diffuse out to less experienced centers, the value of multicenter registries decreases. Such proved to be the case for attempted registries for fetal metabolic diseases and cardiac arrhythmias.

In the 1990s, it became clear that for fetal therapy to progress it would be necessary to determine the efficacy of intervention through properly controlled clinical trials, which have proven incredibly difficult to execute. Two multicenter trials comparing vaginal to cesarean delivery for gastroschisis have not succeeded despite considerable effort. Single-center trials are much easier logistically. The only successful controlled trial to date, comparing open fetal surgery to optimal postnatal care for diaphragmatic hernia, was successfully completed despite incredible logistic and bureaucratic challenges. This trial, although difficult, provided a definitive answer to a difficult question, and prevented further attempts at total repair of diaphragmatic hernias in fetuses without liver herniation. No other trials have succeeded to date. By stopping fetal surgical repair, it directly spurred development of a new approach to reversing pulmonary hypoplasia by temporary tracheal occlusion. The power of properly conducted clinical trials is clear and must be brought to bear on the many therapeutic dilemmas in fetal treatment. The transition from registry data to controlled trials will be a continuing challenge for the international fetal treatment community.

We can find and define many birth defects in utero. As diagnostic abilities improve, so also does our ability to select for treatment only fetuses who will benefit from intervention. We must refine our ability to measure fetal organ function so that we do not have to make important clinical decisions based on morphologic criteria alone. Treatment of several fetal disorders has proved to be feasible, but a great deal of clinical and laboratory expertise will be required to determine which procedures are safe and effective. Treatment of more complicated congenital anomalies will expand as techniques for fetal intervention improve. However, this progress will require a great deal of work, both clinical and experimental.

The short but eventful history of the fetus as a patient reassures us that fetal treatment offers new hope for the fetus with a correctable defect, and reminds us that there is considerable potential for doing harm. We know that innovative fetal treatment must be fully tested in the laboratory, carefully considered in the light of current diagnostic and therapeutic uncertainties, honestly presented to the prospective parents, and finally undertaken only with trepidation. It is now clear that because a procedure can be done does not mean that it should be done and that a fetal abnormality of any type should never be treated simply "because it is there," and never by someone who is unprepared for this fearsome responsibility. In the early harrowing days of fetal treatment, no one could be sure whether the enterprise would succeed or die. At that time, the banner of the fetal treatment center read: "Proceed with caution . . . and enthusiasm." We can now be confident that the enterprise itself has succeeded as reflected in the robustness of professional societies like the International Fetal Medicine and Surgery Society and the Fetus as a Patient Society, the proliferation of professional journals like *Fetal Diagnosis and Therapy* and *Ultrasound in Obstetrics and Gynecology,* and of textbooks like this one. As the number and quality of professionals devoted to fetal treatment increase, and the number and quality of fetal treatment teams and fetal treatment centers around the world continues to grow, the banner for the 21st century should read "Fetal Therapy: Build On a Solid Foundation."

REFERENCES

1. Harrison MR: Unborn: Historical perspective of the fetus as a patient. The Pharos 45:19, 1982.
2. Rosenkrantz JG, Simon RC, Carlisle JH: Fetal surgery in the pig with a review of other mammalian fetal techniques. J Pediatr Surg 3:392, 1965.
3. Jost A: Sur la differenciation sexuelle de l'embryon de lapin. I: Remarques au sujet de certaines operations chirurgicales sur l'embryon. II: Experiences de paraboise. CR Soc Biol 140:461, 1946.
4. Louw JH, Bernard CN: Congenital intestinal atresia: Observations on its origin. Lancet 2:1065, 1955.
5. Jackson BT, Piasecki GJ, Egdahl RH: Experimental production of coarctation of the aorta in utero with prolonged postnatal survival. Surg Forum 14:290, 1963.
6. Blanc WA, Silver LA: Intrauterine abdominal surgery in the rabbit fetus: Production of congenital intestinal atresia. Am J Dis Child 104:548, 1962.
7. deLorimier AA, Tierney DF, Parker HR: Hypoplastic lungs in fetal lambs with surgically produced congenital diaphragmatic hernia. Surgery 62:12, 1967.
8. Thomasson BM, Easterly JR, Ravitch MM: Morphologic changes in the fetal kidney after intrauterine ureteral ligation. Invest Urol 8:261, 1970.
9. Beck AD: The effect of intra-uterine urinary obstruction upon the development of the fetal kidney. J Urol 105:784, 1971.
10. Heymann MA, Rudolph AM: Effects of congenital heart disease on fetal and neonatal circulations. Prog Cardiovasc Dis 15:115, 1972.
11. Assali NS (ed): Biology of Gestation. New York: Academic Press, 1968.
12. Suzuki K, Plentyl AA: Chronic implantation of instruments in the neck of the primate fetus for physiologic studies and production of hydramnios. Am J Obstet Gynecol 103:272, 1969.
13. Harrison MR, Bressack MA, Churg AM, et al: Correction of congenital diaphragmatic hernia in utero. II: Simulated correction permits fetal lung growth with survival at birth. Surgery 88:260, 1980.
14. Liley AW: Intrauterine transfusion of the foetus in haemolytic disease. Br Med J 2:1107, 1963.
15. Adamsons K: Fetal surgery. N Engl J Med 275:204, 1966.
16. Harrison MR, Filly RA, Parer JT, et al: Management of the fetus with a urinary tract malformation. JAMA 246:635, 1981.
17. Harrison MR, Filly RA, Golbus MS: Management of the fetus with a correctable congenital defect. JAMA 246:774, 1981.

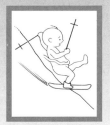

CHAPTER 3

Ethical Considerations

FRANK A. CHERVENAK and LAURENCE B. McCULLOUGH

The bulk of any major textbook such as *The Unborn Patient* is by definition heavily technology laden and technology driven. Whenever dealing with fetal issues, however, there are always ethical concerns that emerge that cannot and should not be ignored. Whether one starts from a theologic, religious, or other perspective, there will also be unreconcilable differences of opinion that are not amenable to satisfactory compromise among all parties. In this chapter, we present the issues so that an ethical framework can be created to identify and manage potential conflicts.

Fetal interventions appear to make the fetus as much a patient as any other patient, save for its locale in utero,[1–5] and so it is no surprise that references to the fetus as a patient are becoming evermore commonplace in the literature and practice of maternal-fetal medicine.[6–12] The concept and language of the fetus as a patient should not, however, develop solely as the effect of technological advances. Clinically grounded, ethical investigation of the concept of the fetus as a patient is also required to guide clinical judgment and practice.

We begin with a brief summary of medical ethics and its principles. We then turn to the task of setting out our ethical framework. On the basis of this framework we address ethical issues in fetal therapy. The chapter closes with a consideration of public policy issues regarding fetal diagnosis and therapy in the context of managed care.

Concepts and Terms of Medical Ethics

Medical ethics involves the disciplined study of the moral obligations of physicians to their patients. This concern for protecting and promoting the interests of human beings when they are patients has been the starting point for medical ethics since the Hippocratic Oath. In the Oath, the physician swore to do what would benefit the sick clinically, while preventing clinical harm to them.[13] In the current language of medical ethics, the Hippocratic Oath should be understood as asserting beneficence-based ethical obligations of the physician to the patient. Beneficence requires the physician to act in such a way as to produce a greater balance of goods over harms for the patient as a result of clinical management, as those goods and harms are understood from, and balanced within, a rigorous, well-informed clinical perspective.[14, 15] The definition of these goods and harms has been clarified over time on the basis of what medicine as a profession can reasonably claim as its competencies: the prevention of premature death; the prevention and management of disease, injury, and handicap; and the prevention and management of unnecessary pain and suffering.[14] Acting on these goods provides concrete, clinically applicable meaning to the fundamental ethical obligation of protecting and promoting the interests of patients. The ethical principle of beneficence translates this perspective into beneficence-based obligations to the pregnant woman and the fetal patient (Fig. 3–1).

Beneficence-based clinical judgment and ethical obligations constituted the whole of medical ethics until the early decades of the 20th century. Since that time, under the influences of United States common law and philosophical ethics, medical ethics in the United States has increasingly come to acknowledge and emphasize the importance of the patient's perspective on her interests and what should count as protecting and promoting her interests.[16] There is growing international debate about an "American" approach to medical ethics that places strong emphasis on respect for the patient's autonomy and rights. European medical ethics, as well as medical ethics in Japan and other Pacific Rim countries, have tended to place greater emphasis on beneficence. In the United States, autonomy has been developed as a bulwark against physician paternalism (i.e., acting on beneficence-based obligations to the patient as the justification for restricting the patient's autonomy).[15, 17] By contrast, European and Asian medical ethics have been more willing to play an important clinical role for medical paternalism.

To implement the principle of respect for autonomy in clinical practice, the pregnant patient should be presumed by her physician to be able to form her judgments about her interests on the basis of her own values and to express those judgments in value-based preferences. The ethical principle of respect for autonomy translates this fact into autonomy-based ethical obligations of the physician to the pregnant woman (Fig. 3–1). Respect for autonomy obligates the physician to acknowledge the integrity of the patient's values in her life; to elicit

PREGNANT WOMAN

Beneficence-based   Autonomy-based
obligations of   obligations of
physician   physician

FETAL PATIENT

Beneficence-   Beneficence-
based obligations   based obligations
of physician   of pregnant woman

F I G U R E 3–1. Ethical obligations in fetal diagnosis and therapy.

the patient's value-based preferences; and to assist the patient to put her preference(s) into effect. Clinically, these obligations are met by carrying out the informed consent process, which is usually understood to have three elements: (1) disclosure by the physician to the patient of clinically salient information about the patient's condition and its management that the patient should not be expected to know; (2) understanding of that information by the patient; and (3) a voluntary decision by the patient to authorize or refuse clinical management.[16]

The concepts of autonomy-based clinical judgment and autonomy-based obligations and of beneficence-based clinical judgment and beneficence-based obligations provide an ethical framework for fetal therapy (Fig. 3–1) within which the concept of the fetus as a patient can be articulated and its clinical implications identified,[14, 18] tasks to which we now turn.

The Concept of the Fetus As a Patient

In the medical ethics literature there are competing ways to think about the concept of the fetus as a patient. This competition has developed around the question of whether or not the fetus has independent moral status[19–31] (Fig. 3–2). Independent moral status for the fetus would mean that one or more characteristics that the fetus possesses in and of itself and, therefore, independently of the pregnant woman or any other factor, generate and therefore ground obligations to the fetus on the part of the pregnant woman and her physician.

There are three main positions about when the fetus might acquire independent moral status that have been predominant ways of analyzing the ethics of fetal diagnosis and therapy (Fig. 3–2). One position is that the fetus possesses *full* independent moral status from the moment of conception or implantation.[32–34] A second position is that the fetus acquires independent moral status in degrees, thus resulting in *graded* moral status.[22, 29] A third position is that the fetus has *no* independent moral status.[25] The first two support *fetal rights* while the third supports *maternal rights.*

Despite an enormous philosophical and theological literature on this subject, there has been no agreement on a single intellectually authoritative position on the independent moral status of the fetus.[35, 36] This is a logical outcome of the intellectual fact that there is no single methodology that is authoritative for all of the markedly diverse theological and philosophical schools of thought involved in this protracted debate, which began with the ancient Greek philosophers about 2,500 years ago.

This debate helped to shape the Hippocratic Oath itself. The framers of the Oath were members of the Pythagorean religious cult, which condemned abortion, a distinctly minority moral view at that time. The dominant view, found in Aristotle, was that abortion was morally unproblematic. This deep division has not closed in the intervening centuries. Throughout these millennia this dominant way of thinking has resulted in *ethical and clinical gridlock,* manifested in the polarizing language of "the right to life" versus the "woman's right to control her body."

In the absence of such an authoritative methodology to bridge this divide, agreement on the independent moral status of the fetus has been, and remains, impossible. For agreement ever to be possible, deep disagreements about such a final authority about the fetus' alleged independent moral status would have to be resolved in a way satisfactory to all, which is intellectually inconceivable. We conclude that it is best to avoid any further, ultimately futile attempts to understand the fetus as a patient by asking whether or not the fetus possesses independent moral status.

We turn, therefore, to an alternative, more clinically and intellectually promising approach, based on the concept of dependent moral status of the fetus, which makes it possible to identify ethically distinct and clinically relevant senses of the fetus as a patient (Fig. 3–2).

We underscore that the ethical framework for fetal therapy set out here means that the language of fetal rights or personhood has no meaning and therefore no application to the fetus in the ethics of fetal diagnosis and therapy, despite its popularity in public and political discourse in many countries. A principal advantage

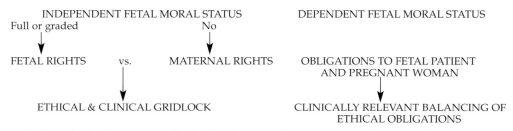

INDEPENDENT FETAL MORAL STATUS
Full or graded   No

FETAL RIGHTS   vs.   MATERNAL RIGHTS

ETHICAL & CLINICAL GRIDLOCK

DEPENDENT FETAL MORAL STATUS

OBLIGATIONS TO FETAL PATIENT
AND PREGNANT WOMAN

CLINICALLY RELEVANT BALANCING OF
ETHICAL OBLIGATIONS

F I G U R E 3–2. Fetal rights or fetal obligations? A fundamental choice for the ethics of fetal diagnosis and therapy.

of this framework, therefore, is that all of the controversy about "right to life" and the "woman's right to control her body" is avoided, along with the gridlock these polarizing positions produce.

This alternative approach starts with the claim that a human being does *not* always have to possess independent moral status in order to be a patient.[21] Instead, being a patient means that one can benefit from the application of the clinical skills of the physician, a form of *dependent moral status*. Put more precisely, a human being without independent moral status is properly regarded as a patient when two conditions are met: that a human being (1) is presented to the physician and (2) there exist clinical interventions that are reliably expected to be efficacious, in that they are reliably expected to result in a greater balance of goods over harms in the future of the human being in question.[14, 18, 37] When the human being has autonomy, a third condition also applies: consent.

We turn now to an account of when there are beneficence-based obligations to the fetus (i.e., when medical interventions reasonably can be expected to result in a greater balance of goods over harms for the child the fetus can become).[14, 18, 37] When the fetus is a patient, both the physician and the pregnant woman have beneficence-based obligations to it (Fig. 3–1). They are the moral fiduciaries of the patient (i.e., they are expected to act primarily to protect and promote the clinical interests of the fetal patient).[14] Those interests are defined by beneficence-based clinical judgment and the woman's judgment about the fetus' interests. This beneficence-based approach to the concept of the fetus as a patient is not distinctively "American," because beneficence is an internationally accepted medical ethical principle.[38]

The concept of the fetus as a patient depends on links that can be established between the fetus and the child it can become and not on the alleged—and always disputable—independent moral status of the fetus (Fig. 3–3). The first such link is viability, providing the basis for the first ethical sense of the fetus as a patient. Viability must be understood in terms of both biological *and* technological factors.[35, 39, 40] Both factors are required for a viable fetus to exist ex utero and become a child with independent moral status.[14] These two factors, therefore, do not exist as a function of the autonomy of the pregnant woman. When a fetus is viable (i.e., when it is of sufficient maturity so that it can survive into the neonatal period and become a child with independent moral status), even if it requires technological support, the fetus is a patient[14] (Fig. 3–3). Beneficence-based obligations to the viable fetus must, of course, be considered together with beneficence-based and autonomy-based obligations to the pregnant woman[14, 18] (Fig. 3–1).

The only possible link between the previable fetus and the child it can become is the pregnant woman's autonomy, providing the basis for the second ethical sense of the fetus as a patient. Technological factors cannot result in the previable fetus becoming a child, because this is what previable means. A link, therefore, between a previable fetus and the child it can become is established only by the pregnant woman's decision to confer the status of being a patient on her previable fetus (Fig. 3–3). The previable fetus, because it cannot reliably be thought to possess independent moral status, has no claim to the status of being a patient independently of the pregnant woman's autonomy. It follows that the previable fetus is a patient solely as a function of the pregnant woman's autonomy to take the pregnancy to viability, at which time the fetus becomes a patient independently of the pregnant woman's autonomy, as explained above.[14]

An important subset of previable embryos comprises in vitro embryos. It might seem that the in vitro embryo is a patient because such an embryo is presented to the physician. However, simply being presented to a physician does not make the in vitro embryo a patient. This is because, in terms of beneficence, whether the fetus is a patient depends as well on links that can be established between the fetus and its future (i.e., the child with independent moral status it can become). Therefore, the reasonableness of medical interventions on the in vitro embryo turns on whether that embryo later becomes viable. Otherwise, no benefit of such intervention can meaningfully be said to result. An in vitro embryo, therefore, becomes viable only when it survives in vitro cell division, transfer, implantation, and subsequent gestation to such a time as it becomes viable.

This process of achieving viability occurs in vivo and is therefore dependent on the woman's decision regarding the status of the fetus(es) as a patient, should assisted conception successfully result in the gestation of the previable fetus(es). Whether an in vitro embryo will become a viable fetus and whether medical intervention on such an embryo will benefit the fetus are both functions of the pregnant woman's autonomy. It therefore is appropriate to regard the in vitro embryo as a previable fetus rather than as a viable fetus. As a consequence, any in vitro embryo(s) should be regarded as a patient only when the woman into whose reproductive tract the embryo(s) will be transferred confers that status.[14] Whether the in vitro embryo is a patient is therefore not a function of her partner's (if there is one) autonomy. The woman is free to confer with her partner as she chooses.

To summarize this analysis of the concept of the fetus as a patient: the viable fetus is a patient; the previable fetus, including the in vitro embryo, is a patient solely

VIABLE FETUS
Patienthood status a function of biological and technological capacity to become a child with independent moral status

PREVIABLE FETUS
Patienthood status a function of pregnant woman's autonomy to take the pregnancy to viability

F I G U R E   3–3. The fetus as a patient.

as a function of the exercise of the woman's autonomy (Fig. 3–3).

An Ethical Framework for Fetal Therapy

Whether fetal therapy can be judged to be standard of care on ethical grounds depends on the clinical implications of the concept of the fetus as a patient. This standard must be understood on both beneficence-based and autonomy-based grounds. Beneficence requires that fetal therapy must reliably be thought, on the basis of documented clinical experience, to benefit the child that the fetus can become. Recall that the ethical content of this concept is to be understood, not simply in terms of physical accessibility, but also in terms of whether clinical interventions on the fetus are reliably thought to be efficacious because they are reliably expected to result in a greater balance of goods over harms for the child the fetus can become.

Autonomy-based considerations include the following. The pregnant woman is under no ethical obligation to confer the status of being a patient on her previable fetus simply because there exists a fetal therapy that meets the preceding beneficence-based condition. Whether such therapy is, on ethical grounds, to be judged standard of care for her previable fetus is also a function of the pregnant woman's autonomy. That is, satisfying both beneficence-based and autonomy-based conditions are necessary for fetal therapy to be reliably judged to be the ethical standard of care for previable fetuses on ethical grounds.

The same is true for fetal therapy on the viable fetus. Such a fetus is properly judged to be a patient. However, as noted above, beneficence-based obligations to the fetal patient must be negotiated with beneficence-based and autonomy-based obligations to the pregnant woman (Fig. 3–1). This is because of a factual consideration—fetal therapy necessarily involves physical (and, perhaps, mental health) risks to the pregnant woman; and an ethical consideration—she is ethically obligated only to accept reasonable risks to herself in order to attempt to benefit her fetus.[14, 18]

This ethical framework for fetal therapy helps to distinguish an ethical from a legal standard of care for fetal therapy. An ethical standard must take account not only of beneficence-based considerations applied to the fetal patient but also of both beneficence-based and autonomy-based considerations applied to the pregnant woman. The law has yet to develop in terms of the ethical concept of the fetus as a patient. A legal standard of care tends to focus on efficacy and safety, which are beneficence-based considerations applied to both the fetus and the pregnant woman. A legal standard of care tends to ignore autonomy-based considerations applied to the pregnant woman. This constitutes the fundamental difference between a legal and an ethical standard of care for fetal therapy.

Given what is at stake in fetal therapy, physicians understandably may have concerns about risks of litigation. The law of each state differs in its development and clinical sophistication in the area of fetal therapy. Developing law is usefully informed by ethical analysis and argument of the sort advanced in this chapter. The physician concerned about litigation should obtain appropriate legal consultation and advocate for the use of the ethical framework of this chapter as a guide for the clinical ethical judgment. After all, practicing medicine on the basis of rigorous clinical ethical judgment should be the physician's primary goal, not the avoidance of litigation. Failure to maintain this priority risks the integrity of the medical profession.

Fetal therapy should be recommended when the intervention will benefit the fetus and the risks of the intervention are those the pregnant woman ought to accept. The authors caution that there is no simple algorithm by which a pregnant woman—or her physician—can conclude that she is obligated to accept risk to herself on behalf of her viable fetus. In the authors' view, such an ethical obligation—which should *not* be automatically equated with a legal obligation—exists when three criteria are satisfied: (1) when invasive therapy of the viable fetus is reliably judged to have a very high probability of being life-saving or of preventing serious and irreversible disease, injury, or handicap for the fetus and for the child the fetus can become; (2) when such therapy is reliably judged to involve low mortality risk and low or manageable risk of serious disease, injury, or handicap to the viable fetus and the child it can become; and (3) when the mortality risk to the pregnant woman is reliably judged to be very low, and when the risk of disease, injury, or handicap to the pregnant woman is reliably judged to be low or manageable.[14, 41]

As required by the above ethical framework for fetal therapy, the justifications for these criteria are both beneficence-based and autonomy-based. When the first two criteria are satisfied there is expected to be a clear and substantial net benefit to the viable fetus and the child it can become. When the third criterion is satisfied there is expected to be no clear and substantial net harm to the pregnant woman. Given the expected net benefit to the viable fetus and the low risk of harm to the pregnant woman, the latter are risks she should reasonably be expected to accept,[14] for example, as in intravascular transfusion for severe isoimmunization. This moral fact shapes how she should exercise her autonomy in response to her beneficence-based fiduciary ethical obligations to her fetus.[14, 37]

Under beneficence-based and autonomy-based clinical judgment, therefore, directive counseling in the form of recommending treatment of the viable fetus is ethically justified when these three criteria are satisfied. The burden of ethical proof rests with those who would propose recommending intervention when one or more of these three criteria cannot be satisfied. This should be a matter of further careful investigation and debate in the ethics of fetal therapy.

Forms of fetal therapy for which an ethical obligation (as defined above on the part of the pregnant woman to accept them) cannot be established should be regarded as experimental. For example, because open abdominal fetal surgery involves risks that no pregnant woman can be understood, at this time, to be *obligated* to accept on behalf of an attempt to benefit her viable fetus, all such surgery must, on ethical grounds, be regarded as experimental. There is no ethical justification for recommending experimental fetal therapy because none of the three conditions above is satisfied.

Investigational invasive fetal therapy should be scientifically sound and meet ethical and legal requirements for research with human subjects. These legal requirements vary internationally, but the clear trend is to require review and approval by an institutional review board. To proceed in the absence of such review not only risks disrespect for the pregnant woman and grave risk to the fetus, but loss of scientific rigor as well. Thus, to proceed with experimental therapy without appropriate institutional review is not ethically justified. So-called innovative therapy is subject to the same stringent ethical requirement.

The physician's response, when the pregnant woman rejects a recommendation of fetal therapy for a viable fetus that satisfies an ethically justified standard of care, should be the strategies of preventive ethics.[42] Certainly, informed consent as an ongoing dialogue with the pregnant woman should be the first response. In undertaking a further response, negotiation, the physician should acknowledge and take into account the pregnant woman's assessment of the risks and benefits of invasive fetal therapy to herself and her fetus. It is justified to go beyond negotiation to respectful persuasion, and perhaps even to an ethics committee, as part of a preventive ethics clinical strategy.[14, 42]

Experimental therapy (i.e., situations in which one or more of the above-mentioned criteria are not satisfied) of the viable fetus can justifiably be *offered* to the pregnant woman only with the approval of an institutional review board. The ethical justification for doing so rests on the three criteria for ethical standard of care defined above. By definition, if the first two criteria are not satisfied, there is no net fetal benefit and therefore there is no beneficence-based obligation to the fetus to offer experimental therapy. If the third criterion is not met (even if the first two are), there is only net harm to the pregnant patient and no beneficence-based obligation to her to offer experimental fetal therapy.

The principal justification for offering fetal therapy that does not meet the three criteria is twofold: (1) to benefit future patients; and (2) to enhance the pregnant woman's autonomy by expanding the range of her options. The first part of this justification appeals to a beneficence-based obligation to provide quality medical care to future fetal patients. This two-part justification must be made clear to the pregnant woman as part of the informed consent process, so she does not subscribe to the mistaken belief that experimental fetal interventions will benefit her fetus or herself. When there are well-developed clinical trials that are requesting referrals from one's geographic area, the authors believe that there is an obligation to offer the opportunity for enrollment as a research subject—again, only on the justification that research benefits future patients, that the woman's autonomy will be enhanced, and that approval is granted by the appropriate institutional review board.

In cases in which the first two criteria are satisfied but the third is not, intervention should be regarded as experimental and only offered, not recommended, to the pregnant woman. This is because respect for her autonomy requires that she be accorded the opportunity to decide for herself whether the unavoidable risk of serious harm to her is warranted for the sake of possibly benefiting the fetus and the child it can become. Medicine has no competence to make this judgment. Thus, a pregnant woman's refusal to enroll as a subject in experimental fetal therapy should always be respected and she should be assured her subsequent care will not be affected by her refusal and this assurance should, in fact, be carried out.

There are two subgroups of previable fetuses. The first comprises those upon whom the pregnant woman has conferred the status of being a patient. When she has done so and the above-mentioned ethical criteria are also satisfied, it is ethically justified to recommend fetal therapy. This situation is directly analogous to informed consent to therapy for the viable fetus and the strategies discussed above apply.

When the pregnant woman withholds or withdraws the status of being a patient from her previable fetus, the situation is directly analogous to experimental fetal therapy. This is so because there is no ethical obligation on the part of the pregnant woman or the physician to regard the previable fetus as a patient. It follows that any discussion of experimental fetal intervention must be strictly nondirective, which is consistent with offering but not recommending enrollment as a research subject in a clinical investigation trial.[14, 43]

Public Policy: Implications for Managed Care

Most of the interventions discussed in this volume are, on the criteria we have defined above, experimental. They are also very costly. It has been public policy to permit insurance companies, and now managed care organizations, not to pay for medical interventions that are clearly experimental. We now argue that this public policy should change.

Medical institutions, and managed care organizations, in particular, as co-fiduciaries or co-trustees of patients, have inescapable ethical obligations to support medical education and research.[50] First, managed care organizations sell knowledge and skills that were created as the result of investment by society, just as physicians do. Reciprocal justice applies in such circumstances and unambiguously requires that, when one has benefited from the investment and sacrifice of others, one owes them proportional recompense. Reciprocal justice also prohibits causing harm to those whose investment and sacrifice benefited one. Society therefore is justified, by virtue of its investment and sacrifice that help to create the fetal therapies described in this volume, in insisting that managed care organizations, for profit or not-for-profit alike, pay their fair share for medical education and research.

Second, should managed care organizations come to dominate the market and fail in their reciprocal-justice-based social responsibility, medical progress in fetal therapy will be impaired. This is inconsistent with continuous quality improvement, which is an explicit commitment of every well-managed care organization. Moreover, fetal patients in the future will suffer or die when they otherwise might have been helped, a failure of the future-oriented, fiduciary obligations of managed care organizations to patients. Academic medical centers have traditionally fulfilled this obligation, to a great extent, by subsidizing research and education from practice-plan revenues. If managed care organizations had been the dominant market force 20 years ago and failed in this social responsibility, as they are currently failing, fetal diagnosis and therapy would most likely be deficient from what we now understand it to be. For example, the present clinical utility of obstetric ultrasound and many of the interventions described in this volume, which have developed, in part, from support from clinical revenues in academic medical centers, would most likely be vestigial.

Third, the failure of managed care organizations to fulfill their social responsibilities to medical education and research might have deleterious consequences for the free flow of scientific information. In business, research and development costs are recovered through patenting and license fees. In order to facilitate its future-oriented fiduciary obligations, medicine has rejected this practice. Should academic medical centers change their moral character in this respect and pursue a business course, the free flow of information that has been a great strength of modern medicine would be impaired and patients injured from restricted access and increased costs associated with patents and licensing.

These three ethical considerations justify in our judgment a comprehensive approach to enforcing through public policy the social responsibilities of managed care organizations, not-for-profit and profit alike, to support research in fetal diagnosis and therapy, as well as research in other clinical specialties and subspecialties. Fulfilling such obligations should not be voluntary but mandatory. Such support should not be selective (e.g., with a medical center targeted for business reasons by the managed care organization) but comprehensive. Support should be directly proportional to the benefit derived, which is considerable. Support should also be immediate because harm is now being done. These considerations support legal enforcement of social responsibility of managed care organizations, perhaps in the form of a corporate income or sales tax. This approach will prevent managed care organizations from segmenting fiduciary responsibility—going after profitable fiduciary activities and ignoring unprofitable ones.

Conclusion

The ability to identify and clinically apply an ethical framework to fetal diagnosis and therapy is an essential clinical skill. The professional integrity of physicians depends on the continuing development of this skill. In this chapter, we have attempted to contribute to this goal by providing an account of the clinical ethical concept of the fetus as a patient. This provides the basis of an ethical framework for fetal therapy. Because the diagnosis of a fetal anomaly is the prerequisite to most of the fetal therapies described in this volume, an analysis is provided of the routine obstetric ultrasound controversy. Because funding for the continuing performance and development of fetal therapy is challenged in today's era of managed care as never before, we have provided an argument for managed care organizations to support research in fetal diagnosis and therapy.

REFERENCES

1. Liley AW: The fetus as a personality. Aust NZJ Psychiatry 6:99–105, 1972.
2. American College of Obstetricians and Gynecologists: Technical Bulletin. Ethical decision-making in obstetrics and gynecology. Washington, DC: American College of Obstetricians and Gynecologists, 1989.
3. American Academy of Pediatrics, Committee on Bioethics: Fetal therapy: Ethical considerations. Pediatrics 81:898–899, 1988.
4. Harrison MR, Golbus MS, Filly RA: The Unborn Patient. New York: Grune & Stratton, 1988.
5. American College of Obstetricians and Gynecologists: Committee on Ethics. Patient choice: Maternal-fetal conflict. Washington, DC: American College of Obstetricians and Gynecologists, 1987.
6. Mahoney MJ: Fetal-maternal relationship. In Reich WT (ed): Encyclopedia of Bioethics. New York: Macmillan, 1978, pp 485–488.
7. Newton ER: The fetus as patient. Med Clin North Am 73:517–540, 1980.
8. Fletcher JC: The fetus as patient: Ethical issues. JAMA 246:772–773, 1981.
9. Pritchard JA, MacDonald PC, Gant NF: Williams Obstetrics, 17th ed. Norwalk, CT: Appleton-Century-Crofts, 1985, p xi.
10. Walters L: Ethical issues in intrauterine diagnosis and therapy. Fetal Ther 1:32–37, 1986.
11. Murray TH: Moral obligations to the not-yet born: The fetus as patient. Clin Perinatol 14:313–328, 1987.
12. Mahoney MJ: The fetus as patient. West J Med 150:517–540, 1989.
13. Edelstein L: The Hippocratic Oath: Text, translation, and interpretation. In Temkin O, Temkin CL (eds): Ancient Medicine: Selected Papers of Ludwig Edelstein. Baltimore: The Johns Hopkins Press, 1967, pp 3–63.
14. McCullough LB, Chervenak FA: Ethics in Obstetrics and Gynecology. New York: Oxford University Press, 1994.
15. Beauchamp TL, Childress JF: Principles of Biomedical Ethics, 3rd ed. New York: Oxford University Press, 1989.
16. Faden R, Beauchamp TL: History and Theory of Informed Consent. New York: Oxford University Press, 1986.
17. Beauchamp TL, McCullough LB: Medical Ethics: The Moral Responsibilities of Physicians. Englewood Cliffs, NJ: Prentice-Hall, 1988.
18. Chervenak FA, McCullough LB: Perinatal ethics: A practical method of analysis of obligations to mother and fetus. Obstet Gynecol 66:442–446, 1985.
19. Hellegers AE: Fetal development. Theological Stud 31:3–9, 1970.
20. Noonan JT (ed): The Morality of Abortion. Cambridge: Harvard University Press, 1970.
21. Ruddick W, Wilcox W: Operating on the fetus. Hastings Cent Rep 12:10–14, 1982.
22. Strong G: Ethics in Reproductive and Perinatal Medicine: A New Framework. New Haven, CT: Yale University Press, 1997.
23. Engelhardt HT Jr: The Foundations of Bioethics. New York: Oxford University Press, 1986.
24. Curran CE: Abortion: Contemporary debate in philosophical and religious ethics. In Reich WT (ed): Encyclopedia of Bioethics. New York: Macmillan, 1987, pp 17–26.
25. Elias S, Annas GJ: Reproductive Genetics and the Law. Chicago: Year Book Medical Publishers, 1987.
26. Fleming L: The moral status of the fetus: A reappraisal. Bioethics 1:15–34, 1987.
27. Strong C: Ethical conflicts between mother and fetus in obstetrics. Clin Perinatol 14:313–328, 1987.

28. Anderson G, Strong C: The premature breech: Cesarean section or trial of labor? J Med Ethics 14:18–24, 1988.
29. Evans MI, Fletcher JC, Zador IE, et al: Selective first-trimester termination in octuplet and quadruplet pregnancies: Clinical and ethical issues. Obstet Gynecol 71:289–296, 1988.
30. Ford NM: When Did I Begin? Conception of the Human Individual in History, Philosophy and Science. Cambridge: Cambridge University Press, 1988.
31. Strong C, Anderson G: The moral status of the near-term fetus. J Med Ethics 15:25–27, 1989.
32. Noonan JT: A Private Choice. Abortion in America in the Seventies. New York: The Free Press, 1979.
33. Bopp J (ed): Restoring the Right to Life: The Human Life Amendment. Provo, UT: Brigham Young University, 1984.
34. Bopp J (ed): Human Life and Health Care Ethics. Frederick, MD: University Publications of America, 1985.
35. Roe v. Wade, 410 US 113 (1973).
36. Callahan S, Callahan D (eds): Abortion: Understanding Differences. New York: Plenum Press, 1984.
37. Chervenak FA, McCullough LB: Does obstetric ethics have any role in the obstetrician's response to the abortion controversy? Am J Obstet Gynecol 163:1425–1429, 1990.
38. Gillon R: Principles of Healthcare Ethics. Chichester: John Wiley, 1994.
39. Fost N, Chudwin D, Wikker D: The limited moral significance of fetal viability. Hastings Cent Rep 10:10–13, 1980.
40. Mahowald M: Beyond abortion: Refusal of cesarean section. Bioethics 3:106–121, 1989.
41. Chervenak FA, McCullough LB: An ethically based standard of care for fetal therapy. J Matern Fetal Invest 1:185–190, 1991.
42. Chervenak FA, McCullough LB: Clinical guides to preventing ethical conflicts between pregnant women and their physicians. Am J Obstet Gynecol 162:303–307, 1990.
43. Chervenak FA, McCullough LB: The fetus as patient: Implications for directive versus nondirective counseling for fetal benefit. Fetal Diagn Ther 6:93–100, 1991.
44. Chervenak FA, McCullough LB, Chervenak JL: Prenatal informed consent for sonogram: An indication for obstetric ultrasonography. Am J Obstet Gynecol 161:857–860, 1989.
45. Ewigman BG, Crane JP, Frigoletto FD, et al: Effect of prenatal ultrasound screening on perinatal outcome. N Engl J Med 329:821–827, 1993.
46. Ewigman BG, Le Fevre M, Bain RP, et al: Ethics and routine ultrasonography in pregnancy [letter]. Am J Obstet Gynecol 163:256–257, 1990.
47. Romero R: Routine obstetric ultrasound. Ultrasound Obstet Gynecol 3:303–307, 1993.
48. Skupski DW, Chervenak FA, McCullough LB: Is routine screening for all patients? Clin Perinatol 21:707–722, 1994.
49. Devore G: The routine antenatal diagnostic imaging with ultrasound study: Another perspective. Obstet Gynecol 84:622–626, 1994.
50. McCullough LB, Chervenak FA: Ethical challenges in the managed practice of obstetrics and gynecology. Obstet Gynecol 93:304–307, 1999.

CHAPTER 4

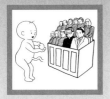

Legal Considerations in Fetal Treatment

HOWARD R. BELKIN

Much progress has been made in the scientific basis and techniques used for fetal treatment over the past 10 years. Along with these medical advances have come legal and ethical controversies. The purpose of this chapter is to examine both the legal and the ethical aspects of the treatment of fetuses. It will examine the obligations, rights, and duties of pregnant women and their physicians. It will also examine the rights and obligations of society at large. This chapter will look at those types of therapy that are not well established or are controversial. This will include a discussion of the controversy generated by the development of mammalian cloning and its implications for therapy. The concept of the preservation of human embryos through freezing techniques and the controversy that can arise over their ownership will be examined. At appropriate points in this discussion specific examples of litigated cases that have involved prenatal fetal treatment will be reviewed.

The notion of mandatory duties during pregnancy for the benefit of offspring is highly controversial. Many persons fail to see how a duty could arise to treat a fetus that could be lawfully aborted. Similarly, there is a percentage of the population who believe that a duty to protect the fetus arises at conception, or shortly thereafter. Although in many instances, the ultimate constitutionality has not been determined, several state legislatures have recently enacted laws imposing both civil and criminal penalties for injuring an unborn child. Physicians, lawyers, and ethicists are concerned that these laws could severely infringe upon the personal freedom of pregnant women. Many physicians are also concerned that these laws could be used against them to impose liability if they inadvertently cause harm to a fetus.

This chapter reviews the moral and legal grounds upon which duties to treat during pregnancy might arise. It is our belief that although both postbirth sanctions and prebirth seizures have been used in the past and may be constitutional in an extremely limited number of instances, they should rarely if ever be used. Society needs instead to concentrate on improving patient knowledge through education of the need for pre-

ventive and other types of prenatal treatment. Pregnant women must also be able to obtain these services when desired. Although it is arguable that some role for criminal statutes punishing the most outrageous cases of prenatal child abuse serve an appropriate state function, laws that force recalcitrant women to undergo medical or surgical treatment for the benefit of an unborn child likely never are justified. Due to the intimate relationship between a mother and fetus, conflict can arise when a mother's refusal to undergo prenatal medical treatment threatens the potential life of the fetus. In several cases, courts have ordered immediate cesarean sections to be performed against the will of the mother. Newly enacted laws purporting to protect fetuses from injury through the criminalization of injuring a fetus will also be examined. The final section in this chapter discusses the relationship between treatment of pregnant women and the legal and ethical obligations of physicians to these women and their unborn children. This includes the legal concepts of wrongful life and wrongful birth, in addition to potential future areas of physician liability. In certain cases, physicians have a legal obligation to report suspected cases of child abuse. They do not, however, have a legal right to intervene and forcibly perform medical or surgical treatment upon a pregnant woman in order to potentially protect an unborn child. Cases in which courts have ordered interventions have often resulted in disaster for all concerned. Prebirth seizures and forced treatment for the benefit of an unborn child should basically be avoided in almost every imaginable circumstance.

The Problem: Maternal Conduct During Pregnancy

The increasing ability to prevent the birth of handicapped infants has raised new issues with regard to the scope of reproductive freedom issues of special concern to women and the physicians who treat them. Most women at risk welcome knowledge about treatment or behavior that will prevent the birth of a child with handicaps. They avoid risky behavior and accept medical treatment or surgery that will ensure a healthy child. If a healthy child is not possible, they may avoid conception or terminate the pregnancy.

However, not all women are aware of the dangers that certain behaviors pose or of the treatments available to minimize congenital defects. Even if they do know, they may lack access to the prenatal screening and treatment that would prevent the handicaps from occurring.

Sometimes, however, women ignore the knowledge or refuse treatment and they act or fail to act in ways that cause children who could have been born healthy to be born handicapped. What is the ethical status of such conduct? What should public policy be with regard to this problem, and what is the physician's role in such situations?

The need for public policies to prevent avoidable prenatal injuries has arisen in several different contexts: prenatal medical or surgical treatment and cesarean section; prenatal abuse of alcohol, heroin, and cocaine; exclusion from workplaces that pose prenatal danger to offspring; and prenatal transmission of herpes and syphilis. As more cases of prenatal harm become known, pressure to change the behavior of pregnant women will increase and will have important implications for physicians who treat pregnant women or who counsel them about reproductive behavior.

Public efforts to modify the behavior of pregnant women are controversial for several reasons. The idea that women could, with impunity, cause or fail to prevent handicapped births is, of course, troubling. However, there is no consensus about the seriousness of the problem and the appropriateness of particular remedies. In addition, many people are suspicious of public control of women's bodies during pregnancy for the sake of the unborn child. They regard any control as constituting a significant intrusion on personal liberty with the potential to accord fetuses a legal status that could diminish the right to have an abortion.[1]

Moral Obligations to Unborn Children During Pregnancy as a Basis for Legal Obligations

Questions of prenatal obligations to offspring are ethically complex because of the prenatal timing of the harmful conduct and the unborn child's location in the mother's uterus when the harmful conduct occurs. The importance of these ethical and legal issues was originally noted in an article written nearly 20 years ago, a time during which both in vitro fertilization and genetic therapy were in their infancy.[2] Taking actions designed to improve or protect an unborn child necessarily requires placing limits on the mother's actions in such a way that would be clearly unthinkable if she were not pregnant. Thus, in any case that places the health of an unborn child in a position that opposes the desires and rights of its mother, the mother's interest in autonomy and bodily integrity automatically has to be balanced against the welfare of her fetus.

Most reasonable people would agree that a mother has a moral duty of some type to the unborn child

that she has decided to take to term. All persons have obligations to refrain from harming children after birth. Third parties certainly may be liable if they do in fact cause harm to an unborn child by prenatal actions. Certainly, a criminal who assaults a woman, causing the death of an unborn but viable child can be held both morally and legally liable for its death. A question arises, however, of whether a mother who has chosen to go to term has a legal duty to prevent harm from occurring to the unborn child or to take affirmative steps to protect that unborn child when she may reasonably do so.

It is important to recognize that the interests of offspring to be free of harm caused prenatally is a completely different issue than that of the right of the fetus to complete gestation. Physicians, attorneys, and ethicists must be consistent and constantly emphasize the distinction between these two concepts. Whether or not we as a society choose to protect offspring against harm caused prenatally, this in no way diminishes the woman's right to terminate a pregnancy, because the issue arises only if the woman chooses to continue the pregnancy. No right of the fetus to be brought to term is at issue.

One can argue that ethically, prenatal duties owed to the planned offspring may even arise before viability. The mother's plans, and not the state of fetal development, determine moral responsibility, because even first-trimester conduct could culpably injure fetuses who are subsequently brought to term. A woman who has not decided or is ambivalent about a first-trimester pregnancy may still be morally, even if not legally, obligated to act as if she will carry the fetus to term if first-trimester conduct poses a serious risk to a baby that is born. Although she is allowed to terminate the pregnancy later, morally, she may not be free to injure offspring prenatally just because she is uncertain about whether to continue the pregnancy (and eventually decides to do so). However, one must clearly distinguish this type of moral responsibility from culpable legal liability for causing potential harm at the nonviability stage to a later-born child.

Ethical analysis must balance the mother's interest in freedom and bodily integrity against the offspring's interest in being born in a healthy condition. This balance varies with the burdens of altering the mother's conduct and the risk of prenatally caused harm to offspring. It also varies with the degree of importance that a society places upon a woman's right to her own bodily integrity. Depending on how one balances the risks and benefits, a certain type of prenatal conduct may be morally discretionary, advisable, or even prudent. It is, however, much less likely that absent extreme circumstances, such conduct would ever become obligatory.

An example of the type of case in which a court might take an interest in the conduct of the mother as it affects the unborn child occurred in Florida several years ago.[3] In this criminal case, the defendant, Jennifer Johnson, was found guilty of violating a state statute criminalizing the delivery of drugs to a minor. The trial court decision was based upon the prosecutor's contention that Ms. Johnson's use of cocaine during the term of her pregnancy amounted to her act of delivering cocaine to her *unborn child* through the umbilical cord connection.

In overturning the conviction, the state supreme court stated that it clearly was not the purpose of this statute to punish pregnant women for using drugs. In this case, whereas Ms. Johnson most certainly had a moral obligation to refrain from drug use during her pregnancy, no legal liability attached to her actions. Although the use of drugs during a pregnancy is morally repugnant, absent clear legislative intent criminalizing such behavior, it is not a crime.

It is clear that a distinction must be made between those acts that are morally proscribed and those that are also illegal. Drug use by a pregnant woman is one of those such acts. A recent law review article examined the problem of prenatal use of drugs and the solution that the State of Minnesota has implemented to deal with the problem.[4] The article noted that previous laws had turned the maternal-fetal dyad into an adversarial relationship. This is diametrically opposed to the actual beneficial relationship that exists physiologically. That shift in the essential nature of the interpretation of the relationship has led to the conflicts that are evident in cases such as the one involving Ms. Johnson. The State of Minnesota has enacted a progressive statute that can address the problem of drug abuse by pregnant women, causing as little legal "harm" to the mother as possible, while at the same time attempting to protect the later-born child from prenatally caused harm. On its surface, this statute appears to be morally acceptable and "abuser-friendly." It provides for the use of drug treatment programs, prenatal care, and medical assistance to the pregnant women. However, it also permits the use of civil commitment in those cases in which the mother who, during her pregnancy, has engaged in "habitual or excessive use, for a nonmedical purpose, of . . . cocaine, heroin, phencyclidine, methamphetamine, or amphetamine."[5] Thus, even in a "medically informed" progressive type of statute, the mother's interests in her own physical bodily integrity and medical decision-making processes can clearly be subrogated to the prenatal rights of her later-born child. Another Minnesota statute includes in its definition of neglect, "prenatal exposure to a controlled substance . . . used by the mother for a nonmedical purpose, as evidenced by withdrawal symptoms in the child at birth, results of a toxicology test performed on the mother at delivery or the child at birth, or medical effects or developmental delays during the child's first year of life that medically indicate prenatal exposure to a controlled substance."[6] This statute is a further example of a state's attempt to erode a woman's interest in her own personal bodily integrity for the benefit of later-born children.[7]

The extreme to which the concept of the protection of a fetus can be taken is seen in a law review article written in 1997.[8] In that lengthy article, the author compares cigarette smoking to maternal cocaine and alcohol abuse and argues for the consideration of prenatal smoking in abuse and neglect hearings. Cigarette smoking is one of the greatest health hazards facing American society today. Physicians need to be hypervigilant about advising patients to discontinue their smoking habits. However, proposing the consideration of cigarette smoking in a hearing to determine whether prenatal child abuse or neglect has occurred is a complete abrogation of the rights of the mother in favor of the later-born child. This is an example of a morally admirable concept, the protection of a helpless fetus, taken to an absurd end.

It should also be noted that moral analysis is more clear when a healthy child cannot be born because of genetic or other factors or because in utero damage, which could have been avoided at one time, has already occurred. Delivery in those situations does not harm offspring, because they have no alternative but to live a damaged life.[9] If the birth is truly wrongful, harm can be minimized by withholding all treatment. Birth, however, may harm persons who bear the burden of rearing the offspring who is now unavoidably damaged. The ethical issue then posed is whether persons have duties to avoid conception or delivery of an unavoidably handicapped offspring in order to avoid imposing rearing costs on others. This is a completely different issue than the issue of forced medical treatment. Forced or coerced pregnancy termination is an action for which society should show virtually no tolerance.

Policy Options: Voluntary Compliance or Compulsion?

Several policy options are available to influence the behavior of women and others during pregnancy for the sake of planned offspring, ranging from voluntary compliance through education and access to services to very infrequently, if ever, used coercive sanctions and seizures.

Relying on voluntary compliance is obviously the most desirable policy, because it raises fewer civil liberties and privacy issues and is more likely to be effective. Most women welcome such knowledge and act accordingly. If they have not been able to avoid the damaging conduct, many choose to have an abortion rather than to bring the damaged fetus to term. The main need here is to ensure that women are informed adequately and that they have access to treatments that can avoid the harm to offspring. A society truly concerned about prenatal harm to offspring can do much in the way of education and services to prevent such harm from occurring. A discussion follows about the physician's role in inducing voluntary compliance.

In any discussion about the policy options involving the compulsory provision of treatment for a pregnant woman, one must consider the cases of forced cesarean sections. Court-ordered cesarean sections have been examined in detail in a paper published several years ago.[10] There have been a few reported instances of courts that have ordered pregnant women to undergo cesarean section deliveries. As time is generally of the essence in this type of treatment, it would seem unusual that any such cases would progress past the trial court level. This is evidenced by the fact that most of the reports of such cases are found in the medical literature.[11, 12] However, at least one such case has reached the level of appellate review.[13] That case, decided in 1981, involved a young woman named Jessie Mae Jefferson. Ms. Jefferson was in her 39th week of pregnancy when she presented to the Griffin Spalding County Hospital for prenatal care. Physical examination demonstrated that the pregnancy was complicated by a complete placenta previa. Because of her religious beliefs, Ms. Jefferson informed the hospital that, at the time of delivery, she would allow neither blood transfusions nor cesarean section delivery of the fetus. The patient was informed by her physicians that without a cesarean delivery, there was a 99 to 100% chance that the fetus would die and a 50% chance that she would die during childbirth. She was also told that if a cesarean section were to be performed, the probability of a successful outcome was nearly 100%. Ms. Jefferson continued to refuse her consent to a cesarean delivery. The hospital immediately petitioned the trial court for the authority to override Ms. Jefferson's stated wishes and deliver the child surgically. The trial court entered an order allowing the hospital to perform the procedure and the patient appealed. In upholding the trial court, the Georgia Supreme Court stated that "this child is a viable human being and entitled to the protection of the Juvenile Court Code of Georgia. The Court concludes that this child is without the proper parental care and subsistence necessary for his or her physical life and health."[14] The court ordered Ms. Jefferson to submit to an ultrasound examination, a cesarean section, and any other procedures deemed necessary by the physicians in order to save the life of the child. The final sentence of the opinion stated that, "[t]he Court finds that the intrusion involved into the life of Jessie Mae Jefferson and her husband, John W. Jefferson, is outweighed by the duty of the State to protect a living, unborn human being from meeting his or her death before being given the opportunity to live."[15] Ironically, 2 days after the court's decision, Ms. Jefferson delivered her baby without the need for the performance of a cesarean section.[16]

A somewhat different factual situation presented in a case that originated in the District of Columbia. In that case, George Washington University Hospital petitioned the court for guidance in the treatment of its patient, Angela Carter. The patient, 26 weeks pregnant, was being treated by the hospital for the final stages of terminal cancer. The patient, her husband, and both of her parents had agreed that no heroic procedures were to be performed to save the life of the unborn child. This included their request to not perform a cesarean section.[17, 18] The attending physician felt that it was his obligation to inform the hospital administration that he intended to comply with the patient's expressed desires. The hospital administration called in legal counsel, who petitioned the trial court for guidance. The trial court judge took the unusual step of holding a hearing at the hospital and subsequently entered an order permitting the hospital to perform a cesarean delivery. The lawyer appointed for the patient field an immediate request for a stay by telephone, but it was denied by a three-judge panel. The cesarean section was performed, but the child died within 2½ hours of delivery. The patient died some 2 days later. In an opinion written several months later,[19] the appellate court upheld the actions of the trial court judge, making the incredible statement that the "Caesarean section would not significantly affect A.C.'s condi-

tion because she had, at best, two days left of sedated life; the complications arising from the surgery would not significantly alter that prognosis. The child, on the other hand, had a chance of surviving delivery, despite the possibility that it would be born handicapped. Accordingly, we concluded that the trial judge did not err in subordinating A.C.'s right against bodily intrusion to the interests of the unborn child and the state."[20] Even though now, with the death of both the mother and the child, the case was moot, the appellate court, reflecting on the importance of this matter, decided to consider the entire matter *en banc.* The full court vacated the decision of the previous appellate panel.[21] It also took pains to distinguish itself from the decision in the *Jefferson* case discussed above. It noted that in that case, the mother had consistently refused to have the procedure performed, while in this case, the mother had expressed conflicting wishes. Furthermore, in *Jefferson,* the surgery was for the benefit of both the mother and the child. In the instant case, there was no possible benefit to the mother, only to the unborn child. The court stated that, "every person has the right, under the common law and the Constitution, to accept or refuse medical treatment. This right of bodily integrity belongs equally to persons who are competent and persons who are not. Further, it matters not what the quality of a patient's life may be; the right of bodily integrity is not extinguished simply because someone is ill, or even at death's door . . . we hold that a court must determine the patient's wishes by any means available and must abide by those wishes unless there are truly extraordinary or compelling reasons to override them. When the patient is incompetent or when the court is unable to determine competency, the substituted judgment procedure must be followed."[22] The court went further and stated that "it would be an extraordinary case indeed in which a court might ever be justified in overriding the patient's wishes and authorizing a major surgical procedure such as a cesarean section . . . some may doubt that there could ever be a situation extraordinary or compelling enough to justify a massive intrusion into a person's body, such as a cesarean section, against that person's will."[23] These are truly extraordinary statements made by the court, and when compared with the decision in *Jefferson,* an example of just how distinctly different two courts' opinions may truly be. As stated by one commentator, In *re A.C.* "provide[s] strong support for the primacy of the woman's rights when her own welfare is endangered by any procedure designed to safeguard the fetus and its potential for life."[24–26]

A case decided in New York in 1990 provides another example of a court's recognition of the importance of patient autonomy.[27] In that case, a blood transfusion was refused by an adult Jehovah's Witness patient, who was both pregnant and facing the need for a cesarean delivery of her child. The trial court ordered the blood transfusion, and the patient appealed. Although the issue was moot as the transfusion was given, the court felt it necessary to examine this important issue. The court clearly stated that it is essential to realize that the patient is an adult and not a child whose parents have refused to give consent to specific medical treatment, nor is the patient an incompetent requiring court intervention for the provision of medical care. The patient was in fact, a nurse and her husband, a radiologist. In emphasizing the importance of patient autonomy in the decision-making process, the court stated that it "will intervene to prevent suicide, or the self-inflicted injuries of the mentally deranged. But merely declining medical care, even essential treatment, is not considered a suicidal act or indication of incompetence . . . . [The court] consistently support[s] the right of the competent adult to make his own decisions by imposing civil liability on those who perform medical treatment without consent, although the treatment may be beneficial or even necessary to preserve the patient's life."[28]

However, women who do not or cannot comply with proper conduct end up injuring a fetus who could have been born healthy. Should the state go beyond education and punish irresponsible maternal behavior during pregnancy by imposing civil or criminal sanctions when actual damage to offspring has occurred? Should the state prevent the harm before it occurs by incarcerating or forcibly treating pregnant women?

Postbirth Civil and Criminal Sanctions

The law has recognized for a long time that actions or omissions during pregnancy can be as harmful to children as actions or omissions after the child is born. Since the 16th century, prenatal actions that cause a child to die after live birth have been prosecuted as homicide.[29] Similarly, under the civil law, damages have been awarded for injuries that occur during pregnancy or before conception when a child who could have been born healthy is born damaged.[30] Recent developments that allow family members to sue each other now permit such suits by children against parents if the latter have culpably caused the children avoidable injury.[31] Because these duties arise only if the woman chooses to continue a pregnancy that she is legally free to end, punishing culpable maternal behavior that unreasonably damages offspring does not conflict with the Supreme Court decision guaranteeing access to abortion.[32]

In theory, a child who is severely retarded as a result of culpable prenatal conduct could sue the mother. However, suits by damaged offspring against mothers occur rarely. In any event, the theoretical possibility of civil suit is not likely to deter harmful prenatal conduct. A more likely scenario for liability is that of the physician to the parent for the wrongful birth of an anomalous child or to the child itself for wrongful life. A wrongful birth claim arises in the case wherein a child is born with an abnormality that could have been detected prenatally.[33] This claim has developed into the right of a parent to seek damages against a physician for failure to provide them with the opportunity to prevent this child's "wrongful birth."[34, 35] It allows them to seek damages for injuries that they themselves have suffered, rather than for any injury suffered by the abnormal child. It is therefore a claim by the parents that had they been properly informed of the child's condition at the appropriate time, they would have chosen to not have continued with the pregnancy. This claim is distinct from the child's claim of "wrongful life." Wrongful life is a claim by the abnormal child that the physician was negligent in allowing it to be born.[36] It is a claim wherein the child states that he or she would have been better off not to have been born than to have been born with this abnormality.

The state might pursue criminal prosecution for culpable prenatal conduct that causes severe damage to offspring. Although only a few prosecutions for prenatal child abuse have been reported, including the example discussed above, this avenue is probably within the state's authority. It is unlikely to become a frequently utilized or an effective means by which we attempt to protect children in any but those rare cases of extremely outrageously harmful prenatal conduct. The application of this type of law may, however, prove to cause a good deal of consternation and confusion to the medical community. One example of a newly enacted statute providing criminal penalties for the death of a fetus was enacted in California in 1997.[37] That statute defines murder as the "unlawful killing of a human being, or a fetus, with malice aforethought."[38] It specifically exempts from the definition of murder if one of three instances apply. These include the act complying with the Therapeutic Abortion Act; the act committed by a physician wherein "to a medical certainty, the result of childbirth would be death of the mother of the fetus or where her death from childbirth, although not medically certain, would be substantially certain or more likely than not"; or in the instance wherein the act was "solicited, aided, abetted, or consented to by the mother of the fetus."[39] The first and most obvious problem with such a statute is that on its face, it appears to permit the prosecution for the death of a fetus at any stage postconception. Thus, a defendant could theoretically be held liable for the death of a fetus that is not only nonviable, but of which the pregnant mother is unaware. It is theoretically possible that a physician could be held liable under this statute in the event that he provided a drug, medication, or treatment for a patient, knowing that a pregnancy loss was a foreseeable side effect. If the doctor did not fully inform his patient of this possibility and thus did not fully receive her consent to treatment and a pregnancy loss did, in fact occur, although unlikely, the physician could, depending upon the court's definition of malice aforethought, be held criminally liable for the death, instead of merely civilly liable in a malpractice suit.[40] Another significant problem with this statute lies in the lack of a definition of what exactly constitutes a fetus. A 1994 case indicated that this fact alone does not invalidate the statute for vagueness.[41] In fact, the court held in that case that it is generally recognized that a fetus is "defined as 'the unborn offspring in the postembryonic period after major structures have been outlined' . . . [at] seven or eight weeks after fertilization . . . [and further agree] that the Legislature could criminalize murder of the postembryonic product without the imposition of a viability requirement."[42, 43]

In a slightly different factual and legal scenario, a highly publicized example of another prosecution occurred in 1986 in San Diego when a full-term pregnant woman with placenta previa allegedly ignored her doctor's advice and took amphetamines, had sex with her husband, and delayed going to the hospital for "many hours" after she began bleeding.[44] Her baby was born alive with severe brain damage and died within 6 weeks in a neonatal intensive care unit. The district attorney filed misdemeanor charges against the mother under a California statute that penalizes a "parent of a minor child who willfully omits, without lawful excuse, to furnish necessary medical attendance or other remedial care for his or her child."[45] The statute included a provision that "a child conceived but not yet born (is) an existing person" within the meaning of the statute. The father, whose knowledge of the risks to the offspring was less clear, was not prosecuted. The charges were dismissed eventually on the ground that the statute had not been intended to apply to prenatal acts and omission.[46]

Another case of great interest was decided in Florida in 1997.[47] The State had charged the defendant, 19-year-old Kawana M. Ashley, with manslaughter and third-degree felony murder for the death of her infant child. In her 25th or 26th week of pregnancy, the defendant shot herself in the abdomen through a pillow. The bullet passed through the fetal wrist. Ashley was taken to a Florida hospital, whereat a cesarean section was performed. The newborn died at age 15 days as a result of her prematurity. Ashley had reportedly indicated to one police officer that she shot herself "in order to hurt the baby." A second officer was allegedly told that the gun had discharged accidentally and that Ashley had actually wanted to continue with the pregnancy. Two questions were posed to the court. The first inquired as to whether or not a pregnant woman may be charged with the death of her newborn child if that death was the result of self-inflicted injuries during the pregnancy. The second question asked the court to determine if felony murder charges apply when the underlying crime is a self-induced abortion.

In its decision, the court reviewed the common law doctrine that although it was a crime for a third party to cause or induce an abortion in a pregnant women, it was not illegal for the pregnant woman herself to either do so herself or consent to such treatment. Such actions on behalf of the pregnant woman made her liable criminally for neither the actual act nor as an accessory. In holding that common law doctrine provided immunity for the actions of a pregnant woman who seeks or assents to an abortion, the court dismissed the criminal charges against the defendant.

It can be argued that through proper police and judicial conduct and investigation, only the most outrageous cases of prenatal abuse and neglect will be punished. This is similar to the situation currently wherein only the worst cases of child abuse are punished with the most severe penalties. However, this comparison is not necessarily valid, as postnatal punishment is much less invasive. Prenatal sanctions of necessity grossly invade a woman's right of bodily integrity. It is quite reasonable to fear that some patients may believe that obstetricians may become agents of the police in their actions toward patients. The fear that an obstetrician may become a "police informant" will most obviously deter some patients from seeking prenatal care.

In a Florida case in which a trial court attempted to act as a member of the "pregnancy police,"[48] T. H., the mother of three children born with cocaine addiction, was ordered by the trial court to undergo bimonthly pregnancy testing and urine drug screening. The court stated that the purpose of these examinations was to ensure that if the defendant did become pregnant she was not using drugs. If the defendant did in fact test positive for pregnancy and for drugs, then the court indicated that it would place the defendant in jail. It is not stated in the opinion, but it is assumed that the court intended to keep the defendant in jail for the duration of her pregnancy. In reversing the trial court's order, the appellate court stated that state law "does not grant . . . the trial court the power to order the mother of the dependent child to undergo the challenged pregnancy testing."[49]

Because of the dubious nature of the imposition of criminal sanctions for prenatal maternal child abuse, we as a society must emphasize the need for education and should make needed services available. It must be realized, however, that any laws enacted to regulate maternal conduct during pregnancy as child abuse must be limited to only the most outrageous cases of parental behavior. Overall, however, postbirth sanctions are much less important than are education and services in limiting harmful maternal conduct during pregnancy. One must develop a policy whereby prebirth sanctions or detention are rarely if ever utilized.

Prebirth Seizures

The most extreme and controversial policy option is incarceration or forced treatment of pregnant women who are unlikely or unwilling to avoid behavior that is damaging to fetuses. From the perspective of the child at risk, this approach is preferable to punishment after the damage occurs, because it may prevent the damage. However, from the perspective of the mother, this approach is highly intrusive and from a civil libertarian point of view, it is reprehensible.

Direct intervention on the mother, however, is an extremely troubling option because it involves bodily seizures of varying duration and risk without the woman's consent. The right to be free of seizure and forced bodily intrusion is a basic human right. Few cases would meet the high standards necessary to justify a direct seizure for the benefit of unborn offspring.

There is an extremely strong case against the use of seizures as a policy to prevent prenatal harm to offspring. Although there may arguably be some role for postbirth sanctions, the role for prebirth seizures in preventing avoidable handicaps is extremely rare. Often, they could not be brought to bear in time to prevent the damage. If they could, there would be major problems in ensuring the fairness and certainty that such an extreme step was required. Policy efforts are better spent in informing women of risks and in making treatment available than in seizing recalcitrant women during pregnancy for the sake of their expected offspring.

Seizures are basically objectionable intrusions upon a person's freedom. Although direct bodily seizures are rare in the law, they are not unknown. They occur in civil commitment, prison sentences, capital punishment, the draft, forced treatment of adults for the sake of minor children, and blood tests and surgery to recover evidence of crime. However, none of these seizures involves the direct violation of one person's physical integrity for the benefit of another. No court would ever order a person to donate a bone marrow to a sibling or a parent to donate a kidney to her child, no matter how urgent the need. Their validity depends on a sufficient state interest to justify the intrusion on protected personal interests in bodily integrity, liberty, and privacy, balanced against the important right to maintain one's own bodily integrity. It is unlikely that such a state interest could be demonstrated in anything but the most extreme cases.

What situations would justify seizure or forced treatment of the pregnant woman (or father) to prevent harm to expected offspring? It is difficult to even imagine the appropriate circumstances wherein a court would be so justified. The only possible case would be when the intrusion or seizure is trivial and when the harm to be prevented is certain and substantial. Even then, considerable doubt and controversy remain about whether the power should be used. The case for seizure weakens rapidly as the length, risk, and burdens of the seizure increase and as the benefit to the offspring diminishes.

Forcing pregnant women to undergo medical treatment is probably never justifiable. The only arguable case for forced treatment would be a one-time minor intervention of miniscule risk that is administered to avert a severe and certain anomaly to the unborn child. This would have to be a procedure so minor that maternal risk is virtually zero and fetal risk is enormous. One of the only examples that readily comes to mind is a RhoGAM injection to prevent fetal hydrops. Virtually any other type of therapy, including just about any type of fetal surgery, involves such a major intrusion into the mother, with great attendant risks, that it seems inconceivable that a court would ever be justified in ordering it.

In practice such cases fortunately occur rarely. When safety and efficacy of other procedures are clearly established, few mothers will refuse the procedure, but those who do will likely still have the right to do so.

Thus, prebirth seizures may fall arguably within the power of the state in a narrow class of compelling cases, yet rarely if ever should be sought. The likelihood of error in predicting benefit, the difficulty in ensuring due process, and the burden of forced treatment and incarceration make such an extreme remedy therefore a dubious method to reduce the number of handicapped children. Given the risks of such an intrusive policy, prebirth education and possibly some type of postbirth sanctions should be the sole coercive remedies used by the state, even though exceptional cases that attain the very high standards for seizures can rarely be justified.

Sanctions, Seizures, and Prenatal Screening Programs

The ethical and legal principles analyzed earlier would also apply to prenatal screening programs. Once again, the main policy should be voluntarism, encouraged by public education and access to essential services. A law mandating that women be informed of screening options (e.g., the California law requiring that women be informed of α-fetoprotein screening) is desirable.[50]

Mandatory screening, enforced by criminal or civil penalties, arguably can be justified when the costs and burdens of screening are *de minimus* and when a great benefit to the offspring or others can be shown. The optimal timing of such interventions is, of course, debatable. However, the appropriate punishment for the failure to comply with such screening requirements would be both difficult to determine and difficult to enforce. Furthermore, mandatory screening raises questions such as, If screening demonstrated a significant prenatal defect, should mandatory abortion or treatment of that defect be required?

Forced screening, like forcing any treatment or making any bodily seizure, is the most difficult of all to justify. However, if an extreme enough situation presented itself, such a policy would be within the constitutional authority of the state. One must, however, never forget that forced screening may be but the first step down the slippery slope to forced treatment of other types. Screening only identifies a problem that may need treatment. Although it may enhance the possibility that treatment or prevention occurs, it does not guarantee it.

Advanced Reproductive Technologies

Cryopreservation

With the advent of advances in reproductive science, legal and ethical questions have arisen that were inconceivable only one or two decades ago. Two of these issues will be discussed here—the legal issues surrounding cryopreservation of human embryos and the cloning of human embryos. Cryopreservation of embryos is a procedure whereby fertilized eggs are stored for later implantation in the female member of the couple. It is a valuable method of preserving a couple's genetic information for the later production of children. However, when a relationship breaks up, issues may arise about the possession and future of the cryopreserved eggs. One such case arose in Tennessee in 1992.[51] Mary Sue Davis sought possession of embryos fertilized by her ex-husband, Junior Davis, during the term of their marriage. Junior Davis objected, claiming that he had not yet decided whether or not he wished to become an unmarried father. Mr. Davis argued for the continued preservation of the embryos in their frozen state. The trial court ruled in favor of Ms. Davis, but the appellate court reversed that order, vesting possession of the embryos in the joint control and custody of both parties. Ms. Davis appealed again and the state supreme court heard the matter.

The court was struck with the importance of this case, in that it reflected an important legal aspect of a new medical technology. It first reviewed the factual changes that had occurred since the initial presentation of the case. Both parties had remarried, and Ms. Davis, although not wanting to personally have the embryos implanted, wished to donate the embryos to a childless couple. Mr. Davis had become adamant in his opposition to this donation and stated that he would rather see the eggs discarded. The court stated that it was initially important to understand that no written agreement was made between the parties or between the parties and the clinic that would have provided for the disposition of the embryos in the case of separation, divorce, or disagreement, nor was there any statute that provided guidance. The court held that the embryos were really neither person nor property, but entities of an in-between nature. As such, they were not entitled to the constitutional protections afforded to persons. The court resolved the dispute by applying a balancing test. In doing so, the court stated that "[o]ne way of resolving these disputes is to consider the positions of the parties, the significance of their interests and the relative burdens that will be imposed by differing resolutions . . . [that is] the right to procreate and the right to avoid procreation."[52] The court, in ruling in favor of Mr. Davis, concluded that in balancing the interests in this case, including Ms. Davis' ability to become a parent in a manner not including the use of these specific fertilized ova, Mr. Davis' interest in not becoming a parent outweighed Ms. Davis' desires to use the fertilized eggs as she wished.[53]

The importance of this case lies in the fact that it acknowledges that the rights of the parents supercede any rights purported to be possessed by the frozen embryo and that the rights of neither parent is superior to those of the other. As a balancing test is utilized by the court, there is no actual veto power vested in the nonconsenting parent. With the proper factual situation, it is quite conceivable that a court could permit the implantation of fertilized ova over the objection of one parent. In such a case, it would be necessary for the court to determine what, if any, rights and obligations attached to the nonconsenting parent in the case that a live birth did, in fact occur. Would there be child support responsibility? Should the nonconsenting father have visitation privileges? In the event of the death of the nonconsenting parent, is the child an heir-at-law?

Cloning

Since the first successful cloning of a sheep in 1997, the topic of mammalian and human cloning has received a great deal of attention. Barely 3 months after the first successfully reported cloning of a sheep, an 18-member panel of experts appointed by the President of the United States recommended that federal legislation be enacted to prevent the cloning of a human being.[54] Indeed, within a week of the announcement of the production of "Dolly," the secretary-general of the 40-nation Council of Europe stated that the successful cloning experiment "demonstrates the need for firmer rules on bioethics."[55] In an editorial that accompanied the publication of the original article reporting the first successful sheep cloning, the editors of the journal *Nature* reported that even prior to its publication, they received e-mail from a "Harvard academic" pleading that the article be withdrawn from publication pending greater consideration being given to bioethical and information access issues.[56]

This controversy was sparked by a short article detailing the procedure by which through the transfer of an adult nucleus to an unfertilized egg, a viable sheep was created.[57] No ethical, legal, or moral issues were raised in that original article. It was the straightforward presentation of a novel scientific technique. Yet the procedure by its very nature raises these issues. No one can deny the potential utility of the cloning procedure. Humans could be born with greater intelligence, greater strength, and fewer genetic abnormalities. Congenital diseases could be reduced or eliminated and resistance to acquired disease could be increased. On the other hand, reprogramming of the genes could go wrong with disastrous consequences. Would late-term abortions be permitted to "correct" erroneous cloning experiments? Would groups of individuals looking to create a population of supermen and women be allowed to clone these "perfect" children? Would those of us who were born in the ordinary way somehow become second-class citizens, closed out of the finest schools and professions? Or will the potential usefulness of this new procedure be, as one biologist puts it, "too exciting to pass up"?[58] Importantly, does the potential criminalization of scientific research take us one more step down the slippery slope of governmental control of the dissemination of knowledge?[59]

Legal Duties of Physicians in Prenatal Situations

The physician has a legal obligation to act with due care toward the offspring who will be born. This duty requires that the fetus who will be brought to term be treated like a "patient," because prenatal acts and omissions can significantly affect the welfare of the resultant child. As noted earlier, the fetus is not a patient for its own sake. Depending on the mother's wishes and the stage of pregnancy, there is no duty to ensure that the fetus is born alive.

Physicians play an important role in implementing voluntary compliance as being the most desirable approach to preventing prenatal harm to offspring. Physicians must inform women of the prenatal risks of certain behaviors and the steps that should be taken to avoid harm to offspring. They must also inform women of damage that has progressed so far that it cannot be avoided, except by termination of the pregnancy.

Failure to inform a woman of risks and alternative procedures violates her right to informed consent and the child's right to be born free of avoidable prenatal harm. A physician who neglects to identify an avoidable source of prenatal harm or to inform the woman of it and ways to avoid it could be legally liable to the parents and offspring for the damages that they suffer. Prenatal negligence on the part of a physician is clearly actionable.

Recovery is also possible when the woman would have had an abortion, because the injury or damage was now unavoidable, even though she could not be punished for refusing to abort. However, as discussed earlier, the concept of a wrongful life suit on behalf of the abnormally born child has not been well received by the courts.

The more difficult question for physicians is their legal duty when they have informed a woman of the risks or harm that she is imposing on her planned offspring, and when she refuses to comply or ignores recommendations that are essential for the child's welfare. Suppose that the physician strenuously urges her to take the necessary steps (e.g., to stop using alcohol, tobacco, heroin, cocaine, or marijuana, or consent to a medical test or treatment), and she still refuses. Should the physician regretfully acquiesce to her refusals? Must he or she report the case to child welfare authorities? What if the mother could not herself be prosecuted because the jurisdiction has not enacted a prenatal child abuse law to apply to pregnant women? In this type of case, does the physician have either an obligation or even a right to report the refusal to social services or does he violate confidentiality by doing so? A close examination of the applicable state law would be warranted, however, before making such a report. Although state laws authorizing disclosure of child abuse do abrogate the physician–patient privilege, if a physician is reporting a matter not covered by the law, liability could arguably attach to his or her actions.

Informing the woman of the risks, urging compliance, and reporting the case to child welfare authorities in the case of further refusals (if legally permissible) is the extent of the physician's legal obligation in cases of prenatal risks to offspring. The physician clearly has no legal or moral right or obligation to seize the woman and force treatment on her or to seek legal authorization (guardianship) to do so, and in fact could be held legally liable if he attempted to do so. At most, the physician may have an obligation to inform the child welfare authorities, who may then decide to take action within the limits of the law. At that point the physician may have to cooperate by providing facts to the authorities or to courts that are investigating the matter, although he or she would not be obligated to administer treatments that have been refused but that have been legally authorized if the mothers have scruples against it.

By applying this analysis to a mother's refusal of a cesarean section, we see that the physician would, of course, have no right to force a cesarean section on an unwilling woman and could arguably have a duty to protect his patients from unwarranted intrusion by the state. Doing so without proper court authorization would most certainly subject the doctor to charges of assault and battery. The action of informing the mother of the risks and, if mandated by law, of reporting damaging refusals to child welfare authorities satisfy the physician's duty. The benefit to the few children who would avoid injury seems to be outweighed by the errors that are likely to occur under forced treatment policies.

Conclusion

While describing legal considerations in fetal treatment, this chapter has examined the ethical, legal, and policy controversy that has arisen over the question of prenatal duties to prevent harm to offspring.

Prenatal duties to offspring may arise, if at all, only after a woman has decided to continue a pregnancy that she is free to terminate. Analysis must also distinguish between postbirth civil and criminal sanctions and forcible seizures before birth; the legal status and desirability of these two policies differ greatly. The use of forcible seizures should be limited to those extremely rare instances of egregiously harmful prenatal conduct. Education, services, and voluntary compliance are still the most desirable policies to pursue. Forcible seizures and treatment coerced through court order must only be permitted in the most extraordinary circumstances. The essential freedoms of our constitution protect the inviolability of one's person. Although the developing fetus does deserve a certain degree of protection, in general and barring extreme or outrageous situations, the rights of the mother must prevail in most maternal–fetal controversy.

The physician plays an important role in minimizing the number of handicapped births that could have been avoided. The physician must explain to pregnant women the options for treating fetuses or avoiding conduct harmful to them and must attempt to persuade them to act for the good of the child. There may also be a legal duty to report refusals or risks to child welfare authorities. At that point physicians have done all that may reasonably be asked to fulfil their legal duty to the unborn child, whose care they have assumed during pregnancy.

Lastly, medical technology in the area of prenatal diagnosis and treatment is advancing at breakneck speed. Unfortunately, as evidenced by the controversy surrounding cryopreservation of embryos and cloning of mammalian cells, ethical and legal consideration of these procedures has sadly lagged behind. It is the duty of all physicians—research scientist and private practitioner alike—to examine the advances in medicine as they appear and critically ask how these procedures can best benefit society medically, morally, and ethically.

Acknowledgment

Acknowledgment is made to John Robertson, author of the previous edition's version of this chapter. This chapter is both based upon and retains significant portions of his work, some portions of which have had their wordings changed to reflect a different viewpoint based upon 10 years' further experience in the field. Our basic hypothesis and conclusions that we have drawn are different than those drawn by him.

The research for this chapter was supported, in part, by the Richard J. Barber Fund for Interdisciplinary Legal Research, Wayne State University Law School, Detroit, Michigan.

REFERENCES

1. Johnsen D: The creation of fetal rights: Conflicts with women's constitutional rights to liberty, privacy, and equal protection. Yale Law Rev 95:599, 614, 1986.
2. Evans MI, Dixler AO: Human in vitro fertilization: Some legal issues. JAMA 245:22, 2324, 1981.
3. *Johnson v. State*, 602 So2d 1288 (Fla 1992).
4. Lencewica M: Article: Don't crack the cradle: Minnesota's effective solution for the prevention of prenatal substance abuse—analysis of Minnesota Statute Section 626.5561. Rev Jur U P R 63:599, 1994.
5. Minn Stat Ann 253B.02 subd.2.
6. Minn Stat Ann 626.556(2)(c).
7. For a discussion of the need to assist, rather than involuntarily intervene with these women, see, Linden PM: Drug addiction during pregnancy: A call for increased social responsibility. Am U J Gender Law 4:105, 1995.
8. Johnson KL. Comments: An argument for consideration of prenatal smoking in neglect and abuse determinations. Emory L J 46:1661, 1997.
9. Robertson J: Embryos, families and procreative liberty: The legal structure of the new reproduction. So Cal Law Rev 59:939, 1986.
10. Kolder VE, Gallagher J, Parsons MT: Court-ordered obstetrical interventions. N Engl J Med 316(19):1192–1196, 1987.
11. Elkins TE, Andersen HF, Barclay M, et al: Court-ordered cesarean section: An analysis of ethical concerns in compelling cases. Am J Obstet Gynecol 161(1):150–154, 1989.
12. Bowles WA, Selgestad B: Fetal versus maternal rights: Medical and legal perspectives. Obstet Gynecol 58:209–214, 1981.
13. *Jefferson v. Griffin Spalding County Hospital Authority* 247 Ga 86, 274 SE2d 457 (1981).
14. *Ibid* at 88, 459.
15. *Ibid* at 89, 460.
16. Annas GJ: Forced cesareans: The most unkindest cut of all. Hastings Cent Rep 12(3):16–17, 45, 1982.
17. Annas GJ: She's going to die: The case of Angela C. Hastings Cent Rep 18(1):23–25, 1988.
18. Annas GJ: Foreclosing the use of force: A.C. reversed. Hastings Cent Rep 20(4):27–29, 1990.
19. *In re A.C.* 533 A2d 611 (1987 D.C. App).
20. *Ibid*, at 617.
21. *In re A.C.* 573 A2d 1235 (1990 D.C. App).
22. *Ibid*, at 1247.
23. *Ibid*, at 1252.
24. Curran WJ: Court-ordered cesarean sections receive judicial defeat. JAMA 323(7):489–492, 1990.
25. Also see, Bourke LH: *In re A.C.* Issues Law Med 6(3):299–304, 1990.
26. However, see Pacheco DA: Court-ordered cesarean sections [letter]. JAMA 324(4):272–273, 1990, for an alternative interpretation of *In re A.C.*
27. *Fosmire v. Nicoleau*, 75 NY2d 218, 551 NE2d 77 (1990).
28. *Ibid*, at 227, 82.
29. 3 E Coke, Institutes 50 (1648).
30. Robertson H: Toward rational boundaries of tort liability for injury to the unborn. Duke Law J 1401, 1978.
31. *Grodin v. Grodin*, 102 Mich. App. 396, 301 N. W. 2d 869 (1980).
32. *Roe v. Wade*, 410 U.S. 113 (1973).
33. See e.g., *Reed v. Campagnolo*, 332 Md 226, 630 A2d 1145, a case in which the defendants failed to inform the plaintiff of the availability of or need for an α-fetoprotein testing of maternal blood. This failure led to the failure to detect several significant genetic defects. Plaintiffs claimed that had the tests been performed, they would have been positive and the plaintiffs would have terminated the pregnancy.
34. Chase RF. Liability for prenatal injuries. 40 ALR3d 1222.
35. Sarno GG: Tort liability for wrongfully causing one to be born. 83 ALR3d 15, 1997.
36. Rockwell HP: What patient claims against doctor, hospital or similar health care provider are not subject to statutes. 89 ALR4th 887, 1998.
37. Cal Pen Code Section 187 (1997).
38. Cal Pen Code Section 187(a) (1997).
39. Cal Pen Code Section 187(b) (1997).
40. For a discussion of the definition of malice, see *People v. Watson*, 30 Cal3d 290, 637 P2d 279 (1981).
41. *People v. Davis*, 7 Cal 4th 797, 872 P2d 591 (Cal 1994).
42. *Ibid*, at 810, 599.
43. Also see, *People v. Dennis*, 17 Cal 4th 468, 950 P2d 1035 (Cal 1998).
44. Chambers M: Dead baby's mother faces criminal charges on acts in pregnancy. New York Times, Sept 9, 1986, p 10.
45. Cal Pen Code, Chap 2, Section 270, (Suppl) 1986.
46. Chambers M: Charges against mother in death of baby are thrown out. New York Times, Feb 27, 1987, p A25.
47. *State v. Ashley*, 701 So2d 338 (Fla 1997).
48. *T.H. v Department of Health and Rehabilitative Services*, 661 So2d 403 (Fla 1995).
49. *Ibid*, at 404.
50. California Health and Welfare Code, 1986.
51. *Davis v. Davis*, 842 SW2d 588 (Tenn 1992).
52. *Ibid*, at 603.
53. For an example of a case in which the preexisting contract between the parties and the clinic was valid and sufficient to determine the disposition of the frozen embryos, see *Kass v. Kass*, 91 NY2d 554, 696 NE2d 174 (NY 1998).
54. Marshall E: Clinton urges outlawing human cloning. Science 276:1640, 1997.
55. Williams N: Cloning sparks calls for new laws. Science 275:1415, 1997.
56. Caught napping by clones. Nature 385:753, 1997.
57. Wilmut I, Schnieke AE, McWhir J, et al: Viable offspring derived from fetal and adult mammalian cells. Nature 385:810, 1997.
58. Pennisi E, Williams N: Will Dolly send in the clones? Science 275:141, 1997.
59. See Carmen IH: Essay: Should human cloning be criminalized? J L Politics 13:745, 1997, for a discussion of the National Bioethics Advisory Counsel's report on cloning and policy and ethical issues that have arisen therefrom.

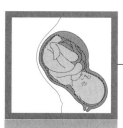

P A R T   II

Diagnostic and Therapeutic Techniques: A View into the Womb

CHAPTER 5

The Rationale for Fetal Treatment: Selection, Feasibility, and Risk

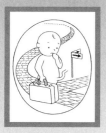

MICHAEL R. HARRISON

The human fetus has for centuries remained a medical recluse in an opaque womb. Now normal and abnormal fetal anatomy can be accurately delineated by sonography, a noninvasive technique that appears to be safe for both the fetus and the mother. The fetal genome can be probed for inherited defects by chorionic villus sampling, amniocentesis, and fetal blood sampling. Some fetal malformations with a known pattern of inheritance may be specifically sought. Others are identified serendipitously during obstetric sonography, sometimes because the obstetric conditions that lead to sonography are associated with underlying fetal malformations. For example, oligohydramnios may be associated with fetal urinary tract obstruction, and polyhydramnios may be related to fetal upper gastrointestinal (GI) tract obstruction.[1-4]

Until recently, the only question raised by the prenatal diagnosis of a fetal malformation was whether to abort the fetus or to await delivery. However, other therapeutic alternatives are becoming available, such as changing the timing, mode, and place of delivery or even treatment before birth (Fig. 5–1). Because perinatal management may be altered, prenatal diagnosis assumes new clinical significance.

The rationale for determining how the prenatal diagnosis of any given fetal defect will affect perinatal management is quite simple (Fig. 5–2). But experience in fetal management is limited, thus optimal management of any given defect is often unknown or is in evolution. Opinions about the management of each fetal lesion must be tentative and must be open to revision in relation to rapidly growing knowledge and experience.

Defects Usually Managed by Termination of Pregnancy

When serious malformations incompatible with postnatal life are diagnosed, the family has the option to terminate the pregnancy. Table 5–1 shows examples of severe defects that may be considered to be indications for selective abortion. Some are chromosomal defects that can be diagnosed by culture of amniotic fluid or chorionic villus cells. Anatomic defects associated with chromosomal abnormalities, such as omphalocele associated with trisomy 18, should routinely have karyotype analysis. Other severe developmental abnormalities may be diagnosed by imaging procedures alone. In all, a long list of severe chromosomal, metabolic, and developmental disorders can be diagnosed in utero and usually lead to selective abortion.[5, 6]

Defects Best Corrected after Delivery at Term

Most correctable malformations that can be diagnosed in utero are best managed by appropriate medical and surgical therapy after delivery at term. The term infant is a better anesthetic and surgical risk than the preterm infant. Examples of malformations that have been diagnosed in utero are given in Table 5–2. Although this list is not complete, most neonatal surgical disorders fall into this category. Knowing that a fetus has one of these anomalies, even if it does not alter the timing or mode of delivery, allows preparation for appropriate prenatal and postnatal care. Therapy for hydramnios and premature labor may be desirable to allow the fetus to remain in utero as long as possible. The delivery can be planned so that appropriate personnel (e.g., neonatologist, anesthesiologist, pediatric surgeon) are available. When the neonate requires highly specialized services, maternal transport is usually preferable to postnatal transport of the fragile newborn.

Defects That Can Influence the Mode of Delivery

Elective cesarean delivery rather than a trial at vaginal delivery may be indicated for the fetal malformations shown in Table 5–3. In most cases, this is because the

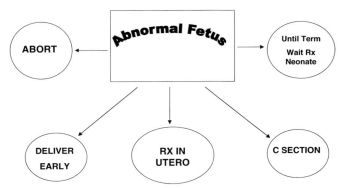

FIGURE 5–1. Prenatal diagnosis of fetal defects would have little clinical significance if the options for management were limited to terminating the pregnancy or to doing nothing until birth. Diagnosis may now alter perinatal management by allowing choices about the timing, mode, and place of delivery. In a few cases, treatment before birth may be appropriate.

malformation would cause dystocia. Another indication for elective cesarean delivery is a malformation that may benefit from immediate surgical correction best performed in a sterile environment. Examples are a ruptured omphalocele or an uncovered meningomyelocele. In this case, the baby can be resuscitated and then undergo immediate surgical correction. Finally, cesarean delivery may be required if preterm delivery of an affected fetus is elected but labor is inadequate or the fetus does not tolerate labor as determined by fetal monitoring.

Defects That Can Influence the Timing of Delivery

Early delivery may be indicated for certain fetal anomalies that require correction as soon as possible after diag-

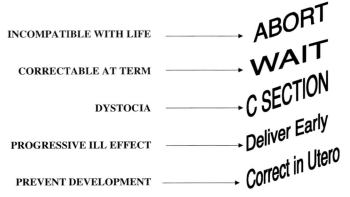

FIGURE 5–2. The nature of the fetal problem determines the management. Very bad defects may lead to abortion. Most lesions that can be corrected by surgery are best treated after birth, and maternal transport to a perinatal center may be advantageous. Lesions that cause dystocia may require a cesarean delivery. Lesions that cause progressive harm may lead to early delivery for immediate repair ex utero. A few lesions that cause progressive harm or that prevent adequate organ development before the time of extrauterine viability may require treatment before birth.

TABLE 5–1. DEFECTS USUALLY MANAGED BY SELECTIVE ABORTION

Anencephaly, hydranencephaly, alobar holoprosencephaly
Severe anomalies associated with chromosomal abnormalities (e.g., trisomy 13)
Bilateral renal agenesis
Severe, untreatable, inherited metabolic disorders (e.g., Tay-Sachs disease)
Lethal bone dysplasias (e.g., thanatophoric dysplasia, recessive osteogenesis Imperfecta)

nosis (Table 5–4). In each of these situations, the risk of premature delivery must be weighed against the risk of continued gestation. This approach has already proved to be beneficial in managing fetuses with immune hydrops fetalis and intrauterine growth retardation. Recent advances in stimulating fetal surfactant production with corticosteroids, and in ventilating small babies, have improved the outcome for premature infants with respiratory distress syndrome.

The reason for early delivery is unique to each anomaly, but the principle remains the same: Continued gestation would have a progressive ill effect on the fetus. In some cases, the function of a specific organ system is compromised by the lesion and will continue to deteriorate until the lesion is corrected. In congenital hydronephrosis, unrelieved urinary tract obstruction results in progressive deterioration of renal function. Preterm delivery for early decompression of the urinary tract may alleviate renal maldevelopment at the earliest possible time and thus may maximize subsequent brain development and may avoid the difficult obstetric problem of delivering a baby with an abnormally large head.[9]

In gastroschisis, the bowel becomes coated with thick, fibrous inflammatory peel and may develop progressive dilatation and wall thickening that may hinder repair and delay resumption of function. Early delivery may minimize this damage.[10] Anomalies associated with progressive organ ischemia should be corrected as soon as possible. Volvulus associated with intestinal malrotation or meconium ileus may lead to intestinal gangrene, perforation, and meconium peritonitis. Early delivery for correction of this type of bowel lesion would be

TABLE 5–2. DEFECTS DETECTABLE IN UTERO BUT BEST CORRECTED AFTER DELIVERY AT TERM

Esophageal, duodenal, jejunoileal, and anorectal atresias
Meconium ileus (cystic fibrosis)
Enteric cysts and duplications
Small intact omphalocele
Small intact meningocele
Unilateral hydronephrosis
Craniofacial, extremity, and chest wall deformities
Cystic hygroma
Small sacrococcygeal teratoma, mesoblastic nephroma, etc.
Benign cysts: ovarian, mesenteric, choledochal, etc.

TABLE 5–3. MALFORMATIONS THAT MAY BENEFIT FROM CESAREAN DELIVERY

Conjoined twins
Giant omphalocele
Severe hydrocephalus, large or ruptured meningomyelocele
Large sacrococcygeal teratoma or cervical cystic hygroma
Malformations requiring preterm delivery in the presence of
 inadequate labor or fetal distress

aimed at minimizing the amount of bowel lost to the ischemic process.

Defects That May Require Intervention *During* Birth

Fetal defects that compromise pulmonary function at the time of birth, particularly those that cause airway obstruction, may benefit from the newly developed technique of the ex utero intrapartum treatment (EXIT) procedure (Fig. 5–3). The at-risk fetus is "partially" delivered and the life-threatening defect (usually airway obstruction) repaired while the "fetus/newborn" is still supported on placental circulation. (An alternative acronym is OOPS—operating on placental support.) After the airway is secured, the cord is divided and cesarean section completed.

This technique was developed to deliver safely fetuses who had undergone tracheal occlusion to treat severe diaphragmatic hernia, but has since been successfully applied to a wide variety of other fetal airway problems (Table 5–5).

Defects That May Require Intervention Before Birth

Fetal Deficiencies That May Require Medical Treatment

Some fetal deficiency states may be alleviated by treatment before birth (Table 5–6). Hydrops fetalis secondary to red blood cell deficiency (usually due to isoimmunization-induced hemolysis) can be treated by transfusing

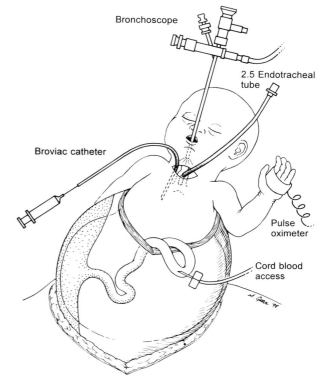

FIGURE 5–3. Technique of the EXIT procedure: Maternal general anesthesia relaxes the uterus and provides fetal anesthesia. A hysterotomy is performed with a specially designed stapling device loaded with absorbable staples to ensure hemostasis. Fetal heart rate and hemoglobin oxygen saturation are continuously monitored by a neonatal pulse oximeter placed on the fetal hand. The baby's airway can be examined with a bronchoscope and secured in a variety of ways. In this drawing, the child was delivered due to hydrops from laryngeal atresia and is undergoing a tracheostomy. Access to the fetal circulation is gained via the umbilical cord or by placing a Broviac catheter in the superior vena cava. Once the airway is secured, the umbilical cord is clamped and divided.

red blood cells into the fetus. Indeed, since Liley's original description more than 20 years ago, fetal transfusion has become standard therapy.[11] With recent advances in percutaneous umbilical cord puncture, blood can be transfused directly into the fetal vascular system, if necessary.[12]

Several deficiency states can be alleviated by transplacental treatment. In the fetus who is born with immature

TABLE 5–4. DEFECTS THAT MAY BENEFIT FROM INDUCED PRETERM DELIVERY FOR EARLY CORRECTION EX UTERO

Some urinary tract obstruction
Some hydrocephalus
Some gastroschisis or ruptured omphalocele
Some intestinal ischemia/necrosis secondary to volvulus, meconium
 ileus, etc.
Some hydrops fetalis
Some intrauterine growth retardation
Some arrhythmias (e.g., supraventricular tachycardia with failure)

TABLE 5–5. DEFECTS THAT MAY BENEFIT FROM THE EXIT PROCEDURE

Cervical teratoma compressing the airway
Cervical cystic hygroma obstructing the larynx
Congenital high airway obstruction syndrome (CHAOS) (laryngeal
 atresia, etc.)
Lung mass preventing chest expansion
Anticipated pulmonary insufficiency requiring extracorporeal
 membrane oxygenation (ECMO)

EXIT, ex utero intrapartum treatment.

TABLE 5–6. DEFICIENCIES AND MALFUNCTIONS THAT MAY BENEFIT FROM MEDICAL TREATMENT BEFORE BIRTH

DISORDER	EXAMPLE	TREATMENT
Anemia	Erythroblastosis	Red blood cells: intraperitoneal or intravenous
Surfactant deficiency	Pulmonary immaturity	Glucocorticoids: transplacental
Metabolic block	Methylmalonic acidemia	Vitamin B_{12}: transplacental
	Multiple carboxylase deficiency	Biotin: transplacental
Cardiac arrhythmia	Supraventricular tachycardia	Digitalis: transplacental
		Propranolol: transplacental
		Procainamide: transplacental
	Heart block	β-Mimetics: transplacental
Endocrine deficiency	Hypothyroidism and goiter	Thyroxin: transamniotic
	Adrenal hyperplasia	Corticosteroids: transplacental
Nutritional deficiency	Intrauterine growth retardation	Protein-calories: transamniotic

lungs, glucocorticoids given to the mother may increase deficient pulmonary surfactant and may alleviate the disease. This form of fetal treatment has become widely used.

A fetus with vitamin B_{12}–responsible methylmalonic acidemia has been treated in utero by giving massive doses of vitamin B_{12} to the mother,[13] and a fetus with biotin-dependent multiple carboxylase deficiency has been treated by giving the mother pharmacologic doses of biotin during the last half of pregnancy.[14]

Cardiac arrhythmias are amenable to medical management. Supraventricular tachycardia, causing fetal congestive heart failure and hydrops, can be converted by giving antiarrhythmic drugs (e.g., digitalis) transplacentally or even directly to the fetus. Fetal heart block associated with maternal collagen-vascular disease can be treated by increasing ventricular rate with β-mimetics.[14, 15]

When the necessary substrate, medication, or nutrient cannot be delivered across the placenta, it may be injected into the amniotic fluid where it can be swallowed and absorbed by the fetus. Intra-amniotic thyroid hormone may be used to treat congenital hypothyroidism and goiter and to help mature the fetal lung.[17, 18] Other endocrine diseases may be treated by providing a specific hormone to the fetus either through the placenta or orally via the amniotic fluid. For example, the masculinization seen in congenital adrenal hyperplasia may be prevented by treatment with steroids throughout gestation.[19] When the fetus is growth-retarded because it cannot derive sufficient nutrients across a damaged placenta, it might be possible to provide oral feedings by instilling nutrients into the amniotic fluid.

In the future, it is possible that deficiencies in cellular function (e.g., hemoglobinopathies, immunodeficiencies) will be corrected by providing the appropriate stem cell graft,[20] and that enzymatic deficiencies will be corrected by gene manipulation.[21]

Life-Threatening Malformations That May Benefit From Surgical Correction

The only anatomic malformations that warrant consideration are those that interfere with fetal organ develop-

ment and that, if alleviated, would allow normal development to proceed (Table 5–7). At present, only a small number of life-threatening malformations have been successfully corrected (the first six conditions listed). A few others should be successfully treated as their pathophysiologic characteristics are unraveled. When less invasive interventional techniques are developed and proved safe, a few nonlethal anomalies may be considered. Finally, fetal stem cell transplantation should open the door to treatment of a variety of inherited disorders and perhaps to inducing tolerance before birth so organs can be transplanted after birth.

Urinary Tract Obstruction

Fetal urethral obstruction produces pulmonary hypoplasia and renal dysplasia, and these often fatal consequences can be ameliorated by urinary tract decompression before birth.[22] The natural history of untreated fetal urinary tract obstruction is well documented, and selection criteria based on fetal urine electrolyte and β_2-microglobulin levels and the sonographic appearance of the fetal kidneys have proven reliable.[23, 24] Of all fetuses with urinary tract dilation, as many as 90% do not require intervention. However, fetuses with bilateral hydronephrosis due to urethral obstruction who develop oligohydramnios require treatment. If the lungs are mature, the fetus can be delivered early for postnatal decompression. If the lungs are immature, the bladder can be decompressed in utero by a catheter shunt placed percutaneously under sonographic guidance,[25] by open fetal vesicostomy,[26] by fetoscopic vesicostomy,[27] by cystoscopic laser ablation of valves, or by placement of an improved wire mesh stent that may solve the technical problems encountered with shunts (malfunction, dislodgement, abdominal wall disruption).[28] Experience treating several hundred fetuses in many institutions suggests that selection is good enough to avoid inappropriate intervention, and that restoration of amniotic fluid can prevent the development of fatal pulmonary hypoplasia. It is not clear that decompression can reverse renal functional damage.

Table 5–8 summarizes the many factors that must be considered in evaluating a fetus with urinary tract obstruction.

T A B L E 5–7. MALFORMATIONS THAT MAY BENEFIT FROM TREATMENT BEFORE BIRTH

	EFFECT ON DEVELOPMENT (RATIONALE FOR TREATMENT)	RESULT WITHOUT TREATMENT	RECOMMENDED TREATMENT
Life-Threatening Defects			
Urinary obstruction (urethral valves)	Hydronephrosis	Renal failure	Percutaneous catheter
	Lung hypoplasia	Pulmonary failure	Fetoscopic vesicostomy
			Open vesicostomy
Cystic adenomatoid malformation	Lung hypoplasia-hydrops	Fetal hydrops, death	Open pulmonary lobectomy
Diaphragmatic hernia	Lung hypoplasia	Pulmonary failure	Open complete repair
			Bowel exteriorization
			Temporary tracheal occlusion
Sacrococcygeal teratoma	High-output failure	Fetal hydrops, death	Resection of tumor
			Fetoscopic vascular occlusion
Twin–twin transfusion syndrome	Vascular "steal" through placenta	Fetal hydrops, death	Open fetectomy
			Fetoscopic division of placenta
Aqueductal stenosis	Hydrocephalus	Brain damage	Ventriculoamniotic shunt
			Open ventriculoperitoneal shunt
Complete heart block	Low-output failure	Fetal hydrops, death	Percutaneous pacemaker
			Open pacemaker
Pulmonary-aortic obstruction	Ventricular hypertrophy	Heart failure	Percutaneous valvuloplasty
			Open valvuloplasty
Tracheal atresia-stenosis-obstruction by tumor	Overdistention by lung fluid	Hydrops, death	Fetoscopic tracheostomy
			Open tracheostomy
			Ex utero intrapartum treatment (EXIT)
Nonlethal Defects			
Myelomeningocele	Spinal cord damage	Paralysis, neurogenic bladder, hydrocephalus, etc.	Fetoscopic coverage
			Open repair
Clefting lip and palate	Facial defect	Persistent deformity	Fetoscopic repair
			Open repair
Metabolic-cellular defects & stem cell–enzyme defects	Hemoglobinopathy	Anemia, hydrops	Fetal stem cell transplant or gene therapy with fetal stem cells (autologous-allogeneic)
	Immunodeficiency	Infection	
	Storage diseases	Retardation	
Predictable organ failure	Hypopastic heart-kidney-lung	Neonatal heart-kidney-lung failure	Induce tolerance for postnatal organ transplant

Cystic Adenomatoid Malformation

Although congenital cystic adenomatoid malformation (CCAM) often presents as a benign pulmonary mass in infancy or childhood, some fetuses with large lesions die in utero or at birth from hydrops and pulmonary hypoplasia.[29] The pathophysiology of hydrops and the feasibility of resecting the fetal lung have been studied in animals.[30,31] Experience managing over 80 cases suggests that most lesions can be successfully treated after birth, and that some lesions resolve before birth.[32] Although only a few fetuses with very large lesions will develop hydrops before 26 weeks, almost all these progress rapidly and die in utero. Careful sonographic surveillance of large lesions is necessary to detect the first signs of hydrops, because fetuses who develop hydrops (< 10% of all fetuses with CCAMs) can be successfully treated by emergency resection of the cystic lobe in utero. Nine fetuses have undergone open surgical resection of the massively enlarged pulmonary lobe. Five of these had rapid resolution of hydrops, impressive in utero lung growth bilaterally, and normal postnatal growth and development with a follow-up of 12 to 45 months.[33,34] Fetal pulmonary lobectomy has proven to be surprisingly simple and quite successful. For lesions with single, large cysts, thoracoamniotic shunting has also been successful.[35]

Table 5–9 summarizes the many factors that must be considered in evaluating a fetus with CCAM. Since reduction of intrathoracic volume is all that is necessary to reverse life-threatening hydrops, a minimally invasive method that reduces mass acutely (e.g., radiofrequency ablation) may eventually replace lung resection by open fetal surgery.

Diaphragmatic Hernia

Congenital diaphragmatic hernia (CDH) is an anatomically simple defect that is correctable after birth by removing the herniated viscera from the chest and closing the diaphragm. Although less severely affected babies survive with modern postnatal surgical care including ECMO, the majority of babies die despite all intervention

T A B L E 5–8. EVALUATION OF THE FETUS WITH OBSTRUCTIVE UROPATHY

ULTRASOUND FINDINGS	FAVORABLE PROGNOSTIC INDICATORS	UNFAVORABLE PROGNOSTIC INDICATORS	PRENATAL WORK-UP	ASSOCIATED ANOMALIES
Anteroposterior diameter of the renal pelvis >10 mm For urethral obstruction: ureterectasis, vesicomegaly, a thickened bladder wall, and posterior urethral dilation Keyhole sign with posterior urethral valves Cystic renal parenchyma Thinning of renal cortex Echogenic renal parenchyma	Normal amniotic fluid volume Normal renal parenchyma on ultrasound Normal fetal urinary electrolytes: Sodium <100 mEq/L Chloride <90 mEq/L Osmolality <210 mOsm/L β_2-Microglobulin <2 mg/L	Oligohydramnios, especially with onset in the second trimester Increased echogenicity and cystic changes of the kidneys (cortical cysts) Abnormal fetal urinary electrolytes: Sodium >100 mEq/L Chloride >90 mEq/L Osmolality >210 mOsm/L β_2-Microglobulin >2 mg/L	Fetal urinary electrolytes (to assess current renal function, bladder tap is performed twice with an interval of 24–48 hr; examine second specimen) Karyotype Detailed sonogram	Ureteropelvic junction obstruction: Other anomalies of the urinary tract in 27% Extraurinary anomalies: neural tube defects, imperforate anus and Hirschsprung's disease Urethral obstruction: Other anomalies of the genitourinary tract such as duplication of the urethra; hypospadias, and megalourethra; an association with chromosomal abnormalities (trisomy 18, 13, del 2q) has been reported in 60%

because their lungs are underdeveloped. Because retrospective estimates of mortality for congenital diaphragmatic hernia vary widely and are flawed by a "hidden mortality" of unknown magnitude, we prospectively studied 52 fetuses with potentially correctable, isolated diaphragmatic hernias diagnosed before 24 weeks. The mortality was 58% despite the best postnatal care including extracorporeal membrane oxygenation (ECMO).[36] Babies who die in utero and soon after birth contribute to a substantial "hidden mortality." Salvage of these severely affected babies remains an unsolved problem.

The pulmonary hypoplasia of diaphragmatic hernia is reversible after repair, but weeks or months are required. After birth, pulmonary support with ECMO is limited to 1 or 2 weeks and cannot save severely affected babies. We have shown experimentally that repair before birth, when the lungs can grow while the fetus remains on placental support, is physiologically sound and technically feasible.[37] Repair in utero has proven to be a formidable challenge, particularly when the left lobe of the liver is incarcerated in the chest, because reduction of the liver compromises umbilical blood

flow.[38, 39] Many technical problems associated with this difficult repair led to the development of the "congenital diaphragmatic hernia two-step," a carefully orchestrated approach that allows the reduction of viscera, reconstruction of the diaphragm, and enlargement of the abdomen to accept the returned viscera.[40] The efficacy, safety, and cost-effectiveness of in utero repair are now being prospectively evaluated in a National Institutes of Health (NIH)-sponsored trial.

When an isolated fetal CDH is diagnosed prior to 24 weeks' gestation, the family has three choices: (1) terminate the pregnancy; (2) carry to term and deliver in a tertiary neonatal center for intensive care with an expected mortality of 58%, considerable morbidity, and an average cost of $161,000; or (3) attempt prenatal intervention. The family's dilemma in choosing management is particularly difficult because the natural history of fetal CDH is quite variable. Although some new sonographic parameters look promising, there are no prognostic criteria that adequately predict which fetus will survive and which will die. We do know that fetuses who herniate late in gestation will do well with modern

T A B L E 5–9. EVALUATION OF THE FETUS WITH CCAM

ULTRASOUND FINDINGS	FAVORABLE PROGNOSTIC INDICATORS	UNFAVORABLE PROGNOSTIC INDICATORS	PRENATAL WORK-UP	ASSOCIATED ANOMALIES
Usually unilateral intrathoracic lesion Cystic or echogenic lung tumor without feeding vessel from the aorta (vs. pulmonary sequestration)	No placentomegaly No hydrops Shrinking or stable lesion Mild mediastinal shift	Placentomegaly Hydrops Polyhydramnios Progressive growth and severe mediastinal shift Everted diaphragm	Echocardiography Level II ultrasound to rule out additional abnormalities Serial ultrasound (every 1–2 wk) for development of hydrops	Sporadic (rare) association with cardiac anomalies, bilateral renal agenesis, renal dysplasia, and other malformations

CCAM, congenital cystic adenomatoid malformation.

postnatal surgical care after delivery at a tertiary center. Conversely, fetuses with early herniation, severe mediastinal shift, and dilated intrathoracic stomach (gastric outlet obstruction produces polyhydramnios and gastric dilation) have a poor outlook. Fetuses without liver herniation may be repaired in utero using the two-step technique. However, fetuses with herniated liver have never been successfully repaired in utero despite extensive efforts using a variety of techniques. Indeed, it took many years to recognize the significance of liver herniation and to be able to reliable predict it sonographically. For fetuses deemed unfixable by virtue of liver herniation, we have developed experimentally and now tested clinically a new approach to improving fetal lung development. We have shown in lamb fetuses that impeding the normal egress of fetal lung fluid by controlled tracheal obstruction enlarges the hypoplastic lungs and pushes the viscera back into the abdomen.[41-43] Initial experience with this new procedure, which we call "plug the lung until it grows" (PLUG), suggests that temporary occlusion of the fetal trachea accelerates fetal lung growth and ameliorates the often fatal pulmonary hypoplasia associated with severe CDH. Techniques for achieving a reversible and controlled temporary tracheal occlusion are still evolving. Recently, a technique for applying a metal clip to the trachea using fetoscopic rather than open fetal surgery has been developed and successfully applied in human fetuses.

Table 5–10 summarizes the many factors that must be considered in evaluating a fetus with CDH.

Sacrococcygeal Teratoma

Most neonates with sacrococcygeal teratoma (SCT) survive and malignant invasion is unusual. However, the outcome for SCT diagnosed prenatally (by sonogram or elevated α-fetoprotein) is less favorable. A subset of fetuses (<20%) with large tumors develop hydrops from high output failure secondary to extremely high blood flow through the tumor. Because hydrops progresses very rapidly to fetal demise, frequent sonographic follow-up is mandatory. Excision of the tumor reverses the pathophysiology and has been successful. Since interruption of the blood flow to the tumor will reverse the pathophysiologic failure, many attempts have been made to embolize or obstruct the tumor vessels by sonographically guided or fetoscopic techniques. We have successfully treated fetal SCT by sonographically guided radiofrequency ablation of the twin stalk.[44]

Table 5–11 summarizes the many factors that must be considered in evaluating a fetus with SCT.

Twin–Twin Transfusion Syndrome

In some twin pregnancies, abnormal chorionic blood vessels in the placenta connect the circulation of the two fetuses. These placental abnormalities are associated with perinatal mortality as high as 75% for twin–twin transfusion syndrome (anatomically normal twins) and for acardiac–acephalus twin syndrome. Serial amniocenteses of the polyhydramniotic sac has proven effective in stabilizing the pathophysiologic imbalance in many cases. Interrupting the abnormal placental vascular connections may improve outcome in severe cases. This has been accomplished by occluding the umbilical circulation percutaneously, by dividing the abnormal placental vessels endoscopically, and by removing the abnormal fetus by hysterotomy.[45, 46] All of these techniques have proven successful in small series, and the optimal approach has not yet been determined.

Heart Block

Most fetuses with structurally normal hearts who develop complete heart block associated with maternal collagen-vascular disease will survive without intervention. A few with very slow rates (<50 bpm) may develop hydrops and die in utero. If low output failure cannot be reversed by increasing the heart rate with β-agonists or by treatment with steroids, a pacemaker can be placed by open or percutaneous techniques. This has proven effective experimentally, but has only been attempted a few times.[47]

TABLE 5–10. EVALUATION OF THE FETUS WITH CDH

ULTRASOUND FINDINGS	FAVORABLE PROGNOSTIC INDICATORS	UNFAVORABLE PROGNOSTIC INDICATORS	PRENATAL WORK-UP	ASSOCIATED ANOMALIES
Bowel in the thorax Liver in the thorax (umbilical and portal vessels above level of the diaphragm) Mediastinal shift Polyhydramnios	Liver down Lung-to-head ratio >1.4 No polyhydramnios Appropriate abdominal circumference Gestational age at diagnosis >25 wk Stomach positioned anterior in thorax (i.e., no liver herniation) or in the abdomen	Liver up Lung-to-head ratio <1.0 Polyhydramnios (appears late) Abdominal circumference <5th percentile Gestational age at diagnosis <25 wk Stomach positioned posterior (i.e., liver up anterior)	Fetal karyotype Fetal echocardiography Level II sonogram to detect additional abnormalities	Chromosomal abnormalities (3.6–9%), usually trisomies 18 and 21 Cardiac anomalies: 23% Urinary anomalies: 15% CNS anomalies: 10% Musculoskeletal: 9% Genital anomalies: 8% GI anomalies: 7% Associated with syndromes: Fryn, Cornelia de Lange, and multiple pterygium syndrome

CDH, congenital diaphragmatic hernia; CNS, central nervous system; GI, gastrointestinal.

TABLE 5–11. EVALUATION OF THE FETUS WITH SACROCOCCYGEAL TERATOMA

ULTRASOUND FINDINGS	FAVORABLE PROGNOSTIC INDICATORS	UNFAVORABLE PROGNOSTIC INDICATORS	PRENATAL WORK-UP	ASSOCIATED ANOMALIES
Caudal or intra-abdominal mass (cystic/solid), calcifications Color flow Doppler may demonstrate high vascularity and solid tumor	Predominantly cystic and external lesion No hydrops No polyhydramnios Late (>30 wk) diagnosis	Placentomegaly Hydrops Polyhydramnios or oligohydramnios Rapid growth Large solid and vascular Large internal component	Serial ultrasound every 1–2 wk to assess growth and development of hydrops Fetal echocardiography to assess cardiac output Level II sonogram to detect additional abnormalities	Anorectal stenosis Sacrococcygeal defects (e.g., myelomeningocele) Polyhydramnios or oligohydramnios rapid growth Urinary tract obstruction Miscellaneous anomalies (no specific pattern: 5–25%)

Aqueductal Stenosis

Obstruction to the flow of cerebrospinal fluid (CSF) dilates the ventricles, compresses the developing brain, and eventually compromises neurologic function. For severe cases with progression in utero, decompressing the ventricles may ameliorate the adverse effects on the developing brain. However, percutaneously placed ventriculoamniotic shunts have not improved outcome,[25] and a moratorium is being observed until the natural history is clarified and selection criteria and better fetal shunting techniques are developed.[48]

Pulmonary/Aortic Obstruction

A few simple structural cardiac defects that interfere with development may benefit from prenatal correction. For example, if obstruction to blood flow across the pulmonary or aortic valve interferes with development of the ventricles or the pulmonary or systemic vasculature, relief of the anatomic obstruction may allow normal development with improved outcome. While this pathophysiology remains to be proven experimentally, stenotic heart valves have been dilated by a balloon catheter placed percutaneously,[49] and several centers are developing experimental techniques to correct fetal heart defects.[50]

Tracheal Atresia/Stenosis

Fetuses with congenital high airway obstruction syndrome (CHAOS) have large echogenic lungs due to overdistention by lung fluid. Fetal tracheostomy may prevent development of fetal hydrops.[51]

At delivery, fetuses with an intrinsic or extrinsic obstruction can have the airway repaired and secured while the fetus remains on placental support before dividing the cord. We developed this EXIT procedure to deliver fetuses with CDH who had their trachea plugged, and have applied it successfully to fetuses with large neck tumors.

Nonlethal Defects That May Benefit From Fetal Correction

Myelomeningocele

Myelomeningocele is becoming less common because it can be detected early in gestation by α-fetoprotein screening or sonography, and may be prevented by vitamin supplementation. Although it has been assumed that the spinal cord is intrinsically defective, recent studies suggest that neurologic impairment after birth may be due to exposure of the spinal cord in utero. We have shown in fetal lambs that exposure of the spinal cord causes neurologic damage that can be prevented or ameliorated by repairing the anatomic defect in utero.[52, 53] Although techniques have been developed to repair the lesions by both open and fetoscopic techniques, and both have been tried clinically, it is not yet clear whether repair improves outcome. The natural history of myelomeningocele in human fetuses, particularly when in gestation the lower extremity neurologic damage occurs, has not been resolved. Another unresolved question is the role of Chiari malformation and the hydrocephalus usually seen after birth. Understanding the developmental pathophysiology is crucial to developing appropriate and effective techniques.

Craniofacial Defects, Cleft Lip and Palate

The observation that fetal wounds heal without scar formation has stimulated interest in the possibility of correcting cleft lip and palate in utero in order to avoid scarring, midfacial growth restriction, and secondary nasal deformity. However, the theoretical benefits of repair are unproven and do not yet justify the risks of intervention.[54]

Inherited Defects Correctable by Fetal Stem Cell Transplantation

A variety of inherited defects potentially curable by hematopoietic stem cell (HSC) transplantation are now detectable early in gestation (e.g., immunodeficiencies, hemoglobinopathies, storage diseases). However, postnatal bone marrow transplantation is limited by donor availability, graft rejection, graft-versus-host disease (GVHD), and patient deterioration prior to transplant, which often starts in utero. Transplantation of fetal hematopoietic stem cells early in gestation may circumvent all these difficulties.

The rationale for in utero rather than postnatal transplantation is summarized in Table 5–3. The preimmune fetus (<15 weeks) will not reject the transplanted cells, and the fetal bone marrow is primed to receive HSCs migrating from the fetal liver. Thus, myeloablation and immunosuppression are not necessary. In addition, in utero transplantation allows treatment before the fetus has been damaged by the underlying disease. The disadvantage of treatment in utero is that the fetus is difficult to access for both diagnosis and treatment. Definitive diagnosis using molecular genetic techniques requires fetal tissue obtained by transvaginal or transabdominal chorionic villus sampling, amniocentesis, or fetal blood sampling. Delivering even a small volume (<1 mL) of cells to an early-gestation fetus by intra-abdominal or intravenous injection requires skill and carries significant risks. The greatest potential problem with in utero transplantation is that the degree of engraftment or chimerism may not be sufficient to cure or palliate some diseases. In diseases like chronic granulomatous disease and severe combined immunodeficiency, a relatively small number of normal donor cells can provide sufficient enzyme activity to alleviate symptoms. However, a significantly higher degree of donor cell engraftment and expression in the periphery might be necessary to change the course of diseases like β-thalassemia or sickle cell disease. For diseases that require a high percentage of donor cells, a promising strategy is to induce tolerance in utero for subsequent postnatal booster injections from a living relative. At the present time, this experimental fetal intervention should be offered only to families who have already chosen to carry the pregnancy and raise the affected child.

The optimal source of donor HSCs for in utero transplantation is not known. Donor HSCs can be obtained from adult bone marrow or peripheral blood, from neonatal umbilical cord blood, and from the liver of aborted fetuses.[55] Table 5–12 summarizes the advantages and disadvantages of different sources of donor cells for fetal transplantation. A major advantage of using a postnatal source of stem cells is that living-related transplantation is possible from the same donor both before and after birth. Repeated booster doses may be particularly important for diseases that require a high degree of engraftment. The obvious disadvantage is that unfractionated cells will cause T-cell–mediated GVHD. T cells can be depleted from the graft by a variety of techniques, but this decreases the efficiency of engraftment. It is presently unclear whether highly purified HSCs will engraft without producing GVHD.

The major advantage of using HSCs obtained from the liver of aborted fetuses is that preimmune (<15 weeks) HSCs do not cause GVHD, so T-cell depletion or purification is not necessary. In addition, unfractionated fetal liver provides stroma and "facilitating" cells, so fetal liver HSCs appear to proliferate and possibly expand more readily both in vivo and in vitro. Fetal liver stem cells also have a homing advantage, as they are primed to travel to the waiting fetal marrow. Finally, because these more primitive embryonic HSCs are programmed to provide a lifetime of self-renewal, they may provide more durable stem cell function. We have transplanted fetal HSCs into early-gestation fetal sheep[56] and monkeys[57] and demonstrated long-lasting hematopoietic chimerism of all cell lines without rejection, GVHD, or the need for marrow ablation or immunosuppression. Indeed, this strategy of in utero fetal stem cell transplantation is powerful enough to allow successful transplantation across species barriers.[58] Major disadvantages of using fetal liver HSCs include the difficulty of separating use of fetal tissue from the issue of abortion, the problem of bacterial and viral contamination, and the small number of cells in a fetal liver. All of these problems have proven surmountable.

Clinical experience with fetal HSC transplantation is limited due in part to restrictions in funding for fetal tissue research. In the few cases attempted, low levels

TABLE 5–12. HSC TRANSPLANTATION FOR GENETIC DISEASE

	ADVANTAGES	DISADVANTAGES
Age of Recipient		
Preimmune fetus (<15 wk)	No rejection of graft Marrow empty and primed to receive HSC, from liver No ablation/immunosuppression Treatment before disease causes irreversible damage	Risks of fetal Dx & Rx Partial engraftment (chimerism) may not "cure" disease
Immunocompetent Neonate (up to adult)	Complete replacement of marrow likely to cure disease	Rejection of donor HSCs Requires marrow ablation/immunosuppression Requires marrow ablation to "make room" for donor HSCs, damage from disease that occurs before treatment
Source of Donor HSC		
Preimmune fetal liver (<15 wk)	No GVHD T-cell depletion not necessary Increased proliferative capacity Increased homing capacity Increased durability (?)	Abortion issues Contamination (bacterial/viral) Number of cells limited
Adult marrow/blood	Living related transplant possible	GVHD varies as T cells; therefore, T-cell depletion necessary
Neonatal cord blood	Repeat transplant from same donor possible Large number of cells	T-cell depletion hinders engraftment

Dx, diagnosis; Rx, treatment; HSCs, hematopoietic stem cells; GVHD, graft-versus-host disease.

of engraftment after injection have limited clinical efficacy.[59] However, several centers in the United States and Europe are embarking on in utero HSC transplantation programs. After a decade of preparation in experimental animal models, we have opened a trial in which fetuses less than 15 weeks' gestation with chronic granulomatous diseases and severe combined immunodeficiencies (SCIDs) will receive HSCs obtained from fetal liver or prepared from parents' marrow. Fetuses with β-thalassemia and selected storage diseases will be studied subsequently.

Pitfalls in Selection

There are two major problems in selecting a fetus for treatment. The first problem involves making an accurate diagnosis not only of the lesion type but also of its severity. This aspect of selection, assessing severity, is discussed for each lesion in the appropriate chapter. The second problem in selecting a fetus for treatment is more difficult: the possibility of another unrecognized defect.

Therapeutic decisions require a thorough evaluation of the fetus beyond an accurate anatomic definition of the malformation being considered for therapy. Because it is known that malformations often occur as part of a syndrome, a search for associated abnormalities is necessary to avoid delivering a neonate with one corrected anomaly but other unrecognized disabling or lethal abnormalities. Real-time sonographic evaluation may yield important information on fetal breathing, fetal movements, and fetal vital functions. Amniocentesis allows culture of amniotic fluid cells for detection of chromosomal defects and inherited metabolic abnormalities, evaluation of fetal pulmonary maturity from lecithin-sphingomyelin analysis, and detection and quantitation of fetal hemolysis. Chorionic villus sampling allows first-trimester diagnosis of many of the same genetic diseases. Fetal tissue sampling, including fetal liver biopsy, fetal skin biopsy, and most important, fetal blood sampling, allows rapid karyotyping, and diagnosis of hemoglobinopathies and other hematologic diseases. Occasionally, imaging modalities other than sonography provide valuable information and include radiography, computed tomography, and magnetic resonance imaging. Amniography, another form of augmented imaging, affords further definition of fetal anatomy, including the fetal GI tract, but is invasive. Finally, fluid collections in the fetus (including blood, urine, ascites, CSF) can be aspirated under real-time sonographic guidance for both diagnosis and therapy. The technique, in our experience, has proved to be safe and relatively simple. Despite these increasingly accurate diagnostic aids, it is still quite possible that a subtle but disabling malformation might be missed, making the decision to treat inappropriate. This possibility should be a deterrent to overenthusiastic intervention.

Assessing Risk and Benefit

Fetal therapy raises complex ethical and legal issues that are discussed in their respective chapters. From the responsible physician's point of view, the principal problem is defining the benefits and risks of fetal diagnosis and treatment (Fig. 5–4). For the fetus, the risk of the procedure is weighed against the possibility of correction or amelioration of the malformation. The benefit to be derived from correction depends on the severity of the malformation and its predictable consequences on survival and quality of life (i.e., on the natural history of the disease). Assessing the risks and benefits for the mother is more difficult. Most fetal malformations do not directly threaten the mother's health; however, she must bear some risk and discomfort from the procedure. She may choose to accept the risk to aid her unborn fetus and to increase the fetus' prospects for a normal life and to alleviate her own burden in carrying and preparing to raise a child with a severe malformation. For example, a mother carrying a fetus with urethral obstruction and severe bilateral hydronephrosis must weigh the risk of correction against not only the risk of neonatal death or severe disability from renal or pulmonary failure, but also the emotional and financial burden of prolonged, arduous, expensive, and sometimes unrewarding treatment of chronic renal failure. The lifelong emotional and financial burden of any given malformation on the person and his or her family should be weighed against the risk of fetal intervention undertaken to ameliorate this burden.

Maternal Risk in Open Fetal Surgery

The risks involved in fetal diagnosis and treatment are generally greater for the fetus and for the mother and vary greatly according to the magnitude and invasiveness of the procedure. Sonography carries no known risk. Amniography poses the slight risk of low-dose radiation exposure. Puncture of the amniotic cavity poses a small risk of fetal injury or loss (estimated to be approximately 0.5%).[5] Chorionic villus sampling has a small risk of spontaneous abortion, which is estimated

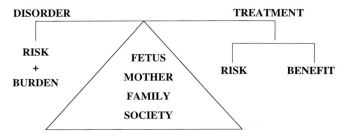

MANAGEMENT OF FETAL DISORDERS

ASSESSING RISK

FIGURE 5–4. In counseling and management, the risk and burden of the untreated disorder on the individual and his or her family is compared with the possible benefit of treatment. The risk of the treatment itself may not be known when a procedure is new. It includes not only the possibility of injury to the fetus and mother, but also the possibility that a fatal lesion will be "corrected" to a nonfatal, but disabling one.

to be 1 to 2%.[6] With appropriate equipment and expertise, sonographically guided aspiration of fetal blood, ascites, pleural fluid, urine, and CSF can be performed with a low risk of fetal loss, probably 1 to 2%. This risk to the fetus and the mother of more extensive therapeutic manipulation (e.g., intravascular intrauterine transfusion or placement of shunt catheters) is significant, although the magnitude of the risk is not yet known. Percutaneous sonographically guided procedures to relieve urinary tract obstruction and hydrocephalus had very significant morbidity in the early experience reported to the Fetal Surgery Registry,[60] but complications have decreased as experience increased and techniques improved.[61]

The risk of hysterotomy and open fetal surgery is unknown but formidable. Initial experience in the 1960s with direct surgical exposure of the fetus to catheterize fetal vessels for exchange transfusion must have been discouraging, because the procedure was quickly abandoned.[62, 63] Recently, newer surgical techniques and im-

proved anesthetic and tocolytic therapy have proved to be effective in the nonhuman primate.[64–66] This experimental work has made possible surgical exposure of fetuses for attempted surgical correction of various anatomic defects. The techniques developed for open fetal surgery are summarized in Figure 5–5.

Because open fetal surgery has only recently been attempted elsewhere, the 50 cases done at the UCSF Fetal Treatment Center through 1994 (Table 5–13) provide the best data on maternal outcome. There have been no maternal deaths and few postoperative maternal complications, but there has been considerable morbidity, primarily related to preterm labor and its treatment.[67, 68] There were no infections. Six patients required blood transfusions. In our early experience, two patients developed amniotic fluid leaks through the hysterotomy site requiring repair, and five patients developed amniotic fluid leaks from the vagina. All patients experienced labor after hysterotomy, and treatment of preterm labor accounted for most of the morbidity. Four patients de-

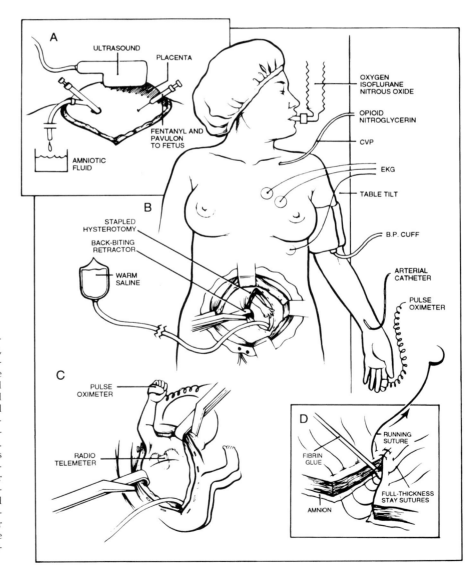

FIGURE 5–5. Summary of fetal surgery techniques. *A,* The uterus is exposed through a low, transverse abdominal incision. Ultrasonography is used to localize the placenta, inject the fetus with narcotic and muscle relaxant, and aspirate amniotic fluid. *B,* The uterus is opened with staples that provide hemostasis and seal the membranes. Warm saline solution is continuously infused around the fetus. Maternal anesthesia, tocolysis, and monitoring are shown. *C,* Absorbable staples and back-biting clamps facilitate hysterotomy exposure of the pertinent fetal part. A miniaturized pulse oximeter records pulse rate and oxygen saturation intraoperatively. A radiotelemeter monitors fetal electrocardiogram and amniotic pressure during and after operation. *D,* After fetal repair the uterine incision is closed with absorbable sutures and fibrin glue. Amniotic fluid is restored with warm lactated Ringer's solution.

T A B L E 5–13. MATERNAL OUTCOME WITH OPEN FETAL SURGERY*

VARIABLE	MEDIAN	RANGE
Maternal age, yr	26	18–43
Gestational age of fetus, wk	25.0	17–28
Operative time, total, min	127.4	69–182
Operative time, fetal repair, min	34	10–92
Blood loss, mL	455	150–1,400
Interval to delivery, wk	4.0	1–15
Gestational age at delivery, wk	28.0	22–36
Subsequent pregnancy history, No.		
Term cesarean delivery, healthy	24†	
Currently pregnant	1	
History of infertility	9	
Not attempted—not desired, too early, etc.	18	

* University of California at San Francisco, Fetal Treatment Center, 50 cases through 1994.
† Two women had two subsequent pregnancies each.

veloped pulmonary edema while receiving high doses of tocolytic drugs. Although reversible, this frightening complication emphasized the need for close monitoring in an intensive care setting.[69, 70] Since the midgestation hysterotomy is not in the lower uterine segment, delivery after fetal surgery and all future deliveries should be by cesarean section. In our series, two uterine disruptions occurred in subsequent pregnancies; uterine closure and neonatal outcome were excellent in both cases. Finally, the ability to carry and deliver subsequent pregnancies does not appear to be jeopardized by fetal surgery; 30 patients have had normal children in subsequent pregnancies.

The risk of fetoscopic or more extensive fetal interventional endoscopic (FETENDO) procedures is unknown, but should be less than hysterotomy and open fetal surgery. This is certainly our experience with the temporary tracheal occlusion procedure, which was first performed by open fetal surgery and then by FETENDO. The morbidity of the procedure, particularly preterm labor, was much less with fetoscopic surgery than with open surgery.

The Future of Fetal Treatment

The pathophysiologic arguments for fetal intervention are compelling, but great care must be exercised in undertaking any new fetal manipulation. Extensive experience with fetal surgery in laboratory animals may not be readily translatable to humans. Survival after fetal surgery is easy to achieve in sheep but is much more hazardous in primates, where premature labor is often difficult to control. Repair of human fetal malformations should not be undertaken until competence and a high degree of success are achieved in a primate model. Recent advances in anesthetic and surgical techniques and pharmacologic control of labor may soon make these repairs feasible.

Because the more invasive diagnostic and therapeutic procedures involve significant risks, a great deal of clinical and laboratory experience is required to establish which procedures are safe and feasible. Until then, we should all maintain a healthy skepticism of fetal treatment. Because a procedure can be done does not mean that it should be done. At this early stage, fetal intervention should be pursued only in centers committed to research and development as well as (and prior to) responsible clinical application. At the present, the minimum requirements for fetal intervention include the cooperative efforts of an obstetrician experienced in prenatal intervention, a sonographer experienced and skilled in fetal diagnosis, a surgeon experienced in operating on tiny preterm infants and in performing fetal procedures in the laboratory, a perinatologist working in a high-risk obstetric unit associated with a tertiary intensive care nursery, a geneticist experienced in syndromology and counseling, a reasonable and compassionate bioethicist, and uninvolved professional colleagues who will monitor such innovative therapy (i.e., a committee on human research). Because there is considerable potential for doing harm, a fetal abnormality of any type should never be treated simply "because it is there" and never by someone who is unprepared for this great responsibility. The responsibility of those undertaking fetal therapy includes an obligation to report all results to the medical profession, whether good or bad, so that the merits and liabilities of fetal treatment can be established as soon as possible.[71]

Our ability to diagnose fetal birth defects has achieved considerable sophistication. Treatment of several fetal disorders has proved to be feasible, and treatment of more complicated lesions will undoubtedly expand as techniques for fetal intervention improve.

R E F E R E N C E S

1. Harrison MR, Golbus MS, Filly RA: Management of the fetus with a correctable congenital defect. JAMA 246:774–777, 1981.
2. Harrison MR: Unborn: Historical perspective of the fetus as a patient. The Pharos 45(1):19–24, 1982.
3. Hobbins JC, Grannum PAT, Berkowitz RL, et al: Ultrasound in the diagnosis of congenital anomalies. Am J Obstet Gynecol 134:331, 1979.
4. Touloukian RJ, Hobbins JC: Maternal ultrasonography in the antenatal diagnosis of surgically correctable fetal abnormalities. J Pediatr Surg 15:373, 1980.
5. Golbus MS, Loughman WD, Epstein CJ, et al: Prenatal genetic diagnosis in 3,000 amniocenteses. N Engl J Med 300:157, 1979.
6. Hogge WA, Schonberg SA, Golbus MS: Chorionic villus sampling: Experience of the first 1000 cases. Am J Obstet Gynecol 154:1249, 1986.
7. Harrison MR, Filly RA, Parer JT, et al: Management of the fetus with a urinary tract malformation. JAMA 246:635–639, 1981.
8. Harrison MR, Golbus MS, Filly RA, et al: Management of the fetus with congenital hydronephrosis. J Pediatr Surg 17:728–742, 1982.
9. Glick PL, Harrison MR, Nakayama DK, et al: Management of the fetus with ventriculomegaly. J Pediatr Surg 105:97–105, 1984.
10. Bond SJ, Harrison MR, Fily RA, et al: Severity of intestinal damage in gastroschisis: Correlation with prenatal sonographic findings. J Pediatr Surg 23(6):520–525, 1988.
11. Queenan JT: Intrauterine transfusion—a comparative study. Am J Obstet Gynecol 104:397, 1969.
12. Grannum PA, Copel JA, Plaxe SC, et al: In utero exchange transfusion by direct intravascular injection in severe erythroblastosis fetalis. N Engl J Med 314:1431, 1986.

13. Ampola MG, Mahoney MJ, Nakamura E, et al: Prenatal therapy of a patient with vitamin B_{12}-responsive methylmalonic acidemia. N Engl J Med 293:313, 1975.
14. Packman S, Cowan MJ, Golbus MS, et al: Prenatal treatment of biotin-responsive multiple carboxylase deficiency. Lancet 1:1435, 1982.
15. Kleinman CS, Donnerstein RL, Jaffe CC, et al: Fetal echocardiography: A tool for evaluation of in utero cardiac arrhythmias and monitoring of in utero therapy: Analysis of 71 patients. Am J Cardiol 51:237, 1983.
16. Devore GR, Brar HS, Platt LD: Doppler ultrasound in the fetus: A review of current applications. J Clin Ultrasound 15:687, 1987.
17. Masiach S, Barkai G, Sack J, et al: The effect of intraamniotic thyroxine administration on fetal lung maturity in man. J Perinat Med 7:161, 1979.
18. Weiner S, Scharf JI, Bolognese RJ, et al: Antenatal diagnosis and treatment of fetal goiter. J Reprod Med 24:39, 1980.
19. Evans MI, Chrousos GP, Mann DL, et al: Pharmacologic suppression of the fetal adrenal gland: Attempted prevention of 21 hydroxylase sufficiency congenital adrenal hypoplasia in utero. JAMA 253:1015, 1985.
20. Harrison MR, Villa R: Transamniotic fetal feeding I. Development of an animal model: Continuous amniotic infusion in rabbits. J Pediatr Surg 17:376–380, 1982.
21. Kantoff PW, Flake AW, Eglitis MA, et al: In utero gene transfer and expression: A sheep transplantation model. Blood 73:1066, 1989.
22. Adzick NS, Harrison MR, Flake AW, Glick PL: Fetal urinary tract obstruction: Experimental pathophysiology. Semin Perinatol 9:79–80, 1985.
23. Nicolaides KH, Cheng HH, Snijders RJM, Moniz CF: Fetal urine biochemistry in the assessment of obstructive uropathy. Am J Obstet Gynecol 166:932–937, 1992.
24. Johnson MP, Bukowski TP, Reitleman C, et al: In utero surgical treatment of fetal obstructive uropathy: A new comprehensive approach to identify appropriate candidates for vesicoamniotic shunt therapy. Am J Obstet Gynecol 170:1770–1779, 1994.
25. Manning FA, Harrison MR, Rodeck CH, et al: Special report: Catheter shunts for fetal hydronephrosis and hydrocephalus. N Engl J Med 315:336–340, 1986.
26. Crombleholme TM, Harrison MR, Langer JC, et al: Early experience with open fetal surgery for congenital hydronephrosis. J Pediatr Surg 23:1114–1121, 1988.
27. MacMahan RA, Renou PM, Shekelton PA, Paterson RJ: In utero cystostomy. Lancet 340:1234, 1992.
28. Estes JM, Harrison MR: Fetal obstructive uropathy. Semin Pediatr Surg 2:129–135, 1993.
29. Adzick NS, Harrison MR, Glick PL, et al: Fetal cystic adenomatoid malformation: Prenatal diagnosis and natural history. J Pediatr Surg 20:483–488, 1985.
30. Rice HE, Estes JM, Hedrick MH, et al: Congenital cystic adenomatoid malformation: A sheep model of fetal hydrops. J Pediatr Surg 29:692–696, 1994.
31. Adzick NS, Hu LM, Davies P, et al: Compensatory lung growth after pneumonectomy in the fetus. Surg Forum 37:648, 1986.
32. MacGillivray TE, Harrison MR, Goldstein RB, Adzick NS: Disappearing fetal lung lesions. J Pediatr Surg 28:1321–1325, 1993.
33. Harrison MR, Adzick NS, Jennings RW, et al: Antenatal intervention for congenital cystic adenomatoid malformation. Lancet 336:965–967, 1990.
34. Adzick NS, Harrison MR, Flake AW, et al: Fetal surgery for cystic adenomatoid malformation of the lung. J Pediatr Surg 28:806–812, 1993.
35. Blott M, Nicolaides KH, Greenough A: Postnatal respiratory function after chronic drainage of fetal pulmonary cyst. Am J Obstet Gynecol 159:858–859, 1988.
36. Harrison MR, Adzick NS, Estes JM, Howell LJ: A prospective study of the outcome of fetuses with congenital diaphragmatic hernia. JAMA 271:382–384, 1994.
37. Harrison MR, Ross NA, deLorimier AA: Correction of congenital diaphragmatic hernia in utero. III. Development of a successful surgical technique using abdominoplasty to avoid compromise of umbilical blood flow. J Pediatr Surg 16:934–942, 1981.
38. Harrison MR, Langer JC, Adzick NS, et al: Correction of congenital diaphragmatic hernia in utero. V. Initial clinical experience. J Pediatr Surg 25:47–57, 1990.
39. Harrison MR, Adzick NS, Flake AW, et al: Correction of congenital diaphragmatic hernia in utero: VI. Hard-earned lessons. J Pediatr Surg 28:1411–1418, 1993.
40. Harrison MR, Adzick NS, Flake AW, Jennings RW: The CDH two-step: A dance of necessity. J Pediatr Surg 28:813–816, 1993.
41. DiFiore JW, Fauza DO, Slavin D, et al: Experimental fetal tracheal ligation reverses the structural and physiologic effects of pulmonary hypoplasia in congenital diaphragmatic hernia. J Pediatr Surg 29:248–257, 1994.
42. Hedrick MH, Estes JM, Sullivan KM, et al: Plug the lung until it grows (PLUG): A new method to treat congenital diaphragmatic hernia in utero. J Pediatr Surg 29:612–617, 1994.
43. Harrison MR, Adzick NS, Flake AW, et al: Correction of congenital diaphragmatic hernia in utero. VIII: Response of the hypoplastic lung to tracheal occlusion. J Pediatr Surg 31:1339–1348, 1996.
44. Langer JC, Harrison MR, Schmidt KG, et al: Fetal hydrops and death from sacrococcygeal teratoma: Rationale for fetal surgery. Am J Obstet Gynecol 160:1145–1150, 1989.
45. De Lia JE, Cruikshank DP, Keye WR: Fetoscopic neodymium: YAG laser occlusion of placental vessels in severe twin-twin fusion syndrome. Obstet Gynecol 75:1046–1053, 1990.
46. Fries MH, Goldberg JD, Golbus MS: Treatment of acardiac-acephalic twin gestations by hysterotomy and selective delivery. Obstet Gynecol 79:601–604, 1992.
47. Estes JM, Silverman NH, Van Hare GS, et al: In utero placement of an epicardial pacemaker for the treatment of congenital heart block. (Submitted for publication.)
48. Hudgins RJ, Edwards MSB, Goldstein RB, et al: Natural history of fetal ventriculomegaly. Pediatrics 82:692, 1988.
49. Allan LD, Maxwell D, Tynan M: Progressive obstructive lesions of the heart—an opportunity for fetal therapy. Fetal Ther 6:173–177, 1991.
50. Hanley FL: Fetal cardiac surgery. Adv Cardiac Surg 5:47–74, 1994.
51. Martinez-Ferro M, Hedrick MH, Flake AW, et al: Prenatal diagnosis of congenital high airway obstruction (CHAOS): Potential for perinatal intervention. J Pediatr Surg 29:271–274, 1994.
52. Meuli M, Meuli-Simmen C, Yingling CD, et al: A new model of myelomeningocele: Studies in the fetal lamb. J Pediatr Surg 30:1034–1037, 1995.
53. Meuli M, Meuli-Simmen C, Hutchins GM, et al: In utero surgery rescues neurologic function at birth in sheep with spina bifida. Nat Med 1:342–347, 1995.
54. Longaker MT, Whitby DJ, Adzick NS, et al: Fetal surgery for cleft lip: A plea for caution. Plast Reconstr Surg 88:1087–1092, 1991.
55. Flake AW, Harrison MR, Zanjani ED: In utero stem cell transplantation. Exp Hematol 19:1061–1064, 1991.
56. Flake AW, Harrison MR, Adzick NS, Zanjani ED: Transplantation of fetal hematopoietic stem cells in utero: The creation of hematopoietic chimeras. Science 233:776–778, 1986.
57. Harrison MR, Slotnick RN, Crombleholme TM, et al: In-utero transplantation of fetal liver haemopoietic stem cells in monkeys. Lancet 1:1425–1427, 1989.
58. Kosteche RA, Ildstad ST: Chimerism and the facilitating cell. Transplant Rev 9:97–110, 1995.
59. Cowan MJ, Golbus MS: In utero hematopoietic stem cell transplants for inherited diseases. Am J Pediatr Hematol Oncol 16:35–42, 1994.
60. Manning F, Harrison MR, Rodeck C, et al: Report of the International Fetal Surgery Registry: Catheter shunts for fetal hydronephrosis and hydrocephalus. N Engl J Med 315:336, 1986.
61. Crombleholme TM, Harrison MR, Golbus MT, et al: Fetal intervention in obstructive uropathy: Prognostic indicators and efficacy of intervention. Am J Obstet Gynecol 162(5):1239–1244, 1990.
62. Asensio SH: Surgical treatment of erythroblastosis fetalis. In Adamson K (ed): Diagnosis and Treatment of Fetal Disorders. New York: Springer-Verlag, 1969, p 264.
63. Adamson K: Fetal surgery. N Engl J Med 275:204, 1966.
64. Harrison MR, Anderson J, Rosen MA, et al: Fetal surgery in the primate. I. Anesthetic, surgical, and tocolytic management to maximize fetal-neonatal survival. J Pediatr Surg 17:115–122, 1982.
65. Nakayama DK, Harrison MR, Seron-Ferre M, Villa RL: Fetal surgery in the primate. II. Uterine electromyographic response to operative procedures and pharmacologic agents. J Pediatr Surg 19(4):333–339, 1984.

66. Adzick NS, Harrison MR, Glick PL, et al: Fetal surgery in the primate. III. Maternal outcome after fetal surgery. J Pediatr Surg 21(6):481–484, 1986.
67. Harrison MR: Fetal surgery. West J Med 159:341–349, 1993.
68. Longaker MT, Golbus MS, Filly RA, et al: Maternal outcome after open fetal surgery. JAMA 265:737–741, 1991.
69. Bealer JF, Rice HE, Adzick NS, Harrison MR: Acute non-cardiac pulmonary edema complicating nitroglycerin tocolysis following open fetal surgery. (Submitted for publication.)
70. Harrison MR, Vander Wall KJ, Bealer JF, et al: Nitroglycerin suppresses preterm labor after hysterotomy and fetal surgery. (Submitted for publication.)
71. Harrison MR, Filly RA, Golbus MS, et al: Fetal treatment 1982. N Engl J Med 307:1651, 1982.

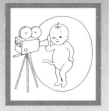

Sonographic Anatomy of the Normal Fetus

ROY A. FILLY

Our understanding of normal fetal anatomy, based on sonograms, continues to be an area of considerable growth. Instrumentation has improved steadily and has yielded both improved and more consistent image quality. Among the most significant advancements for fetal imaging has been the ability to choose the depth of the zone of best focus of the ultrasonic beam. With this capability, the area of anatomy being observed can be inspected consistently with the focused portion of the beam, which is a highly significant advantage.

Further, sonologists have gradually improved their understanding of the anatomy portrayed on in utero sonograms. Unquestionably, clearer images have led the way to our improved understanding, but other factors have been involved. Not the least of these has been the surge in ultrasonic imaging of premature newborns.[1, 2] These tiny newborns are the equivalent of midtrimester fetuses as early, sometimes, as 24 weeks. Visualization of their head and body anatomy in the more ideal ex utero environment, which permits the use of higher frequency transducers, a greater selection of planes of section, and comparison with other imaging modalities, has done much to improve our understanding of fetal anatomy (Figs. 6–1 and 6–2).[1, 2] This newly won information can be extrapolated, to a large extent, to younger fetuses.

The ability of sonography to detect intrafetal structures depends on a balance between spatial resolution and contrast.[3] This balance, however, strongly favors contrast as being the more important aspect of perception. For example, a large white dot on a white wall is difficult or impossible to see, because no contrast differential exists even though the eye can spatially resolve easily a tiny black dot (high contrast) on the same wall. Structures that have high levels of subject contrast can be consistently detected at a smaller size (often equating to an earlier age) than can those displaying poor contrast. Sonologists, unfortunately, do not have agents that can alter contrast of fetal organs and thus are totally dependent on subject contrast (inherent contrast) for visualization of internal fetal morphologic details. Clearly, spatial resolution is also a critical feature in defining morphology, but has not been the limiting factor in demonstrating fetal anatomy.

Other parameters, important in fetal imaging, also cannot be controlled. Ultrasound is a tomographic technique. Appropriate positioning for obtaining the best tomographic plane is always desirable. However, we are unable to control fetal position for this purpose. We also cannot control maternal body habitus or the amount of amniotic fluid, both of which may dramatically alter our ability to discern fetal anatomy. Despite these problems, a large number of fetal structures are consistently visible sonographically.

High-resolution, real-time scanners with their flexible approach to imaging are mandatory for modern fetal sonography.[4–6] In the following sections, various aspects of fetal anatomy are described. An estimate is made of the ability of ultrasound instrumentation to consistently demonstrate the anatomic part under consideration as well as an attempt to estimate when the fetus has attained sufficient size such that the anatomic structure is large enough to be detected. It is important to recall that size and visualization may be relative to any given stage of development. For example, in a small fetus whose urinary bladder is well distended, identification of the bladder is relatively easy. Alternatively, identification of the bladder is difficult or impossible in a term fetus who has recently voided. The urine, in this case, provides the ''contrast'' that usually makes the urinary bladder an easy structure to perceive. If this ''contrast agent'' drains away, the size of the fetus (and thus its bladder) will not rescue one from the loss of contrast. Another important concept is that the human eye sees best in the ''relative'' rather than the ''absolute'' sense of size. Thus, in a young fetus, the cerebral ventricle is seen more readily than that in an older fetus because the relative size of the ventricle, compared with overall size of the brain, is large early (even though the absolute size is larger later).

If the sonographer begins with a specific intent to image a particular fetal part, it is frequently possible to succeed.[3, 7] To accomplish this end, the sonographer must (1) assess the precise fetal position; (2) consider whether the anatomic part of interest is best visualized

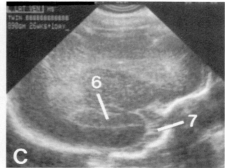
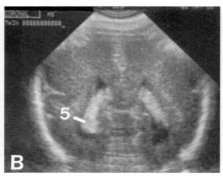
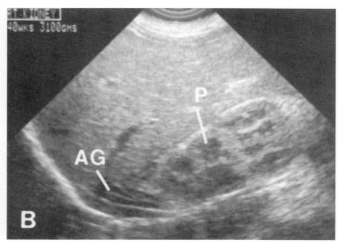

FIGURE 6–1. Neonatal head sonogram. Coronal (*A*), axial (*B*), and parasagittal (*C*) images enable correlation with fetal examinations. (1 = lateral ventricular body; 2 = temporal horn; 3 = ambient cistern; 4 = choroidal fissure; 5 = glomus of choroid plexus; 6 = temporal lobe; 7 = cistern with linear bridging veins.)

in planes perpendicular to the fetal long axis or parallel to the fetal long axis; and (3) adjust time gain compensation (TGC) and transducer angulation to visualize the area to best advantage. Obviously, such rules are the same throughout all of sonography. The challenge of imaging intrafetal structures is to apply these rules when the fetal position is changing such that the current scanning plane is no longer applicable for the part that one wishes to visualize.

The flexibility offered by real-time sonographic systems enables one to quickly survey the fetus to determine its precise position. Second, the sonographic tomograms, which are rapidly generated (virtually "real-time" imaging), enable one to view a large volume of the fetus with closely spaced sections. Such a rapid look at many contiguous tomograms eliminates one of the basic flaws of tomographic imaging of a moving target. Finally, fetal movements are viewed directly, which enables one to quickly reorient the transducer to the optimal plane of section to image the structure of interest.

Fetal parts of interest to the sonologist fall into three major categories of subject contrast that subsequently, then, determine the relative ease with which the structure is sonographically visible. These categories are (1) structures that generate high-amplitude reflections (e.g., ossified bones), (2) structures that generate no internal echoes (e.g., fluid-containing viscera), and (3) those that generate midrange gray echoes (e.g., the parenchymal organs—lungs, brain, spleen, liver, kidneys, and muscles). The categories are listed in terms of being most visible to being least visible. Within the last category one may anticipate seeing a spectrum of gray shades that will enable a distinction to be made between several parenchymal organs and intraorgan components. For example, the medullary portions of the fetal renal parenchyma generate lower amplitude internal echoes than do the surrounding cortical tissues and septa of Bertin, thus enabling recognition of this separate component of renal tissue (Fig. 6–3).[8]

A feature of critical importance for organ imaging is the fetal position. Clearly, a prone fetus is in an optimal position for imaging the kidneys, which are usually difficult to perceive, but is in a poor position to demonstrate the urinary bladder, which is usually easy to image.

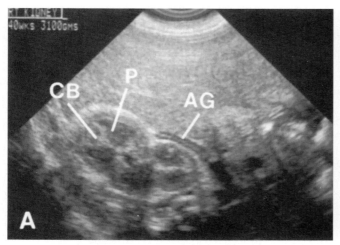
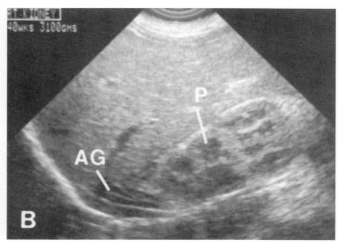

FIGURE 6–2. Neonatal abdominal sonogram: (*A*) transverse; (*B*) parasagittal. (AG = adrenal gland, both cortex [thicker] and medulla [thinner]; CB = Bertin column; P = medullary pyramid of the kidney.)

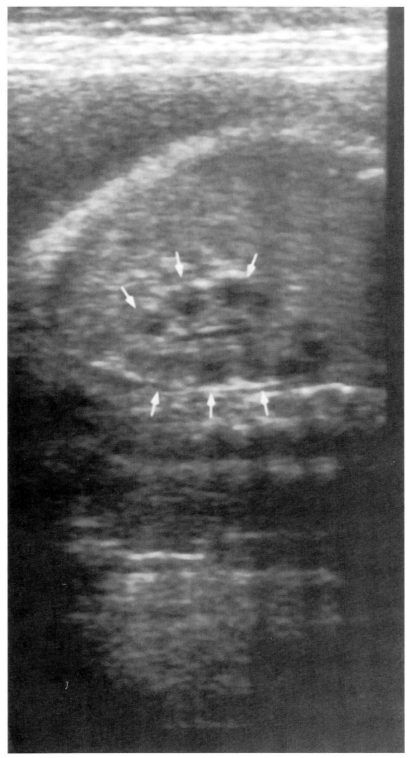

F I G U R E 6–3. Sonogram of a fetal kidney (*arrows*). The medullary pyramids are distinguished from surrounding cortical tissues and septa of Bertin. Bright echos surrounding the kidney represent perirenal fat.

Determination of fetal position should be accomplished in all obstetric sonographic examinations from the second trimester onward. The fetal position should be determined as precisely as possible before an interpretation of fetal anatomy is begun, because the position of a structure often influences our interpretation. The general fetal orientation is first assessed; that is, cephalic, breech, oblique, or transverse. Once this is determined, the location of the fetal spine is noted. If, for example, the fetal spine is on the maternal left side and the fetus is in a cephalic presentation, one can judge that the fetus is lying on its left side (Fig. 6–4). Conversely, if the fetus is in a breech position, then it must be lying on its right side. The reverse is the case for breech and cephalic fetuses when the fetal spine lies on the maternal right side. In the transverse or oblique fetal positions the same rules apply, but with a different orientation.

Such an analysis of fetal position is vital for proper interpretation of abdominal and thoracic situs and for identification of abnormal fetal structures. For instance, a rounded, fluid-filled structure in the left posterior portion of the upper fetal abdomen may be assumed to represent the fundus of the fetal stomach. However, a structure of identical appearance, but located on the right side of the upper fetal abdomen, must be interpreted as being a pathologic lesion.

It is important to recall that pathologic structures are frequently more visible than are their normal counterparts (i.e., dilated small bowel loops are easier to detect than normal small bowel loops). However, it is even more important to keep in mind that the most difficult pathologic observation is to recognize the "absence" of a structure that ordinarily could be visualized (i.e., a missing portion of an extremity, the inability to see the "stomach" when esophageal atresia without tracheo-esophageal fistula is present).

Superficial Anatomy of the Fetus

Routine sonography for obstetric indications rarely requires a survey of the superficial fetal structure. However, when an anomaly is suspected a careful look at superficial features of the fetus becomes important or even mandatory. Superficial anatomy that is considered in this section includes the face, ears, hair, and external genitalia.

The fetal face can be viewed with considerable clarity. Expectant mothers are often surprised to "see" their fetus so clearly (Figs. 6–5 and 6–6). The brow, cheeks, eyelids (and occasionally even eyelashes), nose, lips, and chin can be seen with consistency. The nose and lips

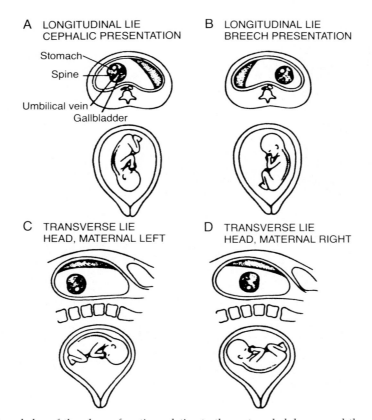

F I G U R E 6–4. Knowledge of the plane of section relative to the maternal abdomen and the position of the fetal head and spine allows one to determine laterality of fetal organs. *A,* The fetus lies on its right side. If, however, the fetal spine were on the maternal left, a cephalic fetus would lie on its left side. The same calculations can be made for images *B, C,* and *D.*

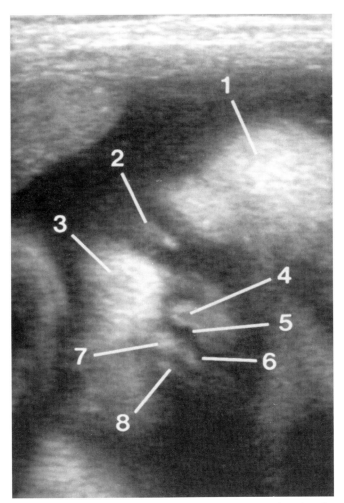

FIGURE 6–5. Sonogram of the fetal face. Despite the fact that this image is a tomogram with relatively little depth, facial features are seen well. (1 = brow; 2 = eyelid; 3 = cheek; 4 = ala of nose; 5 = nostril; 6 = philtrum; 7 = upper lip; 8 = lower lip.) Amniotic fluid surrounding the face provides the "contrast" for visualization.

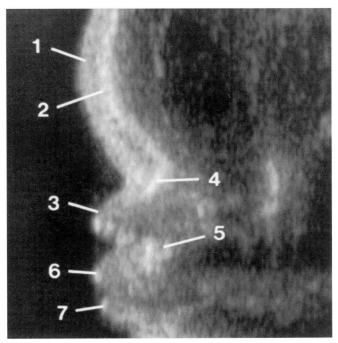

FIGURE 6–6. "Profile" view of the fetal face. Diagnostically, it offers substantially less information than Figure 6–5. (1 = soft tissues of brow; 2 = frontal bone; 3 = soft tissues of nose; 4 = nasal bone; 5 = portion of hard palate; 6 = upper lip; 7 = lower lip.)

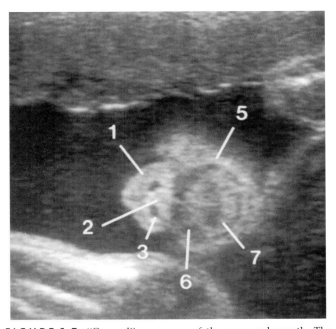

FIGURE 6–7. "Coronal" sonogram of the nose and mouth. The nasal structure is particularly well seen. (1 = ala; 2 = nostril; 3 = column.) The mouth displays less detail, although consistent and characteristic layering of echoes is seen. These layers are (presumably) the subcutaneous (5) and muscular tissue (6), the orbicularis oris muscle, and the mucosal tissue (7).

are the more important features to image in detail (to exclude clefting). The alae, column, and nares can be clearly shown (Figs. 6–7 and 6–8). The upper lip is more important diagnostically than is the lower lip and is fortunately easier to see. Visualization is usually good enough to identify the filtrum. The cheeks are prominent, as expected, and the subcutaneous tissues of the cheek, due to the presence of a large fat pad, are brightly echogenic.

The ears can be visualized quite well, and their progressive maturation is noted.[9] The external auditory canal, helix (and antihelix in older fetuses), lobule, and tragus can be depicted (Fig. 6–9), but the relative position of the ear (i.e., as in "low set" ears) is difficult to judge. The ear may be protuberant and can be mistaken for an abnormality, especially an encephalocele.[10]

Hair on the scalp is readily perceived in late fetuses (that have some). The bright linear echoes protruding from or parallel to the scalp and neck are quite conspicu-

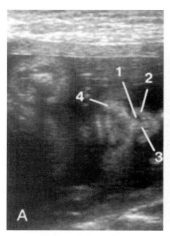 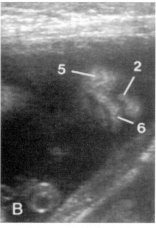

FIGURE 6–8. *A,* True coronal image of the nose and upper lip. (1 = nostril; 2 = column; 3 = ala; 4 = upper lip.) *B,* Inclined coronal image demonstrates a slightly different perspective. (5 = cheek; 6 = philtrum.)

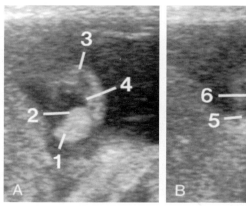

FIGURE 6–9. Fetal ear. (1 = lobule; 2 = antitragus; 3 = helix; 4 = antihelix; 5 = tragus; 6 = fossa triangularis.)

ous. Indeed, the only benefit of recognizing hair is not to mistake long hair for a pathologic process, namely, an encephalocele or cystic hygroma, because longer hair, which is wet and matted by the amniotic fluid, may "trap" some of the fluid between it and the skin of the occiput or neck, creating the false impression of a cystic mass in this location (Fig. 6–10).

The external genitalia can be appreciated from the early second trimester onward. Gender can be quite accurately assigned.[11-13] Ordinarily, this has no clinical consequence. However, gender should always be determined in certain circumstances. These include all living twins where a single placental site is seen, or when monozygotic twinning, other than for reasons of placentation, would be considered to be detrimental to the outcome of pregnancy.[14] All fetuses with suspected lower urinary tract obstruction should have their gender

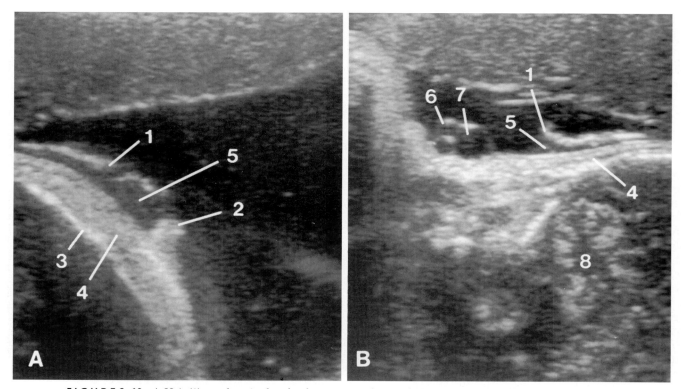

FIGURE 6–10. *A,* Hair (1) may be mistaken for the outer membrane of a cystic mass in an older fetus. (2 = portion of ear; 3 = occipital bone; 4 = subcutaneous tissues and muscles in the occipital region; 5 = "trapped" amniotic fluid.) *B,* Scan at 90 degrees to Figure 6–10A. This image clarifies that the fetus is normal. (6 = umbilical artery; 7 = umbilical vein; 8 = cerebellum.)

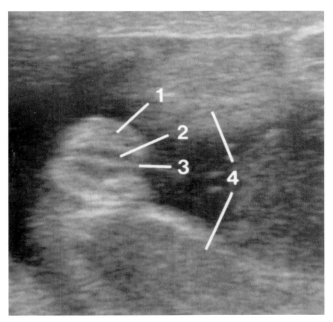

FIGURE 6–11. External female genitalia. (1 = major labium; 2 = minor labium; 3 = vaginal cleft; 4 = thighs.)

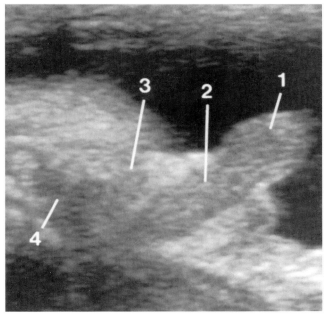

FIGURE 6–12. The penis is seen sonographically. (1 = glans; 2 = shaft; 3 = subcutaneous tissues of the groin; 4 = pubic ramus.)

determined, because the differential diagnosis is different in males and females. Certain other circumstances would require gender determination if karyotyping were refused or impractical to perform. These circumstances would include, but are not limited to, risk for X-linked disorders or when the Turner syndrome is suspected due to a dysmorphic feature (e.g., cystic hygroma).

Female gender should be assigned only by identification of the major and minor labia (Fig. 6–11). Assigning female gender because of an inability to "see" a penis results in many diagnostic errors. Male genitalia are readily seen (Fig. 6–12). The penis and scrotum are most obvious. Testes may be seen in the scrotal sac, sometimes as early as the beginning of the third trimester. Details of the penis, including the glans, urethra, and corpora cavernosa, may be appreciated (Fig. 6–13). Even the foreskin is visible in some cases.

Musculoskeletal System

Real-time ultrasonography provides the most appropriate format for imaging fetal bones. The resolution and flexibility offered by such systems enables one to rapidly survey the fetal skeleton. Of all structures within the fetus, the ossified portions of the skeleton possess the highest level of subject contrast and thus are seen earlier and more consistently than are any other organ system.[4, 15–18] Indeed, sonography surpasses all other imaging modalities in fetal skeletal imaging. Although radiographs of abortuses demonstrate bony morphology more advantageously than would a sonogram,[19, 20] the reverse is true of fetuses in the womb where overlying

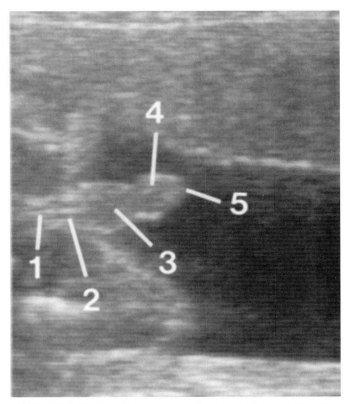

FIGURE 6–13. Details in an erect fetal penis (1 = urethra; 2 = corpus cavernosum; 3 = shaft; 4 = glans; 5 = foreskin.)

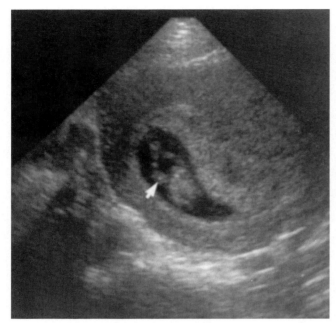

FIGURE 6–14. Sonogram of a 10.5-week embryo demonstrates the tiny (approximately 1 mm) primary ossification center of the femur (*arrow*). (From Mahony BS, Filly RA: High-resolution sonographic assessment of the fetal extremities. J Ultrasound Med 3:489, 1984, Copyright 1984 by the American Institute of Ultrasound in Medicine.)

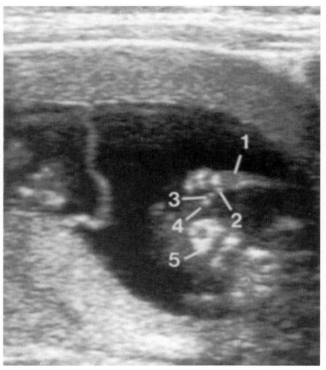

FIGURE 6–15. Sonogram of a 15-week-old fetal hand. (1 = cartilaginous carpal bones seen as a conglomerate; 2 = 1st metacarpal 3 = proximal phalanx of the thumb; 4 = distal phalanx of the thumb; 5 = maxilla.)

maternal soft tissues and bones, fetal movement, and inappropriate fetal position defeat x-ray techniques in visualization of the early fetal skeleton.

Fetal position is extremely important. The posterior elements of the fetal spine may be clearly imaged with the fetus in a prone or decubitus position but are difficult to image when the fetus is supine.[21] Similarly, the extremities are imaged to excellent advantage when floating freely in the amniotic fluid. The same extremity tucked under the fetus will be quite difficult to image.

Despite these potential problems, fetal skeletal structures remain the earliest and most readily recognized. Indeed, the earliest structures seen with consistency are the ossification centers of the maxilla, mandible, and clavicle, the first bones of the human body to ossify.[4] The calvaria can be imaged from the late first trimester onward. The same is true of the long bones of the upper and lower extremities (Fig. 6–14). Visibility of bony detail rapidly increases, and even phalanges can be visualized by 17 to 18 menstrual weeks (sometimes earlier). Bones of only 2 to 3 mm in size can be consistently imaged via sonography if no unusual impediments to the scanning procedure exist (Fig. 6–15). Many specific

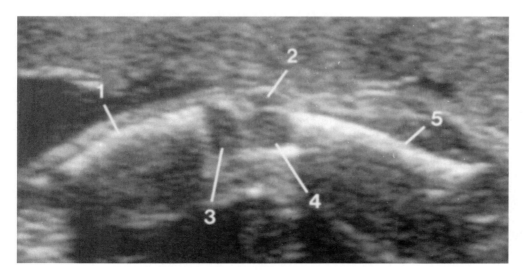

FIGURE 6–16. Midsagittal sonogram through the leg of a fetus with a bone dysplasia (note the bowed tibial diaphysis [1]). The patella (2), which is an entirely cartilaginous bone, is clearly shown. (3 = proximal tibial epiphysis; 4 = distal femoral epiphysis; 5 = femoral diaphysis.)

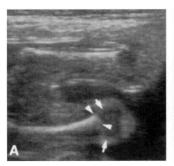 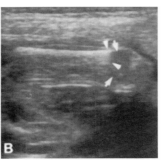

FIGURE 6–17. *A,* Sonogram best demonstrating the femur farther from the transducer. *Arrows* mark the edges of the distal epiphysis. *Arrowheads* mark the apparent "edges" of the distal femoral diaphysis. The more medial edge of the diaphysis matches the edge of the medial condyle, but the lateral edges of "diaphysis" and lateral condyle are widely disparate. *B,* The same exercise can be done on the closer femur. Again *arrows* mark the edges of the distal epiphysis, and *arrowheads* mark the "edges" of the femoral diaphysis. Shadowing, which is caused by the bone and not by the cartilage, causes this deceptive appearance.

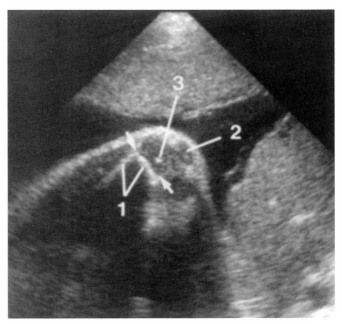

FIGURE 6–18. Sector sonogram of the distal femur taken such that the lines of sight from the transducer intersect the inferior end of the femoral metaphysis at the epiphyseal plate (1). By this maneuver, the full thickness of the distal ossified femur is seen sonographically (compare with Figure 6–17). Now, the thickness of the epiphysis (*arrows*) and ossified femoral shaft match perfectly. (2 = patella; 3 = secondary ossification center of the distal femoral epiphysis.)

bony structures can be depicted. Bones in both the appendicular and axial skeleton are well imaged.

It is important to clarify that sonography has the capacity to visualize not only the ossified portions of the fetal skeleton, but also the cartilaginous portions.[4] Cartilaginous ends of the long bones may be seen by early second trimester. Indeed, bones entirely in cartilage can be seen sonographically (Fig. 6–16). It is equally important to recognize that the full thickness of the ossified diaphysis of long bones is not seen sonographically.[22] This is due to acoustic shadowing. The cartilaginous ends of long bones help us to recognize this aberration. By matching up the width of the epiphysis, the full thickness of which can be seen, with the apparent "width" of the bony diaphysis, it is clear that these are

unequal (Figs. 6–17 and 6–18). This observation helps to correct some perceptual errors that can lead to erroneous diagnoses. For example, the inability to see the full thickness of the femoral diaphysis creates the impression that the fetal femur farther from the transducer is bowed (Fig. 6–19).[22] This error is caused by visualization of

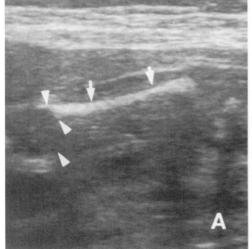 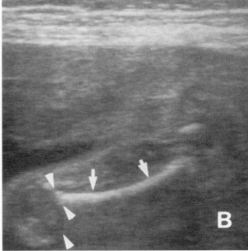

FIGURE 6–19. *A,* The diaphysis of the femur nearer to the transducer appears to be straight (*arrows*). The full thickness of the diaphysis is not seen. (Match the edges of the epiphysis [*arrowheads*] as in Figures 6–17 and 6–18 and to the radiograph in Figure 6–20.) *B,* The diaphysis of the femur farther from the transducer appears to be curved (*arrows*). (Compare with Figure 6–20.) This is a normal shape of this aspect of the bone. However, the curvature is visually compensated by the straight lateral cortex in the radiograph, but not by the sonogram, because the full thickness of bone is not perceived. (Compare again the diaphyseal "thickness" with the epiphyseal thickness.)

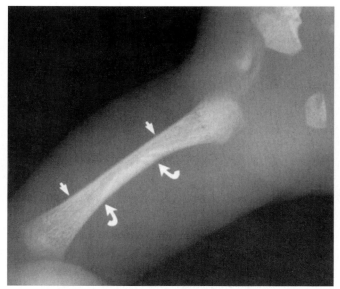

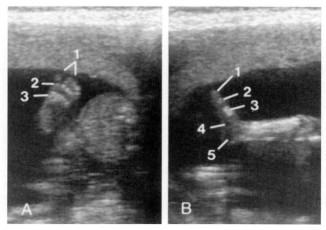

FIGURE 6–21. Fetal foot at 16 weeks in transverse axial (*A*) and parasagittal (*B*) planes. (1 = toes; 2 = proximal phalangeal ossification centers; 3 = metatarsal ossification centers; 4 = tarsal cuboid in cartilage; 5 = tarsal calcaneus in cartilage.)

FIGURE 6–20. Radiograph of a midtrimester fetal femur. Note that the eye compensates for the curvature of the medial diaphyseal cortex (*curved arrows*) by noting the straight lateral diaphyseal cortex (*straight arrows*). (Compare with Figure 6–19.)

only the medial cortex of the femoral diaphysis (which is normally curved) (Fig. 6–20). However, the inability to "visually correct" this normal curvature by simultaneous observation of the "straight" lateral cortex causes the perceptual error.

The majority of the bones of the appendicular skeleton can be seen in early to mid-second trimester, although phalanges may be difficult to perceive in some cases. It is a general rule of appendicular skeletal imaging that the more proximal a bone, the more readily it is identified. This rule in one sense is not true of the hands and feet, where the metacarpals and metatarsals are seen more readily and earlier than are either the carpal or tarsal bones (Fig. 6–21; see also Fig. 6–15), because the metacarpals and metatarsals are well ossified at 4 months, whereas the carpals and tarsals (except for the tarsal calcaneus and talus) remain cartilaginous throughout pregnancy. The tarsal calcaneous and talus ossify between the fifth and sixth months, whereas the remaining tarsals and carpals do not ossify until after birth (Figs. 6–22 and 6–23).

The scapula (Figs. 6–24 and 6–25), clavicle, humerus (Figs. 6–24 and 6–26), radius (Figs. 6–26 and 6–27), ulna (see Figs. 6–26 and 6–27), metacarpals (see Figs. 6–15 and 6–27), and phalanges (see Fig. 6–15) can be imaged in most cases. Interestingly, the clavicle may be difficult to see, presumably because of the flexed position of the fetal neck that draws the calvaria into a position that

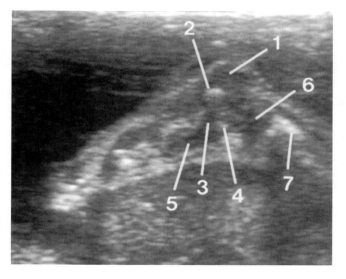

FIGURE 6–22. Midsagittal sonogram of the fetal foot in late midtrimester. (1 = cartilaginous calcaneus; 2 = primary ossification center of calcaneus; 3 = cartilaginous talus; 4 = primary ossification center of talus; 5 = tarsal navicular in cartilage; 6 = distal tibial epiphysis; 7 = distal tibial disphysis.)

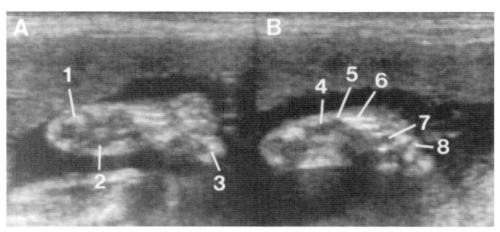

FIGURE 6–23. Transverse axial sonograms (*A* and *B*) of the fetal foot, late second trimester. (1 = calcaneus, both ossified and nonossified; 2 = talus, both ossified and nonossified; 3 = great toe; 4 = tarsal cuboid in cartilage; 5 = proximal epiphysis of fifth metatarsal; 6 = ossified diaphysis of fifth metatarsal; 7 = distal epiphysis of second metatarsal; 8 = ossification center of distal phalanx of second toe.)

obscures the clavicle. Nonetheless, if one desires to see the clavicle, this can almost always be accomplished. Indeed, measurements exist for normal clavicular length at various gestational ages.[23] Similarly, the femur (Figs. 6–28 to 6–31), tibia (Fig. 6–32), fibula (see Fig. 6–32), metatarsals (see Figs. 6–21 to 6–23), and phalanges (see Figs. 6–21 to 6–23) of the lower extremity can be appreciated well sonographically. The figures demonstrating the hip joint, femur, and knee (see Figs. 6–28 to 6–30) may be reviewed to appreciate the remarkably detailed anatomy that can be achieved with high-resolution sonography.

The simplest way to identify the types of long bones of the extremity viewed on the sonogram is to obtain planes of section that traverse the short axis of the limb. Sonograms obtained in such a plane through the forearm and calf demonstrate two bones. In the lower leg, the more lateral bone is the fibula, and the medial bone is the tibia (see Fig. 6–32). This method works as well in the forearm but is less precise because pronation may cause the radius and ulna to "cross." In the normal fetus, the tibia and fibula and the radius and ulna end at the same level distally (see Fig. 6–27). Proximally, of course, the ulna is longer than the radius (see Fig. 6–26). This allows both ready differentiation of these two bony sets and of the radius from the ulna in the upper extremity set. That both paired long bones of the upper and lower extremity end at the same level distally is important in assessing possible limb reduction abnormalities.

The hand can be assessed more critically than can the foot.[24–26] With patience, one can usually discern all four fingers and the thumb. The hand is frequently clenched in a fist-like fashion, which can complicate the counting of fingers. However, even in this case, one can frequently make the necessary observations. The toes, although

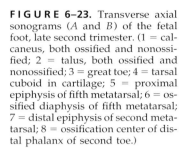

FIGURE 6–24. Coronal sonogram of the shoulder and upper arm. (1 = distal clavicle; 2 = cartilaginous humeral head; 3 = ossified humeral diaphysis; 4 = latissimus dorsi muscle; 5 = scapula.)

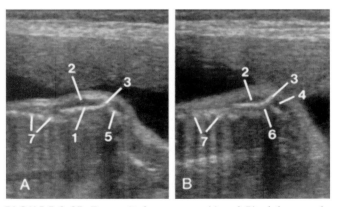

FIGURE 6–25. Parasagittal sonograms (*A* and *B*) of the scapula. (1 = infraspinous fossa; 2 = infraspinatus muscle; 3 = scapular spine; 4 = supraspinatus muscle; 5 = supraspinous fossa; 6 = subscapularis muscle; 7 = ribs in short axis.)

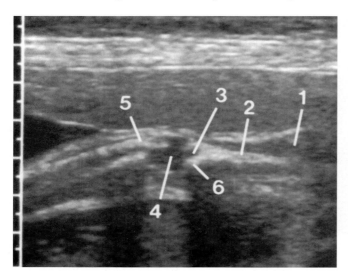

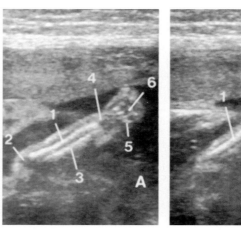

FIGURE 6–26. Fetal elbow, hand pronated, coronal sonogram. (1 = triceps muscle; 2 = ossified humeral diaphysis; 3 = cartilaginous olecranon fossa; 4 = conglomerate cartilages about the elbow joint; 5 = proximal ulnar diaphysis; 7 = medial humeral epicondyle.)

FIGURE 6–27. Coronal sonograms (*A* and *B*) of the forearm and wrist. (1 = ulnar diaphysis; 2 = olecranon in cartilage; 3 = radial diaphysis; 4 = distal ulnar epiphysis; 5 = fifth metacarpal diaphysis; 6 = distal third metacarpal epiphysis; 7 = phalangeal ossification centers; 8 = carpal arch seen as a conglomerate cartilage.)

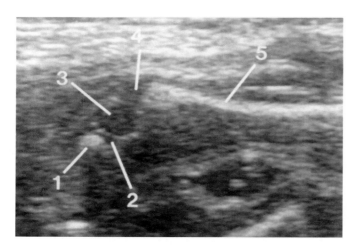

FIGURE 6–28. Coronal image of the fetal hip. (1 = ischial ossification center; 2 = cartilaginous acetabulum; 3 = femoral head in cartilage; 4 = greater trochanter in cartilage; 5 = femoral diaphysis.)

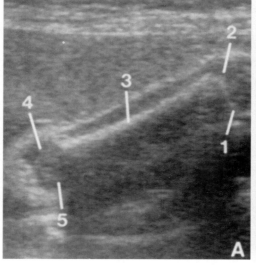

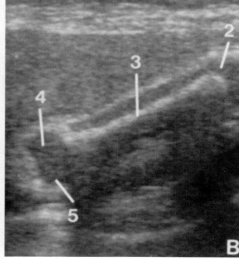

FIGURE 6–29. Longitudinal coronal sonograms (*A* and *B*) of the thigh. (1 = posterior hip joint capsule; 2 = greater trochanter; 3 = femoral diaphysis; 4 = lateral condyle; 5 = medial condyle.)

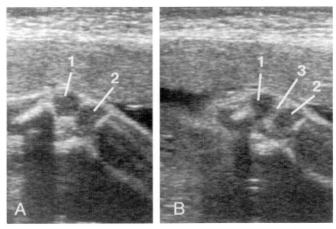

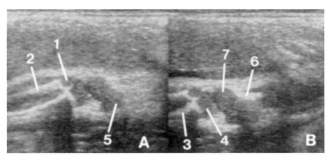

FIGURE 6–32. Coronal sonograms (*A* and *B*) of the knee (off axis). (1 = proximal fibular epiphysis; 2 = fibular diaphysis; 3 = tibial diaphysis; 4 = proximal tibial epiphysis; 5 = patella; 6 = femoral metaphysis; 7 = lateral femoral condyle.)

FIGURE 6–30. *A,* Parasagittal sonogram of the fetal knee. The femoral condyle (1) articulates with the tibial plateau (proximal tibial epiphysis [2]). *B,* Midsagittal sonogram of the fetal knee. Note the gap (3) between the distal femoral epiphysis (1) and the proximal tibial epiphysis (2). This gap is due to the intercondylar notch (see Fig. 6–31).

smaller than the fingers, can be seen relatively well with modern equipment (see Fig. 6–21). If a difficulty arises, it is usually the functionally less important fourth and fifth toes that are unseen.

It is possible in the fetus in the late third trimester to identify the distal femoral (Fig. 6–33; see also Fig. 6–18) and proximal tibial (see Fig. 6–33) epiphyseal ossification centers.[27, 28] Ossification of these epiphyses, as seen on radiographs, is known to be an indicator of fetal maturity. Identification of the epiphyseal ossification centers about the knee provides a different type of parameter that sonologists can use in the assessment of

gestational age in the third trimester of pregnancy. One can obtain a high sensitivity, specificity, and accuracy of a positive prediction if one uses a 33-week cut-off point for the appearance of the distal femoral epiphysis (Figs. 6–34 to 6–36). Similarly, the same data suggest a threshold for the appearance of the proximal tibial epiphysis at 35 weeks. Statistical analysis of this threshold demonstrates that only a positive identification of the proximal tibial epiphysis appears to be clinically useful. A relatively large number of fetuses greater than 35 menstrual weeks do not possess an identifiable proximal tibial epiphysis. These ossification centers appear earlier, on average, in female fetuses (see Fig. 6–35).[28] The size of the distal femoral ossification center correlates with late gestational age (see Fig. 6–36).[28]

As stated earlier, many "bones" of the fetal appendicular skeleton are entirely cartilaginous. Some of these bones can still be imaged sonographically. Indeed, the patella can be seen rather commonly (see Figs. 6–16 and

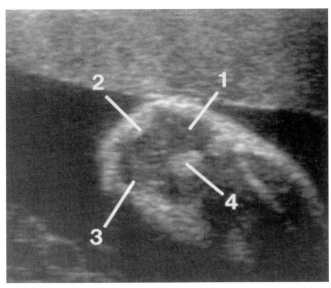

FIGURE 6–31. Transverse axial sonogram through the distal epiphysis of the femur (cartilaginous). (1 = lateral condyle; 2 = patella groove; 3 medial condyle; 4 = intercondylar notch.)

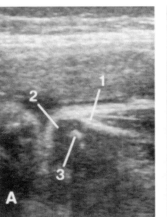

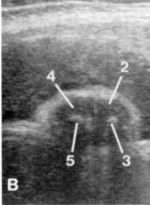

FIGURE 6–33. *A,* Coronal sonogram of the distal thigh in a term fetus. (1 = femoral metaphysis; 2 = lateral condyle; 3 = ossification center of the distal femoral epiphysis.) *B,* Axial sonogram through the knee. (4 = proximate tibial epiphysis; 5 = ossification center of the proximal tibial epiphysis.) Note the large and similar sizes of the ossification centers, which is virtually a certain sign of a near-term fetus.

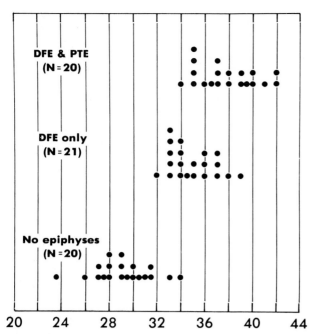

FIGURE 6–34. Appearance time of the distal femoral epiphysis (DFE) and the proximal tibial epiphysis (PTE) in a mixed group of 61 fetuses in which two of the following three dating parameters agreed: LMP, early sonogram, Dubowitz scores. (From Chinn DH, Bolding DB, Callen PW, et al: Ultrasonographic identification of fetal lower extremity epiphyseal ossification centers. Radiology 147:815, 1983, with permission.)

6–18). This bone does not begin to ossify until after birth. All of the carpal bones and most of the tarsal bones are entirely cartilaginous (see Figs. 6–15, 6–21 to 6–23, and 6–27). The carpals cannot be seen discretely. Rather, they are perceived as a conglomerate hypoechoic band that bridges the gap from the distal radius and ulna to the proximal metacarpal ossification centers (see Fig. 6–27). Of course, this "gap" also includes the cartilaginous epiphyses of the long bones. Conversely, some of the tarsal bones can sometimes be discretely identified (see Figs. 6–21 to 6–23). These bones include, most notably, the early tarsal calcaneus and talus (before 24 weeks) and the tarsal navicular and cuboid throughout gestation.

Visualization of the cartilaginous ends of the long bones assists in their measurement in two ways. The measurement of fetal long bones is confined to the ossified portion. A potential error is to foreshorten the bone by failing to obtain the plane of section through the true long axis of the bone. To avoid underestimating the length, this shortcoming is often compensated for by assuming that the "longest" measurement obtained in several attempts is the most accurate, which is an assumption that can lead to serious overestimates. However, if both cartilaginous ends of the desired bone to be measured are seen, this guarantees that the plane of section has passed through the longest axis of the bone (Fig. 6–37). The only remaining task to minimize error is to accurately position measurement cursors at the end of the bone.

Another common misconception in measurement of the femur is that no other tissue in proximity to the bony termination will yield an echo of equal brightness to the bone. Thus, one "should always place measurement cursors" from the edge of the distal brightest reflection to the edge of the proximal brightest reflection. This longstanding belief is unfortunately erroneous, especially in the case of older fetuses, although younger fetuses are not exempt from this potentially significant error in femur length estimation.[29] Figure 6–38 demonstrates that a nonosseous, but nonetheless equally bright, reflection is returned from tissues that are distal to the epiphyseal plate but are in immediate contiguity with the distal femoral metaphysis. We call this the "distal femoral point" for lack of a more precise anatomic term.[29] The fact that this "point" is not part of the ossified femur can be determined by noting its relationship to the cartilaginous lateral condyle. The femoral metaphysis ends at the beginning of the distal femoral epiphysis and does not overlap the edge of the epiphysis. Compare the radiograph of the fetal femur (see Fig.

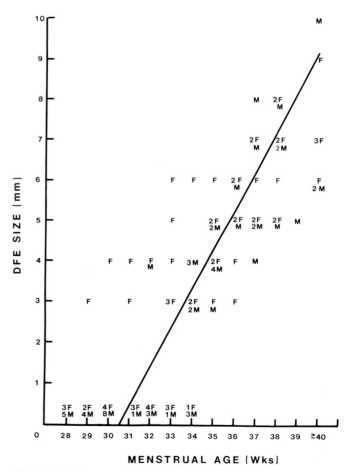

FIGURE 6–35. Variation in appearance of the DFE appearance time and size in male and female fetuses. (From Mahony BS, Callen PW, Filly RA: The distal femoral epiphyseal ossification center in the assessment of third trimester menstrual age: Sonographic identification and measurement. Radiology 155:201, 1985, with permission.)

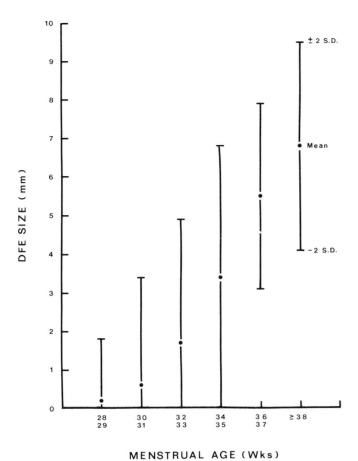

FIGURE 6-36. Mean diameter of the DFE with increasing age. (From Mahony SB, Callen PW, Filly RA: The distal femoral epiphyseal ossification center in the assessment of third trimester menstrual age: Sonographic identification and measurement. Radiology 155:201, 1985, with permission.)

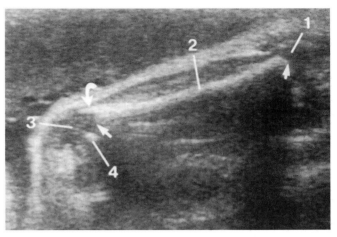

FIGURE 6-38. A view of the fetal femur in the third trimester. A bright reflector (*curved arrow*) is seen in continuity with the lateral femoral metaphysis. This structure is not part of the ossified femur. End points of femur measurement are marked by *straight arrows* (1 = greater trochanter; 2 = femoral diaphysis; 3 = lateral condyle; 4 = ossification center of the distal epiphysis.)

6-20) with Figure 6-38. No such *ossified* femoral point exists.

Sonography sometimes demonstrates rather extraordinary features of the musculoskeletal system of the extremities. At present, no known diagnostic usefulness for this information has been established nor is it possible to demonstrate such structures with the consistency necessary to use their visualization in diagnostic pursuits. However, Figures 6-39 to 6-41 demonstrate several of these remarkable features.

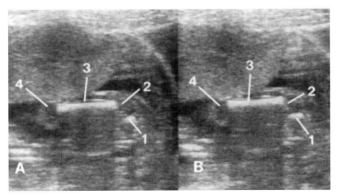

FIGURE 6-37. *A* and *B*, Two views of femur for measurement. Visualization of the proximal (2) and distal (4) cartilaginous bone ensures that the plane of section is through the long axis of the diaphysis (3). Only proper positioning of the cursors remains to ensure an accurate measurement. (1 = ischial ossification center.)

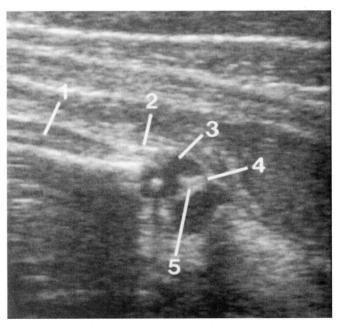

FIGURE 6-39. Midsagittal sonogram of the extended knee. In addition to structures pointed out in earlier figures, note the quadriceps muscle (1), the quadriceps tendon (2), the patella (3), the patella ligament (4), and the synovium (5) contained by the knee joint.

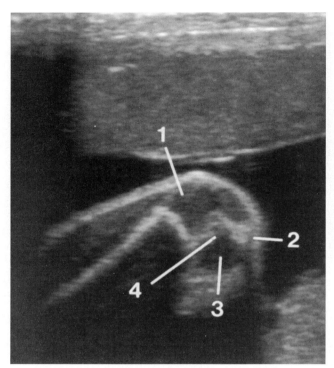

FIGURE 6-40. Midsagittal sonogram of the fetal knee in flexion. The distal femoral epiphysis (1), patella, patella ligament (2), and proximal tibial epiphysis (3) define the knee joint boundaries. Within the knee joint is a large quantity of highly echogenic tissue, presumably synovium. The cruciate ligament (4) is clearly outlined by the bright "synovium."

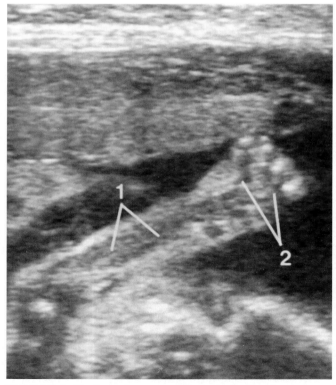

FIGURE 6-41. Coronal sonogram through the dorsal soft tissues of the forearm and hand. (1 = extensor muscle group; 2 = extensor tendons.)

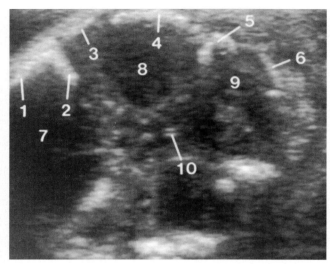

FIGURE 6-42. Transverse axial sonogram near the skull base. (1 = frontal bone; 2 = greater wing of sphenoid bone; 3 = parietal bone; 4 = temporal bone; 5 = petrous ridge; 6 = occipital bone; 7 = anterior cranial fossa; 8 = middle cranial fossa; 9 = posterior cranial fossa; 10 = basilar artery.)

Many bones or components of bones of the axial skeleton are also routinely visualized. In the skull region one can perceive a number of bones individually or as a conglomerate. The greater wing of the sphenoid and petrous ridge are easily identified and define the anterior, middle, and posterior cranial fossae (Fig. 6–42). The orbits can be visualized without difficulty, unless the more anteriorly positioned orbit severely shadows the more posteriorly positioned orbit (Fig. 6–43). Standards have been established for fetal interorbital distances to evaluate hypotelorism and hypertelorism.[30] In older fetuses, surprising detail of the intraorbital contents can be appreciated, including the wall of the globe, lens, retrobulbar fat, optic nerve, and rectus muscles

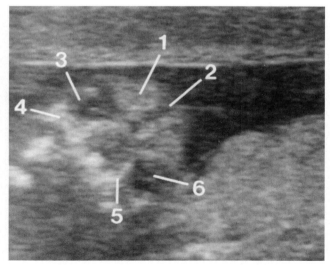

FIGURE 6-43. Fetal orbits in the early second trimester. (1 = frontal bone; 2 = metopic suture; 3 = orbit; 4 = maxilla; 5 = nasal bone; 6 = lens.)

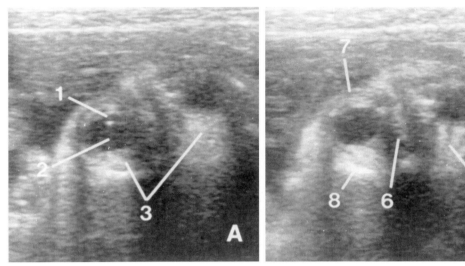

FIGURE 6–44. Orbits and contents (*A* and *B*). (1 = lens; 2 = globe; 3 = retrobulbar fat; 5 = optic nerve; 6 = lateral rectus muscle; 7 = eyelid; 8 = lateral orbit wall.)

(Fig. 6–44). Portions of the maxilla and almost all of the mandible can be identified, as well as the bony nasal ridge (see Fig. 6–43). Similarly, the frontal, parietal, and squama of the temporal and occipital bones, which comprise the calvaria, can be seen clearly. The cartilaginous zones of articulation of these bones, the coronal, sagittal, and lambdoid sutures, are commonly visible (Fig. 6–45). The fontanelles may also be seen (Fig. 6–46) and are used as windows for brain imaging (Fig. 6–47).

The ribs, spine, and pelvis are easily imaged and serve as excellent anatomic landmarks. In the pelvis, the iliac ossification centers are easily observed from early sec-

ond trimester onward (ossified at 2.5 to 3 fetal months). Ischial ossification (see Fig. 6–28) is present at 4 months, but pubic ossification is not present until 6 months.

The spine is an important structure in fetal diagnosis.[21, 31-33] With the advent of maternal serum α-fetoprotein screening, as well as the concurrent development of sophisticated high-resolution ultrasound imaging technology, the potential currently exists to diagnose almost all spina bifida lesions before the 20th week of pregnancy.[34] These changes in obstetric care mandate that the morphology of the fetal spine be well understood by sonologists. The sequence of development of ossification centers in the fetal vertebral column has been studied extensively in the past with radiologic and histologic methods.[19, 20] Each vertebra usually has

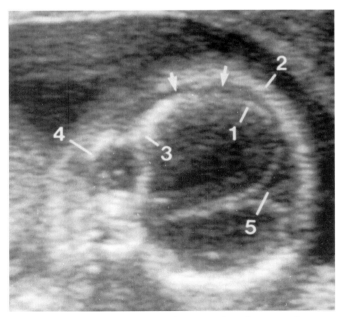

FIGURE 6–45. Oblique view demonstrating the coronal suture (*arrows*). (1 = frontal bone; 2 = parietal bone; 3 = greater wing of sphenoid bone; 4 = maxilla; 5 = interhemispheric fissure with brain edges showing the brightly reflective pia-arachnoid covering.)

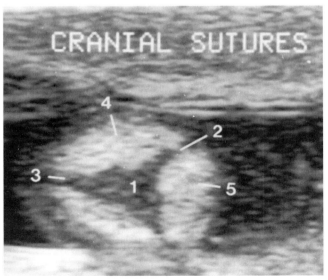

FIGURE 6–46. Transverse axial sonogram of the posterior fontanelle (1). (2 = lambdoid suture; 3 = sagittal suture; 4 = parietal bone; 5 = occipital bone.)

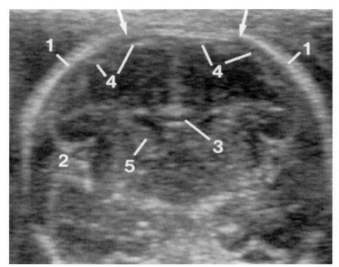

FIGURE 6–47. The sonographic beam was directed through the anterior fontanelle (*arrows*) in a midtrimester fetus, enabling recognition of striking detail in the fetal brain due to the "bone-free window." (1 = parietal bone; 2 = lateral fissure; 3 = corpus callosum; 4 = brain edges over the most cephalic portions of the parietal lobes; 5 = head of caudate nucleus.)

three primary ossification centers, one for the body (centrum) and one on each side of the posterior neural arch. The centra are ossified first in the lower thoracic and upper lumbar regions, followed by progressive ossification in both the cephalic and caudal directions. By contrast and in general, the ossification centers for the posterior neural arch appear in a more standard cephalocaudal direction. the posterior neural arch first begins to ossify (sonographically recognizable high-amplitude reflections) at the base of the transverse process (Fig. 6–48). Ossification proceeds from this center to progressively include the laminae and pedicles. The progression of ossification of the laminae is the more

important for the diagnosis of neural tube defects, because spina bifida is the most consistently demonstrable dysmorphic lesion in open spinal defects. This abnormality is recognized sonographically by an abnormal outward flaring of the posterior neural arch ossification centers.

Various degrees of maturation of spinal ossification are present at different levels of the spine when we are most frequently required to assess the normalcy of the fetal spine.[21] Although there are some exceptions, such as those noted earlier, ossification in the neural arch first appears at the base of the transverse process. Early posterior neural arch ossification then progresses anteriorly into the pedicles, also contributing a portion of the vertebral body, and posteriorly into the laminae. Additionally, craniocaudal extension into the articular processes and lateral extension into the transverse process occur. Because the critical observation in the diagnosis of open spinal neural tube defects is the demonstration of spina bifida (seen as an outward flaring of the posterior arch ossification centers), the ideal situation to confirm normalcy would be to observe the antithesis of this pathologic state (i.e., inward angulation of the laminae). This indeed is the case when visible ossification is present in the normal laminae (Fig. 6–49). Unfortunately, there is insufficient ossification of the laminae to perceive inward angulation of the posterior neural arch ossification centers in the lower spine to confirm normalcy of the fetal spine during the crucial stage of gestation when this sonographic diagnosis must be made (18 to 22 menstrual weeks) (see Fig. 6–48).[31, 34] This is particularly important when considering the most common locations of these lesions (i.e., lumbar and sacral regions).[31] Easily identifiable ossification of the laminae is visible in the cervical region in all fetuses by 18 to 19 menstrual weeks, whereas thoracic ossification of

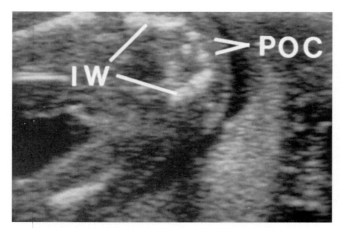

FIGURE 6–48. Early ossification centers in the sacral spine. The centrum is found anteriorly, and the ossifications of the posterior arch appear posteriorly (POC) near the base of the transverse processes. (IW = iliac wings.) (From Filly RA, Simpson GF, Linkowski G: Fetal spine morphology and maturation during the second trimester: Sonographic evaluation. J Ultrasound Med 6:631, 1987. Copyright 1987, by the American Institute of Ultrasound in Medicine.)

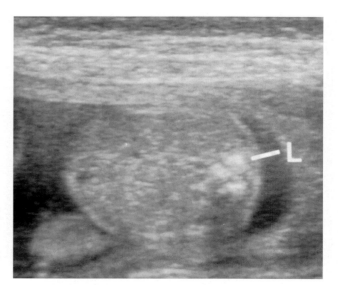

FIGURE 6–49. Lumbar vertebra on axial sonogram. The laminae (L) demonstrate early ossification, causing the appearance of "inward angulation" of the posterior arch. (From Filly RA, Simpson GF, Linkowski G: Fetal spine morphology and maturation during the second trimester: Sonographic evaluation. J Ultrasound in Med 6:631, 1987. Copyright 1987 by the American Institute of Ultrasound in Medicine.)

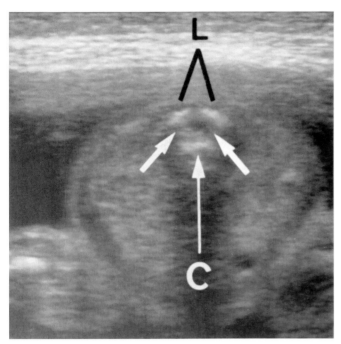

FIGURE 6–50. Lumbar spine on axial sonogram at 23 weeks. Well-defined ossification of the laminae (L). (C = centrum; *arrows* = neuro-central synchondroses.) (From Filly RA, Simpson GF, Linkowski G: Fetal spine morphology and maturation during the second trimester: Sonographic evaluation. J Ultrasound Med 6:631, 1987. Copyright 1987 by the American Institute of Ultrasound in Medicine.)

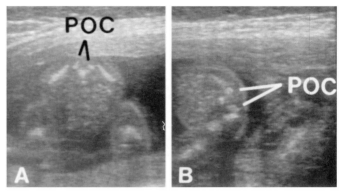

FIGURE 6–52. Axial sonograms, sacral spine, same fetus in prone (*A*) and decubitus (*B*) positions. The posterior arch (POC) anatomy is seen well in either position. (From Filly RA, Simpson GF, Linkowski G: Fetal spine morphology and maturation during the second trimester: Sonographic evaluation. J Ultrasound Med 6:631, 1987. Copyright 1987 by the American Institute of Ultrasound in Medicine.)

there consistently recognizable ossification of the arch in the sacral region (Fig. 6–51). Fetal position (either prone or decubitus) does not appear to affect appreciably the ability to discern the degree of neural arch ossification, although the prone position usually results in the clearest images (Fig. 6–52). If the fetus is in a supine position, a critical examination of the posterior neural arch cannot be carried out (Fig. 6–53).[21]

The spine may be seen in both longitudinal and transverse axial planes. Although both planes are important,

the laminae is only partially visible during the 18th to 19th menstrual week period.[21] There is no ossification of the laminae in the lumbar or sacral regions of fetuses examined before 19 menstrual weeks (see Fig. 6–48). The thoracic vertebrae consistently demonstrate partial ossification of the laminae in the range of 20 to 22 weeks, whereas the lumbar region does not demonstrate a similar degree of ossification until 22 to 24 weeks (Fig. 6–50). The sacral spine reveals no evidence of ossification in the laminae before 22 weeks. Only after 25 weeks is

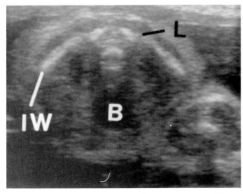

FIGURE 6–51. Sacral spine on axial sonogram at 26 weeks. (B = bladder; IW = iliac wing; L = laminae.) (From Filly RA, Simpson GF, Linkowski G: Fetal spine morphology and maturation during the second trimester: Sonographic evaluation. J Ultrasound Med 6:631, 1987. Copyright 1987 by the American Institute of Ultrasound in Medicine.)

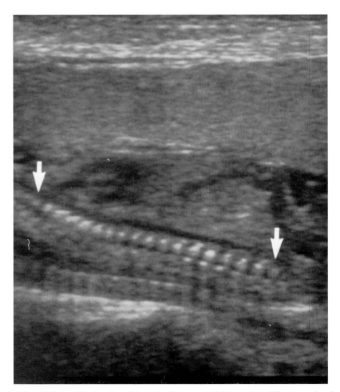

FIGURE 6–53. Supine fetus in the second trimester. The vertebral bodies (lying between the *arrows*) are clearly seen, but the posterior neural arch cannot be well appreciated.

the transverse axial plane demonstrates the anatomy to best advantage. On longitudinal planes of a section the posterior elements are seen as "parallel" bands of echos. In fact, they are not precisely parallel because they flair in the upper cervical region and converge in the sacrum and, in addition, careful scanning usually discloses a slight widening of the lumbar area. It is important not to mistake this slight lumbar widening as being a pathologic event. Because the fetal spine is normally kyphotic, usually one cannot visualize the entire spine in a single longitudinal coronal plane. Thus, transverse axial planes of section are necessary to be certain that the entirety of the spine has been imaged on a segment-by-segment basis. Care must also be taken to ensure that the spine has been thoroughly examined on transverse planes. At the cephalic end, no problem arises because one encounters the calvaria. However, the caudal end poses a more difficult problem. One can successfully use the ischial ossification centers as landmarks to ensure that the caudal end of the spine has been reached. In older fetuses, both spinal and spinal canal anatomy can often be quite dramatically depicted (Fig. 6–54).

Cartilaginous structure in the axial skeleton is less conspicuous than in the appendicular skeleton; nonetheless, it is visible in almost all fetuses. The sutures of the calvarial vault have already been noted. The cartilaginous neurocentral synchondrosis of the spine (the junction of the centrum and the posterior ossification centers) is visible in all fetuses from the end of the first trimester onward (see Figs. 6–48 to 6–52).[21] Similarly, the gaps between the vertebral body ossification centers is a composite of the unossified margin of the adjoining vertebral bodies plus the intervertebral discs (see Fig. 6–53). The margin of cartilage in the verebral body is best appreciated posteriorly, lying between the ossification center and the dura of the spinal canal (see the section on the central nervous system) (see Fig. 6–54C and D). The spinous processes of the posterior neural arch are also occasionally seen, these structures again consisting entirely of cartilage in fetal life (see Fig. 6–54C).

One feature that cannot be well judged on sonograms is the degree of ossification of the bones. Thus, increased ossification, such as in osteopetrosis, goes completely

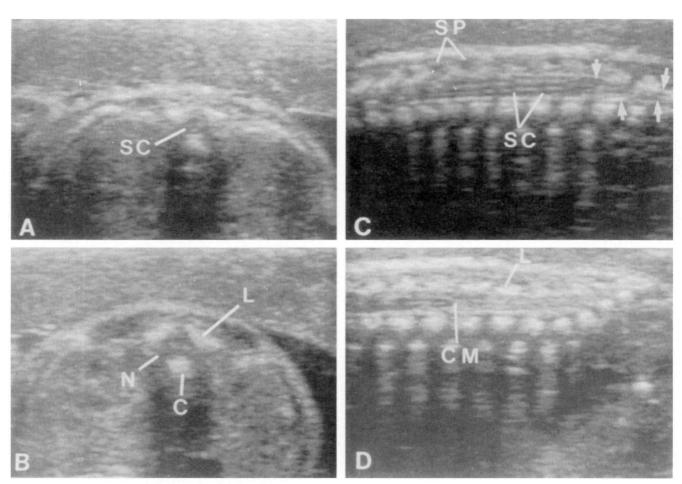

FIGURE 6–54. *A* and *B,* The lumbar spine on axial sections of a 27-week-old fetus are shown. (C = centrum; L = 0 + 2 laminae; N = neurocentral synchondrosis; SC = spinal cord.) *C* and *D,* Longitudinal scans of the thoracolumbar (C) and lumbosacral (D) regions. (*arrows* = dura; CM = conus medullaris; L = laminae; SC = spinal cord [note the bright linear echo from the central canal]; SP = spinous process [in cartilage]). (From Filly RA, Simpson GF, Linkowsid G: Fetal spine morphology and maturation during the second trimester: Sonographic evaluation. J Ultrasound Med 6:631, 1987. Copyright 1987 by the American Institute of Ultrasound in Medicine.)

unrecognized on sonograms. Similarly, diminished ossification is poorly judged. Only in the most extremely osteopenic bone can one appreciate diminished ossification on sonograms. Examples would be the almost non-ossified calvaria in fetuses with recessive osteogenesis imperfecta or recessive hypophosphatasia[35-37] or the spine in fetuses with achondrogenesis.[38]

Little space is devoted to the fetal muscular system even though many muscles and muscle groups may be seen-quite well (see Fig. 6–24 and 6–25). In general, normal muscles are quite hypoechoic, at times so much so that they simulate fluid collections. This is most notable of the abdominal wall musculature, which may simulate ascites (pseudoascites) (Fig. 6–55).[39] Currently, high-resolution sonographic equipment decreases the propensity to "overcall" ascites caused by this artifactual situation, because the layers of the abdominal wall can be seen quite clearly.[40]

The abdominal wall muscles, the internal and external oblique and the transversus abdominis, are sometimes so clearly visible that the individual layers can be detected (Fig. 6–56). More commonly seen as a "single" layer of muscles, this tissue is easily recognized as lying within the abdominal wall by noting its position between the subcutaneous fat and the properitoneal fat. The latter is traced from the paranephric fat as it curves onto the flank. Further, the abdominal wall muscles "meet" the ends of the lower thoracic ribs, whereas ascites would pass "between" the ribs and the abdominal viscera.[40]

Cardiovascular System

The anatomy of the heart and great vessels is discussed in detail in Chapter 5. This section deals with the fetal

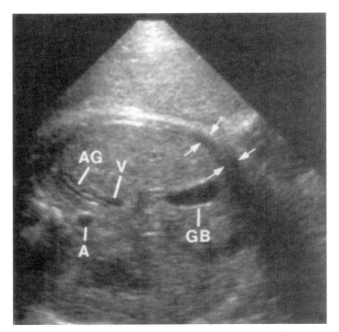

FIGURE 6–55. Transverse axial sonogram or a retal abdomen. Lucent abdominal wall musculature (*arrows*) may erroneously give the impression that ascites is present. (A = aorta; AG = adrenal gland; GB = gallbladder; V = vena cava.)

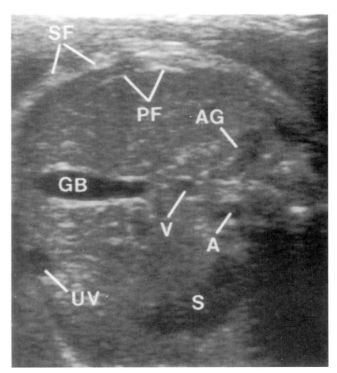

FIGURE 6–56. Abdominal wall musculature lies between the subcutaneous fat (SF) and the properitoneal fat (PF). Individual layers can be appreciated. (A = aorta; AG = adrenal gland; GB = gallbladder; S = stomach; UV = umbilical vein; V = vena cava.)

vessels visible within the uterus and fetal corpus that are not covered elsewhere. Indeed, a surprisingly large number of individual fetal blood vessels can be seen. The list could be expanded substantially if one were to include arteries that are recognized only by the location of their pulsation, although the wall and lumen of the vessel are still undetected or their color signature on color Doppler sonography.

The fetal circulation begins in the placenta. In almost all second- and third-trimester fetuses one can detect the surface (fetal) vessels of the placenta, and one can even appreciate that these vessels penetrate the placental substance. The surface vessels coalesce at the cord "insertion." The identification of the cord insertion has become important since the advent of percutaneous fetal blood sampling (FBS) for diagnosis and management (see Chapter 9).[41] The "insertion" of the cord is often easily seen, but if not, it is worthwhile to search for large placental surface vessels and trace these to the cord.

The normal umbilical cord consists of two arteries and a vein (Fig. 6–57). The cord is almost always coiled and sometimes extremely so. This leads to a variety of appearances of the cord when viewed with tomographic sections as generated by sonography. Indeed, the "simple" task of counting cord vessels can be made quite frustrating by the coils. To consistently obtain the correct count of cord vessels, one must rely on a true transverse axial section of the cord vessels. Longitudinal or oblique views can be misleading.

These vessels enter the fetus, by definition, at the umbilicus and there immediately diverge.[42] The umbili-

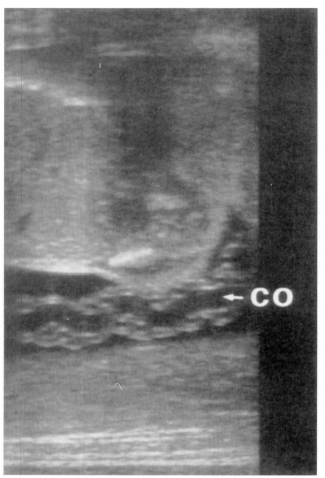

F I G U R E 6–57. Longitudinal sonogram of a three-vessel umbilical cord (CO).

tal anatomy.[43] Because there are no blood-diverting branches of the umbilical vein, the volume of placental blood entering the left portal venous system is equal to that in the umbilical vein. Thus, the umbilical vein and the initial portion (umbilical segment) of the left portal vein have the same diameter (see Fig. 6–58). Thus, the left portal vein of the fetus is larger than the right portal vein, which is the reverse of the situation seen in the child and adult. From this point, there are several avenues via which blood may reach the right atrium. A common misconception of the maternal–fetal circulation is that the bulk of umbilical venous blood bypasses the liver capillary bed via a large patent ductus venosus. However, in utero, the ductus venosus averages only one seventh of the diameter of the umbilical vein[44] and may even be closed (see Fig. 6–58).[45] It should be remembered, however, that the peripheral resistance of the hepatic vascular bed is not present in the ductus venosus, enabling this smaller caliber vessel to carry a larger quantity of blood than might be expected. Nonetheless, a significant portion of umbilical venous blood, which carries the highest concentration of nutrients and oxygen in the fetus, actually circulates through the left lobe of the fetal liver via branches supplying the medial and lateral segments before entering the systemic venous system through the left and middle hepatic veins (Fig. 6–60). Although the right lobe of the liver receives a small amount of umbilical venous blood from the left portal vein, the bulk of blood entering the right portal vein is derived from the main portal vein, which, in the fetus, contains low concentrations of both nutrients and oxygen.[45] The unequal distribution of nutrients to the

cal vein proceeds cephalically (Fig. 6–58); the umbilical arteries egress from a caudal direction. The umbilical arteries proceed along the margin of the urinary bladder from their origin at the iliac arteries in their course toward the umbilicus (Fig. 6–59). As they course along the bladder margin, they should not be mistaken for dilated ureters, a distinction that can be made easily by taking a moment to notice their pulsation or by interrogation with color Doppler sonography.

The umbilical vein joins the fetal portal circulation. The fetal portal circulation is seen with a high degree of consistency on ultrasonograms. Obviously, the larger the fetus, the more readily one will see the smaller elements of this system. Importantly, many of the illustrations seen in the ultrasonic literature incorrectly interpret the fetal umbilical and portal venous anatomy. Confusion has led not only to improper nomenclature, but also to the use of inappropriate landmarks for obtaining important fetal measurements. With a clear understanding of fetal portal vein anatomy, one can avoid these drawbacks and can better appreciate fetal and adult segmental hepatic anatomy.

The dynamics of maternal-fetal circulation determine the details of fetal hepatic portal venous and segmen-

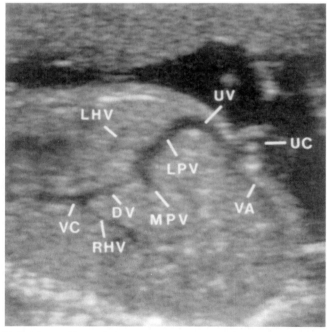

F I G U R E 6–58. Midsagittal sonogram of the umbilical circulation. (DV = ductus venosus; LHV = left hepatic vein; LPV = umbilical segment of left portal vein; MPV = main portal vein; RHV = right hepatic vein; UA = umbilical artery; UC = umbilical cord; VC = inferior vena cava.)

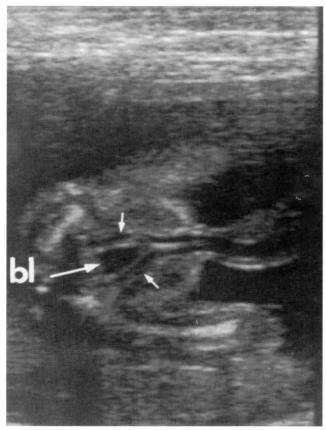

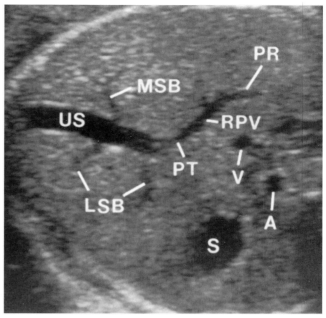

FIGURE 6–60. Fetal portal circulation. (A = aorta; LSB = lateral segmental branches; MSB = medial segmental branch; PR = posterior division of the right portal vein; PT = pars transversa of the left portal vein; RPV = right portal vein; US = umbilical segment of the left portal vein; V = vena cava.)

FIGURE 6–59. Umbilical cord insertion into the fetus. The umbilical arteries (arrows) egress from a caudal direction and course along the margin of the urinary bladder (bl).

fetal liver partially accounts for the relatively large size of the left lobe of the fetal liver. After closure of the umbilical vein at birth, the supply of nutrients to the entire liver equalizes, and the relative size of the left lobe decreases.

In the fetus, the umbilical vein courses cephalically in the free margin of the falciform ligament (see Fig.

6–58). As noted earlier, it joins the umbilical portion of the left portal vein at the caudal margin of the left intersegmental fissure of the liver.[46] After birth, the umbilical vein thromboses, collapses, and ultimately becomes the ligamentum teres hepatis.

The umbilical portion of the left portal vein has a predominantly posterior route but also courses superiorly in the left intersegmental fissure (see Fig. 6–58). Its branches supply the medial and lateral segments of the left lobe of the liver.[47] The left portal vein then courses abruptly to the right, leaving the left intersegmental fissure, and forms the transverse portion (pars transversa) of the left portal vein (Fig. 6–61; see also Fig.

FIGURE 6–61. Transverse axial sonograms (A and B) of fetal liver. (AR = anterior division of the right portal vein; DV = ductus venosus; LC = left diaphragmatic crus; LS = lateral segmental branch; MH = middle hepatic vein; PR = posterior division of the right portal vein; RC = right diaphragmatic crus; RH = right hepatic vein; RP = right portal vein; S = stomach; SP = spleen; US = umbilical segment of the left portal vein.)

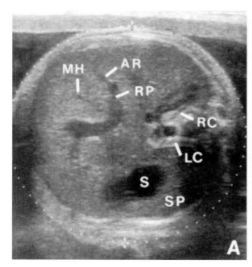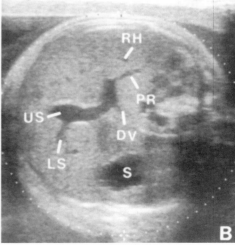

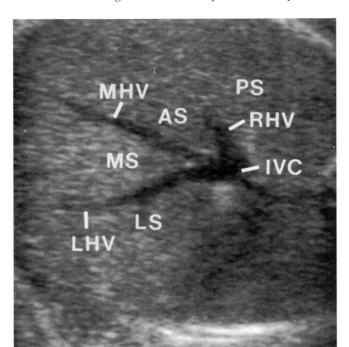

FIGURE 6-62. Sonogram through the long axis of the proximal fetal hepatic veins. (IVC = inferior vena cava; LHV = left hepatic vein; MHV = middle hepatic vein; RHV = right hepatic vein.) These veins divide the liver into lobes and segments. (AS and PS = anterior and posterior segments of the right hepatic lobe; MS and LS = medial and lateral segments of the left hepatic lobe.)

6-60). The pars transversa joins imperceptibly with the right portal vein at the main lobar fissure. The ductus venosus originates from the pars transversa (but occasionally more rightward).[48] The ductus continues posteriorly, but assumes a more cephalad course than that of the umbilical portion of the left portal vein (see Fig. 6-61). It continues as an unbranched structure to join the left or, less commonly, the middle hepatic vein. In this position, it lies in the superior extension of the gastrohepatic ligament that separates the developing caudate lobe posteriorly from the medial and lateral segments of the left hepatic lobe anteriorly. After birth, the ductus venosus closes and becomes the fibrous ligamentum venosum.[46]

Ultrasonograms of the upper portion of the fetal abdomen clearly demonstrate the anatomy described earlier (see Fig. 6-58 to 6-61). Because the umbilical vein courses cephalically, transversely oriented planes of section intersect this vessel's short axis (see Fig. 6-56). Slight cephalad movement of the transducer demonstrates a position at which this venous structure abruptly courses posteriorly (see Fig. 6-60 and 6-61). This posteriorly coursing vein represents the umbilical portion of the left portal vein rather than the cephalic portion of the umbilical vein, which is commonly mislabeled in the ultrasound literature. This vessel can easily be seen as being the left portal vein, because branches to the medial and lateral segments of the left lobe arise from this vein (see Fig. 6-60 and 6-61). Recall that the umbilical vein has no branches. When the umbilical portion of the left portal vein is seen throughout its entire course,

one can be certain that some angulation has been introduced into the scan plane, because this venous structure courses not only posterior but slightly cephalad (see Fig. 6-58). Various branches of the umbilical segment of the left portal vein are occasionally imaged; these branches include the medial, superolateral, and inferolateral branches (see Fig. 6-60).

The right portal vein divides into anterior and posterior segmental branches, such as in the adult (see Fig. 6-61). Each branch supplies a respective segment of the right hepatic lobe. The hepatic veins can be recognized by their relationship with the portal veins[46] and can be seen to radiate toward the inferior vena cava, coalescing with this venous channel immediately before it enters the right atrium (Fig. 6-62). These veins divide the liver into lobes and segments. The hepatic veins are most easily sought near the level of the diaphragm where their caliber is the largest.[49] Nonetheless, the middle and right hepatic veins are commonly seen in more inferior planes of section by noting their relative position compared with the right portal vein divisions (see Fig. 6-61). The right hepatic vein (anterior branch) passes between the anterior and posterior divisions of the right portal vein, while the middle hepatic vein always crosses anterior to the right portal vein (in the main lobar fissure). The aorta and inferior vena cava (IVC) have a similar course in the lower abdomen, but diverge in the upper abdomen where the aorta penetrates the diaphragm posteriorly (in contact with the spine) while the IVC turns anteriorly to join the right atrium (Fig. 6-63).

The great vessels near and around the heart are described in Chapter 9. The vessels arising from the transverse aorta are frequently visible and include the brachiocephalic, left common carotid, and left subclavian arteries. The common carotid arteries and jugular veins are also commonly seen in the neck of older fetuses. The brachial artery and vein are less frequently seen adjacent to the humerus when the arterial pulsation or the color Doppler signature is sought.

Certain intracranial arterial structures are occasionally perceived as being tubular vessels (Fig. 6-64). More commonly, they are recognized because of the location of their pulsation or color Doppler signature. These structures include the middle cerebral artery in the sylvian cistern, the posterior cerebral artery in the ambient cistern, the anterior cerebral arteries in the interhemispheric cistern (near the genu of the corpus callosum), and the basilar artery in the interpeduncular cistern. The

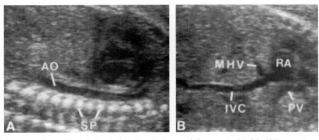

FIGURE 6-63. A, Longitudinal view of the aorta (AO). (SP = spine.) B, Longitudinal view of the inferior vena cava (IVC). (MHV = middle hepatic vein; PV = pulmonic vein; RA = right atrium.)

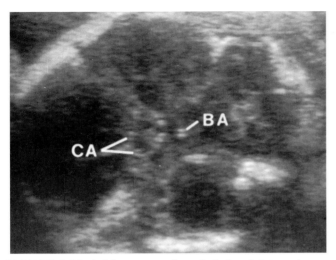

FIGURE 6–64. Axial sonogram through the basal cisterns demonstrates the internal carotid arteries (CA) and the basilar artery (BA).

circle of Willis is seen in the basilar cisterns caudal to the third ventricle.

The abdominal aorta and inferior vena cava are easily identified, as are the common iliac arteries and veins. Other branches of the abdominal aorta can be visualized, although inconsistently, and include the celiac axis, the superior mesenteric artery, and the renal arteries. Similarly, the renal veins are seen from time to time. These vessels are seen consistently with color Doppler sonography.

In the leg, the superficial femoral artery and vein (Fig. 6–65) may be visualized in older fetuses. When the knee is extended, it is not difficult to trace these vessels to the level of the popliteal artery and vein (Fig. 6–66), which is an almost impossible task when the knee is flexed.

Gastrointestinal System

Many components of the gastrointestinal (GI) system can be seen sonographically, some as early as the end of the first trimester.[50] The largest parenchymal organ of the system and of the torso, the liver, is seen consistently from the second trimester onward, although its margins are often indistinct in the earlier phases of pregnancy. Conversely, the other major parenchymal organ of the GI system, the pancreas, is only uncommonly seen, even in third-trimester fetuses. For lack of a better section in which to include it, the spleen is considered with the GI tract. This organ is also visible consistently in the second trimester, however, like the liver, each of its margins are rarely distinct. Conversely, those portions of the fetal GI system that consistently contain fluid, the stomach (see Figs. 6–56, 6–60, and 6–61) and gallbladder (see Figs. 6–55 and 6–56), are among the earliest and most consistently seen fetal structures.

The components within and about the oral cavity are seen relatively well on sonography.[51] The lips and cheeks have been described in the section on superficial anatomy (see Figs. 6–7 and 6–8). The tongue is also consistently seen (Fig. 6–67) and is viewed to best advantage during the swallowing movements. The gingival ridge with tooth buds is seen not uncommonly in older fetuses (see Fig. 6–67A). The hard palate is difficult to define consistently but can be detected with practice (see Fig. 6–6). Thus, cleft palate is a difficult diagnosis to establish sonographically. The soft palate cannot be recognized discretely. The oropharynx and laryngeal pharynx frequently contain fluid and thus are seen relatively often when sought (Fig. 6–68; see also Fig. 6–67). Transverse axial scans through the upper neck are quite successful for visualization of the pharynx; however, longitudinal coronal images, which are more difficult to obtain, display the anatomy to greater advantage. In longitudinal coronal planes, the continuity of the pharyngeal zones

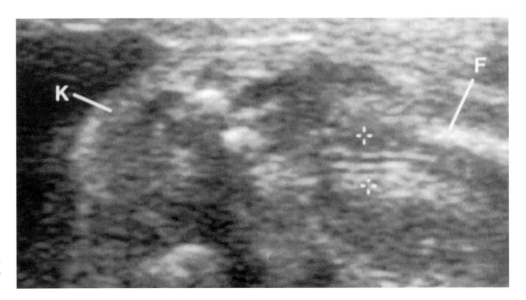

FIGURE 6–65. Superficial femoral artery and vein are marked by cursors. (F = femur; K = knee.)

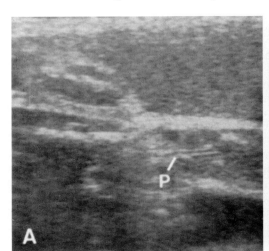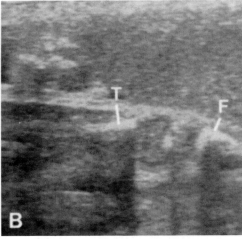

FIGURE 6–66. *A,* Posterior aspect (P) of the knee is shown in extension. The popliteal artery and the vein are visible. *B,* A more anterior plane is shown for reference. (F = femur; T = tibia.)

can be appreciated, as well as the larynx protruding into the pharynx (see Fig. 6–68). The pyriform sinuses, valleculae, and glottis may be appreciated.

The midesophagus and distal esophagus may be seen surprisingly often when sought (Fig. 6–69).[51] The proximal esophagus is extraordinarily difficult, if not impossible, to visualize in the normal fetus. The midesophagus and distal esophagus may be seen, although inconsistently, in both longitudinal coronal and transverse axial images. The key to identification of this structure is the descending thoracic aorta, which is a structure that can be easily seen. The midesophagus and distal esophagus lie immediately anterior to the descending thoracic aorta. The aorta is first visualized in a longitudinal coronal plane. The transducer is then slowly moved anteriorly. As the aorta disappears from view, the esophagus comes into "view" but cannot be recognized so easily. It is seen as five parallel linear echoes that are created by the hyperechoic serosa and lumen and the hypoechoic muscular wall (see Fig. 6–69). Conceptually, one could apply a similar strategy to visualization of the upper third of the esophagus. In this case, one would image the trachea (see the subsequent section) in a longitudinal coronal plane, then slowly move the transducer pos-

teriorly. As the trachea disappears, the esophagus should again come into "view." Unfortunately, this concept, although anatomically correct, is practically unsuccessful.

The stomach and gallbladder are the only portions of the subdiaphragmatic fetal GI system that normally contain fluid (see Figs. 6–55, 6–56, 6–60, and 6–61).[50, 52, 53] Thus, any fluid-containing small bowel should be considered with suspicion, although in late fetuses one may occasionally see very small amounts of normal succus entericus in the small bowel lumen, which is usually made more obvious by accompanying peristalsis.

Fluid contained within the normal fetal stomach is almost entirely imbided. The fetus begins to swallow amniotic fluid at approximately 16 weeks.[52, 53] The volume that the fetus swallows increases dramatically throughout pregnancy and reaches 400 to 500 mL by term. There is a relative proportionality between the volume of urine produced and the amount of amniotic fluid imbibed by the fetus. In the absence of a patent esophagus the stomach will be empty (invisible), except in two circumstances. First, and most common, is the concomitant presence of a tracheoesophageal fistula (TEF) enabling the fetus to leak fluid produced by the

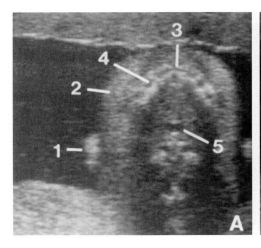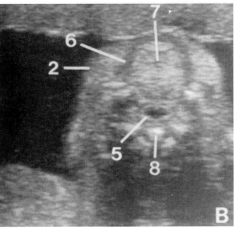

FIGURE 6–67. Transverse axial sonograms of the oral cavity. (1 = ear; 2 = cheek fat pads (Bichat's); 3 = mandible; 4 = tooth buds; 5 = oropharynx; 6 = buccal musculature; 7 = tongue; 8 = cervical vertebral centrum.)

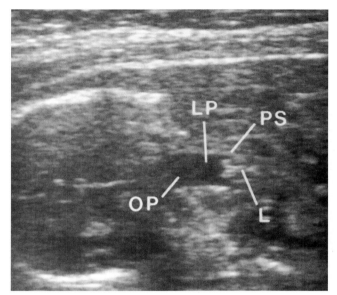

FIGURE 6–68. Coronal sonogram of the fetal hypopharynx. The fluid-filled oropharynx (OP) and laryngopharynx (LP) are well seen. Fluid slightly distends the pyriform sinuses. (L = larynx.)

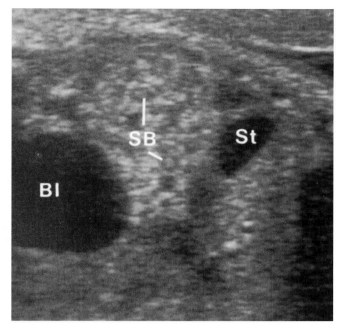

FIGURE 6–70. Small bowel (SB) in a late third-trimester fetus. (Bl = bladder; St = stomach.)

lung into the distal esophagus and from there to the stomach.[54] This inefficient method is almost universally associated with polyhydramnios in late pregnancy but does not always occur before 24 weeks. Second, the association of esophageal atresia wihout TEF, but with a second proximal GI tract atresia or obstruction, will allow secretions from the stomach to accumulate within the gastric lumen.

The stomach varies considerably in size depending, presumably, on how much amniotic fluid has been recently imbided by the fetus.[52, 53] A prominent stomach should never be taken as being sole evidence of obstruction. When well distended, the various parts of the stomach can be identified (i.e., the fundus, body, and antrum). The fundus is most posterior, whereas the antrum is most anterior. The incisura angularis can be noted when the stomach is well distended. The incisura angularis is a notch of variable depth that is usually found along the lesser curvature between the body and antrum of the stomach.[55]

The small bowel becomes progressively more visible through the second and third trimesters. Fat accumulat-ing in the small bowel mesentery during early and mid-second trimester and increased conspicuity of the submucosa begins to impart an appearance of a "conglomerate" zone of increased echogenicity in the mid- and lower abdomen of the fetus. This should not be mistaken either for an abnormal mass (pseudomass of bowel)[56-58] or for a bowel abnormality. With time, and somewhat dependent on the ease of imaging, discrete small bowel loops become visible (Fig. 6–70). As with the esophagus, the lumen tends to be brighter relative to the hypoechoic muscular wall. The serosa is again greater in echogenicity than is the muscular layer. Late in pregnancy, the deposition of small amounts of fat in the mesentery probably accentuates this feature. Ultimately, in late pregnancy, discrete small bowel containing small amounts of fluid (succus entericus) can be visualized in almost all fetuses.[59]

The colon tends to become visible near the beginning of the third trimester and, again, is seen progressively better with increasing gestational age.[59, 60] The colon tends to be relatively hypoechoic (Figs. 6–71 and 6–72).

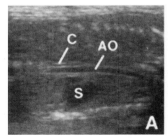 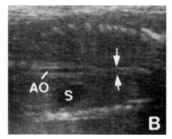 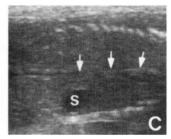

FIGURE 6–69. Three (A, B, C) coronal sonograms depict the esophagus. First (A), the descending aorta (AO) is localized. (C = diaphragmatic crura; S = stomach.) As the transducer is moved anteriorly (B and C), the esophagus (*arrows*) comes into view.

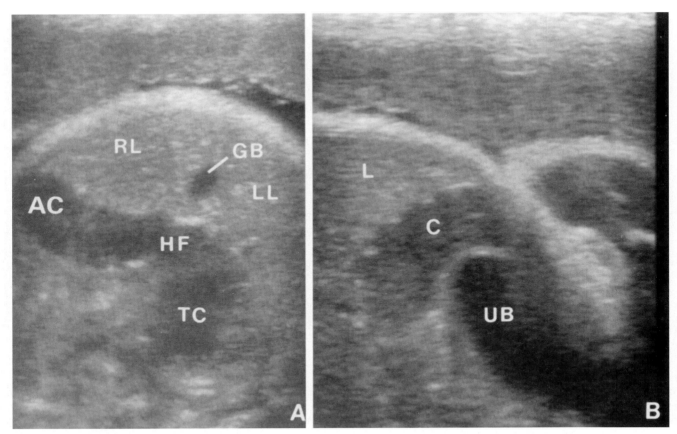

FIGURE 6–71. *A,* Transverse axial sonogram of the fetal abdomen demonstrates, by position, the ascending colon (AC) and the transverse colon (TC) with the hepatic flexure (HF) between them. (GB = gallbladder; LL = left hepatic lobe; RL = right hepatic lobe.) *B,* Off-axis coronal sonogram of the lower abdomen. The sigmoid colon (C) arches over the urinary bladder (UB). Note the haustral markings at the edge of the bowel loop. (L = liver.)

As such, the colon should not be mistaken for a dilated small bowel loop. The characteristic course of the colon most readily permits the distinction from the pathologically dilated small bowel. The ascending colon courses along the right flank (see Fig. 6–71*A*) in relation to the right kidney. As it approaches the liver it bends to the left, the hepatic flexure (see Fig. 6–71*A*). The transverse colon courses along the free edge of the liver (see Figs. 6–71*A* and 6–72*A*) and passes inferior to the stomach. At the splenic flexure the colon turns posteriorly and

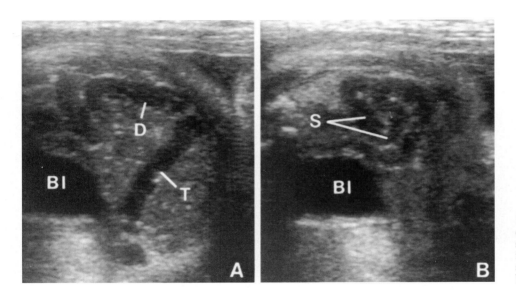

FIGURE 6–72. *A,* Coronal sonogram demonstrates the transverse (T) and descending (D) colon. The splenic flexure is not labeled. *B,* A markedly looped sigmoid colon (S) is noted. (Bl = bladder.)

again comes into intimate relationship with the kidney; of course in this case it is the left kidney. Frequently, when imaging the kidneys, the colon is detected. Indeed, when a kidney is absent, the colon occupies the renal fossa and should not be misinterpreted as being a normal or abnormal kidney. Finally, the sigmoid colon arcs over the urinary bladder to join the rectum (see Figs. 6–71B and 6–72B). Occasionally, haustral markings can be noted in the colon wall. A redundant sigmoid colon (see Fig. 6–72B) should not be mistaken for dilated small bowel.

The liver, as noted earlier, is proportionately larger in the fetus than in the child or adult.[61] Similarly, in the early second trimester, the liver constitutes 10% of the total fetal weight but is only 5% of the total weight at term. The fetal liver, in addition, has a substantially larger left lobe. Indeed, the fetal liver spans the entire width of the abdomen throughout pregnancy, and the left lobe always has contact with the left abdominal wall. This would be unusual in an adult, although this relationship can also be seen in adults.

The two major segments of each hepatic lobe can be seen in older fetuses (see Fig. 6–62) and to some extent even in early second-trimester fetuses.[43, 46] The lateral segment of the left lobe extends to the left of the umbilical segment of the left portal vein (see Figs. 6–60 and 6–61). The medial segment of the left lobe is the tissue lying between the gallbladder (or middle hepatic vein more superiorly) and the umbilical segment of the left portal vein or the intersegmental fissure more caudally (Fig. 6–73). The right lobe consists of all of the hepatic

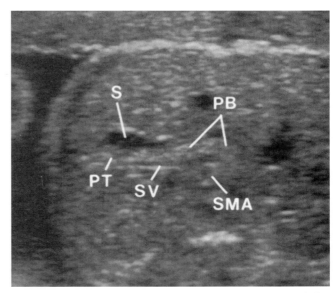

FIGURE 6–74. Fetal pancreas is not commonly seen discretely but, as shown in this unusual example, lies between the splenic vein (SV) and the posterior stomach wall (S). (PB = pancreatic body; PT = pancreatic tail; SMA = superior mesenteric artery.)

tissue lying to the right of the gallbladder, middle hepatic vein, and the inferior vena cava (see Figs. 6–56 and 6–61). These latter three structures all reside in the main lobar fissure. The left portal vein and left hepatic vein mark the left intersegmental fissure. Finally, the right intersegmental fissure is marked by the right hepatic vein cephalically and its anterior branch inferiorly.

The pancreas, as noted, is difficult to perceive at any gestational age. The pancreatic tissue lies posterior to the stomach, which is an area that can be visualized consistently in the fetus. However, discrete perception of the pancreas requires the demonstration of the splenic vein and the origin of the superior mesenteric artery in a transverse axial plane of section (Fig. 6–74). The pancreas is then the band of tissue between these vessels and the posterior gastric wall.

The spleen is not truly a GI organ (see Fig. 6–61). The spleen is bounded superiorly by the diaphragm, laterally by the lower ribs, medially by the stomach, and posteriorly by both the diaphragm and kidney. It is only the inferior margin that is difficult to delimit. In the fetus, the echogenicity of the spleen is similar to that of the liver. In the adult, the liver is slightly less echogenic than is the spleen.[62–65] The spleen grows progressively through fetal life, and nomograms of splenic size are available in the literature.[62]

Respiratory System

The upper respiratory system is seen partially. The nose has been previously illustrated (see Figs. 6–7 and 6–8). The nasal cavity, septum and palate can be detected with practice. As noted earlier, portions of the pharynx and hypopharynx are commonly visible because of the presence of fluid.[51] The pyriform sinuses are seen when

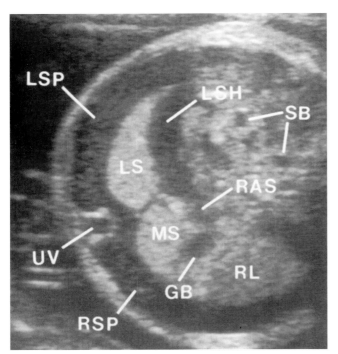

FIGURE 6–73. Axial sonogram of the fetal abdomen after an intraperitoneal transfusion of Rh isoimmunization enables recognition of many peritoneal spaces, including the right (RSP) and left (LSP) subphrenic spaces and the right anterior (RAS) and left subhepatic spaces. Segmental anatomy of the fetal liver is also well seen, including the medial (MS) and lateral (LS) segments of the left hepatic lobe. (GB = gallbladder; RL = right hepatic lobe; SB = small bowel.)

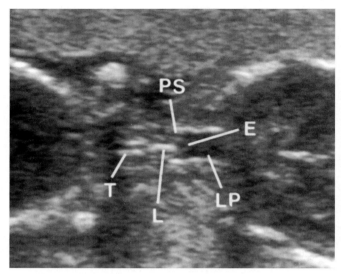

FIGURE 6–75. Fetal larynx (L) and epiglottis (E). (LP = laryngo-pharynx; PS = pyriform sinus; T = trachea.)

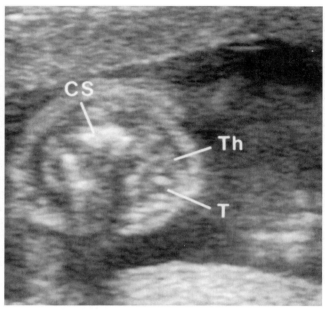

FIGURE 6–77. Transverse axial sonogram of the fetal neck. (CS = cervical spine; T = traches; Th = thyroid lobe.)

they are filled with fluid (see Fig. 6–68). When relatively large amounts of fluid are present in the pharynx of an older fetus, the epiglottis may be seen protruding into the fluid (Fig. 6–75). The epiglottis is particularly visible during swallowing.

The larynx is almost always visible when the hypopharynx is filled with fluid (see Figs. 6–68 and 6–75). Details of laryngeal anatomy are not particularly evident, but the larynx itself is easily recognized as a superior constriction of the tracheal fluid column protruding into the hypopharynx and flanked by the pyriform sinuses. If the head is markedly flexed, the overlying mandible frequently defeats efforts to visualize the larynx and hypopharynx.

The trachea is a relatively easy structure to visualize (Figs. 6–76 and 6–77; see also Fig. 6–75).[51] Again, this is predominantly due to the fact that it is consistently filled with fluid. The lungs produce fluid that is expelled into the amniotic sac via the trachea. Additionally, the

trachea, along most of its length, is flanked by the conspicuous pulsations of the common carotid arteries. The trachea can usually be traced to its distal end, passing posterior to the aortic arch (see Fig. 6–76A), but the carina and bronchi are quite difficult to perceive. Because mainstem bronchi are usually invisible, smaller ramifications of the bronchi are, for all intents and purposes, universally invisible at this time in the development of fetal sonography.

The right and left pulmonary arteries and several pulmonary veins (Fig. 6–78 see also Fig. 6–63) are visible in a large percentage of older fetuses. However, one generally pursues visualization of these major vessels during examination of the heart rather than of the lungs. Details of the pulmonary arterial and venous anatomy are found in Chapter 9.

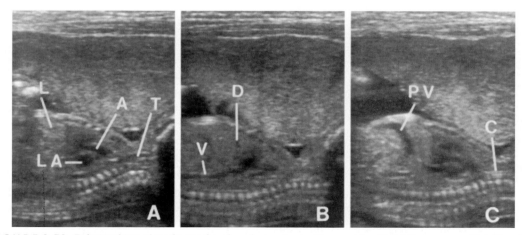

FIGURE 6–76. Relationships of mediastinal and neck structures. Three midsagittal (*A*) or parasagittal (*B* and *C*) sonograms demonstrate the trachea (T) down to the level of the aortic arch (A). The carotid (C) arteries lie adjacent to the trachea in the neck. (D = diaphragm; L = liver; LA = left atrium; PV = left portal vein; V = inferior vena cava.)

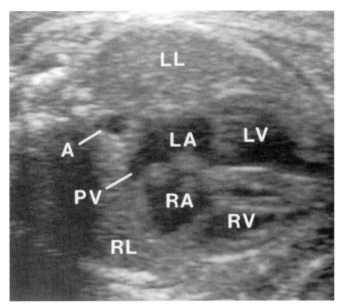

FIGURE 6–78. Transverse axial sonogram of the fetal thorax. (A = descending aorta; LA = left atrium; LL = left lung; LV = left ventricle; PV = pulmonary vein; RA = right atrium; RL = right lung; RV = right ventricle.)

The lung (at least lung tissue) can be seen from late first trimester onward. Early in pregnancy, definition of the lung is drawn more from the structures that surround it. These include, predominantly, the ribs superolaterally and the heart (and to a lesser extent other mediastinal structures) medially. Inferiorly, the early lung blends imperceptibly with the liver. These two organs may be equal in echogenicity throughout the second trimester and the early third trimester.

As pregnancy progresses, the lung becomes more echogenic than does the liver (Fig. 6–79). The reason for this is unknown. This difference may indicate pulmonary maturity, a notion that has never been proved and

that is likely to be erroneous.[66, 67] Furthermore, the muscular portion of the diaphragm becomes progressively more visible with fetal growth (Fig. 6–80). These markers of the inferior extent of the lung improve the visibility of pulmonary tissue with advancing gestational age. Discrete pulmonary lobes are not visible in the normal fetus, but when a pleural effusion is present, insinuation of fluid into the major fissures (and the minor fissure on the right) marks lobar boundaries.

Genitourinary System

Although the extreme variability of fetal positioning and the lack of subject contrast between kidney and the surrounding tissues do not permit consistent identification of both fetal kidneys, normal fetal kidneys may be identified in their paraspinous location as early as 15 to 16 menstrual weeks. Visualization does not become consistent until the 20th week.[68] In longitudinal section, fetal kidneys appear as bilateral elliptic structures. In transverse section, they have a circular appearance adjacent to the lumbar spinal ossification centers bilaterally. Later in pregnancy echogenic retroperitoneal fat, which surrounds the kidneys, assists in their sonographic visualization (Fig. 6–81; see also Fig. 6–3). The echopenic fetal renal pyramids can frequently be discriminated from the surrounding cortex and columns of Bertin in older fetuses and are arranged in an anterior and posterior row (see Fig. 6–3) in a configuration corresponding

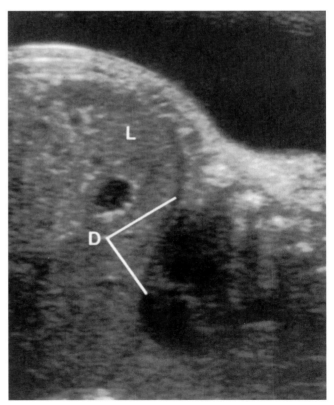

FIGURE 6–80. The muscular diaphragm (D) is relatively hypoechoic. (L = liver.)

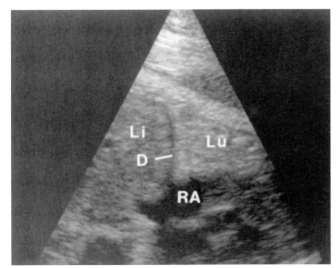

FIGURE 6–79. Echogenicity difference between the lung (Lu) and the liver (Li) in an older fetus. (D = diaphragm; RA = right atrium.)

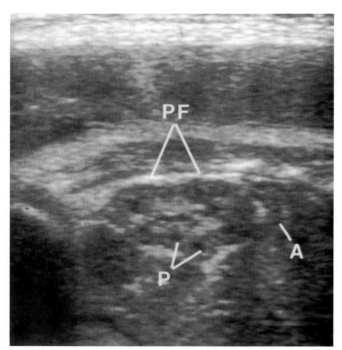

FIGURE 6–81. Sagittal sonogram of the fetal kidney marginated by perirenal fat (PF). Pyramids (P) can be discretely seen. The adrenal (A) gland caps the upper pole.

to the calices that contact the apices of the pyramids (the papillae).[69] The echotexture of the normal fetal renal cortex, which usually approximates or may even be slightly greater than that of the surrounding tissues, highlights the relatively echopenic pyramids. The characteristic position of the pyramids avoids any potential confusion with renal parenchymal cysts. Confusion with dilated calices is avoided by noting the interspaced columns of Bertin and the lack of communication with dilated infundibulae and the pelvis. Within the renal sinus of fetuses there is generally a paucity of fat. Intrarenal collecting structures, the pelvis and infundibulae, are commonly seen in fetuses because they frequently contain fluid[70, 71].

The fetal kidneys grow throughout gestation. Standards for renal length, width, thickness, volume, and circumference have been established as a function of menstrual age and correspond with measurements of renal size obtained for stillborn fetuses postnatally.[72–74] Throughout pregnancy, the ratio of kidney circumference to abdominal circumference is relatively constant at 0.27 to 0.30. Such measurements are more efficient for detecting enlarged kidneys that for small ones. Diminution in renal size is more difficult to detect because the exact renal border, especially of small kidneys, may be partially obscured, the plane of section may not be through the longest renal axis, and because of the wide standard deviation in renal size.[72–74]

The normal fetal ureter cannot be identified. Rarely, one may see a normal ureter, but visualization of a fetal ureter should always suggest pathologic dilatation. However, as early as 15 menstrual weeks the normal

fetal urinary bladder can be identified (see Fig. 6–59). Only a few cubic centimeters of bladder urine would be needed to allow ready visualization in such a young fetus. Because the fetus normally fills and empties the urinary bladder every 30 to 45 minutes, the bladder will frequently be seen to increase in size and to empty during the course of a sonographic examination.[75–77] Similarly, fetuses in whom the urinary bladder is not visualized can be examined at intervals for bladder filling. If the bladder cannot be seen in the presence of oligohydramnios, sequential imaging to test for bladder filling is mandatory.

At 32 weeks of gestation the maximum fetal bladder volume measures 10 mL. By term the normal fetal bladder volume quadruples (see Fig. 6–70). Similarly, production of fetal urine, which is calculated by a determination of the change in bladder volume with time, increases from 9.6 mL/hr at 30 weeks to 27.3 mL/hr at 40 weeks' menstrual age.[75, 76] Of course, term fetuses void, thus the bladder may be empty.[77] Filling and emptying of the fetal urinary bladder confirms that the fetus produces urine but does not indicate the "quality" of urine produced. The normal fetal urinary bladder, the wall of which is very thin and almost invisible when the bladder is well distended (see Fig. 6–70), occupies a midline position within the fetal pelvis. Changes in volume of the urinary bladder with time differentiate it from cystic pathologic pelvic structures.

The normal fetal urethra may be identified occasionally as an echogenic line that extends the length of an erect penis (see Fig. 6–13). In females and males examined at a time when the penis is flaccid, the normal urethra is difficult or impossible to identify. The uterus and ovaries cannot be visualized in normal female fetuses. The testes can be visualized in male fetuses only after they have descended into the scrotum. The prostate cannot be visualized. The external genitalia were discussed earlier in the section on superficial anatomy.

The fetal adrenal gland, although not part of the genitourinary system, is seen routinely when searching for the kidneys (Fig. 6–82; see also Fig. 6–81).[78, 79] Indeed, even in the presence of agenesis of one or both kidneys, the adrenal glands can be appreciated in their expected paraspinous locations. Lewis and associates consider that the fetal adrenal glands can be consistently imaged after 30 menstrual weeks. The adrenal glands have a specific size, shape, and echogenicity. The echo pattern is so characteristic that the cortex and medulla can be appreciated separately (see Fig. 6–55, 6–56, 6–61A, and 6–82). In the fetus, both adrenal glands cap the upper renal poles (in the adult the left adrenal gland lies more often anterior to the upper pole).[79] The right adrenal gland is seen more consistently. Its upper portion lies immediately posterior to the proximal inferior vena cava (see Fig. 6–82).

Central Nervous System

The fetal brain was one of the first areas of investigational interest in the diagnosis of fetal anomalies.[80] This was a result of two factors: the fetal head was imaged

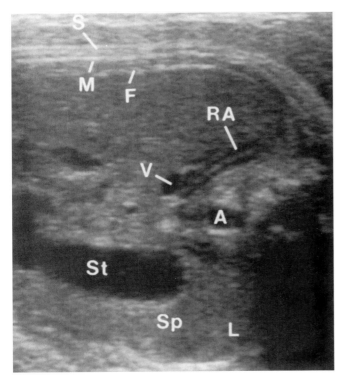

FIGURE 6–82. Sonogram of the right adrenal gland (RA), although much anatomy can be seen on this image of the upper fetal abdomen. Note both limbs of the right adrenal gland immediately posterior to the inferior vena cava (V) and a portion of the left adrenal gland (unlabeled) to the left of the aorta (A). The spleen (Sp) is well seen posterior and lateral to the stomach (St). A slight change in echogenicity discriminates the lung (L) lying above the diaphragm in the posterior costophrenic sulcus from the spleen below the diaphragm. The abdominal wall, including the subcutaneous (S) fat, muscle layers (M), and properitoneal fat (F), is well seen.

proved to the present day, many malformations of the brain can be diagnosed with accuracy, even before 20 weeks of development.[81–86]

The diagnosis of anomalous development, as always, begins with a firm grasp of normal developmental anatomy. Initially, many errors were made when interpreting normal fetal intracranial anatomy as seen by sonography.[87–89] This was due to the unusual circumstance that "fluid" and "solid" areas of the brain did not behave in an anticipated fashion. It was expected initially that the sonographic appearance of the lateral ventricles would be dominated by cerebrospinal fluid (CSF), which would render them echolucent. Instead, their appearance was dominated by highly echogenic choroid plexus (Figs. 6–83 to 6–85).[90, 91] Conversely, the bulk of neural tissue, the telencephalon, diencephalon, and mesencephalon, is quite echopenic compared with other solid tissues in the human body (see Fig. 6–83).[90, 92] The more recent entrant into the area of diagnostic sonography can well imagine the potential for misinterpretation among early researchers when the largest fluid-containing areas of the brain yielded the greatest amplitude echoes, whereas the solid tissue yielded the lowest amplitude echoes. To complicate matters even more, dramatic changes occur as the development of the brain progresses, which result in ever-changing positions of certain "landmarks." These changes had never been observed in vivo, and postmortem examination of the brain can be at variance with its appearance during life.

A series of important observations led to the clear delineation of normal developmental neuroanatomy as viewed by ultrasound. These observations included recognition of the fetal third ventricle, the brightly echogenic choroid plexus,[90] and pulsating vasculature in several cisterns.[92] The first two identified the supratentorial ventricular system. The last enabled identification of the sylvian cistern (middle cerebral artery pulsation), interpeduncular cistern (basilar artery pulsation), and ambient cisterns (posterior cerebral artery pulsations). The landmarks established by these observations provided a framework for subsequent identification of other specific neural structures.

routinely to obtain a biparietal diameter (BPD) for the determination of gestational age; and central nervous system anomalies are among the most common birth defects. At first, only gross morphologic aberrations such as anencephaly or advanced hydrocephalus were discovered prenatally. As instrumentation has im-

FIGURE 6–83. *A,* Axial scan at the level of the lateral ventricular atria. The brain parenchyma (P) is very lucent. (C = choroid plexus; IF = interhemispheric fissure.) *B,* A slightly lower scan demonstrates the well-developed thalami (T) and the midbrain (M) (27-mm BPD at 14 weeks). The frontal horns (F) are large and filled with CSF.

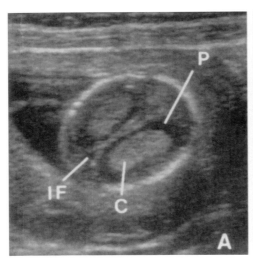

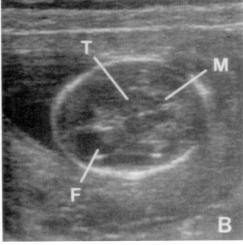

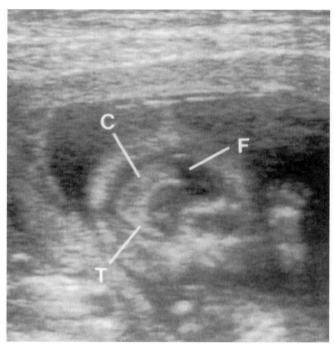

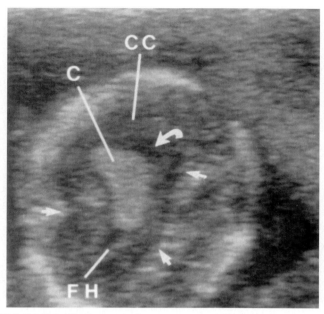

FIGURE 6–84. Parasagittal sonogram taken early in the second trimester shows choroid filling the early ventricle. The frontal horn (F) is demarcated by specular reflectors. The early temporal horn is seen (T). Note the absence of an occipital horn. Choroid (C) fills the body, atrium, and early temporal horn.

FIGURE 6–85. Parasagittal sonogram through the ventricle of an 18-week-old fetus. The choroid (C) defines the ventricular size. Note the substantial increase in cortical brain (CC) thickness compared with fetuses only a few weeks younger (see Fig. 6–84). Bright echoes marginate the edge of the telencephalon (*straight arrows*). Note the beginnings of an occipital horn (*curved arrows*). (FH = frontal horn.)

Later in the course of the development of sonography, the neonatal brain was studied (Fig. 6–86; see also Fig. 6–1).[1, 2, 91] Interestingly, this resulted in much greater understanding of the appearance of the *fetal* brain, because examination of "newborn children" now begins commonly at 25 to 26 weeks of development (essentially a second-trimester fetus). Investigators then began to apply neuroanatomy as learned from the neonatal brain, which was imaged with great clarity through the anterior fontanelle, to the developing fetal brain. The following analysis of fetal intracranial anatomy is presented on the basis of these observations.

The fetal head can be clearly discriminated from the fetal torso when an embryo reaches a crown-rump

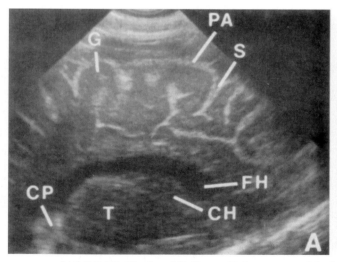

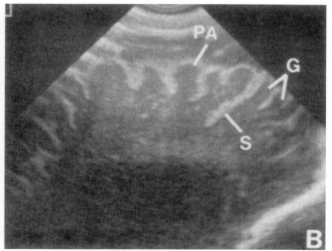

FIGURE 6–86. *A* and *B,* Parasagittal sonogram of the brain of a 6-month-old child. Gyri (G) are well developed. pia-arachnoid (PA) tissues cover the surface of the brain and make the sulci (S) highly conspicuous. Careful inspection of gyri shows that cortical gray matter is less echogenic than the white matter. (CH = caudate head; CP = choroid plexus; FH = frontal horn; T = thalamus.)

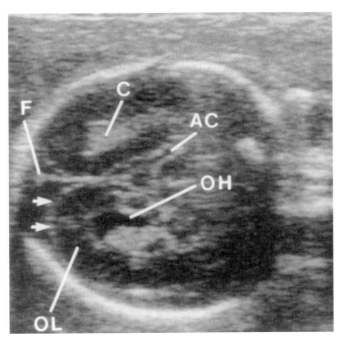

FIGURE 6–87. Transverse axial sonogram of the occipital lobes (OL) and occipital horn (OH). The brain edge is marginated by bright echoes (pia-arachnoid) (*arrows*). The cisterns over the brain surface have visible CSF. (AC = ambient cistern; C = choroid plexus; F = falx.)

is the easiest structure to recognize because of its size and high-amplitude echogenicity. Conversely, the mantle of developing cerebral cortex surrounding the lateral ventricle is more difficult to delineate because of its low-amplitude echogenicity, but a demarcation between the lateral ventricle and the cerebral mantle can be appreciated from specular reflections that arise from the walls of the lateral ventricle (see Fig. 6–84). These reflections, of course, are seen where the acoustic beam intersects the ventricular wall perpendicularly. By 18 weeks the mantle of developing cortical tissue has thickened appreciably (compare Figs. 6–84 and 6–85).

The relative echogenicity of structures, which is seen throughout the remainder of gestation, is established at this time. Two types of tissue are brightly echogenic and are, therefore, most easily seen during the examination of the fetal brain. These tissues are the choroid plexus, as noted earlier, and the brain covering: the dura (*pachymeninx*) and pia-arachnoid (*leptomeninx*). Interestingly, the choroid develops from vascular pia. The leptomeninges demarcate the edges of the brain with a brightly reflective margin of echoes (Fig. 6–87; see also Fig. 6–86). Peripheral to this echogenic margin are the subarachnoid spaces that contain CSF (Fig. 6–88; see also Fig. 6–87). A feature that confounds the inexperienced sonologist is the relative lack of change in echogenicity

length of approximately 10 to 16 mm. By the 10th to 11th weeks after the last normal menstrual period, one can already begin to appreciate symmetric anatomy inside of the developing fetal calvaria. At this time, the intracranial tissue components consist almost entirely of the thalamus and corpus striatum, which yield the symmetric appearance of the brain as these structures narrow the developing third ventricle into a midline specular reflector.

By the end of the first trimester, the thalamus, third ventricle, midbrain, brain stem, and cerebellar hemispheres have achieved an appearance that remains largely unchanged, other than progressive enlargement, throughout the remaining period of sonographic observation of the fetus (see Fig. 6–83). Therefore, most of the changes that are observed (and they are substantial) relate to the growth and development of the telencephalon. As mentioned, by the end of the first and the beginning of the second trimesters, the sonographic appearance of the telencephalon is dominated by the lateral ventricles (see Figs. 6–83A, 6–84, and 6–85), which, in turn, are dominated by the brightly echogenic choroid plexus. By 12 to 13 weeks, the lateral ventricles can be clearly seen, appear ovoid in shape, and are filled mainly with choroid plexus. Only the frontal horns are devoid of choroid plexus, as they are throughout life (see Figs. 6–83B, 6–84, and 6–86). At this stage of development, only the rudiments of a temporal horn (see Fig. 6–84) and no occipital horn (see Fig. 6–85) are present. The frontal horn, the body of the ventricle, and the atrium of the ventricle are large and easily detected. The choroid

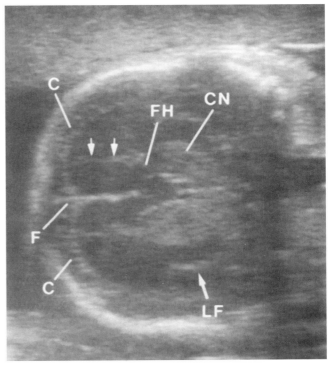

FIGURE 6–88. Coronal section through the heads of the caudate nuclei (CN). The frontal horn (FH), which is not well seen, drapes over the caudate. Extending between the ventricular margin and the edge of the brain are linear echoing structures that were previously mistaken for ventricles (*arrows*). Also seen are bridging strands of pia-arachnoid through the cistern (C) over the convexities (probably bridging veins covered with pia-arachnoid). (F = falx; LF = lateral fissure.)

between the peripheral (i.e., cortical brain) tissue and the CSF space, such as that seen across the brightly reflecting marginal echo from the pia-arachnoid (indeed, the CSF-containing space may be more echogenic) (Fig. 6–89; see also Fig. 6–88). This perceptual problem originates from the anticipation that the subarachnoid spaces should be anechoic whereas the brain parenchyma should be echogenic. This reasonable assumption is untrue in many cases. These spaces have both CSF and pia-arachnoid tissue within them. *It is the relative amount of these two components that determines the sonographic appearance of the subarachnoid spaces.* Small subarachnoid cisterns (e.g., the basal and perimesencephalic cisterns) have an appearance dominated by pia-arachnoid and thus are seen as brightly echogenic spaces (see Fig. 6–89). This is not to say that these cisterns are devoid of CSF, but the fluid does not significantly influence their sonographic appearance. Conversely, larger subarachnoid spaces, such as those over the convexities of the hemispheres (see Fig. 6–87) and the cisterna magna (see Fig. 6–89), have an appearance dominated by CSF. Thus, they behave, in the sonographic sense, as one would anticipate for a fluid-containing cavity. Intermediate-sized subarachnoid spaces have both anechoic zones from visible CSF and brightly echogenic zones from visible pia-arachnoid tissues (Fig. 6–90A).

As noted earlier, brightly reflecting structures dominate the appearance of the fetal brain as seen by the sonologist. The choroid plexus and brain coverings (pia-arachnoid and dura) are the two major components within the developing calvaria that produce bright reflections. The important dural structures from the perspective of sonographic fetal brain anatomy are the falx

and tentorium (see Fig. 6–88 to 6–90). Specular reflections from the walls of the ventricular system are also important as high-amplitude echoing structures (see Figs. 6–84 and 6–87). Such reflections occur when the ultrasonic beam strikes the smooth ventricular wall perpendicularly or almost perpendicularly. Thus, one would assume that points and lines of brightness produced in this way might vary from one moment to another, depending on the direction in which the transducer was pointed. This, however, is not the case for two reasons. First, fetal brain images are produced predominantly in axial planes (appropriate for both BPD and head circumference measurements) and less commonly in coronal planes. In both of these planes, the beam tends to intersect the ventricular system perpendicularly at the same interfaces. Second, the curvature of the bony calvaria limits the number of axial and coronal planes that can be achieved due to significant beam divergence when curved portions of calvaria are intersected by the beam. Thus, the specular reflections from the ventricular walls tend to be seen in stable locations and can be used as important and reproducible anatomic landmarks.

Additionally, within the substance of the brain, most notably in the region of the tracts of the cerebral white matter, other bright reflections are noted (see Figs. 6–88 to 6–90). Earlier, these reflectors were mistaken for the lateral ventricular walls with which they are contiguous.[89, 92, 93] These reflections originate from the deep medullary veins which drain blood from the periventricular white matter. The vessels have a sheath of pia which results in the high-amplitude signals they return.

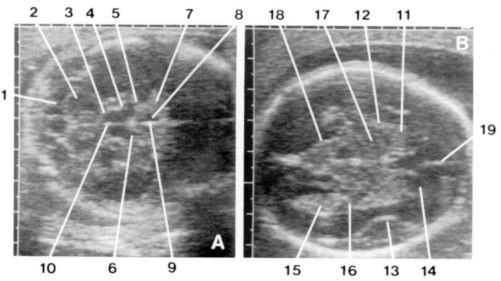

FIGURE 6–89. *A* and *B,* Transverse axial sonograms demonstrating many discrete neural structures. Note the varying echogenicities of the cisterns. Large cisterns (1 = cisterna magna) have an appearance dominated by CSF. Small cisterns (7 = basal cisterns) are dominated by a pia-arachnoid. (2 = cerebellar hemisphere; 3 = quadrigeminal cistern; 4 = ambient cistern; 5 = crural cistern; 6 = interpeduncular cistern [note the walls of basilar artery centrally in this cistern]: 8 = hypothalamus; 9 = inferior recess of the third ventricle; 10 = sylvian aqueduct; 11 = head of caudate; 12 = lentiform nuclei; 13 = lateral fissure; 14 = frontal horn; 15 = atrial choroid; 16 = posterior limb of internal capsule; 17 = thalamus; 18 = tentorial hiatus; 19 = falx.)

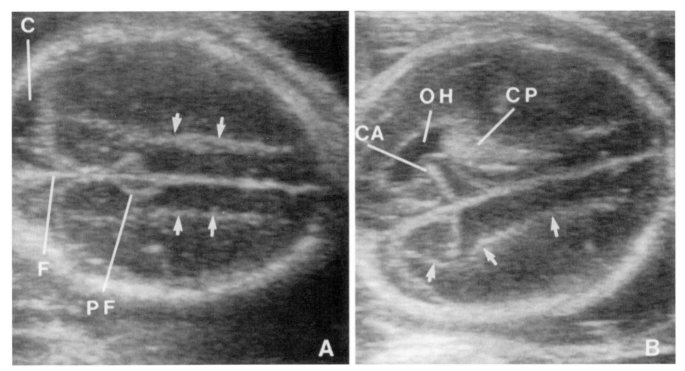

FIGURE 6–90. *A,* Transverse axial sonogram near the vertex. Bright linear echoes (*arrows*) often mistaken for lateral ventricles are clearly seen. Note that these echoes extend to the edge of the brain. (C = convexity cistern with CSF and hair-like bridging veins covered by brightly echogenic pia-arachnoid; F = falx; PF = parieto-occipital fissure.) *B,* Off-axis scan through both the lateral ventricle and the linear echo (*arrow*) seen in Figure 6–90A. The occipital horn (OH) is now well seen. Note again that the linear echo extends to the brain edge, whereas the occipital horn is entirely marginated by brain tissue. (CA = calcar avis; CP = choroid.)

Brightly Reflective Structures in the Developing Fetal Brain

1. Choroid plexus
2. Brain coverings
   a. Pia-arachnoid (leptomeninges)
   b. Dura (pachymeninges)
3. Specular reflections from ventricular walls

The sonographic "skeleton" of the developing fetal brain originates from the brightly reflective structures just considered. By using these structures as the framework, numerous discrete neural tissue areas can be discerned sonographically (Figs. 6–91 to 6–95; see also Fig. 6–89).[1, 2] As the brain develops, multiple areas of the telencephalon, diencephalon, midbrain, pons, and cerebellum become anatomically identifiable. These are recognized by variations in the echogenicity of specific nuclei and tracts that pass through these zones. Several brain nuclei, as well as some other areas of neural tissue, demonstrate a moderate increase in echo amplitude compared with surrounding brain elements. These nuclei demonstrate lower amplitude signals than do choroid or leptomeninges. Among these structures are the caudate and lenticular nuclei, which are separated by the internal capsule. Less commonly, the claustrum, marginated by the extreme and external capsules, is visible. Similarly, the substantia nigra in the midbrain and dentate nuclei of the cerebellum can be discerned.

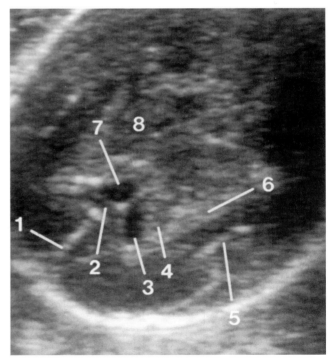

FIGURE 6–91. Transverse axial sonogram. (1 = falx; 2 = corpus callosum; 3 = frontal horn; 4 = caudate nucleus; 5 = lateral fissure; 6 = lentiform nuclei; 7 = cavum septi pellucidi; 8 = thalamus.)

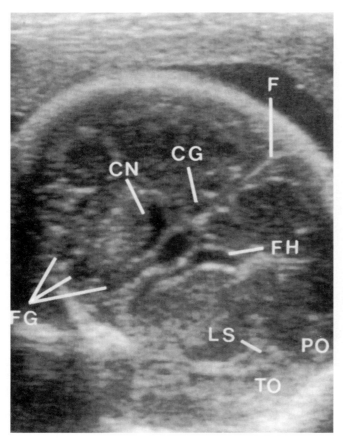

FIGURE 6–92. Coronal sonogram, anteriorly.

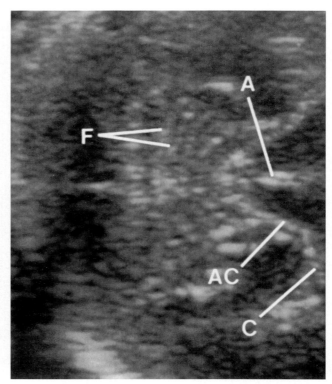

FIGURE 6–94. Posterior fossa view (axial) demonstrating folla (F) of the cerebellum. (A = sylvian aqueduct; AC = ambient cistern; C = choroidal fissure.)

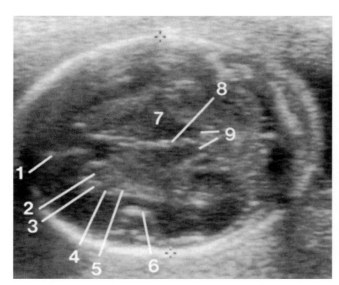

FIGURE 6–93. Transverse axial sonogram. (1 = falx; 2 = frontal horn; 3 = caudate head; 4 = anterior limb of internal capsule; 5 = lentiform nuclei; 6 = lateral sulcus; 7 = thalamus; 8 = third ventricle; 9 = quadrigeminal bodies.)

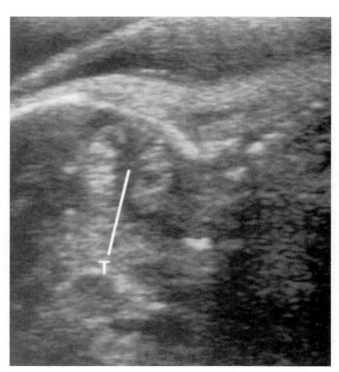

FIGURE 6–95. Parasagittal sonogram of the posterior fossa. Cerebellar white matter tracts (T) are well seen. Bright margin is most likely due to reflections from pia-arachnoid drawn into the cerebellum by folia formation. (Gray matter is hypoechoic.)

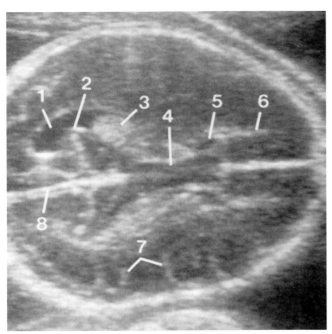

FIGURE 6–96. Transverse axial sonogram. (1 = occipital horn; 2 = calcar avis; 3 = atrial choroid; 4 = corpus callosum; 5 = frontal horn; 6 = linear echo in white matter [see Figs. 6–88 and 6–90A]; 7 = sulci; 8 = falx.)

The pars ventralis (belly) of the pons is also seen as a zone of moderate echogenicity, compared with the pars dorsalis (tegmentum) that returns low-amplitude echoes.[1]

It is important for sonologists to be familiar with the appearance of the lateral ventricles as they change throughout growth and development of the fetal brain. By 18 to 20 weeks, easily recognizable occipital horns and temporal horns are visible. The lateral ventricles have achieved their adult components. From this point onward, the lateral ventricles change in shape and proportion. They are reshaped by neural tissues growing adjacent to their walls. For example, the growth of the caudate nucleus markedly reshapes the lateral ventricles.[94] However, throughout the period of observation of fetal lateral ventricles (from 13 to 40 weeks), the size of the atria remains largely unchanged. The transverse diameter of the ventricular atrium at the level of the glomus of the choroid plexus shows an average dimension of 6 to 7 mm and a range of 5 to 10 mm throughout the second and third trimesters.[95] This is the most convenient area to recognize fetal ventricular enlargement, which is discussed in detail in the section on ventriculomegaly.[90, 91, 95] It is important to note that the anterior and occipital horns of the lateral ventricles do not possess choroid plexus. Between 24 weeks and term, the telencephalon undergoes little structural change other than increased cortical growth and the consequent increase in convolutions (and thus sulcal markings) that can be recognized adjacent to the convexities (Fig. 6–96).[96] The increase in brain volume causes the lateral ventricles, which are more stable in volume, to become progressively less conspicuous.

Compared with sulci, which are narrow and develop later as gyri form, fissures are present earlier in development and can be seen prior to 20 weeks. Of the two that are commonly seen, the parieto-occipital fissure is smaller and is less important (see Fig. 6–90). The lateral fissure is a deep groove in the margin of the developing telencephalon.[95, 97, 98] This important fissure results in frequent confusion, because it causes a portion of the brain surface to be invaginated deeply into the hemisphere (see Figs. 6–88, 6–89, and 6–93). The pia-arachnoid on the surface of the insula, the tissue at the base of the lateral fissure, generates a curvilinear reflection that appears to lie within the brain substance rather than at its "edge." This echo is often mistaken for a specular reflection from the lateral wall of the lateral ventricle, which is an error that leads to the misdiagnosis of hydrocephalus. With progressive growth of the temporal and parietal lobes, this fissure progressively closes and buries the previously exposed insular cortex behind the developing temporal and parietal opercula (see Fig. 6–92). By term (38 to 42 weeks), the lateral fissure closes and ultimately becomes the sylvian cistern complex.

One of the difficulties in mastering the sonographic anatomy of intracranial structures is the usual inability to see both hemispheres of the brain symmetrically.[99] The hemisphere nearest to the transducer is almost always "clouded" over by reverberation artifacts generated as the acoustic beam passes through the near calvarial wall. Calvarial ossification appears to be at the root of this artifact because the artifact is greatly reduced in fetuses with recessive osteogenesis imperfecta or other bone dysplasias wherein calvarial ossification is almost absent (Fig. 6–97). Unfortunately, essentially all other

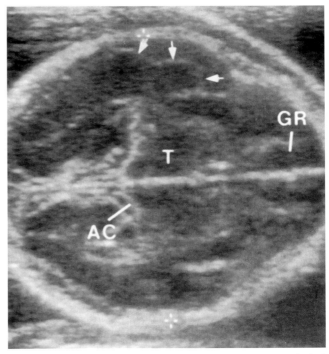

FIGURE 6–97. Transverse axial sonogram of a fetus with little calcification of the calvaria (recessive osteogenesis imperfecta). Note the lack of near-calvarial reverberation artifact. (*arrows* = near edge of temporal lobe; AC = ambient cistern; GR = gyrus rectus; T = thalamus.)

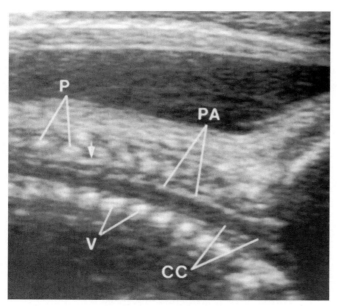

FIGURE 6–98. Longitudinal sonogram at the craniocervical junction demonstrating the cervical cord (CC). (*arrow* = dura; P = posterior arch ossification centers; PA = pia-arachnoid; V = vertebral body ossification centers.)

fetuses possess calvarial ossification. The following rule should always be applied: *The sonologist must assume that a fetus' intracranial anatomy is symmetric, whether normal or abnormal, unless images document an asymmetry.*

As noted earlier, the fetal spine is seen well from 15 to 16 weeks onward. However, evaluation for suspected myelomeningocele is often delayed until 18 to 22 weeks of gestation. This is due to significant and favorable maturational changes in the spine that occur during this period. The posterior ossification centers begin at the base of the transverse processes (see Figs. 6–48 to 6–54). As ossification progresses, the laminae become visible (see Figs. 6–49 to 6–51 and 6–54). The inward angulation of the normal laminae is the opposite of the outward splaying of the laminae that is seen in spina bifida, an optimal situation for detecting this anomaly. Spina bifida, of course, is the bony anomaly seen in all myelomeningoceles. The spinal cord neural tissue, like that of most brain tissue, is echopenic (see Fig. 6–54). The conus medullaris (see Fig. 6–54*D*) and the craniocervical junction (Fig. 6–98) can be seen, albeit inconsistently, in older fetuses. The tissues surrounding the cord (leptomeninges) are brightly echogenic, as are those that surround the brain, and the dura is usually also seen discretely as a linear bright reflector (see Fig. 6–54*C* and *D*).

REFERENCES

1. Yousefzadeh DK, Naidich TP: US anatomy of the posterior fossa in children: Correlation with brain sections. Radiology 156:353, 1985.
2. Naidich TP, Gusnard DA, Yousefzadeh DK: Sonography of the internal capsule and basal ganglia in infants. 1: coronal sections. AJNR Am J Neuroradiol 6:909, 1985.
3. Filly RA, Callen PW: Ultrasonographic evaluation of normal fetal anatomy. *In* Sanders R, James E (eds): Ultrasonography in Obstetrics and Gynecology, 2nd ed. New York: Appleton-Century-Crofts, 1980.
4. Mahony BS, Filly RA: High-resolution sonographic assessment of the fetal extremities. J Ultrasound Med 3:489, 1984.
5. Cooperberg PL, Chow T, Kite V, et al: Biparietal diameter: A comparison of real-time and conventional B-scan techniques. J Clin Ultrasound 4:421, 1976.
6. Docher MF, Sellatree RS: Comparison between linear array, real-time ultrasonic scanning and conventional compound scanning in the measurement of the fetal biparietal diameter. Br J Obstet Gynecol 84:924, 1977.
7. Johnson ML, Reese GK, Hattan RA: Normal fetal anatomy. *In* Callen PW (ed): Ultrasonography in Obstetrics and Gynecology. Philadelphia: WB Saunders Company, 1983.
8. Bowle JD, Rosenberg ER, Andreotti MD, et al: The changing sonographic appearance of the fetal kidneys during pregnancy. J Ultrasound Med 2:505, 1983.
9. Bimholz JC: The fetal external ear. Radiology 147:819, 1983.
10. Fink IJ, Chinn DH, Callen PW: A potential pitfall in the ultrasonographic diagnosis of fetal encephalocele. J Ultrasound Med 2:313, 1983.
11. Elejalde BR, de Elejalde MM, Heitman T: Visualization of the fetal genitalia by ultrasonography: A review of the literature and analysis of its accuracy and ethical implications. J Ultrasound Med 4:633, 1985.
12. Bimholz JC: Determination of fetal sex. N Engl J Med 309:942, 1983.
13. Natsuyama E: Sonographic determination of fetal sex from 12 weeks of gestation. Am J Obstet Gynecol 149:748, 1984.
14. Mahony BS, Filly RA, Callen PW: Amnionicity and chorionicity in twin pregnancies: Prediction using ultrasound. Radiology 155:205, 1985.
15. Filly RA, Golbus MS: Ultrasonography of the normal and pathologic fetal skeleton. Radiol Clin North Am 20:311, 1982.
16. Filly RA, Golbus MS, Carey JC, et al: Short-limbed dwarfism: Ultrasonic diagnosis by mensuration of fetal femoral length. Radiology 138:653, 1981.
17. O'Brien GB, Queenan JT, Campbell S: Assessment of gestation age in the second trimester by real-time ultrasound measurement of the femur length. Am J Obstet Gynecol 139:540, 1981.
18. Jeanty P, Kirkpatrick C, Dramaix-Wilmet M, et al: Ultrasonic evaluation of fetal limb growth. Radiology 140:165, 1981.
19. O'Rahilly R, Meyer DB: Roentgenographic investigation of the human skeleton during early fetal life. AJR Am J Roentgenol 76:455, 1956.
20. Bagnall KM, Harris PF, James RM: A radiographic study of the human fetal spine. 2: The sequence of development of ossification centers in the vertebral column. J Anat 124:791, 1977.
21. Filly RA, Simpson GF, Linkowsid G: Fetal spine morphology and maturation during the second trimester: Sonographic evaluation. J Ultrasound Med 6:631, 1987.
22. Abrams SL, Filly RA: Curvature of the fetal femur: A normal sonographic finding. Radiology 156:490, 1985.
23. Yarkonis J, Schmidt W, Jeanty P, et al: Clavicular measurement: A new biometric parameter for fetal evaluation. J Ultrasound Med 4:467, 1985.
24. Jeanty P, Romero R, d'Alton M, et al: In utero sonographic detection of hand and foot deformities. J Ultrasound Med 4:595, 1985.
25. Bemacerraf BR, Frigoletto FD: Prenatal ultrasound diagnosis of clubfoot. Radiology 155:211, 1985.
26. Hashimoto BE, Filly RA, Callen PW: Sonographic diagnosis of clubfoot in utero. J Ultrasound Med 5:81, 1986.
27. Chinn DH, Bolding DB, Callen PW, et al: Ultrasonographic identification of fetal lower extremity epiphyseal ossification centers. Radiology 147:815, 1983.
28. Mahony BS, Callen PW, Filly RA: The distal femoral epiphyseal ossification center in the assessment of third trimester menstrual age: Sonographic identification and measurement. Radiology 155:201, 1985.
29. Goldstein RB, Filly RA, Simpson G: Pitfalls in femur length measurement. J Ultrasound Med 6:203, 1987.
30. Jeanty P, Cantraine F, Cousaert E, et al: The binocular distance: A new way to estimate fetal age. J Ultrasound Med 3:241, 1984.
31. Dennis MA, Drose JA, Pretorius DH, Manco-Johnson ML: Normal fetal sacrum simulating spina bifida: Pseudodysraphism. Radiology 155:751, 1985.
32. Abrams SL, Filly RA: Congenital vertebral malformations: Prenatal diagnosis using ultrasonography. Radiology 155:762, 1985.

33. Birnholz JC: Fetal lumbar spine: Measuring axial growth with ultrasound. Radiology 158:805, 1986.

34. Hashimoto BE, Mahony BS, Filly RA, et al: Sonography, a complementary examination of alpha-fetoprotein testing for neural tube defects. J Ultrasound Med 4:307, 1985.

35. Brown BS: The prenatal diagnosis of osteogenesis imperfecta lethalis. J Can Assoc Radiol 35:63, 1984.

36. Kousseff BG, Mulivor RA: Prenatal diagnosis of hypophosphatasia. Obstet Gynecol 57:9, 1981.

37. Merz E, Goldhofer W: Sonographic diagnosis of lethal osteogenesis imperfecta in the second trimester: Case report and review. J Clin Ultrasound 14:380, 1986.

38. Mahony BS, Filly RA, Cooperberg PL: Antenatal sonographic diagnosis of achondrogenesis. J Ultrasound Med 3:333, 1984.

39. Rosenthal SJ, Filly RA, Callen PW, et al: Fetal pseudoascites. Radiology 131:195, 1979.

40. Hashimoto BE, Filly RA, Callen PW: Fetal pseudoascites: Further observations. J Ultrasound Med 5:151, 1986.

41. Daffos F: Fetal blood sampling under ultrasound guidance. In Harrison MR, Golbus MS, Filly RA (eds): The Unborn Patient: Prenatal Diagnosis and Treatment, 2nd ed. Philadelphia, WB Saunders Company, 1990.

42. Moore KL: The Placenta and Fetal Membranes. The Developing Human: Clinically Oriented Embryology, 4th ed. Philadelphia, WB Saunders Company, 1988.

43. Chinn DH, Filly RA, Callen PW: Ultrasonic evaluation of fetal umbilical and hepatic vascular anatomy. Radiology 144:153, 1982.

44. Barron DH: The changes in the fetal circulation at birth. Physiol Rev 24:277, 1944.

45. Emery JL: Functional asymmetry of the liver. Ann NY Acad Sci 111:37, 1963.

46. Marks WM, Filly RA, Callen PW: Ultrasonic anatomy of the liver: A review with new applications. J Clin Ultrasound 7:137, 1979.

47. Gupta SC, Gupta CD, Arora AK: Intrahepatic branching patterns of portal veins: A study by corrosion cast. Gastroenterology 72:621, 1977.

48. Rosen MS, Reich SB: Umbilical venous catheterization in the newborn: Identification of correct positioning. Radiology 95:335, 1970.

49. Hattan RA, Rees GK, Johnson ML: Normal fetal anatomy. Radiol Clin North Am 20:271, 1982.

50. Goldstein RB, Callen PW: Ultrasound evaluation of the fetal thorax and abdomen. In Callen PW (ed): Ultrasonography in Obstetrics and Gynecology, 2nd ed. Philadelphia, WB Saunders Company, 1988.

51. Cooper C, Mahony BS, Bowie JD, et al: Ultrasound evaluation of the normal fetal upper airway and esophagus. J Ultrasound Med 4:343, 1985.

52. Pritchard JA: Fetal swallowing and amniotic fluid volume. Obstet Gynecol 28:606, 1966.

53. Abramovich DR: Fetal factors influencing the volume and composition of liquor amnii. J Obstet Gynecol Br Commonw 77:865, 1970.

54. Pretorius DH, Meier PR, Johnson ML: Diagnosis of esophageal atresia in utero. J Ultrasound Med 2:475, 1983.

55. Gross BH, Filly RA: Potential for a normal fetal stomach to simulate the sonographic "double bubble" sign. J Can Assoc Radiol 33:39, 1982.

56. Grand RJ, Watkins JB, Torti FM: Development of the human gastrointestinal tract. Gastroenterology 70:790, 1976.

57. Manco LG, Nunan FA, Sohnen H, et al: Fetal small bowel simulating abdominal mass at sonography. J Clin Ultrasound 14:404, 1986.

58. Fakhry J, Reiser M, Shapiro LR, et al: Increased echogenicity in the lower fetal abdomen: A common normal variant in the second trimester. J Ultrasound Med 5:489, 1986.

59. Zilianti M, Fernandez A: Correlation of ultrasonic images of fetal intestine with gestational age and fetal maturity. Obstet Gynecol 62:569, 1983.

60. Nygerg DA, Mack LA, Patten RM, et al: Fetal bowel, normal sonographic findings. J Ultrasound Med 6:3, 1987.

61. Crelin ES: Functional anatomy of the newborn. New Haven, Yale University Press, 1973, pp 47–69.

62. Schmidt W, Yarkoni S, Jeanty P, et al: Sonographic measurements of the fetal spleen: Clinical implications. J Ultrasound Med 4:667, 1985.

63. Potter EL: Pathology of the fetus and infant. Chicago, Yearbook Medical Publishers, 1961, p 14.

64. Gruenwald P, Minh HN: Evaluation of body and organ weights in perinatal pathology. Am J Clin Pathol 34:247, 1960.

65. Mittlestaedt CA: Ultrasound of the spleen. Semin Ultrasound 2:233, 1981.

66. Fried AM, Loh FK, Umer MA, et al: Echogenicity of fetal lung: Relation to fetal age and maturity. AJR 145:591, 1985.

67. Gayea PD, Grant DC, Doubilet PM, et al: Prediction of fetal lung maturity: Inaccuracy of study using conventional ultrasound instruments. Radiology 155:473, 1985.

68. Lawson TL, Foley WD, Berland LL, et al: Ultrasonic evaluation of fetal kidneys: Analysis of normal size and frequency of visualization as related to stage of pregnancy. Radiology 138:153, 1981.

69. Bowie JD, Rosenberg ER, Andreotti MD, et al: The changing sonographic appearance of fetal kidneys during pregnancy. J Ultrasound Med 2:505, 1983.

70. Hoddick WK, Filly RA, Mahony BS, Callen PW: Minimal fetal renal pyelectasis. J Ultrasound Med 4:85, 1985.

71. Arger PH, Coleman BG, Mintz MD, et al: Routine fetal genitourinary tract screening. Radiology 156:485, 1985.

72. Grannum P, Bracken M, Silverman R, et al: Assessment of fetal kidney size in normal gestation by comparison of ratio of kidney circumference. Am J Obstet Gynecol 136:249, 1980.

73. Jeanty P, Dramaix-Wilmet M, Elkhazen N: Measurement of fetal kidney growth on ultrasound. Radiology 144:159, 1982.

74. Bertagnoli L, Lalatta F, Gallicchio MD, et al: Quantitative characterization of the growth of the fetal kidney. J Clin Ultrasound 11:349, 1983.

75. Wladimiroff JW, Campbell S: Fetal urine-production rates in normal and complicated pregnancy. Lancet 1:151, 1974.

76. Campbell S, Wladimiroff JW, Dewhurst CJ: The antenatal measurement of fetal urine production. J Obstet Gynecol Br Commonw 80:680, 1973.

77. Chamberlain P, Manning FA, Morrison I, et al: Circadian rhythm in bladder volumes in the term human fetus. Obstet Gynecol 64:657, 1984.

78. Rosenberg ER, Bowie JD, Andreotti RF, et al: Sonographic evaluation of fetal adrenal glands. AJR 139:1145, 1982.

79. Co S, Filly RA: Normal fetal adrenal gland location. J Ultrasound Med 5:117, 1986.

80. Goldberg BB, Isard HJ, Gershon-Cohen J, et al: Ultrasonic fetal cephalometry. Radiology 87:328, 1966.

81. Hidalgo H, Bowie J, Rosenberg ER, et al: In utero sonographic diagnosis of fetal cerebral anomalies. AJR 139:143, 1982.

82. Fiske CE, Filly RA: Ultrasound evaluation of the normal and abnormal fetal neural axis. Radiol Clin North Am 20:285, 1982.

83. Pasto ME, Kurtz AB: The prenatal examination of the fetal cranium, spine, and central nervous system. Semin Ultrasound CT MR 5:170, 1984.

84. Filly RA: Ultrasonography. In Harrison MR, Golbus MS, Filly RA (eds): The Unborn Patient: Prenatal Diagnosis and Treatment, 1st ed. Orlando, Grune & Stratton, 1984, pp 33–123.

85. Carrasco CR, Stierman ED, Harnsberger HR, Lee TG: An algorithm for prenatal ultrasound diagnosis of congenital CNS abnormalities. J Ultrasound Med 4:163, 1985.

86. Edwards MSD, Filly RA: Diagnosis and management of fetal disorders of the central nervous system. In Hoffman HJ, Epstein F (eds): Disorders of the Developing Nervous System: Diagnosis and Treatment. Boston, Blackwell Scientific Publications, 1986, pp 55–73.

87. Young GB: The arrow pattern: A new anatomical fetal biparietal diameter. Radiology 137:445, 1980.

88. Jeanty P, Chervenak FA, Romero R, et al: The Sylvian fissure: A commonly mislabeled cranial landmark. J Ultrasound Med 3:15, 1984.

89. Denkhaus H, Winseberg F: Ultrasonic measurement of the fetal ventricular system. Radiology 131:781, 1979.

90. Chinn DH, Callen PW, Filly RA: The lateral cerebral ventricle in early second trimester. Radiology 148:529, 1983.

91. Fiske CE, Filly RA, Callen PW: The normal choroid plexus; ultrasonographic appearance of the neonatal head. Radiology 141:467, 1981.

92. Johnson ML, Dunne MG, Mack LA, Rashbaum CL: Evaluation of fetal intracranial anatomy by static and real-time ultrasound. J Clin Ultrasound 8:311, 1980.

93. Jeanty P, Dramaix-Wilmet M, Delbeke D, et al: Ultrasonic evaluation of fetal ventricular growth. Neuroradiology 21:127, 1981.
94. Day WR: Casts of the foetal lateral ventricles. Brain 82:109, 1959.
95. Seidler DE, Filly RA: Relative growth of the higher fetal brain structures. J Ultrasound Med 6:573, 1987.
96. Worthen NJ, Gilbertson V, Lau C: Cortical sulcal development seen on sonography: Relationship to gestational parameters. J Ultrasound Med 5:153, 1986.
97. Pilu G, DePalma L, Romero R, et al: The fetal subarachnoid cisterns: An ultrasound study with report of a case of congenital communicating hydrocephalus. J Ultrasound Med 5:365, 1986.
98. Laing FC, Stamler CE, Jeffrey RB: Ultrasonography of the fetal subarachnoid space. J Ultrasound Med 2:29, 1983.
99. Reuter KL, D'Orsi CJ, Raptopoulos VD, et al: Sonographic pseudo-asymmetry of the prenatal cerebral hemispheres. J Ultrasound Med 1:91, 1982.

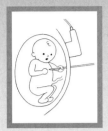

7

Sonography for Fetal Thoracic Intervention

BRYAN J. GUSHIKEN and ROY A. FILLY

Fetal surgery for thoracic masses has now been performed for more than a decade. Three chest anomalies are considered to be appropriate for consideration for in utero surgical correction. These are congenital diaphragmatic hernia (CDH), congenital cystic adenomatoid malformation (CCAM), and pulmonary sequestration. Each of these abnormalities can produce an intrathoracic mass of sufficient size to cause life-threatening pulmonary hypoplasia, hydrops fetalis, or both.[1] These lesions differ dramatically in the likelihood that they will produce life-threatening disease. Each has a different natural history. It is common for CDH to produce pulmonary hypoplasia and rare for a sequestration to do so even though both commonly present as a large intrathoracic fetal mass.[1] Sonography plays a pivotal role in the preoperative assessment of etiology and prognosis. It provides invaluable intraoperative assistance and is the most important tool in postoperative monitoring.

Advances in sonography now allow accurate prenatal diagnosis of CDH,[2-4] CCAM,[5] and pulmonary sequestration.[5] Given the dismal prognosis associated with certain cases of these pathologies in the newborn, recent therapy has focused on fetal intervention for a select few.[2, 6-8] Once the prenatal diagnosis is made, families currently may choose between termination, postnatal management, or fetal intervention. In order to provide families with as much information as possible, sonography has focused on accurate characterization of these thoracic masses and identification of potential prognostic findings. This chapter will also describe sonography's role in the operative setting and in postoperative monitoring of the fetus.

Congenital Diaphragmatic Hernia

Diagnosis and Evaluation

CDH occurs in approximately 1 per 2,000 to 3,000 births.[9] CDH results from embryologic failure to completely form the diaphragm with resultant herniation of abdominal viscera into the thorax.[1] While the diaphragmatic defect is a relatively simple and easily correctable defect, mortality remains high (approximately 58%) even with optimal postnatal care.[10] The true mortality is probably higher due to the substantial "hidden mortality," comprised of infants who die in utero or soon after birth with unrecognized CDH.[11] The mortality in CDH has been attributed to the severe pulmonary hypoplasia that occurs as a result of compression of the growing fetal lung by the intrathoracic herniated viscera.[1, 2, 6, 7]

The sonographic diagnosis of CDH is commonly made before 24 weeks' gestation and has been made as early as 15 weeks' gestation.[12-14] This defect results from a failure of fusion of a portion of the diaphragm during formation between the sixth and 14th weeks of gestation.[1] The diagnosis is usually suspected during routine sonographic scanning when a mediastinal shift is noted. Occasionally the diagnosis is specifically sought in patients being evaluated because of polyhydramnios or hydrops fetalis, both of which can be secondary to CDH.[1, 2] Visualizing abdominal organs in the fetal thorax makes the definitive diagnosis. Typically the fluid-filled stomach is the most conspicuous herniated viscus in the more common left CDH.[1] Small bowel and liver are also commonly identified within the chest[2] (Figs. 7–1 and 7–2). Occasionally, however, specific herniated abdominal viscera may not be initially evident and secondary features such as mediastinal shift, absence of an intraabdominal stomach, or polyhydramnios raise a strong suspicion of a CDH.[1] The herniated stomach in left-sided CDH usually is the most conspicuous herniated viscus given the anechogenicity of gastric fluid. Right-sided CDH is far less common. The hernia in right CDH can be more difficult to detect due to the subtle intrinsic difference in echogenicity between the right lung and liver.[2] Identification of an intrathoracic gallbladder, however, can be helpful in diagnosing right-sided hernias[1] (Fig. 7–3).

When assessing gastric herniation into the chest, it is essential that true transverse axial images be obtained, preferably the standard four-chambered heart view, as a slight oblique section through a normal fetal chest may make infradiaphragmatic structures appear as though they are in the thorax. Examination in orthogonal (coronal and parasagittal) planes helps to avoid this

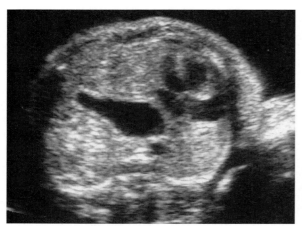

FIGURE 7–1. Left CDH. Transaxial image through the fetal thorax shows herniation of the stomach, liver, and small bowel into the left hemithorax. The heart is markedly displaced into the right hemithorax.

problem. In addition, identifying a diaphragmatic leaf does not exclude a diagnosis of CDH, as most defects involve only a portion of the hemidiaphragm.[1, 2]

Several studies have confirmed the accuracy of sonography in the diagnosis of CDH. In a review of 20 cases of CDH, review of prenatal sonograms made the diagnosis in all but one case.[15] In a larger series of 94 cases, the prenatal diagnosis was correctly made in 97% of cases.[3] The high accuracy of sonographic diagnosis has been reconfirmed in a more recent series.[14] False-negative diagnoses can occur when there are lesser degrees of visceral herniation. Indeed, Stringer found a better prognosis in neonates with isolated left-sided CDHs who were not detected on ultrasound in the second trimester, hypothesizing that these patients without sonographic evidence of in utero visceral herniation likely have less mediastinal shift with less resultant pulmonary hypoplasia and thus higher survival rates.[16] On a more disappointing note, however, a study by Lewis found that

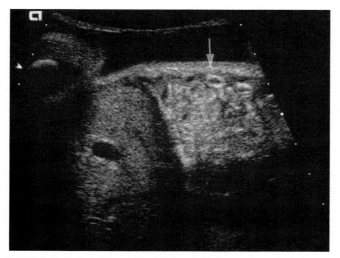

FIGURE 7–2. Left CDH. High-resolution parasagittal image through the fetal thorax and abdomen shows bowel loops (*arrow*) within the thorax.

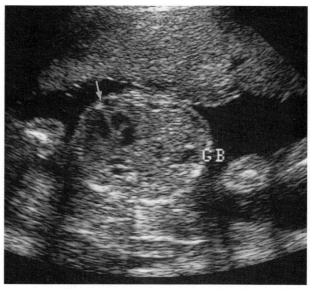

FIGURE 7–3. Right CDH. Transaxial image through the fetal thorax shows displacement of the heart (*arrow*) to the left by liver herniated into the right hemithorax. Note the gallbladder (GB) herniated into the right hemithorax.

in spite of a relative increase in prenatal ultrasound utilization over a 10-year period from 33% to 100%, the false-negative rate for CDH diagnosis remained at 55%. A review of the nondiagnostic cases revealed technical difficulties in 25%, failure to follow established guidelines (stomach localization and four-chamber heart view) in 57%, and missed findings suggestive of CDH in 33%. Not unexpectedly in the setting of poor quality imaging, the authors found no significant difference in survival between neonates with diagnostic and nondiagnostic scans.[17]

False-positive diagnosis is a less common occurrence, and in such instances another serious intrathoracic abnormality is generally mistaken for CDH. In a series of 94 cases, six false-positive cases proved to be cystic adenomatoid malformations in four, lung leiomyosarcoma in one, and mediastinal cystic teratoma in one.[3] It is imperative to consider a differential diagnosis when encountering a fetus with an intrathoracic mass, including lung masses such as cystic adenomatoid malformation or congenital lobar emphysema and cystic mediastinal masses such as neuroenteric cysts, bronchogenic cysts, thymic cysts, and cystic germ cell neoplasms. Unlike in cases of CDH, with these other pathologies, the fetal abdominal viscera are normally located within the abdomen.[1, 2]

Prognostic Assessment

The sonographic characteristics and accuracy of CDH diagnosis have been well established. However, the sonographic assessment of CDH severity and prognostic predictors has not. Given the recent advances in fetal intervention, the family with an affected fetus must now make the difficult choice between ''watchful waiting'' with standard postnatal treatment, pregnancy termination, or fetal intervention. While the natural history of untreated isolated CDH is poor (58% mortality for isolated CDH), fetal intervention has not yet been shown to improve the mortality rate. In addition, fetal surgery carries physical risks to the mother, as well as high financial and emotional costs.[3, 6, 10]

One of the most important roles of sonography in the prenatal evaluation of CDH, especially when fetal intervention is being considered, is the detection of other concomitant anomalies.[2] Associated malformations are frequent and have been reported to occur in 20 to 53% of fetuses with CDH.[1] The most common sites include cardiac (23%), urinary (15%), central nervous system (CNS) (10%), musculoskeletal (9%), genital (8%), and gastrointestinal (7%) malformations.[9] Over 30 multiple malformation syndromes have been described in association with CDH. These include the Fryn and Cornelia de Lange syndromes.[18] Importantly, chromosomal abnormalities have been found in 3.6 to 9% of cases, especially trisomies 18 and 21.[1, 3, 14, 15] Several series confirm an increased mortality in the presence of other associated anomalies.[14, 18–20] Thus, prenatal evaluation of CDH should include a detailed fetal anatomic survey, genetic amniocentesis, and fetal echocardiography in order to detect as many associated abnormalities as possible.

The high mortality of isolated CDH is thought to occur due to visceral herniation into the fetal thorax with fetal lung compression and resultant pulmonary hypoplasia. Pulmonary hypoplasia is thought to be the principal cause of neonatal death.[1, 2, 6, 7] Unfortunately, determining the function of fetal organs is difficult. This is particularly true of fetal lung function (i.e., gas exchange capability), which does not become operational until birth and thus cannot be assessed in utero.[2] Numerous studies have focused on methods to directly or indirectly assess the degree of pulmonary hypoplasia but many of these indicators remain of questionable value and are not widely accepted. We retrospectively reviewed 55 cases of isolated left-sided CDH referred to our fetal treatment center between 1990 and 1994. The predictive value of various fetal sonographic parameters was studied, with the principal outcome being survival.[21]

The influence of gestational age at the time of CDH diagnosis has been extensively studied. CDH is believed to have a dynamic variation in the timing and degree of visceral herniation.[3, 16] Intuitively, early identification (i.e., before 24 weeks) would be expected to detect fetuses with more severe herniation and earlier onset of pulmonary compression with greater resultant hypoplasia.[4] An early survey of 94 fetuses with CDH from across North America showed no significant difference in survival comparing gestational age at the time of diagnosis (mean age, 29 weeks). A later series by the same author examined 38 fetuses that were evaluated and treated by a single surgical team. They found that none of the 14 fetuses diagnosed before 25 weeks survived whereas 9 of the 24 fetuses diagnosed at or after 25 weeks survived.[3, 4] Other, more recent, series by Guibaud and Dillon, however, have not shown a statistical association between early diagnosis and outcome after birth.[14, 22] Our series

demonstrated differences in survival based on gestational age at diagnosis, with 100% survival for diagnosis made after 25 weeks and 56% survival for diagnosis made at or earlier than 25 weeks. These differences, however, were influenced by the exclusion of fetuses with other anomalies, which reflects the population in which fetal intervention is considered.[21] In addition, Stringer demonstrated 100% survival in neonates with isolated left CDH not detectable in detailed second-trimester studies, again suggesting better prognosis for fetuses with later herniation and subsequently less pulmonary hypoplasia.[16] While the data on the influence of gestational age at the time of diagnosis is not uniform, possibly due to differences in sample populations and inclusion of fetuses with other anomalies, the grave prognosis of the fetus with an early diagnosis (i.e., 25 weeks or less) appears difficult to ignore.

The predictive value of the presence of polyhydramnios complicating CDH on survival has also been extensively studied. Polyhydramnios in CDH is thought to result from gastric outlet obstruction secondary to herniation into the chest, a finding frequently noted at autopsy.[2] Polyhydramnios may be the initial reason for sonographic referral when a CDH is discovered.[1, 2] The incidence of polyhydramnios varies from 30% to 76%.[3, 4, 14, 19] Two early studies demonstrated a significant difference in survival (11% and 18% survival with polyhydramnios vs. 55% and 50% survival without polyhydramnios, respectively).[3, 4] However, these studies also suggested that polyhydramnios tended to occur in the third trimester.[4] Another series also confirmed a statistically significant difference in survival based on the presence or absence of polyhydramnios.[19] Other series, however, including our own more recent work, do not show an influence on survival.[21] In a 1995 series by Guibaud, although no significant association was demonstrated, note was made that none of the three fetuses with polyhydramnios before 24 weeks survived.[14] In our series, polyhydramnios was evaluated only at the time of initial diagnosis, which is when decisions about fetal intervention need to be made. Under this circumstance, polyhydramnios did not appear to influence outcome, but was uncommon. We speculate that the differences in results between series reflect different study populations as some series contained more referrals for polyhydramnios. The tendency for polyhydramnios to develop during the third trimester also likely influences results. Although still controversial, the fetus with early (25 weeks or less) onset of polyhydramnios should probably be viewed as having a poor prognosis.

Herniation of the fetal stomach into the thorax is also thought to indirectly predict pulmonary hypoplasia by serving as a marker for abdominal visceral herniation. Goodfellow[23] and Burge[24] both found better survival in neonates when the stomach was located within the abdomen on plain films. Respectively, these authors demonstrate 58.8% mortality for thoracic stomach versus 6.2% mortality for abdominal stomach and 75% mortality for thoracic stomach versus 0% mortality for abdominal stomach.[23, 24] These two studies were performed on postnatal films, however, and are less applicable to the evaluation for potential fetal intervention. A prenatal ultrasound series of 135 cases found 71% mortality for thoracic stomachs versus 7% mortality for abdominal stomachs; however, the incidence of intrathoracic stomach was 92%.[19] Our series failed to confirm a statistical association for stomach position given that 94% of our cases had an intrathoracic stomach.[21] Because most cases of CDH are suspected or confirmed by detecting an intrathoracic stomach, it is likely that stomach position in itself may not be as helpful in predicting outcome given its high incidence, especially in cases of early diagnosis where fetal intervention is a consideration. It is also likely that CDH fetuses with an intra-abdominal stomach often go undetected on sonograms, a feature, which we have already noted, has a better prognosis.

Position of the fetal liver is another marker thought to help assess severity of herniation. Detection of liver herniation is unfortunately technically challenging.[25] In our fetal treatment program, at a time when in utero surgical diaphragmatic defect closure was our primary method of surgical therapy offered, experience showed that reduction of the herniated liver was difficult due to kinking of the umbilical vessels and subsequent fetal bradycardia and possible fetal death.[6] It thus became imperative that the position of liver, completely below versus partially above the diaphragm, be accurately determined preoperatively. We retrospectively reviewed 16 prenatal preoperative ultrasounds with a diagnosis of CDH using operative findings as a comparison to determine sonographic features suggestive of liver herniation into the thorax. Analysis was based on the predicted anatomic alteration of hepatic and portal venous anatomy in the setting of herniation. Identification of these vessels was facilitated by the use of color Doppler imaging (Fig. 7–4). We found that visualization of the lateral segment branches of the left portal vein (LPV) coursing toward the diaphragmatic ridge (Fig. 7–5A and B) had a 75% sensitivity, 100% specificity, and 100% positive predictive value (PPV) for detecting liver herniation. Visualization of the umbilical segment of the LPV deviated to the left of midline (Fig. 7–5C) had a 92% sensitivity, 52% specificity, and 85% PPV for detecting liver herniation. Interestingly, we also noted an indirect correlation for relative position of the herniated stomach within the thorax. Stomachs located in the posterior or mid hemithorax had a 100% specificity and 100% PPV for predicting liver herniation but only a 58% sensitiv-

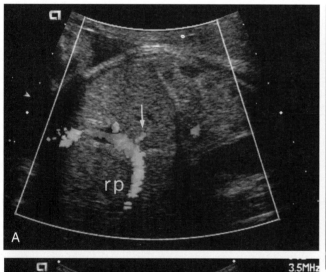

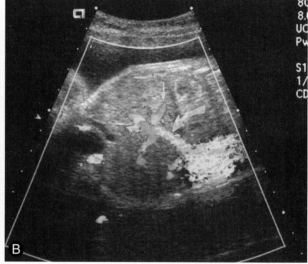

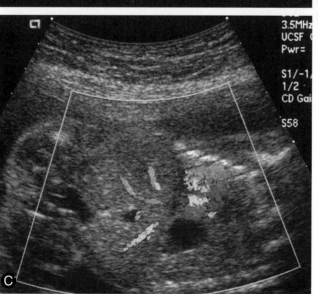

FIGURE 7–4. *A,* Left CDH without liver in the thorax. Color Doppler image in the coronal plane through the fetal thorax and abdomen shows normal hepatic vasculature: right portal vein (rp) and left portal venous branch (*arrow*) remaining below the expected region of the diaphragm. *B,* Color Doppler image in the coronal plane through the fetal thorax and abdomen shows normal hepatic vasculature: ductus venosus (*curved arrow*) and left lateral segment portal branches (*straight arrow*) remaining below the expected region of the diaphragm. *C,* Color Doppler image in the coronal plane through the fetal thorax and abdomen shows normal hepatic veins coursing toward but not above the diaphragm. *See Color Plate 1*

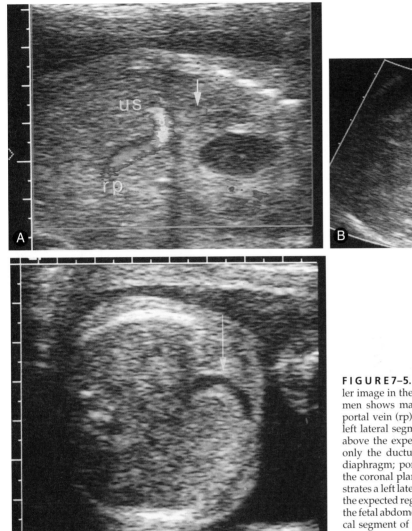

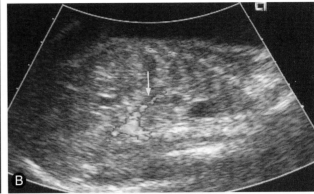

FIGURE 7–5. *A*, Left CDH with liver in the thorax. Color Doppler image in the coronal plane through the fetal thorax and abdomen shows marked distortion of the hepatic vasculature: right portal vein (rp), umbilical segment of the portal vein (us), and a left lateral segmental portal branch (*arrow*) coursing toward and above the expected region of the diaphragm. In normal fetuses only the ductus venosus and hepatic veins course toward the diaphragm; portal branches do not. *B*, Color Doppler image in the coronal plane through the fetal thorax and abdomen demonstrates a left lateral segmental portal branch (*arrow*) coursing above the expected region of the diaphragm. *C*, Transaxial image through the fetal abdomen shows marked deviation (bowing) of the umbilical segment of the portal vein (*arrow*) toward the left side of the fetus. In normal fetuses, the vessel courses straight posteriorly toward the spine.

ity.[26] In our more recent series evaluating factors associated with survival in CDH, there was 100% survival if the liver was not herniated versus 56% survival if a portion of the liver was herniated into the chest.[21] In contrast, a prenatal series that did not employ Doppler analysis showed no significant association for liver position.[14]

On a similar note, Teixeira (1997) found that an abdominal circumference (AC) below the fifth centile during the second trimester predicted a poor prognosis (100% mortality compared to only 43% mortality if the AC was above the fifth centile). A significant association between an AC below the fifth centile and liver herniated into the chest was found, as well.[25] The major determinant of the AC is the liver. Although we did not find AC to have predictive value in our series, an AC below the fifth centile is likely seen in the setting of a large volume of herniated liver.[21]

Cardiac ventricular disproportion as seen on a four-chamber view of the heart is another indirect predictor of the mortality.[20] Ventricular disproportion first detected during the second trimester was associated with 100% mortality. On the other hand, absence of ventricular disproportion in the third trimester suggests a good prognosis, while ventricular disproportion first noted during the third trimester was associated with an intermediate survival rate. We speculate that ventricular disproportion is due to mass effect of the herniated organs on the left ventricle or due to altered hemodynamics.[20] Although potentially promising, assessment of ventricular disproportion is not widely performed.

The above-described predictors indirectly assess the degree of lung hypoplasia. More recent work has focused on direct quantification of residual lung. Two earlier series[27,28] assessed lung hypoplasia by measuring the area of the residual lungs bilaterally and divided the lung area by the area of the thorax on the four-chamber heart view, creating the lung/thorax (L/T) ratio. The L/T ratio taken at 35 to 38 weeks' gestation was found to correlate with postnatal blood-gas data but not with survival.[27,28] Quantifying bilateral lung area on earlier second-trimester fetuses however, and especially quantifying ipsilateral lung area, proved to be difficult due to the similar echogenicity of bowel, liver, and lung.[14, 21] In contrast, the contralateral lung is relatively easy to identify and quantitate, as it sonographically contrasts with the heart and chest wall. One approach quantified the area of the contralateral lung, taking the ratio of the lung area to the hemithorax area on an axial four-chamber heart view.[14] If the ratio was greater than or equal to 0.5, there was 86% survival compared with only 25% survival for ratios less than 0.5. This was the only statistically significant predictive factor in their series.[14] We similarly quantified the contralateral lung on a transverse axial sonogram of the thorax at the level of the atria, calculating lung area as the product of two perpendicular linear measurements (Fig. 7–6). We divided the area by the head circumference to adjust for differences in gestational age. The resultant lung/head circumference ratio (LHR) was found to be statistically significant when compared to survival with 100% survival for LHR greater than 1.35, 61% survival for LHR between 0.6 and 1.35, and 0% survival for LHR less than 0.6.[21] To date, direct sonographic quantification of residual lung area may be our best available predictor of pulmonary hypoplasia. Volumetric quantification of residual lung size utilizing echo-planar magnetic resonance imaging (MRI) techniques is a promising new area of research.[29]

It should be noted that the value of prenatal sonographic prognosis of congenital diaphragmatic hernia has been questioned. In a series by Wilson in 1994, no significant difference in survival was seen in patients with isolated CDH diagnosed antenatally versus postnatally. In addition, the timing of diagnosis had no value on predicting outcome.[30]

From a practical standpoint, it becomes difficult to decide which predictors are the most useful. In essence, however, they all attempt to either directly or indirectly assess the same parameter, the degree of pulmonary hypoplasia. At our fetal treatment center, prospective candidates for fetal interventions receive a detailed fetal anatomic survey and fetal echocardiogram primarily to exclude other associated anomalies. Attention then focuses on sonographic confirmation and assessment of the diaphragmatic hernia. Although factors such as polyhydramnios, gestational age at diagnosis, and stomach position are noted, our attention primarily focuses on the position of the liver and the quantity of remaining contralateral lung (LHR). Doppler evaluation is utilized to search for left portal vein segmental branches coursing abnormally to or above the diaphragmatic ridge and bowing of the umbilical segment of the LPV to the left, as we have found these signs to be the most predictive of liver position. A favorable prognosis is given when the liver is positioned in the abdomen and an LHR is greater than 1.35. Conversely, a poor prognosis with possible benefit from fetal intervention is discussed when a portion of liver is herniated into the thorax and an LHR is less than 1.35. The value of these indicators in selecting candidates for fetal intervention, specifically fetal tracheal occlusion, and outcomes for those with or without fetal intervention is currently under investigation. Unpublished prospective data indicate that fetuses with liver herniated into the chest and an LHR of less than 1.0 have a very poor prognosis, even with extracorporeal membrane oxygenation (ECMO) support if they have not undergone in utero intervention.

Intraoperative and Postoperative Evaluation

The most effective treatment for the fetus with CDH is not known. This is especially true in fetuses with an expected poor prognosis based on sonographic evaluation such as a portion of liver herniated into the chest.[21] Years of attempted primary in utero repair of CDH with herniated liver have been largely unsuccessful in spite of a variety of technique modifications.[6, 31] In utero fetal tracheal occlusion has been shown experimentally to correct pulmonary hypoplasia associated with CDH by blocking the normal egress of fetal lung fluid, expanding the lung resulting in pulmonary hyperplasia, and subsequently reducing herniated abdominal viscera.[7] Presently, in utero tracheal occlusion appears to be the most promising treatment for fetuses with a large CDH.[8]

Sonography plays an integral role in the operative treatment of CDH.[6, 8, 31] This has become especially true given the recent trend towards endoscopic treatment rather than open hysterotomy to ameliorate or repair the lesion. Prior to preparation of the operative field sonography assesses the fetus for any unexpected change (e.g., death, and development of hydrops fetalis, development of polyhydramnios). After sterilization of the operative field, preliminary sonographic evaluation focuses on mapping the in utero operative field. The placenta is specifically mapped on the uterine surface prior to selection of incision sites or port punctures for endoscopic instruments. The fetal position is assessed for optimizing the position relative to the available operative field. The lie and specifically the fetal neck position are determined. The fetal shoulder is identified and a sonographically guided intramuscular injection of a paralytic agent and narcotic is performed. The quantity of

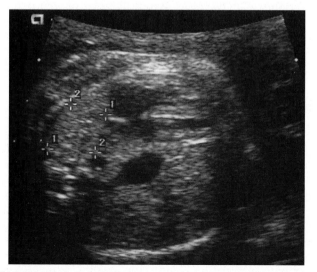

FIGURE 7–6. Left CDH. Transaxial image through the thorax in a fetus with a left CDH demonstrates measurements of the remaining contralateral right lung. The calculated lung area is divided by the head circumference to obtain the lung/head circumference ratio (LHR).

amniotic fluid is monitored to ensure that an appropriate amount is present for adequate manipulation. Once the fetus is positioned, sonography guides a puncture of the trachea for deployment of a T-bar posterior to the trachea. The attached suture guides the position of the neck incision. The T-bar helps to elevate the trachea for easier dissection.

The sonographer may play an active role by guiding endoscopic instruments to the operative field under direct continuous sonographic visualization. Throughout the course of the operation, sonography also plays a role in fetal monitoring. Such monitoring includes heart rate, resistance in the umbilical artery, and visual assessment of cardiac stroke volume.

Sonography plays an important role in the postoperative evaluation and monitoring of both the fetus and mother. Frequent interval postoperative sonography may help in documenting fetal lung expansion in response to tracheal occlusion. In our early experience with fetuses treated with tracheal occlusion, fetuses usually do not demonstrate a visible sonographic response (Fig. 7–7) until 1 week postoperatively. Subsequent exams continue to demonstrate lung enlargement, decreased shift of the mediastinum, and reduction of herniated abdominal viscera. Some dilatation of the fetal trachea and mainstem bronchi may be noted.[8]

Postoperative sonographic evaluation is also important in assessing complications, some of which may require early delivery. Amniotic fluid volume is frequently assessed as it often reflects the general well-being of the fetus and may provide an early clue to poor fetal or maternal status. A theoretical risk of tracheal occlusion is the development of hydrops given the expansion of the lungs and increase in thoracic pressure causing compromise of venous return and cardiac compression. This is believed not to occur in cases of CDH due to decompression of the expanding lung by return of herniated viscera into the abdomen. Nevertheless, a case of postoperative hydrops prompting early delivery was found at our institution that began on the third postoperative day. Of note, unlike previous cases, in this case visible lung expansion was evident as early as the second postoperative day.[32] In addition to hydrops, we have observed a few cases of fetal intracranial hemorrhage, the etiology of which is unclear.[8]

Congenital Cystic Adenomatoid Malformation of the Lung and Pulmonary Sequestration

Diagnosis and Evaluation

In contrast to CDH, survival is significantly higher for intrathoracic masses of pulmonary origin; as high as 90% in the absence of hydrops or other anomalies.[33] Fetal intrathoracic masses are most commonly either a CCAM of the lung or a pulmonary sequestration. Although these lesions are embryologically and pathologically quite different, they both present sonographically as thoracic masses and can be very similar in appearance. The natural history in the fetus and considerations for in utero therapy are remarkably similar for these two lesions, but very different than CDH. Thus, we will con-

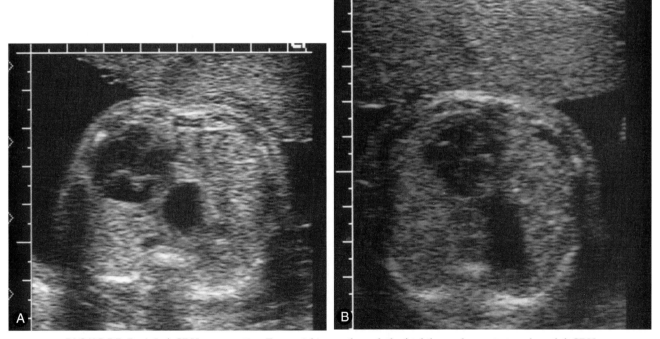

FIGURE 7–7. *A,* Left CDH preoperative. Transaxial image through the fetal thorax demonstrates a large left CDH with marked cardiac shift to the right. *B,* Left CDH postoperative day 4. Transaxial image through the fetal thorax 4 days after fetal surgery shows interval increase in size of the contralateral right lung and decreased cardiac shift to the right.

sider them simultaneously, contrasting them with one another and with CDH where appropriate.

Both of these intrathoracic pulmonary masses are relatively commonly encountered in fetuses. CCAM is the most common type of fetal thoracic mass diagnosed in utero.[5] It is thought to occur as a result of failure of maturation of bronchiolar structures during the 5th or 6th week of gestation.[34, 35] Some have speculated a hamartomatous origin to CCAM.[36] Stocker and associates have divided these lesions into three pathologic categories. Type I masses present with large cysts (>2 cm) that are usually few in number. Type II masses present with multiple smaller cysts (<2 cm). Type III masses present with tiny usually unresolvable cysts and appear to be a solid mass.[35] These definitions are somewhat impractical from an imaging perspective as "large" and "small" are not generally separated by a cutoff of 2 cm. Pragmatically, type I CCAM is generally diagnosed when the mass is predominantly comprised of a single large cyst, usually much larger than 2 cm (Fig. 7–8). Type II CCAM is diagnosed when multiple relatively small cysts are seen, although commonly one or more of the cysts is larger than 2 cm. Type III CCAM is considered an appropriate diagnosis when no cysts are seen or there is a large mass with only one or two small cysts (Fig. 7–9). The matter of precise terminology might be of greater concern if these categories were employed prognostically. As we will see later, they are not. Therefore, overzealous adherence to an older schema of categorization is valueless.

Most CCAMs have a small communication with the tracheobronchial tree and can fill with air postnatally.[34] CCAMs obtain their arterial blood supply and venous drainage from the pulmonary arterial and venous systems, respectively. Cases of anomalous arterial supply

and venous drainage of CCAMs have, however, been reported.[34] Most CCAMs are unilateral and occur more commonly in the lower lobes.[37] They can occur in any pulmonary lobe and can occur in an extrapulmonary location as well; for example, within the upper abdomen.

In contrast to CCAMs, pulmonary sequestrations represent nonfunctioning but histologically normal lung that is isolated or "sequestered" from the tracheobronchial and pulmonary vascular tree.[34] Importantly, arterial blood supply is from an anomalous systemic artery arising from the aorta (Fig. 7–10). Pulmonary sequestrations fall under the general category of bronchopulmonary foregut malformations and are thought to arise from a supernumerary lung bud in a caudal location relative to the normal lung bud.[34] Ninety percent of pulmonary sequestrations occur posteriorly near the diaphragm in the left costophrenic sulcus. Pulmonary sequestration can also occur in the abdomen, usually just below the diaphragm.[38]

Two forms of pulmonary sequestration are recognized: intralobar and extralobar. Intralobar pulmonary sequestration shares a common pleural investment with the rest of the lung, while extralobar pulmonary sequestration has a separate pleural envelope. In addition, intralobar pulmonary sequestration generally has venous drainage to the pulmonary veins, while extralobar pulmonary sequestration has venous drainage to the systemic veins (hemiazygous or portal). For reasons unknown, while 75% of pulmonary sequestrations in children and adults are intralobar, nearly all pulmonary sequestrations detected in utero are extralobar.[39]

Sonographically, both CCAM and pulmonary sequestration are usually incidentally detected as fetal lung masses. Mediastinal shift is the observation that often first draws attention to the presence of a pulmonary

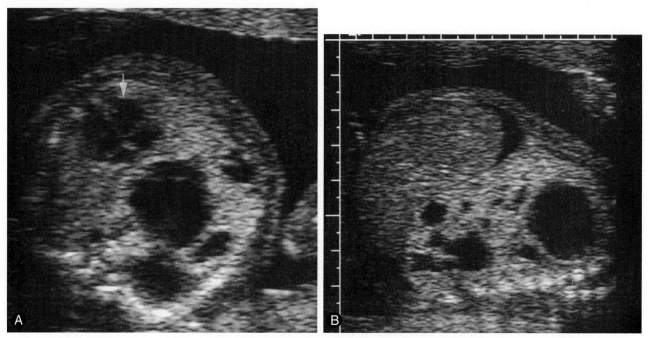

F I G U R E 7–8. *A,* CCAM type I. Transaxial image through the fetal thorax demonstrates a large cystic and solid mass in the right hemithorax with cardiac (*arrow*) shift to the left. The cysts are relatively large, compatible with a type I CCAM. *B,* Parasagittal image through the fetal thorax and abdomen shows the large CCAM everting the diaphragm. Note the fetal ascites.

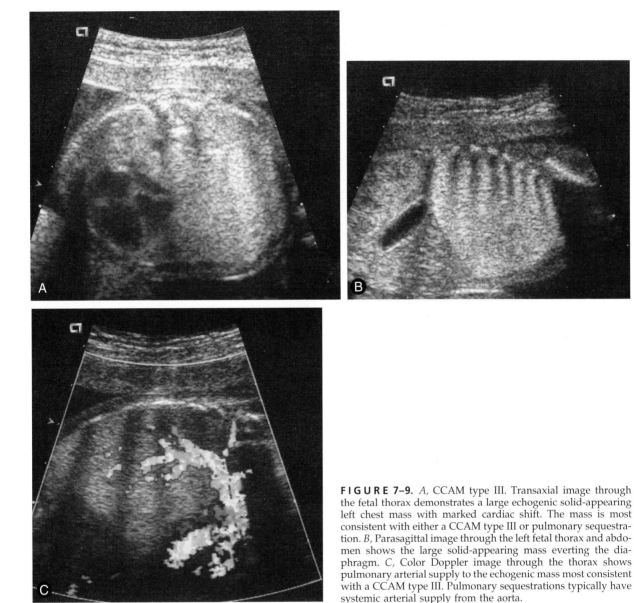

FIGURE 7–9. *A,* CCAM type III. Transaxial image through the fetal thorax demonstrates a large echogenic solid-appearing left chest mass with marked cardiac shift. The mass is most consistent with either a CCAM type III or pulmonary sequestration. *B,* Parasagittal image through the left fetal thorax and abdomen shows the large solid-appearing mass everting the diaphragm. *C,* Color Doppler image through the thorax shows pulmonary arterial supply to the echogenic mass most consistent with a CCAM type III. Pulmonary sequestrations typically have systemic arterial supply from the aorta.

mass. Polyhydramnios may be present. Both lesions can be diagnosed as early as 16 weeks, with the majority of cases in some series being diagnosed before 22 weeks of gestation.[40] The presence of cysts within the mass favors a type I or II CCAM, depending on the size and number of the cysts. An echogenic mass without resolvable cysts, however, may represent either a type III CCAM or a pulmonary sequestration. Differentiation between these two can be difficult. One should make an effort to demonstrate a feeding arterial vessel to the mass from the aorta with color Doppler sonography, as this finding overwhelmingly favors a diagnosis of pulmonary sequestration.[1] The presence of cysts does not exclude the diagnosis of sequestration, as "cysts" may be seen in the bronchiectatic form of intralobar pulmonary sequestration,[39] but cysts strongly favor a CCAM. While accurate diagnosis is desirable, the histology of the mass is usually not the crucial prognostic feature, as will be discussed later.

It can be difficult at times to differentiate between a CCAM and pulmonary sequestration and not uncommonly the two coexist. Focal areas of microscopic CCAM have been found in 15 to 28% of pulmonary sequestration pathology specimens.[38, 41, 42] In fact, any of the bronchopulmonary foregut malformations may occur in combination with CCAM. In addition, bronchopulmonary foregut malformations may be seen in association with CDH, especially extralobar pulmonary sequestration (Fig. 7–11). CCAM and pulmonary sequestration may also occur intra-abdominally, where they need to be differentiated from other abdominal masses such as neuroblastoma. It is important to exclude a CDH by confirming the presence of normal abdominal anatomy. An intra-abdominal stomach position should be confirmed in all cases.[1]

Other less common thoracic masses should also be considered. An obstructed segment of lung may present as an echogenic lung mass. Bronchial atresia may pre-

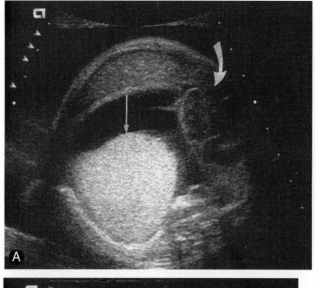

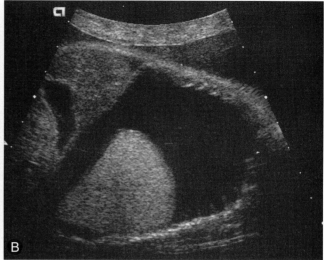

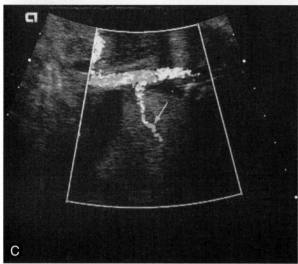

FIGURE 7–10. *A,* Sequestration. Transaxial image through the fetal thorax shows marked cardiac (*curved arrow*) shift to the right by the combination of a large echogenic mass (*straight arrow*) and surrounding pleural effusion. *B,* Parasagittal image through the left fetal thorax and abdomen shows that the echogenic mass is solid-appearing and wedge-shaped in the region of the left lower lobe, a common location for sequestrations. A large left pleural effusion is noted as well. *C,* Parasagittal image with color Doppler shows systemic arterial supply to the mass from the aorta, most consistent with a pulmonary sequestration.

sent as an upper lobe large echogenic fetal lung mass, occasionally with a dilated fluid-filled bronchus.[1] Bronchogenic cysts are rarely detected in utero but may present as a single unilocular cyst or an echogenic distended lung obstructed by a small cyst.[1] Other bronchopulmonary foregut abnormalities such as enteric or neuroenteric cysts should be considered. A neuroenteric cyst should be suggested in the presence of associated thoracic spinal dysraphism.[1] Calcifications in a cystic or solid mass are atypical of CCAM or pulmonary sequestration and other diagnoses such as mediastinal teratomas, neuroblastoma, or CDH with meconium peritonitis should be considered.[1]

Thoracic masses may occur bilaterally as well. Mediastinal shift may be absent in the setting of symmetric masses. CCAM, pulmonary sequestration, and CDH all rarely can occur bilaterally[43] (Fig. 7–12). More commonly, bilaterally echogenic masses represent fluid-filled obstructed lungs from upper respiratory tract obstruction (laryngeal or tracheal atresia).[1]

The overall sonographic sensitivity for detection of significant echogenic lung masses is likely very high.

The true sensitivity may be difficult to determine, as many of the smaller missed masses are likely insignificant and may not come to clinical attention. The accuracy of sonography in determining the specific type of echogenic lung mass, however, is variable. In one series of masses prenatally diagnosed as CCAM, only 38% were correct, with 15% likely correct without pathologic proof. Forty-six percent of masses that were erroneously diagnosed in utero as CCAM were pulmonary sequestrations at pathology.[44] In a more recent and larger series, the prenatal diagnosis of CCAM was correct in 88% of cases. The misdiagnoses (12%) again were all pulmonary sequestrations.[33]

Prognosis and Assessment

While accurate detection of echogenic lung masses is important, specific differentiation between CCAM and pulmonary sequestration is not critical, as both lesions have similar natural histories. In addition, considerations for in utero therapy are usually the same.

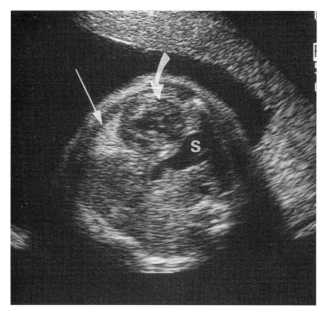

FIGURE 7–11. Left CDH with sequestration. Transaxial image through the fetal thorax shows a left CDH with stomach (s) and heart (*curved arrow*) displaced into the right hemithorax. Incidentally noted is a region of echogenic tissue (*straight arrow*) most compatible with concurrent sequestration.

Like CDH, echogenic lung masses have the potential to be life threatening by causing pulmonary hypoplasia and hydrops. Pulmonary hypoplasia is likely secondary to compression by the mass. Hydrops may occur from excessive mediastinal shift with resultant vena caval obstruction or cardiac compression.[45]

In contrast to CDH, however, CCAM and pulmonary sequestration have been observed to spontaneously regress in utero. Prenatal detection of these masses has allowed observation of their natural histories. Budorick and co-workers reported regression of lung masses in 5 of 14 fetuses (36%).[46] In a recent series, 13 of 17 (76%) fetal lung masses without hydrops decreased during the course of gestation, with two resolving completely.[5] Among 40 fetuses with lung masses studied at our institution, 12 (four CCAMs and eight pulmonary sequestrations) demonstrated a decrease in mass size or resolution of hydrops and polyhydramnios during gestation (Fig. 7–13). Congenital chest masses are likely more common than previously reported, as many of these children with regressing masses are asymptomatic at birth.[2] In addition, surgical studies report pulmonary sequestration as an incidental finding in 1 to 2% of all patients undergoing pulmonary resection.[47]

The potential for regression greatly impacts counseling offered to the parents of a fetus with a CCAM or pulmonary sequestration compared to that of a fetus with a CDH. Regression may not occur until the third trimester, making decisions about termination or in utero treatment difficult. Several sonographically evaluated potential prognostic factors have been evaluated.

As with CDH, before any intervention is considered, it is critical to evaluate the fetus for associated anomalies. Stocker reported a high frequency of associated anomalies with CCAM type II, particularly genitourinary, cardiac, and chromosomal.[35] In a series by Bromely and co-workers, 2 of 25 fetuses with lung masses had trisomies, both with CCAM type II.[40] These associations have not been confirmed by all investigators.[1]

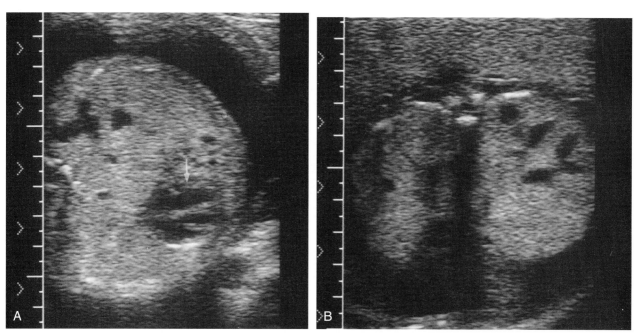

FIGURE 7–12. *A,* Bilateral CCAM. Transaxial image through the fetal chest shows large bilateral echogenic intrathoracic masses containing several cysts. There is anterior displacement of the heart (*arrow*) from the mass effect. *B,* Transaxial image more caudal to *A* further demonstrates the large bilateral masses. Autopsy revealed predominantly type III CCAM involving all lobes of the lungs.

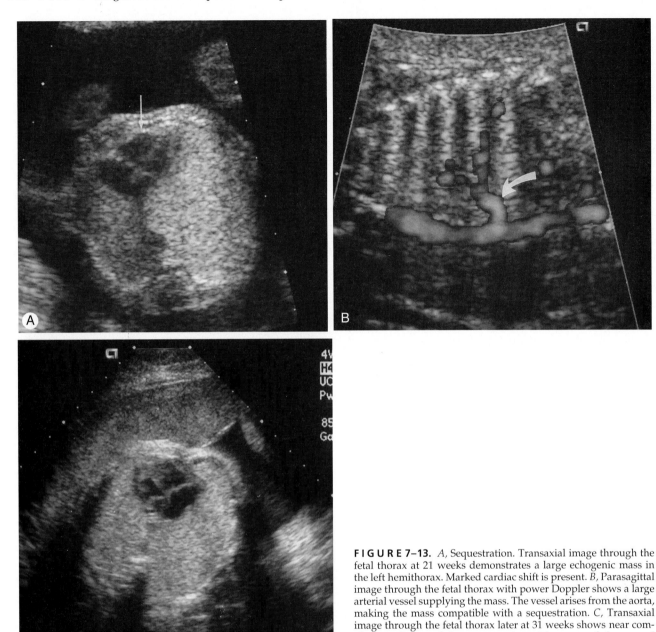

F I G U R E 7–13. *A*, Sequestration. Transaxial image through the fetal thorax at 21 weeks demonstrates a large echogenic mass in the left hemithorax. Marked cardiac shift is present. *B*, Parasagittal image through the fetal thorax with power Doppler shows a large arterial vessel supplying the mass. The vessel arises from the aorta, making the mass compatible with a sequestration. *C*, Transaxial image through the fetal thorax later at 31 weeks shows near complete resolution of the sequestration with return of the normal cardiac axis.

In contrast, associated anomalies with extralobar pulmonary sequestration have been well described in the postnatal literature, occurring in 15 to 60%.[1] While the most common associated anomaly is a CDH, cardiac and gastrointestinal anomalies also occur. In a review of 18 cases of prenatal pulmonary sequestration by Dolkhart (17 cases from the literature), however, no associated anomalies were found. The discrepancy between the antenatal and postnatal literature is unclear.[48]

All fetuses with an echogenic lung mass should undergo a careful anatomic survey including a fetal echocardiogram. It may be prudent as well to consider genetic amniocentesis, particularly if fetal intervention is a consideration.

The majority of the series evaluating the natural history of echogenic lung masses have evaluated potential prognostic factors and their ability to predict in utero or perinatal mortality. Perhaps the most ominous sign evaluated to date is the development of hydrops fetalis. Hydrops is thought to occur secondary to mediastinal shift with resultant venous and cardiac compression.[45] It has also been suggested that the loss of protein from a CCAM may reduce fetal colloid oncotic pressure, exacerbating hydrops.[34]

The reported incidence of hydrops in the setting of an echogenic lung mass ranges from 23 to 47%, likely due to differences in study populations.[5,33,42,49] Nevertheless, nearly all series confirm a significantly increased incidence of poor outcome in the setting of hydrops. Several series have demonstrated a 100% mortality for fetuses with CCAM in the setting of hydrops from in utero death, perinatal death, or pregnancy termination.[42, 45] It is important to note, however, that while the chance of a poor outcome is dramatically increased in the setting of hydrops, it is not a uniformly fatal sign. Several reports have documented the spontaneous resolution of hydrops in fetuses with echogenic lung masses managed conservatively.[43] In a series of fetuses with CCAM by Thorpe-Beeston and Nicolaides, for nonterminated pregnancies, survival was 6 per 28 (21%) for hydropic compared to 55 per 60 (92%) for nonhydropic fetuses.[49]

As noted above, in the absence of hydrops, the outcome is very favorable. Indeed, nearly all series report survival rates of over 90% in the absence of hydrops, with many neonates appearing normal at birth. In a series by Miller and co-workers, all 12 fetuses with CCAM but without hydrops survived, with only four requiring some form of neonatal respiratory support at birth.[42] Frequent periodic sonographic evaluation of the fetus should be performed to detect developing hydrops. Fortunately, in the absence of hydrops at the time of diagnosis of an echogenic lung mass, the chance of hydrops developing later in gestation is reported to be only 6%.[33]

Thus the development of hydrops in the fetus with an echogenic lung mass, while not uniformly fatal, should be looked upon as an ominous sign, perhaps identifying a group of fetuses that could benefit from in utero intervention. The fetus without hydrops, however, is likely to do well.

Polyhydramnios may occur in the setting of a thoracic mass due to decreased swallowing of amniotic fluid from esophageal compression by the mass. Increased fetal lung fluid production by the mass may also contribute the polyhydramnios. The incidence ranges from 17 to 42%, again likely due to differences in study populations.[5, 40, 49]

Polyhydramnios is reported to adversely influence outcome. Bromley and co-workers demonstrated survival in 50% versus 100% for affected fetuses with polyhydramnios and normal amniotic fluid, respectively.[40] While often seen together, polyhydramnios and hydrops may occur independently.[45] Miller and co-workers demonstrated that isolated polyhydramnios (unassociated with hydrops) was not a poor prognostic indicator.[42] While isolated polyhydramnios may not be useful in predicting outcome, its effect on the pregnancy management, mainly threatened premature labor, should not be ignored.[5]

The proposed mechanisms of polyhydramnios and hydrops secondary to a thoracic mass are likely closely related to the degree of mediastinal shift. The series by Bromley and co-workers reported a 37% survival with moderate or severe shift compared to a 76% survival with no or mild shift.[40] In contrast, no significant difference in survival according to degree of mediastinal shift was seen in another series.[42] One should take caution in using the degree of mediastinal shift to predict outcome, especially when intervention is being considered, as dramatic improvement in shift may occur in the setting of spontaneous regression of a CCAM or pulmonary sequestration.

Occasionally, an extralobar pulmonary sequestration may be associated with a large, tension hydrothorax resulting in severe mediastinal shift. It has been proposed that this hydrothorax is the result of torsion of the pulmonary sequestration on its pedicle[50] (Fig. 7–10). These cases may respond to thoracoamniotic shunt placement.

As mentioned above, sonographic discrimination of the histology of an echogenic lung mass, particularly between CCAM type III and pulmonary sequestration, is poor when the blood supply cannot be demonstrated. Sonography can, however, classify lung masses into broad categories based on the Stocker classification, namely, CCAM type I for large cysts, CCAM type II for small to medium cysts, and CCAM type III (or pulmonary sequestration) for solid appearing masses. Earlier series suggested an almost uniformly fatal outcome for solid appearing masses.[45] More recent series, however, demonstrate no significant difference in survival based on sonographic classification of the type of mass.[40, 42] The sonographic category is also unable to predict the likelihood of mass regression. Sonographic characterization of the mass may be important, however, in determining the type of fetal intervention to be performed. For example, a mass comprised primarily of a large cyst is best treated with a thoracoamniotic shunt.

In summary, when an echogenic fetal lung mass is detected a careful fetal anatomic survey and echocardiogram should be performed. Genetic amniocentesis should be considered as well. While not critical in predicting outcome, the characteristics of the mass, particularly the size and number of cysts, should be documented. The degree of mediastinal shift should be documented for future evaluation of potential mass regression. Polyhydramnios should be addressed primarily as it relates to the threat of premature delivery. Perhaps our best predictor of poor outcome is hydrops. While the likelihood that a fetus without hydrops at the time of diagnosis will later develop hydrops is low, periodic sonographic evaluation should be performed. Unfortunately, we are currently unable to predict which lesions are likely to undergo spontaneous regression.

Fetal Intervention, Intraoperative Evaluation, and Postoperative Evaluation

The current treatment options for fetal lung masses are observation with postnatal treatment, single in utero thoracic aspiration, multiple in utero thoracic aspirations, in utero thoracoamniotic shunt placement, and operative resection[51–54] (Fig. 7–14). Sonography plays an important role in each of these options.

For percutaneous thoracic aspiration or shunt placement, sonography is utilized to guide puncture into the fetal thoracic cavity and assist with catheter manipulation. The optimal entry site into the uterine cavity is determined to avoid placental tissue and to enter the

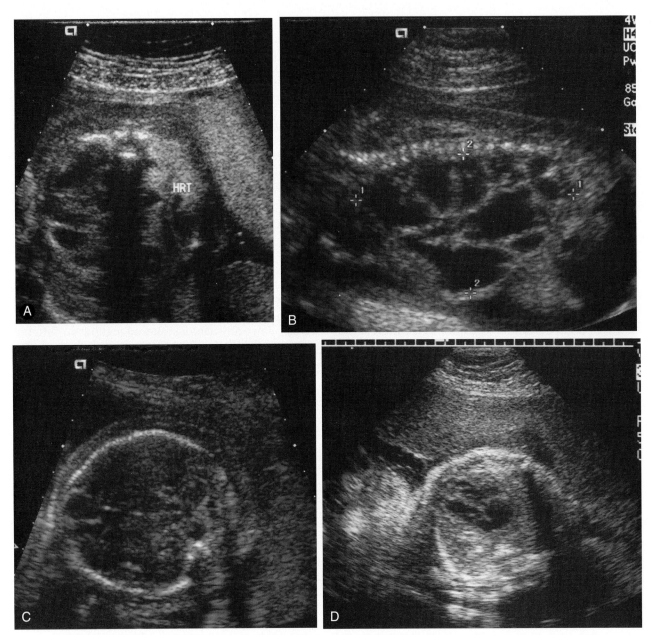

FIGURE 7–14. *A,* CCAM type I (preoperative). Transaxial image through the lower fetal thorax at 23 weeks' gestation demonstrates a large left predominantly cystic mass most compatible with a CCAM type I. *B,* Parasagittal image through the left fetal thorax at 23 weeks' gestation shows the large multicystic mass. Note the fetal ascites. *C,* Transaxial image through the fetal posterior fossa demonstrates diffuse scalp edema. This finding is supportive of fetal hydrops. The fetus subsequently underwent in utero surgery for excision of the CCAM. *D,* Transaxial image through the fetal thorax on postoperative day 49 shows absence of the cystic mass as well as interval left lung growth. The cardiac axis is nearly normal.

fetal thorax in a safe location. Cyst decompression can be monitored with real-time observation. Sonography is also useful in postprocedure follow-up of the fetus to ensure appropriate shunt position. Follow-up studies can also document reaccumulation of cyst fluid.

In the event that operative therapy is chosen, sonography may assist in mapping the operative field before entry into the uterus. Postoperative sonographic evaluation may be useful in monitoring hydrops, mediastinal shift, and amniotic fluid volume.

REFERENCES

1. Goldstein RB: Ultrasound evaluation of the fetal thorax. *In* Callen PW (ed): Ultrasonography in Obstetrics and Gynecology. Philadelphia: WB Saunders Company, 1994, pp 338–341.
2. Harrison MR, Globus MS, Filly RA: The fetus with a diaphragmatic hernia: Pathophysiology, natural history, and surgical management. *In* Harrison MR, Globus MS, Filly RA (eds): The Unborn Patient: Prenatal Diagnosis and Treatment. Philadelphia: WB Saunders Company, 1990, pp 295–313.
3. Adzick NS, Harrison MR, Glick PL, et al: Diaphragmatic hernia in the fetus: Prenatal diagnosis and outcome in 94 cases. J Pediatr Surg 20:357, 1985.

4. Adzick NS, Vacanti JP, Lillehei CW, et al: Fetal diaphragmatic hernia: Ultrasound diagnosis and clinical outcome in 38 cases. J Pediatr Surg 24:654, 1989.

5. Dommergues M, Louis-Sylvestre C, Mandelbrot L, et al: Congenital adenomatoid malformation of the lung: When is active fetal therapy indicated? Am J Obstet Gynecol 177:953, 1997.

6. Harrison MR, Adzick NS, Flake AW, et al: Correction of congenital diaphragmatic hernia in utero: VI. Hard-earned lessons. J Pediatr Surg 28:1411, 1993.

7. Hedrick MH, Estes JM, Sullivan KM, et al: Plug the lung until it grows (PLUG): A new method to treat congenital diaphragmatic hernia in utero. J Pediatr Surg 29:612, 1994.

8. Harrison MR, Adzick NS, Estes JM, Howell LJ: A prospective study of the outcome for fetuses with diaphragmatic hernia. JAMA 271:382, 1994.

9. Nyberg DA, Mahony BS, Pretorius DH: The thorax. *In* Diagnostic Ultrasound of Fetal Anomalies: Text and Atlas. Chicago: Year Book Medical Publishers, Inc, 1992, pp 283–288.

10. Harrison MR, Adzick NS, Flake AW, et al: Correction of congenital diaphragmatic hernia in utero VIII: Response of the hypoplastic lung to tracheal occlusion. J Pediatr Surg 31:1339, 1996.

11. Harrison MR, Bjordal RI, Langmark F: Congenital diaphragmatic hernia: The hidden mortality. J Pediatr Surg 13:227, 1978.

12. Benacerraf BR, Greene MF: Congenital diaphragmatic hernia: US diagnosis prior to 22 week gestation. Radiology 158:809, 1986.

13. Benacerraf BR, Adzick NS: Fetal diaphragmatic hernia: Ultrasound diagnosis and clinical outcome in 19 cases. Am J Obstet Gynecol 156:573, 1987.

14. Guibaud L, Filiatrault D, Garel L, et al: Fetal congenital diaphragmatic hernia: Accuracy of sonography in the diagnosis and prediction of the outcome after birth. AJR Am J Roentgenol 166:1195, 1996.

15. Nakayama DK, Harrison MR, Chinn DH, et al: Prenatal diagnosis and natural history of the fetus with a congenital diaphragmatic hernia: Initial clinical experience. J Pediatr Surg 20:118, 1985.

16. Stringer MD, Goldstein RB, Filly RA, et al: Fetal diaphragmatic hernia without visceral herniation. J Pediatr Surg 30:1264, 1995.

17. Lewis DA, Reickert C, Bowerman R, Hirshcl RB: Prenatal ultrasonography frequently fails to diagnose congenital diaphragmatic hernia. J Pediatr Surg 32:352, 1997.

18. Puri P, Gorman F: Lethal nonpulmonary anomalies associated with congenital diaphragmatic hernia: Implications for early intrauterine surgery. J Pediatr Surg 19:29, 1984.

19. Dommergues M, Louis-Sylvestre C, Mandelbrot L, et al: Congenital diaphragmatic hernia: Can prenatal ultrasonography predict outcome? Am J Obstet Gynecol 174:1377, 1996.

20. Crawford DC, Wright VM, Drake DP, Allan LD: Fetal diaphragmatic hernia: The value of fetal echocardiography in the prediction of postnatal outcome. Br J Obstet Gynecol 96:705, 1989.

21. Metkus AP, Filly RA, Stringer MD, et al: Sonographic predictors of survival in fetal diaphragmatic hernia. J Pediatr Surg 31:148, 1996.

22. Dillon E, Renwick M: Antenatal detection of congenital diaphragmatic hernias: The northern regional experience. Clin Radiol 48:264, 1993.

23. Goodfellow T, Hyde I, Burge DM, Freeman NV: Congenital diaphragmatic hernia: The prognostic significance of the site of the stomach. Br J Radiol 60:993, 1987.

24. Burge DM, Atwell JD, Freman NV: Could the stomach site help predict outcome in babies with left sided congenital diaphragmatic hernia diagnosed antenatally? J Pediatr Surg 24:567, 1989.

25. Teixeira J, Sepulveda W, Hassan J, et al: Abdomnial circumference in fetuses with congenital diaphragmatic hernia: Correlation with hernia content and pregnancy outcome. J Ultrasound Med 16:407, 1997.

26. Bootstaylor BS, Filly RA, Harrison MR, Adzick NS: Prenatal sonographic predictors of liver herniation in congenital diaphragmatic hernia. J Ultrasound Med 14:515, 1995.

27. Hasegawa T, Kamata SK, Imura K: Use of lung-thorax transverse area ratio in the antenatal evaluation of lung hypoplasia in congenital diaphragmatic hernia. J Clin Ultrasound 18:705, 1990.

28. Kamata S, Hasegawa T, Ishikawa S, et al: Prenatal diagnosis of congenital diaphragmatic hernia and perinatal care: Assessment of lung hypoplasia. Early Hum Dev 29:375, 1992.

29. Baker PN, Johnson IR, Gowland PA, et al: Estimation of fetal lung volume using echo-planar MRI. Obstet Gynecol 83:951, 1994.

30. Wilson JM, Fauza DO, Lund DP, et al: Antenatal diagnosis of isolated congenital diaphragmatic hernia is not an indicator of outcome. J Pediatr Surg 29:815, 1994.

31. MacGillivray TE, Jennings RW, Rudolph AM, et al: Vascular changes with in utero correction of diaphragmatic hernia. J Pediatr Surg 29:992, 1994.

32. Graf JL, Gibbs DL, Adzick NS, Harrison MR: Fetal hydrops after in utero tracheal occlusion. J Pediatr Surg 32:214, 1997.

33. Barret J, Chitayat D, Sermer M, et al: The prognostic factors in the prenatal diagnosis of the echogenic fetal lung. Prenat Diagn 15:849, 1995.

34. Morin L, Crombleholme TM, D'Alton ME: Prenatal diagnosis and management of fetal thoracic lesions. Semin Perinatol 18:228, 1994.

35. Stocker JT, Madewell JE, Drake RM: Congenital cystic adenomatoid malformation of the lung. Hum Pathol 8:155, 1977.

36. Chin KY, Tang MY: Congenital adenomatoid malformation of one lobe of a lung with general anasarca. Arch Pathol 48:221, 1949.

37. Morcos SF, Lobb MO: The antenatal diagnosis by ultrasonography of type III congenital cystic adenomatoid malformation of the lung. Br J Obstet Gynaecol 93:1065, 1983.

38. Rosado-de-Christenson ML, Stocker JT: Congenital cystic adenomatoid malformation. Radiographics 11:865, 1991.

39. Maulik D, Robinson L, Daily DK, et al: Prenatal sonographic depiction of intralobar pulmonary sequestration. J Ultrasound Med 6:703, 1987.

40. Bromely B, Parad R, Etroff JA, Benacerraf BR: Fetal lung masses: Prenatal course and outcome. J Ultrasound Med 14:927, 1995.

41. Revillon Y, Plattner JV, Sonigo P, et al: Congenital cystic adenomatoid malformation of the lung: Prenatal management and prognosis. J Pediatr Surg 28:1009, 1993.

42. Miller JA, Corteville JE, Langer JC: Congenital cystic adenomatoid malformation in the fetus: Natural history and predictors of outcome. J Pediatr Surg 31:805, 1996.

43. Maas KL, Feldstein VA, Goldstein RB, Filly RA: Sonographic detection of bilateral chest masses: Report of three cases. J Ultrasound Med 16:647, 1997.

44. McCullagh M, MacConnachie I, Garvie D, Dykes E: Accuracy of prenatal diagnosis of congenital cystic adenomatoid malformation. Arch Dis Child 71:111, 1994.

45. Adzick NS, Harrison MR, Glick PL, et al: Fetal cystic adenomatoid malformation: Prenatal diagnosis and natural history. J Pediatr Surg 20:483, 1985.

46. Budorick NE, Pretorius DH, Leopold GR, Stamm ER: Spontaneous improvement of intrathoracic masses diagnosed in utero. J Ultrasound Med 11:653, 1992.

47. Carter R: Pulmonary sequestration. Ann Thorac Surg 7:68, 1969.

48. Dolkhart LA, Reimers FT, Helmuth WV, et al: Antenatal diagnosis of pulmonary sequestration: A review. Obstet Gynecol Surv 47:515, 1992.

49. Thorpe-Beeston JG, Nicolaides KH: Cystic adenomatoid malformation of the lung: Prenatal diagnosis and outcome. Prenat Diagn 14:677, 1994.

50. Hernanz-Schulman M, Stein SM, Neblett WW: Pulmonary sequestrations: Diagnosis with color Doppler sonography and a new theory of associated hydrothorax. Radiology 180:818, 1991.

51. Adzick NS, Harrison MR, Flake AW, et al: Fetal surgery for cystic adenomatoid malformation of the lung. J Pediatr Surg 28:806, 1993.

52. Kyle PM, Lange IR, Menticoglou SM, et al: Intrauterine thoracentesis of fetal cystic lung malformations. Fetal Diagn Ther 9:84, 1994.

53. Brown MF, Lewis D, Brouillette RM, et al: Successful prenatal management of hydrops, caused by congenital cystic adenomatoid malformation, using serial aspirations. J Pediatr Surg 30:1098, 1995.

54. Clark SL, Vitale DJ, Minton SD, et al: Successful fetal therapy for cystic adenomatoid malformation associated with second-trimester hydrops. Am J Obstet Gynecol 157:294, 1987.

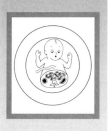

Magnetic Resonance Imaging and Computed Tomography of the Fetus

FERGUS V. COAKLEY and VICKIE A. FELDSTEIN

Ultrasound (US) is the primary modality for fetal imaging, because of relatively low cost, widespread availability, and proven utility. Ultrasound has revolutionized prenatal diagnosis, without subjecting the mother or fetus to any known deleterious effects. Advantageous imaging characteristics of ultrasound include multiplanar capability, availability of Doppler to depict flow, high spatial resolution, and real-time display. However, ultrasound has some drawbacks, including a relatively small field of view and limited acoustic contrast between soft tissue structures. Particular limitations in obstetric imaging include beam attenuation by maternal adipose tissue, poor acoustic access to the fetal head that has deeply engaged in the maternal pelvis, poor image quality in oligohydramnios, and limited visualization of the posterior fossa due to calvarial calcification after 33 weeks of gestation.[1] Experienced sonologists and obstetricians are well aware that ultrasound may be inconclusive or unhelpful in certain difficult diagnostic situations. In these cases, complementary imaging techniques are desirable. The development of fetal medicine as a recognized subspecialty has been an additional impetus to the expansion of imaging techniques other than ultrasound. The major nonsonographic techniques for imaging the fetus are magnetic resonance imaging (MRI) and computed tomography (CT), and these will be described below. While MRI in pregnancy was first described in 1983,[2] it has only been in recent years that MRI technology has evolved sufficiently to routinely allow high-quality imaging of the fetus. Consequently, the discussion will focus particularly on MRI, since this is emerging as an exciting and powerful tool in fetal diagnostic imaging. Advantages of MRI include absence of ionizing radiation, multiplanar capability, multiparameter contrast, and large field of view. Multiparameter contrast refers to the ability to select different MRI pulse sequences so that signal intensity in the image reflects different physical characteristics (see below). It should be noted that CT and MRI have other applications in pregnancy, such as pelvimetry, assessment of indeterminate adnexal or uterine lesions

detected on prenatal ultrasound, diagnosis of pelvic deep venous thrombosis, staging of gynecologic malignancy detected in pregnancy, and evaluation of placenta previa.[3–7] Also, indications for CT or MRI may arise for reasons that are entirely unrelated to pregnancy. These primarily maternal applications are not discussed further in this chapter.

MRI Physics: Critical Concepts in Fetal Imaging

MRI is an evolving field, driven by rapid technical developments in scanner hardware and software. New sequences and applications have resulted in an alphabet soup of acronyms, often designed more for market appeal than clarity. These factors are a common cause of confusion in understanding MRI physics. As a result, clinicians can be forgiven for thinking of an MRI scanner as a black box, which magically produces images of a patient placed in the scanner. However, this view fails to appreciate the essential simplicity of MRI physics, and may also result in unrealistic expectations of the modality. Briefly stated, MRI works because the protons in hydrogen atoms act like tiny bar magnets. The MRI scanner has a strong static magnetic field, which is always active. When a patient is placed in the scanner, the protons in the hydrogen atoms of the patient align in the direction of the main magnetic field, like the needle of a compass aligning with the earth's static magnetic field. This longitudinal magnetization cannot be directly measured, so short radiofrequency pulses are used to disturb the longitudinal magnetization of the protons. After these radiofrequency pulses, the protons return to their alignment with the main field. This process of relaxation results in a detectable electromagnetic signal, which is used to generate the MR image. Depending on the choice of radiofrequency pulses, the signal intensities in the resulting image reflect different physical characteristics. Usually, images are acquired to reflect the so-called T1 or T2 relaxation times of the protons, giving rise to images that are said to be T1 or T2 weighted, respectively. However, other characteristics can also be imaged, such as proton density, T2* (pronounced T2 "star"), flow (i.e., MR angiography), or metabolite levels (i.e., MR spectroscopy). The complexity of MRI arises from the almost endless variety of pulse sequences that can be chosen.

The main practical difference between MRI sequences is speed. Image acquisition time can be divided into slow (several minutes), fast (few minutes), and ultrafast (seconds). In general, image quality decreases with faster acquisition times. Currently, the major pulse sequences used in MRI are spin echo (SE), gradient-echo (GE, also known as gradient-recalled echo, or GRE), and echo-planar imaging (EPI). Conventional SE sequences are slow, fast SE (FSE) sequences are fast, and single-shot fast spin echo (SSFSE) sequences are ultrafast. Conventional GRE sequences are fast, and rapid GRE sequences are ultrafast. There are two basic types of GRE sequence, known as spoiled or steady-state, depending on the particular choice of radiofrequency pulses. EPI is inherently ultrafast. The relationship between sequence choice, imaging speed, and image quality is shown schematically in Table 8–1. It should be noted that SSFSE is a General Electric acronym, and is equivalent to the HASTE sequence marketed by Siemens.

Acquisition time is of critical importance in fetal MRI, because of image degradation by fetal motion and, to a lesser extent, by maternal respiratory motion. Standard slow MRI sequences that produce exquisitely detailed images of the stationary adult brain are of no use in fetal MRI, because nothing degrades image quality more than a moving fetus. Motion artifact has been the greatest barrier to uniformly successful fetal MR imaging. Attempts to eliminate fetal motion artifact have included the administration of muscle relaxants directly into the umbilical vein.[8] However, such invasive methods are not advisable or applicable in routine practice. Advances in MRI hardware and software have produced increasingly fast sequences, which generate images of diagnostic quality. The recent growth in fetal MRI has been largely driven by the emergence of these ultrafast sequences, particularly the development of SSFSE and HASTE.[9] SSFSE and HASTE are analogous ultrafast T2-weighted sequences, with an acquisition time of under a second per slice. This rapid acquisition essentially "freezes" fetal motion, making it possible to routinely obtain detailed and diagnostically useful images of the fetus during maternal breath-holding.[10, 11] SSFSE and HASTE are available as software upgrades from major manufacturers. Hardware requirements include a medium to high field strength (0.5 T [tesla] or greater) and high performance gradients. A fundamental concept of clinical relevance is that the spatial resolution of MRI is usually less than ultrasound (Fig. 8–1). The images produced by MRI are impressive because of high contrast resolution and large field of view, rather than high spatial detail. As a result, with currently available technology, MRI of the fetus is probably not worth undertaking before 18 to 20 weeks' gestation. Limitations in the visualization of cerebral and extracerebral fetal structures before 20 weeks has been systematically demonstrated.[10]

Technique of Fetal MRI

No maternal preparation is required, though it may be prudent to have the mother arrive fasting, to reduce bowel peristalsis artifact, and to instruct the mother to empty her bladder prior to scanning, to prevent interruptions for voiding in a patient whose bladder capacity may already be functionally reduced by pregnancy. The mother should undergo the normal MRI screening procedure, to ensure there are no maternal contraindications to scanning, such as a cardiac pacemaker, intracranial ferromagnetic surgical clips, or intraocular metallic foreign body. Written consent is not obligatory, but may be wise in view of the lack of Food and Drug Administration (FDA) approval for fetal MRI. In our experience, parental concern regarding the suspected fetal abnormality far exceeds any anxiety about the scan itself. Fetal sedation, by maternal administration of 1 mg of flunitrazepam (Rohypnol; Hoffmann-LaRoche) orally prior to scanning has been advocated to reduce fetal movement.[1] The sedative effect lasts for approximately 45 minutes. If necessary, the dose can be repeated. We have not found sedation necessary as a routine, though it may be helpful in cases where the fetus is very mobile. Fetal motion is more marked in the second trimester, and decreases as the fetus becomes more confined in the third trimester. Fetal motion is also greatly reduced by oligohydramnios, which is therefore beneficial to image quality in fetal MRI, whereas oligohydramnios is detrimental to sonographic image quality. A surface phased-array multicoil should be used for imaging, because the resulting improvement in signal/noise ratio increases spatial resolution.[12] We have found a two-element coil is suitable in small patients who are not advanced in gestation, while larger patients are more appropriately imaged with a four-element coil. The mother can usually be scanned in a supine position, but a semidecubitus position may be required in late pregnancy, in order to prevent compression of the inferior vena cava by the gravid uterus.

A scout sequence is used to localize the fetus. Subsequent sequences and imaging planes are chosen accord-

T A B L E 8–1. COMMONLY USED MRI PULSE SEQUENCES, AND ASSOCIATED ACRONYMS*

IMAGE QUALITY	High	Intermediate	Low
	SEQUENCE SPEED		
	Slow	Fast	Ultrafast
High	Spin echo/SE	Fast spin echo/ FSE	Single shot FSE (SSFSE, HASTE)
Intermediate		Gradient-echo/GE (SPGR, FLASH)	Fast GE (FMPSPGR, TurboFLASH)
Low			Echo-planar imaging (EPI).

* The relationship between sequence choice, image quality, and acquisition time is schematically indicated. Note that the relative rating with respect to image quality is strictly applicable only to stationary objects, since motion severely degrades image quality. In such cases faster sequences, which freeze motion, will be of better quality.

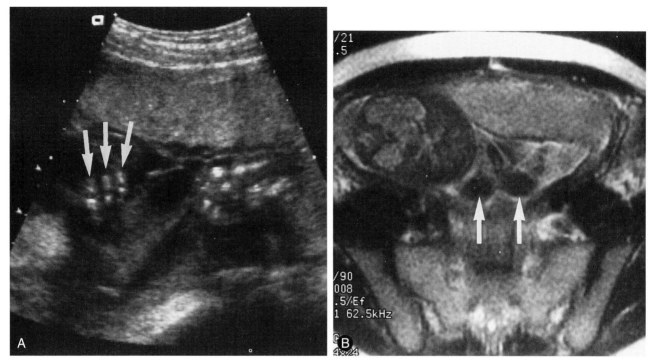

FIGURE 8–1. Comparison of the spatial resolution of ultrasound and MRI in a fetus with amniotic band syndrome and partial amputation of the fingers. Ultrasound image of the clenched hand (*A*) shows only three digits (*arrows*), where visualization of four digits would be expected. Both hands (*arrows*) are depicted by MRI (*B*), but the spatial resolution is insufficient to allow assessment of individual fingers. The spatial resolution of MRI is generally inferior to that of US, and the main imaging advantages of MRI are large field of view and excellent soft tissue contrast. Failure to appreciate this principle may result in unrealistic expectations of fetal MRI.

ing to the particular clinical concern. It is helpful to acquire images in planes that are anatomic to the fetus. This can be done by careful attention to the fetal position on the scout view, and by graphical prescription of subsequent imaging planes. These planes may be oblique to the mother, but are anatomic to the fetus. For fetal brain studies, we acquire T1- and T2-weighted images in the axial, coronal, and sagittal planes. For nonneurologic studies, imaging planes and weighting are chosen as appropriate to the clinical question. Fetal movement between acquisitions may require repetition of some sequences, to acquire images in true anatomic planes. Note that this potential interacquisition motion is different from the intra-acquisition degradation of images caused by fetal motion occurring during the sequences. Another practical difficulty is the lateralization of fetal anatomy as right or left. Careful analysis of fetal position relative to the mother allows distinction of the right and left side of the fetus. It may help to label the images accordingly. Magnification of the images, either on the hard copies or on the viewing monitor, is also useful, although it is important that the entire image is scrutinized, even if the final hard copy is cropped, since there may be unexpected pathology present outside the fetus (Fig. 8–2).

T1-weighted images are useful to assess cerebral tissue and to look for intracranial hemorrhage, which is typically bright on T1-weighted images during the subacute and chronic phases.[13] Satisfactory T1-weighted images can be difficult to obtain, and we have found

spoiled fast GRE sequences to be the most useful. Such sequences are marketed as FMPSPGR by General Electric and FLASH by Siemens. T2-weighted images are extremely useful to assess both anatomy and pathology, in both neurologic and nonneurologic cases. SSFSE (General Electric) or HASTE (Siemens) sequences result in T2-weighted images that are generally of a very high diagnostic quality. It is noteworthy that other investigators have also found that visualization of fetal structures is better on T2-weighted SSFSE sequences than T1-weighted spoiled GRE sequences.[11] The technical parameters used at our institution are shown in Table 8–2. Other sequences may occasionally be helpful. EPI T2-weighted sequences are generally of inferior image quality, but have been used for simple volumetric measurements of the fetus as a whole[14] and of individual fetal organs.[15, 16] Maternally administered intravenous gadolinium chelates cross the placenta, and are not approved for use in pregnancy. To date, no role for intravenous contrast has been shown or suggested in fetal MRI. Total imaging time should not exceed 1 hour, and in most cases will be between 30 and 45 minutes.

Safety of MRI During Pregnancy

The issue of safety of MRI exposure during pregnancy is clearly of major importance, and is often a question parents raise prior to scanning. The current guidelines

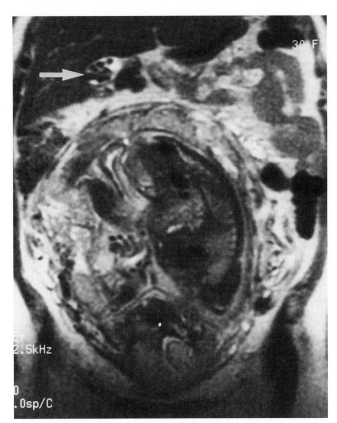

FIGURE 8–2. Maternal gallstones (*arrow*) detected incidentally by MRI in a pregnancy complicated by severe oligohydramnios. Virtually no amniotic fluid is visible around the fetus, which is in cephalic presentation. While image magnification and framing may be helpful, it is important that significant extrafetal pathology is not overlooked.

of the FDA require labeling of the MRI devices to indicate that the safety of MRI with respect to the fetus "has not been established."[17] Safety concerns arise with respect to both mother and fetus. Maternal safety concerns are the same as for a nonpregnant patient, and are addressed by prescan screening, to ensure there are no maternal contraindications to MRI. Fetal concerns are twofold; first, the possibility of teratogenetic effects, and second, the possibility of acoustic damage.

Most studies evaluating MRI safety during pregnancy show no ill effects.[18–21] However, a number of studies have raised the possibility of teratogenetic effects of MRI exposure in early pregnancy. A reduction in crown-rump length was seen in mice exposed to MRI in mid-gestation.[22] Exposure to the electromagnetic fields simulating a clinical study caused eye malformations in a genetically predisposed mouse strain.[23] Several hours of exposure of chick embryos in the first 48 hours of life to a strong static magnetic field and rapid electromagnetic gradient fluctuations resulted in an excess number of dead or abnormal chick embryos, when examined at day 5.[24] Possible mechanisms for apparent deleterious effects include the heating effect of MR gradient changes, and direct nonthermal interaction of the electromagnetic field with biologic structures. Tissue heating is greatest at the maternal body surface, and approaches negligible levels near the body center,[25] making

it unlikely that thermal damage to the fetus is a serious risk. A possible criticism of many of these studies is that they are not applicable to humans. However, they provide sufficient cause for concern such that a cautionary approach should be taken regarding fetal MRI in

TABLE 8–2. UNIVERSITY OF CALIFORNIA, SAN FRANCISCO PROTOCOL FOR FETAL MRI*

PARAMETER	TECHNICAL CHOICE	COMMENTS
1. Localizer		
Sequence	FMPSPGR	General Electric equivalent of Siemens TurboFLASH
Plane	Coronal (relative to mother)	Useful plane for localization of the fetus
TR/TE/flip angle	90–120 msec/ 4.2 msec/70 degrees	In-phase T1-weighted images
Slice thickness and gap	8 mm/1 mm	Thick slices—adequate for localizer
FOV/Matrix/NEX/ BW	32–40 cm/256 × 160/1/30 kHz	
2. T2-weighted images		
Sequence	SSFSE	General Electric equivalent of Siemens HASTE
Plane	Axial, coronal, and sagittal	Relative to fetus, through region of interest
TR/Effective TE	∞/100 msec	Moderately T2-weighted images, with good SNR
Slice thickness and gap	4 mm/0 mm	
FOV/Matrix/NEX/ BW	20–30 cm/ 256 × 192/ 0.5/31 kHz	
3. T1-weighted images		
Sequence	FMPSPGR	General Electric equivalent of Siemens TurboFLASH
Plane	Axial, coronal, and sagittal	Relative to fetus, through region of interest
TR/TE/flip angle	90–120 msec/ 4.2 msec/70 degrees	Provides in-phase T1-weighted images
Slice thickness and gap	5 mm/0 mm	Thinner slices may be too grainy
FOV/Matrix/NEX/ BW	20–30 cm/256 × 128–160/ 1/16 kHz	

* Our protocol is designed for a 1.5 T Signa superconducting magnet (General Electric Medical Systems, Milwaukee, WI). Appropriate modifications may be required for other MR imaging systems.
General comments
1. A phased array surface coil should always be used. The two-element pelvic coil is appropriate for smaller patients earlier in pregnancy, and the four-element torso coil for larger patients later in pregnancy.
2. Within reason, a small FOV is preferred, because it increases spatial resolution. However, a smaller FOV also reduces SNR, causing image graininess, and may cause image wrap.
3. Careful prescription of slice number and thickness should result in all sequences being short enough to acquire during maternal breath-holding. Split acquisitions are suboptimal, because the fetus may move between the acquisitions.
4. T2-weighted images are usually of better quality than T1-weighted images, and therefore are acquired first.
5. The FMPSPGR sequence is prone to poor SNR. Parameters should be tailored to prevent signal starvation. Therefore, relative to SSFSE T2-weighted images, the slice thickness is larger, the number of phase-encoding steps is lower, and the bandwidth is lower.
FOV, field of view; NEX, number of excitations; BW, bandwidth; SNR, signal/noise ratio.

the first trimester. Accordingly, the guidelines of the National Radiological Protection Board in the United Kingdom state that "it might be prudent to exclude pregnant women during the first three months of pregnancy."[26] An additional concern in the first trimester is the underlying relatively high rate of spontaneous abortion in this period. An MRI study could be coincidentally followed by a spontaneous abortion, but might give rise to parental concerns regarding causal effect. From a practical viewpoint, first-trimester MRI will usually be performed for maternal rather than fetal indications, and in this context MRI is still preferable to any imaging study involving ionizing radiation.[27]

A less obvious concern is the potential risk of acoustic damage to the fetus, due to the loud tapping noises generated by the coils of the MR scanner as they are subjected to rapidly oscillating electromagnetic currents, especially with EPI, which is the noisiest sequence in current clinical use. This issue has been addressed in two reports from the United Kingdom. A follow-up study of 18 patients who had undergone EPI as fetuses showed that 16 passed their 8-month hearing test, compared to 16.7 expected.[28] In a second study, a microphone was passed through the esophagus into the fluid-filled stomach of a volunteer.[29] The aim was to simulate the acoustic environment of the gravid uterus. The sound intensity in the stomach was measured within an MRI scanner, across a range of radiofrequencies. The attenuation of the transmitted sound was greater than 30 dB, sufficient to reduce sound intensity from near the dangerous level of 120 dB to an acceptable level of under 90 dB. The results of these studies provide reassuring clinical and experimental evidence that there is no significant risk of acoustic injury to the fetus during prenatal MRI.

In summary, pregnant women in the second and third trimesters can be reassured that MRI poses no known risk to the fetus, and while the safety has not been positively established, any hazard appears negligible and is outweighed by the possible diagnostic benefit of the study. A more cautious approach should be taken in those cases where an MRI scan is required in the first trimester.

Clinical Applications of Fetal MRI

Overview

The primary indication for fetal MRI is to assess abnormalities that are not detectable by ultrasound, or to evaluate equivocal or indeterminate sonographic findings. Ultrasound remains the imaging modality of choice for screening studies of the fetus. Much of the existing work in fetal MRI relates to assessment of cerebral abnormalities, though nonneurologic applications have also been described. MRI is particularly useful in the assessment of fetal brain anomalies, because calvarial calcification may limit sonographic evaluation of portions of the brain and posterior fossa, and because subtle parenchymal abnormalities such as migrational anomalies, ischemic lesions, or white matter disease may not be sonographically detectable.[7, 30] Specific cerebral and extracerebral applications are described below. Multiple case reports and small series have described a wide variety of uses for fetal MRI outside the brain, but systematic studies of large numbers of patients are lacking. Therefore, extracerebral applications of fetal MRI remain under investigation. Several specific extracerebral applications are described below, and represent a selection of cases encountered at our institution. In general, we have found fetal MRI to be particularly useful in cases where fetal therapy is being considered, since confirmation of sonographic diagnoses by complementary imaging may increase diagnostic confidence prior to undertaking high-risk fetal intervention. It is possible that as fetal medicine develops, fetal MRI will be more widely used to confirm sonographic diagnoses and evaluate cases with inconclusive ultrasound findings.

The acquisition of multiple contiguous slices using MRI allows for easy and accurate measurement of fetal volumes, both of the entire fetus and of individual fetal organs.[14–16] The cross-sectional area of the fetus or organ of interest can be measured on each slice by using a computerized outline tracing tool. The volume per slice is calculated by multiplying the cross-sectional area by the slice thickness. The total volume is the sum of the volumes per slice. Accurate assessment of fetal weight before delivery is useful in clinical management, particularly by allowing identification of intrauterine growth retardation (IUGR). It is known that IUGR is difficult to accurately diagnose by clinical assessment or sonographic evaluation. Fetal weight estimation by MRI is very accurate. In a study of 11 fetuses 1 week prior to delivery, fetal weight was estimated by volumetric analysis of contiguous T2-weighted EPI images through the fetus.[14] The estimated fetal weight as determined by MRI correlated closely with the actual birthweight, with a median difference between the two measurements of only 3%. The median difference between estimated fetal weight as determined by ultrasound and actual birthweight was 6.5%. In a further study of 32 high-risk pregnancies, 11 resulted in birth of a fetus with an individualized birthweight ratio (i.e., the ratio of the actual birthweight to the expected birthweight, with adjustments for gestational age at delivery, fetal gender, maternal parity, maternal ethnic origin, and maternal weight and booking weight) below the tenth centile, representing IUGR.[16] Ten of these 11 fetuses had an abnormally small liver volume at prenatal MRI, while the remaining 21 fetuses all had normal liver volumes. These results suggest antenatal measurement of liver volume by MRI may be a useful predictor of growth retardation.

Perinatal necropsy frequently provides useful additional information in cases of stillbirth or spontaneous abortion, but is often not performed because of reluctance on the part of obstetricians, pathologists, and parents, and because of the lack of subspecialized perinatal pathologists.[31] It has been shown that MRI of stillborn or aborted fetuses provides similar, and sometimes additional, information to perinatal necropsy,[31] and this is an application of fetal MRI that should be considered when warranted by clinical circumstances.

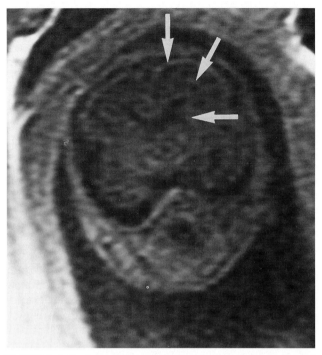

FIGURE 8–3. Coronal T1-weighted spoiled GRE image through the fetal brain at 24 weeks' gestation. The five layers of the brain parenchyma can be seen. From internal to external, these are the germinal matrix (hyperintense), deep intermediate zone (hypointense), migrating cell layer (hyperintense), superficial intermediate zone (hypointense), and the cortex (hyperintense). The three hyperintense layers are arrowed.

Brain Parenchyma

The gyral pattern of the fetal brain is best studied between 28 and 32 weeks of gestation.[1] Before 28 weeks, spatial resolution does not allow for optimal assessment. After 32 weeks, the subarachnoid space narrows, and the gyri are not as well seen. The pattern of sulcation can be compared to anatomic atlases[32] and published timetables,[33] although there is considerable variability in sulcal development.[33] The developing cerebrum has multiple parenchymal layers, which are best appreciated on T1-weighted images, and can be detected from 23 to 28 weeks[34] (Fig. 8–3). The germinal matrix appears as a high-signal-intensity rim around the ventricles. This is surrounded by a hypointense layer, the deep intermediate zone. Next is a second hyperintense layer, which represents the migrating cells. Fourth is a second hypointense layer, which is the superficial intermediate zone. Finally, there is the hyperintense layer of the cortex peripherally. MRI may be particularly helpful in late pregnancy, when calvarial calcification limits sonographic evaluation of the fetal brain. Near-field parenchymal abnormalities may be especially difficult to evaluate, because of sound beam reverberation artifact arising from the calvarial wall nearest to the transducer. In cases with a suspected but inconclusive sonographic abnormality, MRI can be useful for further assessment (Fig. 8–4). The corpus callosum can be detected from 20 weeks of gestation, and is best seen on coronal images.[1] Failure to detect the corpus callosum before this time is not indicative of pathology. In a series of 20 fetuses with

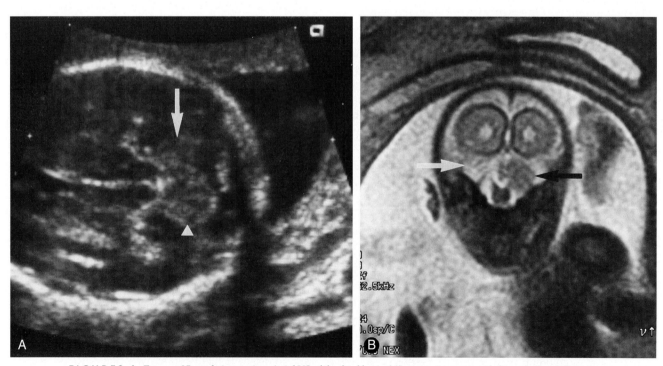

FIGURE 8–4. Fetus at 25 weeks' gestation. Axial US of the fetal brain (*A*) suggests apparent left cerebellar deficiency (*arrow*), when compared with the normal appearance of the right cerebellar hemisphere (*arrowhead*). However, this assessment is equivocal because the abnormality is subtle, and in the near field, where reverberation artifact from the calvarium can limit assessment. Coronal SSFSE T2-weighted 4-mm section of the fetal brain (*B*) confirms left cerebellar deficiency (*white arrow*). The normal right cerebellar hemisphere is indicated (*black arrow*).

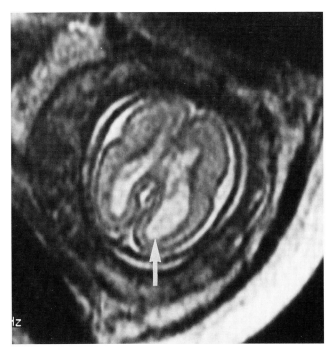

FIGURE 8–5. Fetus at 24 weeks' gestation. Routine antenatal ultrasound revealed unilateral isolated lateral ventriculomegaly. SSFSE T2-weighted 4-mm axial MRI section confirms unilateral dilatation of the lateral ventricle, predominantly involving the occipital horn (*arrow*), and does not demonstrate any additional parenchymal abnormality.

callosal agenesis, the diagnosis was made by ultrasound in 80% of cases and by MRI in 95%.[1] There are very few published reports examining the use of MRI in ischemic or hemorrhagic intracranial abnormalities. In one study, MRI demonstrated such lesions in 7 of 13 cases, using neuropathologic or postnatal MRI findings as the standard of reference.[1] Migrational disorders can be detected by fetal MRI, but may not be seen until after 30 to 32 weeks of gestation.[1] In a series of 20 fetuses with an established diagnosis of a migrational disorder, prenatal MRI detected 54% of neuronal heterotopias, 80% of lissencephalies, 73% of polymicrogyrias, and 100% of schizencephalies.[30]

Ventricular Size

The cerebral ventricles are relatively large in early fetal life, and remain so until the 25th week of gestation. Relative enlargement of the occipital horns persists until the 30th week.[35] On axial US images of the fetal brain, a diameter of the ventricular atrium that measures greater than 10 mm after is considered abnormal.[36] In cases of hydrocephalus, the choroid plexuses appear small relative to the dilated ventricles, and the medial and lateral walls of the ventricles are convex.[1] Occasionally, isolated lateral ventriculomegaly is detected by US. Causes include ischemia with periventricular leukomalacia, malformations of cortical development, agenesis of the corpus callosum, mild forms of holoprosencephaly, and congenital infection. Approximately 20% of such fetuses will demonstrate delayed neurologic devel-

opment by 1 year of age.[37] Unfortunately, US cannot reliably distinguish the various etiologies, and prediction of prognosis in an individual patient is often not possible. It may be that fetal MRI may help in this setting, by identifying additional intracranial abnormalities not seen by US (Fig. 8–5) that have prognostic significance. However, this application remains theoretical and is an area of ongoing research. Fetal ventriculomegaly is well demonstrated by MRI (Fig. 8–6), although any incremental benefit over imaging by US has not been determined.

Congenital Diaphragmatic Hernia

The overall mortality of congenital diaphragmatic hernia (CDH) is approximately 68%, due to lethal pulmonary hypoplasia resulting from the space-occupying effect of herniated abdominal contents in the thorax (Fig. 8–7). Accurate prediction of prognosis is desirable, both to guide therapeutic planning and because novel techniques now exist for potential in utero treatment of this condition. The lung/head ratio (LHR), which is the ratio of the cross-sectional area of the right lung to head circumference as measured by ultrasound, has been shown to be a predictor of prognosis.[38] When the LHR measures less than 0.6, the prognosis is very poor. When the LHR is greater than 1.35, the prognosis is very good. However, most fetuses with CDH have an LHR between

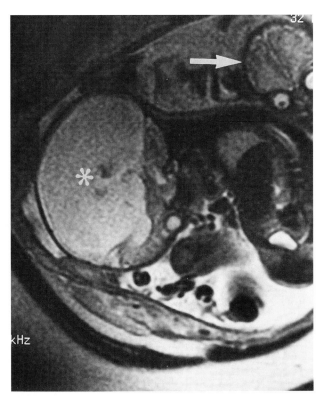

FIGURE 8–6. Twin fetuses at 30 weeks' gestation. Antenatal ultrasound demonstrated severe hydrocephalus (*asterisk*) in one of the twins. SSFSE T2-weighted 4-mm sagittal MRI section confirms the diagnosis. The degree of ventriculomegaly can be appreciated by comparison with the cranial size of the normal twin (*arrow*).

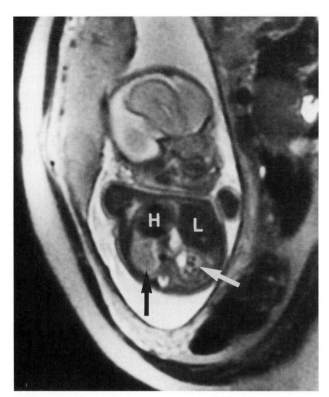

FIGURE 8–7. SSFSE T2-weighted 5-mm axial MRI section of a fetus with a left congenital diaphragmatic hernia. Herniation of stomach and small bowel (*white arrow*) and of the left hepatic lobe (L) into the left hemithorax is evident. The left lung is not visible, likely due to severe hypoplasia. The right lung (*black arrow*) and heart (H) are markedly displaced to the right side.

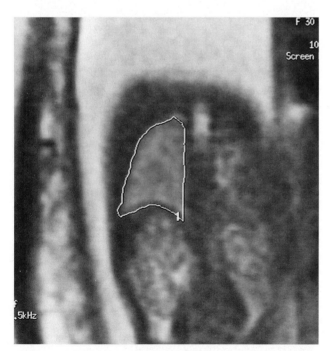

FIGURE 8–8. SSFSE T2-weighted 5-mm coronal MRI section of a fetus with a left congenital diaphragmatic hernia. The cross-sectional area of the right lung has been measured. The volume of right lung on this slice is calculated by multiplying the area by the slice thickness. This process is repeated for each slice that contains right lung tissue, and in this way the total lung right volume can be calculated. The prognostic significance of such volumetric measurements is not yet known, but may prove more predictive than currently available sonographic techniques.

these outlying values, and have an indeterminate prognosis, with a reported 57% overall survival rate. Therefore, a more accurate predictor of prognosis is desirable. It is possible that morphologic assessment of CDH by MRI may provide more precise prognostic information.[39] For example, volumetric measurement of the fetal right lung (Fig. 8–8) may be more predictive of outcome than the measurement of the lung cross-sectional area. A further potential application of MRI in fetuses with CDH is in the identification of the position of the left hepatic lobe. Liver position is known to be a useful secondary prognostic indicator in fetuses with CDH. Patients in whom the left hepatic lobe remains in the abdomen usually have a high LHR, and have a relatively good prognosis. In contrast, herniation of the left hepatic lobe into the chest is often associated with a lower LHR and a higher neonatal mortality rate. However, ultrasound signs of liver herniation are subtle, and considerable operator experience is required for optimal results.[40] Demonstration of liver position by MRI may be more straightforward for general radiologists without special-

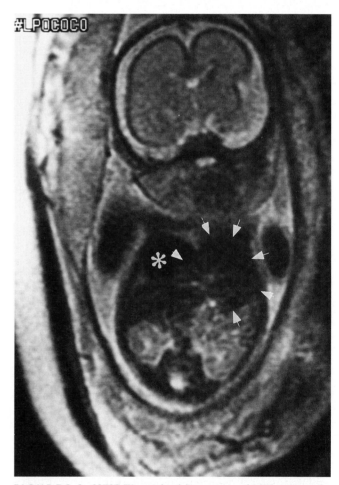

FIGURE 8–9. SSFSE T2-weighted 5-mm coronal MRI section of a fetus with a left congenital diaphragmatic hernia. Herniation of the left hepatic lobe into the left hemithorax is readily demonstrated (*arrows*). The heart (*asterisk*) is deviated to the right. Determination of the left hepatic lobe position by ultrasound may be difficult and requires considerable operator experience. Centers without experienced sonologists may find MRI helpful in the assessment of left hepatic lobe position.

ist experience in the sonographic evaluation of CDHs (Fig. 8–9).

Congenital High Airway Obstruction Syndrome

Congenital high airway obstruction syndrome (CHAOS) is a very rare condition characterized by developmental obstruction of the upper airway, either the fetal larynx or upper trachea.[41] The exact pathology has not been well described, because of the rarity of the condition, and because previously reported cases have resulted in fetal or neonatal demise. Upper airway obstruction results in retention of bronchial secretions and pulmonary distention by the retained fluid. Overinflation of the lungs, with flattening or eversion of the diaphragm, is thought to impair venous return to the heart, resulting in fetal hydrops and ascites. This results in a characteristic constellation of sonographic findings, including large bilateral echogenic fetal lungs, flattening or eversion of the diaphragm, dilated fluid-filled airways below the level of obstruction, and fetal hydrops or ascites. We have utilized MRI to confirm the diagnosis

antenatally (Fig. 8–10). This fetus subsequently underwent in utero tracheostomy. The patient survived, and postnatal assessment demonstrated a focal web in the larynx, without evidence of segmental laryngeal atresia.

Congenital Hemochromatosis

Congenital (perinatal, neonatal) hemochromatosis is characterized clinically by severe neonatal liver failure, and histologically by prominent stainable iron in the parenchymal cells of the liver and other viscera.[42] The condition is rare, but is probably the second most common cause of neonatal liver failure, after sepsis.[43] The condition is not precisely defined, because a specific etiology or metabolic defect has not been identified.[42] Familial and recurrent cases have been described, but a definite pattern of inheritance has not been established. Oligohydramnios is a recognized finding.[44] It has been suggested that abnormally high transfer of iron from the mother to the fetus across the placenta may be the underlying abnormality.[45] We have used a T2*-weighted GRE sequence to prenatally diagnose congenital hemochromatosis. This sequence is very sensitive to causes

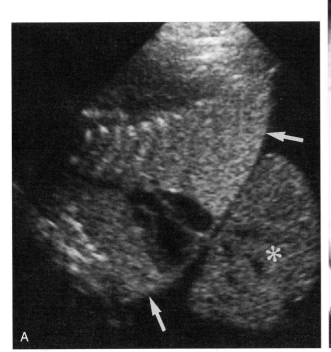

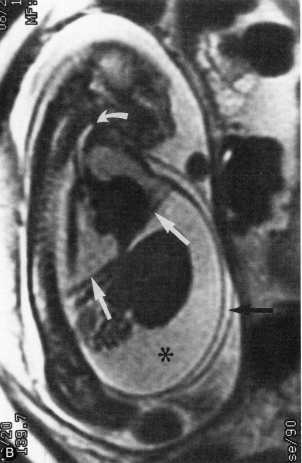

FIGURE 8–10. Fetus at 25 weeks' gestation. Coronal US of the fetal thorax (*A*) demonstrates bilaterally enlarged echogenic lungs causing eversion of the diaphragm (*arrows*), with associated ascites outlining the fetal liver (*asterisk*). Oblique longitudinal SSFSE T2-weighted 4-mm MRI section (*B*) of the fetal torso confirms diaphragmatic eversion (*white arrows*), with a large volume of fetal ascites (*asterisk*), marked subcutaneous edema (*black arrow*), and a blind-ending fluid-filled upper airway (*curved white arrow*). The findings are consistent with CHAOS.

of T2* dephasing, such as parenchymal iron deposition, and has been used to assess hemochromatosis in adults.[46] There has been one previous report describing the antenatal diagnosis of congenital hemochromatosis by MRI.[47] The iron-laden liver appears darker than expected on T2*-weighted images (Fig. 8–11). The maternal liver, maternal spleen, and fetal spleen can be used as internal controls to assess the relative signal intensity of the fetal liver.

Amniotic Band Syndrome

The amniotic band syndrome is a known cause of severe fetal malformations, and is estimated to occur in 1 per 1,200 live births.[48] The condition is believed to be due to rupture of the amnion, with the result that the fetus becomes trapped in the fibrous septae of the chorionic

space.[49] Entanglement of fetal parts in these fibrous septae results in random nonembryologic slash defects and amputations, which are variable in severity and distribution. The head, trunk, and extremities are frequently involved. In the extremities, the combination of a constriction ring with distal lymphedema is virtually diagnostic. The diagnosis can be made with US, but the abnormalities can also be well shown by MRI (Fig. 8–12).

CT of the Fetus

Risks of CT During Pregnancy

CT is the second major nonsonographic modality available for fetal imaging. Risks to the fetus due to in utero MRI are theoretical and unproved. In contrast, fetal exposure to ionizing radiation during pregnancy is undoubtedly harmful, with risks of teratogenesis and carcinogenesis. The International Commission on Radiologic Protection has recommended that the radiation dose to the fetus should not exceed 1 rad during a known pregnancy. It is agreed that every effort should be made to limit to a minimum the radiation that a fetus receives. Organogenesis occurs predominantly between 2 and 15 weeks of gestation, and this is the period when the fetus is susceptible to the teratogenetic effects of ionizing radiation. Teratogenetic effects are extremely unlikely in fetuses before 2 weeks of gestation and after 15 weeks of gestation.[50] The radiation dose below which no deleterious effects on the fetus occur even in the most sensitive developmental phase is not known, but is estimated to range from 5 to 15 rad.[51] The radiation dose to the fetus from a spiral CT study of the pelvis using typical technical parameters is 5 to 10 rad.[52] Therefore, even if pelvic CT is performed during organogenesis, the radiation dose is at the estimated threshold level for induction of congenital malformations. The incidence of malformations is not measurably increased after in utero irradiation in humans.[53] In practice, fetal CT is usually performed later in gestation, when any remote risk of teratogenesis should be outweighed by the clinical benefit of the study. For these reasons, teratogenesis is not a significant risk in fetal CT. However, cancer induction is a real consideration. The risk of a fatal childhood cancer between 0 and 15 years of age after radiation exposure in the third trimester has been estimated at 4.6×10^{-4} per rad of fetal whole body dose.[54] Using a fetal dose estimate of 5 to 10 rad for a standard pelvic CT, this implies an excess risk of death from childhood cancer of 1 in 220 to 1 in 440. A review of 11 retrospective studies determined the risk of childhood cancer doubled with a fetal radiation exposure of 5 rad.[55] These risks are small, but not negligible, and should be discussed with parents prior to fetal CT.

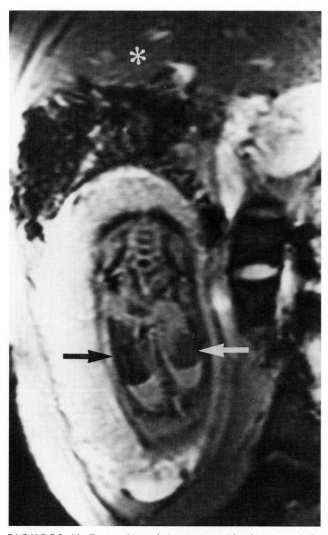

FIGURE 8–11. Fetus at 31 weeks' gestation, with a fetus in cephalic presentation. Coronal GE T2*-weighted 6-mm MRI section demonstrates markedly reduced signal intensity in the fetal liver (*black arrow*), particularly in comparison with the fetal spleen (*white arrow*) and the maternal liver (*asterisk*). The findings suggest hemochromatosis. This sequence is extremely sensitive to iron deposition, which manifests as reduced signal intensity. The diagnosis of congenital hemochromatosis was confirmed postnatally.

Clinical Applications

In current obstetric practice, the use of CT is limited. The most common obstetric indications are pelvimetry and amniography. Pelvimetry is performed to determine maternal pelvic dimensions, particularly in cases

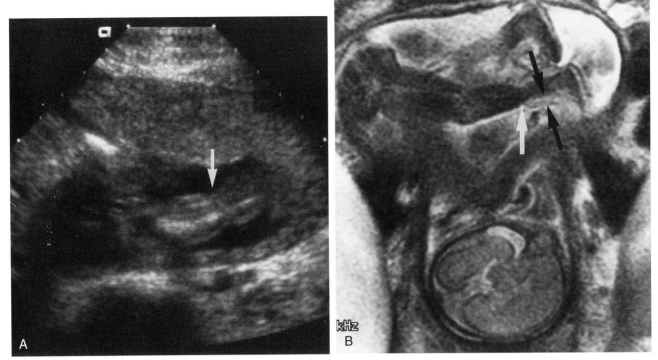

FIGURE 8–12. Fetus at 24 weeks' gestation. Longitudinal US of the fetal right lower extremity (*A*) indicates a constriction ring in the midcalf (*arrow*). Sagittal SSFSE T2-weighted 4-mm MRI section (*B*) of the fetal body and right lower extremity also demonstrates a constriction ring in the midcalf (*white arrow*) and marked distal subcutaneous edema (*black arrows*), confirming the diagnosis of amniotic band syndrome.

of breech presentation when vaginal delivery is being considered. Presently, pelvimetry is the major single source of fetal radiation exposure. CT amniography is occasionally performed as a means of confirming monoamnionicity.[56–58] This technique should be used only after extensive attempts to determine amnionicity by sonography have been performed. Monoamnionicity can be excluded with ultrasound by demonstrating a membrane separating the fetuses, separate placental sites, different fetal sexes, or a "stuck twin." For CT amniography, ultrasound is used to select a transverse plane of section and this location is marked. A single transverse axial precontrast CT section may be obtained at this level. Under sonographic guidance, the amniotic sac is punctured and water-soluble iodinated contrast material is instilled. Using a contrast agent with a concentration of approximately 300 mg of iodine per mL of solution, 1 mL per 100 mL of anticipated amniotic fluid volume provides adequate opacification. Typically, approximately 8 to 10 mL of contrast are used in a third-trimester pregnancy with normal amniotic fluid volume. A postcontrast transverse axial CT scan at the same level is obtained (Fig. 8–13). Monoamnionicity is indicated by the presence of contrast material completely surrounding each twin, though rarely this appearance may be mimicked by a diamniotic pregnancy with a "stuck twin." Finberg[59] has reported that the presence of contrast material within the gastrointestinal tract of both twins, after a delay of approximately 4 hours, is a reliable, unambiguous sign of monoamnionicity.

CT has several potential applications in the evaluation of fetal anatomy and structural abnormalities.[60] For example, in the past, CT has been used at our institution to further evaluate fetal cerebral abnormalities, initially detected by ultrasound (Figs. 8–14 and 8–15). However, with the refinement of MRI, CT of the fetus has become a fairly rare examination. Still, CT has certain advantages for fetal imaging. For example, as described above, iodinated contrast material can be instilled into the amniotic cavity. It is swallowed by the fetus with subsequent opacification of the fetal gastrointestinal tract. In this way, CT can be used to confirm and quantitate the degree of bowel herniation in cases of congenital diaphragmatic hernia.

A fairly recent form of CT imaging, termed spiral CT, is ideally suited to three-dimensional reconstruction of fetal bony anatomy (Fig. 8–16). This is because bone detail is well imaged by CT, the scan speed of spiral CT is such that it effectively freezes fetal motion, and the technique is inherently volumetric. Finally, it should be remembered that CT of the fetus remains an option in those cases where further assessment of sonographic findings, which suggest a fetal morphologic abnormality, is required, but MRI cannot be performed because of maternal contraindications, such as the presence of a cardiac pacemaker or ferromagnetic intracranial clips.

Summary

Ultrasound remains the established primary modality for fetal imaging, especially for obstetric screening ex-

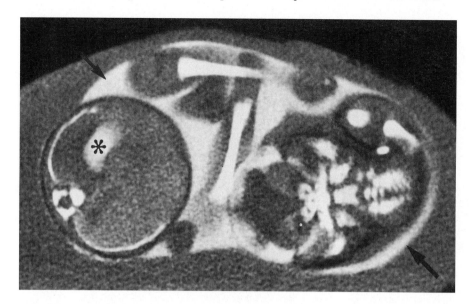

FIGURE 8–13. CT amniogram. Transverse CT section obtained following contrast instillation showing opacified amniotic fluid (*arrows*) completely surrounding both fetuses, confirming monoamnionicity. In addition, ingested contrast is seen within the stomach (*asterisk*) of the fetus on the maternal right.

aminations. MRI is emerging as a powerful supplementary technique for fetal imaging, because modern ultrafast sequences and technology now allow for the noninvasive acquisition of images that both freeze fetal motion and are of diagnostic quality. Fetal MRI should be regarded as an imaging technique that is complementary to ultrasound, rather than an alternative or replacement modality. The primary indications for fetal MRI include assessment of equivocal or indeterminate ultrasound findings, and the evaluation of specific clinical concerns that ultrasound cannot address. Fetal MRI has predominantly been used to assess fetal cerebral abnormalities. Extracerebral applications have been described, and are currently being systematically explored. Such extracerebral applications are likely to be more clearly defined in the future. Volumetric measurements of fetal size and fetal organ size by MRI appear particularly promising. CT of the fetus is rarely performed, and is likely to become even rarer with the continuing evolution of fetal MRI. However, certain specific applications remain, including cases where MRI cannot be performed because of maternal contraindications.

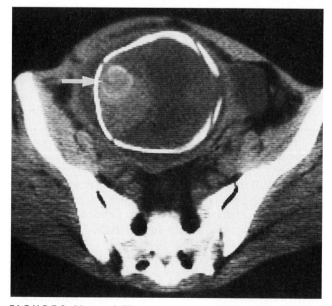

FIGURE 8–14. Axial CT section of the fetal brain, performed after ultrasound demonstrated moderate ventriculomegaly and a poorly characterized abnormality in the posterior fossa. CT section shows a hyperdense lesion (*arrow*) in the posterior fossa, suggestive of hematoma. Gradual resolution on serial sonograms confirmed the presumptive diagnosis.

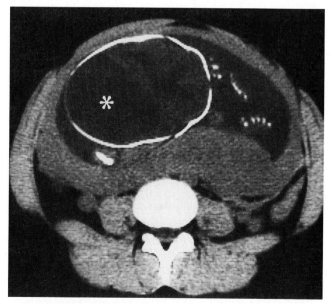

FIGURE 8–15. Axial CT section of the fetal brain, performed because ultrasound suggested the diagnosis of Dandy-Walker malformation, but was limited by multiple technical problems. A large posterior fossa cyst (*asterisk*) is clearly identified, confirming the diagnosis.

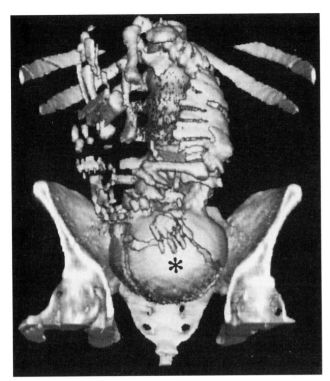

FIGURE 8–16. Three-dimensional reconstruction of the fetal skeleton using spiral CT. The study was performed because of suspected maternal nephrolithiasis. The rapid volumetric data acquisition during spiral CT makes this an ideal technique for such three-dimensional reconstruction. Note the clear depiction of the relationship between the maternal pelvis (*arrow*) and the fetal skull (*asterisk*).

REFERENCES

1. Garel C, Brisse H, Sebag G, et al: Magnetic resonance imaging of the fetus. Pediatr Radiol 28:201–211, 1998.
2. Smith FW, Adam AH, Phillips WDP: NMR imaging in pregnancy. Lancet 1:61–62, 1983.
3. Federle MP, Cohen HA, Rosenwein MF, et al: Pelvimetry by digital radiography: A low-dose examination. Radiology 143:733–735, 1982.
4. Stark DD, McCarthy SM, Filly RA, et al: Pelvimetry by magnetic resonance imaging. AJR Am J Roentgenol 144:947–950, 1985.
5. Forstner R, Kalbhen CL, Filly RA, Hricak H: Abdominopelvic MR imaging in the nonobstetric evaluation of pregnant patients. AJR Am J Roentgenol 166:1139–1144, 1996.
6. Angtuaco T, Shah H, Mattison D, Quirk J: MR imaging in high risk obstetric patients: A valuable complement to US. Radiographics 12:91–109, 1992.
7. Levine D, Edelman RR: Fast MRI and its application in obstetrics. Abdom Imaging 22:589–596, 1997.
8. Seeds JW, Corke BC, Spielman FJ: Prevention of fetal movement during invasive procedures with pancuronium bromide. Am J Obstet Gynecol 155:818–819, 1986.
9. Kiefer B, Grassner J, Hausman R: Image acquisition in a second with half Fourier acquisition single-shot turbo spin-echo. J Magn Reson Imaging 4(P):86–87, 1994.
10. Levine D, Barnes PD, Sher S, et al: Fetal fast MR imaging: Reproducibility, technical quality, and conspicuity of anatomy. Radiology 206:549–554, 1998.
11. Yamashita Y, Namimoto T, Abe Y, et al: MR imaging of the fetus by a HASTE sequence. AJR Am J Roentgenol 168:513–519, 1997.
12. Campeau NG, Johnson CD, Felmlee JP, et al: MR imaging of the abdomen with a phased-array multicoil: Prospective clinical evaluation. Radiology 195:769–776, 1995.
13. Barkovich AJ, Atlas SW: Magnetic resonance imaging of intracranial hemorrhage. Radiol Clin North Am 26:801–820, 1988.
14. Baker PN, Johnson IR, Gowland PA, et al: Fetal weight estimation by echo-planar magnetic resonance imaging. Lancet 343:644–645, 1994.
15. Baker PN, Johnson IR, Gowland PA, et al: Estimation of fetal lung volume using echo-planar magnetic resonance imaging. Obstet Gynecol 83:951–954, 1994.
16. Baker PN, Johnson IR, Gowland PA, et al: Measurement of fetal liver, brain, and placental volumes with echo-planar magnetic resonance imaging. Br J Obstet Gynecol 102:35–39, 1995.
17. Food and Drug Administration: Magnetic resonance diagnostic device: Panel recommendation and reports on petitions for MR reclassification. Federal Register 53:7575–7579, 1988.
18. Mevissen M, Buntenkotter S, Loscher W: Effects of static and time-varying (50 Hz) magnetic fields on reproduction and fetal development in rats. Teratology 50:229–237, 1994.
19. Beers GJ: Biological effects of weak electromagnetic fields from 0 Hz to 200 Hz: A survey of the literature with special emphasis on possible magnetic resonance effects. Magn Reson Imaging 7:309–331, 1989.
20. Schwartz JL, Crooks LE: NMR imaging produces no observable mutations or cytotoxicity in mammalian cells. AJR Am J Roentgenol 139:583–585, 1982.
21. Wolff S, Crooks LE, Brown P, et al: Test for DNA and chromosomal damage induced by nuclear magnetic resonance imaging. Radiology 136:707–710, 1980.
22. Heinrichs WL, Fong P, Flannery M, et al: Midgestational exposure of pregnant balb/c mice to magnetic resonance imaging. Magn Reson Imaging 8:65–69, 1986.
23. Tyndall DA, Sulik KK: Effects of magnetic resonance imaging on eye development in the C57BL/6J mouse. Teratology 43:263–275, 1991.
24. Yip YP, Capriotti C, Talagala SL, Yip JW: Effects of MR exposure at 1.5T on early embryonic development of the chick. J Magn Reson Imaging 4:742–748, 1994.
25. Kanal E, Shellock FG, Talagala L: Safety considerations in MR imaging. Radiology 176:593–606, 1990.
26. National Radiological Protection Board: Principles for the Protection of Patients and Volunteers During Clinical Magnetic Resonance Diagnostic Procedures. Documents of the NRPB, Volume 2, no 1. London: HM Stationery Office, 1991.
27. Shellock FG, Kanal E: Policies, guidelines, and recommendations for MR imaging safety and patient management. J Magn Reson Imaging 1:97–101, 1991.
28. Baker PN, Johnson IR, Harvey PR, et al: A three year follow-up of children imaged in utero with echo-planar magnetic resonance. Am J Obstet Gynecol 170:32–33, 1994.
29. Gover P, Hykin J, Gowland P, et al: An assessment of the intrauterine sound intensity level during obstetric echo-planar magnetic resonance imaging. Br J Radiol 68:1090–1094, 1995.
30. Sonigo PC, Rypens FF, Carteret M, et al: MR imaging of fetal cerebral anomalies. Pediatr Radiol 28:212–222, 1998.
31. Brookes JAS, Hall-Craggs MA, Sams VR, Lees WR: Non-invasive perinatal necropsy by magnetic resonance imaging. Lancet 348:1139–1141, 1996.
32. Feess-Higgins A, Larroche JC: Development of the Human Fetal Brain. An Anatomical Atlas. Paris: Masson, 1987.
33. Chi JG, Dooling EC, Gilles FH: Gyral development of the human brain. Ann Neurol 1:86–93, 1977.
34. Girard N, Raybaud C, Poncet M: In vivo MR study of brain maturation in normal fetuses. AJNR Am J Neuroradiol 16:407–413, 1995.
35. Larroche JC: Morphological criteria of central nervous system development in the human fetus. J Neuroradiol 8:93–108, 1981.
36. Farrell TA, Hertzberg BS, Kliewer MA, et al: Fetal lateral ventricles: Reassessment of normal values for atrial diameter seen at US. Radiology 193:409–411, 1994.
37. Patel MD, Filly RA, Hersh DR, Goldstein RB: Isolated mild fetal cerebral ventriculomegaly: Clinical course and outcome. Radiology 192:759–764, 1994.
38. Metkus AP, Filly RA, Stringer MD, et al: Sonographic predictors of survival in fetal diaphragmatic hernia. J Pediatr Surg 31:148–152, 1996.

39. Hubbard AM, Adzick NS, Crombleholme TM, Haselgrove JC: Left-sided diaphragmatic hernia: Value of prenatal MR imaging in preparation for fetal surgery. Radiology 203:636–640, 1997.

40. Bootstaylor BS, Filly RA, Harrison MR, Adzick NS: Prenatal sonographic predictors of liver herniation in congenital diaphragmatic hernia. J Ultrasound Med 14:515–520, 1995.

41. Hedrick MH, Ferro MM, Filly RA, et al: Congenital high airway obstruction syndrome (CHAOS): A potential for perinatal intervention. J Pediatr Surg 29:271–274, 1994.

42. Witzleben CL, Uri A: Perinatal hemochromatosis: Entity or end result? Hum Pathol 20:335–340, 1989.

43. Silver MM, Cave CT, Kirpalani H: Case 6. Perinatal hemochromatosis. Pediatr Pathol 9:203–210, 1989.

44. Singh S, Sills JH, Waffarn F: Interesting case presentation: Neonatal hemochromatosis as a cause of ascites. J Perinatol 10:214–216, 1990.

45. Knisely AS, Grady RW, Kramer EE, Jones RL: Cytoferrin, maternofetal iron transport, and neonatal hemochromatosis. Am J Clin Pathol 42:755–759, 1989.

46. Gandon Y, Guyader D, Heautot JF, et al: Hemochromatosis: Diagnosis and quantification of liver iron with gradient-echo MR imaging. Radiology 193:533–538, 1994.

47. Marti-Bonmatti L, Baamonde A, Poyatos CR, Monteagudo E: Prenatal diagnosis of idiopathic neonatal hemochromatosis with MRI. Abdom Imaging 19:55–56, 1994.

48. Seeds JW, Cefalo RC, Herbert WNP: Amniotic band syndrome. Am J Obstet Gynecol 144:243–248, 1982.

49. Burton DJ, Filly RA: Sonographic diagnosis of the amniotic band syndrome. AJR Am J Roentgenol 156:555–558, 1991.

50. Wagner LK, Lester RG, Saldana LR: Exposure of the Pregnant Patient to Diagnostic Radiations: A Guide to Medical Management. Philadelphia: JB Lippincott Company, 1985, pp 19–223.

51. Berlin L: Radiation exposure and the pregnant patient. AJR Am J Roentgenol 167:1377–1379, 1996.

52. Wagner LK, Archer BR, Zeck OF: Conceptus dose from two state-of-the-art CT scanners. Radiology 159:787–792, 1986.

53. Mole RH: Irradiation of the embryo and fetus. Br J Radiol 60:17–31, 1987.

54. Mole RH: Childhood cancer after prenatal exposure to diagnostic x-ray examinations in Britain. Br J Cancer 62:152–168, 1990.

55. Ginsberg JS, Hirsh J, Rainbow AJ, Coates G: Risks to the fetus of radiologic procedures used in the diagnosis of maternal venous thromboembolic disease. Thromb Haemost 61:189–196, 1989.

56. Carlan SJ, Angel JL, Sawai SK, Vaughn V: Late diagnosis of non-conjoined monoamniotic twins using computed tomographic imaging: A case report. Obstet Gynecol 76:504–506, 1990.

57. Sargent SK, Young W, Crow P, Simpson W: CT amniography: Value in detecting a monoamniotic pair in a triplet pregnancy. AJR Am J Roentgenol 156:559–560, 1991.

58. Wax JR, Smith JF, Floyd RC: Monoamniotic twins discordant for anencephaly: Diagnosis by CT amniography. J Comput Assist Tomogr 18:152–154, 1994.

59. Finberg HJ, Clewell WH: Definitive prenatal diagnosis of monoamniotic twins. Swallowed amniotic contrast agent detected in both twins on sonographically selected CT images. J Ultrasound Med 10:513–516, 1991.

60. Siegal H, Seltzer S, Miller S: Prenatal computed tomography: Are there indications? J Comput Assist Tomogr 8:871–876, 1984.

9

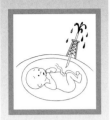

Prenatal Diagnostic Techniques

JAMES D. GOLDBERG and MARY E. NORTON

dvances in prenatal diagnosis have significantly contributed to the management of the fetal patient. Invasive fetal diagnostic techniques provide fetal cells and tissue for the diagnosis of karyotype abnormalities and a wide range of molecular and biochemical defects. Population screening approaches are useful in identifying abnormal fetuses in general, low-risk populations. Genetic counseling is an extremely important aspect of any prenatal diagnostic procedure to provide patients with information regarding their fetuses in a nondirective manner. This chapter reviews the various approaches to invasive prenatal diagnosis and population screening, including the reproductive genetic issues. In addition, advances in molecular biology will be discussed as they relate to prenatal diagnosis.

Birth Defects and Genetic Counseling

Approximately 3% of pregnancies result in delivery of an infant with a birth defect or genetic disease. Such congenital anomalies have become the single largest cause of infant mortality in the United States.[1] Genetic factors are involved in the etiology of many such disorders, although the numerous causes include chromosomal abnormalities, contiguous gene deletion syndromes, single gene disorders, teratogen exposure (drugs and environmental chemicals, maternal metabolic imbalance, infections, and radiation), and multifactorial disorders due to interactions or combinations of these factors. In addition, many other reproductive complications, including infertility, early pregnancy loss, late stillbirth, or neonatal demise, can have a genetic cause. Indeed, the more our ability to diagnose genetic disease increases, the more disorders are found to have a detectable genetic basis.

Genetic Counseling

Genetic counseling has been defined by an ad hoc committee of the American Society of Human Genetics as a communication process dealing with the occurrence, or risk of recurrence, of a genetic disorder. This process includes helping the individual or family (1) to understand the medical facts, including diagnosis, prognosis, and therapy; (2) to understand the role of genetics in the disorder and the risk of recurrence; (3) to understand the reproductive options; (4) to choose an appropriate course of action; and (5) to adjust as well as possible to the disorder or to the risk of its recurrence.

Most geneticists believe that a counselor should provide information as objectively as possible, and avoid judgmental or directive advice. Of course, completely nondirective counseling is probably a myth, and it has been noted that merely offering antenatal diagnostic services implies approval. Nevertheless, one should attempt to provide a variety of viewpoints objectively, and to encourage couples to make their own decisions. Families must weigh many concerns, including the perceived burden of the disorder, their capacity to withstand adversity, the level of family support, the impact on existing children, their financial status, and moral commitments.

Genetic counseling in any setting has many components, including the confirmation of a diagnosis, and discussion of the natural history, therapeutic options, recurrence risk, and psychological and social issues raised by the disorder. The importance of an accurate diagnosis cannot be overemphasized, and confirmation is always obligatory. If a diagnosis has been made in another child or family member, it is important to obtain and review the relevant medical data. A diagnosis given to a patient as a "possibility" is often later reported as definitive, although it may never have been confirmed. A patient who has male relatives with a bleeding disorder, for example, may report a family history of hemophilia if either family members or their physicians have assumed this. Before carrier testing or prenatal diagnosis can be performed or recurrence risks determined, medical records must be reviewed to ensure that the diagnosis is accurate.

Genetic counseling also involves discussion of the natural history of a disorder. This discussion may be simplified in a patient with a family history and first-hand experience with a particular condition. Many disorders have a broad range of severity, which can be significant even within a family, and this should be described to the patient. With prenatal diagnoses, couples are often frustrated that molecular testing results and the genetic counselors who interpret them cannot be more definitive in providing specific prognostic information other than the range of outcomes seen in other affected individuals. This should be discussed when offering prenatal diagnosis for conditions with a variable range of severity.

Another aspect of genetic counseling is discussion of available treatment options. While our ability to detect genetic disease has advanced more quickly than our capability for prevention or treatment, there are increasing options available for intervention both prenatally and after birth, and for avoiding recurrence in the future. This is true of metabolic as well as structural disorders, and all available options should be discussed with the couple. In some situations, there are options for experimental therapies or prenatal interventions that must be weighed against a less aggressive approach. In circumstances in which there is controversy regarding which treatment affords the most favorable outcome, the family must be carefully and objectively counseled, and a nondirective approach should be taken.

Recurrence risk is a concern that also must be addressed, although often not in the acute setting of a recent diagnosis. Again, discussion of recurrence risk rests on the accuracy of the diagnosis. In families in which a diagnosis is unknown or uncertain, clinicians can estimate risk using principles of genetic inheritance, empiric information from analysis of population data, information from the pedigree, and laboratory data including biochemical and other analyses as well as any available DNA data. In some situations, preventive therapies may be helpful, such as folic acid supplementation in the avoidance of neural tube defects, and this should be discussed as soon as possible so that therapy is instituted before there is another pregnancy. In other cases, preimplantation diagnosis, sperm or ovum donation, or adoption may be options in preventing recurrence of a particular genetic disease.

Finally, the psychological aspect of the disorder must be addressed. Couples often feel guilt surrounding an inherited disorder. For patients who experience anxiety or depression, referral to resources such as psychologists or social workers is important. Many prenatal diagnostic centers now offer support groups, which are helpful for some couples. In acute situations, family members will not retain complicated details. One of the fine arts of genetic counseling lies in determining the best time and circumstances in which to convey complex but essential information.

Genetic Counseling in a Prenatal Setting

In a prenatal setting, patients may be seen before, during, or after a pregnancy complicated by a problem which may have a genetic basis or place them at increased risk (Table 9–1). Most patients are seen because age, biochemical screening tests, or family history places them at increased risk to have a child with a birth defect, and most of these patients will ultimately deliver normal, healthy infants. A smaller percentage of patients are seen because they have been found to be carrying a fetus with sonographically detected anomalies or a

TABLE 9–1. COMMON INDICATIONS FOR PRENATAL GENETIC COUNSELING

Advanced maternal age (≥35 years old)
Abnormal maternal serum screening
Family history
    Single-gene disorder
    Birth defects
    Chromosome abnormality
    Mental retardation
Teratogen exposure
Consanguinity
Repeated pregnancy loss or infertility
Abnormal ultrasound findings
    Fetal anomalies
    Subtle features suggestive of aneuploidy

specific genetic disease. The role of the geneticist in this setting is to determine a diagnosis, where possible, and to explain this to a family in light of their options for pregnancy management. Again, an accurate diagnosis is critically important in predicting outcome to the family. While patients presenting for postnatal genetic counseling after the birth of a child with a genetic disease or birth defect will most often have some personal experience with the disorder of concern, parents learning of such a problem prenatally often have no knowledge of the diagnosis under consideration. Patients frequently over- or underestimate the severity of the condition affecting their unborn children, and must be carefully counseled regarding the full spectrum of the disorder and potential impact on their family.

The need for information in prenatal genetic counseling falls into several general time frames. First, prior to any prenatal testing, the couple must decide whether to pursue any evaluation. Later, a genetic counselor may see a patient after a sonographic diagnosis of a congenital anomaly or a positive result on an invasive prenatal test. At that point, decision-making often involves whether to continue the pregnancy. If the pregnancy is continued, they must decide on the extent of usual or extraordinary care that will be provided during the pregnancy and for the infant after delivery. Concerns for the mother's health must always be considered. A third situation occurs when a child is born with unexpected anomalies and a decision must be made immediately regarding how aggressively to support the child. Finally, genetic counselors are often involved after the pregnancy, when the family is trying to make later reproductive decisions.

Preprocedure Counseling

Primary providers of obstetric care, including obstetricians, midwives, and family practitioners, typically provide the initial counseling regarding advanced maternal age, biochemical screening, ultrasound, and options for prenatal fetal evaluation, as well as screening for genetic disorders such as Tay-Sachs disease, cystic fibrosis, and the hemoglobinopathies. Genetic counselors commonly see patients who are greater than 34 years old to discuss the options for karyotype analysis for advanced maternal age. They may also meet with patients with a significant family history, again to discuss the options for prenatal testing and whether such testing is desired. Again, a nondirective approach is important, even at the initial discussions regarding screening test options.

Prior to any prenatal diagnostic procedure, patients must be counseled as to the risks and benefits of the procedure, as well as the information to be gained and the limitations of testing. It is important that women understand that an amniocentesis or chorionic villus sampling (CVS) for advanced maternal age will provide very accurate information regarding chromosome abnormalities, but not other causes of birth defects or mental retardation.

A family history and other risk factors should also be reviewed prior to prenatal diagnostic testing, to ensure that there are no other issues in the history that should be addressed. In some patients, ethnic background may indicate screening for disorders such as cystic fibrosis, Tay-Sachs disease, or the hemoglobinopathies. In others, the family history may include relatives with mental retardation, and fragile X testing may be appropriate. The cells obtained from a CVS or amniocentesis can be used to test for these other genetic disorders, in the event the patient is found to be at risk.

Prenatal Management of Congenital Anomalies

When a fetal anomaly is detected by ultrasound, the genetic counseling approach should be similar to that used in the postnatal setting. The sonographic diagnosis must be as complete and accurate as possible, and the fetus thoroughly evaluated for the presence of other anomalies or minor dysmorphic features that might give clues as to a syndromic diagnosis. Research in tertiary centers has found that a large number of abnormal findings were not consistent with the initial indication for referral. While some of the inconsistencies were simply an incorrect sonographic diagnosis, often the correct diagnosis was made due to the increased information provided by genetic pedigree analysis and recognition of syndromes.[2] Diligence in the search for associated anomalies, careful pedigree analysis, and knowledge of syndromic abnormalities are critical components of the differential diagnosis.

A detailed history is imperative in all cases in which a fetal anomaly is detected. Issues to be discussed include medication exposures, maternal medical disorders, pregnancy history or complications, previous pregnancies and outcomes, and any family history of birth defects or genetic disease. Genetic counselors also typically inquire about family history of renal disease or other medical disorders, children requiring surgery soon after birth, and persons dying in infancy or childhood. A relevant family history can often aid in making a precise diagnosis in a case in which the sonographic findings suggest a broad differential diagnosis or be suggestive of a genetic syndrome in the setting of an isolated fetal anomaly. Under such circumstances, the prognosis may

be very different than that given without the added information provided by the family pedigree.

Once a family history has been recorded, determination of which prental tests are indicated is appropriate. In most cases in which a fetal abnormality is detected, discussion of karyotyping is warranted. Fetal structural abnormalities identified with ultrasound are more likely to be associated with chromosomal aneuploidy than similar abnormalities in the newborn. This is in part because a fetus that appears to have a single major malformation by ultrasound examination may in fact have multiple congenital anomalies not identifiable until birth. In addition, fetuses with structural malformations and/or chromosomal abnormalities have a high intrauterine death rate.

The likelihood of a chromosomal aneuploidy in a fetus with anomalies depends on the number, as well as the type and severity of structural defects. Rizzo et al. found that the incidence of chromosomal abnormalities increased from 10% in fetuses with one malformation to 35% with two or more.[3] The type of defect also frequently suggests a particular aneuploidy syndrome. For example, trisomy 21 is frequently diagnosed after the sonographic identification of an atrioventricular canal defect or duodenal atresia, whereas alobar holoprosencephaly and clefting are typically associated with trisomy 13, and cystic hygroma with monosomy X.

With improvement in prenatal ultrasound as well as in our understanding of the etiology of various birth defects, we can provide patients with more specific information regarding the risk of a chromosome abnormality and the option of other types of testing. Whereas previously only karyotyping was available for further evaluation of the fetus with a prenatally detected birth defect, the application of advances in medical genetics now allows more accurate counseling and more sophisticated and discriminatory testing in many circumstances (Table 9–2).

TABLE 9–2. CAUSES OF ELEVATED MSAFP

Multiple gestation
Fetal demise
Fetomaternal hemorrhage
Placental abnormalities
Uterine abnormalities
Maternal ovarian or hepatic tumors

Fetal structural defects
Neural tube defects
  Spina bifida
  Anencephaly
  Encephalocele
Open ventral wall defects
  Omphalocele
  Gastroschisis
Congenital nephrosis
Triploidy
Bilateral renal agenesis
Congenital skin disorders
  Epidermolysis bullosa
  Aplasia cutis
Infantile polycystic kidney disease
Sacrococcygeal teratoma
Cystic adenomatoid malformation of the lung

MSAFP, maternal serum α-fetoprotein.

For some structural anomalies, such as gastroschisis, it is now recognized that a vascular etiology is responsible for most cases. Reported risk factors for gastroschisis include young maternal age and maternal smoking,[4] and this disorder is not felt to be associated with an increased risk of aneuploidy.[5] This contrasts with omphalocele, which is associated with a risk of fetal aneuploidy as high as 30 to 40%. This high risk varies in part with the size of the omphalocele, with smaller defects associated with a higher risk and larger, liver containing defects associated with a lower risk.[6] In addition, an apparently isolated omphalocele has been associated with Beckwith-Weidemann syndrome (BWS) in up to 22% of cases.[7] BWS is an autosomal dominant disorder in some families, and a careful family history may reveal other members with findings such as large birth weight, hypoglycemia at birth, macroglossia, or hemihypertrophy. Molecular testing can determine the DNA basis for BWS in some cases in which the disorder is associated with a duplication on the short arm of chromosome 11. BWS might also be suggested sonographically in the fetus with a relatively large size, a persistently protruding tongue, or large echogenic kidneys.

Karyotyping in the setting of a fetal anomaly is most commonly accomplished on amniocytes, as these patients are typically seen in the second trimester. Occasionally a late CVS or placental biopsy may be performed (i.e., in the setting of oligohydramnios precluding a straightforward amniocentesis). As karyotyping of amniocytes can take as long as 14 days, umbilical blood sampling is sometimes performed with preliminary results available in 24 to 48 hours. In some cases, karyotype results from amniocytes and lymphocytes may be different, and this can have important implications. For example, tetrasomy 12p (Killian/Teschler-Nicola syndrome) can be associated with congenital diaphragmatic hernia (CDH). This particular chromosome abnormality is usually seen only in fibroblasts, but is not usually present in blood.[8] Therefore, the fetus with a CDH is better evaluated through amniocentesis than percutaneous umbilical cord blood sampling (PUBS), and a newborn with a CDH and suspicion of tetrasomy 12p should undergo a skin biopsy as opposed to routine lymphocyte karyotype.

When a family history suggests a particular diagnosis, determining which prenatal tests are appropriate is usually straightforward. In the absence of a family history, a genetic consultation can aid in determining which genetic syndromes are in the differential diagnosis, and which tests are available with a high enough yield to be warranted. For some studies, such as DNA-based linkage analysis, testing can only be done in the setting of a positive family history and the availability of other family members. For others, direct mutation analysis may be available and suggested by a particular constellation of findings.

In the patient who ultimately terminates her pregnancy, or whose pregnancy ends in stillbirth or neonatal demise, it is important that the option of autopsy be discussed. Although the concept of autopsy may be distressing, it is important to explain that carefully performed studies will allow more accurate recurrence risk counseling and prenatal diagnosis in the future. Studies of perinatal autopsy have found that, in those cases in which autopsy was performed, 45% changed or added to the prenatal diagnosis,[9] a high enough percentage to warrant consideration of autopsy in most cases.

Optimal evaluation and care of the fetus with one or more anomalies is best accomplished with a multidisciplinary approach. With advances in the fields of obstetric sonography, neonatal care, pediatric surgery, and genetic testing, each member of the team provides valuable information for the family faced with difficult decisions. It is impossible for one individual to keep abreast of all developments in these rapidly changing fields, and it is in our patients' best interest to provide the most accurate and up-to-date information.

The role of the sonologist and geneticist is in ensuring an accurate diagnosis. The sonologist provides the details of the "physical exam," which may provide clues as to a syndromic diagnosis and lead to other testing options. The geneticist, neonatologist, and pediatric surgical team can then describe the likely outcome and options for further management of the pregnancy. The perinatologist coordinates the obstetric care and can discuss ways in which a diagnosis might lead to pregnancy complications, such as premature delivery or need for cesarean section.

The genetic counselor helps the couple synthesize the complicated medical facts, and with the social worker, helps the family place them in perspective of their own values and beliefs to aid in decision-making. The experience of coping with an abnormality in a pregnancy is among the most difficult many people will encounter, and it is important to address this psychological component. The stress of caring for a disabled child is reflected in a divorce rate twice that of the general population.[10] Long after the pregnancy is over and the family has left our care, they may be struggling to care for a child with disabilities or may be coping with the memories of pregnancy loss. It is critically important that these families feel that the highest quality of medical care available was provided in a compassionate way. In addition, we must respect the families' perspective and decisions, which ultimately they live with much longer than we will.

Invasive Prenatal Diagnostic Techniques

Amniocentesis

Midtrimester amniocentesis is currently the most commonly performed invasive prenatal diagnostic test. The diagnosis of Down syndrome from cultured amniotic fluid cells obtained by amniocentesis was first reported in 1968.[11] Since that time, amniocentesis has evolved into the "gold standard" against which all other invasive prenatal diagnostic procedures are compared.

The procedure is most commonly performed between 16 and 18 weeks of gestation. Following ultrasound evaluation of the fetus, including placental localization, an insertion site is marked on the maternal abdomen. The site should be chosen to avoid traversing the placenta if possible. However, it appears the fetal loss rate is not increased following transplacental passage of the amniocentesis needle.[12] The abdomen is then prepped with povidone-iodine and alcohol. A local anesthetic may then be used, although many practitioners feel this is unnecessary. Under direct, real-time ultrasound guidance, a 22-gauge needle is inserted into the amniotic fluid. The use of ultrasound guidance has been shown to reduce the number of needle insertions and to reduce the incidence of bloody taps.[13] In addition, patient anxiety appears to be reduced by the use of ultrasound guidance. Approximately 20 mL of amniotic fluid is then aspirated. If bloody fluid is aspirated, a small amount of heparin should be added to reduce clumping of the amniocytes in clotted blood. The first 1 to 2 mL of amniotic fluid should be discarded to reduce the incidence of maternal cell contamination. Rh-negative women with an Rh-positive partner should be given Rh immune globulin following the procedure.

The amniotic fluid obtained from amniocentesis may be used for a variety of analyses. The most common one is karyotype analysis following long-term culture. This process typically takes 1 to 2 weeks to obtain a result. In an effort to shorten this procedure to result interval, fluorescent in situ hybridization (FISH) has been used for rapid analysis of interphase amniocytes. Recently, multicolor FISH has been used to identify the most common aneuploidies found at the time of amniocentesis utilizing probes for chromosomes 13, 18, 21, X, and Y.[14] There have been no large prospective studies looking at the sensitivity and specificity of this approach. The American College of Medical Genetics policy currently states that FISH should be used as an adjunct to other testing. The cells obtained from long-term culture may also be used as a source of DNA for molecular analysis or for biochemical analysis of metabolic disorders. If a molecular analysis can be performed by DNA amplification, cells from uncultured amniotic fluid may be used.

Several studies in the 1970s looked at the safety of midtrimester amniocentesis. A National Institutes of Health (NIH)-sponsored, prospective, nonrandomized, collaborative study found an overall loss rate of 3.5% between the time of the procedure and delivery compared to a loss rate of 3.2% in matched controls.[15] A Canadian prospective study, which did not include a control group, found a similar loss rate of 3.2% following midtrimester amniocentesis.[16] A British collaborative study, however, found a higher loss rate following amniocentesis compared to controls (2.6% vs. 1%).[17] The British study included many patients whose indication for amniocentesis was an elevated maternal serum α-fetoprotein (AFP), which in subsequent studies has been shown to be associated with adverse perinatal outcome. A Danish study published in 1986 was the first prospective randomized study of outcome following amniocentesis. The study group consisted of 4,606 women aged 25 to 34 years of age who had no known risk factors to increase their risk of pregnancy loss.[18] The loss rate in the amniocentesis group was 1.7% compared to 0.7% in controls, which was significant. The procedures in this

study were performed with a 20-gauge needle (as compared with a 22-gauge needle in most of the other studies), which may be a factor in the increased loss rate. Based on these studies, most practitioners in the United States quote a procedure-related loss rate of 0.5%.

Because of the gestational age at which amniocentesis has traditionally been performed and the need for long-term culture of the amniocytes, there has been significant interest in developing procedures that could be performed earlier in gestation. Historically, the reason that amniocentesis was not performed earlier in pregnancy had been the difficulty in obtaining amniotic fluid. This was most likely due to the poor quality of ultrasound that was then available. With modern ultrasound equipment this is not an issue, and several investigators have reported their experience with amniocentesis as early as 10 weeks of gestation.[19, 20] Until recently, however, there has been no large prospective trial looking at the safety of this approach.

Results of a Canadian prospective, randomized trial of early amniocentesis (between 11 [+0] and 12 [+6] gestational weeks [days]) versus midtrimester amniocentesis (between 15 [+0] and 16 [+6] gestational weeks [days]) revealed a significantly increased loss rate in the early amniocentesis group (7.6% vs. 5.9%).[21] In addition, there was a significantly increased incidence of talipes equinovarus in the early amniocentesis group (1.3% vs. 0.1%). Thus, it appears that early amniocentesis does carry an increased risk as compared to midtrimester amniocentesis. Currently, there are few data regarding the risk of amniocentesis between 13 and 15 weeks of gestation.

Chorionic Villus Sampling

As mentioned above, because of the time in gestation when patients usually receive amniocentesis results there has been a desire to develop an earlier approach for prenatal diagnosis. CVS has developed into a first-trimester prenatal diagnosis option. The first successful report of chorionic villus sampling being used for prenatal diagnosis was reported from China in 1975.[22] The procedure was performed by passing a small catheter next to the gestational sac and aspirating chorionic villi without ultrasound guidance. The villi were analyzed by sex chromatin evaluation without full karyotyping being performed. The procedure has evolved into an ultrasound-guided procedure performed either transcervically or transabdominally under direct ultrasound guidance.[23] The type of procedure is dictated by the location of the implantation site and the position of the uterus. Typically, with an anterior placental implantation site the procedure is most easily performed transabdominally. With a posterior implantation or a retroflexed uterus the transcervical approach is easiest. Centers performing CVS should have the capability of performing both types of procedures. The procedure is performed between 10 and 12 gestational weeks, at which time the background spontaneous abortion rate has significantly decreased. Earlier procedures have been shown to be associated with an increased incidence of adverse outcome (see below).

Prior to performing either a transcervical or transabdominal CVS an ultrasound examination is performed to assess fetal anatomy and heart rate and to identify the implantation site. Frequently, by having the patient fill or empty her bladder the position of the uterus can be optimized for the sampling procedure. At our center, patients are counseled that the practitioner at the time of the ultrasound will suggest which approach is preferable.

If a transcervical procedure is to be performed, the patient is put in lithotomy position. A sterile speculum is inserted and the cervix visualized. The cervix and vagina are prepped with an iodine solution. Generally, a tenaculum is not necessary but may be helpful in some cases to rotate the uterus or apply traction. A thin (approximately 16-gauge) polyethylene catheter with a malleable stainless steel obturator is then guided to the area of the trophoblast under direct ultrasound vision. The catheter can be curved to facilitate placement. Care is taken to avoid an insertion site close to the fetal membranes or maternal decidua. A small amount of cramping may be felt by the patient as the catheter passes the internal os. No anesthesia is necessary. Communication between the sonologist and the person inserting the catheter is critical for successful placement of the catheter. A 20-mL syringe is then attached to the catheter after removing the obturator, negative pressure is applied, and the catheter is slowly withdrawn. The sample is then aspirated into transport media and immediately examined under a low-power dissecting microscope to determine its adequacy.

Transabdominal CVS is performed in a similar manner to amniocentesis. The insertion site is marked on the maternal abdomen and the abdomen is prepped with iodine and alcohol. A local anesthetic is injected. Under ultrasound guidance a 20-gauge spinal needle is inserted into the long axis of the trophoblast. Some practitioners utilize a two-needle technique where an 18-gauge needle is inserted into the myometrium and a smaller needle inserted through this needle to obtain a sample. The advantage to this technique is that a second needle insertion is not needed if the sample is inadequate. However, in over 90% of cases in most centers, a second insertion is not necessary and thus most centers use the single-needle approach. A 20-mL syringe is attached and negative pressure applied. The needle is moved up and down several times in the villi and removed. The sample is then examined for adequacy.

The chorionic villi obtained are composed of three cell types, syncytiotrophoblast, cytotrophoblast, and a central mensenchymal core. The cytotrophoblast cells are actively dividing and may be analyzed for karyotyping after short-term (24 to 48 hour) culture. The mesenchymal core is grown out in long-term culture and produces a fibroblast-like cell type similar to amniocytes. While the short-term culture produces a rapid result, there have been more discrepancies with the true fetal karyotype with this approach.[24] Thus, most centers rely on the long-term culture result.

The incidence of chromosomal mosaicism is higher in chorionic villi as compared to amniocytes (1.3% vs. 0.25%).[25] Several large series have reported that in most of these cases the mosiacism is confined to the trophoblast only.[24, 25] This is most likely due to postzygotic nondisjunction in the trophoblast or trisomic rescue in the fetus. In the case of trisomic rescue, uniparental disomy can occur resulting in an abnormal outcome for chromosomes that have been shown to be imprinted.[26] Because some of these cases might truly represent mosaicism in the fetus, follow-up should include amniocentesis. Percutaneous umbilical blood sampling may also be helpful in providing an additional tissue for karyotyping. The effect of confined placental mosaicism on the developing embryo is somewhat controversial, although some studies have shown an increased incidence of intrauterine growth restriction and perinatal death.[27] Follow-up ultrasound evaluation may be helpful in assessing this.

The procedure-related risk of pregnancy loss following chorionic villus sampling appears to be the same as midtrimester amniocentesis when performed in experienced centers. The Canadian collaborative experience, published in 1989, showed no significant increase in fetal loss following CVS when compared to midtrimester amniocentesis.[28] Shortly thereafter, data from the American collaborative series were reported that also showed no significant difference in loss between CVS and amniocentesis.[29] In contrast to this, a collaborative European trial (MRC Working Party on the Evaluation of CVS) reported a 4.6% increased loss rate following CVS as compared to midtrimester amniocentesis.[30] Examining the studies, it appears that the MRC study was performed at a greater number of centers and with more practitioners than the other studies. In addition, each practitioner performed fewer procedures than in the North American trials. Thus, it has been suggested that the relative lack of experience might have contributed to the increased loss rate in the MRC study.

There has been much discussion in the literature regarding the association of CVS and fetal limb reduction defects following the report by Firth in 1991 of five infants born with limb reduction defects following CVS in a series of 539 women.[31] Four of the infants had the oromandibular–limb hypogenesis syndrome and one had a terminal transverse limb reduction defect. All of the CVS procedures in the affected infants were between 55 and 66 days of gestation and were done by transabdominal sampling. Several other small series have also reported an increased incidence of limb reduction defects following CVS. The most common association seems to be with procedures performed early (prior to 70 days of gestation), although not all reports have found this.[32–34] In an effort to further study this association, over 140,000 cases submitted to the World Health Organization (WHO) registry were analyzed with no increase in limb reduction defects over baseline being found.[35] Thus, it appears that procedures performed after 10 weeks of gestation in experienced centers carry no increased risk of limb reduction defects. All patients considering CVS, however, should have these data reviewed with them, since it remains somewhat controversial.

The tissue obtained from chorionic villus sampling can also be used for a variety of biochemical and DNA diagnoses. The quantity of tissue is usually sufficient to allow an analysis without the need for tissue culture. In this type of analyses there is the concern of maternal cell contamination. This can be minimized by careful initial separation of the tissue by a technician experienced in handling chorionic villi.

Fetal Blood Sampling

The indications for fetal blood sampling have dramatically changed over the past several years. In the past, fetal blood was needed for the prenatal diagnosis of thalassemia, one of the most common indications for prenatal diagnosis in many Mediterranean countries.[36, 37] Fetal blood was necessary to perform globin chain synthesis studies to diagnoses both α- and β-thalassemia. Molecular DNA diagnosis has essentially done away with this indication for fetal blood sampling. Currently, the most common indication for fetal blood sampling is for karyotype analysis of fetal lymphocytes. This is primarily done for two reasons. The first is for a rapid result. Cytogenetic results from fetal lymphocytes are available in 48 to 72 hours as compared to the 7 to 10 days required for amniocytes or chorionic villi. The second indication is for further evaluation of unusual results on amniocentesis or chorionic villi which usually involves mosaicism. Other rarer indications for fetal blood sampling include the diagnosis of hematologic disorders where a molecular defect has not been defined.

Fetal blood was initially obtained by a fetoscopic procedure.[38] The umbilical cord was directly visualized and a small needle (27-gauge) inserted into the cord and blood aspirated. This procedure was technically difficult to perform and available in only a few centers around the world. It has been replaced by PUBS, developed and described by Daffos.[39] The procedure is performed in a similar manner to amniocentesis. Under direct ultrasound guidance, a 20- or 22-gauge needle is inserted into the umbilical vein. The area of the cord near to the cord insertion into the placenta is usually chosen because the cord is most fixed at this location. The aspirated fetal blood is immediately analyzed in a Coulter channelizer to confirm that it is fetal. This can be done because the fetal cells have a larger mean cell volume as compared to maternal cells. The procedure is generally performed after 18 weeks of gestation.

The risk of fetal blood sampling is significantly dependent on the indication for the procedure.[40] In well-grown, structurally normal fetuses several large studies have shown the risk for fetal loss to be 1 to 2%. This risk rises substantially in the growth-restricted or structurally abnormal fetus. Excessive bleeding from the cord puncture site is extremely rare; however, exsanguination has been reported in cases of fetuses affected with hemophilia A, Glanzmann thrombasthenia, and severe thrombocytopenia secondary to alloimmune thrombocytopenia.

Biochemical Screening in Pregnancy

One of the great advances in genetics over the past two decades has been the development of biochemical screening for birth defects. In 1972, scientists in Edinborough, Scotland, first discovered that AFP levels are elevated in amniotic fluid in patients carrying a fetus with anencephaly or open spina bifida.[41] Two years later, it was reported that AFP is also elevated in maternal serum in these patients.[42, 43] After confirmation in large, multicenter studies, population-based screening became a possibility.[44] Soon after such screening was introduced in the early 1980s, it was recognized that fetuses with Down syndrome had a lower mean maternal serum AFP (MSAFP) in the second trimester,[45, 46] and that this same test could be used to screen for Down syndrome in women younger than 35. Later research resulted in development of multiple marker screening, in which AFP, unconjugated estriol, and human chorionic gonadotropin are all used in calculating Down syndrome risk. It has been shown that multiple marker screening for Down syndrome is safer and more financially cost effective than screening based on age alone,[47] and screening for neural tube defects has also been shown to be cost effective.[48] At present, there is active research into ways to improve these tests, with attempts to increase the detection rate and decrease the false-positive rate.

α-Fetoprotein

AFP is an oncofetal protein produced by the fetal yolk sac and liver, and is the major serum protein in early fetal life.[49] AFP initially enters the amniotic fluid through diffusion across the immature fetal skin, and later through fetal urination. Much lower concentrations of AFP diffuse across the placenta and amnion into the maternal circulation. Nonpregnant women have levels of AFP that are barely detectable (approximately 1 μg/L), while normal median levels at 16 to 18 weeks of gestation range from 18 to 40 μg/L. When the fetal serum level is 2,000,000 μg/L, the corresponding amniotic fluid AFP is 20,000 μg/L, and the maternal serum level is 20 μg/L.[50] Fetal plasma and amniotic fluid levels of AFP peak in the midtrimester of pregnancy,[51] while maternal serum AFP continues to increase until 28 to 32 weeks of gestation[52] (Fig. 9–1). The discrepancy between amniotic fluid and maternal serum levels of AFP is not completely understood, but may be due to the rapidly expanding placental and amniotic interfaces.

In the fetus with a defect such as anencephaly or spina bifida, AFP will leak into the amniotic fluid in increased amounts, leading to higher levels in the maternal serum as well. Levels of AFP are elevated in amniotic fluid and in maternal serum only when such lesions are "open" (i.e., when the neural tissue is exposed or covered by only a thin membrane). When neural tube defects are skin-covered, AFP does not escape from the fetal circulation, and closed lesions are generally not detected by MSAFP screening. While virtually 100% of cases of anencephaly are open, approximately 20% of spina bifida lesions are closed, as are about 82% of en-

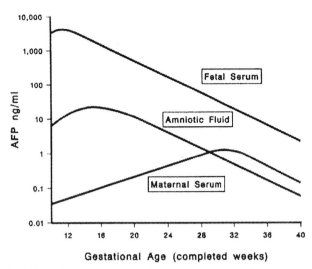

FIGURE 9–1. Mean concentrations of AFP in maternal serum, amniotic fluid, and fetal serum.

cephaloceles.[50] Discussions of the sensitivity and specificity of MSAFP screening and amniotic fluid AFP (AFAFP) testing are generally restricted to open lesions, as it is assumed that closed lesions will not be detected.

Approximately 99% of anencephaly cases are associated with elevated AFP in the amniotic fluid, and about 90% with an elevated MSAFP. Among open spina bifida cases, 75 to 85% have an elevated MSAFP, while 97% have an elevated AFAFP.[50] The most likely explanation for this lower sensitivity is that open spina bifida is usually a smaller lesion, and therefore smaller amounts of AFP gain access to amniotic fluid and maternal serum. Encephalocele is diagnosed much less frequently in the presence of an elevated AFP, due to both a lower incidence and a higher frequency of closed lesions.

In laboratories providing AFP screening, results are expressed as multiples of the median (MoM) for each gestational week, which allows expression of measurements in a common way. The distribution of MSAFP is log gaussian, with median values of 1.0 for normal pregnancies, 3.8 for pregnancies with open spina bifida, and 6.5 for pregnancies affected with anencephaly[50] (Fig. 9–2). There is significant overlap between affected and unaffected pregnancies, and choosing an MSAFP cutoff requires consideration of both detection rates and false-positive rates. The two most commonly used cutoffs are 2.0 and 2.5 MoM. At 2.0 MoM, the false-positive rate ranges from 4 to 6%, and the detection rate for open spina bifida ranges from 85 to 90%. With a higher cutoff of 2.5 MoM, the false-positive rate decreases to 2 to 3%, while the detection rate also decreases to 75 to 80%.[50] Given the extent of overlap between affected and unaffected pregnancies, it is not possible to detect all cases of open spina bifida with MSAFP screening, and, likewise, most cases of elevated MSAFP will ultimately be determined to be normal.

The original studies of MSAFP screening utilized dating based on last menstrual period (LMP). Such dates have been shown to be reliable in only approximately 80% of cases, and the performance of MSAFP screening is improved when sonographic dating is used. In addition, because biparietal diameter (BPD) measurements are, on average, smaller during the second trimester in cases of spina bifida, this will make the MSAFP appear higher, and this artifact actually improves the detection rate for open spina bifida.

There are a number of variables that must be considered when reporting MSAFP values. These include not only gestational age but also maternal weight,[53] race,[54, 55] the presence of insulin-dependent diabetes,[56] and the number of fetuses. Because heavier women have a larger volume of distribution, their MSAFP concentration will be lower, and formulas have been developed to correct for maternal weight. Black and Asian women have levels approximately 10 to 15% higher than women from other racial groups and have a lower prior risk than the general population for neural tube defects. Because the amount of AFP entering the maternal circulation is directly proportional to the number of fetuses, it is twice as high with a twin gestation.[52] In pregnancies in which first-trimester multifetal pregnancy reduction has been performed, MSAFP is virtually always elevated, and therefore cannot be used to screen for neural tube defects or aneuploidy.[57]

Women with insulin-dependent diabetes mellitus (IDDM) have MSAFP values that average 20% lower in the second trimester than nondiabetics. Women with IDDM also have a higher prior risk for neural tube defects (NTDs), and these factors are taken into account when interpreting MSAFP levels. There are some data that women with well-controlled diabetes, as determined by HbA_{1C} levels in the first trimester, may actually have MSAFP values similar to the nondiabetic population.[58] At present, however, MSAFP is corrected in women with IDDM without regard to diabetic control. Although average MSAFP levels in women who smoke cigarettes are 3% higher when compared with nonsmokers, this difference is not significant enough to warrant risk adjustment.[59]

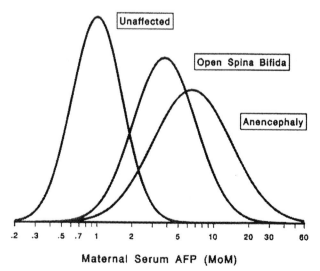

FIGURE 9–2. Distribution of second-trimester MSAFP levels in unaffected pregnancies and those affected by open spina bifida and anencephaly. The median for open spina bifida is 3.8 MoM, and for anencephaly is 6.5 MoM.

Follow-up when MSAFP is Elevated

When the MSAFP is above the cut-off, the accuracy of dating is assessed. If the LMP was used for the original calculation, an ultrasound should be performed. A screening ultrasound at this point will confirm dating, and rule out multiple gestation and fetal demise, both of which can cause an elevated AFP. In addition, most cases of anencephaly will be detected. Each program determines the discrepancy in dates at which recalculation of risk is performed, generally between 7 and 14 days.

If the screening ultrasound does not identify a cause of the elevated AFP, further assessment with more sophisticated sonography and/or amniocentesis is indicated. Amniocentesis allows measurement of both AFAFP and acetylcholinesterase (AChE). AChE is generally measured only in samples with an AFAFP greater than 2.0 MoM, an approach that provides the best balance between sensitivity and specificity.[60] Measurement of AFAFP and AChE has a 97% detection rate for neural tube defects, with a false-positive rate of 0.5%,[61] although such testing requires amniocentesis with a small but definite risk of pregnancy loss. Of note, the false-positive rate of AChE at the time of early amniocentesis (from 10 to 15 weeks) has been found to be four times higher than with amniocentesis after 15 weeks, a limitation of early amniocentesis in screening for neural tube defects.[62]

The sensitivity of ultrasound for the detection of neural tube defects and other significant structural anomalies associated with increased MSAFP has been reported to be as high as 94%,[63, 64] although this is somewhat operator dependent. Ultrasound is less expensive than amniocentesis, and does not carry the risk of pregnancy loss. Many centers now routinely offer targeted ultrasound without amniocentesis as standard evaluation of an elevated MSAFP. One study comparing strategies for evaluation of elevated MSAFP indicated that a program using targeted ultrasound and an MSAFP cut-off of 2.0 MoM would detect 90 of 110 structurally abnormal fetuses, without iatrogenic fetal loss, at a cost of $5,700 per anomalous fetus. The authors contrast this with a strategy of amniocentesis with karyotyping for MSAFP of 2.5 MoM or greater, which will detect 15 additional abnormal fetuses (including some autosomal as well as sex chromosomal aneuploidies), but with nine iatrogenic fetal losses and incremental cost of $46,100 per anomalous fetus.[65]

Several investigators have reported an association of elevated MSAFP with an increased risk of fetal aneuploidy,[66, 67] an additional argument for amniocentesis. These studies have estimated the prevalence of clinically significant aneuploidy in this setting at 1%, with approximately 55% of these being autosomal aneuploidies and 45% sex chromosome abnormalities.[68, 69]

Other Abnormalities Associated with Elevated MSAFP

An elevated MSAFP can be associated with other fetal abnormalities (Table 9–3), including other open fetal defects, such as omphalocele and gastroschisis (Fig. 9–3). In addition, some fetal skin disorders allow increased diffusion of AFP into the amniotic fluid, resulting in an elevated MSAFP. Congenital nephrosis can cause extremely high levels of AFP due to fetal proteinuria, and is suspected with a normal ultrasound and markedly elevated MSAFP. This autosomal recessive disorder results in renal failure early in life, and children generally die in infancy or early childhood. It is relatively rare except in Finland, where the reported incidence of 1 per 2,600 makes the disease a primary focus of AFP screening programs.[50, 70]

Elevated Amniotic Fluid AFP

A number of studies have addressed the residual risk of an abnormality after an elevated AFAFP in a structurally normal fetus. Because the concentration gradient between fetal plasma and amniotic fluid AFP is about 200:1, fetal blood contamination can result in a mislead-

TABLE 9–3. PRENATAL FINDINGS THAT CAN BE EVALUATED WITH DNA BASED OR BIOCHEMICAL TESTING

ABNORMALITY	POSSIBLE DIAGNOSIS	TEST TO BE CONSIDERED
Congenital heart defect, microcephaly	Maternal PKU	Maternal phenylalanine level
Ambiguous genitalia	Congenital adrenal hyperplasia (21-hydroxylase deficiency)	DNA-based mutation analysis
	Smith-Lemli-Opitz syndrome	Amniotic fluid dehydrocholesterol
Conotruncal cardiac defect	Velocardiofacial syndrome	22q deletion studies (FISH)
Aqueductal stenosis (male fetus)	X-linked aqueductal stenosis	MASA syndrome gene mutation studies
Low estriol on second-trimester screen	Smith-Lemli-Opitz syndrome	Amniotic fluid dehydrocholesterol
	Placental sulfatase deficiency	Amniotic fluid steroid sulfatase
		Xq deletion studies
Markedly elevated MSAFP	Finnish nephrosis	DNA-based mutation analysis
		Fetal renal biopsy
Phocomelia	Roberts SC syndrome	Centromere separation studies
Bilateral renal agenesis	Familial renal dysgenesis	Renal ultrasound of first-degree relatives
Radial abnormality	Fanconi anemia	Chromosome breakage studies
	Thrombocytopenia absent radius	PUBS
Echogenic bowel	Cystic fibrosis	CFTR mutation studies

DNA, deoxyribonucleic acid; PKU, phenylketonuria; FISH, fluorescent in situ hybridization; MSAFP, maternal serum α-fetoprotein; PUBS, percutaneous umbilical cord blood sampling; CFTR, cystic fibrosis transmembrane conductance regulator.

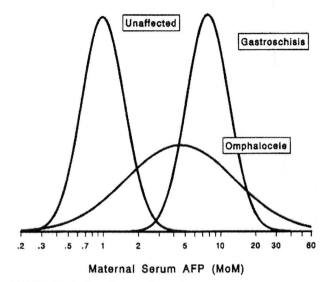

Maternal Serum AFP (MoM)

F I G U R E 9–3. Distribution of second-trimester MSAFP levels in un-affected pregnancies and those affected by gastroschisis and omphalocele. The median for gastroschisis pregnancies is 7.0 MoM, and for omphalocele is 4.1 MoM.

ingly high AFAFP value. In one study of 85,000 consecutive samples from the California screening program, 2.2% had an AFAFP greater than 2.0 MoM. Half measured 2.0 to 2.4 MoM, and 93% had a normal outcome. Sixty-seven percent of those with higher levels had abnormalities. With a positive AChE, the chance of an abnormal fetus was 67% for levels between 2.0 and 2.4 MoM and 99% at greater than 5.0 MoM. After a normal ultrasound and karyotype, the risk for a fetal abnormality was 1% for AFAFP measuring 2.0 to 2.4 MoM and 3% for higher levels.[71] Like MSAFP, an unexplained AFAFP has also been associated with pre-eclampsia and preterm delivery.[72]

While there are numerous disorders that can result in an elevated AFAFP level, AChE is more specific to neural tissue and enhances the specificity of testing for neural tube defects. Detection of AChE in the amniotic fluid generally signifies that an open neural tube defect is present, although a positive AChE has also been reported with omphalocele, gastroschisis, cystic hygroma, fetal hydrops, and blood-stained amniotic fluid. There are also a limited number of reports of false-positive AChE results.[73]

Screening for Aneuploidy

Since the introduction of AFP screening, a large number of studies have confirmed that MSAFP levels in Down syndrome pregnancies are lower, averaging 0.74 MoM.[74] Other investigations have reported that maternal serum, amniotic fluid,[46] and fetal cord serum[75] levels of AFP are also lower in pregnancies in which the fetus has Down syndrome. This may be due to either decreased production of AFP by the fetal liver, or more rapid removal of AFP from the fetal circulation. Two distinct forms of AFP have been identified, one produced by the fetal liver and the other by the yolk sac. Both fractions

have been found to be decreased in pregnancies with Down syndrome.[76]

Because AFP levels are independent of maternal age, they can be used to screen for Down syndrome in women younger than 35 years old. As first described by Cuckle et al., MSAFP and maternal age are combined to establish an individual Down syndrome risk.[46] Most screening programs in the United States select a risk of 1 per 270, comparable with that of a 35-year-old woman, as "screen positive."[77, 78] When applied to the younger population, this cut-off value will select 3 to 5% of patients as candidates for amniocentesis. The test will detect 20 to 25% of Down syndrome fetuses in the under-35 age group.[77,78] Combining MSAFP screening for patients younger than 35, together with the practice of offering amniocentesis to all patients older than 35, will yield a Down syndrome detection rate of 45%. This practice will result in recommending amniocentesis to 9 to 13% of the pregnant population. As with screening for neural tube defects, the extensive overlap in the distribution of MSAFP in normal and affected pregnancies implies that selecting a cut-off in which patients are considered at higher risk for fetal Down syndrome involves a compromise between the detection rate and the false-positive rate. No specific MSAFP value will accurately separate all affected from unaffected pregnancies.

In general, study protocols require that MSAFP be drawn between 15 and 20 weeks. A second sample is not drawn in patients with a positive low result, as MSAFP levels increase in both affected and unaffected populations, and such "regression to the mean" confounds the interpretation of a second result.[79] An important exception to this is when a blood sample is obtained before 15 weeks of gestation, in which case a new sample should be obtained when the patient reaches the appropriate gestational age.

Unconjugated Estriol and Human Chorionic Gonadotropin

A number of other biochemical markers have now been studied for use in aneuploidy screening. Although some of these analytes have not been found to be useful, both unconjugated estriol (uE3) and human chorionic gonadotropin (hCG) add specificity and sensitivity to second-trimester biochemical screening for Down syndrome.[80] Like AFP, uE3 is 25 to 30% lower in Down syndrome pregnancies,[80, 81] whereas hCG levels in affected pregnancies have a median value about twice that of normal controls.[78]

Estriol is a steroid hormone produced by the syncytiotrophoblast. Dehydroepiandrosterone sulfate (DHEAS) produced by the fetal adrenal gland is converted to 16α-OH-DHEAS in the fetal liver. In the placenta, 16α-OH-DHEAS is deconjugated by a sulfatase and then aromatized to yield unconjugated estriol.[78] In 1987, Canick et al. found lower second-trimester levels of maternal serum unconjugated estriol in Down syndrome pregnancies, with a median MoM value of 0.79. Neither direct measurement of DHEAS nor conjugated estriol appear to be as discriminating as unconjugated estriol in

Down syndrome detection.[82] Very low levels of uE3 have been reported when the fetus is affected with placental sulfatase deficiency, a relatively minor, X-linked disorder that usually manifests only as mild to moderate ichthyosis.[83] In 5 to 10% of cases, the disorder is due to a contiguous gene deletion syndrome that may include mental retardation, hypogonadism, anosmia, and/or chondrodysplasia punctata.[84, 85] It has been suggested that amniocentesis and testing for steroid sulfatase deficiency as well as the gene deletion should be considered in such cases.

Human chorionic gonadotropin is secreted by the syncytiotrophoblast, and is higher in maternal samples from Down syndrome pregnancies, as are almost all of the other placental secretory products studied, including progesterone, human placental lactogen (hPL), and pregnancy-specific β-glycoprotein. These findings suggest that a hypersecretory or immature placenta may be a characteristic of fetal Down syndrome.[86, 87]

In 1984, Chard et al. suggested that hCG might be a useful biochemical marker in the detection of Down syndrome.[88] Bogart et al. later reported that 11 of 17 Down syndrome pregnancies studied had second-trimester hCG levels of 2.5 MoM or greater.[86] A number of other investigators have confirmed that the median hCG value in Down syndrome pregnancies is twice that of normal controls,[80, 87, 89] making it the most sensitive biochemical marker for Down syndrome detection.

Human chorionic gonadotropin is composed of two, nonidentical subunits (α and β). Most hCG circulates in its intact form, with less than 1% of hCG present in maternal serum as the free β-subunit.[90] Both the free α- and β-subunits are elevated in Down syndrome pregnancies, and some studies have implied that specific measurements of either might be more sensitive in the detection of Down syndrome.[91] The degree of overlap of these two subunits and thus the difference in performance if either were used in screening is the subject of ongoing investigation.

Triple Marker Screening

AFP, uE3, and hCG are all independent of maternal age and only weakly correlated with each other, and can therefore be used in combination to estimate fetal Down syndrome risk. Such screening is now routinely offered in pregnancy. The weight given each marker in the statistical analysis will vary with its sensitivity, and the calculated risk depends on maternal age. Multiple marker screening has a significantly higher sensitivity than MSAFP screening alone, and has been shown to detect 58 to 91% of Down syndrome with a 5 to 6% false-positive rate and a positive predictive value of 1 in 23 to 1 in 38[92, 93] (Fig. 9–4).

As with AFP screening alone, maternal weight, race, diabetes, and the number of fetuses present are all considered in the risk calculation. In addition, parity is negatively associated with hCG levels, which decrease by about 3% for each previous birth. The reason for this decline is unknown, and as the effect on screening performance is negligible, no adjustment is made for maternal parity.[94]

It has been shown that women who were screen positive in a previous pregnancy are more likely to be screen positive in subsequent pregnancies. This increased risk is age related, and greater in younger than in older women. Until more data are available, however, it is not possible to accurately adjust risks for patients who have a recurrent screen-positive test.[94–96] Assisted reproduction seems to have a small effect on levels, with hCG 9% higher, uE3 levels 8% lower, and AFP unchanged. This magnitude of difference is insufficient to warrant risk adjustment.[94, 97, 98] Abnormal renal function has also been shown to cause false-positive biochemical screening, due to an abnormally elevated hCG in these patients.[51]

Trisomy 18 Screening

In pregnancies in which the fetus is affected with trisomy 18, all three serum markers are lower than normal, with the following median values: AFP, 0.6 MoM; uE3, 0.5 MoM; and hCG, 0.3 MoM. Because hCG levels are low (as opposed to the high levels seen in Down syndrome pregnancy), trisomy 18 will not be detected unless this particular pattern is specifically assessed. Use of this protocol is associated with an 80% detection rate for trisomy 18, with a false-positive rate of only 0.5%. Thus, one case of trisomy 18 will be detected for every 15 amniocenteses offered.[99]

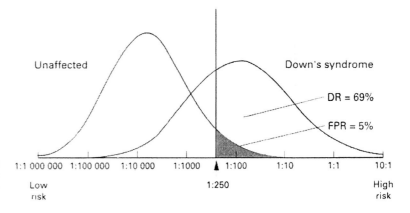

FIGURE 9–4. Distribution of Down syndrome risk based on triple marker screening in affected and unaffected pregnancies. (DR = detection rate; FPR = false-positive rate.)

Twin Pregnancies

Serum markers in twins are approximately twice as high as in singleton pregnancies. Observed maternal serum levels of AFP and hCG are actually slightly more than doubled, while uE3 is slightly less.[94] Because there are limited data available on observed values of these markers in women with twin pregnancies in which one or both fetuses has Down syndrome, a risk is calculated by dividing the observed MoM in a twin pregnancy by the median MoM in twin pregnancies without Down syndrome. Patients are usually classified as screen positive or negative using the same cut-off level as with singleton pregnancies, but without reporting a risk estimate.[94] In one large series of multiple marker screening in twin pregnancies, it was found that 5.5% had a false-positive test, a result that did not differ significantly from singleton pregnancies. While there were no cases of Down syndrome detected, it was estimated based on modeling that 73% of monozygous twins and 43% of dizygous twins would have been identified, with an overall detection rate of 53%.[100]

Pregnancy Outcome after Unexplained Abnormal Biochemical Screening

With the introduction of MSAFP screening, it was noted that women with an elevated MSAFP but a normal fetus had an increased risk of preterm delivery, fetal death, intrauterine growth restriction, and hypertension. The magnitude of this risk increases with increasing maternal serum levels, from a risk of 19% with levels of 2.5 to 2.9 MoM, to 67% with an MSAFP of greater than 6.0 MoM.[101]

With unexplained increased MSAFP, it is felt that increased transplacental transfer of AFP is responsible for the elevated value. Such increased transfer occurs with various abnormalities of placental implantation, which later result in poor fetal growth, abruption, preterm labor, preeclampsia, and other pregnancy complications. Abnormalities such as placenta accreta, increta, and percreta have been reported in association with an elevated MSAFP,[102] and uterine anomalies have been reported to be 22 times more common in these patients as well. Because of the very large concentration gradient between fetal and maternal serum, a slight compromise in uteroplacental integrity will allow detectably increased transport of AFP across the placenta.[103]

Other biochemical markers and combinations of markers have also been studied with respect to adverse outcome in late pregnancy. Elevated hCG in particular has been associated with an increased risk of intrauterine growth retardation,[104] hypertension/preeclampsia,[105] fetal malformations,[106] chromosomal abnormalities,[107] and adverse perinatal outcome generally.[108, 109] Optimal management of these patients, however, remains controversial.

Other Biochemical Markers

Dimeric inhibin is a placental protein which, like hCG, has been shown to be elevated in Down syndrome pregnancies.[110, 111] In 1996, dimeric inhibin A was shown to increase the detection rate for Down syndrome to 76%, with the same false-positive rate when used in combination with standard triple screening with AFP, uE3, and hCG[112, 113] (Fig. 9–5). hCG and free β-hCG have been shown to be increased in maternal urine as well as serum, with a pooled median of 3.67 MoM, and urinary core β-hCG, a breakdown product of hCG, has been investigated as a potential screening test. Estimates of the effectiveness of this marker when combined with maternal age range from 41 to 80%, with a 5% false-positive rate.[94] The potential for altering present screening methods by addition of either of these tests is under study.

First-Trimester Biochemical Screening

Although biochemical screening has significantly improved the detection rate of neural tube defects and Down syndrome, follow-up evaluation is still required, and diagnosis is usually delayed until the mid-second

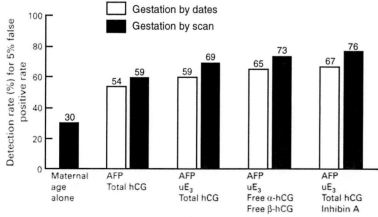

All with maternal age

FIGURE 9–5. Detection rate for various combinations of serum markers based on a 5% false-positive rate.

trimester. Several investigators have thus looked at the efficacy of first-trimester biochemical screening. While the same general pattern of lower AFP and uE3 and increased hCG is seen as with second-trimester screening, the overlap with normal pregnancies is greater and the detection rate lower than with later screening.[94]

Other biochemical markers may be of greater utility in first-trimester screening, and investigators have evaluated such markers as free β-hCG,[114] pregnancy-associated plasma protein-A (PAPP-A),[114, 115] placental protein 14,[116] CA-125,[117, 118] α and dimeric inhibin,[94] schwangerschaftsprotein 1 (SP1),[119] and neutrophil alkaline phosphatase.[120] PAPP-A and free β-hCG seem to be the most effective markers at this time in pregnancy. When used together with maternal age, these two markers have an estimated detection rate of 65%, with a false-positive rate of 5%.[121] The addition of ultrasound screening using nuchal translucency in the first trimester has been reported to yield a detection rate of 80%, with a false-positive rate of 5%,[122] and future programs may use a combination of these approaches to optimize screening effectiveness.

Fetal Cells in Maternal Circulation

Walknowska et al. in 1969 first reported the detection of lymphocytes in the circulation of pregnant women.[123] Following mitogen stimulation, they found rare lymphocytes having a small acrocentric chromosome consistent with a Y chromosome. These findings were highly correlated with women who were carrying a male fetus. This report stimulated a wide range of investigations in the area of fetal cells in maternal circulation. These investigations have focused primarily in two areas. The first has been the identification and enrichment of fetal cells in the maternal circulation. The other area has been in the analysis of these fetal cells.

Several fetal cell types have been reported to exist in the maternal circulation. These include fetal trophoblasts, lymphocytes, granulocytes, nucleated erythrocytes, and platelets. Except for platelets (which do not contain genomic DNA), all of the above cell types have been investigated as a source of fetal cells for prenatal diagnosis.

The number of investigators that have utilized trophoblast cells as a source of fetal cells in maternal circulation has been relatively small, probably due to the difficulty in developing monoclonal antibodies to trophoblast specific antigens. Various antibodies have been used in an attempt to enrich for fetal cells with varying degrees of success.[124, 125] The diagnosis by FISH analysis of a 47, XYY fetus by enrichment using antitrophoblast antibodies has been described.[126] A concern about using trophoblasts for noninvasive prenatal diagnosis is the fact that these cells are frequently multinucleate, which would make interphase cytogenetic analysis by FISH difficult. In addition, extensive experience with analysis of chorionic villi from CVS has demonstrated the presence of confined placental mosaicism (CPM) in villus tissue.[25] Thus, results obtained from trophoblast cells might not truly reflect the fetal status.

Many studies have confirmed the report of Walknowska et al. regarding the presence of fetal lymphocytes in the maternal circulation. Herzenberg et al. were the first to attempt to enrich for the population of fetal lymphocytes.[127] They utilized flow sorting to identify fetal cells using an antibody against a paternally inherited HLA antigen followed by Y chromatin identification. Unfortunately, this type of approach requires an informative polymorphic couple and known paternity, making this approach not universally applicable. Another potential problem with this approach is the persistence of fetal lymphocytes in maternal circulation for long periods of time.

Fetal nucleated red cells have been the most commonly studied cell type for several reasons. Based on studies of staining for fetal hemoglobin, it has been known for many years that fetal red cells cross into the maternal circulation.[128] In addition, the frequency of nucleated red cells in the fetus early in gestation is relatively high, thus increasing the possibility of recovering these cell in the maternal circulation.[129] These cells are also fairly well differentiated and likely to have a limited life span in the fetal circulation.

The presence of fetal nucleated red cells was first described by Bianchi et al. in 1990.[130] The cells were identified by a combination of morphologic features, staining for the presence of fetal hemoglobin by the Kleihauer-Betke technique, and the demonstration of Y-chromosome–specific sequences in women who were carrying male fetuses. Enrichment for fetal cells was performed using an antibody to the transferrin receptor CD71. This antibody is expressed on all cells incorporating iron and will thus identify all nucleated red cells in maternal blood. Unfortunately, evidence suggests that a significant proportion of nucleated red cells in maternal blood are of maternal origin, having increased during pregnancy as compared to nonpregnant controls.[131]

It is clear that the frequency of fetal cells in the maternal circulation is very low. There has been significant controversy on what the frequency is, with ranges of 1 in 10^5 to 1 in 10^9 maternal cells. Most of the studies that have attempted to answer this question have utilized fetal cell enrichment techniques and have had an unknown rate of loss due to the enrichment steps. Hamada et al. used a direct approach using FISH analysis of Y-probe positivity on unsorted cells.[132] They were able to demonstrate the frequency of Y-probe positivity to be less than 1 per 10^5 in the first trimester to 1 per 10^4 at term. Bianchi et al. utilized quantitative polymerase chain reaction (PCR) to quantitate the number of male fetal cell DNA equivalents in the blood of pregnant women.[133] The found the mean number of male fetal cell DNA equivalents amplified from 16 mL of maternal blood to be 19 (range, 0 to 91), with male DNA detected in 99.3% of pregnant women carrying a male fetus. There was a sixfold increase in the number of DNA cell equivalents in pregnancies where the fetus had trisomy 21.

Another important issue is the timing of passage of fetal cells into the maternal circulation. Investigators have demonstrated by PCR the presence of Y sequences in mothers carrying male fetuses as early as 33 and 40 days of gestation in dated pregnancies following in vitro fertilization.[134] The cell type is unlikely to be fetal red cells, since fetal vessels are not present in the villous stroma until about 8 weeks' gestation. A more likely candidate would be circulating trophoblasts. Investigators looking at flow-sorted nucleated red blood cells (NRBC) could not demonstrate the presence of fetal cells after 16 weeks of gestation.[135] While this window remains to be better defined, it suggests that a first-trimester approach might be feasible.

Because of the rarity of fetal cells in maternal circulation, most investigators have utilized a variety of enrichment techniques. Most investigators begin with approximately 20 mL of maternal venous blood that is put through an initial enrichment step to remove maternal nonnucleated erythrocytes. This is usually accomplished through density gradient centrifugation. Following this step, various "positive" and "negative" selection techniques have been used following specific antibody conjugation. These techniques have included fluorescence-activated cell sorting, magnetic activated cell sorting, immunomagnetic beads, and antibody conjugated columns. There is no clear consensus at present on what techniques produce the best separation as judged by the total number of fetal cells recovered and the ratio of fetal/maternal cells obtained. Recently, several investigators have utilized immunostaining with fetal hemoglobin antibodies to specifically identify fetal cells in sorted samples of NRBCs. Zheng et al. utilized a mouse antifetal hemoglobin antibody (UCHγ) and FISH analysis to identify fetal gender on sorted cells.[136] There is some concern with this approach because some mothers will have elevated fetal hemoglobin levels leading to misidentification. To avoid this, Cheung et al. utilized an antiembryonic (ζ) antibody to identify sorted fetal cells.[137]

The small number of fetal cells obtained has been a significant limitation with this type of analysis. If the small number of cells could be cultured, expanded numbers of cells would be available for analysis. Initial investigations into culturing of fetal erythroid progenitor cells have shown the feasibility of this approach.[138, 139] Further research in this area is warranted to provide increased numbers of fetal cells for analysis.

The analysis of fetal cells in maternal circulation has primarily relied on PCR and FISH techniques. PCR has been used both for the amplification of sequences in nonenriched and enriched maternal blood. Lo et al. were able to show, by a nested PCR technique, the amplification of Y sequences in nonenriched maternal blood from women carrying male pregnancies.[140] They were able to detect all 12 of 19 women who later gave birth to boys. The diagnosis of single-gene disorders is also possible if the father carries a mutation or polymorphism that the mother lacks. For example, the detection of fetal hemoglobin Lepore-Boston and the Rh D gene have been reported by this strategy.[141, 142] At present, the accuracy of this approach is unknown.

Recently, Lo et al. have reported the presence of fetal DNA in maternal serum and plasma.[143] By utilizing a real-time quantitative PCR technique, these investigators were able to demonstrate high concentrations of fetal DNA, with a mean of 25.4 genome equivalents per milliliter of maternal plasma.[144] Fetal DNA was detected as early as 7 weeks of gestation and increased in concentration as pregnancy progressed.

FISH technology has been used for the diagnosis of aneuploidy in maternal blood samples enriched for fetal cells. Simpson and Elias, following enrichment for fetal NRBCs, successfully reported the diagnosis of 47, XXY, trisomy 18, and trisomy 21.[145] The percentage of fetal aneuploid cells detected ranged from 0% to 74%. Other groups have reported similar results.[146] Because of the significant background of maternal cells, this current approach will probably only be useful as an improved population screen with the use of chorionic villus sampling or amniocentesis as a diagnostic test. Only if pure fetal cells could reliably be obtained would this become a primary diagnostic test.

Another approach to obtaining pure fetal cells has been described by Takabayashi et al.[147] They retrieved single cells by use of a micromanipulator under a microscope and analyzed them for Y sequences. Cheung et al. applied this technique to CD71-positive sorted cells that had been stained for embryonic hemoglobin.[137] The retrieved cells were then pooled and used for the PCR-based diagnosis of sickle cell anemia and thalassemia. These investigators were able to identify 7 to 22 fetal cells from 16 to 18 mL of maternal blood.

While significant advances have been made in the isolation and analysis of fetal cells from maternal blood, very few data have been generated regarding the sensitivity and specificity of this approach. The main reason for this has been that separation and analysis techniques are still evolving. Until a large prospective study is performed, this approach will not be ready for clinical application.

Prenatal Diagnosis by DNA Analysis

Advances in molecular biology have revolutionized our understanding of the structure and function of human genes. The advent of recombinant DNA technology has not only improved our ability to diagnose individuals affected with genetic diseases but has greatly advanced the areas of carrier detection and presymptomatic and prenatal diagnosis.

Until the availability of molecular tools, clinical criteria and biochemical studies were the primary means for diagnosis of genetic disorders. These methods are often not definitive, and are limited in their ability to identify carriers or provide prenatal testing. Molecular methods avoid the uncertainty of clinical diagnosis by directly determining the presence or absence of a gene mutation in an affected person or carrier. DNA testing can be performed before the appearance of clinical symptoms (or prenatally), and can distinguish between disorders with similar phenotypes. Molecular diagnosis requires only a sample of DNA, which can be obtained from any nucleated cell, including chorionic villus cells or amniocytes, as well as lymphocytes in blood.

There are limitations to molecular diagnosis, due to the number and complexity of genetic mutations that underlie inherited disorders. A wide variety of changes, from single amino acid substitutions to deletion of an entire gene, can disrupt genetic function[148] (Fig. 9–6). While some disorders, such as sickle cell disease and achondroplasia, are caused by one or a very limited number of genetic mutations, in other conditions almost no two people carry the same gene change. Different individuals with tuberous sclerosis may actually have mutations in entirely different genes, further complicating molecular diagnosis. In conditions such as Gaucher

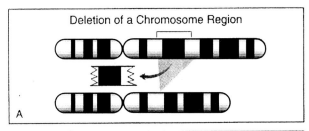

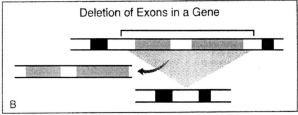

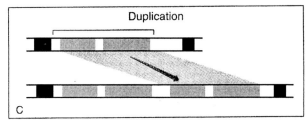

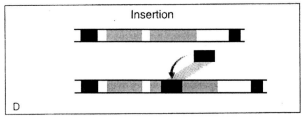

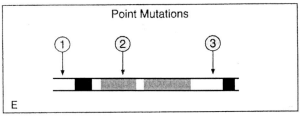

FIGURE 9–6. Types of genetic mutations. *A,* A chromosome region containing many genes is deleted (contiguous gene syndrome). *B,* Two exons of a gene are deleted. *C,* Duplication of two exons of a gene. *D,* Insertion of genetic material from another part of the genome into an exon of the gene. *E,* Locations of point mutations which can lead to gene disruption. A mutation at site 1, the promoter region of the gene, causes aberrant levels of gene expression. A mutation at site 2, within an exon, causes amino acid substitution or chain termination. And a point mutation at site 3, in an intron, can cause gene disruption if it alters the pattern of splicing and leads to exon skipping or the inclusion of some intron sequence in the processed messenger RNA.

disease, there is such heterogeneity of clinical expression that it is difficult to provide a prognosis for the individual carrying the genetic mutation, especially in a prenatal case.

The Human Genome

There are approximately 3 billion base pairs of DNA that encode the estimated 50,000 to 100,000 genes in the human genome. The genes themselves range in length from hundreds to millions of base pairs, but compose a relatively small fraction of the genome. The majority of DNA exists as intergenic sequences that serve little or no known function.

Genes are composed of alternating exons and introns that vary widely in size and number. Exons compose the DNA coding region of a structural gene and are transcribed into RNA and translated into protein. The intervening sequences, or introns, are not part of the coding region. These sequences are included in the primary RNA transcription product, but are subsequently spliced out before translation occurs. It is within the exons that the majority of detectable mutations producing phenotypic change are found.

Polymorphisms

Molecular biology provides the ability to visualize sequence differences in DNA. Such differences are referred to as polymorphisms, and may occur in coding regions (exons) or noncoding regions (introns) of genes. The ability to visualize DNA differences has made it possible to locate and identify genes for many diseases. The most useful polymorphisms are those with numerous forms. At sites with many different polymorphisms, a person is most likely to carry two distinguishable DNA sequences, thus accurately marking the two alternative chromosomes.[149]

Within the human genome are many sequences of nucleotides that occur repeatedly from a few to thousands of times. Unique sequences, encoding the structural genes, are generally represented only twice, once on each of a pair of chromosomes. Repeated sequences vary in complexity, from repetition of an entire gene, to recurring sequences of one or two base pairs. The entire α-globin gene is normally repeated twice on each chromosome 16; therefore, most people have four copies of this gene. Tandem repeats, such as the dinucleotide repeat AC (adenosine and cytosine), can be repeated from a few up to about 50 times, and occur in an estimated 50,000 to 100,000 locations within the genome. Such repeats frequently occur as polymorphisms, which may be near enough to important genes to be used for linkage studies.[150]

While most dinucleotide repeats are located outside of structural genes, a group of trinucleotide repeats are located within genes and can increase in copy number and cause human disease. This mechanism of mutation is responsible for a number of neurologic diseases, including fragile X syndrome, myotonic dystrophy, and Huntington's disease.

Molecular Diagnosis

To study a gene and its mutations, it is necessary to distinguish that gene from the remainder of the DNA. Direct detection of genetic disorders is now possible using recombinant DNA technology for the many diseases in which the precise mutation(s) are known. The use of polymorphisms within and around these genes as indirect markers allows the tracking of disease alleles in some affected pedigrees in which direct analysis is not yet possible.

When a gene mutation is first identified in the research laboratory, it is analyzed to determine whether the genetic change is truly a pathogenic mutation, or merely a benign polymorphism with no deleterious effect on structure or function. A pathogenic mutation will segregate with the disease in a family, and will only occur in affected persons or carriers. Careful analysis is required, as a polymorphism may be near the gene and therefore segregate with the disorder. With a pathogenic mutation, it should be possible to predict the effects of the mutation on the expression of a protein. Mutations that abolish the expression of a protein are likely to be pathogenic. Obviously, a great deal of study is required to determine with certainty that a change seen at the molecular level is truly responsible for the disease in a population or family.

Direct Detection

Direct analysis of mutations can be used in disorders in which a limited number of well-known mutations account for the majority of cases. This often occurs due to the founder effect, in which one member introduced a mutation into a small population, leading to a high prevalence of that mutation in the population. This is why, in many cases, mutations are specific to a particular population or ethnic group.[151] Such analysis for specific mutations can be performed in an affected individual to confirm a diagnosis, in an asymptomatic person to determine carrier status, or in a fetus in whom a particular diagnosis is suspected (i.e., a fetus with echogenic bowel might be tested for the common mutations causing cystic fibrosis). Direct detection can be used in prenatal diagnosis for disorders such as sickle cell anemia, which are consistently caused by the same base pair mutation, without the need for DNA testing of both parents. With most diseases, however, it is necessary to determine which mutation(s) are carried by the affected family member(s), to be certain that they are identifiable and therefore conducive to prenatal diagnosis.

In pedigrees in which a genetic disease is present but analysis does not identify a known mutation, other available options to allow DNA-based prenatal diagnosis include sequencing of the gene to identify the mutation in the individual or family, or utilization of linkage analysis. Direct detection provides the most ac-

curate molecular diagnosis, and is preferable to linkage analysis when the genetic mutation is known. In some cases in which the commonly encountered genetic mutations are not identified, the gene can be sequenced to determine that individual's unique mutation. While this technique will allow accurate prenatal testing, it is time consuming and frequently not practical for clinical purposes, especially in a prenatal setting in which time is limited by advancing gestational age.

Linkage

In some affected pedigrees in which the mutation has not been identified, linkage analysis can be used for prenatal diagnosis. Polymorphic DNA sequences that are near or within the gene are used to track it through the family. Linkage can only be used if multiple family members are available, and requires extensive analysis. It cannot be used in an individual to confirm a diagnosis in the absence of a family history or other affected relatives. The approach is limited by potential errors due to genetic recombination, which may separate the polymorphic markers being followed from the disease gene in some family members. The clinical diagnosis must be reliable, and it must be certain the suspected gene is responsible for the disease in the family, which is less clear when the mutation itself is not identified. For example, many, but not all, cases of autosomal dominant polycystic kidney disease (ADPKD) are due to a mutation in a gene on chromosome 16. In a family with ADPKD due to a mutation in a different gene, following chromosome 16 markers through affected and unaffected family members would provide misleading information with regard to presymptomatic or prenatal diagnosis.

DNA probes used for linkage analysis may be intragenic, or may merely be near the gene on the chromosome. Depending on the genetic distance, recombination may be more or less likely to occur between the gene itself and the marker probe being used. This recombination must be taken into account when counseling couples regarding the accuracy of this type of approach. In general, linkage using intragenic probes is more accurate, and the risk of recombination is very small (<1%). However, for very large genes, such as the dystrophin gene of Duchenne muscular dystrophy (DMD), the recombination risk of even an intragenic probe may be significant.

Even in disorders where intragenic probes are available, they may not be useful in all families. Individuals in whom there are not distinguishable polymorphisms at sites for which probes are available are said to not be informative. Different polymorphisms have varying degrees of being informative in a population, but if an individual is not informative, linkage analysis using DNA diagnostic techniques is not possible.

If an individual is informative, it is necessary to identify which of a chromosome pair carries the mutated disease gene. For an autosomal recessive disorder, an affected individual must be present to identify the two mutant alleles. For an X-linked disorder in which the mother is a known carrier, an affected or unaffected male may be used to determine which polymorphism is linked to the mutant gene. Unfortunately, for many X-linked disorders it is not known whether the mother is a carrier, as one third of affected males with no family history are affected due to new mutations. In such cases, extensive family DNA analysis may be helpful in allowing linkage analysis.

Techniques of Molecular Analysis

A variety of approaches are used to detect and study gene mutations. The common tools of diagnostic molecular genetics include restriction endonucleases and DNA oligonucleotide probes, which are used in conjunction with PCR and Southern blotting, as well as other techniques.

A gene-specific probe is a recombinant DNA molecule used to detect the presence of a particular sequence in the genome. Such a probe, when mixed with denatured (single-stranded) human DNA, will hybridize only to its complementary sequence. Probes are typically labeled with a radioisotope or fluorescence for subsequent detection.

Restriction endonucleases are enzymes that recognize and cut precise DNA sequences from any source. A mutation at such a site will prevent enzyme cutting, or, conversely, a mutation may create a new enzyme recognition site and lead to cutting where it should not occur. If the enzyme cuts, two shorter fragments will result; otherwise there will be a single, longer fragment (Fig. 9–7).

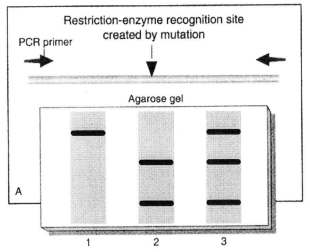

FIGURE 9–7. Mutation detection using restriction enzymes. In this figure, there is a point mutation in the DNA leading to creation of a new enzyme recognition site. The region surrounding the mutation is amplified by PCR, and the resulting product is incubated with the restriction enzyme and studied with electrophoresis. Lane 1 contains DNA from a person without the mutation; there is only one band because the enzyme does not cut the DNA. Lane 2 contains DNA from a person homozygous for the mutation; the two bands represent the two fragments obtained after enzyme digestion. Lane 3 contains DNA from a person heterozygous for the mutation; there is one cut and one uncut fragment.

Southern Blotting

Southern blotting,[152] named for the investigator who described the technique, takes the many fragments produced by restriction enzyme digestion and applies them to an electrophoretic gel. The negatively charged DNA migrates toward the positive pole set at the other end. Smaller DNA fragments travel through the gel more quickly than larger fragments, thus separating the fragments by size. The DNA is then denatured, transferred to a nitrocellulose or nylon filter, and hybridized to labeled DNA probe. The signal can then be detected using autoradiography or fluorescence, depending on the type of label attached to the probe. Identification, localization, and fine restriction mapping of a particular gene can be performed with Southern blotting. In addition, gene deletions and insertions, as well as single base substitutions within a restriction enzyme recognition site, can be identified with this technique.

While Southern blotting is a powerful technique for studying genetic mutations, it is time consuming, typically requiring 2 or more weeks to complete a study. In addition, relatively large quantities of DNA are needed, which means that cells obtained by amniocentesis may need to be cultured for several weeks to obtain the necessary amount of DNA.

Polymerase Chain Reaction

The development of the PCR revolutionized the field of molecular biology.[153] PCR is an enzymatic technique that uses a DNA polymerase to amplify short sequences of DNA, producing 10^6 to 10^7 copies of the target sequence. Minute amount of DNA isolated from cells can be used as a template, eliminating the need for the large amounts of DNA required for Southern blotting.

To perform PCR, the nucleotide sequences that flank the target DNA must be known, and DNA primers that are complementary to these sequences are needed. The DNA to be amplified is first denatured into single strands, the primers are then annealed, and a polymerase is added. The polymerase synthesizes a DNA strand between the two primers, creating a duplication of the target DNA region. The cycle of denaturation, annealing, and synthesis is repeated multiple times to create a logarithmic increase in the DNA sequence of interest. After 30 cycles, there is about a 1 billionfold amplification in the quantity of DNA.

In the simplest use of PCR to study a specific gene mutation, the DNA product is incubated with a restriction enzyme, and analyzed by electrophoresis. The specificity of the PCR reaction itself can also be used for mutation detection (Fig. 9–8). If a primer is used that corresponds to the normal gene sequence, the PCR product cannot be made if that sequence is not present. A separate reaction is carried out using a primer that corresponds to the mutant sequence, which will produce the gene product when those sequences are present. An agarose gel pattern can determine the presence of the normal gene, the mutant gene, or both. Multiplex PCR is another modification of the PCR technique that can be used to study genes in which different deletions may

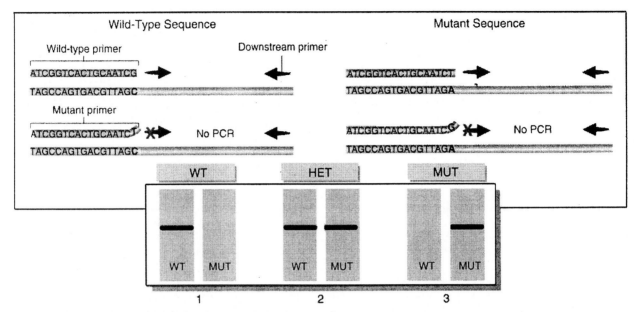

F I G U R E 9–8. Mutation detection using allele-specific PCR. Two PCR primers are necessary, one corresponding to the wild-type sequence (WT) and one to the mutant (MUT) sequence. A common downstream primer is used for the two reactions. With a wild-type gene, only the primer corresponding to the wild-type sequence yields a PCR product. Similarly, with a mutant sequence, only the primer corresponding to the mutant sequence yields a product. DNA from a heterozygote will yield both products.

be responsible for the disorder in different individuals (Fig. 9–9).

Dot Blot and Reverse Dot Blot Hybridization

Other variations of PCR have been developed to look for multiple mutations simultaneously. In dot blot hybridization, DNA is studied without restriction enzyme digest. Amplified DNA is directly loaded onto a mem-

brane and denatured. Labeled probes (allele-specific oligonucleotides [ASOs]) are then hybridized to the membrane, and indirectly visualized (Fig. 9–10). This technique allows one to distinguish between normal and mutant alleles, and is useful in analysis of mutations that do not involve a restriction site.

Reverse dot blot was also developed to analyze single-gene disorders caused by a number of different mutations.[154] Here, filter membranes are fixed with labeled

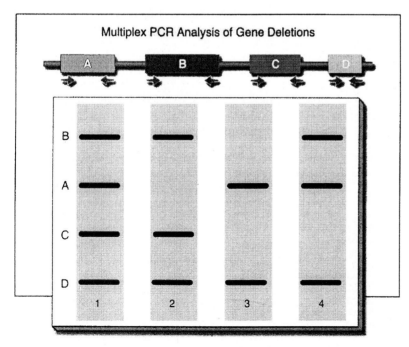

F I G U R E 9–9. Detection of gene deletions using multiplex PCR. The rectangles labeled A, B, C, and D represent exons in a gene on the X-chromosome in a male. The four exons are simultaneously amplified by PCR in the same reaction tube; the *arrows* represent primers. The products are separated by gel electrophoresis. Lane 1 shows a control sequence with no deletion, while deletions of various exons are demonstrated in lanes 2 through 4. This method can be used to detect deletions in the dystrophin gene causing Duchenne muscular dystrophy.

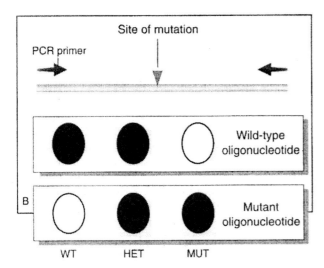

FIGURE 9–10. Mutation detection using dot blot hybridization. The segment of DNA is amplified by PCR, and spotted onto separate filter membranes. Each filter membrane is hybridized with a labeled oligonucleotide corresponding to the wild-type (normal) or mutant sequence. The amplified DNA from a person with the wild-type sequence (WT) hybridizes only with the wild-type oligonucleotide, while the DNA from a person homozygous for the mutant (MUT) sequence hybridizes only with the mutant oligonucleotide. DNA from a heterozygote (HET) hybridizes with both oligonucleotides.

oligonucleotides corresponding to either the normal gene, or the mutant sequence. DNA to be studied is amplified with PCR, divided into aliquots, and spotted onto separate filter membranes. The amplified segment of DNA from a person with the normal sequence will hybridize with the normal oligonucleotide, leaving an identifiable blot on the membrane. DNA from a person with the mutation will hybridize with the mutant oligonucleotide, and a person with both sequences (i.e., a heterozygote or carrier) will hybridize with both.[151]

Fluorescence In Situ Hybridization

With this technique, a large piece of cloned DNA labeled with a fluorescent tag is hybridized to chromosomal DNA on a microscope slide. The region corresponding to the cloned DNA lights up under fluorescence illumination, and the number of fluorescent sites can be counted (Fig. 9–11). FISH can be used to identify deletions, in which one fluorescent site will not be present, and is also used to study chromosomal aneuploidies, in which three targets will be present instead of the normal two. There are several microdeletion syndromes that have been characterized using FISH, including Prader-Willi and Angelman syndromes (chromosome 15), Di-George and velocardiofacial syndromes (chromosome 22), aniridia/Wilms tumor (chromosome 11), and Williams syndrome (chromosome 7). These disorders result from the simultaneous deletion of a group of genes, rather than the mutation of a single gene.[148]

Many more mutation detection technologies have now been developed. Some of these are used to scan for mutations within a gene, including single-strand conformational polymorphism (SSCP), denaturing gradient gel electrophoresis (DGGE), heteroduplex analysis

(HET), chemical cleavage analysis (CCM), and ribonuclease cleavage (Rnase). More direct mutation analysis is provided with such techniques as oligonucleotide ligation assay (OLA), primer extension, and artificial introduction of restriction sites (AIRS), as well as other variations of these.[155] Commercial laboratories have developed techniques such as multiplex allele-specific diagnostic assay (MASDA), to allow analysis of large numbers of samples (>500) simultaneously for a large number of known mutations (>100) in a single assay.[155]

Sources of DNA

DNA can be obtained from any nucleated cell, and in a prenatal setting is commonly obtained from chorionic villi, amniocytes, or lymphocytes from the parents, or from the fetus through umbilical blood sampling. DNA can also be obtained from single cells isolated by blastomere biopsy, a technique that allows genetic testing prior to embryo transfer in patients undergoing in vitro fertilization. Such preimplantation diagnosis is used to avoid transfer of affected embryos in couples at risk for specific genetic disorders. DNA can also be obtained from cheek cells obtained by a buccal smear with a cotton-tipped swab. This will capture enough nucleated cells for PCR analysis, and is used in carrier testing for some genetic diseases.

For Southern blot analysis, approximately 5 μg of DNA per analysis is required, and laboratories typically request 15 to 20 μg to allow all necessary analyses. For PCR testing only, less DNA is needed, as amplification can take place from very small samples. Because amplification will indiscriminately amplify all DNA in a sample, it is important in prenatal specimens that maternal cell contamination be avoided. With CVS specimens, the chorionic villi must be meticulously separated from the maternal decidua. With amniotic fluid, evidence of maternal blood in the sample must be noted, and the initial aliquot of fluid (approximately 1 mL) obtained at the time of amniocentesis should be discarded.

When amniotic fluid is used as a source of DNA, cells are most often cultured for 2 to 3 weeks to allow growth to sufficient numbers. On uncultured amniotic fluid, approximately 7 μg of DNA can be obtained from 20 mL of fluid, the typical volume taken at the time of a second-trimester amniocentesis. Some cells must also be saved for backup culture and karyotype. Therefore, if direct DNA testing on amniotic fluid is planned, approximately 30 mL must be obtained. Direct amniotic fluid specimens can be used for some PCR analyses, but culturing is required to provide sufficient quantities of DNA for tests that require Southern blot analysis.

Chorionic villus sampling provides approximately 1 μg of DNA per milligram of villi. A typical CVS procedure produces 25 to 50 mg of villi, and can provide sufficient DNA for analysis without waiting for culture, thereby decreasing the time interval for results. As Southern blot analysis can take as long as 2 to 3 weeks, the time interval from procedure to result averages 4 to 6 weeks when cultured cells are required. If an amniocentesis is performed at 16 weeks, this means a result may not be available until 22 weeks, a time frame that

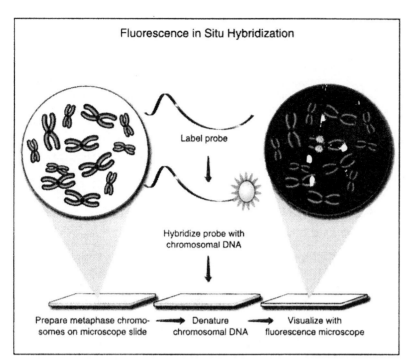

Fluorescence in Situ Hybridization

Label probe

Hybridize probe with chromosomal DNA

Prepare metaphase chromo-somes on microscope slide → Denature chromosomal DNA → Visualize with fluorescence microscope

F I G U R E 9–11. Technique of fluorescence in situ hybridization (FISH). Chromosomes in metaphase are fixed onto a microscope slide, and the chromosomal DNA denatured into single strands. The slide is then hybridized with a piece of DNA labeled with a fluorescent marker, and the marker will light up under ultraviolet light. If there is a deletion, only one copy of the chromosome will show hybridization, while three copies will be identified in cases of trisomy.

is unacceptable to many couples with a 25% risk of an autosomal recessive disorder. With CVS, the procedure is performed many weeks earlier in pregnancy, and culturing time is generally eliminated, meaning that results can be available in 2 to 3 weeks, usually corresponding to 12 to 13 weeks of gestation. Therefore, for many couples at risk of disorders diagnosable through DNA testing, CVS provides an enormous advantage.

Indications for DNA Testing

As more molecular DNA tests become available, there are an increasing number of patients who are candidates for such testing. Many are those with a genetic diagnosis themselves, or a family history of a particular genetic disease. In such cases, the challenge for the geneticist is to ensure an accurate diagnosis, determine the risk to the fetus, and investigate the availability of DNA testing. Because DNA tests are complex and specialized, each clinical diagnostic DNA laboratory will typically provide testing for a limited number of disorders. Conversely, only one or two laboratories may provide testing for a specific genetic disease. In addition, laboratories may vary in the testing that is provided for a given disorder. For example, one laboratory may test for the 70 most common mutations causing cystic fibrosis, while another may test for just 30. There are now on-line databases that are helpful both in determining the status of each genetic disorder with regard to localization and characterization of the genetic defect, and also the availability of DNA diagnostic testing. Many labs will provide testing on a research basis only, and not all will perform prenatal diagnosis.

DNA analysis is used in forensics to evaluate polymorphisms and identify individuals. These same techniques can be applied to prenatal testing in areas such as paternity testing. In addition, such testing can be used to determine zygosity in complicated twin gestations in which chorionicity is a concern in evaluating obstetric management options.[156] Twins that are dizygotic must be dichorionic, essentially ruling out placental vascular anastamoses, and this information can occasionally be useful in difficult obstetric situations.

It is important to remember that in cases in which DNA analysis is to be considered for prenatal diagnosis, extensive family studies or testing of possible carriers has not always been completed. In some cases, testing has been performed in the past, but newer, more sophisticated or accurate probes may have been cloned. In the majority of cases, preconception evaluation is preferable to allow the counseling, identification, contacting, and testing of needed family members. In patients in whom preconception genetic counseling does not occur, a referral for genetic counseling should be made at the first prenatal visit, to allow the maximum amount of time for arrangements to be made. If patients are not seen until 16 weeks, the time of a midtrimester amniocentesis, the full evaluation of a family and performance of testing of individuals becomes more problematic. In some cases, it may be determined that the gene has not been identified, and that linkage is not possible. In other families, a disorder may be under current investigation, with a definitive test available within a short time frame, making it preferable to wait before attempting pregnancy. With the very rapid advances in genetics and prenatal diagnosis, there are very frequently changes in testing options and procedures between pregnancies even for a family that has undergone prenatal diagnosis in a prior pregnancy.

REFERENCES

1. CDC: Contribution of birth defects to infant mortality—United States, 1986. MMWR Morb Mortal Wkly Rep 38:633, 1989.
2. Evans MI, Hume RF, Johnson MP, et al: Integration of genetics and ultrasonography in prenatal diagnosis: Just looking is not enough. Am J Obstet Gynecol 174:1925–1233, 1996.
3. Rizzo N, Pittalis MC, Pilu G, et al: Prenatal karyotype in malformed fetuses. Prenat Diagn 10:17, 1990.
4. Haddow JE, Palomaki GE, Holman MS: Young maternal age and smoking during pregnancy as risk factors for gastroschisis. Teratology 47:225–228, 1993.
5. Curry CJR, Honore L, Boyd E: The ventral wall of the trunk. In Stevenson RE, Hall JG, Goodman RM (eds): Human Malformations and Related Anomalies. New York: Oxford University Press, 1993, pp 869–891.
6. De Veciana M, Major CA, Porto M: Prediction of an abnormal karyotype in fetuses with omphalocele. Prenat Diagn 14:487–492, 1994.
7. Boyd PA, Bhattacharjee A, Gould S, et al: Outcome of prenatally diagnosed anterior abdominal wall defects. Arch Dis Child Fetal Neonatal Ed 78:F209–F213, 1998.
8. Jones KL: Killian/Teschler-Nicola syndrome. In Jones KL (ed): Smith's Recognizable Patterns of Human Malformation, 5th ed. Philadelphia: W. B. Saunders Company, 1997, pp 208–209.
9. Saller DN, Lesser KB, Harrel U, et al: The clinical utility of the perinatal autopsy. JAMA 273:663–665, 1995.
10. Tew BJ, Payne H, Laurence KM: Must a family with a handicapped child be a handicapped family? Dev Med Child Neurol 16(Suppl 32):95, 1974.
11. Valenti C, Schutta EJ, Kehaty T: Prenatal diagnosis of Down syndrome. Lancet 2:220, 1968.
12. Bombard AT, Powers JF, Carter S, et al: Procedure-related fetal losses in transplacental versus nontransplacental genetic amniocentesis. Am J Obstet Gynecol 172:868–872, 1995.
13. Romero R, Jeanty P, Reece EA, et al: Sonographically monitored amniocentesis to decrease intraoperative complications. Obstet Gynecol 65:426–430, 1985.
14. Ried T, Landes G, Dackowski W, et al: Multicolor fluorescence in situ hybridization for the simultaneous detection of probe sets for chromosomes 13, 18, 21, X and Y in uncultured amniotic fluid cells. Hum Mol Genet 1:307–313, 1992.
15. National Institute of Child Health Development National Registry for Amniocentesis Study Group: Midtrimester amniocentesis for prenatal diagnosis: Safety and accuracy. JAMA 236:1471–1476, 1976.
16. Simpson NE, Dellaire L, Miller JR, et al: Prenatal diagnosis of genetic disease in Canada: Report of a collaborative study. Can Med Assoc J 15:739–748, 1976.
17. United Kingdom Medical Research Council: Working Party on amniocentesis. An assessment of the hazards of amniocentesis. Br J Obstet Gynaecol 85(Suppl 2):1–41, 1978.
18. Tabor A, Philip J, Madsen MI, et al: Randomized controlled trial of genetic amniocentesis in 4,606 low-risk women. Lancet 1:1287–1293, 1986.
19. Hanson FW, Tennant F, Hune S, Brookhyser K: Early amniocentesis: Outcome, risks, and technical problems at less than or equal to 12.8 weeks. Am J Obstet Gynecol 166:1707–1711, 1992.
20. Diaz Vega M, De La Cueva P, Leal C, Aisa F: Early amniocentesis at 10–12 weeks gestation. Prenat Diagn 16:307–312, 1996.
21. The Canadian Early and Mid-trimester Amniocentesis Trial (CEMAT) Group: Randomised trial to assess safety and fetal outcome of early and midtrimester amniocentesis. Lancet 351:242–247, 1998.
22. Department of Obstetrics and Gynecology THoAIaSCA, China: Fetal sex prediction by sex chromatin of chorionic villi during early pregnancy. Chin Med J 1:117–126, 1975.
23. Wapner RJ: Chorionic villus sampling. Obstet Gynecol Clin North Am 24:83–110, 1997.
24. Phillips OP, Tharapel AT, Lerner JL, et al: Risk of fetal mosaicism when placental mosaicism is diagnosed by chorionic villus sampling. Am J Obstet Gynecol 174:850–855, 1996.
25. Goldberg JD, Wohlferd MM: Incidence and outcome of chromosomal mosaicism found at the time of chorionic villus sampling. Am J Obstet Gynecol 176:1349–1353, 1997.
26. Ledbetter DH, Engel E: Uniparental disomy in humans: Development of an imprinting map and its implications for prenatal diagnosis. Hum Mol Genet 4:1757–1764, 1995.
27. Johnson A, Wapner RJ: Mosaicism: Implications for postnatal outcome. Curr Opin Obstet Gynecol 9:126–135, 1997.
28. Canadian Collaborative CVS-Amniocentesis Clinical Trial Group Multicentre randomised clinical trial of chorion villus sampling and amniocentesis. First report. [see comments]. Lancet 1:1–6, 1989.
29. Rhoads GG, Jackson LG, Schlesselman SE, et al: The safety and efficacy of chorionic villus sampling for early prenatal diagnosis of cytogenetic abnormalities. N Engl J Med 320:609–617, 1989.
30. Medical Research Council European trial of chorion villus sampling. MRC working party on the evaluation of chorion villus sampling [see comments]. Lancet 337:1491–1499, 1991.
31. Firth HV, Boyd PA, Chamberlain P, et al: Severe limb abnormalities after chorion villus sampling at 56–66 days' gestation [see comments]. Lancet 337:762–763, 1991.
32. Brambati B, Simoni G, Travi M, et al: Genetic diagnosis by chorionic villus sampling before 8 gestational weeks: Efficiency, reliability, and risks on 317 completed pregnancies. Prenat Diagn 12:789–799, 1992.
33. Hsieh FJ, Shyu MK, Sheu BC, et al: Limb defects after chorionic villus sampling [see comments]. Obstet Gynecol 85:84–88, 1995.
34. Mastroiacovo P, Tozzi AE, Agosti S, et al: Transverse limb reduction defects after chorion villus sampling: A retrospective cohort study. GIDEF—Gruppo Italiano Diagnosi Embrio- Fetali. Prenat Diagn 13:1051–1056, 1993.
35. Froster UG, Jackson L: Limb defects and chorionic villus sampling: Results from an international registry, 1992–94 [see comments]. Lancet 347:489–494, 1996.
36. Loukopoulos D, Hadji A, Papadakis M, et al: Prenatal diagnosis of thalassemia and of the sickle cell syndromes in Greece. Ann N Y Acad Sci 612:226–236, 1990.
37. Cao A, Rosatelli MC, Leoni GB, et al: Antenatal diagnosis of beta-thalassemia in Sardinia. Ann N Y Acad Sci 612:215–225, 1990.
38. Hobbins JC, Mahoney MJ: Fetoscopy in continuing pregnancies. Am J Obstet Gynecol 129:440–442, 1977.
39. Daffos F, Capella-Pavlovsky M, Forestier F: Fetal blood sampling during pregnancy with use of a needle guided by ultrasound: A study of 606 consecutive cases. Am J Obstet Gynecol 153:655–660, 1985.
40. Maxwell DJ, Johnson P, Hurley P, et al: Fetal blood sampling and pregnancy loss in relation to indication [see comments]. Br J Obstet Gynaecol 98:892–897, 1991.
41. Brock DJH, Sutcliffe RG: Alpha-fetoprotein in the antenatal diagnosis of anencephaly and spina bifida. Lancet 2:197–199, 1972.
42. Wald NJ, Brock DJH, Bonnar J: Prenatal diagnosis of spina bifida and anencephaly by maternal serum alpha-fetoprotein measurement. Lancet 1:765–767, 1974.
43. Brock DJH, Bolton AE, Scrimgeour JB: Prenatal diagnosis of spina bifida and anencephaly through maternal plasma alpha-fetoprotein measurement. Lancet 1:767–769, 1974.
44. Wald NJ, Cuckle HS: Maternal serum alpha-fetoprotein measurement in antenatal screening for anencephaly and spina bifida in early pregnancy. Report of the U.K. Collaborative Study on alpha-fetoprotein in relation to neural tube defects. Lancet 1:1323–1332, 1977.
45. Merkatz IR, Nitowsky HM, Macri JN, Johnson WE: An association between low maternal serum alpha-fetoprotein and fetal chromosome abnormalities. Am J Obstet Gynecol 148:886–894, 1984.
46. Cuckle HS, Wald NJ, Lindenbaum RH: Maternal serum alpha-fetoprotein measurement: A screening test for Down's syndrome. Lancet 1:926, 1984.
47. Shackley P, McGuire A, Boyd PA, et al: An economic appraisal of alternative prenatal screening programmes for Down's syndrome. J Public Health Med 15:175–184, 1993.
48. Sadovnick AD, Baird PA: A cost-benefit analysis of a population screening programme for neural tube defects. Prenat Diagn 3:117–126, 1983.
49. Bergstrand CG, Czar B: Demonstration of a new protein fraction in serum from the human fetus. Scand J Clin Lab Invest 8:174, 1956.

50. Haddow JE: Prenatal screening for open neural tube defects, Down's syndrome, and other major fetal disorders. Semin Perinatol 14:488–503, 1990.

51. Wathen NC, Campbell DJ, Kitau MJ, Chard T: Alphafetoprotein levels in amniotic fluid from 8 to 18 weeks of pregnancy. Br J Obstet Gynaecol 100:380–382, 1993.

52. Report of the United Kingdom Collaborative Study on Alpha-Fetoprotein in Relation to Neural Tube Defects: Maternal serum alpha-fetoprotein measurement in antenatal screening for anencephaly and spina bifida, 1977.

53. Haddow JE, Knight GJ, Kloza EM: Relation between maternal weight and serum alpha-fetoprotein concentration during the second trimester. Clin Chem 27:133, 1981.

54. Johnson AM: Racial differences in MSAFP screening. In Mizejewski GJ, Porter IH (eds): Alpha-Fetoprotein and Congenital Disorders. New York: Academic Press, 1985, p 183.

55. O'Brien JE, Drugan A, Chervenak F: Maternal serum alpha-fetoprotein screening: The need to use race/ethnic specific medians in Asians. Fetal Diagn Ther 8:367–370, 1993.

56. Wald NJ, Cuckle HS, Boreham J, et al: Maternal serum alpha-fetoprotein and diabetes mellitus. Br J Obstet Gynaecol 86:101, 1979.

57. Lynch L, Berkowitz RL: Maternal serum alpha-fetoprotein and coagulation profiles after multifetal pregnancy reduction. Am J Obstet Gynecol 169:987–990, 1993.

58. Baumgarten A, Reece EA, Davis N, Mahoney MJ: A reassessment of maternal serum alpha-fetoprotein in diabetic pregnancy. Eur J Obstet Gynecol Reprod Biol 28:289–295, 1988.

59. Palomaki GE, Knight GJ, Haddow JE, et al: Cigarette smoking and levels of maternal serum alpha-fetoprotein, unconjugated estriol, and hCG: Impact on Down syndrome screening. Obstet Gynecol 81:675–678, 1993.

60. Wald NJ, Cuckle HS, Nanchahal K: Amniotic fluid acetylcholinesterase measurement in the prenatal diagnosis of open neural tube defects. Second Report of the Collaborative Acetylcholinesterase Study. Prenat Diagn 9:813–829, 1989.

61. Milunsky A, Sapirstein VS: Prenatal diagnosis of open neural tube defects using the amniotic fluid acetylcholinesterase assay. Obstet Gynecol 59:1–5, 1982.

62. Drugan A, Syner FN, Greb A, Evans MI: Amniotic fluid alpha-fetoprotein and acetylcholinesterase in early genetic amniocentesis. Obstet Gynecol 72:35–38, 1988.

63. Nadel AS, Green JK, Holmes LB, et al: Absence of need for amniocentesis in patients with elevated levels of maternal serum alpha-fetoprotein and normal ultrasonographic examinations. N Engl J Med 323:557–561, 1990.

64. Watson WJ, Chescheir NC, Katz VL, Seeds JW: The role of ultrasound in evaluation of patients with elevated maternal serum alpha-fetoprotein: A review. Obstet Gynecol 78:123–128, 1991.

65. Nadel AS, Norton ME, Wilkins-Haug L: Cost-effectiveness of strategies used in the evaluation of pregnancies complicated by elevated maternal serum alpha-fetoprotein. Obstet Gynecol 89:660–665, 1997.

66. Feuchtbaum LB, Cunningham G, Waller DK, et al: Fetal karyotyping for chromosome abnormalities after an unexplained elevated maternal serum alpha-fetoprotein screening. Obstet Gynecol 86:248–254, 1995.

67. Warner AA, Pettanati MJ, Burton BK: Risk of fetal chromosomal anomalies in patients with elevated maternal serum alpha-fetoprotein. Obstet Gynecol 75:64–66, 1990.

68. Megerian G, Godmilow L, Donnenfeld A: Ultrasound-adjusted risk and spectrum of fetal chromosomal abnormality in women with elevated materal serum alpha-fetoprotein. Obstet Gynecol 85:952–956, 1995.

69. Feuchtbaum LB, Cunningham G, Waller DK, et al: Fetal karyotyping for chromosome abnormalities after unexplained maternal serum alpha-fetoprotein screening. Obstet Gynecol 86:248–254, 1995.

70. Ryynanen M, Seppaala M, Kuusela P, et al: Antenatal screening for congenital nephrosis in Finland by maternal serum alpha-fetoprotein. Br J Obstet Gynecol 90:437–442, 1983.

71. Crandall BF, Matsumoto M: Risks associated with an elevated amniotic fluid alpha-fetoprotein level. Am J Med Genet 39:64–67, 1991.

72. Wenstrom KD, Owen J, Davis RO, Brumfield CG: Prognostic significance of unexplained elevated amniotic fluid alpha-fetoprotein. Obstet Gynecol 87:213–216, 1996.

73. Kelly JC, Petrocik E, Wassman ER: Amniotic fluid acetylcholinesterase ratios in prenatal diagnosis of fetal abnormalities. Am J Obstet Gynecol 161:703–705, 1989.

74. Wald NJ, Cuckle HS: Biochemical screening. In Brock DJH, Rodeck CH, Ferguson-Smith MA (eds): Prenatal Diagnosis and Screening. London: Churchill Livingstone, 1992, p 566.

75. Cuckle HS, Wald NJ, Lindenbaum RH: Cord serum alpha-fetoprotein and Down syndrome. Br J Obstet Gynecol 93:407, 1986.

76. Jones SR, Evans SE, Gillan L: Amniotic fluid alpha-fetoprotein subfractions in fetal trisomy 21 affected pregnancies. Br J Obstet Gynecol 95:327–329, 1988.

77. The New England Regional Genetics Group Collaborative Study of Down Syndrome Screening: Combining maternal serum alpha-fetoprotein measurements and age to screen for Down syndrome in pregnant women under age 35. Am J Obstet Gynecol 160: 575, 1989.

78. DiMaio MS, Baumgarten A, Greenstein RM, et al: Screening for fetal Down's syndrome in pregnancy by measuring maternal serum alpha-fetoprotein levels. N Engl J Med 317:342–346, 1987.

79. Haddow JE, Palomaki GE, Wald NJ, et al: Maternal serum alpha-fetoprotein screening for Down syndrome and repeat testing. Lancet 2:1460, 1986.

80. Wald NJ, Cuckle HS, Densem JW, et al: Maternal serum screening for Down's syndrome in early pregnancy. BMJ 297:297, 1988.

81. Jorgensen PI, Trolle D: Low urinary oestriol excretion during pregnancy in women giving birth to infants with Down's syndrome. Lancet 2:782, 1972.

82. Canick JA, Knight GJ, Palomaki GE: Low second trimester maternal serum unconjugated estriol in Down syndrome pregnancies. Am J Hum Genet 41:A269, 1987.

83. Schleifer RA, Bradley LA, Richards DS, Ponting NR: Pregnancy outcome for women with very low levels of maternal serum unconjugated estriol on second-trimester screening. Am J Obstet Gynecol 173:1152–1156, 1995.

84. Ballabio A, Shapiro LJ: Steroid sulfatase deficiency and X-linked ichthyosis. In Scriver CR, Beaudet AL, Sly WS, Valle D (eds): The Metabolic and Molecular Bases of Inherited Disease, 7th ed. New York: McGraw-Hill, 1995, pp 2999–3022.

85. Zalel Y, Kedar I, Tepper R, et al: Differential diagnosis and management of very low second trimester maternal serum unconjugated estriol levels, with special emphasis on the diagnosis of X-linked ichthyosis. Obstet Gynecol Surv 51:200–203, 1996.

86. Bogart MH, Pandia MR, Jones CW: Abnormal maternal serum chorionic gonadotropin levels in pregnancies with fetal chromosome abnormalities. Prenat Diagn 7:623–630, 1987.

87. Knight GJ, Palomaki GE, Haddow JE, et al: Maternal serum levels of placental products hCG, hPL, SP1, and progesterone are all elevated in case of fetal Down syndrome. Am J Hum Genet 45:A263, 1989.

88. Chard T, Lowings C, Kitau MJ: Alpha-fetoprotein and chorionic gonadotropin levels in relation to Down syndrome. Lancet 2:750, 1984.

89. Bogart MH, Golbus MS, Sorg ND, et al: Human chorionic gonadotropin levels in pregnancies with aneuploid fetuses. Prenat Diagn 9:379–384, 1989.

90. Ozturk M, Berkowitz R, Goldstein D, et al: Differential production of human chorionic gonadotropin and free subunits in gestational trophoblastic disease. Am J Obstet Gynecol 158:193–198, 1988.

91. Macri JN, Kasturi RV, Drantz DA, et al: Free beta-protein is a more effective marker than human chorionic gonadotropin. Am J Obstet Gynecol 163:1248–1253, 1990.

92. Haddow JE, Palomaki GE, Knight GJ, et al: Prenatal screening for Down's syndrome with use of maternal serum markers. N Engl J Med 327:588–593, 1992.

93. Cheng EY, Luthy DA, Zebelman AM: A prospective evaluation of a second-trimester screening test for fetal Down syndrome. Obstet Gynecol 81:72–77, 1993.

94. Wald NJ, Kennard A, Hackshaw A, McGuire A: Antenatal screening for Down's syndrome. J Med Screen 4:181–246, 1997.

95. Holding S, Cuckle H: Maternal serum screening for Down's syndrome taking account of the result in a previous pregnancy. Prenat Diagn 14:321–324, 1994.

96. Spencer K: Between-pregnancy biologic variability of maternal serum AFP and free alpha-hCG: Implications for Down syndrome screening in subsequent pregnancies. Prenat Diagn 17:39–45, 1997.

97. Barkai G, Goldman B, Ries L, et al: Down's syndrome screening marker levels following assisted reproduction. Prenat Diagn 16:1111–1114, 1996.

98. Ribbet LSM, Kornman LH, De Wolf BTHM, et al: Maternal serum screening for fetal Down's syndrome in IVF pregnancies. Prenat Diagn 16:35–38, 1996.

99. Palomaki GE, Knight GJ, Haddow JE, et al: Prospective trial of a screening protocol to identify trisomy 18 using maternal serum alpha fetoprotein, unconjugated estriol, and human chorionic gonadotropin. Prenat Diagn 49(Suppl):227, 1991.

100. Neveux LM, Palomaki GE, Knight GJ, Haddow JE: Multiple marker screening for Down syndrome in twin pregnancies. Prenat Diagn 16:29–34, 1996.

101. Robinson L, Grau P, Crandall BF: Pregnancy outcomes after increasing levels of maternal serum alpha-fetoprotein. Obstet Gynecol 74:17–20, 1989.

102. Zelop C, Nadel AS, Frigoletto F, et al: Placenta accreta, percreta, and increta: A cause of elevated increased maternal serum alpha-fetoprotein. Obstet Gynecol 80:693–694, 1992.

103. Heinonen S, Ryynanen M, Kirkinen P, Saarikoski S: Uterine malformation: A cause of elevated maternal serum alpha-fetoprotein concentrations. Prenat Diagn 16:635–639, 1996.

104. Tanaka M, Natori M, Kohno H, et al: Fetal growth with elevated maternal serum hCG levels. Obstet Gynecol 81:341–343, 1993.

105. Fejgin MD, Kedar I, Amiel A, et al: Elevated hCG as an isolated finding during the second trimester biochemical screen: Genetic, ultrasonic and perinatal significance. Prenat Diagn 17:1027–1031, 1997.

106. Schmidt D, Rose E, Greenberg F: An association between fetal abdominal wall defects and elevated levels of human chorionic gonadotropin in mid-trimester. Prenat Diagn 13:9–12, 1993.

107. Muller F, Aegerter P, Boue A: Prospective maternal serum human chorionic gonadotropin screening for the risk of fetal chromosome abnormalities and subsequent fetal and neonatal death. Prenat Diagn 13:29–43, 1993.

108. Gravett CP, Buckmaster JG, Watson PT, Gravett MG: Elevated second trimester maternal serum beta-hCG concentration and subsequent adverse pregnancy outcome. Am J Med Genet 44:485–486, 1992.

109. Wenstrom KD, Owen J, Boots LD, et al: Elevated second trimester hCG is associated with poor pregnancy outcome. Am J Obstet Gynecol 171:1038–1041, 1994.

110. Lambert-Messerlian GM, Canick JA, et al: Second trimester levels of maternal serum inhibin A, total inhibin, alpha inhibin precursor, and activin in Down's syndrome pregnancy. J Med Screen 3:58–62, 1996.

111. Wallace EM, Swanston IA, McNeilly AS, et al: Second trimester screening for Down's syndrome using maternal serum dimeric inhibin A. Clin Endocrinol 44:17–21, 1996.

112. Van Lith JM, Pratt JJ, Beekhuis JR, Mantinga A: Second trimester maternal serum immuno-reactive inhibin as a marker for fetal Down's syndrome. Prenat Diagn 12:801–806, 1992.

113. Wald NJ, Densem JW, George L, et al: Prenatal screening for Down's syndrome using inhibin-A as a serum marker. Prenat Diagn 16:143–153, 1996.

114. Wald NJ, George L, Smith D, et al: On behalf of the International Prenatal Screening Research Group. Serum screening for Down's syndrome between 8 and 14 weeks of pregnancy. Br J Obstet Gynaecol 103:407–412, 1996.

115. Casals E, Fortuny A, Grudzinskas JG, et al: First-trimester biochemical screening for Down syndrome with the use of PAPP-A, AFP, and beta-hCG. Prenat Diagn 16:405–410, 1996.

116. Wald NJ, Stone R, Cuckle HS, et al: First trimester concentrations of pregnancy associated plasma protein A and placental protein 14 in Down's syndrome. BMJ 305:28, 1992.

117. Norton ME, Golbus MS: Maternal serum CA 125 for aneuploidy detection in early pregnancy. Prenat Diagn 12:779–781, 1992.

118. Van Lith JMM, Mantinga LA, Beekhuis JR, et al: First trimester CA 125 and Down's syndrome. Br J Obstet Gynaecol 98:493–494, 1991.

119. Qin QP, Christiansen M, Nguyen TH, et al: Schwangerschaftsprotein 1 (SP1) as a maternal serum marker for Down syndrome in the first and second trimester. Prenat Diagn 17:101–108, 1996.

120. Cuckle HS, Wald NJ, Goodburn FS, et al: Measurement of activity of urea resistant neutrophil alkaline phosphatase as an antenatal screening test for Down's syndrome. BMJ 301:1024–1026, 1990.

121. Wald NJ, Kennard A, Hackshaw AK: First trimester serum screening for Down's syndrome. Prenat Diagn 15:1227–1240, 1995.

122. Wald NJ, Hackshaw AK: Combining ultrasound screening and biochemistry in first-trimester screening for Down syndrome. Prenat Diagn 17:821–829, 1997.

123. Walknowska J, Conte FA, Grumbach MM: Practical and theoretical implication of fetal/maternal lymphocyte transfer. Lancet 1:1119–1122, 1969.

124. Mueller UW, Hawes CS, Wright AE, et al: Isolation of fetal trophoblasts cells from peripheral blood of pregnant women. Lancet 336:197–200, 1990.

125. Durrant LG, Martin WL, McDowall KM, Liu DTY: Isolation of fetal trophoblasts and nucleated erythrocytes from the peripheral blood of pregnant women for prenatal diagnosis of fetal aneuploides. Early Hum Dev 47(Suppl):S79–S83, 1996.

126. Cacheux V, Milesi-Fluet C, Tachdjian G, et al: Detection of 47,XYY trophoblast fetal cells in maternal blood by fluorescence in situ hybridization after immunomagnetic lymphocyte depletion and flow cytometric sorting. Fetal Diagn Ther 7:190–194, 1992.

127. Herzenberg LA, Bianchi DW, Schröder J, et al: Fetal cells in the blood of pregnant women: Detection and enrichment by fluorescence-activated cell sorting. Proc Natl Acad Sci U S A 73:1453–1455, 1979.

128. Clayton EM, Feldhaus MT, Whitacre FE: Fetal erythrocytes in the maternal circulation of pregnant women. Obstet Gynecol 23:915–919, 1964.

129. Thomas DB, Yoffey JM: Human foetal haemopoiesis I. The cellular composition of foetal blood. Br J Haematol 8:290–295, 1962.

130. Bianchi DW, Flint AF, Pizzimenti MF, et al: Isolation of fetal DNA from nucleated erythrocytes in maternal blood. Proc Natl Acad Sci U S A 87:3279–3283, 1990.

131. Slunga-Talberg A, El-Rifai W, Keinänen M, et al: Maternal origin of nucleated erythrocytes in peripheral venous blood of pregnant women. Hum Genet 96:53–57, 1995.

132. Hamada H, Arinami T, Kubo T, et al: Fetal nucleated cells in maternal peripheral blood: Frequency and relationship to gestational age. Hum Genet 91:427–432, 1993.

133. Bianchi DW, Williams JM, Sullivan LM, et al: PCR quantitation of fetal cells in maternal blood in normal and aneuploid pregnancies. Am J Hum Genet 61:822–829, 1997.

134. Thomas MR, Williamson R, Craft I, et al: Y chromosome sequence DNA amplified from peripheral blood of women in early pregnancy. Lancet 343:413–414, 1994.

135. Bianchi DW, Stewart JE, Garber MF, et al: Possible effect of gestational age on the detection of fetal nucleated erythrocytes in maternal blood. Prenat Diagn 11:523–528, 1991.

136. Zheng Y, Carter NP, Price CM, et al: Prenatal diagnosis from maternal blood: Simultaneous immunophenotyping and FISH of fetal nucleated erythrocytes isolated by negative magnetic cell sorting. J Med Genet 30:1051–1056, 1993.

137. Cheung M-C, Goldberg JD, Kan YW: Prenatal diagnosis of sickle cell anaemia and thalassaemia by analysis of fetal cells in maternal circulation. Nat Genet 14:264–268, 1996.

138. Lo YMD, Morey AL, Wainscoat JS, Flemming KA: Culture of fetal erythroid cells from maternal peripheral blood. Lancet 344:264–265, 1994.

139. Valerio D, Aiello R, Altieri V, et al: Culture of fetal erythroid progenitor cells from maternal blood for non-invasive prenatal genetic diagnosis. Prenat Diagn 16:1073–1082, 1996.

140. Lo YMD, Patel P, Wainscoat JS, et al: Prenatal sex determination by DNA amplification from maternal peripheral blood. Lancet 2:1363–1365, 1989.

141. Camaschella C, Alfarano A, Gottardi E, et al: Prenatal diagnosis of fetal hemoglobin Lepore-Boston disease on maternal peripheral blood. Blood 75:2102–2106, 1990.

142. Lo YMD, Bowell PJ, Selinger M, et al: Prenatal determination of fetal RhD status by analysis of peripheral blood of rhesus negative mothers. Lancet 341:1147–1148, 1993.

143. Lo YM, Corbetta N, Chamberlain PF, et al: Presence of fetal DNA in maternal plasma and serum. Lancet 350:485–487, 1997.

144. Lo YM, Tein MS, Lau TK, et al: Quantitative analysis of fetal DNA in maternal plasma and serum: Implications for noninvasive prenatal diagnosis. Am J Hum Genet 62:768–775, 1998.

145. Simpson JL, Elias S: Isolating fetal cells from maternal blood: Advances in prenatal diagnosis through molecular technology. JAMA 270:2357–2361, 1993.

146. Gänshirt-Ahlert D, Börjesson-Stoll R, Burschyk M, et al: Detection of fetal trisomies 21 and 18 from maternal blood using triple gradient and magnetic cell sorting. Am J Reprod Immun 30:194–201, 1993.

147. Takabayashi H, Kuwabara S, Ukita T, et al: Development of noninvasive fetal DNA diagnosis from maternal blood. Prenat Diagn 15:74–77, 1995.

148. Korf B: Molecular medicine: Molecular diagnosis (Part 1). N Engl J Med 332:1218–1220, 1995.

149. Housman D: Molecular medicine: Human DNA polymorphisms. N Engl J Med 332:318–320, 1995.

150. Sutherland GR, Richards RI: DNA repeats—a treasury of human variation. N Engl J Med 331:191–193, 1994.

151. Korf B: Molecular medicine: Molecular diagnosis (Part 2). N Engl J Med 332:1499–1502, 1995.

152. Southern EM: Detection of specific sequences among DNA fragments separated by gel electrophoresis. J Mol Biol 98:503–517, 1975.

153. Saiki RK, Scharf S, Faloona F, et al: Enzymatic amplification of beta-globin genomic sequences and restriction site analysis for the diagnosis of sickle cell anemia. Science 1985:1350–1354, 1985.

154. Saiki RK, Walsh PS, Levenson CH, Erlich HA: Genetic analysis of amplified DNA with immobilized sequence-specific oligonucleotide probes. Proc Natl Acad Sci U S A 74:6230, 1989.

155. Shuber AP, Michalowsky LA, Nass GS, et al: High throughput parallel analysis of hundreds of patient samples for more than 100 mutations in multiple disease genes. Hum Mol Genet 6:337–347, 1997.

156. Norton ME, D'Alton ME, Bianchi DW: Molecular zygosity studies aid in the management of discordant multiple gestations. J Perinatol 17:202–207, 1997.

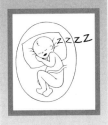

CHAPTER 10

Anesthesia and Monitoring for Fetal Intervention

CHARLES B. CAULDWELL, MARK A. ROSEN, and RUSSELL W. JENNINGS

Providing anesthesia for fetal intervention poses several unique challenges, as there are two patients for whom the anesthesiologist and surgeon must provide care. The challenges and risks associated with surgery during pregnancy are combined with the potential for direct fetal intervention, varying from minimal fetoscopic manipulation to hysterotomy and invasive procedures on the fetus itself. The nature and invasiveness of fetal surgery have continued to undergo evolutionary changes since its inception almost two decades ago, and the procedure has major effects on the requirements and goals of anesthesia. There are six basic objectives of anesthetic management that remain important: (1) maternal safety; (2) avoidance of teratogenic agents, (3) avoidance of fetal asphyxia; (4) fetal anesthesia and monitoring; (5) uterine relaxation; and (6) prevention of preterm labor.

Maternal Safety

Anesthesia during pregnancy is associated with increased risk to the mother because of the physiologic changes that occur with pregnancy, and to the fetus because of the potential adverse effects of surgery and anesthesia. There are physiologic changes that occur to almost every organ system in the pregnant woman, attributable to either placental hormones or to the mechanical effects of the enlarging uterus. Many of these changes begin early, in the first or second trimester. An appreciation of these changes and how they alter anesthetic management is crucial for the safe delivery of care to the pregnant woman.

Respiratory changes are complex. Oxygen consumption increases by 20% during pregnancy, due to the growth and metabolic demands of the fetus, placenta, and the uterus.[1] This leads to increases in alveolar ventilation of 25% by the fourth month of gestation and 70% at term, manifested primarily by increased tidal volumes and small increases in respiratory rate (Fig. 10–1).[2, 3] Vital capacity remains unchanged, but the upward displacement of the diaphragm by the growing uterus leads to a decrease in expiratory reserve volume, producing a decrease in the functional residual capacity (FRC) of 10% by 16 weeks' gestation, and 20% at term (Fig. 10–2).[2] The increased alveolar ventilation is associated with a decrease in the normal $Paco_2$ to 32 mm Hg (respiratory alkalosis), but a compensatory change in the serum bicarbonate to 22 mEq/L (metabolic acidosis) maintains the maternal pH close to 7.4 (Fig. 10–3).[4–6] The decreased FRC and the increased alveolar ventilation lead to an increase in the speed of induction with inhaled anesthetics, although this is partially offset by the increased cardiac output.[7]

The decreased FRC combined with increased oxygen consumption can lead to the more rapid development of hypoxia in a pregnant woman during the apnea accompanying endotracheal intubation or if respiratory obstruction develops. Intubation is considered more challenging and potentially more difficult in a pregnant woman due to the airway mucosal edema that accompanies pregnancy. To prevent hypoxia, the administration of 100% oxygen for several minutes prior to induction and intubation is standard practice. The Pao_2 can fall to 50 mm Hg in only 30 seconds without preoxygenation.[8]

There are multiple cardiovascular changes occurring during pregnancy as well. The maternal blood volume increases starting in the first trimester.[9] The increase in plasma volume is greater than the increase in red blood cell (RBC) volume, leading to the physiologic anemia of pregnancy (Fig. 10–4). The plasma volume increases by 40% by term and the red blood cell volume increases by 20%.[10]

The increases in blood and plasma volumes are associated with an increase in cardiac output, 30 to 40% in the first trimester, and remaining elevated throughout pregnancy (Fig. 10–4).[11] However, blood pressure normally does not rise, implying that there is a decrease in peripheral vascular resistance.

The gravid uterus during the second and third trimesters, can produce aortocaval compression and consequent hypotension in the pregnant woman in the supine position (Fig. 10–5).[12, 13] Compression of the vena cava can decrease venous return leading to a decrease in cardiac output. Uterine arterial hypotension or a rise in uterine venous pressure can lead to a decrease in uterine

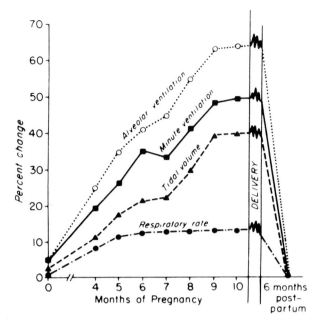

FIGURE 10-1. Changes in respiratory parameters during pregnancy.

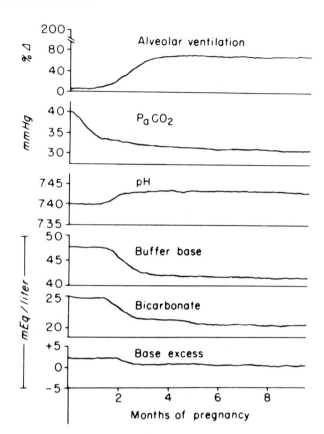

FIGURE 10-3. Alveolar ventilation, arterial CO_2, pH, and buffer-base changes during pregnancy.

blood flow.[14] Compression of the aorta by the gravid uterus can also directly decrease uterine blood flow. General anesthetic agents like isoflurane and thiopental can accentuate these hemodynamic changes by producing vasodilation. Regional anesthesia, either epidural or spinal, can lead to a sympathectomy. Both mechanisms can decrease venous return and promote hypotension and uterine hypoperfusion, as well as compromising

the maternal autonomic nervous system and the ability to compensate for these changes. For the above reasons it is important to avoid the supine position in the pregnant

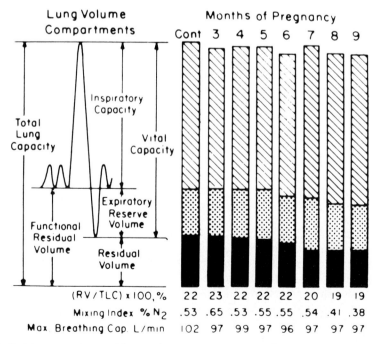

FIGURE 10-2. Serial measurements of lung volume compartments, pulmonary mixing index, and maximum breathing capacity during pregnancy.

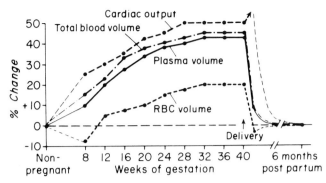

FIGURE 10–4. Changes in blood volume, plasma volume, RBC volume, and cardiac output during pregnancy.

woman undergoing fetal surgery. Tilting the operating room (OR) table and shifting the uterus off the great vessels can prevent supine hypotension and uterine hypoperfusion. Mechanical compression of the aorta and vena cava can occur when the uterus is manipulated during surgery, especially when the uterus is returned to the abdomen or the abdomen is packed to position the uterus, leading to maternal hypotension. Uterine manipulation and positioning can lead to compression of the uterine vessels, particularly during procedures on the back of the uterus.

The enlarging uterus displaces the stomach to a more cephalic and horizontal position during pregnancy. This changes the angle of the gastroesophageal junction and predisposes the patient to passive regurgitation.[15] There is, in addition, an increase in gastric acid production.[16]

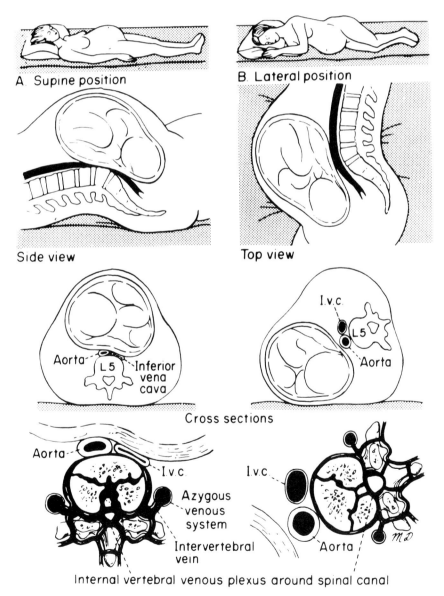

FIGURE 10–5. The effects of the pregnant uterus on the inferior vena cava (IVC) and the aorta in the supine position (*left*) and the lateral position (*right*). The marked aortocaval compression in the supine position causes venous blood to be diverted to and through the vertebral venous plexus, which becomes engorged and thus reduces the size of the epidural and subarachnoid spaces.

The increased risk of regurgitation and the increased acid production make the pregnant patient more susceptible to the aspiration of acidic gastric contents and development of aspiration pneumonitis during the induction of general anesthesia. It has been known for some time that the aspiration of gastric contents during pregnancy is associated with increased morbidity and mortality.[17] The prophylactic administration of an oral nonparticulate antacid immediately prior to the induction of anesthesia is recommended for all pregnant women undergoing surgery. The safety and efficacy of other drugs, such as cimetidine or metoclopramide, to decrease gastric acidity or volume, respectively, is still under scrutiny. For any pregnant woman with symptoms of gastroesophageal reflux, or during the second half of pregnancy for anyone, a rapid sequence induction of anesthesia should take place, involving the use of a cuffed endotracheal tube and the use of cricoid pressure provided by an assistant to occlude the esophagus.[18]

The pregnant woman is more sensitive to the volatile anesthetic agents. The potency of these agents is measured by the minimum alveolar concentration (MAC). MAC is decreased by 25 to 40% during pregnancy.[19] This means that doses that would be safe in the nonpregnant patient may produce an overdose in the pregnant patient, with associated cardiac depression and hypotension.

Increased intra-abdominal pressure and increased femoral venous pressure lead to engorgement of the epidural veins and a decrease in the epidural space. This increases the risk of encountering bleeding during placement of an epidural catheter for labor analgesia or for fetal surgery. The increased epidural pressure, transmitted to the subarachnoid space, decreases the volume of the cerebrospinal fluid (CSF) in the vertebral column, though CSF pressure is not elevated. There is a 30% decrease in the amount of local anesthetic required to achieve a certain level of block for both epidural and spinal anesthesia in the pregnant patient compared to the nonpregnant one.[20]

The increased cardiac output during pregnancy leads to increased renal plasma flow, glomerular filtration rate, tubular reabsorption of water and electrolytes, and an increase in creatinine clearance.[21] The normal blood urea nitrogen (BUN) is 8 to 9 mg/dL, and serum creatinine is 0.6 mg/dL, but serum electrolytes are unchanged.[22]

Some liver enzyme serum concentrations can be elevated during normal pregnancy, including serum glutamic-oxaloacetic transaminase (SGOT), lactate dehydrogenase (LDH), and alkaline phosphatase; bilirubin levels and hepatic blood flow remain unchanged.[23] There is a decrease in total protein concentration and the albumin/globulin ratio. Serum cholinesterase is decreased, which is usually clinically insignificant, but may prolong the neuromuscular blockade from succinylcholine.[24–26]

Uterine blood flow at term is about 700 mL/min. This is about 10% of the maternal cardiac output. The placenta receives 70 to 90% of the uterine blood flow, with myometrium getting the rest.[27,28] The uterine vasculature is normally almost maximally dilated and has little capacity for further dilation. The uterine vasculature is capable of vasoconstriction, however. Due to the lack of autoregulation, uterine blood flow is proportional to the mean perfusion pressure, making the uterus particularly sensitive to maternal blood pressure.

Reduction in uterine blood flow can cause serious fetal hypoxia with disastrous results. Factors that can reduce uterine blood flow relevant to anesthetic management are the following:

A. Hypotension (decreased uterine artery pressure) due to:
   1. Sympathetic blockade (spinal or epidural anesthesia)
   2. Hypovolemic shock
   3. Supine hypotension syndrome or aortic compression
   4. Iatrogenic hypotension secondary to vasodilators (e.g., nitroprusside) or deep general anesthesia
B. Vasoconstriction (increased uterine vascular resistance) due to:
   1. Endogenous sympathetic discharge (pain, anxiety, stress, hypoxia, hypercarbia)
   2. Essential hypertension
   3. Toxemia
   4. Exogenous α-adrenergic drugs
   5. Uterine vascular compression due to surgical manipulation
C. Increased uterine venous pressure due to:
   1. Uterine contractions
   2. Supine position with vena caval compression
   3. Excessive positive-pressure ventilation (by decreasing venous return and cardiac output)
   4. Uterine vessel compression due to positioning or surgical manipulation

Avoidance of Teratogenic Agents

The administration of a drug to a pregnant woman at any time during gestation may produce teratogenic effects. To produce an effect, the drug must be given to an individual who is genetically susceptible during a particular developmental stage of gestation. The drug must be able to cross the placenta and achieve concentrations adequate to bring about the teratogenic effect. Each organ or system, during its development, has a stage of differentiation at which it is most vulnerable to the effects of teratogenic agents and during which it is most likely to produce a specific malformation. In humans, it is generally felt that the first trimester is the most vulnerable period.

In order to evaluate the literature and counsel patients appropriately, several distinctions should be made. Many studies have been performed in animal models, but there remain serious questions about their applicability to humans. Anesthetic agents should be considered separately from other agents, like tranquilizers.

In animal studies virtually all anesthetic and premedication drugs have been shown to be teratogenic in some species. Barbiturates, antipsychotics, and some opioids have all been associated with increased fetal anomalies.[29–38] Nitrous oxide has been investigated because of its known inhibition of methionine synthetase and possible subsequent interference with DNA synthesis.[39, 40] In rodents and chickens, very high exposure levels of nitrous oxide are associated with teratogenesis, but exposures up to 12 hours a day do not seem to have an effect.[32–34, 41, 42] One study showed prevention of anomalies by isoflurane or halothane anesthetic agents, without reversing the inhibition of the enzyme methionine synthetase, and failure to prevent the effect of the nitrous by administration of folinic acid, which should bypass the metabolic block caused by the nitrous oxide.[43, 44] Other studies with halothane and isoflurane have not consistently shown teratogenic effects on several different model systems. It should be noted that in animal studies hypoxia,[45, 46] hyperoxia,[47] and hypercarbia[48] may be associated with teratogenesis.

There are several studies that have shown an association between minor tranquilizers (e.g., meprobamate and chlordiazepoxide) and increased risk of congenital anomalies.[49] Though the results are not conclusive, in 1975 the Food and Drug Administration (FDA) recommended that minor tranquilizers be avoided in the first trimester of pregnancy.[50] However, in 1998, this was challenged by further studies with more solid scientific foundation.[51]

Human reports of exposure to anesthetic agents fall into two categories: studies looking at chronic occupational exposure to the agents, and studies involving women who underwent surgery during pregnancy. Several large retrospective studies have looked at women with chronic occupational exposure to anesthetic agents. For example, female anesthesiologists, operating room nurses, and dental assistants compared, respectively, to female pediatricians, ward nurses, and dental assistants without anesthetic exposure. Anesthetic exposure is associated with increased rates of spontaneous abortion.[52–54] However, the increases are small and may be due to confounding variables. The association between exposure to anesthetic agents and major congenital anomalies is far less certain. Although two studies—one on operating room personnel and the other from the American Dental Association—showed borderline statistically significant increases in the rates of congenital anomalies, those results have been challenged.[55] These retrospective studies have significant limitations due to the lack of control groups, lack of confirmation of reported adverse outcomes, low response rate to survey questionnaires, lack of details on duration and amounts of anesthetic gas exposure, and lack of information on the numerous other potentially teratogenic confounding variables associated with work in an operating room or dental office. Scavenging systems to remove these anesthetic compounds have been introduced into most operating rooms, and future surveys may indicate whether removal of trace concentration of drugs has reduced the incidence of abortion and anomalies.

The second major group of women exposed to anesthetic agents during pregnancy consists of those women who underwent surgery during pregnancy. Most early studies were hampered by small size. Duncan et al. looked at data from Canada in the early 1970s and found no difference in the rate of birth defects. However, this study did not differentiate among the trimesters during which the operation occurred.[56] Mazze and Kallen examined the data from three linked Swedish health care registries.[57] Over 5,000 women received surgery during pregnancy. There were no differences in the rates of anomalies or stillbirths, but there was a difference in the incidence of low-birth-weight infants delivered. However, Kallen and Mazze reexamined their data and noted that there may be an elevated risk of neural tube defects in women having surgery during the first trimester.[59] Subsequently, Sylvester et al. in a case-control study from Atlanta claimed that there may be an increased risk of hydrocephalus, especially with other defects, in the offspring of women having surgery during the first trimester.[59] Despite these recent suggestive results, the numbers remain small; no agent has been shown to be safer than another; and they have failed to list types of anesthetics, indications for surgery, operations performed, or exposure to other drugs and toxins.

With the available data, it is not possible to separate the effects of surgery or the underlying medical condition from those of anesthetic exposure. Therefore, a categorical statement regarding anesthetic agents and teratogenicity is not warranted. As a general rule, however, it is prudent to postpone elective surgery until after delivery, and to delay urgent surgery until the second trimester (when feasible and safe) to limit exposure of the developing fetus to drugs during the first trimester when it is the most vulnerable. If maternal surgery is necessary during the first trimester, then a local or a regional anesthetic technique probably carries with it the least risk for the fetus.

Avoidance of Fetal Asphyxia

Fetal oxygenation depends on maternal arterial oxygen content and placental blood flow. Fetal asphyxia is avoided by maintaining normal maternal Pa_{O_2} and Pa_{CO_2} concentrations and normal uterine blood flow.

The causes of maternal hypoxia during general anesthesia do not differ from those of any intubated and ventilated patient. Elevated maternal oxygen tensions that commonly occur during anesthesia are safe for the fetus.[60, 61] Even a rise of maternal Pa_{O_2} to 600 mm Hg seldom produces a fetal Pa_{O_2} above 45 mm Hg and never above 60 mm Hg. Thus, premature closure of the ductus arteriosus or retrolental fibroplasia cannot be produced in utero with normobaric maternal hyperoxia.

Fetal Pa_{CO_2} is directly related to maternal Pa_{CO_2}. Maternal hypercapnia causes fetal respiratory acidosis. Maternal hypocapnia produced by excessive positive-pressure ventilation increases mean intrathoracic pressure and decreases venous return, thereby decreasing cardiac output.[62] This action causes a fall in the uterine blood flow, which is deleterious to the fetus. Maternal alkalosis also reduces umbilical blood flow by direct vasoconstriction and shifts the oxygen-hemoglobin dissociation curve to the left.[63] This shift increases the affinity of maternal hemoglobin for oxygen and decreases the transfer of oxygen to the fetus via the placenta. Thus, fetal hypoxia and acidosis can result from maternal hyperventilation.

Since uterine arterial flow depends directly on maternal blood pressure, maternal hypotension should be avoided or corrected promptly with fluid administration, reduction of the anesthetic concentration, or, if necessary, an appropriate vasopressor (e.g., ephedrine) given to prevent the development of fetal asphyxia. A slight fall in blood pressure due to high concentrations of volatile anesthetic agent is not associated with significant reduction of uterine vascular resistance.[64] Deep halothane anesthesia, which results in maternal hypotension (30% decrease from control levels), will produce fetal asphyxia, however.

Uterine vasoconstriction from endogenous or exogenous sympathomimetics increases uterine vascular resistance and decreases uterine blood flow, potentially resulting in fetal asphyxia.[65, 66] Maternal anxiety, inadequate anesthesia for surgical stimuli, and many vasoactive drugs (e.g., dopamine, methoxamine, phenylephrine, or systemic absorption of epinephrine, which is commonly infiltrated with local anesthetics) may produce uterine vasoconstriction. When hypotension requires vasopressor administration, drugs with predominant central-adrenergic stimulant activity (e.g., ephedrine, mephentermine, or metaraminol) restore normal uterine blood flow and should be preferred.[67]

Fetal Anesthesia

Surgery during pregnancy is performed to produce the least possible effect on the uterus and fetus. The nature of fetal surgery, however, requires that the fetus be subjected to a variety of noxious stimuli.

It is known that later in gestation a fetus will respond to environmental stimuli, such as noise, light, music, pressure, touch, and cold.[68, 69] Surgical manipulation of an unanesthetized fetus will stimulate its autonomic nervous sysyem.[69, 70] Several studies of premature infants undergoing surgery with minimal anesthesia have demonstrated increased levels of catecholamines, growth hormone, glucagon, cortisol, aldosterone, and corticosteroids, and decreased levels of insulin, endocrine, and metabolic markers associated with the stress response.[71-73] Provision of adequate anesthesia has been shown to abolish these changes.[74]

Because one of the goals of anesthesia for adults is to attenuate or abolish autonomic and stress responses, it seems reasonable to conclude that the fetal anesthesia would carry some benefit and, in conjunction with fetal immobility during a surgical procedure, may be an important goal of fetal anesthesia.[75] However, it must be said that the necessity and benefit of fetal anesthesia has not been documented.

Various fetal procedures and techniques may affect fetal physiologic functions to an unknown extent because of etiologic factors that are not yet precisely understood. Uterine incision, fetal manipulation, or anesthetic management may affect fetal and placental circulation by several mechanisms potentially leading to fetal compromise. Increased uterine activity, maternal hypoten-

sion, maternal hypocarbia, or hyperventilation may interfere with uterine or umbilical blood flow by direct compression or may induce fetal responses that affect the fetal circulation. The impact of some of these procedures on the fetal cardiovascular system, the distribution of fetal cardiac output, and fetal well-being is still under investigation.

The fetal cardiovascular system is adapted for use of the placenta as the organ for oxygen uptake and carbon dioxide elimination. The placenta receives a large amount of blood flow, whereas the pulmonary circulation receives very little blood flow. The cardiovascular system is also adapted for existence in a low-oxygen environment and provides the cerebral circulation with blood that has greater oxygen content than that perfusing the lower body. Fetal cardiovascular circulation allows the mixing of blood between the right and left sides of the heart (Figs. 10–6 and 10–7). Approximately one third of the relatively well-oxygenated inferior vena caval blood (which includes the blood returning from the placenta) is deflected by the crista dividens in the right atrium and is shunted through the foramen ovale into the left side of the heart. Two thirds of the inferior vena caval blood passes from the right atrium to the right ventricle. Almost all poorly oxygenated superior vena caval blood also passes from the right atrium to the right ventricle. Approximately 90% of the right ventricular output, ejected into the pulmonary artery, is shunted by the ductus arteriosus into the descending

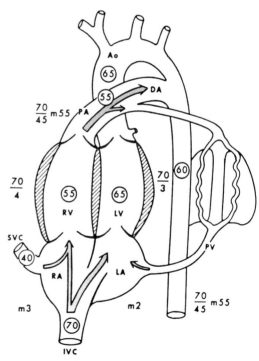

F I G U R E 10–6. Depiction of the fetal circulation. The numbers in *circles* within the chambers and vessels represent percentage oxygen saturation levels. The numbers beside the chambers and vessels are pressures in millimeters of mercury relative to an amniotic pressure level of zero. (Ao = aorta; DA = ductus arteriosus; IVC = inferior vena cava; m = mean pressure; PA = pulmonary artery; RA,LA = right and left atrium; RV,LV = right and left ventricle.) Data are obtained from late-gestation lambs.

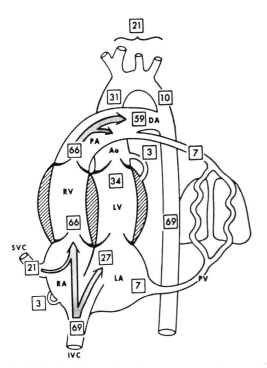

FIGURE 10–7. Depiction of the fetal circulation. The numbers in *squares* within the chambers and vessels represent percentages of the combined ventricular output that return to the fetal heart, percentages ejected by each ventricle, and percentages flowing through the main vascular channels. (Ao = aorta; DA = ductus arteriosus; IVC = inferior vena cava; m = mean pressure; PA = pulmonary artery; RA,LA = right and left artrium; RV,LV = right and left ventricle.) Data are obtained from late-gestation lambs.

aorta, reflecting the high pulmonary vascular resistance. The left ventricular output, which includes the relatively well-oxygenated inferior vena caval blood deflected through the foramen ovale plus the small amount of blood that perfuses the pulmonary circulation, is ejected into the aorta and perfuses the cerebral and coronary circulations and the upper extremities.

Cardiac output has two determinants: heart rate and stroke volume. Fetal cardiac output, measured in terms of combined left and right ventricular output, is directly related to and is more dependent on heart rate.[76] Stroke volume is a function of preload, afterload, and myocardial contractility. Fetal myocardial contractility is probably maximally stimulated, with limited capacity to increase stroke volume. Fetal myocardial muscle strips are less compliant than are those of adult hearts and have not only a greater resting tension but also a decreased ability to develop tension when stimulated.[77] In fetal lambs, augmentation of preload has little effect on increasing cardiac output. Volume loading increases fetal cardiac output only 15 to 20%.[78]

Because the fetus has limited capacity to increase cardiac output in response to stress, oxygen delivery to vital organs must be maintained by redistribution of blood flow. Cerebral blood flow in the fetal lamb is twice that in the adult, although both cerebral metabolic rates are similar.[79, 80] Among the factors that may modulate cerebral blood flow are cerebral metabolic rate, Pa_{CO_2}, arterial oxygen content, blood pressure, and autoregulation.[81–83] In fetal lambs, increases in arterial oxygen content are associated with increased cerebral blood flow. Cerebral blood flow autoregulation has been demonstrated to preserve cerebral blood flow in normoxic fetal lambs when systemic blood pressures are 20% above or below normal values. However, autoregulation in response to hypotension may be incomplete, and the mechanism of autoregulation may depend on arterial oxygen concentration.[84]

In fetal lambs, the concentration of halothane required to prevent movement in response to painful stimuli is much lower than is that for adult sheep or newborn lambs.[85] Although placental transfer of inhaled agents occurs rapidly, fetal levels of the halogenated agents remain lower than maternal levels for a significant period after the administration of these agents to the mother (Figs. 10–8 and 10–9). Studies on the fetal effects of maternal administration of halothane or isoflurane have been performed and demonstrate some inconsistencies. Maternal anesthesia with 0.7% halothane or 1% isoflurane (1.0 MAC for sheep) caused a mild decrease in fetal blood pressure with no change in fetal pulse

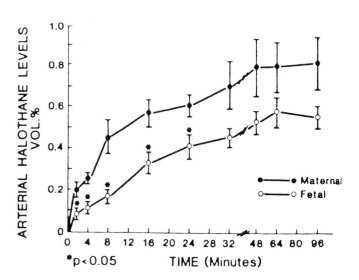

FIGURE 10–8. Maternal and fetal arterial halothane levels in sheep during maternal administration of 1.5% halothane (mean ± SE).

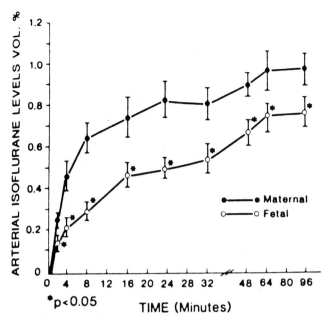

FIGURE 10–9. Maternal and fetal arterial isoflurance levels in sheep during maternal administration of 2% isoflurane (mean ± SE).

sive fetal acidosis, which was not seen after only a 30-minute exposure.[88] A recent study looked at the response to halothane for intrauterine cardiac surgery and found that this inhaled agent produced a negative effect on contractility.[89]

It seems that exposure of the unstressed fetus to light levels of inhaled anesthetics does not lead to fetal compromise, whereas prolonged, deep levels of inhaled agents may result in progressive fetal acidosis. The acidosis may be the result of direct negative inotropy or redistribution of blood flow. However, the combined effects of fetal anesthesia, uterine manipulation, and fetal stress are unknown.

Studies on the effects of maternal halothane administration on the asphyxiated fetus are not consistent. In unanesthetized animals, fetal asphyxia induced by occlusion of the umbilical circulation results in fetal bradycardia and hypertension, with decreased cardiac output and increased cerebral blood flow mediated partially by the fetal α-adrenergic and β-adrenergic systems.[90–94] In one study looking at the effects of halothane, maternal administration did not further compromise fetal well-being. The blood pressure of the anesthetized fetus declined to values that were normal compared with those of the awake asphyxiated fetus. However, because the pulse rate increased, the cardiac output remained unchanged. Oxygenation did not deteriorate, and the cerebral blood flow remained elevated.[95] In another study, halothane administered to the mother of a severely acidotic fetus caused further aggravation of fetal acidosis and oxygen desaturation.[96] Cerebral blood flow decreased as the fetal blood pressure decreased.

For all but percutaneous procedures, uterine relaxation is an important goal of the anesthetic technique chosen for fetal surgery. Inhaled halogenated volatile anesthetics are the author's choice for tocolysis during surgery. At the beginning of the clinical experience with fetal surgery at the University of California at San Francisco (UCSF), halothane was the preferred agent,[97] but for the last several years isoflurane has become the stan-

rate, oxygen, or acid-base status; however, anesthesia with 1.5% halothane or 2.0% isoflurane caused decreases in fetal blood pressure, heart rate, oxygen saturation, and base excess, with progressive fetal acidosis (Fig. 10–10).[64] Other studies demonstrated that maternal anesthesia with 1.5% halothane caused a decrease in fetal arterial blood pressure after a few minutes (primarily because of a decrease in peripheral vascular resistance), with no change in pulse rate, cardiac output, oxygen, acid-base status, or blood flow to the fetal brain or other major organs (Figs. 10–11 and 10–12).[86, 87] Yet another study demonstrated that maternal anesthesia with 2% isoflurane for 90 minutes produced no significant decline in fetal blood pressure but did produce a decrease in fetal cardiac index and the development of progres-

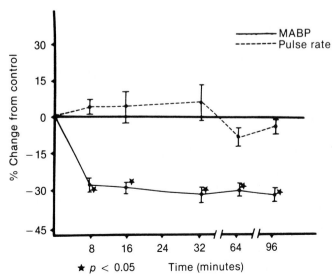

FIGURE 10–10. Changes in the mean arterial blood pressure (MABP) in fetal sheep and the pulse rate during maternal administration of 1.5% halothane, expressed as a percentage change from control levels (mean ± SE).

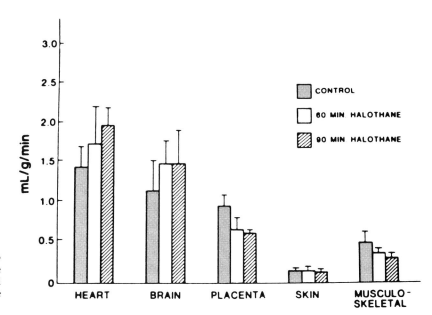

FIGURE 10–11. Regional blood flow in fetal sheep during maternal administration of 1.5% halothane (mean ± SE). Values were obtained at control and after 60 and 90 minutes of anesthesia with halothane by using labeled microsphere injection technique.

dard anesthetic. It is delivered in 100% oxygen with muscle relaxants to provide unconsciousness, amnesia, and analgesia for the mother, as well as fetal and maternal immobility and uterine relaxation for the surgeon.

We avoid anesthetic premedications or other adjuvant anesthetic agents to allow the maximal administration of isoflurane for uterine relaxation. The dose of isoflurane is limited by the maternal cardiovascular response. Maternal hypotension may lead to fetal compromise. Treatment consists of either maintaining the level of isoflurane and supporting the maternal blood pressure with a sympathomimetic agent that preserves uterine blood flow, such as ephedrine, or decreasing the isoflurane concentration and treating with an additional tocolytic agent, usually intravenous doses of nitroglyc-

erin or terbutaline. (At one time, our anesthetic technique consisted of nitrous oxide, fentanyl, and low doses of isoflurane, with tocolysis achieved with an intravenous infusion of nitroglycerin, up to 20 μg/kg/min.[98] Maternal hypotension was treated with doses of ephedrine. Although the technique was useful, it did not offer any advantage and was abandoned.)

Because there are no data describing human fetal response to inhaled agents and the occasional need for additional tocolysis, there has been some concern about our ability to adequately block the fetal autonomic response with inhaled agents, particularly in cases involving direct fetal manipulation. For these cases, we have chosen to deliver to the fetus an intramuscular injection of fentanyl, an opioid, and pancuronium, a muscle relaxant. These are delivered prior to hysterotomy, or placement of trocars for laparoscopic operations, by one of the perinatologists under ultrasound guidance. Pancuronium is used for its vagolytic properties, to help prevent fetal bradycardia.

When the uterus is being closed, the maternal anesthetic is changed to promote a smooth awakening. The isoflurane is decreased, fentanyl is given, nitrous oxide is started, and if an epidural catheter is in place, a dose of local anesthetic and opioid is administered. The patient's trachea is extubated in the operating room with the patient awake and able to respond to commands.

Prevention of Preterm Labor

Because uterine stimulation may increase the likelihood of inducing uterine contraction, the risk of preterm labor accompanies all invasive fetal intervention, and prevention and treatment assume crucial clinical importance. Fortunately, there has been an attempt to perform more fetal surgery fetoscopically, but hysterotomy may still be necessary. The uterine wall of primates has a thick, muscular layer. In experimental preparations using pri-

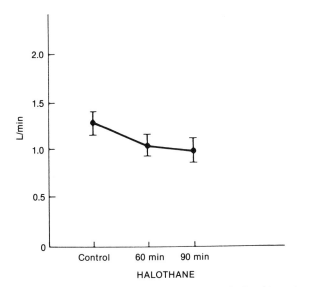

FIGURE 10–12. Cardiac output in fetal sheep calculated by using a labeled microsphere injection technique during maternal administration of 1.5% halothane (mean ± SE). Values were obtained at control and after 60 and 90 minutes of anesthesia with halothane.

mate fetuses, uterine incision can produce uterine contractions, resulting in a high incidence of postoperative abortion. Strong uterine contractions may impede uterine blood flow or induce partial placental separation that interferes with umbilicoplacental blood flow; both of these may compromise fetal well-being.

Prevention and treatment of preterm labor are paramount for the success of fetal surgery. Our current approach to tocolysis consists of multiple drugs, including preoperative indomethacin, intraoperative halogenated agents, intraoperative and postoperative magnesium sulfate, and intraoperative and postoperative β-adrenergic agents and indomethacin. We have also investigated the place of nitric oxide donors for the control of uterine contractions. There is experimental work with primates suggesting efficacy of such agents for tocolysis,[99] as well as numerous clinical reports of uterine relaxation provided by nitric oxide donors for the removal of a retained placenta, reduction of an inverted uterus, or delivery of an entrapped fetal head during vaginal breech delivery.[100, 101]

Maternal and Fetal Monitoring

The fetus is deep within the mother's body and extremely difficult to access for assessment of fetal well-being, as well as for intervention. While this inaccessibility provides a measure of safety for the normally developing fetus, this barrier to fetal access can prevent detection and inhibit therapy for those fetuses that need medical assistance. Remarkable advances have been made in the last few years in both fetal diagnosis and in fetal intervention. The quest to give the fetus access to medical therapy and surgical intervention necessarily imposes an obligation on the physicians to detect anomalies, provide appropriate medical or surgical therapy, and to closely monitor the fetus' well-being throughout the period of intervention.

Assessing the fetus in a noninterventional manner within the womb is now very successful using fetal ultrasonography. While the demands of equipment and manpower limit fetal ultrasonography to once or twice a day, it is increasingly accurate at assessing fetal and placental conditions. Unfortunately, the infrequency of the ultrasonographic examinations limits the physician's ability to continously monitor the fetus prior to, during, and after a medical or surgical intervention. Continuous monitoring of the fetus with a rapidly changing condition is optimal in order to provide enough time to assess and treat any problems. Just as a neonate who undergoes a major intervention is carefully monitored in an intensive care setting in the neonatal intensive care unit, a fetus who undergoes a major intervention should be monitored as closely as possible. While the physician's intentions are good, the technology still significantly lags behind the need.

A few tenets underlie the needs for maternal and fetal monitoring. In the uncompromised fetus, maternal well-being optimizes delivery of nutrients and removal of waste products from the fetus. It is only in the situation of maternal illness or a compromised fetus that intervention may become important. These are the conditions where continuous fetal monitoring can be life saving.

Animal Studies

All studies to investigate fetal physiology and surgery use animal models that do not have preterm labor as a major effect after surgery on the uterus and fetus. These animal models provide the opportunity to investigate the development of fetal anomalies and their surgical correction without the hurdle of uterine irritability. For this reason, the rabbit is a common small animal model and the sheep is the most commonly used large animal model. However, even extensive experience with fetal surgery using sheep and rabbits cannot be translated to human conditions because of the difference in uterine activity after surgery. The best model for posthysterotomy preterm labor is the nonhuman primate that has a similar rate of preterm labor and uterine contractions as the human.

The Fetal Treatment Center at UCSF has extensive experience over 20 years with fetal surgery in the sheep model and rabbit model. In addition, we have performed over 500 fetal surgical procedures on pregnant monkeys in the last 15 years.[97, 102–104] The nonhuman primate uterus is very susceptible to postoperative irritability and preterm labor with late-gestation fetal loss. The rhesus monkey has a spontaneous rate of preterm labor and fetal loss comparable to that of humans.[105, 106] We and others have learned that preterm labor makes maintaining a viable pregnancy with neonatal survival after fetal surgery in the monkey very challenging.[107, 108] This severe test makes fetal surgery experiments in the nonhuman primate model mandatory before progressing to humans.

The Monkey as Teacher

Early studies of the maternal response to fetal surgery provide us with the raw data to investigate fetal surgery in humans. A key component of this series of experiments was close monitoring of mother and uterus. Fetal surgery was performed on 25 time-mated pregnant monkeys at 100 to 147 days' gestation.[97] Twelve cynomolgus (*Macaca fasicularis*) and 13 rhesus (*Macaca mulatta*) underwent late second-trimester and third-trimester fetal surgery. They were compared to normal unoperated, control monkeys of similar gestational age. All experiments were carried out under veterinarian supervision at the University of California Primate Research Center at Davis. Early lessons learned included the importance of nonsteroidal anti-inflammatory drugs (especially indomethacin) for controlling immediate perioperative uterine irritability, and prevention of inferior vena cava compression by the gravid uterus by tilting the operating table to the side. Close maternal monitoring was essential, including arterial blood pressure, maternal core temperature, and maternal hydration status. Anesthesia was induced after ketamine sedation, using 60% nitrous oxide and 1% halothane.

Maternal hypotension had to be avoided in order to minimize the insult to uterine and placental perfusion (Table 10–1).

Fetal surgery always entailed complete exposure of the gravid uterus, and after assessment for fetal and placental positioning, the uterus was opened with a staple system (GIA) to minimize bleeding. The fetus was monitored by a fetal scalp electrode that revealed the fetal heart rate and beat-to-beat variability. The fetal surgical procedure was performed by exposing the fetus while avoiding compression of the umbilical cord. Most fetuses underwent urinary tract surgery (Fig. 10–13). The fetus was then returned to the amniotic cavity and the uterus filled with warm saline solution. In these early studies the uterus was closed with a TA-90 stapler after everting and removing the set of staples placed during the opening of the uterus.

All animals were returned to the breeding colony after recovery with no further attempts at controlling labor. Ultrasound examinations of the fetus were performed every 2 weeks under ketamine sedation. Near-term cesarean sections were performed for delivery and all neonates resuscitated and placed in a nursery.

Table 10–1 illustrates the learning curve for fetal surgery in the primate. The survival of group 1 was only 4 of 15 operated fetuses (26.7%), while in group 2, 8 of 10 fetuses were born alive (80%). Significantly, the 20% mortality in group 2 was about the same as the spontaneous late-gestation and early neonate mortality of 21.4% in a control group of 56 monkeys in the same institution.[109] While this study was closely analyzed for operative and surgical variables to correlate with fetal outcome, close monitoring of both fetus and mother identified several problem areas. The use of the β-mimetic drug isoxsuprine was halted early in the study because of difficulty with maternal tachycardia, despite its tocolytic effects. Close intraoperative monitoring of mother and fetus validated the use of inhaled halothane as the anesthetic. Halothane provided excellent maternal anesthesia and uterine relaxation, and provided fetal anesthesia as well. The depth of fetal anesthesia was assessed by both the absence of fetal movement and the fetal heart rate response during surgery.

These initial fetal surgical procedures were performed in monkeys that were returned to the breeding colony after surgery. We could not therefore monitor the fetus or the uterus after surgery, as this requires continuous cage monitoring with a vested monkey, or chair-restrained monitoring. Since it was clear that preterm labor is the limiting factor in outcome for these fetal surgical cases, we turned our attention to studying the perioperative monkey uterus. We studied both the electromyographic (EMG) and mechanical effects causing elevation of intra-amniotic pressure (IAP) of uterine activity. This required chronic implantation of electrodes into the uterine muscle to monitor the EMGs and catheterization of the amniotic sac to measure IAP.[110] This preparation was used to study the uterine response to nonobstetric surgery on the mother, surgical opening of the uterus, and operations on the fetus. We studied the effects of anesthetic and tocolytic agents in preventing preterm delivery and fetal loss.[102]

We wanted to investigate the response of the gravid uterus to both anesthetic and tocolytic agents during and after surgical procedures; 34 third-trimester pregnant rhesus monkeys were restrained in chairs (123 to 153 days' gestation, term = 168 days). Seven rhesus monkeys had electrodes placed to monitor the uterine EMG activity, while another seven rhesus monkeys had electrodes placed at the time of hysterotomy for placement of IAP catheters without operating on the fetus (Fig. 10–14). Another 12 rhesus monkeys had electrodes placed as well as intra-amniotic catheters after operating on the fetus for placement of carotid and jugular catheters. Eight additional rhesus monkeys had electrodes placed to study the uterine EMG response to surgery. These procedures included amniocentesis, maternal laparotomy without uterine manipulation, hysterotomy without fetal surgery, and hysterotomy with fetal surgery (Fig. 10–15).

This careful monitoring of the uterus provided a lot of information. Preterm labor and subsequent delivery occurred in 1 monkey of the 14 who underwent procedures with minimal manipulation of uterus, which included amniocentesis, electrode placement, and nonobstetric maternal laparotomy. Preterm delivery occurred in three of eight monkeys (37.5%) that had hysterotomies without fetal surgery, and 9 of 19 monkeys (47.7%) that had hysterotomies with fetal surgery. The EMG monitoring provided insight into the uterine response to surgery. In monkeys undergoing hysterotomy, emergence from anesthesia was associated with rapid and coordinated EMGs that generated large increases in IAP (type I EMG pattern). This uterine activity could be halted by deep halothane anesthesia, but was not controlled well by indomethacin given preoperatively or by ritodrine infusion postoperatively (Fig. 10–16). Chair-restrained monkeys are severely stressed, and this maternal stress likely accounts for the 90% fetal loss in this study.

This and similar studies clearly demonstrate that uterine injury caused by uterine and fetal surgical procedures results in patterns of EMG and IAP activity identical to contractions at term. In the monkey, these electrically and mechanically organized uterine contractions are called type I events and generate IAPs of 45 to 60 mm Hg. There is a clear nocturnal effect present in the monkey, with contractions becoming more frequent and more intense at night and decreasing during the day. Regular uterine contractions precede delivery by several days, to become progressively more frequent and vigorous with each successive night until labor and delivery occurs. Operating on the fetus and uterus accelerates this time course dramatically.

The uterus responds to surgical injury with the same type I EMG activity as occurs near term. There is a spectrum of postoperative responses of the uterus to injury. The most severe response is the rapid highly organized type I bursts that result in preterm delivery of the fetus 12 to 48 hours after surgery. This appears to be a rapidly progressive, nonperiodic, unstoppable series of contractions. Medications seem to have no effect on either the EMG or the IAP. A less severe response of the uterus to surgical injury occurs with maximal uterine intensity immediately postoperatively, but with

TABLE 10–1. FETAL SURGERY IN THE PRIMATE: DEVELOPMENT OF ANESTHETIC AND SURGICAL TECHNIQUE

MONKEY NUMBER	TYPE	GESTATIONAL AGE AT OPERATION	ANESTHESIA/TOCOLYSIS N₂O/O₂ Halo	Indomethacin Pre-	Indomethacin Post	Isoxsuprine	Diazepam Post	Intraoperative Fluid	TOTAL TIME (MIN)	Hysterotomy Uterine Incision	Open	Close	Fetal Procedure Operation	Time (min)	OUTCOME Pregnancy	Delivery	Neonatal	Pe Mc
Group 1																		
1-7535	MMU	147	+	–	–	+	–	450	90	Fundus	GIA	Suture	Ligate urethra	40	Abortion day 150	–	–	–
2-4748	MMU	117	+	–	–	–	–	250	120	Ant. high	GIA	TA-90	Dissect perineum	40	Uneventful	Vaginal on day 170	–	–
3-17868	MCY	104	+	–	–	–	–	250	65	Ant. low	GIA	TA-90	Dissect perineum	20	Abortion day 109	–	–	–
4-18227	MCY	101	+	–	–	–	–	300	30	Post. high	GIA	TA-90	Dissect perineum	10	Uneventful	C-section at term	Viable male, 390 g	–
5-17962	MCY	111	+	–	–	–	–	250	60	Ant. low	GIA	TA-90	Dissect perineum	35	Uneventful	C-section at term	Viable female, 271 g	–
6-18157	MCY	109	+	–	–	–	–	250	90	Fundus	GIA	TA-90	Dissect perineum	50	Abortion day 110	–	–	–
7-17798	MCY	113	+	–	–	–	–	250	90	Ant. high	GIA	TA-90	Dissect perineum	12	Abortion day 115	–	–	73.3%
8-18237	MCY	102	+	–	–	–	–	300	80	Post. high	GIA	TA-90	Dissect perineum	5	Abortion day 104	–	–	–
9-17777	MCY	118	+	–	–	+	+	150	70	Ant. high	GIA	TA-90	Urethral cath.	29	Mat. death (toxemia) day 12	–	–	–
10-17961	MCY	124	+	+	–	+	+	200	35	Post. low	GIA	Suture	Suprapubic cath.	23	Abortion day 125	–	–	–
11-18168	MCY	114	+	+	–	+	+	100	54	Ant. low	GIA	TA-90	Suprapubic cath.	24	Uneventful	Vaginal on day 137	Viable male, 170 g	–
12-17088	MMU	126	+	+	+	–	+	100	50	Post. high	GIA	TA-90	Suprapubic cath.	10	Uneventful	C-section day 168	Viable female, 548 g	–
13-18163	MCY	120	+	+	+	–	+	100	49	Ant. low	GIA	TA-90	Suprapubic cath.	22	Fetal death on day 125	–	–	–

14-18162	MCY	122	+	+	+	−	100	Ant. high	GIA	TA-90	Obstruct urethra*	9	Abortion day 124	—	—
15-5737	MMU	120	+	+	+	−	250	Ant. low	Suture	Suture	Suprapubic cath.	21	Fectectomy on day 126	—	—
Group 2															
16-17867	MCY-	124	+	+	+	−	200	Fundus	Suture	Suture	Cystostomy†	18	Labor disrupts the uterus	C-section day 159	Viable male, 285 g
17-6388	MMU	106	+	+	+	−	450	Ant. low	GIA	TA-90	Cystostomy†	20	Uneventful	C-section day 159	Viable female, 400 g†
13-4853	MMU	105	+	+	+	−	250	Post. high	GIA	TA-90	Obstruct urethra*	9	Uneventful	Vaginal on day 156	Viable male, 385 g
19-8166	MMU	103	+	+	+	−	300	Ant. low	GIA	TA-90	Obstruct urethra*	28	Abortion day 105	—	—
20-7797	MMU	119	+	+	+	−	350	Ant. low	GIA	TA-90	Suprapubic cath.	26	Uneventful	C-section day 161	Viable female, 450 g
21-17063	MMU	104	+	+	+	−	300	Fundus	GIA	TA-90	Cystostomy	17	Uneventful	C-section day 158	Viable female, 360 g†
22-4010	MMU	105	+	+	+	−	400	Post. high	GIA	TA-90	Obstruct urethra*	7	Uneventful	C-section day 160	Viable male, 460 g
23-8150	MMU	100	+	+	−	−	400	Ant. low	GIA	TA-90	Cystostomy	18	Uneventful	Vaginal on day 159	Stillborn female, 340 g
24-7400	MMU	109	+	+	−	−	250	Post. high	GIA	TA-90	Obstruct urethra*	22	Uneventful	C-section day	Viable male, 400 g†
25-7376	MMU	107	+	+	−	−	200	Ant. low	GIA	TA-90	Obstruct urethra†	13	Uneventful	Vaginal on day 161	Viable male, 456 g‡

20.0%

Spontaneous perinatal loss from 2nd half of pregnancy through neonatal period — 21.4%

Controls: 56 normal pregnancies from same breeding colony

* Ameroid constrictor or Silastic band around perineal urethra.
† Marsupialization of the bladder to the abdominal wall.
‡ Neonates catheterized.
MMU, rhesus; MCY, cynomolgus; Ant., anterior; Post., posterior; Cath., catheterization; Halo, halothane.

161

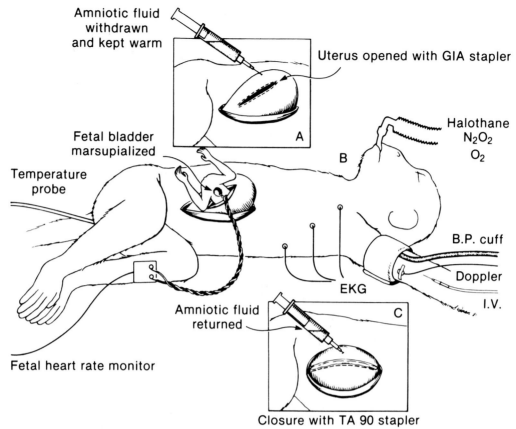

FIGURE 10–13. Technique for fetal surgery in the nonhuman primate. Mother and fetus are closely monitored. Indomethacin and antibiotics are given intravenously before surgery. Halothane (Fluothane) anesthesia provides uterine relaxation. The uterus is opened and closed with staples.

maintenance of circadian nocturnal rhythmicity. This labor tends to become progressively less frequent on each succeeding night, although fetal loss may still occur. Tocolysis has little effect on EMG or IAP during this postoperative pattern. In procedures were the uterus is minimally manipulated, such as electrode placement, amniocentesis, and nonobstetric laparotomy, type I activity occurs only briefly if at all, and preterm delivery occurs rarely.

Uterine incision appears to be the inciting event in preterm labor and delivery. Inhaled anesthetics such as halothane depress the uterine irritability during anesthesia, but do not affect uterine activity in the postoperative period. Use of the β-mimetic ritodrine was not effective in the postoperative period at stopping uterine contractions. Indomethacin was used to stop prostaglandin synthesis induced by surgery on the uterus and fetal membranes. Preoperative intravenous bolus of 10 mg indomethacin did not stop postoperative labor, although others have devised techniques using indomethacin with more success on a continuous infusion basis.[111] However, while effectively decreasing uterine contractions, this regimen was associated with oligohydramnios, maternal anemia, and increased fetal mortality rate. The potential for adverse derangements in the fetal circulation limits the use of indomethacin for tocolysis after fetal surgery.

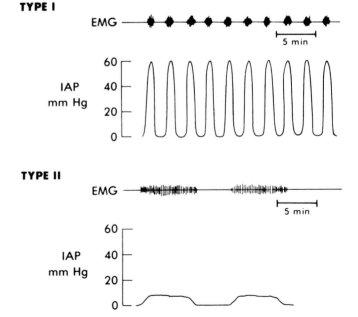

FIGURE 10–14. Electromyographic (EMG) patterns and intra-amniotic pressure (IAP) recordings in the gravid monkey uterus. In type I activity, short bursts of activity at regular intervals correlate with uterine contractions. Type II is the normal resting activity of the gravid uterus.

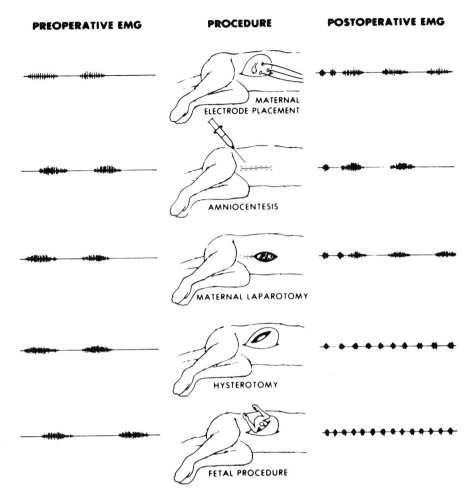

PREOPERATIVE EMG

PROCEDURE

POSTOPERATIVE EMG

MATERNAL ELECTRODE PLACEMENT

AMNIOCENTESIS

MATERNAL LAPAROTOMY

HYSTEROTOMY

FETAL PROCEDURE

FIGURE 10–15. Experiments designed to study the electromyographic response of the gravid uterus to surgical procedures. EMG electrodes were placed at an initial procedure, and the EMG response recorded continuously before, during, and after the increasingly invasive procedures listed.

These early monkey experiments demonstrated the incredible complexity of the system that maintains pregnancy. Performing fetal surgery and then releasing the mother to the breeding colony did not appear to increase the spontaneous abortion rates. However, operating on a monkey and then keeping them chair restrained causes such a high level of stress that a preterm fetal loss rate of 90 to 100% despite tocolytic medications can be expected. While we did not find an effective tocolytic regimen in this rigorous system, we did learn that hysterotomy and fetal surgery primes the uterus for labor and preterm delivery. This effect is amplified by maternal

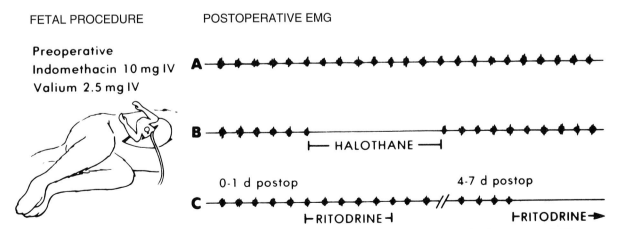

FETAL PROCEDURE

POSTOPERATIVE EMG

Preoperative
Indomethacin 10 mg IV
Valium 2.5 mg IV

A

B

├— HALOTHANE —┤

0-1 d postop   4-7 d postop

C

├RITODRINE┤   ├RITODRINE➤

FIGURE 10–16. Hysterotomy and fetal surgery results in type I activity that persists for days untreated (*A*). Halothane can completely suppress the activity (*B*), but ritodrine has little effect until the uterine irritability begins to resolve (*C*).

stress. It is therefore very important to monitor both the fetus and the uterus, in addition to maternal monitoring, in a stress-free and minimally invasive manner.

Preoperative Monitoring of the Human Uterus

Early in gestation, reliable noninvasive monitoring of the human uterus is difficult. Questioning of the mother about sensations of pelvic fullness, contractions, and cramping can provide some information, but it is very subjective both on the mother's part and in the clinician's interpretation. The diagnosis of preterm labor based on maternal sensations of contractions is very inaccurate, with errors in diagnosing preterm labor of 40 to 70%.[99] The most common objective assessment of labor is the digital examination of the cervix. Preterm labor is therefore usually diagnosed in the face of cervical dilation and/or effacement. Obvious uterine contractions with spontaneous rupture of the membranes is also an indicator of preterm labor.[113] These are relatively late indicators of labor that has progressed to the stage of cervical changes that are currently irreversible. It would be much better to have a noninterventional or minimally invasive objective assessment of uterine irritability and contractility prior to the onset of cervical dilation and membrane bulging.

Intraoperative Monitoring of the Uterus

Any type of uterine stimulation can induce uterine contractions. Surgical stimulation of the uterus inevitably leads to the immediate induction of uterine contractions and preterm labor. Intraoperative and postoperative uterine irritability and preterm labor remain the single biggest hurdle to prolonging the pregnancy after surgery. Accurate monitoring of the uterus and cervix during and after surgery provides the best objective information to allow control of the preterm labor. It is important to intervene early in the positive feedback loop of preterm labor in order to break the cycle before the preterm labor becomes irreversible. We have seen unstoppable uterine contractions during fetal surgery, which have resulted in the delivery of a nonviable fetus intraoperatively. It is for precisely these reasons that an accurate assessment of uterine irritability early in the cycle of labor is mandatory.

During a surgical procedure where the uterus is exposed we have the opportunity to directly evaluate the myometrium. This provides a reliable method of assessing the degree of myometrial contractions and the resultant intrauterine pressure. Prior to performing a hysterotomy, we can quickly detect a contraction of the uterus, which causes an increase in intrauterine pressure. This method is also reliable in assessing uterine contractions after the hysterotomy has been closed. While subject to some interpretation, a soft compliant uterus during fetal surgery is reassuring for both the anesthesiologists and the fetal surgeons. Interestingly, we often find that the myometrium has local contractility around the regions of the uterus that have been injured by the surgical

procedure—either by an incision or trocar site for fetoscopic surgery. While this technique does not provide us with a precise measurement of intrauterine pressure, it does detect contractions of the uterus with stimulation and relaxation of the uterus with deepening of inhaled anesthesia or administration of intravenous nitroglycerin.

We currently have no clinically useful methods of monitoring cervical dilation during surgery. Cervical sonocrystals may provide a reliable monitoring technique in the future. Since membrane rupture is always a potential problem during surgery, we do monitor the maternal perineum very closely for passage of fluid during surgery. Such a leakage of intrauterine fluid onto the perineum would indicate that the cervix has opened and that the membranes have ruptured. This mandates strict bed rest and intravenous tocolysis in the postoperative period, and inevitably leads to preterm delivery of the fetus.

We have developed a technique for precise and objective measurement of myometrial electrical and mechanical contractility during and after fetal surgery using implantable radiotelemeters.[99] The technique involved the use of tiny battery-powered radiotelemeters, which can detect and transmit data to an outside antenna (Data Sciences, Inc.; Minneapolis, MN) (Fig. 10–17). The data acquired includes an electrical signal from the uterus, and a pressure tracing from the amniotic fluid space. By placing the detection leads 1 cm apart within the muscle of the uterus, we were able to receive a very clean electromyogram from the myometrium. Combining these data with intrauterine pressure, which reflect the mechanical properties of uterine contraction, we are able to get a very clear picture of the start of labor and its progression to delivery. We have not yet tried either of these techniques in humans.

Intraoperative Monitoring of the Fetus

The goal during fetal intervention, be it a percutaneous needle procedure or a major tumor resection, is to optimize the fetal condition. This implies knowledge of optimal fetal physiology, and the variables that may perturb the system. It is essential during the fetal operation to avoid fetal hypoxia, hypothermia, and fetal asphyxia by kinking of the umbilical cord. During an open fetal operation we have our best opportunity to assess the condition of the fetus, but once returned to the confines of the closed uterus all direct contact with the fetus is lost.

While monitoring of the fetus during open fetal surgery is intuitively obvious, in practice it is extremely difficult. We and others have found that the single most useful monitor to assess the condition of the fetus is the pulse oximeter. A sterile pulse oximeter probe, usually used for the micropremature infant, is placed around the fetal hand and connected to sterile cabling and passed off to the anesthesiologists. Due to the bright intraoperative lighting, the fetal hand and pulse oximeter must be covered by aluminum foil held in place with a dressing to avoid interference by the OR lights.

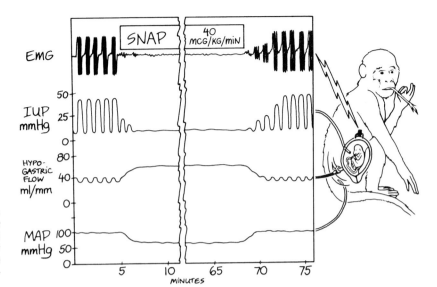

FIGURE 10–17. Effect of nitric oxide donor on postoperative uterine activity. Radiotelemeter monitored uterine electromyograms (EMGs) and intrauterine pressure (IUP), hypogastric artery flow probe monitors mean arterial blood pressure (MAP). (SNAP = S-nitroso-N-acetyl-penicillamine, a spontaneous nitric oxide donor.)

The thin skin and fetal hemoglobin alter the usual readings of the pulse oximeter. We have found that the pulse oximeter provides fairly reliable measurements of the fetal heart rate, although the signal is almost always relatively intermittent due to the ongoing surgical procedure. The oxygen saturation readings of the pulse oximeter typically read 50 to 60% saturation. Desaturation usually indicates a kinking or pressure on the umbilical cord, which can then be relieved prior to fetal bradycardia.

The fetal pulse oximeter is useful also for detecting fetal oxygenation problems that can lead to umbilical cord spasm. During the ex utero intrapartum treatment (EXIT) procedure for control of the fetal airway, we rely heavily on the use of the fetal pulse oximeter to determine the point at which the umbilical cord is clamped and divided. The EXIT procedure, discussed elsewhere in this text, can proceed for 90 minutes or more safely as long as the fetal oximeter is closely monitored. Access to the fetal trachea and ventilation with oxygen inevitably is followed by a rising fetal saturation to 90% or greater in those fetuses with adequate lung function. This high oxygen tension in the fetal blood induces spasm of the umbilical cord vessels very rapidly. We use the combination of fetal saturation greater than 90% and no pulse in the umbilical cord as the indication for clamping and dividing the umbilical cord. The pulse oximeter is then disconnected from its sterile connecting cables and handed off still connected to the neonate so that the pulse oximeter can be used during the subsequent neonatal resuscitation by the neonatologists.

The intermittent information provided by the fetal pulse oximeter can be frustrating. The fetal heart rate variability is a well-established and well-studied technique to monitor and assess fetal condition. Attempts at monitoring the fetal electrocardiogram both by surface electrodes and percutaneously placed skin electrodes have met with frustration. The surface electrodes simply do not pick up the tiny electrocardiogram signal of the fetus. The etiology of this failure is probably multifacto-

rial, but includes the inability of these electrodes to maintain contact with the fetal skin in the amniotic fluid environment, as well as the electrolyte content of the amniotic fluid, which disburses the tiny electrical signal. Placement of skin electrodes under the skin of the fetus is only slightly more effective, but is still unreliable. The problem stems from shorting of the individual electrodes in the amniotic fluid when the conducting portion of the electrodes becomes exposed, and manipulation of the fetus during surgery inevitably leads to loss of the fetal electrocardiogram signal.

Open fetal surgery provides the opportunity to use specially designed implantable radiotelemeters. Placing the entire telemeter including the sensory leads under the skin of the fetus avoids the complications of amniotic fluid shorting out the signal. In addition, this allows an excellent method to assess the radiotelemeter function during surgery, and then to leave it within the fetus in the postoperative period to provide postoperative fetal monitoring. Later modifications of the radiotelemeters have permitted continuous monitoring of the amniotic fluid pressure, and facilitate precise monitoring of uterine contractility after the uterus is closed.

Reliable monitoring of the fetal electrocardiogram during surgery provides a measure of assurance to the surgeons and anesthesiologists. The deep anesthesia required to perform the surgery ablates the fetal heart rate variability; however, bradycardia is still a sign of fetal distress. Use of a radiotelemeter, which provides a rapid readout of temperature, revealed that fetal hypothermia is a very real and very serious issue during open fetal surgery. Soon after using the implantable radiotelemeters, we documented fetal temperatures dropping from 37° C down to as low as 31° C in as little as 10 minutes. It is this rapid drop in fetal temperature due to fetal exposure that necessitates keeping the operating room warm, keeping exposure of the fetus minimal, wrapping the exposed portions of the fetus in warm towels, and using a system of continuous irrigation with warm saline to prevent fetal hypothermia. Fortunately, the fetal temperature quickly returns to normal with these measures.

The advent of minimally invasive fetoscopic surgery (FETENDO) has raised new problems in monitoring the fetus. The advantages of fetoscopic surgery including minimal injury to the uterus, less fetal manipulation, and less postoperative preterm labor are all strong reasons for its use. The small trocars used for fetoscopic surgery currently prohibit the use of implantable radiotelemeters and fetal pulse oximetry. The only technique to monitor a fetus undergoing fetoscopic surgery is intraoperative ultrasonography, and the use of ultrasonography requires the avoidance of gas insufflation of the uterus. We found ultrasound to be a very reliable and effective monitoring tool during surgery. Ultrasonography is manpower intensive in that an ultrasonographer must be scrubbed and present at the operating table during the entire procedure.

We are currently working with the Sensors 2000! development group at the National Aeronautics and Space Administration (NASA) to develop even smaller radiotelemeters. Investigational working models are now functioning for months at a time and are able to sense several things including intra-amniotic pressure and temperature. These devices are small enough that they can be inserted into the uterus through a 5-mm trocar used during fetoscopic surgery. While they do not detect the fetal electrocardiogram, they will provide accurate and reliable monitoring of uterine activity.

Fetal Intravascular Access

Access to the fetal vascular system is difficult during and after fetal surgery. We have tried many techniques to gain access to the fetal circulation during surgery while the fetus is exposed. Placement of central lines has resulted in prolongation of fetal exposure and excessive manipulation of the fetus. Catheters or lines left attached to a fetus when the fetus is returned to the uterus become a potential source of umbilical cord entanglement and fetal strangulation. Efforts at accessing the umbilical cord during fetal surgery have met with mixed results, frequently leading to umbilical cord hematoma, umbilical vessel spasm, and fetal demise. Experimental techniques have successfully allowed placement of catheters in the fetal blood vessels on the surface of the placenta in the rhesus monkey.[114] We have been able to achieve reliable long-term vascular access in the fetal circulation in the monkey model using fetoscopic guidance.[115] While this technique shows promise, it is technically very challenging and is a fetal surgical procedure in itself.

Occasionally during fetal surgery we have needed access to the fetal circulation for blood sampling or to replace blood loss during resection of a tumor or other surgical procedure. Despite our attempts at alternative techniques including intraosseous access,[116] the most reliable technique remains either a saphenous vein angiocatheter placed by a skilled neonatologist, or a central venous catheter placed by the surgeon. We have been able to use hand veins several times. This approach allows withdrawal of blood for electrolytes, hematocrit,

and blood gas analysis. The additional advantages of vascular access are that it allows for infusion of packed red blood cells in the case of blood loss–induced anemia, and that the catheter can be removed at the end of the procedure and the fetus returned to the uterus. The disadvantage, of course, is that access to the fetal circulation is lost.

Postoperative Monitoring of the Uterus and Mother

Monitoring of the postsurgical uterus for preterm labor is mandatory. All postsurgical women are in preterm labor, and tocolysis is required to prolong the pregnancy. The progression of labor from early contractions to irreversible and unstoppable labor can be rapid. It is important to intervene early in order to minimize the uterine irritability in an attempt to break the positive feedback cycle of labor.

The techniques to monitor labor are probably less sensitive after fetal surgery. The mother is on pain medications and has decreased uterine sensations. The low transverse incision used for uterine exposure is tender and makes placement of the tocodynamometer more difficult. The utility of the tocodynamometer to detect uterine contractions is arguable. The design of the system is such that it detects changes in shape of the abdomen. The tracings are subject to interpretation as to the magnitude of the uterine contraction, but the system is moderately accurate at detecting the frequency of contractions. The system is most useful for detecting uterine contractions and the fetal heart rate response to contractions, electronic fetal monitoring (EFM).

The anesthetic used during surgery, and the pain medications used immediately after surgery, tend to decrease the fetal heart rate variability and therefore the usefulness of EFM. However, the Doppler fetal heart rate is reassuring if within the normal range for the gestational age. Bradycardia is still an indicator of fetal distress.

Use of the implantable radiotelemeters to monitor intra-amniotic fluid pressure provides precise measurements of uterine contractility. Rather than subjective interpretations as to the magnitude of a contraction, the radiotelemeter system provides intra-aminotic fluid pressures measured extremely precisely and in real time. These data combined with real-time fetal electrocardiogram and reliable beat-to-beat variability provide a high-fidelity version of the tocodynamometer. This is particularly useful during the postoperative period in the midgestation fetus, a time when the fetus is often difficult to detect by the Doppler and the uterine contractions are difficult to detect and hard to interpret. These data are still supplemented by the use of digital cervical examinations to assess the cervical response to uterine contractions. Additional close monitoring for premature rupture of membranes is mandatory, as premature rupture of membranes occurs at some point in all patients who undergo fetal surgery.

In an attempt to provide similarly precise and objective monitoring of cervical dilation and effacement, we have tested the use of sonomicrometers to monitor the cervix. Tiny sonocrystals have been placed across the cervix in the vaginal fornix, and another in the cervical os. These sonocrystals provide continuous real-time data on uterine contractions as evidenced by cervical changes, cervical dilation, and cervical effacement. These sonomicrometers have only been tested in the pregnant, nonhuman primate and require careful suture of the sonocrystals to the cervix. Wires attached to the sonocrystals exit the vagina and are connected to the monitoring equipment. While very promising, this system needs further improvements prior to human application.

Even though our ability to detect postoperative labor is ripe for improvement, our need to control postoperative labor is mandatory. Control of postoperative labor begins before the end of anesthesia. It is helpful to think of labor as two separate but dependent processes: cervical dilation and effacement, which are dependent upon prostaglandins and myometrial contraction.

Control of the cervical changes is most effectively managed with indomethacin. All patients are given up to 50 mg of indomethacin rectally the night before surgery, and then again just prior to the start of the procedure. Postoperatively, indomethacin is continued at a high dose of 50 mg rectally every 4 to 6 hours, with dosage and frequency gradually tapered over 3 to 5 days. The fetus must be monitored daily with fetal echocardiogram to assess ductus arteriosus closure and right heart dilation with tricuspid valve regurgitation. These changes may force discontinuation of the indomethacin.

Because myometrial contractions begin at the end of anesthesia, prior to the emergence, the patient is administered magnesium sulfate and then started immediately on a continuous infusion of magnesium sulfate at 1 to 2 g/hr. If labor is controlled easily, the tocolytic is changed to either a calcium channel blocker or a β-agonist that will be continued until delivery. Occasionally, postoperative fetal surgery patients will require a combination of drugs to control postoperative labor.

Postoperative Monitoring of the Fetus

Continuous reliable monitoring of the fetus immediately after a fetal surgical procedure is extremely important. However, at midgestation monitoring the uterus using standard tocodynamometer and Doppler techniques (EFM) is often unreliable and difficult. Particularly in the scenario where the fetus moves into a position where the heart is difficult to access with the Doppler, or the fetal heart rate becomes slow or irregular, fetal monitoring becomes very manpower intensive and often frustratingly inadequate. There are few data to support the conclusion that EFM in term and preterm labor has any effect on long-term outcome.[116-118] These are exactly the times when precise and continuous fetal monitoring can be critical and make a difference in fetal outcome.

The only available recourse for the fetus that cannot be monitored well is intermittent ultrasound examinations. Due to manpower restrictions and equipment availability, this examination cannot be carried out on a continuous basis. The use of intermittent ultrasound examinations does, however, provide information on the fetal condition at the moment of the examination. We unfortunately have experienced episodes where unreliable Doppler monitoring of the fetus has led to an ultrasound examination that revealed no fetal heart rate. In these situations it is difficult to retrospectively assess whether or not rapid and early intervention would have changed the course of events.

These types of situations have motivated us to develop improved methods of monitoring the fetus after fetal surgery. We have developed and tested in sheep the use of an implantable radiotelemeter that can continuously detect and transmit to a local antenna the fetal electrocardiogram as well as intra-amniotic pressure as an indication of uterine contraction.[119] The implanted radiotelemeters enable continuous intraoperative and postoperative monitoring of the fetal electrocardiogram. Detection of the electrocardiogram and input into a computer data acquisition system (LabVIEW, National Instruments) allows precise detection of the beat-to-beat heart rate variability as well as an opportunity to interpret the electrocardiogram signals.

REFERENCES

1. Pernoll ML, Metcalf J, Schlenker TL, et al: Oxygen consumption at rest and during exercise in pregnancy. Respir Physiol 25:285–293, 1975.
2. Cugell DW, Frank HR, Gaensler A, et al: Pulmonary function in pregnancy. I: Serial observations in normal women. Am Rev Tuberc 67:568, 1953.
3. Pernoll ML, Metcalf J, Kovach PA, et al: Ventilation during rest and exercise in pregnancy and postpartum. Respir Physiol 25:295–310, 1975.
4. Prowse CM, Gaensler EA: Respiratory and acid base changes during pregnancy. Anesthesiology 26:381, 1965.
5. Bonica JJ: Principles and Practice of Obstetric Analgesia and Anesthesia. Philadelphia: FA Davis, 1969, p 22.
6. Bonica JJ: Obstetric Analgesia and Anesthesia, 2nd ed. Amersterdam: World Federation of Societies of Anesthesiologists, 1980, pp 2–17.
7. Eger EI II: Anesthetic Update and Action. Baltimore: Williams & Wilkins, 1974.
8. Archer GW Jr, Marx GF: Arterial oxygen tension during apnoea in parturient women. Br J Anaesthesiol 46:358–360, 1974.
9. Pritchard JA: Changes in blood volume during pregnancy and delivery. Anesthesiology 26:393, 1965.
10. Ueland K: Maternal cardiovascular dynamics. VII: Intrapartum blood volume changes. Am J Obstet Gynecol 126:671–677, 1976.
11. Lees MM, Taylor SH, Scott DB, Kerr MG: A study of cardiac output at rest throughout pregnancy. J Obstet Gynaecol Br Commonw 74:319–328, 1967.
12. Howard BK, Goddson JG, Mengert WF: Supine hypotension syndrome in late pregnancy. Obstet Gynecol 1:371, 1953.
13. Kerr MG, Scott DB: Inferior vena caval occlusion in late pregnancy. In Marx G (ed): Clinical Anesthesia. Philadelphia: FA Davis, 1973.
14. Bieniarz J, Crotto JJ, Curachet E, et al: Aortocaval compression by the uterus in late human pregnancy. II: An arteriographic study. Am J Obstet Gynecol 100:203, 1968.
15. William NH: Variable significance of heartburn. Am J Obstet Gynecol 42:814, 1941.
16. Murray FA, Erskine JP, Fielding J: Gastric secretion in pregnancy. J Obstet Gynaecol Br Commonw 64:373, 1957.
17. Tindall VR, Beard RW, Sykes MK, et al: Confidential Enquiries into Maternal Deaths in the United Kingdom, 1985–1987. London: Her Majesty's Stationery Office, 1991.
18. Sellick BA: Cricoid pressure to control regurgitation of stomach contents during induction of anesthesia. Lancet 2:404, 1961.

19. Palahniuk RJ, Shnider SM, Eger EI II: Pregnancy decreases the requirement of inhaled anesthetic agents. Anesthesiology 41:82–83, 1974.
20. Bromage PL: Continuous lumbar epidural analgesia for obstetrics. Can Med Assoc J 85:1136, 1961.
21. Dignam WJ, Titus P, Assali NS: Renal function in human pregnancy, I: Changes in glomerular filtration rate and renal plasma flow. Proc Soc Exp Biol Med 97:512, 1958.
22. Dunlop W: Renal physiology in pregnancy. Postgrad Med J 55:329–332, 1979.
23. McNair RD, Jaynes RU: Alterations in liver function during normal pregnancy. Am J Obstet Gynecol 80:500, 1960.
24. Shnider SM: Serum cholinesterase activity during pregnancy, labor, and puerperium. Anesthesiology 26:335, 1965.
25. Blitt CD, Petty WC, Alberternst EE: Correlation of plasma cholinesterase activity duration and action of succinylcholine during pregnancy. Anesth Analg 556:78–83, 1977.
26. Evans RJ, Wroe JM: Plasma cholinesterase changes during pregnancy. Anaesthesia 35:651–654, 1980.
27. Huackabee WE: Uterine blood flow. Am J Obstet Gynecol 84:1623, 1962.
28. Assali NS, Rauramo L, Peltonen T: Measurement of uterine blood flow and uterine metabolism. Am J Obstet Gynecol 79:86, 1960.
29. Setala K, Nyyssonen O: Hypnotic sodium pentobarbital as a teratogen for mice. Naturwissenschaften 51:413, 1964.
30. Tanimura T: The effects of thiamylal sodium administration to pregnant mice upon the development of their offspring. Acta Anat Nippon 40:323, 1965.
31. Geber WF, Schramm LC: Congenital malformations of the nervous system produced by narcotic analgesics in the hamster. Am J Obstet Gynecol 123:705–713, 1975.
32. Smith BE, Gaub MI, Moya F: Teratogenic effects of anesthetic agents: Nitrous oxide. Anesth Analg 44:726, 1965.
33. Fink BR, Shepard TH, Blandau RJ: Teratogenic activity of nitrous oxide. Nature 214:146–198, 1967.
34. Lane GA, Nahrwold ML, Tart AR: Anesthetics as teratogens: Nitrous oxide is fetotoxic; xenon is not. Science 210:899–901, 1980.
35. Koblin DD, Watson JF, Deady JE, et al: Inactivation of methionine synthetase by nitrous oxide in mice. Anesthesiology 54:318–324, 1981.
36. Basford AB, Fink BR: The teratogenicity of halothane in the rat. Anesthesiology 29:1167–1173, 1968.
37. Smith BE, Usubiaga LE, Lehrer SB: Cleft palate induced by halothane anesthesia in C-57 black mice. Teratology 4:242, 1971.
38. Drachman DB, Coulombre AJ: Experimental clubfoot and arthrogryposis multiplex congenita. Lancet 2:523, 1962.
39. Baden JM, Rice SA, Serra M, et al: Thymidine and methionine syntheses in pregnant rats exposed to nitrous oxide. Anesth Analg 62:738–741, 1983.
40. Baden JM, Serra M, Mazze RI: Inhibition of fetal methionine synthetase by nitrous oxide. Br J Anaesth 56:523–526, 1984.
41. Lane GA, DuBoulay PM, Tait AR, et al: Nitrous oxide is teratogenic; halothane is not. Anesthesiology 55:A252, 1981.
42. Mazze RI, Wilson AI, Rice SA, Baden JM: Reproduction and fetal development in mice chronically exposed to nitrous oxide. Teratology 26:11–16, 1982.
43. Mazze RI, Fujinaga M, Baden JM: Halothane prevents nitrous oxide teratogenicity in rats; folinic acid does not. Teratology 38:121–127, 1988.
44. Fujinaga M, Baden JM, Mazze RI: Halothane and isoflurane prevent the teratogenic effects of nitrous oxide; folinic acid does not. Anesthesiology 67:A456, 1987.
45. Ingals TH, Curley FJ, Princle RA: Anoxia as a cause of fetal death and congenital defect in the mouse. Am J Dis Child 80:34, 1960.
46. Grabowski CT: Teratogenic significance of ionic and fluid imbalance. Science 142:1064, 1963.
47. Fujikura T: Retrolental fibroplasia and prematurity in newborn rabbits induced by maternal hyperoxia. Am J Obstet Gynecol 90:854, 1954.
48. Haring OM: Cardiac malformations in rats induced by exposure of the mother to carbon dioxide during pregnancy. Circ Res 8:1218, 1960.
49. Milkovich L, van den Berg BJ: Effects of prenatal meprobamate and chlordiazepoxide hydrochloride on human embryonic and fetal development. N Engl J Med 291:1268–1271, 1974.
50. FDA Drug Bulletin, Volume 5, Number 4, September–November 1975.
51. Koren G, Pastuszak A, Ito S: Drugs in pregnancy. N Engl J Med 338:1128–1137, 1998.
52. Spence AA, Cohen EN, Brown BW Jr, et al: Occupational hazards for operating room-based physicians: Analyses of data from the United States and the United Kingdom. JAMA 238:955–959, 1977.
53. Cohen EN, Brown BW, Bruce DL: Occupational disease among operating room personnel: A national study. Anesthesiology 41:321, 1974.
54. Cohen EN, Gift HC, Brown BW, et al: Occupational disease in dentistry and chronic exposure to trace anesthetic gases. J Am Dental Assoc 101:21–31, 1980.
55. Baden JM: Mutagenicity, carcinogenicity, and teratogenicity of nitrous oxide. In Eger EI II (ed): Nitrous Oxide/N₂O. New York: Elsevier Scientific Publishing, 1985, pp 235–247.
56. Duncan PG, Pope WDB, Cohen MM, Greer N: Fetal risk of anesthesia and surgery during pregnancy. Anesthesiology 64:790–794, 1986.
57. Mazze RI, Källén B: Reproductive outcome after anesthesia and operation during pregnancy: A registry study of 5405 cases. Am J Obstet Gynecol 161:1178–1185, 1989.
58. Källén B, Mazze RI: Neural tube defects and first trimester operations. Teratology 41:717–720, 1990.
59. Sylvester GC, Khoury MJ, Lu X, Erickson JD: First-trimester anesthesia exposure and the risk of central nervous system defects: A population-based case-control study. Am J Public Health 84:1757–1760, 1994.
60. Khazin AF, Hon EH, Hehre FW: Effects of maternal hyperoxia on the fetus. I: Oxygen tension. Am J Obstet Gynecol 109:628–637, 1971.
61. Walker A, Madderin L, Day E, et al: Fetal scalp tissue oxygen measurements in relation to maternal dermal oxygen tension and fetal heart rate. J Obstet Gynaecol Br Commonw 78:1–12, 1971.
62. Levinson G, Shnider SM, DeLorimier AA, Steffenson JL: Effects of maternal hyperventilation on uterine blood flow and fetal oxygenation and acid-base status. Anesthesiology 40:340–348, 1974.
63. Motoyama EK, Rivard G, Acheson F, Cook CD: The effect of changes in maternal pH and pCO2 on the pO2 of foetal lambs. Anesthesiology 28:891–903, 1967.
64. Palahniuk RJ, Shnider SM: Maternal and fetal cardiovascular and acid-base changes during halothane and isoflurane anesthesia in the pregnant ewe. Anesthesiology 41:462–472, 1974.
65. Shnider SM, Wright RG, Levinson G, et al: Uterine blood flow and plasma norepinephrine changes during maternal stress in the pregnant ewe. Anesthesiology 50:524–528, 1979.
66. Adamsons K, Mueller-Heuback E, Myers RE: Production of fetal asphyxia in the rhesus monkey by administration of catecholamines to the mother. Am J Obstet Gynecol 109:248–262, 1971.
67. Ralston OH, Shnider SM, DeLorimier AA: Effects of equipotent ephedrine, metaraminol, mephentermine, and methoxamine on uterine blood flow in the pregnant ewe. Anesthesiology 40:354–370, 1974.
68. Smyth CN: Experimental methods for testing the integrity of the foetus and neonate. J Obstet Gynaecol Br Commonw 72:920, 1965.
69. Liley AW: The foetus as a personality. Aust N Z J Psychiatry 6:99–105, 1972.
70. Rose JC, Macdonald AA, Heymann MA, Rudolph AM: Developmental aspects of the pituitary-adrenal axis response to hemorrhagic stress in lamb fetuses in utero. J Clin Invest 61:4–32, 1978.
71. Anand KJS: Hormonal and metabolic function of neonates and infants undergoing surgery. Curr Opin Cardiol 1:681, 1986.
72. Anand KJS, Brown JJ, Bloom SR, Ansley-Green A: Studies on the hormonal regulation of fuel metabolism in the human newborn infant undergoing anaesthesia and surgery. Horm Res 22:115–128, 1985.
73. Anand KJS, Brown MJ, Causon RC, et al: Can the human neonate mount an endocrine and metabolic response to surgery? J Pediatr Surg 20:41–48, 1985.
74. Anand KJS, Sippell WG, Aynsley-Green A: Randomized trial of fentanyl anaesthesia in preterm neonates undergoing surgery: Effects on the stress response. Lancet 1:62–66, 1987.
75. Anand KJS, Hickey PR: Pain and its effects in the human neonate and fetus. N Engl J Med 317:1321–1329, 1987.

76. Rudolph AM, Heymann MA: Cardiac output in the fetal lamb: The effects of spontaneous and induced changes of heart rate on right and left ventricular output. Am J Obstet Gynecol 124:183–192, 1976.

77. Friedman WF: The intrinsic physiologic properties of the developing heart. Prog Cardiovasc Dis 15:87–111, 1972.

78. Gilbert RD: Control of fetal cardiac output during changes in blood volume. Am J Physiol 238:H80–H86, 1980.

79. Jones MD, Rosenberg AA, Simmons MA: Oxygen delivery to the brain before and after birth. Science 216:324–325, 1982.

80. Makowski EL, Schneider JM, Tsoulos NG, et al: Cerebral blood flow, oxygen consumption, glucose utilization of fetal lambs in utero. Am J Obstet Gynecol 114:292–303, 1972.

81. Rosenberg AA, Jones MD, Traystman RJ, et al: Response of cerebral blood flow to changes in PCO2 in fetal, newborn, and adult sheep. Am J Physiol 242:H862–H866, 1982.

82. Jones MD Jr, Sheldon RE, Peeters LL, et al: Fetal cerebral oxygen consumption at different levels of oxygenation. J Appl Physiol 43:1080–1084, 1977.

83. Tweed WA, Cote J, Wade JG, et al: Preservation of fetal brain blood flow relative to other organs during hypovolemic hypotension. Pediatr Res 16:137–140, 1982.

84. Tweed WA, Cote J, Pash M, Lou H: Arterial oxygenation determines autoregulation of cerebral blood flow in the fetal lamb. Pediatr Res 17:246–249, 1983.

85. Gregory GA, Wade JG, Biehl DR, et al: Fetal anesthetic requirement (MAC) for halothane. Anesth Analg 62:9–14, 1983.

86. Biehl DR, Tweed WA, Cote J, et al: Effect of halothane by the foetal lamb in utero. Can Anaesth Soc J 30:24–92, 1983.

87. Biehl DR, Cote J, Wade JG, et al: Uptake of halothane by the foetal lamb in utero. Can Anaesth Soc J 30:24–27, 1983.

88. Biehl DR, Yarnell R, Wade JG, Sitar D: The uptake of isoflurane by the foetal lamb in utero: Effect on regional blood flow. Can Anaesth Soc J 30:581–586, 1983.

89. Sabik JF, Assad RS, Hanley FL: Halothane as an anesthetic for fetal surgery. J Pediatr Surg 28:542–546, 1993.

90. Cohn HE, Sacks EJ, Heymann MA, Rudolph AM: Cardiovascular responses to hypoxemia and acidemia in fetal lambs. Am J Obstet Gynecol 120:817–824, 1974.

91. Peeters LLH, Sheldon RE, Jones MD, et al: Blood flow to organs as a function of arterial oxygen content. Am J Obstet Gynecol 135:637–646, 1979.

92. Reuss ML, Parer JT, Harris JL, Krueger TR: Hemodynamic effects of alpha-adrenergic blockade during hypoxia in fetal sheep. Am J Obstet Gynecol 142:410–415, 1982.

93. Court DJ, Parer JT, Block BSB, Llanos AJ: Effects of beta-adrenergic blockade on blood flow distribution during hypoxaemia in fetal sheep. J Dev Physiol 6:349–358, 1984.

94. Johnson GN, Palahniuk RJ, Tweed WA, et al: Regional cerebral blood flow changes curing severe fetal asphyxia produced by slow partial umbilical cord compression. Am J Obstet Gynecol 135:48–52, 1979.

95. Yarnell R, Biehl DR, Tweed WA, et al: The effect of halothane anesthesia on the asphyxiated foetal lamb in utero. Can Anesth Soc J 30:474–479, 1983.

96. Palahniuk RJ, Doig GA, Johnson GN, Pash MP: Maternal halothane anesthesia reduces cerebral blood flow in the acidotic sheep fetus. Anesth Analg 59:35–39, 1980.

97. Harrison MR, Anderson J, Rosen MA, et al: Fetal surgery in the primate. I. Anesthetic surgical, and tocolytic management to maximize fetal-neonatal survival. J Pediatr Surg 17:115–122, 1982.

98. Cauldwell CB, Rosen MA, Harrison MR: The use of nitroglycerin for uterine relaxation during fetal surgery. Anesthesiology 83:A929, 1995.

99. Jennings RW, MacGillivray TE, Harrison MR: Nitric oxide inhibits preterm labor in the rhesus monkey. J Matern Fetal Med 2:170–175, 1993.

100. Peng ATC, Gorman RS, Shulman SM, et al: Intravenous nitroglycerine for uterine relaxation in the postpartum patient with retained placenta. Anesthesiology 71:172–173, 1989.

101. Altabef KM, Spencer JT, Zinberg S: Intravenous nitroglycerine for uterine relaxation of an inverted uterus. Am J Obstet Gynecol 166:1237–1238, 1992.

102. Nakayama DK, Harrison MR, Seron-Ferre M, Villa RL: Fetal surgery in the primate. II: Uterine electromyographic response to operative procedures and pharmacologic agents. J Pediatr Surg 19:333–339, 1984.

103. Adzick NS, Harrison MR, Glick PL, et al: Fetal surgery in the primate. III: Maternal outcome after fetal surgery. J Pediatr Surg 21:477–480, 1986.

104. Nakayama DK, Harrison MR, Berger MS, et al: Correction of congenital hydrocephalus in utero. I: The model: Intracisternal kaolin produces hydrocephalus in fetal lambs and rhesus monkeys. J Pediatr Surg 18:331–338, 1983.

105. Hendrick AG, Binkerd PE: Fetal death in nonhuman primates. In Porter IH, Hook EB (eds): Embryonic and Fetal Death. New York: Academic Press, 1980, pp 45–69.

106. Davidson HC, Morris JA, O'Grady JP, et al: Sampling the fetoplacental circulation. III: Combined laparoscopy-fetoscopy in the pregnant macaque for hemoglobin identification. Am J Obstet Gynecol 132:833–844, 1978.

107. Challis JR, Manning FA: Control of parturition in subhuman primates. Semin Perinatol 2:247–260, 1978.

108. Novy MJ: Endocrine and pharmacological factors which influence the onset of labour in rhesus monkeys. In CIBA Foundation Symposium No. 47: The Fetus and Birth. Amsterdam: Elsevier/Excerpa Medica/North Holland, 1977, pp 259–295.

109. Glick PL, Harrison MR, Halks-Miller M, et al: Correction of congenital hydrocephalus in utero. II: Efficacy of in utero shunting. J Pediatr Surg 19:870–881, 1984.

110. Taylor NJ, Martin MC, Nathanielsz PW, et al: The fetus regulates the circadian increases of uterine activity that precedes labor in the rhesus monkey. Presented at the Meeting of the Society for Gynecologic Investigation, 1982.

111. Novy MJ: Effects of indomethacin on labor, fetal oxygenation, and fetal development in rhesus monkeys. In Coceani F, Olley PM (eds): Advances in Prostaglandin and Thromboxane Research, Vol 4. New York: Raven Press, 1978, pp 285–350.

112. Caritis SN, Lin LS, Toig G, Wong LK: Pharmacodynamics of ritodrine in pregnant women during preterm labor. Am J Obstet Gynecol 147:752–759, 1983.

113. Creasy RK: Preterm delivery and delivery. In Creasy RK, Resnik R (eds): Maternal-Fetal Medicine: Principles and Practice. Philadelphia: WB Saunders Company, 1989.

114. Hedrick MH, Jennings RW, MacGillivray TE, et al: Chronic fetal vascular access. Lancet 342(8879):1086–1087, 1993.

115. Hedrick MH, Jennings RW, MacGillivray TE, et al: Endoscopic placental vessel catheterization for chronic fetal vascular access. Surg Forum 43:504–505, 1992.

116. Chagalmers I: Randomized control trials of intrapartum monitoring. In Thalhammer O, Baumgarten KV, Polaka A (eds): Perinatal Medicine. Stuttgart: George Thieme Publishers, 1979, pp 260–265.

117. Langendoerfer S, Haverkamp AD, Murphy J, et al: Pediatric follow-up of a randomized controlled trial of intrapartum fetal monitoring techniques. Pediatrics 97:103–107, 1980.

118. MacDonald D, Grant A, Sheridan-Pereira M, et al: The Dublin randomized controlled trial of intrapartum fetal heart rate monitoring. Am J Obstet Gynecol 152:524–539, 1985.

119. Jennings RW, Adzick NS, Longaker MT, et al: New techniques in fetal surgery. J Pediatr Surg 27(10):1329–1333, 1992.

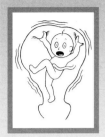

Preterm Labor: The Achilles Heel of Fetal Intervention

WILLIAM J. B. DENNES and PHILLIP R. BENNETT

The management of preterm labor represents a major challenge to obstetricians. Whilst the neonatal care of very preterm infants has improved significantly in the last decade, there has been little concomitant advance in the obstetric management of preterm labor. Preterm delivery affects up to 10% of pregnancies, but causes some 60% of neonatal morbidity and mortality. The impact of preterm delivery on neonatal outcome is significant, notwithstanding the social, financial, and emotional implications.

The fundamental problem in the management of preterm delivery is that the factors responsible for the onset of "normal" labor at term remain poorly understood. However, in the context of fetal intervention specific factors can be identified as potential initiators of uterine contractions and preterm labor. Whilst this provides the theoretical basis for tocolytic regimens, currently therapy is associated with significant side effects. The management of tocolysis in fetal surgery has been referred to as "the Achilles heel of fetal intervention,"[1] in the same manner that rejection was considered in relation to transplantation surgery. As problems with rejection were overcome, the field of transplantation was opened, and similarly once effective tocolysis can be achieved fetal surgery will be able to realize its full potential.

In this chapter we review the current concepts of the biochemistry involved in labor onset, the therapeutic options available in the management of preterm labor, and the specific factors complicating fetal intervention.

The Phases of Parturition

We currently consider pregnancy to be divided into four parturitional phases. The first phase, phase 0, during the first and second trimesters, is dominated by "pro-pregnancy factors" and is the period of myometrial growth and quiescence. The second phase, phase I, during the early and mid third trimester, is also a phase of myometrial quiescence, but during which preparation for labor is made by up-regulation of myometrial, cervical and fetal membrane proteins which will be needed for labor. The third phase, phase II, is the phase of labor itself and has the character of an inflammatory reaction. During this phase of pregnancy, the "brake" on myometrial contractility caused by pro-pregnancy factors is released and the spontaneous contractility of the uterus is augmented by oxytocic compounds such as prostaglandins and possibly oxytocin itself. The fourth parturitional phase, phase III, represents the state of the intrauterine tissues after the process of labor.

Phase 0: Pro-pregnancy Factors

Progesterone

Progesterone, as its name suggests, is the principal pro-pregnancy factor. In the human, maintenance of pregnancy in the first trimester is through release of progesterone by the corpus luteum, whose regression is inhibited by human chorionic gonadotropin (hCG). By about 7 weeks, progesterone production is taken over by the placenta, with subsequent luteal regression. Progesterone has a negative regulatory effect upon many of the "contraction-associated proteins," for example, those associated with the formation of myometrial gap junctions (connexons), and the modulation of cervical ripening (interleukin-8 [IL-8]). Progesterone also decreases uterine sensitivity to oxytocin. Progesterone is therefore probably important in mediating enlargement of the uterus without increasing contractility.

In many species a withdrawal of progesterone immediately precedes the onset of labor. There is no obvious systemic withdrawal of progesterone prior to labor in the human; however, pharmacologic inhibition of the action of progesterone using mifepristone (RU486) increases myometrial contractility[2] and up-regulates cervical IL-8 expression, leading to cervical ripening. It is possible that in the human there is no actual or functional withdrawal of progesterone prior to labor, rather its pro-pregnancy action is simply overwhelmed by "pro-labor" factors. Other theories to explain apparent progesterone withdrawal in the human include changes in progesterone receptor subtypes, modulation of receptor function by cortisol or transcription factors, or local rather than systemic changes in progesterone concentrations.

Nitric Oxide

Nitric oxide (NO) has been proposed as a putative mediator of uterine smooth muscle relaxation and myometrial quiescence,[3] and to have a pro-pregnancy function. NO is a highly reactive free radical with diverse biologic activities and is synthesized from L-arginine by nitric oxide synthase (NOS). NOS exists in at least three isoforms: type I, a constitutive, calcium-dependent neuronal form (nNOS); type II, an inducible, calcium-independent form (iNOS); and type III, a constitutive, calcium-dependent endothelial form (e/cNOS). Nitric oxide donors have an inhibitory effect on pregnant human uterine contractility.[4,5] Whilst exogenous NO therefore appears to relax the uterus, the role of endogenous NO, and generation of NO within the human myometrium is less clear.

NO exerts its effect on smooth muscle by stimulation of the guanylate cyclase pathway. Animal[6] and human studies[3] have suggested that a NO-cGMP relaxation pathway exists in the pregnant uterus, with decreased responsiveness to NO at term. In both rabbits[7] and rats,[8] NOS activity within the uterus has been reported to fall on the last day of pregnancy and with the onset of labor. Human studies have demonstrated expression of e/cNOS in the nonpregnant uterus,[9] and both e/cNOS and iNOS have been reported in the uterus in early pregnancy.[10] Bansal et al.[11] have shown, using immunostaining and Western analysis, that iNOS is expressed in human myometrial cells, and that expression falls significantly at term, and again with the onset of labor. In contrast, using reverse transcriptase polymerase chain reaction (RT-PCR) we found no correlation between gestational age and expression of any of the NOS isoforms in either human fetal membranes, placenta, or myometrium, and no change with the onset of labor.[12] Jones and Poston,[13] studying human myometrial strips in vitro, were unable to demonstrate any effect on spontaneous myometrial contractions following the addition of either L-arginine, the substrate for NOS, or L-NAME, a NOS inhibitor, and concluded that NO was unlikely to be involved in the maintenance of uterine quiescence. Recently, there has been some evidence to suggest that topical glyceryl trinitrate, an NO donor, might ripen the cervix, suggesting that NO in the human at least, might be a pro-labor, rather than a pro-pregnancy factor.[14]

Phase I: Pro-labor Factors

The Placental Clock

Both McLean et al.[15] and Challis et al.[16] have suggested that the timing of labor is mediated through placental release of corticotropin releasing hormone (CRH), whose concentration in maternal plasma begins to rise about 90 days prior to the onset of labor. Circulating CRH is principally in an inactive form, bound to a binding protein CRH-BP, derived from the maternal liver. CRH-BP is itself negatively regulated by CRH, so that as placental release of CRH increases, maternal liver release of CRH-BP decreases. At about 37 weeks in the average pregnancy, CRH concentrations began to exceed those of CRH-BP with effectively, a large increase in the concentration of biologic active CRH. An important difference between pituitary CRH and placental CRH is that whilst pituitary CRH is under the negative feedback control of cortisol, placental release of CRH is increased by cortisol. Free CRH up-regulates expression of the central prostaglandin synthetic enzyme cyclooxygenase type 2 (COX-2),[17] and stimulates prostaglandin synthesis in both fetal membranes[18] and decidua.[19] CRH has also been shown to directly stimulate myometrial contractility.[16]

Although maternal estrogen concentrations do not rise acutely before human labor, as they do in the sheep, there is a gradual rise in both estriol and estradiol concentrations during the third trimester, reaching a plateau at about 38 weeks.[20] Estradiol up-regulates oxytocin receptors and oxytocin synthesis within the uterus.[21] Placental CRH may increase dehydroepiandrosterone production within the fetus via increased placental and fetal adrenocorticotropic hormone (ACTH).[16] It is therefore possible that CRH not only up-regulates COX, but also indirectly up-regulates other pro-labor genes, such as the oxytocin receptor, via fetal androgens, and estrogen.

The role of oxytocin probably varies from species to species. In the monkey, oxytocin controls the switch from prelabor contractures to labor contractions ensuring that labor occurs at night. In the human, no changes have been found in the concentrations of either maternal or fetal oxytocin, with either the onset or the progress of labor.[22] This suggests that oxytocin does not play a role in either the onset or the maintenance of human labor. The density of myometrial oxytocin receptors does, however, increase towards term.[23]

Phase II: Labor—An Inflammatory Reaction

The Cervix

The cervix is composed mainly of a connective tissue of collagen and elastin embedded in a proteoglycan matrix with very little smooth muscle. At term, near to labor, the collagen of the cervix changes, the fibrils become dissociated from their tightly organized bundles and are more widely scattered in an increased amount of ground substance, and there is loosening of the collagen bundles in the cervical stroma. Much of the change in the cervix at term is due to increased collagenase activity. Fibroblasts present in the cervix synthesize collagenase, but there is also an accumulation of neutrophils that release collagenase into the cervix, around the time of parturition. Cervical ripening therefore resembles an inflammatory reaction.

Cytokines and Prostaglandins

Labor is associated with increased prostaglandin synthesis within both the uterus[24] and the fetal membranes.[25]

Prostaglandins mediate cervical ripening and stimulate uterine contractions,[26] and act indirectly to increase fundally dominant myometrial contractility, by up-regulation of oxytocin receptors and synchronization of contractions.[27] Similarly, there is a strong association between both term and preterm labor and increased production of the inflammatory cytokine IL-1β within the uterus. IL-1β concentrations have been shown to be elevated in amniotic fluid in term labor and just prior to labor in patients with chorion amnionitis.[28] Expression of IL-1β at the mRNA level is higher in fetal membranes after labor than before.[29] IL-1β expression, like COX-2, increases throughout the third trimester (unpublished data).

Prostaglandins are formed from the precursor arachidonic acid. The cyclo-oxygenase (COX) pathway produces prostaglandins. Prior to labor, endogenous arachidonic acid metabolism in amnion is principally via the lipoxygenase enzyme pathways. With labor, there is an increase in arachidonic acid metabolism and a change in the ratio of COX to lipoxygenase metabolism to favor synthesis of prostaglandin E_2.[30, 31]

The switch from lipoxygenase to cyclo-oxygenase (COX) metabolism implies up-regulation of COX. There are two COX genes, the constitutively expressed COX-1 and the inducible COX-2.[32, 33] In situ hybridization has localized expression of COX-1 and COX-2 mRNA in the fetal membranes.[34] In amnion at term, expression of the COX-2 mRNA is some 100-fold higher than COX-1 mRNA. COX-1 expression does not change throughout pregnancy or labor. The expression of COX-2 in the fetal membranes increases throughout the third trimester and then doubles in association with labor.[35, 36] In the myometrium there is expression of COX-1 and COX-2 at similar levels, but only COX-2 expression increases near to term and with the onset of labor.[37] The increases in COX-2 expression in the fetal membranes closely mirror the concentration of free CRH in the maternal circulation, and CRH increases both expression of COX-2 and prostaglandin synthesis in fetal membranes in tissue culture.[17]

Phase III: Postlabor

Following labor and delivery both the fetal membranes and the myometrium appear to have undergone irreversible change. In any subsequent pregnancy, the speed and length of labor is significantly different. Pregnancy length tends to be shorter and labor more rapid in a multiparous population when compared to a matched primigravid group.[37] This is probably a reflection not only of anatomic changes but also changes in the sensitivity of gestation-associated tissues to pro-labor factors.

The Biochemical Mechanisms of Preterm Labor

Multiple Pregnancy and Uterine Distention

The concept that the length of pregnancy is controlled by placental products, CRH, and estrogens helps to explain the onset of preterm labor in the case of multiple pregnancy. It would be expected that a larger placental mass would generate higher levels of CRH. Down-regulation of CRH-BP would then occur earlier, leading to an early rise in free active CRH in the maternal circulation. If parturitional phase III is signaled simply by a certain threshold of CRH, or of IL-1β stimulated by CRH, then labor onset would occur earlier. Although progesterone protects the uterus against the effects of stretch, it is probable that in severe polyhydramnios the degree of stretch is such that up-regulation of contraction-associated proteins nevertheless occurs early. It is likely that in addition to gap junction proteins, other contraction-associated proteins will be found to be stretch sensitive.

Infection

It is thought that in most cases infection ascends from the vagina, although it may also be transplacental or introduced during invasive procedures. It is probable that many cases of early preterm labor, thought to be associated with cervical incompetence, occur because vaginal pathogens enter the lower pole of the uterus through a modestly open cervix, where they set up an inflammatory reaction.

It seems logical that bacterial infection would initiate preterm labor by causing an inflammatory reaction within the uterus, and effectively switching on parturitional phase III at an earlier stage. The mechanisms by which bacteria initiate infections are probably mutifactorial. Bacteria do not directly synthesize prostaglandins,[39] but they do release phospholipases, which may liberate arachidonic acid from intracellular lipid pools, therefore increasing synthesis of prostaglandins. Lamont et al.[40] have demonstrated that bacteria release a substance that increases prostaglandin synthesis in amnion cells. This effect is probably mediated by phospholipase release.[41]

Another important mechanism by which bacteria might activate inflammatory mediators within the uterus is by the action of endotoxin. Endotoxin has been shown to stimulate prostaglandin production by monocytes. Romero et al.[42] found that early spontaneous labor in preterm premature rupture of membrane was more likely when endotoxin was detected. Endotoxin stimulates synthesis of inflammatory cytokines including IL-1β and IL-6, tumor necrosis factor, and prostaglandins[43] in amnion cells and in intact fetal membranes through up-regulation of cPLA2 and COX-2.[44]

Stress

There is growing evidence that either maternal or fetal stress may be associated with preterm labor. Major life events have an association with prematurity,[45] as does the fetal stress of intrauterine growth retardation. A premature rise in CRH concentrations in maternal plasma has been associated with preterm labor.[46] Since placental CRH is up-regulated by corticosteroids, chronic up-regulation of maternal or fetal corticosteroid concentrations would lead to an early rise in CRH, signaling the early onset of labor.

Fetal Interventions

Amniocentesis and fetal blood sampling (percutaneous umbilical cord blood sampling [PUBS]) are associated with a pregnancy loss rate of some 0.5%. The two principal causes of pregnancy loss are infection and preterm premature rupture of membranes (PPROM). In general, pregnancy loss associated with chorioamnionitis following amniocentesis occurs 1 to 2 weeks following the procedure. This time interval presumably reflects the time taken for a small bacterial inoculum to incubate to a full-blown infection. The clinical scenario for pregnancy loss is then very similar to that of preterm labor associated with infection, and the biochemical mechanisms are likely to be the same. Infection may also cause PPROM, although this may occur some weeks before there is clinical evidence of, presumably, secondary infection. Why amniocentesis should occasionally cause PPROM without any other apparent complication is unknown, although we hypothesize that when amniocentesis causes a small myometrial or submembrane hemorrhage, subsequent enzymatic lysis of the clot may also cause erosion of the fetal membranes themselves, leading to PPROM. This hypothesis is consistent with our experience that when PPROM follows amniocentesis it becomes clinically apparent 1 to 2 weeks after the procedure, and secondary chorioamnionitis, if it occurs, becomes apparent 1 to 2 weeks after that.

Amnioreduction is often performed partly to reduce the risk of the onset of preterm labor, but occasionally labor follows shortly after the procedure. It is probable that a large reduction in amniotic fluid, particularly if it occurs quickly, will lead to a disruption in the relationship between the maternal decidua and the fetal membranes and therefore to increased synthesis of pro-labor prostaglandins and/or cytokines.

Hysterotomy for fetal surgery in the human has a high associated incidence of preterm labor, which occurs within a very short time of surgery. This is not the case with hysterotomy in the sheep, where preterm labor is rare. This is probably a reflection of the differing sites of prostaglandin (and possibly other inflammatory cytokine) synthesis within the human and sheep uterus. The prostaglandin synthesis, which is associated with the onset of human labor, is principally within the fetal membranes, with the amnion and decidua in particular having a high synthetic capacity. In the sheep, however, it is the placental cotyledons which are the source of prostaglandins. Hysterotomy in the human therefore cuts through and disrupts the principal tissue sources of prostaglandins, whereas in the sheep, provided cotyledons are avoided, prostaglandin synthesis is not stimulated. The stimulation of prostaglandin synthesis by hysterotomy or by the stimulation associated with complex and lengthy fetoscopic procedures is presumably a major cause of the associated preterm labor. As discussed above, there are also mechanisms whereby fetal and/or maternal stress can lead to a premature rise

in CRH and this may augment the effects of physical disruption of the fetal membranes in causing preterm contractions.

Management of Preterm Labor

Supportive Management

Nonspecific supportive management is often provided in preterm labor. Its effectiveness has not been clearly defined due to the placebo effect associated with any treatment regimen in preterm labor. A combination of intravenous hydration and sedation is commonly advocated.

Arginine vasopressin (AVP) is a nine-amino-acid peptide, sharing close homology with oxytocin. AVP is released by the posterior pituitary in response to fluid depletion. There is evidence from both animal[47] and human[48] studies that arginine vasopressin receptors (V1A) are present in the myometrium, and that AVP is capable of stimulating uterine activity by binding to both oxytocin and V1A receptors. A theoretical basis therefore exists for prehydration therapy of patients in threatened preterm labor, to reduce AVP levels and hence potential uterine activity. Clinical studies, however, have shown that there is no advantage in prehydration,[49] and that the use of intravenous hydration in the management of preterm contractions appears to be of no benefit.[50] While pretherapy rehydration may prevent ketoacidosis and possibly improve uteroplacental blood flow, intravenous hydration should be limited to 500 mL, to avoid the potential risks of fluid overload and pulmonary edema associated with subsequent tocolytic therapy.

Sedation with narcotics or barbiturates does not result in myometrial relaxation, but may achieve a transitory decrease in uterine activity.[51] Their use should be cautioned by their profound effect on neonatal respiratory and central nervous system depression.

Tocolysis

Analysis of Effectiveness of Management

The potential problem in analyzing the effectiveness of tocolytics in the management of preterm labor is the establishment of the diagnosis. Preterm labor may be defined as uterine contractions before 37 weeks' gestation, leading to cervical change. Clinically, the differentiation between false and true labor may make diagnosis difficult. Even if the diagnosis is made, up to 60% of patients with painful uterine contractions and cervical change, if left untreated, will resolve spontaneously and will not deliver until term,[52] resulting in a significant placebo effect. Tocolytics are not without significant side effects, and their clinical use must therefore be balanced by their perceived benefit. The decision as to whether to treat preterm labor is largely dependent on gestational age, clinical scenario, and the level of neonatal care available. It is generally accepted that tocolytic intervention between 24 and 26 weeks is acceptable, although some might advocate tocolysis between 20 and 24 weeks. The upper limit of therapy is more equivocal. There is some evidence to suggest that there may be maternal–fetal benefit if tocoloytics are used up to 32 weeks, but at gestational ages of 34 weeks or more this benefit is lost.[53]

Modern Tocolytics

β-Sympathomimetics

β-Sympathomimetics exert their action on the uterus by β-adrenergic receptor stimulation. Intramembranous β-adrenergic receptors activate adenylate cyclase, resulting in an increase in intracellular cAMP.[54] cAMP reduces intracellular calcium and decreases the sensitivity of actin–myosin complexes to the uterotonic effects of calcium and prostaglandins.[55] The first agent proposed for use in preterm labor was isoxsuprine, a nonselective β-mimetic.[56] Its use was limited by its nonselective β-adrenergic side effects. Modern sympathomimetics used for tocolysis all have β-adrenergic selectivity.

Ritodrine

Ritodrine is the most widely used tocolytic in the United States. It was first introduced in 1972. Initial studies compared its use against ethanol and placebo.[57] This study formed the basis of a phase III Food and Drug Administration (FDA) trial and found that ritodrine was significantly better than either ethanol or placebo in its ability to prolong pregnancy. Ritodrine was associated with a 2- to 3-week prolongation in pregnancy. While the FDA was aware of potential complications of pulmonary edema and fluid overload, in this trial, the incidence of these complications was no higher than in the other treatment groups,[58] and as a result the FDA awarded ritodrine a license for use in pregnancy in 1980. This is the only tocolytic currently licensed for use by the FDA. Following these original studies it became apparent that the incidence of maternal cardiovascular complications, and pulmonary edema in particular, were being underreported. With the release of an FDA alert bulletin, increasing the level of awareness of potential maternal complications, the true incidence of complications was established. Currently, the incidence of β-sympathomimetic pulmonary edema is estimated between 0.01 and 9%.[59, 60]

β-Mimetics cause a generalized vasodilatation, with resultant hypotension and compensatory increased cardiac output. Maternal heart rate, stroke volume, and systolic blood pressure all increase. Cardiac output increases by up to 60% with β-sympathomimetic therapy.[61] Antidiuretic effects of tocolytic therapy potentiate the risks of fluid overload and pulmonary edema. Although fatal pulmonary edema associated with ritodrine infusion is almost certainly multifactorial, the balance of evidence suggests that fluid overload is the most important single factor. There is some evidence that the incidence of cardiovascular complications is increased in higher order pregnancies.[62] Metabolic complications include hyperglycemia, primarily due to β-adrenergic stimulation of glucagon release by the pancreas,[63] and reactive hypoglycemia is sometimes seen in fasting patients following cessation of treatment.[64] Hypokalemia may also be associated with β-sympathomimetic treatment, contributing to the risk of pulmonary edema, and is attributable to tocolytic-induced intracellular shift of potassium by insulin.[65]

Fetal side effects of β-sympathomimetics are widely recognized. Fetal tachycardia is a direct result of myocardial β-adrenergic stimulation, resulting in increased fetal cardiac output.[66] Ritodrine stimulates placental prostacyclin production,[67] resulting in increased uteroplacental blood flow.[68] Long-term follow-up of β-mimetics used in pregnancy has shown no evidence of any significant growth disorders or neurodevelopmental or social developmental alterations.

Notwithstanding its complications, ritodrine's efficacy as a tocolytic is by no means conclusive. Recent studies have failed to confirm its effectiveness at prolonging pregnancy. The Canadian Preterm Labor Investigation Group demonstrated only a 24- to 48-hour delay in delivery, with intravenous and oral ritodrine therapy. There was, however, no significant difference in birth weight, perinatal mortality, or neonatal morbidity between treatment and control groups. Meta-analysis of existing studies suggests that ritodrine is only successful at short-term prolongation of pregnancy, and it is unlikely that the FDA would award ritodrine a license for its use in pregnancy today.

Long-term administration of β-sympathomimetics is associated with tolerance to smooth muscle relaxation. This is probably mediated through adrenoreceptor down-regulation, and provides the basis for the clinical observation that the ability of these tocolytic agents to arrest preterm labor is transitory. The possibility of reducing tolerance by pulsatile subcutaneous administration of β-sympathomimetics has been explored[69]; however, evidence for its efficacy is limited and only available from small, uncontrolled studies.[70]

Terbutaline

Terbutaline is a selective β-sympathomimetic, with similar efficacy and side-effect profiles to ritodrine.[71] Comparative studies comparing tocolytic effects of intravenous terbutaline against intravenous magnesium sulfate, and subsequent oral maintenance therapy, failed to show any difference in delivery rates at either 48 hours[72] or after 1 week of therapy.[73] Terbutaline is usually administered intravenously at a dose of 10 μg/min, until contractions stop, unacceptable side effects develop, or a maximal dose of 25 μg/min is reached. Similar efficacy and incidence of side effects have been observed when terbutaline is administered either subcutaneously or intravenously.[74]

Salbutamol

Salbutamol is another selective β-sympathomimetic whose efficacy, side effects, and administration are similar to the other β-mimetic agents. Comparative studies with terbutaline[75] and ethanol[76] confirm no significant difference in side effects or efficacy. Anecdotally, salbutamol is sometimes used when alternative β-sympathomimetics have failed to abolish uterine contractions, although its efficacy in this context has not been proven. Salbutamol is administered intravenously at 10 μg/min, and gradually increased to a maximum of 45 μg/min or until contractions stop or side effects intervene.

Magnesium Sulfate

Magnesium sulfate has been used by physicians in the United States in the management of pre-eclampsia for many years, a result of which its additional ability to effect uterine relaxation is well known.[77,78] Although the actual mechanism of uterine smooth muscle relaxation by magnesium sulfate remains largely unknown, it is likely that magnesium competes with calcium for entry into the cell via voltage operated calcium gates.[79] Placebo-controlled trials of magnesium sulfate are limited. Randomized comparative trials with ethanol,[80] ritodrine,[79] and terbutaline[81] have shown no significant difference in delay in delivery at 48 hours. The incidence of maternal side effects was significantly lower with magnesium sulfate therapy compared with intravenous β-sympathomimetics (2% cf 38%).[72] As a result of the comparable efficacy of magnesium sulfate and β-sympathomimetics, in the United States, magnesium sulfate represents first-line tocolytic therapy. In Europe, magnesium sulfate use is relatively uncommon and is generally confined to cases where first-line β-sympathomimetic treatment has failed, if it is used at all.

Side effects of magnesium sulfate therapy are limited if serum levels are maintained in the therapeutic range (5 to 6 mEq/L). Maternal tachycardia is not associated with magnesium therapy and cardiac output remains unchanged.[82] Serum calcium concentrations have been shown to fall with magnesium therapy,[83] and decreased bone density has been reported with long-term therapy.[84] Nonspecific side effects such as nausea, vomiting, constipation, and generalized muscle weakness are associated with higher levels of magnesium and long-term therapy.

Significant complications of magnesium therapy are associated with magnesium toxicity. Levels above 8 mEq/L may result in loss of deep tendon reflexes; at levels between 12 and 15 mEq/L respiratory depression occurs, and at levels in excess of 15 mEq/L cardiac arrest may occur. These complications are thought to be due to competition between magnesium and calcium at voltage-dependent calcium channels in muscle cells. Magnesium sulfate is usually administered intravenously, with a loading dose of 4 g (40 mL of 10% MgSO$_4$), infused over 2 minutes, followed by a maintenance dose of 2 g/hr. Serum magnesium levels should be measured 1 hour after the start of the maintenance dose, and 6 hourly thereafter. Renal function should be measured and deep tendon reflexes elicited regularly. Fetal side effects are limited. There is no evidence of changes in uteroplacental blood flow.[85] Neonatal hypermagnese-

mia has been reported with prolonged therapy and following delivery during infusion.[86]

Prostaglandin Synthetase Inhibitors

Prostaglandins play a pivotal role in the onset of labor. The use of prostaglandin synthetase inhibitors should theoretically provide a useful therapeutic option in the management of preterm labor. Both placebo-controlled[87] and comparative studies with β-sympathomimetics[88] and magnesium sulfate[89] have shown that prostaglandin synthetase inhibitors are effective at delaying delivery. Unfortunately, the widespread maternal and fetal side effects have limited their application. More recently, the use of selective prostaglandin synthetase inhibitors has offered the potential of abolishing uterine contractions, with the absence of marked side effects.

Prostaglandins ripen the cervix, modulate calcium release from the sarcoplasmic reticulum, and directly activate myometrial calcium channels. As already discussed, prostaglandins are generated from arachidonic acid by cyclo-oxygenase. Currently, two isoforms have been identified, the constitutively expressed type 1 (COX-1) and the inducible type 2 (COX-2). It is the inducible isoform that is largely responsible for the increased synthesis of prostaglandins seen in the fetal membranes and myometrium at term, and with the onset of labor.[37] The constitutive isoform is the isoform predominately found in fetal cardiovascular tissue.[90] Nonselective prostaglandin synthetase inhibitors inhibit both COX-1 and COX-2. The "beneficial" effects of decreased prostaglandin synthesis are the result of COX-2 inhibition, whilst the side effects seen with prostaglandin synthetase inhibitors are largely a result of COX-1 inhibition. Gastrointestinal irritation is commonly reported. Platelet dysfunction, whilst theoretically reversible, may result in prolonged bleeding times. Renal dysfunction and an altered immune response have also been reported. Whilst these complications may be undesirable, it is the fetal side effects that are more profound and that have limited the application of nonselective prostaglandin synthetase inhibitors.

Oligohydramnios results from decreased fetal urine output. It complicates between 10 and 30% of cases of indomethacin therapy. In the presence of normal renal blood flow, it is thought that oligohydramnios is a result of a prostaglandin-mediated alteration in tubular function.[91] Urine output may fall by up to 50%. Oligohydramnios appears to be dose-dependent and resolves on stopping treatment. Isolated cases of fetal renal failure have been reported with indomethacin therapy.[92] Prostaglandin E$_1$ is responsible for maintaining dilatation of the fetal ductus arteriosus. Inhibition of prostaglandin E$_1$ by indomethacin results in ductal constriction. Constriction of the ductus arteriosus complicates between 20 and 50% of fetuses exposed to indomethacin therapy. Ductal constriction can be visualized ultrasonically within 2 hours of treatment and resolves after 24 hours. Ductal effects of indomethacin appear to be gestationally related and most significant after 32 weeks.[93] Chronic constriction of the ductus arteriosus has been associated with fetal pulmonary hypertrophy, pulmonary hypertension, and hydrops. Persistent fetal pulmonary hypertension may also result in neonatal pulmonary hypertension.[94] Indomethacin is usually administered orally, with a 50-mg loading dose followed by 25 mg every 6 hours. Amniotic fluid indices and ductal blood flows should be measured ultrasonically at least twice weekly during treatment with prostaglandin synthetase inhibitors.

Sulindac

Adverse fetal side effects of nonspecific prostaglandin synthetase inhibitors has prompted the use of agents with limited placental transfer. Sulindac (Clinoril) is a prodrug closely resembling indomethacin. It is oxidized to a sulfinyl group and subsequently reduced in the liver to the active sulfide form of the drug. While fetal blood levels of the prodrug are similar to those in the maternal circulation, levels of the active sulfide are lower in the fetus, due to decreased reduction of sulindac to the active sulfide in the fetal liver.[95] Evidence available from comparative studies suggest that sulindac is as effective as indomethacin at controlling preterm contractions, without associated changes in amniotic fluid indices (AFI) and ductal flows,[96] although this effect is not seen in placebo-controlled studies.[97] Theoretically, sulindac has some benefits over indomethacin, with an improved side-effect profile; however, it does inhibit both the constitutive and inducible COX isoforms.

Selective COX-2 Inhibitors

Indomethacin has roughly equal efficacy at inhibiting both COX-1 and COX-2. The advent of specific inhibitors of COX-2 has provided a potential development in tocolytic agents. Nimesulide is a selective COX-2 inhibitor, with approximately 10- to 100-fold lower IC50 for inhibition of COX-2 than for COX-1. There is early evidence that nimesulide is successful at preventing preterm delivery, with limited effects on AFI and ductal flow.[98] As further highly COX-2–specific compounds are developed, this group of drugs may supersede β-sympathomimetics as first-line therapy for preterm labor.

Oxytocin Receptor Antagonists

Whilst no changes have been found in the concentrations of oxytocin with either the onset or the progress of labor,[22] the density of myometrial oxytocin receptors does increase towards term.[23] Oxytocin antagonists, such as atosiban, competitively bind with cell surface oxytocin receptors, inhibiting the uterotonic effects of oxytocin in a dose-dependent manner.[99] Atosiban has been shown to decrease uterine contractions in threatened preterm labor.[100] Atosiban is usually administered intravenously. Atosiban crosses the placenta, although fetal levels are only 10% of maternal,[99] and this results in minimal fetal side effects. Placebo-controlled trials of atosiban in pre-

term labor are currently being carried out and their results are awaited.

Calcium Channel Blockers

Calcium channel blockers such as nifedipine and nicardipine have a theoretical role in the management of preterm labor. They appear to block voltage-dependent calcium channels in myometrial cells.[101] Calcium channel blockers cause uterine relaxation, and although clinical trials are limited, there is some evidence that calcium channel blockers are able to delay delivery in excess of 48 hours.[102] While their action is complicated by maternal hypotension and reflex tachycardia, the incidence of cardiovascular side effects is lower than that associated with the β-sympathomimetics.[102] The effects of calcium channel blockers on placental blood flow appear equivocal. Loss of placental autoregulation has been reported with nifedipine treatment.[103] Nifedipine is usually administered either sublingually or orally, at a dose of 20 mg, 6 hourly.

Nitric Oxide Donors

NO is a potent mediator of smooth muscle relaxation. NO interacts with cyclic guanosine monophosphate (cGMP), resulting in a fall in intracellular calcium. The effects of nitric oxide donors on uterine smooth muscle have been known for many years, and have been used to achieve uterine smooth muscle relaxation with oxytocin-induced contractions[4] and retained placenta.[5, 104] While NO donors relax the human uterus, the role of endogenous NO in the maintenance of uterine quiesence and in the onset of labor is equivocal. Glyceryl trinitrate (GTN) has been used in the management of preterm labor. In an observational study, Lees et al.[105] reported a prolongation of pregnancy using 10-mg glyceryl trinitrate patches. They went on to carry out a multicenter, prospective, randomized controlled study comparing GTN with intravenous ritodrine, in the management of preterm labor.[106] There was no significant difference in efficacy between GTN and ritodrine in the acute tocolysis of preterm labor. More recently, there has been some evidence to suggest that topical GTN applied to the cervix reduces the force required to dilate the cervix prior to termination of pregnancy,[14] implying that NO may be capable of ripening the cervix. While there may be some differential effects of systemic and topical applications, the use of NO donors in preterm labor should be seriously questioned.

Methylxanthines

Methylxanthines such as aminophylline are capable of decreasing uterine activity by inhibiting phosphodiesterase degradation of cAMP. Clinical studies are limited but suggest some prolongation of pregnancy with aminophylline.[107] Inhibition of cAMP is more marked in association with β-adrenergic stimulation. There is, therefore, a theoretical indication for combining methylxanthines with β-sympathomimetics, although this combination therapy has not been evaluated clinically. Evidence to date suggests less maternal side effects associated with aminophylline compared with ritodrine. Currently its use as a tocolytic is limited to experimental protocols.

Tocolytic Management of Fetal Intervention

Fetal Surgery

The development of appropriate tocolytic management for fetal surgery in humans was largely developed from experimental work on primates.[108] Monkeys provide a good model for examining the effects of hysterotomy, compared with sheep, where hysterotomy seldom results in the initiation of uterine contractions. The perinatal loss rates in fetal surgery are as high as 50% in some series,[109] although this is decreasing with advances in surgical techniques. Nevertheless, a significant element of this loss rate is associated with high rates of prematurity associated with preterm labor. Initial studies suggested a combined approach to tocolysis, involving a regimen of preoperative indomethacin; intraoperative deep halothane anesthesia; and postoperative indomethacin, magnesium sulfate, and β-sympathomimetics.[108, 109] Although halothane is capable of achieving uterine relaxation at high concentrations, this is associated with a fall in fetal cardiac output and placental blood flow associated with an increase in placental vascular resistance.[110] Indomethacin as discussed previously can result in premature closure of the ductus arteriosus, and both magnesium sulfate and the β-sympathomimetics are associated with significant maternal and fetal side effects.

More recently, intravenous nitroglycerin (an NO donor) has been used with apparent success for perioperative tocolysis. NO donors, as previously discussed, are well-known mediators of uterine relaxation, although when administered topically they are thought to ripen the cervix.[14] Their use is also associated with maternal systemic hypotension, increasing the risks of diminished uteroplacental blood flow, and there have been case reports of pulmonary edema associated with intravenous nitroglycerin following fetal surgery.[111] Lung damage may have resulted from the combination of NO with exogenous oxygen, to form peroxynitrite, a known inhibitor of alveolar epithelial cell function. Intravenous nitroglycerin, however, appears to be the current drug of choice for perioperative tocolysis for fetal surgery.

Fetal Endoscopic Surgery

Much of the difficulty associated with tocolysis and fetal surgery is the result of hysterotomy and potential initiation of uterine contractions and fetal membrane separation. These problems appear to be directly related to the size of the uterine incision. Fetal endoscopic surgery (FETENDO) avoids the requirement for a large uterine incision and therefore provides an opportunity to reduce uterine trauma and associated preterm labor.[112] While reducing the uterine incision, endoscopic fetal surgery involves the use of surgical techniques that are significantly less aggressive than those associated with hysterotomy. The tocolytic regimens currently used for FETENDO are similar to those used with hysterotomy.

Cervical Cerclage

Cervical cerclage is a technique to close the external cervical os when there is evidence of cervical incompetence or a history of previous preterm delivery, associated with cervical incompetence. It is usually performed vaginally, although sutures may be inserted transabdominally. Instrumental stimulation of the cervix during the procedure results in local prostaglandin synthesis, which may result in further cervical change and the onset of uterine contractions. Perioperative tocolysis may therefore involve a combination regimen of rectal diclofenac, oral sulindac, and oral antibiotics.

Conclusion

The factors responsible for the onset of labor are both complex and multiple, but provide a theoretical basis for a number of tocolytic therapeutic options. Currently, tocolytics are only successful in prolonging pregnancy in the short term, and are associated with widespread side effects. Fetal surgery provides specific challenges to successful tocolysis, although recent advances in endoscopic surgery have reduced the incidence of perioperative preterm delivery. The development of new tocolytics such as the selective prostaglandin synthetase inhibitors, calcium channel blockers, and possibly oxytocin antagonists may provide real advances in this field. With the ability to successfully prevent preterm delivery, fetal surgery, as a specialty, will be able to fully realize its considerable potential.

R E F E R E N C E S

1. Harrison MR: Fetal surgery. Am J Obstet Gynecol 174:1255–1264, 1996.
2. Haluska GJ, Stanczyk FZ, Cook MJ, et al: Temporal changes in uterine activity and prostaglandin response to RU486 in rhesus macaques in late gestation. Am J Obstet Gynecol 157:1487–1495, 1987.
3. Buhimschi I, Yallampalli C, Dong YL, et al: Involvement of a nitric oxide-cyclic guanosine monophosphate pathway in control of human uterine contractility during pregnancy. Am J Obstet Gynecol 172:1577–1584, 1995.
4. Kumar D, Zourlas PA, Barnes AC: In vivo effect of amyl nitrite on human pregnant uterine contractility. Am J Obstet Gynecol 91:1066–1068, 1965.
5. Peng AT, Gorman RS, Shulman SM, et al: Intravenous nitroglycerin for uterine relaxation in the postpartum patient with retained placenta [letter]. Anesthesiology 71:172–1731, 1989.
6. Yallampalli C, Izumi H, Byam SM, et al: An L-arginine-nitric oxide-cyclic guanosine monophosphate system exists in the uterus and inhibits contractility during pregnancy. Am J Obstet Gynecol 170(1 Pt 1):175–185, 1994.

7. Sladek SM, Regenstein AC, Lykins D, et al: Nitric oxide synthase activity in pregnant rabbit uterus decreases on the last day of pregnancy. Am J Obstet Gynecol 169:1285–1291, 1993.

8. Natuzzi ES, Ursell PC, Harrison MR, et al: Nitric oxide synthase activity in the pregnant uterus decreases at parturition. Biochem Biophys Res Commun 194:1–8, 1993.

9. Telfer JF, Lyall F, Norman JE, et al: Identification of nitric oxide synthase in human uterus. Hum Reprod 10:19–231, 1995.

10. Telfer JF, Irvine GA, Kohnen G, et al: Expression of endothelial and inducible nitric oxide synthase in non-pregnant and decidualized human endometrium. Mol Hum Reprod 3:69–75, 1997.

11. Bansal RK, Goldsmith PC, He Y, et al: A decline in myometrial nitric oxide synthase expression is associated with labor and delivery. J Clin Invest 99:2502–2508, 1997.

12. Dennes WJB, Slater DM, Jones GD, et al: Nitric oxide—a role in parturition? Br J Obstet Gynaecol 105:21, 1998.

13. Jones GD, Poston L: The role of endogenous nitric oxide synthesis in contractility of term or preterm human myometrium. Br J Obstet Gynaecol 104:241–245, 1997.

14. Thomson AJ, Lunan CB, Cameron AD, et al: Nitric oxide donors induce ripening of the human uterine cervix: A randomised controlled trial. Br J Obstet Gynaecol 104:1054–1057, 1997.

15. McLean M, Bisits A, Davies J, et al: A placental clock controlling the length of human pregnancy. Nat Med 1:460–463, 1995.

16. Challis JR, Matthews SG, Van MC, et al: Current topic: The placental corticotrophin-releasing hormone-adrenocorticotrophin axis. Placenta 16:481–502, 1995.

17. Alvi SA, Brown NL, Bennett PR, et al: Corticotrophin-releasing hormone and platelet-activating factor induce transcription of the type-2 cyclo-oxygenase gene in human fetal membranes. Mol Hum Reprod 5:476–480, 1999.

18. Jones SA, Challis JR: Effects of corticotropin-releasing hormone and adrenocorticotropin on prostaglandin output by human placenta and fetal membranes. Gynecol Obstet Invest 29:165–168, 1990.

19. Petraglia F, Benedetto C, Florio P, et al: Effect of corticotropin-releasing factor-binding protein on prostaglandin release from cultured maternal decidua and on contractile activity of human myometrium in vitro. J Clin Endocrinol Metab 80:3073–3076, 1995.

20. Buster JE, Chang RJ, Preston DL, et al: Interrelationships of circulating maternal steroid concentrations in third trimester pregnancies. I. C21 steroids: Progesterone, 16 alpha-hydroxyprogesterone, 17 alpha-hydroxyprogesterone, 20 alpha-dihydroprogesterone, delta 5-pregnenolone, delta 5-pregnenolone sulfate, and 17-hydroxy delta 5-pregnenolone. J Clin Endocrinol Metab 48:133–138, 1979.

21. Fuchs AR, Periyasamy S, Alexandrova M, et al: Correlation between oxytocin receptor concentration and responsiveness to oxytocin in pregnant rat myometrium: Effects of ovarian steroids. Endocrinology 113:742–749, 1983.

22. Thornton S, Davison JM, Baylis PH: Plasma oxytocin during the first and second stages of spontaneous human labor. Acta Endocrinol Copenh 126:425–429, 1992.

23. Fuchs AR, Fuchs F, Husslein P, et al: Oxytocin receptors in the human uterus during pregnancy and parturition. Am J Obstet Gynecol 150:734–741, 1984.

24. Turnbull A: The Fetus and Birth. London: Elsevier, 1977.

25. Skinner KA, Challis JR: Changes in the synthesis and metabolism of prostaglandins by human fetal membranes and decidua at labor. Am J Obstet Gynecol 151:519–523, 1985.

26. Crankshaw DJ, Dyal R: Effects of some naturally occurring prostanoids and some cyclooxygenase inhibitors on the contractility of the human lower uterine segment in vitro. Can J Physiol Pharmacol 72:870–874, 1994.

27. Garfield RE, Hertzberg EL: Cell-to-cell coupling in the myometrium: Emil Bozler's prediction. Prog Clin Biol Res 327:673–681, 1990.

28. Romero R, Parvizi ST, Oyarzun E, et al: Amniotic fluid interleukin-1 in spontaneous labor at term. J Reprod Med 35:235–238, 1990.

29. Ammala M, Nyman T, Salmi A, et al: The interleukin-1 system in gestational tissues at term: Effect of labor. Placenta 18:717–723, 1997.

30. Saeed SA, Mitchell MD: Conversion of arachidonic acid to lipoxygenase products by human fetal tissues. Biochem Med 30:322–327, 1983.

31. Bennett PR, Slater D, Sullivan M, et al: Changes in amniotic arachidonic acid metabolism associated with increased cyclooxygenase gene expression. Br J Obstet Gynaecol 100:1037–1042, 1993.

32. Hla T, Farrell M, Kumar A, et al: Isolation of the cDNA for human prostaglandin H synthase. Prostaglandins 32:829–845, 1986.

33. Hla T, Neilson K: Human cyclooxygenase-2 cDNA. Proc Natl Acad Sci U S A 89:7384–7388, 1992.

34. Slater DM, Berger LC, Newton R, et al: Expression of cyclooxygenase types 1 and 2 in human fetal membranes at term. Am J Obstet Gynecol 172(1 Pt 1):77–82, 1995.

35. Slater D, Berger L, Newton R, et al: The relative abundance of type 1 to type 2 cyclo-oxygenase mRNA in human amnion at term. Biochem Biophys Res Commun 98:304–308, 1994.

36. Hirst JJ, Teixeira FJ, Zakar T, et al: Prostaglandin endoperoxide-H synthase-1 and -2 messenger ribonucleic acid levels in human amnion with spontaneous labor onset. J Clin Endocrinol Metab 80:517–523, 1995.

37. Slater DM, Dennes WJB, Jones GD, et al: Expression of COX-1 and COX-2 in human myometrium: Changes in relation to gestational age and labor onset. J Soc Gynecol Invest 4:115A, 1997.

38. Kieler H, Axelsson O, Nilsson S, et al: The length of human pregnancy as calculated by ultrasonographic measurement of the fetal biparietal diameter. Ultrasound Obstet Gynecol 6:353–357, 1995.

39. Bennett PR, Elder MG: The mechanisms of preterm labor: Common genital tract pathogens do not metabolize arachidonic acid to prostaglandins or to other eicosanoids. Am J Obstet Gynecol 166:1541–1545, 1992.

40. Lamont RF, Rose M, Elder MG: Effect of bacterial products on prostaglandin E production in amnion cells. Lancet 2:1331–1337, 1985.

41. Bennett PR, Elder MG, Myatt L: Secretion of phospholipases by bacterial pathogens may initiate preterm labor. Am J Obstet Gynecol 163(1 Pt 1):241–242, 1990.

42. Romero R, Kadar N, Hobbins JC, et al: Infection and labor: The detection of endotoxin in amniotic fluid. Am J Obstet Gynecol 157(4 Pt 1):815–819, 1987.

43. Romero R, Hobbins JC, Mitchell MD: Endotoxin stimulates prostaglandin E2 production by human amnion. Obstet Gynecol 71:227–228, 1988.

44. Rajasingam D, Bennett PR, Alvi SA, et al: Stimulation of prostaglandin production from intact human fetal membranes by bacteria and bacterial products. Placenta 19:301–306, 1998.

45. Newton RW, Hunt LP: Psychosocial stress in pregnancy and its relation to low birth weight. Br Med J Clin Res Educ 288:1191–1194, 1984.

46. Sandman CA, Wadhwa PD, Chicz DA, et al: Maternal stress, HPA activity, and fetal/infant outcome. Ann N Y Acad Sci 814:266–275, 1997.

47. Chan WY, Wo NC, Manning M: The role of oxytocin receptors and vasopressin V1a receptors in uterine contractions in rats: Implications for tocolytic therapy with oxytocin antagonists. Am J Obstet Gynecol 175:1331–1335, 1996.

48. Maggi M, Del CP, Fantoni G, et al: Human myometrium during pregnancy contains and responds to V1 vasopressin receptors as well as oxytocin receptors. J Clin Endocrinol Metab 70:1142–1154, 1990.

49. Freda MC, DeVore N: Should intravenous hydration be the first line of defense with threatened preterm labor? A critical review of the literature. J Perinatol 16:385–389, 1996.

50. Guinn DA, Goepfert AR, Owen J, et al: Management options in women with preterm uterine contractions: A randomized clinical trial. Am J Obstet Gynecol 177:814–818, 1997.

51. Petrie RH, Wu R, Miller FC, et al: The effect of drugs on uterine activity. Obstet Gynecol 48:431–435, 1976.

52. King JF, Grant A, Keirse MJ, et al: Beta-mimetics in preterm labor: An overview of the randomized controlled trials. Br J Obstet Gynaecol 95:211–222, 1988.

53. Macones GA, Bader TJ, Asch DA: Optimising maternal-fetal outcomes in preterm labour: A decision analysis. Br J Obstet Gynaecol 105:541–550, 1998.

54. Scheid CR, Honeyman TW, Fay FS: Mechanism of beta-adrenergic relaxation of smooth muscle. Nature 277:32–36, 1979.

55. Carsten ME, Miller JD: A new look at uterine muscle contraction. Am J Obstet Gynecol 157:1303–1315, 1987.

56. Bishop EH, Wouterxz TB: Isoxsuprine, a myometrial relaxant. Obstet Gynecol 17:442–446, 1961.

57. Merkatz IR, Peter JB, Barden TP: Ritodrine hydrochloride: A betamimetic agent for use in preterm labor. II. Evidence of efficacy. Obstet Gynecol 56:7–12, 1980.

58. Barden TP, Peter JB, Merkatz IR: Ritodrine hydrochloride: A betamimetic agent for use in preterm labor. I. Pharmacology, clinical history, administration, side effects, and safety. Obstet Gynecol 56:1–6, 1980.

59. Leveno KJ, Cunningham FG: Beta-adrenergic agonists for preterm labor. N Engl J Med 327:349–351, 1992.

60. Benedetti TJ: Treatment of preterm labor with the beta-adrenergic agonist ritodrine. N Engl J Med 327:1758–1760, 1992.

61. Schwarz R, Retzke U: Cardiovascular effects of terbutalin in pregnant women. Acta Obstet Gynecol Scand 62:419–423, 1983.

62. Gabriel R, Harika G, Saniez D, et al: Prolonged intravenous ritodrine therapy: A comparison between multiple and singleton pregnancies. Eur J Obstet Gynecol Reprod Biol 57:65–71, 1994.

63. Spellacy WN, Cruz AC, Buhi WC, et al: The acute effects of ritodrine infusion on maternal metabolism: Measurements of levels of glucose, insulin, glucagon, triglycerides, cholesterol, placental lactogen and chorionic gonadotropin. Am J Obstet Gynecol 131:637–642, 1978.

64. Caldwell G, Scougall I, Boddy K, et al: Fasting hyperinsulinemic hypoglycemia after ritodrine therapy for premature labor. Obstet Gynecol 70(3 Pt 2):478–480, 1987.

65. Cano A, Tovar I, Parrilla JJ, et al: Metabolic disturbances during intravenous use of ritodrine: Increased insulin levels and hypokalemia. Obstet Gynecol 65:356–360, 1985.

66. Sharif DS, Huhta JC, Moise KJ, et al: Changes in fetal hemodynamics with terbutaline treatment and premature labor. J Clin Ultrasound 18:85–89, 1990.

67. Jouppila P, Kirkinen P, Koivula A, et al: Ritodrine infusion during late pregnancy: Effects on fetal and placental blood flow, prostacyclin, and thromboxane. Am J Obstet Gynecol 151:1028–1032, 1985.

68. Ylikorkala O, Jouppila P, Kirkinen P, et al: Maternal prostacyclin, thromboxane, and placental blood flow. Am J Obstet Gynecol 145:730–732, 1983.

69. Casper RF, Lye SJ: Myometrial desensitization to continuous but not to intermittent beta-adrenergic agonist infusion in the sheep. Am J Obstet Gynecol 154:301–305, 1986.

70. Lam F, Gill P, Smith M, et al: Use of the subcutaneous terbutaline pump for long-term tocolysis. Obstet Gynecol 72:810–813, 1988.

71. Caritis SN, Toig G, Heddinger LA, et al: A double-blind study comparing ritodrine and terbutaline in the treatment of preterm labor. Am J Obstet Gynecol 150:7–14, 1984.

72. Beall MH, Edgar BW, Paul RH, et al: A comparison of ritodrine, terbutaline, and magnesium sulfate for the suppression of preterm labor. Am J Obstet Gynecol 153:854–859, 1985.

73. Chau AC, Gabert HA, Miller JJ: A prospective comparison of terbutaline and magnesium for tocolysis. Obstet Gynecol 80:847–851, 1992.

74. Haspedis L: Terbutaline in the treatment of preterm labor: A comparison of intravenous and subcutaneous administration. J Am Osteopath Assoc 88:489–493, 1988.

75. Ryden G: The effect of salbutamol and terbutaline in the management of premature labor. Acta Obstet Gynecol Scand 56:293–296, 1977.

76. Sims CD, Chamberlain GV, Boyd IE, et al: A comparison of salbutamol and ethanol in the treatment of preterm labor. Br J Obstet Gynaecol 85:761–766, 1978.

77. Hall DG, McGaughery HSJ, Corey EL, et al: The effects of magnesium therapy on the duration of labor. Am J Obstet Gynecol 78:27–32, 1959.

78. Hutchinson HT, Nichols MM, Kuhn CR, et al: Effects of magnesium sulfate on uterine contractility, intrauterine fetus and infant. Am J Obstet Gynecol 88:747–758, 1965.

79. Guiet BA, Bara M, Durlach J: Comparative study of the effects of two tocolytic agents (magnesium sulfate and alcohol) on the ionic transfer through the isolated human amnion. Eur J Obstet Gynecol Reprod Biol 20:297–304, 1985.

80. Steer CM, Petrie RH: A comparison of magnesium sulfate and alcohol for the prevention of premature labor. Am J Obstet Gynecol 129:1–4, 1977.

81. Cotton DB, Strassner HT, Hill LM, et al: Comparison of magnesium sulfate, terbutaline and a placebo for inhibition of preterm labor. A randomized study. J Reprod Med 29:92–97, 1984.

82. Hollander DI, Nagey DA, Pupkin MJ: Magnesium sulfate and ritodrine hydrochloride: A randomized comparison. Am J Obstet Gynecol 156:631–637, 1987.

83. Cruikshank DP, Pitkin RM, Donnelly E, et al: Urinary magnesium, calcium, and phosphate excretion during magnesium sulfate infusion. Obstet Gynecol 58:430–434, 1981.

84. Smith LJ, Burns PA, Schanler RJ: Calcium homeostasis in pregnant women receiving long-term magnesium sulfate therapy for preterm labor. Am J Obstet Gynecol 167:45–51, 1992.

85. Keeley MM, Wade RV, Laurent SL, et al: Alterations in maternal-fetal Doppler flow velocity waveforms in preterm labor patients undergoing magnesium sulfate tocolysis. Obstet Gynecol 81:191–194, 1993.

86. Lipsitz PJ: The clinical and biochemical effects of excess magnesium in the newborn. Pediatrics 47:501–509, 1971.

87. Zuckerman H, Shalev E, Gilad G, et al: Further study of the inhibition of premature labor by indomethacin. Part II double-blind study. J Perinat Med 12:25–29, 1984.

88. Morales WJ, Smith SG, Angel JL, et al: Efficacy and safety of indomethacin versus ritodrine in the management of preterm labor: A randomized study. Obstet Gynecol 74:567–572, 1989.

89. Morales WJ, Madhav H: Efficacy and safety of indomethacin compared with magnesium sulfate in the management of preterm labor: A randomized study. Am J Obstet Gynecol 169:97–102, 1993.

90. Bennett PR, Slater DM: Cyclo-oxygenase-2 enzyme in labor. In Vane J, Botting J, Botting R (eds): Improved Non-steroidal Anti-Inflammatory drugs: COX-2 Enzyme Inhibitors. London: Kluwer Academic Publications, 1996, p 167.

91. Mari G, Moise KJ, Deter RL, et al: Doppler assessment of the renal blood flow velocity waveform during indomethacin therapy for preterm labor and polyhydramnios. Obstet Gynecol 75:199–201, 1990.

92. Buderus S, Thomas B, Fahnenstich H, et al: Renal failure in two preterm infants: Toxic effect of prenatal maternal indomethacin treatment? Br J Obstet Gynaecol 100:97–98, 1993.

93. Huhta JC, Moise KJ, Fisher DJ, et al: Detection and quantitation of constriction of the fetal ductus arteriosus by Doppler echocardiography. Circulation 75:406–412, 1987.

94. Levin DL, Fixler DE, Morriss FC, et al: Morphologic analysis of the pulmonary vascular bed in infants exposed in utero to prostaglandin synthetase inhibitors. J Pediatr 92:478–483, 1978.

95. Kramer WB, Saade G, Ou CN, et al: Placental transfer of sulindac and its active sulfide metabolite in humans. Am J Obstet Gynecol 172:886–890, 1995.

96. Carlan SJ, O'Brien WF, O'Leary TD, et al: Randomized comparative trial of indomethacin and sulindac for the treatment of refractory preterm labor. Obstet Gynecol 79:223–228, 1992.

97. Carlan SJ, O'Brien WF, Jones MH, et al: Outpatient oral sulindac to prevent recurrence of preterm labor. Obstet Gynecol 85(5 Pt 1):769–774, 1995.

98. Sawdy R, Slater D, Fisk N, et al: Use of a cyclo-oxygenase type-2-selective non-steroidal anti-inflammatory agent to prevent preterm delivery. Lancet 350:265–266, 1997.

99. Akerlund M, Stromberg P, Hauksson A, et al: Inhibition of uterine contractions of premature labor with an oxytocin analogue. Results from a pilot study. Br J Obstet Gynaecol 94:1040–1044, 1987.

100. Goodwin TM, Paul R, Silver H, et al: The effect of the oxytocin antagonist atosiban on preterm uterine activity in the human. Am J Obstet Gynecol 170:474–478, 1994.

101. Braunwald E: Mechanisms of action of calcium channel blocking agents. N Engl J Med 307:1618–1627, 1982.

102. Read MD, Wellby DE: The use of a calcium antagonist (nifedipine) to suppress preterm labor. Br J Obstet Gynaecol 93:933–937, 1986.

103. Maigaard S, Forman A, Andersson KE: Effects of nifedipine on human placental arteries. Gynecol Obstet Invest 18:217–224, 1984.

104. Barnes F: Hour-glass contraction of the uterus treated with nitrite of amyl. BMJ 1:377, 1992.
105. Lees C, Campbell S, Jauniaux E, et al: Arrest of preterm labor and prolongation of gestation with glyceryl trinitrate, a nitric oxide donor. Lancet 343:1325–1326, 1994.
106. Lee CC, Lojacono A, Thompson C, et al: Glyceryl trinitrate and ritodrine in tocolysis: An international multicenter randomized study. GIN preterm labor intervention group. Obstet Gynecol 3: 403–408, 1999.
107. Liu DT, Blackwell RJ: The value of a scoring system in predicting outcome of pre-term labor and comparing the efficacy of treatment with aminophylline and salbutamol. Br J Obstet Gynaecol 85:418–424, 1978.
108. Harrison MR, Anderson J, Rosen MA: Fetal surgery in the primate I. Anesthetic, surgical, and tocolytic management to maximize fetal-neonatal survival. J Pediatr Surg 17:115–122, 1982.
109. Adzick NS, Harrison MR: Fetal surgical therapy. Lancet 348:897–902, 1994.
110. Sabik JF, Assad RS, Hanley FL: Halothane as an anaesthetic for fetal surgery. J Paediatr Surg 28:542–546, 1993.
111. DiFederico EM, Harrison MR, Matthay MA: Pulmonary edema in a woman following fetal surgery. Chest 109:1114–1117, 1996.
112. VanderWall KJ, Bruch, SW, Meuli M, et al: Fetal endoscopic ('Fetendo') tracheal clip. J Pediatr Surg 31:1101–1103, 1996.

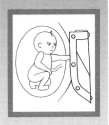

New Tocolytic Strategies for Fetal Surgery

EFFICACY AND FETOMATERNAL SAFETY OF NITROGLYCERIN

ERIK D. SKARSGARD and YASSER Y. EL-SAYED

Premature labor following fetal surgery remains a significant management issue because of the virulent labor caused by hysterotomy in the preterm uterus. The magnitude of postoperative premature labor appears to be proportional to the size of the uterine incision and degree of fetal manipulation necessary for exposure and operation. The advent of minimally invasive approaches to select malformations, such as fetal endoscopic (FETENDO) tracheal occlusion for congenital diaphragmatic hernia (CDH),[1] and endoscopic umbilical cord occlusion for twin reversed arterial perfusion (TRAP) sequence,[2] has led to a significant reduction in preterm labor. However, for fetal lesions not yet amenable to minimally invasive treatment (such as congenital cystic adenomatoid malformation and sacrococcygeal teratoma), posthysterotomy labor remains the principal determinant of fetal outcome.

The high rate of uncontrollable labor (up to 50%) after hysterotomy for fetal intervention with traditional agents such as β-agonists and magnesium sulfate has inspired a search for more potent tocolytic drugs.[3] Nitroglycerin, long known for its vasodilatory properties in the treatment of cardiovascular disease,[4] also causes uterine smooth muscle relaxation and shows considerable promise as a tocolytic agent. The obstetric experience with nitroglycerin has been largely anecdotal, with reports of successful uterine relaxation facilitating manual extraction of retained placenta,[5–7] reduction of uterine prolapse[5, 8] and intrapartum external version,[9–11] and breech extraction.[12]

In this chapter, we discuss the biochemical rationale for the use of nitroglycerin as a tocolytic, and review clinical and animal data relevant to the efficacy and safety of nitroglycerin as a tocolytic for all preterm labor patients and, in particular, those undergoing fetal surgery.

Biochemistry and Mechanism of Action of Nitric Oxide

Endogenous nitric oxide (NO) is synthesized during the oxidation of L-arginine to L-citrulline.[13] Nitric oxide is formed from the guanadino nitrogen of L-arginine by the action of nitric oxide synthase (NOS).[14] Three distinct isoforms of NOS (NOS1, NOS2, NOS3) have been identified, each representing the product of a separate gene. NOS2 is a cytokine-inducible isoform widely expressed following stimulation with inflammatory mediators.[15] NOS1 and NOS3 are constitutively active isoforms that are calcium sensitive.

Several studies using different techniques have provided biochemical evidence of NOS activity in the pregnant uterus. The conversion of radiolabeled L-arginine to L-citrulline has been found to occur in the pregnant human myometrium,[16] and NOS activity observed. Measurement of nitric oxide metabolites (nitrite and nitrate) has also been used to confirm NOS activity in rat whole-uterus explants[17] and rabbit decidual homogenates.[18] Two immunoblotting studies have suggested the presence of all three NOS isoforms in the cervix and uterus.[19, 20] Of note, a 50% reduction in NOS activity has been described in samples from human uteri between 34 and 39 weeks' gestation.[21]

The three potential mechanisms by which NO may cause smooth muscle relaxation are activation of guanylate cyclase, stimulation of calcium-dependent potassium channels, and adenosine diphosphate (ADP) ribosylation.[22] Currently the mechanism most widely accepted for the smooth muscle relaxant property of nitric oxide is via activation of guanylate cyclase, which catalyzes the formation of cyclic guanosine monophosphate (cGMP) from guanosine 5'-triphosphate (Fig. 12–1).[22, 23] Three forms of guanylate cyclase have been described: a membrane-bound particulate

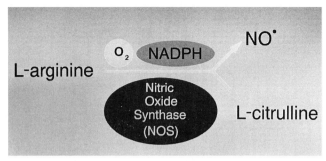

F I G U R E   12–1. Mechanism of action of nitric oxide by activation of guanylate cyclase and formation of cyclic GMP (cGMP).

guanylate cyclase, a cytoskeleton-associated form, and a soluble form. It is the soluble form that is the main target for activation by organic nitrate esters such as nitroglycerin.[23] The cGMP produced by soluble guanylate cyclase activates cGMP-dependent protein kinase (cG-Pk) that activates sarcoplasmic reticulum Ca^{2+}-ATPase, which then leads to increased uptake by the sarcoplasmic reticulum and decreased concentration in cytosolic free calcium.[23, 24] Cyclic GMP is inactivated by phosphodiesterases that open the 3',5'-cyclic phosphoester bond, yielding GMP. GMP cannot activate cG-Pk.[23]

Nitroglycerin, an organic nitrate ester, is a nitric oxide donor. In order for nitric oxide to be liberated, an organic nitrate ester must be catalyzed by enzymes such as glutathione s-transferase, cytochrome P-450, and possibly esterases.[23] Other organic nitrate esters include isosorbide dinitrate and isosorbide-5-mononitrate.

Nitric Oxide Tocolytic Efficacy: Animal Studies

Primates

The rate and magnitude of preterm labor after hysterotomy has made the nonhuman primate an ideal model for the study of tocolytic efficacy. Jennings et al. investigated the efficacy of the nitric oxide donor S-nitroso-N-acetylpenicillamine (SNAP) in controlling surgically induced preterm labor in the rhesus monkey (Fig. 12–2).[25] When no therapy was given, labor progressed to delivery within 32 hours. Administration of SNAP by continuous maternal systemic venous infusion in doses ranging from 0.625 to 40 $\mu g/kg/min$ resulted in a dose-dependent suppression of preterm labor. As the SNAP dose was increased, contractions decreased in frequency and amplitude, and were eventually obliterated completely. There was also a dose-dependent reduction in maternal mean arterial pressure with SNAP infusion that existed whether SNAP was infused into the systemic venous circulation or directly into the uterine circulation via the hypogastric artery. Interestingly, SNAP infusion resulted in a modest increase in uterine artery blood flow, as estimated by a flow transducer on the hypogastric artery. Whether this decrease in vascular resistance was the direct result of nitric oxide–mediated vasodilation, or resulted indirectly from reduced uterine contractions, could not be determined by this study.

Nitroglycerin infusion of doses as high as 2,000 $\mu g/kg/min$ had essentially no effect on either uterine contractility or maternal hemodynamics, suggesting that the rhesus monkey lacks the tissue enzymes necessary to form the S-nitrosothiol intermediates required for NO release.[26]

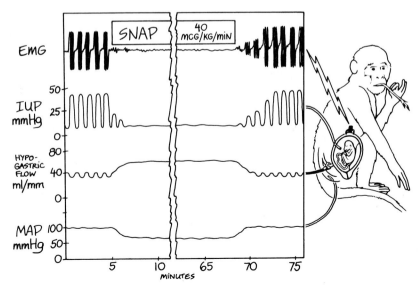

F I G U R E   12–2. Schematic strip chart recording from invasively monitored and actively laboring primate, demonstrating the tocolytic and maternal hemodynamic effects of S-nitroso-N-acetylpenicillamine (SNAP). (EMG = electromyography; IUP = intrauterine pressure; MAP = mean arterial pressure.)

Sheep

Although less prone than the nonhuman primate, late gestation sheep instrumented with amniotic and fetal catheters often develop spontaneous labor. Heymann et al. reported the efficacy of low-dose infusions of nitroglycerin (1 to 3 μg/kg/min) in abolishing established uterine contractions in sheep developing "preterm" labor several days after surgical intervention.[27]

Nitroglycerin Tocolytic Efficacy: Clinical Trials

Clinical data on the tocolytic and uterine relaxant efficacy of nitroglycerin are limited. Most available data are in the form of case reports and case series describing anecdotal experience. Successful uterine relaxation with nitroglycerin has been described for external cephalic version,[9-11] facilitating fetal extraction during cesarean delivery,[5, 28, 29] internal podalic version,[5, 8] and uterine relaxation during fetal surgery.[31] Nitroglycerin delivery systems have included the intravenous, sublingual, and aerosolized routes, with doses ranging from 50 to 1,850 μg.[5, 6, 30]

The uncontrolled nature of these reports has made difficult an accurate assessment of nitroglycerin's efficacy for uterine relaxation. David et al.[32] conducted one of the few randomized trials involving the use of nitroglycerin for uterine relaxation. In this double-blind study, women undergoing elective cesarean delivery under general anesthesia were randomly assigned either 0.25 or 0.5 mg of nitroglycerin or a physiologic saline solution at the time of uterine incision. The surgeons then estimated reduction in uterine tone and the ease of fetal extraction; no clinically relevant easing of fetal extraction was noted. The median maternal–fetal venous nitroglycerin concentration was 400:1 in the 0.25-mg group and 160:1 in the 0.5-mg group. A randomized trial comparing subcutaneous terbutaline and intravenous nitroglycerin for external cephalic version is currently in progress.[33]

The use of nitroglycerin patches for preterm labor has been reported in two small case series,[34, 35] as well as one placebo-controlled trial.[13] The study by Lees et al. was an observational trial involving 13 women with uterine contractions. Nitroglycerin patches delivering 10 mg over 24 hours were used, and up to two patches were applied simultaneously. The reported mean prolongation of pregnancy was 34 days. The second observational study by Rowlands et al. involved 10 subjects in which 50-mg nitroglycerin patches were used. Pregnancy was prolonged for a mean of 46.2 days. However, Smith et al., in placebo-controlled trial of nitroglycerin involving 33 subjects in active preterm labor, showed no statistically significant difference in the number of deliveries within 48 hours.

The use of intravenous nitroglycerin for the treatment of preterm labor has also been investigated in two randomized trials.[36, 37] Clavin et al.[36] reported in abstract form an 89.5% tocolytic success rate with magnesium sulfate compared to 53.3% with intravenous nitroglyc-

erin. Information regarding duration of tocolysis, exact criteria for successful tocolysis, and administered doses was not included in the abstract. El-Sayed et al. performed a study investigating the use of high-dose intravenous nitroglycerin compared to magnesium sulfate for preterm labor tocolysis, and reported that nitroglycerin was associated with more tocolytic failures than magnesium sulfate (62.5% vs. 21.4%).[37]

Nitric Oxide Tocolysis for Fetal Surgery: Safety Issues for Mother and Fetus

Though apparently efficacious in primate and sheep studies, the use of nitric oxide donors for tocolysis following fetal surgery has raised safety concerns based mostly on anecdotal clinical observations. Nonhydrostatic pulmonary edema requiring intubation and 5 days of mechanical ventilation was observed in a young pregnant woman following fetal diaphragmatic hernia repair.[38] Her postoperative labor was particularly difficult to manage, requiring indomethacin, nitroglycerin (up to 17 μg/kg/min), terbutaline, and magnesium sulfate. It was hypothesized that her pulmonary edema was the result of alveolar cell dysfunction caused by the nitroglycerin metabolite, peroxynitrite.

Safety issues pertaining to the fetus are second in import to those of the mother and her subsequent reproductive potential. However, among fetal safety issues associated with maternal tocolysis, few are more important than the prevention of a debilitating cerebral injury in the gestationally predisposed infant. Neonatal cerebral injuries, both hyperemic (intraventricular hemorrhage [IVH] and periventricular hemorrhage [PVH]) and ischemic (periventricular leukomalacia [PVL], result from changes in cerebral blood flow,[39] and it is therefore likely that tocolytic drugs capable of modulating vascular tone might predispose to such injuries in the fetus. This concern was raised by the observation of serious central nervous system (CNS) injuries in 7 of 33 human fetuses with known neurologic outcome after fetal surgery (Table 12–1).[40] Three of these fetuses survived and, in two fetuses, the CNS injury was detectable by ultrasound before birth. Whether these injuries were the result of fetal circulatory disturbances associated with maternal factors (hypotension, anemia, placental membrane separation), fetal factors (bradycardia), or tocolysis could not be elucidated, but it did provide impetus for the investigation of the effects of tocolytics on fetomaternal circulation and on fetal cerebral blood flow and metabolism in sheep.[41]

Sheep Studies: Effects of Maternal Nitroglycerin on Fetomaternal Hemodynamics and Fetal Cerebral Blood Flow and Metabolism

Using chronic invasive monitoring, we administered intravenous nitroglycerin to pregnant sheep and mea-

T A B L E 12–1. SUMMARY OF CNS INJURY IN FETAL SURGICAL PATIENTS

PATIENT NO.	DIAGNOSIS	PROCEDURE	SURVIVAL	FETAL FACTORS	MATERNAL FACTORS	TOCOLYTIC DRUGS	PATHOLOGY
1	CDH	Open repair	No	Fetal bradycardia	None	MS,I	PVL
2	CDH	Open repair	No	None	Respiratory failure and hypotension	NTG,I, TERB	PVL, PVH, IVH
3	CDH	Open repair	No	Fetal bradycardia	2,000-mL blood loss	NTG, I, TERB	PVL
4	CDH	PLUG	Yes	Postnatal hypotension	None	NTG, I, TERG	PVL
5	CDH	Open repair	Yes	None	UC POD 5; I restarted	NTG, I, TERB	PVH and hydrocephalus
6	CDH	PLUG	No	None	UC POD 5; I restarted	NTG, I, TERB	PVH and hydrocephalus
7	CDH	Open repair	Yes	Fetal bradycardia	Membrane separation	NTG, I, TERB	PVH (subependymal hemorrhage)

CDH, congenital diaphragmatic hernia; IVH, intraventricular hemorrhage; NTG, nitroglycerin; PLUG, tracheal plug; PVH, periventricular hemorrhage; I, indomethacin; UC, uterine contrations; PVL, periventricular hemorrhage; TERB, terbutaline; POD, postoperative day; MS, magnesium sulfate.

sured maternal and fetal hemodynamics and arterial blood gases as well as ultrasonic fetal carotid blood flow, and cerebral metabolism of the substrates oxygen, glucose, and lactate. Nitroglycerin infusions were given to pregnant sheep at doses of 5, 10, and 20 μg/kg/min and caused increases in maternal and fetal heart rate (HR), and decreases in maternal and fetal mean arterial pressure (MAP), which were significant at the higher doses (Fig. 12–3). Despite these hemodynamic changes,

fetal arterial pH, P_{CO_2}, and P_{O_2} were not altered (Table 12–2).

In our study, fetal cerebral blood flow and cerebrovascular resistance, as estimated by ultrasonic total carotid flow, did not change significantly during maternal infusion of nitroglycerin, although we did note a trend towards increased flow and decreased resistance at all three dose infusions. That these changes were insignificant despite fetal hypotension suggests that endogenous

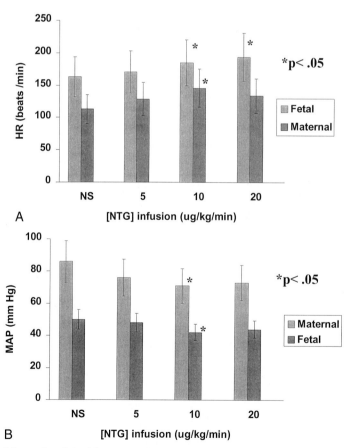

F I G U R E 12–3. *A,* Maternal and fetal heart rate during 30-minute maternal infusion of normal saline (NS) and nitroglycerin. Maternal and fetal heart rate increases during nitroglycerin infusion were significant at the 10-μg/kg/min (maternal) and 10- and 20-μg/kg/min (fetal) doses, respectively. *B,* Maternal and fetal mean arterial pressure (MAP) during 30-minute infusions of normal saline (NS) and nitroglycerin. Maternal and fetal hypotension during nitroglycerin infusion was significant during the 10-μg/kg/min dose only.

T A B L E 12–2. FETAL ARTERIAL BLOOD GASES AND CEREBRAL METABOLIC RATE FOR OXYGEN, GLUCOSE, AND LACTATE DURING MATERNAL INFUSIONS OF NORMAL SALINE, NITROGLYCERIN (10 μg/kg/min), AND INDOMETHACIN

	NS (n = 10)	NTG-10 (n = 11)	Indo (n = 10)
pH	7.37 ± 0.02	7.36 ± 0.02	7.40 ± 0.02
P_{CO_2} (mm Hg)	47.4 ± 3.4	46.4 ± 3.6	44.4 ± 2.9
P_{O_2} (mm Hg)	21.6 ± 1.7	19.8 ± 1.1	19.7 ± 0.88
[Hgb] (mg/dL)	11.1 ± 0.44	11.1 ± 0.49	11.0 ± 0.45
CMR_{O_2} (mL/kg/min)	45.5 ± 7.0	40.9 ± 3.9	47.9 ± 5.7
CMR_{glu} (mL/kg/min)	1.34 ± 0.22	1.92 ± 0.41	1.22 ± 0.24
CMR_{lac} (mL/kg/min)	0.018 ± 0.03	0.019 ± 0.03	0.038 ± 0.02

NS, normal saline; NTG-10, nitroglycerin; Indo, indomethacin; CMR, cerebral metabolic rate.

regulation of fetal cerebral blood flow overrides any direct effect transplacental nitroglycerin might have on the cerebral vessels. The transit time technique of regional blood flow measurement enabled us to measure flow variability, which might be an important predisposing variable for injury, since it may be the amplitude of the flow "flux" that results in either hyperemia or ischemia, rather than mean flow. Although not statistically significant, we did notice an increase in flow variability with nitroglycerin compared to control saline infusion.

Fetal cerebral metabolic rates for oxygen, glucose, and lactate were calculated using the Fick equation, and there was no significant difference in cerebral oxygen, glucose, or lactate utilization during nitroglycerin infusion compared to saline controls.

Bootstaylor et al. reported, also in sheep, similar maternal hemodynamic changes in response to nitroglycerin infusions at doses lower than those used in our study.[42] Fetal heart rate, blood pressure, arterial blood gases, and umbilical consumption of oxygen, glucose, and lactate were unchanged. They also measured regional blood flow (using radioactive microspheres) to a number of organs including the brain, and observed no change in flow before and during nitroglycerin infusion.

Two earlier studies evaluated the effects of nitroglycerin in a sheep model of preeclampsia. Wheeler et al.[43] showed that nitroglycerin infusion at a mean dose of 19 μg/kg/min reduced maternal mean arterial pressure by 20%, without compromise of uterine blood flow, while de Rosayro et al., using a comparable dose of maternal nitroglycerin, demonstrated identical maternal hemodynamic changes, and a significant reduction in uterine artery blood flow. There was, however, no significant hemodynamic or blood gas change in the fetuses.[44]

These studies suggest that, in sheep, the administration of nitroglycerin in doses approximating those used for fetal surgery tocolysis appears to be safe for mother and fetus from a hemodynamic perspective. Fetal regional blood flow and, in particular, cerebral blood flow does not change significantly during nitroglycerin infusion. Flow variability, which could predispose to hyper-

emic or ischemic injury, and cerebral substrate metabolism also remain stable in sheep over a range of nitroglycerin dose.

Nitroglycerin and Safety Issues for Mother and Fetus: Observations in Humans

Nitroglycerin relaxes vascular smooth muscle, resulting in dilation of peripheral arteries and veins, especially the latter.[45] It has a rapid onset and a short duration (half-life of approximately 2 minutes). Bolus administration of intravenous nitroglycerin has been associated with mild maternal hypotension in several case reports.[7, 8] One episode of transient hypotension using nitroglycerin patches was described in the study by Less et al. using transdermal patches for tocolysis.[34] However, up to a 25% incidence of severe maternal hypotension was noted in clinical trials of intravenous nitroglycerin infusion for preterm labor.[36, 37] Other reported maternal side effects include headache, lightheadedness, flushing, palpitations, nausea, vomiting, and redness at the nitroglycerin patch site (Table 12–3).[34–37] Maternal methemoglobinemia has not been reported in clinical trials of nitroglycerin in obstetrics.

Nitroglycerin has a low molecular weight, is lipid soluble, and appears to rapidly cross the placenta, although only a fraction of maternally administered nitroglycerin volume is detected in the fetal circulation.[13, 32] This low ratio may be secondary to placental and fetal nitroglycerin biotransformation.[44] No adverse fetal effects have been described in the case reports and clinical studies involving nitroglycerin for uterine relaxation and tocolysis. Doppler ultrasound has been used to investigate the effect of nitric oxide donors on uteroplacental perfusion.[46–49] In five pregnant women at 34 to 38 weeks' gestation with abnormally elevated umbilical artery velocity ratios, a mean reduction in umbilical systolic/diastolic velocity ratio of 21% was noted 20 minutes following administration of 300 μg sublingual nitroglycerin.[46] The authors suggest that the absence of any fetal heart rate changes indicate minimal hemodynamic alterations in the fetus. In another study, infusion of intravenous nitroglycerin (0.5 to 5.0 μg/kg/min) in 12 women with severe preeclampsia (mean gestational age, 33 weeks) resulted in a mean decrement in the umbilical artery pulsatility index of approximately

T A B L E 12–3. HUMAN MATERNAL SIDE-EFFECT PROFILE OF NITROGLYCERIN

Headache
Lightheadedness
Hypotension
Contact dermatitis
Flushing
Palpitations
Nausea and vomiting
Methemoglobinemia
Anaphylaxis

11%.[47] No change in uterine artery pulsatility indices were noted. The authors state that although their results suggest vasodilation of the umbilical circulation, the unchanged fetal heart rate indicates minimal influences on fetal blood pressure. Ramsey et al.[48] noted declines in the uterine artery pulsatility index in women at 8 to 10 and 24 to 26 weeks' gestation receiving 10 to 20 $\mu g/$ min intravenous nitroglycerin, and no significant changes in umbilical artery pulsatility indices. Thaler et al.[49] administered a single 5-mg dose of sublingual isosorbide dinitrate (a nitric oxider donor) to 18 women with low-risk pregnancies at 17 to 24 weeks' gestation, and found a significant reduction in Doppler impedance in both the umbilical and uterine arteries. Although no detrimental effect on the fetal heart rate has been described in these studies, the effect on uterine and umbilical artery resistance indices has been inconsistent.

Myatt et al. have investigated the vascular resistance effects of nitric oxide in an in vitro, perfused human placental model.[50, 51] In these studies, isolated human placental cotyledons were perfused with the nonmetabolizable NOS substrate analogues N-monomethyl-L-arginine and N-nitro-L-arginine as well as nitroglycerin, and the effects on perfusion pressure were recorded at rest and after pretreatment with a vasoconstrictor. Perfusion with both endogenous NOS antagonists resulted in significantly increased vascular resistance in the fetoplacental circulation, both at rest and following preconstriction, while perfusion with nitroglycerin attenuated the effects of exogenous vasoconstrictor, but did not alter baseline vascular resistance. In a similar study by the same investigator, administration of methylene blue, which inhibits the activation of guanylate cyclase by nitric oxide, resulted in an increase in resting vascular tone. Administration of nitroglycerin and SNAP caused a dose-dependent vasodilation, but only in the presence of previously administered vasoconstrictor. These in vitro, placental perfusion studies support the concept of endogenous NO regulation of placental blood flow which is not affected by exogenous administration of NO donors (except in the presence of vasoconstrictors). From this, one might extrapolate that the administration of nitroglycerin for tocolysis should not adversely affect placental perfusion.

Conclusion

Nitric oxide donors like nitroglycerin have found clinical application as tocolytic and uterine relaxant agents. Although there are considerable human scientific data substantiating the role of endogenous nitric oxide in parturition, and animal data (nonhuman primates) that document its tocolytic efficacy, there are still some unanswered questions regarding the efficacy of nitroglycerin in arresting human preterm labor, as well as questions pertaining to dosage and route of administration. The existing experimental and clinical data suggest that the maternal administration of nitroglycerin for tocolysis is safe from the perspective of both mother and fetus. As with all new therapies, there must be an ongoing critical assessment of both efficacy and untoward effects of nitroglycerin as a tocolytic following fetal surgery.

REFERENCES

1. Harrison MR, Mychalski GB, Albanese CT, et al: Correction of congenital diaphragmatic hernia in utero IX: Fetuses with poor prognosis (liver herniation and low lung-to-head ratio) can be saved by fetoscopic temporary tracheal occlusion. J Pediatr Surg 33:1017–1022, 1998.
2. Quintero RA, Reich H, Puder KS, et al: Brief report: Umbilical cord ligation of an acardiac twin by fetoscopy at 19 weeks gestation. N Engl J Med 330:469–471, 1994.
3. Adzick NS, Harrison MR: Fetal surgical therapy. Lancet 348:897–902, 1994.
4. Abrams J: Mechanisms of action of the organic nitrates in the treatment of myocardial ischemia. Am J Cardiol 70:30–42B, 1992.
5. Riley ET, Flanagan B, Cohen SE, Chitkara U: Intravenous nitroglycerin: A potent uterine relaxant for emergency obstetric procedures. Review of the literature and report of three cases. Int J Obstet Anesth 5:264–268, 1996.
6. DeSimone CA, Norris MC, Leighton BL: Intravenous nitroglycerin aids manual extraction of a retained placenta [letter]. Anesthesiology 73:787, 1990.
7. Peng ATC, Gorman RS, Shulman SM, et al: Intravenous nitroglycerin for uterine relaxation in the post partum patient with retained placenta. Anesthesiology 71:172–173, 1989.
8. Altabef KM, Spencer JT, Zinberg S: Intravenous nitroglycerin for uterine relaxation of an inverted uterus. Am J Obstet Gynecol 166:1237–1238, 1992.
9. Abouleish AE, Corn SB: Intravenous nitroglycerin for intrapartum external version of the second twin. Anesth Analg 78:808–809, 1994.
10. Belfort MA: Intravenous nitroglycerin as a tocolytic agent for intrapartum external cephalic version. S Afr Med J 83:656, 1993.
11. Redick LF, Livingstone E, Bell E: Sublingual aerosol nitroglycerin for uterine relaxation in attempted external version. Am J Obstet Gynecol 176:496–497, 1997.
12. Greenspoon JS, Kovacic A: Breech extraction facilitated by glyceryl trinitrate spray. Lancet 338:124–125, 1991.
13. Smith GN, Brien JF: Use of nitroglycerin for uterine relaxation. Obstet Gynecol Surv 53:559–565, 1998.
14. Norman JE, Ward LM, Martin W, et al: Effects of cGMP and the nitric oxide donors glyceryl trinitrate and sodium nitroprusside on contractions in vitro of isolated myometrial tissue from pregnant women. J Reprod Fertil 110:249–254, 1997.
15. Kelly RA, Smith TW: Nitric oxide and nitrovasodilators: Similarities, differences, and interactions. Am J Cardiol 77:2C–7C, 1996.
16. Ramsay B, Soorana SR, Johnson MR: Nitric oxide synthase activities in human myometrium and villous trophoblast throughout pregnancy. Obstet Gynecol 87:249–253, 1996.
17. Yallampalli C, Garfield RE, Byam-Smith M: Nitric oxide inhibits uterine contractility during pregnancy but not during pregnancy. Endocrinology 133:1899–1902, 1993.
18. Sladek SM, Regenstein AC, Lykins D, Roberts JM: Nitric oxide synthase activity in pregnant rabbit uterus decreases on the last day of pregnancy. Am J Obstet Gynecol 169:1285–1291, 1993.
19. Buhimschi I, Ali M, Jain V, et al: Differential regulation of nitric oxide in the rat uterus and cervix during pregnancy and labour. Hum Reprod 11:1755–1766, 1996.
20. Dong YL, Gangula PRR, Yallampalli C: Nitric oxide synthase isoforms in the rat uterus: Differential regulation during pregnancy and labour. J Reprod Fertil 107:249–254, 1996.
21. Sladek SM, Stranko CP, Roberts JM: Human decidual nitric oxide synthase activity decreases by the last week of gestation but not with labor [abstract P422]. Soc Gynecol Invest 41st Annual Mtg., Chicago, IL, 1994.
22. Norman J: Nitric oxide and the myometrium. Pharmacol Ther 70:91–100, 1996.
23. Torfgard KE, Ahlner J: Mechanism of action of nitrates. Cardiovasc Drugs Ther 8:701–717, 1994.
24. Morgan RO, Newby CA: Nitroprusside differentially inhibits ADP-stimulated calcium influx and mobilization in human platelets. Biochem J 258:447–454, 1989.

25. Jennings RW, MacGillivray TE, Harrison MR: Nitric oxide inhibits preterm labor in the rhesus monkey. J Matern Fet Med 2:170–175, 1993.
26. Ignarro L, Barry B, Gruetter D, et al: Guanylate cyclase activation by nitroprusside and nitroguanidine is related to the formation of S-nitrosothiol intermediates. Biochem Biophys Res Commun 94:93–100, 1980.
27. Heymann MA, Bootstaylor B, Roman C, et al: Glyceryl trinitrate stops active labour in sheep. *In* Moncada S, Feelisch M, Busse R, Higgs EA (eds): The Biology of Nitric Oxide, Vol 3. London: Portland Press, 1994, pp 201–203.
28. Rolbin SH, Hew EM, Bernstein A: Uterine relaxation can be life saving [letter]. Can J Anaesth 38:939–940, 1991.
29. Bayhi DA, Sherwood CD, Campbell CE: Intravenous nitroglycerin for uterine inversion. J Clin Anesth 4:487–488, 1992.
30. Redick LF, Livingstone E: A new preparation of nitroglycerin for uterine relaxation. Int J Obstet Anesth 4:14–16, 1995.
31. Harrison MR: Fetal surgery. Am J Obstet Gynecol 174:1255–1264, 1996.
32. David H, Halle H, Lichtennegger W, et al: Nitroglycerin to facilitate fetal extraction during cesarean delivery. Obstet Gynecol 901:119–124, 1998.
33. El-Sayed Y, Chitkara U, Riley ET, et al: Nitroglycerin versus terbutaline for external cephalic version [abstract 222]. Presented at the 18th Annual Meeting of Society of Perinatal Obstetricians, Miami Beach, FL, 1988.
34. Lees C, Campbell S, Jauniaux E, et al: Arrest of preterm labour and prolongation of gestation with glyceryl trinitrate, a nitric oxide donor. Lancet 343:1325–1326, 1994.
35. Rowlands S, Trudinger B, Visva-Lingam S: Treatment of preterm labor cervical dilation with glyceryl trinitrate, a nitric oxide donor. Aust N Z J Obstet Gynecol 36:377–381, 1996.
36. Clavin DK, Bayhi DA, Nolan TE, et al: Comparison of intravenous magnesium sulfate and nitroglycerin for preterm labor [abstract 15]. Presented at 16th Annual Meeting of Society of Perinatal Obstetricians, Kamuela HI, 1996.
37. El-Sayed YY, Riley ET, Holbrook RH Jr, et al: Randomized comparison of intravenous nitroglycerin and magnesium sulfate for treatment of preterm labor. Obstet Gynecol 93:79–83, 1999.
38. DiFederico EM, Harrison MR, Matthay MA: Pulmonary edema in a woman following fetal surgery. Chest 109:1114–1117, 1996.
39. Allan WC, Volpe JJ: Periventricular-intraventricular hemorrhage. Pediatr Clin North Am 36:47–63, 1986.
40. Bealer JB, Raisanen J, Skarsgard ED, et al: The incidence and spectrum of neurological injury after open fetal surgery. J Pediatr Surg 30:1150–1154, 1995.
41. Skarsgard ED, Vanderwall KJ, Morris JA, et al: The effects of nitroglycerin and indomethacin on fetomaternal circulation and on fetal cerebral blood flow and metabolism in sheep. Am J Obstet Gynecol 181:440–445, 1999.
42. Bootstaylor BS, Roman C, Parer JT, Heymann MA: Fetal and maternal hemodynamic and metabolic effects of maternal nitroglycerin infusions in sheep. Am J Obstet Gynecol 176:644–650, 1997.
43. Wheeler AS, James FM III, Meis PJ, et al: Effects of nitroglycerin and nitroprusside on the uterine vasculature of gravid ewes. Anesthesiology 52:390–394, 1980.
44. De Rosayro M, Nahrwold ML, Hill AB, et al: Plasma levels and cardiovascular effect of nitroglycerin in pregnant sheep. Can Anaesth Soc J 27:560–564, 1980.
45. Physician's Desk Reference, 50th ed. Montvale, NJ: Medical Economics Data, 1996, pp 1523–1524.
46. Giles W, O'Callaghan S, Boura A, Walters W: Reduction in human fetal umbilical-placental vascular resistance by glyceryl trinitrate. Lancet 340:856, 1992.
47. Grunewald C, Kublickas M, Carlstrom K, et al: Effects of nitroglycerin on the uterine and umbilical circulation in severe preeclampsia. Obstet Gynecol 86:600–604, 1995.
48. Ramsay B, De Belder A, Campbell S, et al: A nitric oxide donor improves uterine artery diastolic blood flow in normal early pregnancy and in women at high risk of preeclampsia. Eur J Clin Invest 24:76–78, 1994.
49. Thaler I, Amit A, Jakobi P, Itskovitz-Eldor J: The effects of isosorbide dinitrate on uterine artery and umbilical artery flow velocity waveforms at mid-pregnancy. Obstet Gynecol 88:838–843, 1996.
50. Myatt L, Brewer AS, Langdon G, et al: Attenuation of the vasoconstrictor effects of thromboxane and endothelin by nitric oxide in the human fetal-placental circulation. Am J Obstet Gynecol 166:224–230, 1992.
51. Myatt L, Brewer A, Brockman DE: The action of nitric oxide in the perfused human fetal-placental circulation. Am J Obstet Gynecol 164:687–692, 1991.

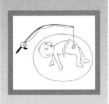

Percutaneous Sonographically Guided Interventions: Catheters and Shunts

PRANAV P. PANDYA and CHARLES H. RODECK

In conjunction with recent advances in the antenatal detection of fetal structural abnormalities by ultrasound, there is now growing experience in the management of these conditions. A number of invasive treatments have been developed for specific abnormalities and these include the insertion of percutaneous shunts and catheters.[1-5]

Fetal shunting in utero should only be considered if the natural history of the abnormality is frequently associated with significant neonatal mortality or morbidity, there is sufficient evidence that the natural progression can be alleviated by the procedure, and the maternal risks are minimal. Furthermore, appropriate patient selection is imperative to prevent unnecessary intervention in cases where either the prognosis is poor or there would be a satisfactory outcome if left alone. The selection of cases for treatment is influenced by the absence of major associated anomalies and the results of appropriate tests to evaluate organ function. Fetal shunting should only be offered in centers with appropriate expertise, where ongoing research is being done and where a multidisciplinary team approach is available. The principles governing fetal therapy are summarized in Table 13–1 and the variety of problems for which shunting has been performed, including obstructive uropathy, pleural effusions, pulmonary cysts, ventriculomegaly, and fetal ascites (Table 13–2). Contraindications for fetal shunting are listed in Table 13–3.

Vesicoamniotic Shunts

Lower urinary tract obstructive uropathy is most commonly due to posterior urethral valves (PUVs) or rarely urethral atresia and occurs in about 1 in 1,000 pregnancies.[10] Ultrasound features include an enlarged bladder (megacystis) which may be detectable as early as 11 weeks,[11] thickening of the bladder wall, dilatation of the upper urethra, a variable degree of hydroureter with or without hydronephrosis, which is often asymmetric, and oligohydramnios. A diagnostic amnioinfusion may aid the detection of associated anomalies.[12] There may also be vesicoureteric reflux, which frequently accompanies gross obstruction. PUV occurs almost exclusively in the male fetus.[13] If a female fetus is found to have an enlarged bladder, the differential diagnosis should be considered and includes cloacal anomalies, megacystis-microcolon-intestinal hypoperistalsis syndrome (MMIH), and the prune-belly syndrome.[3] Most of these cases are unlikely to benefit from any type of prenatal decompression and shunting is usually not indicated. The sonographic recognition of the typically dilated proximal urethra in PUV is of crucial importance.

Assessment

Experimental studies in animal models have provided the theoretical basis for human fetal intervention.[14-17] However, their relevance to spontaneous disease remains controversial. The rationale for vesicoamniotic shunting is to prevent progressive renal damage and correct the associated oligohydramnios, which may in turn prevent pulmonary hypoplasia.

Fetal intervention is usually not required for hydronephrosis, unless hydronephrosis is present in a solitary kidney in conjunction with oligohydramnios. The presence of a normal amount of amniotic fluid has been regarded as a contraindication to shunting, although this may change in the future.[17]

Ultrasound

The prenatal assessment of renal function is important in the selection of fetuses for shunting and in providing realistic counseling for patients. Although the sonographic finding of oligohydramnios before 20 weeks is

T A B L E 13–1. PRINCIPLES OF INVASIVE FETAL THERAPY

The natural history of the condition should be known
The condition should be severe enough to interfere with normal development and cause death or disability
The treatment should be capable of improving the natural history of the condition
Evidence from an animal model should support this
Other fetal abnormalities should be excluded as far as possible
Reliable prognostic tests should be available, to detect appropriate cases for treatment
The fetus should be too immature for delivery and postnatal treatment
The benefits to the fetus should outweigh the risks to the mother and fetus
The parents must be counseled and informed
After treatment antenatal monitoring must continue
Postnatal follow-up is essential
The treatment should be evaluated scientifically

a very poor prognostic sign, both this feature and the degree of pelvicalyceal dilatation are poor predictors of renal dysplasia, chronic renal failure, and fetal or neonatal death. Ultrasound findings of renal cysts are visualized in only 44% of dysplastic kidneys, and hyperechogenicity of the renal parenchyma only predicts dysplasia with a sensitivity and specificity of 73% and 80%, respectively.[18]

Fetal Urine

In view of the inaccuracy of ultrasound, biochemical analysis of fetal urine obtained by ultrasonographically guided aspiration of urine from the fetal bladder[19] and/or from each renal pelvis[20] has been recommended. The healthy fetus produces hypotonic urine, progressive renal damage effects proximal tubular function resulting in the urine becoming isotonic. However, some values are dependent on gestational age, and this must be taken into account during assessment of renal function. Sodium, calcium, phosphate, and sodium/creatine levels show a significant correlation with the degree of renal impairment, with the best sensitivity achieved by calcium and the highest specificity by sodium.[21] β_2-Microglobulin is a low-molecular-weight protein that passes through the glomerular basement membrane and is almost entirely reabsorbed by the proximal renal tubular cells. Elevated urinary levels of β_2-microglobulin have been suggested to be predictive of renal dysplasia.[22] A

T A B L E 13–2. FETAL SHUNTING

PATHOLOGY	TYPE OF SHUNT
Obstructive uropathy	
Posterior urethral valves	Vesicoamniotic
Hydronephrosis	Pyeloamniotic
Hydrothorax or chylothorax	Pleuroamniotic
Pulmonary cyst (CAM type 1)	Cystoamniotic
Ascites	Peritoneoamniotic
Cerebral ventriculomegaly	Ventriculoamniotic

CAM, cystic adenomatoid malformation.

T A B L E 13–3. CONTRAINDICATIONS FOR SHUNT INSERTION

There are associated ultrasonically detectable lethal abnormalities or aneuploidy
The parents wish a termination of pregnancy
The pregnancy is early (<16 weeks) and the fetus is physically too small for the shunt
The fetus is mature and postnatal treatment is a better option

single evaluation of fetal urine may not accurately reflect current or long-term renal function and serial sampling at intervals of 1 to 2 days[23] or 1- to 2-week intervals may give a better idea of the degree of renal damage.[20, 24]

Fetal Intervention

Percutaneous Bladder Aspiration

Rarely, simple percutaneous bladder aspiration with a 22-gauge spinal needle may be enough to open up a urethral obstruction. Renal function may also improve after bladder decompression and this should be the first attempt at interventional therapy. We have also seen significant improvement in fetuses that have undergone serial bladder decompression. Since bladder aspiration is technically easier than shunt insertion and also not associated with the same long-term complications, serial sampling as both a diagnostic and theraputic procedure should be considered in a fetus, especially at gestations less than 20 weeks. Another reason for initial conservative management is that megacystitis sometimes resolves spontaneously. This appears to happen in fetuses with muscular, thick-walled bladders that may be able to generate the pressures required to overcome the urethral obstruction.

Chronic Antenatal Drainage

The aims of vesicoamniotic shunting are summarized in Table 13–4. Vesicoamniotic shunting should be reserved for cases with persistent megacystitis, who have ultrasound and biochemical evidence of adequate renal function.[25] Intervention in a fetus with significantly impaired renal function is unlikely to be beneficial and is not advisable.[26] Antenatal detection of pulmonary hypoplasia remains difficult and it is not yet possible to accurately predict those fetuses at risk.[3] Persistent early-onset oligohydramnios is associated with poor pulmonary

T A B L E 13–4. AIMS OF VESICOAMNIOTIC SHUNTING

Reduce pressure in the urinary tract
Prevent further damage due to raised pressure
Promote normal growth and maturation of nephrons
Allow the formation of amniotic fluid
Improve the freedom of fetal movements and reduce compression
Promote pulmonary growth and maturation
Prevent gross distention of the urinary tract and abdominal wall (prune belly)

function and should be regarded as a poor prognostic sign.

The importance of prevention of gross overdistention of the bladder has been previously underestimated. The atonic, dilated urinary tract may present more management difficulties postnatally than renal failure, for which dialysis and transplantation are available and successful. Some patients with poor fetal prognosis decline termination of pregnancy and insist on shunting in order to give the fetus every chance. This requires careful consideration, because of three possible outcomes: (1) it may not prevent death, (2) it may prevent death but at the cost of survival with severe renal failure, or (3) it occasionally leads to a surprisingly good result.

Outcome

Obstructive uropathy is treated surgically by urinary bypass or diversion in postnatal life and it is illogical to assume that this should not be appropriate in prenatal life. Indeed, if it is believed that treatment is more successful at an early stage of the pathologic process, then prenatal treatment is to be preferred to postnatal. The difficulty, as stated earlier, is in the selection of cases. There are some in whom surgical treatment is not required, and others in whom the pathology is so severe that treatment is hopeless.

In a review of five series involving 169 cases of vesicoamniotic shunting, including cases reported to the International Fetal Medicine and Surgery Society (IFMSS) registry,[7] 79 fetuses (47%) survived and there were seven (4%) procedure-related deaths.[17] Unfortunately, 40% of survivors have end-stage renal disease. However, indications for shunting, ultrasound findings, timing of interventions, and postnatal confirmation of presumed diagnosis were not always reported. In addition, some patients were inappropriately chosen for surgery, including five cases with an abnormal karyotype. At present there are no prospective, randomized trials comparing survival and morbidity in fetuses with and without in utero decompression. Such a trial has proved difficult to implement because of the medical, ethical, and emotional considerations in individual cases. There is always the concern that shunting may prevent in utero death but result in a chronically ill infant.

Some follow-up information is now available through our collaboration with the Department of Paediatric Urology at Great Ormond Street, London. A number of fetuses with urinary tract dilatation but normal amniotic fluid volume have done worse than expected. This would argue for in utero shunting at an earlier stage of pregnancy and in fetuses less severely affected than before. However, if such a policy were to be adopted, randomization into treated and untreated groups would be important.

Thoracoamniotic Shunts

Pleural Effusions and Cysts

Fetal pleural effusions, found in about 1 in 15,000 pregnancies,[27] may be an isolated finding or may occur in association with hydrops fetalis. The causes are similar to those of hydrops such as cardiac defects, anemia, infection, or chromosomal abnormality.[28] Prenatal series report aneuploidy in approximately 10% of fetuses with isolated pleural effusions.[29, 30] In neonates, the commonest cause of an isolated pleural effusion is chylothorax, which is diagnosed by demonstrating chylomicrons in a milky colored pleural fluid after the first feed.[31] The effusion may be primary (chylothorax) or secondary to specific lesions such as cystic adenomatoid malformation (CAM), bronchopulmonary sequestration, or congenital diaphragmatic hernia. Pulmonary cysts may also be seen in cases of CAM, bronchopulmonary sequestration, bronchogenic cysts, and mediastinal teratomas.[32] Large pleural effusions and/or pulmonary cysts causing mediastinal compression may result in fetal or neonatal death due to pulmonary hypoplasia, hydrops, or prematurity as a consequence of polyhydramnios.[33, 34] Thoracoamniotic shunting may be effective in relieving lung compression and any coexisting mediastinal shift. This may prevent pulmonary hypoplasia and reverse fetal hydrops and resolve the polyhydramnios, thereby reducing the risk of fetal death or preterm delivery.[4, 29]

Assessment

Detailed investigation is essential to establish the primary etiology, as this will affect the prognosis. Ultrasonography, including fetal echocardiography, is performed to exclude structural abnormalities associated with pleural effusions and hydrops fetalis. Further investigation of the mother and fetus is similar to that performed for fetal hydrops.[35]

Fetal Intervention

Conservative Management

Serial ultrasound assessment is important because isolated pleural effusions or pulmonary cysts may resolve spontaneously in utero.[36–38] In some cases they have been treated effectively during labor[39] or after birth.[40]

Thoracocentesis

Simple percutaneous aspiration with a 22-gauge spinal needle may be both diagnostic and therapeutic.[41] The diagnosis of an underlying cardiac or lung defect may only become clear after normal mediastinal anatomy is restored. The presence of pulmonary hypoplasia may be indicated by failure of the lungs to expand after decompression.[29] Resolution has been demonstrated following single or repeated aspirations.[34] However, in view of the nature of the underlying condition, the fluid usually reaccumulates within 24 hours after thoracocentesis, necessitating repeated aspiration, which is likely to be more traumatic than thoracoamniotic shunting. Nevertheless, thoracocentesis may be useful in fetuses at early gestations when the chest is too small for a shunt.

Chronic Antenatal Drainage

The aims of thoracoamniotic shunting are summarized in Table 13–5. Thoracoamniotic shunt insertion should be considered, irrespective of the cause, in cases where the fluid reaccumulates following thoracocentesis, and is large enough to produce significant pulmonary compression and/or mediastinal shift that has resulted in hydrops and polyhydramnios. In addition to possible prevention of pulmonary hypoplasia, shunting would facilitate neonatal resuscitation and could potentially reverse hydrops and polyhydramnios.

Outcome

Petterson and Nicolaides[38] compared the perinatal survival of fetuses after conservative management, thoracocentesis, and thoracoamniotic shunting in fetuses with pleural effusions. The data from uncontrolled studies showed that overall shunting was associated with higher survival rates (58 of 85; 68%) than thoracocentesis (7 of 17; 41%) or conservative management (32 of 61; 52%). In addition, the survival rates were worse in those fetuses with hydrops (50%) compared to the nonhydropic fetus (100%), presumably the consequence of the underlying disease causing the hydrops.

Ventriculoamniotic Shunts

Obstructive Hydrocephalus

Ventriculomegaly develops when there is an imbalance of cerebrospinal fluid production and drainage. The most frequent causes of obstructive hydrocephalus include spina bifida, aqueduct stenosis, Dandy-Walker syndrome, chromosomal abnormalities, viral infections, and isolated (idiopathic) cases.[42] The rationale for chronic cerebral ventricular decompression was to reduce ventricular pressure and size, thus preserving cerebral tissue.[2, 5, 43]

Unfortunately, the results of ventriculoamniotic shunting for obstructive hydrocephalus are poor. In the IFMSS registry, although 34 of 44 fetuses (83%) survived, 18 of the 34 survivors had serious neurologic handicap (53%) and only 12 (35%) were neurologically normal at follow-up.[7] In addition, the procedure-related death rate was 10%. It is therefore possible that shunting may not improve survivor morbidity and may have increased survival in the severely handicapped infants.[7] As a result, shunting is not indicated for ventriculomegaly in utero.

Techniques of Shunt Insertion

Shunting procedures should only be performed in referral centers with sufficient expertise and workload to maintain the necessary skills. Consultation with appropriate specialists including pediatricians and counselors may be helpful. Parents must be fully counseled about the procedure and understand the risks and benefits before giving written consent.

Fetal shunting is performed as an outpatient ultrasound-guided procedure and only rarely is maternal and fetal sedation required. Diazemuls (5 to 10 mg intravenously) may be administered to the mother, and if fetal movements are vigorous fetal paralysis can be achieved with pancuronium (1 to 2 mg) injected into the umbilical vein. Some centers give prophylactic antibiotics and tocolytic agents, but this has not been our practice. Whether the fetus should specifically be given some form of analgesia may also require consideration.[44]

Types of Shunts

We use the Rocket fetal catheter developed in 1982[45] (Rocket of London Ltd, Watford, UK). It is a double-pigtail Silastic catheter with external and internal diameters of 2.1 and 1.5 mm, respectively. The ends of the catheter are radiopaque as a result of stainless steel inserts at each end and have lateral holes around the coils. The amniotic coil is at right angles to the rest of the catheter and is therefore less likely to be removed by the fetus or become entangled with the umbilical cord. This shunt is available in one size and we have found it suitable for both thoracoamniotic and vesicoamniotic shunting. It is introduced down an 18-cm-long cannula with an external diameter of 2.5 mm, now made by de Elles Instruments.* The trocar has a very sharp tip in order to make introduction through the maternal and fetal abdominal walls easier and less painful.

Alternative shunts include the following.

1. Harrison fetal bladder stent (Cook Urological, Spencer, IN), a polyethylene catheter that is introduced over the outside of a needle. It has side holes at both ends, a flare at the amniotic cavity end, and resumes a curled end once inserted.[16] It is available in different lengths and calibers, but there have been many technical problems with this catheter.
2. The Denver shunt was developed for the treatment of ventriculomegaly. It is made of silicone rubber and has a rubber flange to maintain its position within the ventricle. Unlike other shunts, it has a one-way valve to prevent reverse flow.[43] However, the manufacturer has discontinued production in view of shunt occlusion and decreasing demands for its use.

TABLE 13–5. AIMS OF THORACOAMNIOTIC SHUNTING

Remove fluid and reduce intrathoracic pressure
Promote resolution of hydrops and polyhydramnios, reducing risk of preterm delivery and fetal death
Prevent development of hydrops and polyhydramnios
Promote pulmonary growth and development
Prevent pulmonary hypoplasia
Assist respiration and ventilation in the neonate

*20 Stagbury Avenue, Surrey, CR5 3PA, UK.

Procedure

1. High-resolution ultrasound scanning should be used to obtain the best transverse section of the fetal target. Curvilinear transducers are particularly convenient.
2. Holding the transducer in one hand, parallel to the intended course of the cannula, an entry site in the maternal abdomen is chosen. The placenta should not be traversed and the site should be away from the maternal uterine vessels, with the needle trajectory as short as possible.
3. The site is cleaned with antiseptic solution (chlorhexidine 0.5% in spirit) and the mother's lower abdomen draped with sterile towels. Local anesthetic (1% lidocaine) is infiltrated into the maternal skin and subcutaneous tissue, down to the myometrium. If there is oligohydramnios, a 20-gauge needle is first passed into the amniotic cavity and an amnioinfusion given with 150 to 200 mL of warmed normal saline. This may improve the image and allow the anomaly scan to be completed, but the main purpose is to facilitate the deposition of the intra-amniotic end of the catheter.
4. Under continuous ultrasound guidance the fetal target is fixed on one side of the ultrasound screen and the metal trocar and cannula are introduced into the amniotic cavity and then inserted through the chest or abdominal wall into the target fluid collection. After ensuring that the cannula is in the correct position, the trocar is removed and drainage of fluid confirms the correct positioning of the cannula. Only minimal drainage should be allowed, as decompression will reduce the size of the target and may result in the cannula becoming dislodged. To prevent this, the end of the catheter can be blocked temporarily with the operator's thumb.
5. The fetal catheter is straightened out on its guidewire and inserted into the cannula. After the guidewire has been withdrawn, the shorter obturator pushes half of the catheter out, and this coils up in the fetal fluid collection. The cannula is then slowly withdrawn out of the fetus into the amniotic cavity, where the other half of the catheter is deposited by the longer obturator. This is the most difficult part of the procedure and requires the presence of fluid in the amniotic cavity.

Bladder Shunting

Oligohydramnios is a frequent finding in cases of obstructive uropathy; in severe cases, prior amnioinfusion facilitates the procedure and avoids the outer end of the catheter being inadvertently left extra-amniotically. To avoid other anatomic structures, the site of fetal insertion should ideally be suprapubic and away from the midline. After the shunt has been inserted there should be rapid decompression of the bladder, which subsequently cannot be identified; indeed, only the presence of the inner tip of the shunt allows its localization. A sample of urine should be sent for appropriate analysis, as described earlier.

Thorax Shunting

Amniodrainage may need to be performed in cases of polyhydramnios to improve both visualization and access to the fetal target. The shunt should be inserted in the midthoracic region, extreme caution being taken to avoid the fetal heart, which ideally should be on the side farthest away from the cannula. In cases of bilateral hydrothorax, if drainage of the contralateral lung is required, the appropriate fetal position may be achieved by rotation of the fetal body using the tip of the cannula, avoiding a repeat puncture of the mother. This is usually possible because polyhydramnios is frequently associated with hydrothorax. A sample of pleural fluid should be sent for lymphocyte count and/or karyotyping.

Complications

The procedure-related death rate of vesicoamniotic shunting has been reported by the International Fetal Medicine and Surgery Society to be on the order of 4% and that of ventriculoamniotic shunting 10.25%.[15, 17] No multicenter figures are available for thoracoamniotic shunting, but in our center the procedure is associated with a 2% fetal loss rate, which is similar to that of vesicoamniotic shunting.

Elder et al.[46] reported a complication rate of 44% following shunting for obstructive uropathy. However, this report was a collection of several small series and case reports and reflects poor case selection and inexperience with the technique. The most common complications were inadequate shunt drainage or migration (19%), followed by preterm labor (12%), urinary ascites (7%), and chorioamnionitis (5%). Other specific complications have been described in the literature and include the formation of fetal urinary ascites, which can be managed by insertion of a peritoneoamniotic shunt.[1] Uteroperitoneal amniotic fluid leakage following thoracoamniotic shunting has been reported.[47] This can result in gross maternal ascites and acute fetal distress due to oligohydramnios and cord compression. Vesicoamniotic shunting has also been associated with a fetal paramedian abdominal wall defect with herniation of small bowel an iatrogenic gastroschisis.[48, 49] Shunts are occasionally drawn into the peritoneal or thoracic cavities and may have to be removed surgically postnatally. These problems and fetal trauma are minimized by operator experience, careful site selection, and continuous monitoring throughout the procedure. Poor drainage and blockage of the shunt may occur due to vernix, blood, or protein exudate. Fetal movement and growth may also result in shunt displacement. Our experience with the technical performance of the Rocket shunt has been very good and complications have been rare. Intrauterine infection is uncommon and may be reduced by ensuring a "sterile" nontouch technique. Prophylactic antibiotics are unlikely to be helpful. The use of tocolytic therapy to inhibit premature uterine contractions is unlikely to be beneficial unless there is considerable polyhydramnios.

Follow-up

Once the shunt has been sited, close observation with serial ultrasound scans is essential. This can be performed at the referring hospital with reassessment in the treatment center as required. The scans should be performed at weekly intervals to determine whether the fluid collections have reaccumulated and also to monitor other features such as improvement of the fetal hydrops and normalization of the amniotic fluid volume. If there are signs of shunt malfunction (due to migration or blockage), such as reaccumulation of fluid, a further shunt placement will have to be considered.

After vesicoamniotic shunting, fetal hydroureter and hydronephrosis frequently persist. Renal parenchymal hyperechogenicity tends to progressively reduce and amniotic fluid reaccumulates, although neither necessarily indicates good renal function.[3] Improvement in the amniotic fluid volume is likely to be an important factor in fetal lung development and maturation.[24] Failure of amniotic fluid to collect indicates severe irreversible renal failure.

Thoracoamniotic shunting should result in a rapid resolution of pulmonary compression, mediastinal shift, polyhydramnios, and fetal hydrops within 1 to 3 weeks. It may help to differentiate between hydrops due to a primary pleural effusion, in which the ascites and skin edema may resolve after shunting, and other causes of hydrops, in which drainage does not necessarily prevent worsening hydrops. Poor prognosis has been associated with the presence of fetal malformations, bilateral effusions, hydrops, and polyhydramnios that has not resolved within 1 to 3 weeks of shunt insertion.[29] Persistence of the pleural effusion with failure of the lungs to expand and fill the chest indicates pulmonary hypoplasia and a poor prognosis, whereas the reverse suggests normal-sized lungs and a good prognosis.[29, 50]

Delivery and Shunt Removal

Provided no serious complications arise after shunt insertion, the pathology is corrected, and the fetus continues to grow normally, delivery should be by spontaneous vaginal delivery at term. If pediatric surgery is required soon after birth, then an elective delivery may be more appropriate either by induction of labor or cesarean section. An experienced neonatologist should always be present at birth.

The neonate with urinary problems may need immediate ventilatory support, but the urinary tract and renal function can usually be investigated at leisure.

There is only limited experience with chest drains at delivery, and the management remains controversial. Immediate clamping and removal to avoid the development of pneumothoraces has been advocated.[1] In our hospital the baby is electively intubated and transferred

to the neonatal unit, where a chest x-ray is performed. Once position of the shunt is confirmed, it is removed in a more controlled manner with local anesthetic. We have found a very low incidence of pneumothoraces using this protocol. Postnatally, the shunt may be used to drain further collections of pleural fluid. A shunt that is not found at birth may be in the baby, in the mother, or it may have been thrown away inadvertently. The mother and baby should undergo radiography, as the steel tips of the shunt are radiopaque.

Conclusions

In utero shunting can be effective therapy for obstructive uropathy, pleural effusions, and thoracic cysts. However, the same cannot be said for the intrauterine treatment of ventriculomegaly, which has now been abandoned. The selection of cases for treatment is determined by the absence of major associated anomalies and the results of appropriate tests to evaluate organ function. The appropriateness of treatment must be individualized for each case, and the decision to intervene must be based on a careful evaluation of the maternal and fetal risks associated with the procedure and its influence on the chances of fetal survival and handicap.

In an attempt to achieve better results, open fetal surgery has been applied in the treatment of some life-threatening conditions.[51, 52] New developments incorporating a minimal access approach using videoendoscopic surgery and laser have been developed. An Angiocath fiberoptic bundle of 0.8-mm diameter can now be passed down an 18-gauge needle for investigation. A laser has been used to create a suprapubic cystotomy.[53] Fetal suprapubic cystoscopy has been performed to enable fulguration of the valves and insertion of a stent into the posterior urethra.[54] We are also hopeful that proton nuclear magnetic resonance spectroscopy of urine will be useful in the future for the assessment of renal function.[55]

Further research to understand the pathophysiology of the individual conditions is required to optimize patient selection prior to fetal shunting. In addition, studies in basic developmental biology may open up possibilities for treating dysplastic kidneys and hypoplastic lungs with embryonic precursor cells and growth factors.

R E F E R E N C E S

1. Lynch L, Mehalek K, Berkowitz RL: Invasive fetal therapy. In Rodeck CH (ed): Fetal Medicine, Vol 1. Oxford: Blackwell Scientific Publications, 1989, pp 118–153.
2. Fisk NM, Kyle P, Rodeck CH: Antenatal diagnosis and fetal medicine. In Rennie J, Robertson NRC (eds): Textbook of Neonatology, 3rd ed. London: Chuchill Livingstone, 1991, pp 121–150.
3. Nicolini U, Rodeck CH: Fetal urinary diversion. In Chervenak FA, Isaacson GC, Campbell S (eds): Ultrasound in Obstetrics and Gynaecology. Boston: Little, Brown & Co, 1993, pp 1277–1282.
4. Nicolaides KH, Azar GB: Thoracoamniotic shunting. In Chervenak FA, Isaacson GC, Campbell S (eds): Ultrasound in Obstetrics and Gynaecology. Boston: Little, Brown & Co, 1993, pp 1289–1293.
5. Clewell WH: Hydrocephalus shunts. In Chervenak FA, Isaacson GC, Campbell S (eds): Ultrasound in Obstetrics and Gynaecology. Boston: Little, Brown & Co, 1993, pp 1283–1287.

6. Potter EL, Craig JM: Pathology of the fetus and infant. Chicago: Year Book Medical Publishers, 1976, pp 434–475.

7. Manning FA, Harrison MR, Rodeck CH, and members of the International Fetal Medicine and Surgery Society: Catheter shunts for fetal hydronephrosis and hydrocephalus. N Engl J Med 315:336–340, 1986.

8. Nicolaides KH, Rodeck CH, Gosden CM: Rapid karyotyping in non-lethal fetal malformations. Lancet i:283–287, 1986.

9. Lipitz S, Robson SC, Ryan G, et al: Management and outcome of obstructive uropathy in twin pregnancies. Br J Obstet Gynaecol 100:879–880, 1993.

10. Estes JM, MacGillivray TE, Hedrick MH, et al: Fetoscopic surgery for the treatment of congenital anomalies. J Pediatr Surg 27:950–954, 1992.

11. Stiller RJ: Early ultrasound appearance of fetal bladder outlet obstruction. Am J Obstet Gynecol 160:584–585, 1989.

12. Gembruch U, Hansmann M: Artificial instillation of amniotic fluid as a new technique for the diagnostic evaluation of cases of oligohydramnios. Prenat Diagn 8:33, 1988.

13. Lebowitz RL, Griscom NT: Neonatal hydronephrosis: 146 cases. Radiol Clin North Am 15:49–59, 1977.

14. Harrison MR, Nakayama DK, Noall RA, de Lorimier AA: Correction of congenital hydronephrosis in utero II. Decompression reverses the effects of obstruction on the fetal lung and urinary tract. J Pediatr Surg 17:965–974, 1982.

15. Harrison MR, Ross NA, Noall RA, de Lorimier AA: Correction of congenital hydronephrosis in utero I. The model: Fetal urethral obstruction produces hydronephrosis and pulmonary hypoplasia in fetal lambs. J Pediatr Surg 18:247–256, 1983.

16. Glick, PL, Harrison MR, Adzick NS, et al: Correction of congenital hydronephrosis in utero IV. In utero decompression prevents renal dysplasia. J Pediatr Surg 19:649–657, 1984.

17. Coplen DE: Prenatal intervention for hydronephrosis. J Urol 157:2270–2277, 1997.

18. Mahoney BS, Filly RA, Callen PW, et al: Fetal renal dysplasia: Sonographic evaluation. Radiology 152:143–146, 1984.

19. Glick PL, Harrison MR, Golbus MS, et al: Management of the fetus with congenital hydronephrosis II. Prognostic criteria and selection for treatment. J Pediatr Surg 20:376–387, 1985.

20. Nicolini U, Rodeck CH, Fisk NM: Shunt treatment for fetal obstructive uropathy. Lancet ii:1338–1339, 1987.

21. Nicolini U, Fisk NM, Rodeck CH, Beachum J: Fetal urine biochemistry: An index of fetal maturation and dysfunction. Br J Obstet Gynaecol 99:46–50, 1992.

22. Lipitz S, Ryan G, Samuell C, et al: Fetal urine analysis for the assessment of renal function in obstructive uropathy. Am J Obstet Gynecol 168:174–179, 1993.

23. Nicolini U, Tannirandorn Y, Vaughan J, et al: Further predictors of renal dysplasia in fetal obstructive uropathy: Bladder pressure and biochemistry of fresh urine. Prenat Diagn 11:159–166, 1991.

24. Evans MI, Sacks AJ, Johnson MP, et al: Sequential invasive assessment of fetal renal function and intrauterine treatment of fetal obstructive uropathies. Obstet Gynecol 77:54–55, 1991.

25. Bewley S, Rodeck CH: Fetal intervention: In Thomas DFM (ed): Urological Disease in the Fetus and Infant: Diagnosis and Management. New York: Butterworth Heinmann, 1997, pp 96–114.

26. Harrison MR, Golbus MS, Filly RA, et al: Management of the fetus with congenital hydronephrosis. J Pediatr Surg 17:728–742, 1982.

27. Watson WJ, Munson DP, Christensen MW: Bilateral fetal chylothorax: Results of unilateral in utero therapy. Am J Perinatol 13:115–117, 1996.

28. Keeling JW, Gough DJ, Iliff PJ: The pathology of non-rhesus hydrops. Diagn Histopathol 6:89–111, 1983.

29. Rodeck CH, Fisk NM, Fraser DI, Nicolini U: Long-term in utero drainage of fetal hydrothorax. N Engl J Med 319:1135–1138, 1988.

30. Nicolaides KH, Azar GB: Thoraco-amniotic shunting. Fetal Diagn Ther 5:153–164, 1990.

31. Chernick V, Reed MH: Pneumothorax and chylothorax in the neonatal period. J Pediatr 76:624–632, 1970.

32. Adzick NS, Harrison MR: Management of the fetus with cystic adenomatoid malformation. World J Surg 17:342–349, 1993.

33. Petres RE, Redwine FO, Cruickshank DP: Congenital bilateral chylothorax. Antepartum diagnosis and successful intrauterine surgical management. JAMA 248:1360–1361, 1982.

34. Benacerraf BR, Frigoletto FD: Mid trimester fetal thoracocentesis. J Clin Ultrasound 13:202–204, 1985.

35. Jauniaux E: Diagnosis and management of early non-immune hydrops fetalis. Prenat Diagn 17:1261–1268, 1997.

36. Lien JM, Colmorgan GHC, Gehret JF, Evantash AB: Spontaneous resolution of fetal pleural effusion diagnosed during the second trimester. J Clin Ultrasound 18:54–56, 1990.

37. Jaffe R, Di Segni E, Altaras M, et al: Ultrasonic real-time diagnosis of transitory fetal pleural and pericardial effusions. Diagn Imag Clin Med 55:373–375, 1986.

38. Pettersen HN, Nicolaides KH: In Fisk MN, Moise KJ (eds): Fetal Therapy: Invasive and Transplacental. Cambridge: Cambridge University Press, 1997, pp 261–272.

39. Schmidt W, Harms F, Wolf D: Successful prenatal treatment of non-immune hydrops fetalis due to congenital chylothorax. Br J Obstet Gynaecol 92:686–687, 1985.

40. Pijpers L, Reuss A, Stewart PA, Wladimiroff JW: Noninvasive management of isolated bilateral hydrothorax. Am J Obstet Gynecol 161:330–332, 1989.

41. Holzgreve W, Evans MI: Nonvascular needle and shunt placements for fetal therapy. West J Med 159:333–340, 1993.

42. Vintzileos AM, Ingardia CJ, Nochimson DJ: Congenital hydrocephalus: A review and protocol for perinatal management. Obstet Gynecol 62:539–549, 1983.

43. Clewell WH, Johnson ML, Meier PR: A surgical approach to the treatment of the fetal hydrocephalus. N Engl J Med 306:1320–1325, 1982.

44. Giannakoulopoulos X, Sepulveda W, Kourlis P, et al: Fetal plasma cortisol and B endorphin response to intrauterine needling. Lancet 344:77–81, 1994.

45. Rodeck CH, Nicolaides KH: Ultrasound guided invasive procedures in obstetrics. Clin Obstet Gynecol 10:515–540, 1983.

46. Elder JS, Duckett JW, Synder HM: Intervention for fetal obstructive uropathy: Has it been effective. Lancet i:1007–1010, 1987.

47. Ronderos-Dumit D, Nicolini U, Vaughan J, et al: Uterine-peritoneal amniotic fluid leakage; an unusual complication of intrauterine shunting. Obstet Gynecol 78:913–915, 1991.

48. Robichaux AG III, Mandell J, Greene MF, et al: Fetal abdominal wall defects. A new complication of vesico-amniotic shunting. Fetal Diagn Ther 6:11–13, 1991.

49. Lewis KM, Pinckert TL, Cain MP, Ghidini A: Complications of intrauterine placement of a vesicoamniotic shunt. Obstet Gynecol 91:825–827, 1998.

50. Thompson PJ, Greenough A, Nicolaides KH: Respiratory function in infancy following pleuro-amniotic shunting. Fetal Diagn Ther 8:79–83, 1993.

51. Harrison MR, Adzick NS, Flake AW: Prenatal management of the fetus with a correctable defect. In Callen PW (ed): Ultrasonography in Obstetrics and Gynaecology, 3rd ed: Philadelphia: WB Saunders Company 1994, pp 536–547.

52. Evans MRI, Drugan A, Manning FA, Harrison MR: Fetal surgery in the 1990's. Am J Dis Child 143:1431–1436, 1989.

53. MacMahon RA, Renou PM, Shekelton PA, Paterson PJ: In utero cystotomy. Lancet 340:1234, 1992.

54. Quintero RA, Hume R, Smith C, et al: Percutaneous fetal cystoscopy and endoscopic fulguration of posterior urethral valves. Am J Obstet Gynecol 172:206, 1995.

55. Foxall PJD, Bewley S, Rodeck CH, et al: High resolution NMR spectroscopic measurements of fetal urine: A novel method to monitor renal abnormalities in utero. J Am Soc Nephrol 3:468, 1992.

CHAPTER *14*

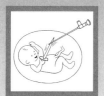

Percutaneous Fetoscopically Guided Intervention

RUBÉN A. QUINTERO and WALTER J. MORALES

T he treatment of congenital anomalies in utero is still viewed as a somewhat utopic or fantastic task given the obstacles posed by the intrauterine location of the fetus. Behind this view stands the feeling of lack of control of the uterine activity and the relative lack of understanding of the mechanisms responsible for the preservation of intact fetal membranes. Indeed, trauma to the uterus is always surrounded by the fear of initiating labor or causing fetal demise. From a historical perspective, this situation is perhaps not too dissimilar to the preantibiotic era in surgery, when infection was a poorly understood and difficult-to-manage complication, and surgical outcome was in part due to skill, speed, and good luck. Thus, minimization of uterine trauma or control of uterine activity is to fetal surgery what control of infection was for general surgery.

Despite the limitations posed by the intrauterine location of the fetus, great strides have been made in the diagnosis of medically and surgically correctable fetal conditions with advances in ultrasound technology, in particular, as well as in reproductive genetics, pathology, and microbiology. As a result, the view of the unhealthy fetus has changed steadily from a distant ailing being to a closer, albeit still relatively inaccessible, patient.

Due to the lack of control of all of the surgical variables, the decision to treat the fetus hinges on a fine balance between the potential risks or benefits to both the fetus and the mother. For example, therapy is indicated in conditions that may result in fetal demise or severe handicap, such as twin–twin transfusion syndrome or select cases of acardiac twins or fetal lower obstructive uropathy, as long as the risks to the mother can be minimized. On the other hand, therapy is not warranted in transient or insignificant fetal disorders, or when the risks to the mother are considered excessive. At the crux of this decision process lies the knowledge of the so-called natural history of the disease. Indeed, knowledge of the in utero and postnatal course of a particular fetal disease helps determine the indication for therapy and the timing of the intervention. In addition to these general concepts, objective diagnostic and prognostic criteria are used within each set of conditions to select those fetuses who would clearly benefit from prenatal intervention. In some disorders, such as twin–twin transfusion syndrome (TTTS), the selection is more easily established once the diagnosis is made. In others, such as lower obstructive uropathy, a complex preoperative work-up is needed before fetal therapy is offered.[1]

Although transplacental medical therapy can be used to treat certain fetal disorders, most conditions require direct access to the fetus. It is here where the concept of least disrupting the uterus and membranes is paramount if loss of the pregnancy is to be avoided. Ultrasound-guided percutaneous needling of the umbilical cord for the treatment of fetal anemia and vesicoamniotic or pleuroamniotic shunting adhere to this concept. By way of their simpler nature and ready availability, these forms of fetal therapy have gained the most popularity. On the other hand, complex fetal anomalies may require more complicated surgical tasks, for which a more express access to the fetus (i.e., open fetal surgery) may be required.

Many of the concepts in fetal surgery stem from the work in open fetal surgery.[2] Among the most significant are the role of healing within the amniotic cavity[3] and the importance of preserving uterine quiescence and membrane integrity. Of interest, however, extrapolation of experimental animal work to human clinical experiences met with important differences in terms of uterine behavior. Thus, whereas the uterus of the pregnant ewe is relatively thin and tolerant of surgical injury, the uterus of human and nonhuman primates is thicker and responds vehemently to injury. Thus, the "unforgiving" nature of the human uterus to the insult of the scalpel has limited the scope and acceptability of this approach for human work.

As revolutionary as ultrasound has been to obstetrics, so has endoscopy been to all surgical fields. The impact of this technology is increasingly greater, reaching specialties like dermatology where a virtual cavity to place the endoscope does not even exist. The fundamental principle of endoscopic surgery is to accomplish a similar surgical task as with open surgery (e.g., a hysterectomy), but through a minimal skin incision and with

199

lesser morbidity. Indeed, the size of the skin incision is a major determinant of morbidity in surgery. Given the above considerations about the implications of surgical trauma to the uterus, it is only logical to conclude that an endoscopic approach to fetal surgery would be more likely to be tolerated by the human myometrium. In parallel to operative laparoscopy, we have called this new approach operative fetoscopy.[4, 5]

Development of Operative Fetoscopy

Given the unique physiologic and anatomic characteristics of the intrauterine environment, the development of operative fetoscopy amounts almost to the development of a whole new surgical field. Indeed, surgery within the amniotic fluid, the access to the amniotic cavity, the operating instruments, and the specific surgical techniques for each particular fetal condition, all constitute areas that require much research and development. In addition to these inherent problems, the new challenges posed by a changing health care system add to the difficulties in making progress in this new surgical field.

Imaging

One of the most unique and distinctive characteristics of operative fetoscopy is the combined and often simultaneous use of two imaging modalities (i.e., ultrasound and endoscopy). Ultrasound provides a panoramic view of the placenta, the amniotic cavity, and the fetus so that the surgical instruments can be placed safely inside the cavity. The delivery of the instruments to the specific intrauterine target is also aided by the wider span of view of ultrasound. Ultrasound also serves an intraoperative monitoring role, allowing assessment of the fetal heart rate and aiding in the assessment of complications such as bleeding and subchorionic membrane dissection. Endoscopy provides a detailed view of the surgical target that is beyond the resolution of ultrasound, allowing the performance of delicate surgical tasks at high magnification. Because both ultrasound and endoscopy are essential for surgery, expertise with both imaging modalities is necessary.

Access

The maximum diameter of the instrument that can be safely used in operative fetoscopy has not been determined. From clinical experience, most surgeries can be accomplished without complications with instruments with a diameter of 3 mm or less. Occasionally, 5-mm instruments may also be used, but the risk of uterine bleeding or rupture of the membranes may be higher.[6] The small caliber of the instruments used allows them to be inserted percutaneously into the amniotic cavity. This procedure is not too dissimilar to an amniocentesis or cordocentesis, although a minimal skin incision (1 to 2 mm) with the scalpel is required. The tip of the trocar must be very sharp to penetrate the uterine wall and membranes swiftly, avoiding dragging or dissection of the membranes. Depending on the type of surgery, one to three trocars may be required, but usually not more than two. Upon completion of the surgery, the trocars are removed and the entry site is monitored with ultrasound for any evidence of bleeding. Leakage of fluid around the membranes or through the skin is not typical, such that no special sealing or suturing is required. The trocars can also be inserted via a minilaparotomy, although this technique is not commonly favored.

There are no trocars designed specifically for operative fetoscopy. Currently available trocars for adult or pediatric laparoscopy are usually 5 mm in inner diameter (6 to 7 mm outer diameter). We have developed special 2- to 3-mm trocars in varying lengths. A check-flow valve at the hub of the trocar prevents amniotic fluid leakage. In addition, a plastic side arm with a valve allows the infusion of fluid or removal of amniotic fluid as desired. Recently, 3-mm trocars have been developed for office laparoscopy. These trocars are within the range of the diameter that can be used safely in the pregnant human uterus.

The Working Environment: Fluid or Gas

Standard laparoscopy uses gas as a distention medium. Ideally, fetal surgery within a gas medium would have several advantages over the liquid environment of the amniotic fluid. Indeed, the techniques used in laparoscopy would be more easily extrapolated, without the need to learn new ones. Visualization would be better, as it is superior within gas over that under fluid, particularly if the amniotic fluid cavity is turbid or if intra-amniotic bleeding has occurred. Lastly, electrosurgery, CO_2 laser, and other laparoscopic tools could be used. Unfortunately, fetuses have been shown to develop acidosis when exposed to a CO_2/fluid medium in an experimental model.[7] In addition, gas does not allow adequate transmission of ultrasound, which is an essential tool in operative fetoscopy. Therefore, operating within a fluid environment appears to be necessary, demanding a unique set of adaptations needed to operate within this medium.

Visualization

The amniotic cavity is typically turbid, particularly with advancing gestational age. Visualization may be further hindered by bloody discoloration from previous procedures such as amniocentesis or cordocentesis, from intra-amniotic bleeding during surgery, or from excessive vernix. Because of this, objects more than 2 cm away typically cannot be seen. To overcome this limitation, we have developed techniques to exchange the amniotic fluid for Ringer's lactate or 0.9 saline solution and thus provide an improved medium for visualization. A suction/irrigation pump with manual pressure calibration is attached to a side port of the trocar. If two trocars are being used, different ports are preferred for irrigation and suction. The system can exchange the amniotic fluid at a maximum rate of 2,250 mL/min without altering the total amniotic fluid volume.

If intraoperative bleeding occurs prior to any fluid exchange, the blood clots rapidly and does not mix readily with the amniotic fluid. However, if the fluid has been exchanged, mixing of blood with fluid occurs quickly and the visualization is rapidly impaired. Therefore, under certain circumstances, we prefer not to exchange the amniotic fluid if minor bleeding occurs. This allows the blood to clot momentarily, while we complete the particular surgical task.

Endoscopes

There are no endoscopes specifically designed for fetoscopic surgery at the present time. Table 14–1 shows a classification of available endoscopes according to their characteristics. From experience, we have determined that different endoscopes need to be available for any given procedure. Whenever possible, the smallest endoscope is always chosen. For diagnostic procedures we prefer to use either a 0.7-mm flexible endoscope (Intramed Laboratories, San Diego, CA), or a 1.9-mm rigid scope (Richard Wolf Inc, Vernon Hills, IL), but we have used endoscopes as large as 5 mm. Normally, we use 2.4- to 2.7-mm endoscopes, which fit within the 3-mm trocars. Diagnostic endoscopes of this caliber provide an excellent view of the intrauterine contents. Operating endoscopes of similar size are associated with less resolution, as they need to accommodate both an optic component and a channel through which instruments are inserted. Therefore, we often combine operating and diagnostic endoscopes during the same procedure, taking advantage of the improved resolution of the diagnostic endoscope and of the working channel of the operating endoscope.

The length of the endoscope is also important. It must be longer than the trocars, so that it can reach the amniotic cavity, and preferably be able to span the whole length of the amniotic cavity. This is particularly important if the fetus changes position during surgery. Our current endoscopes are 18 cm in length. However, 30-cm endoscopes are sometimes useful in patients with difficult access, severe polyhydramnios, or marked obesity. Figure 14–1 shows some of the endoscopes we currently use.

Surgical Instruments

As with the endoscopes, there are currently no given set of instruments specifically designed for operative

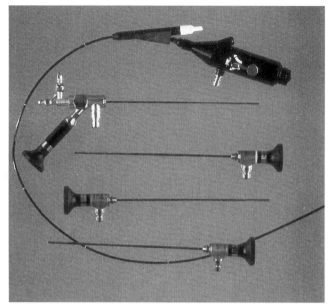

FIGURE 14–1. Endoscopes used in operative fetoscopy. The rigid diagnostic endoscopes have different angles of view to allow better visualization of difficult targets. The operating endoscopes have an off-set eyepiece that allows laser fibers and other instruments to be passed more easily.

fetoscopy. Therefore, a significant amount of research time is devoted to either identifying available products that can be adapted to this type of surgery or in actually designing them. Unfortunately, only a small selection of instruments at or below the 3-mm range are currently available. If the instruments are 1 mm or less in diameter, they can be introduced through the working channel of some endoscopes (operating endoscopes). Figure 14–2 shows some of the instruments we currently use.

Pressure/Volume Regulation

The amniotic fluid pressure rises linearly by 1 mm Hg/L of physiologic fluid infused.[8] This is typically of no clinical significance in operative fetoscopy, as the amount of fluid infused rarely reaches 1,000 mL without being exchanged. An even exchange of amniotic fluid diminishes the likelihood of significant pressure changes. We maintain a normal amount of amniotic fluid, unless it is abnormally high or low to begin with. We have not noticed significant pressure variations (1 to 2 mm Hg) during surgery. Therefore, we measure the amniotic pressure at the beginning and at the end of surgery. We have noticed that the intra-amniotic pressure may vary even under general anesthesia, particularly if uterine contractions occur. As we typically do not administer tocolytic agents during surgery, uterine contractions may alter the pressure readings.

Safety

Before the current development of operative fetoscopy, data regarding pregnancy loss was limited to a few

T A B L E 14–1. GENERAL CHARACTERISTICS OF AVAILABLE ENDOSCOPES

CONSTITUTION	CONSISTENCY	FUNCTION	MANEUVERABILITY
Fiberoptic	Flexible	Diagnostic	Passive
Solid rod lens	Rigid	Operating	Steerable
Multilens			

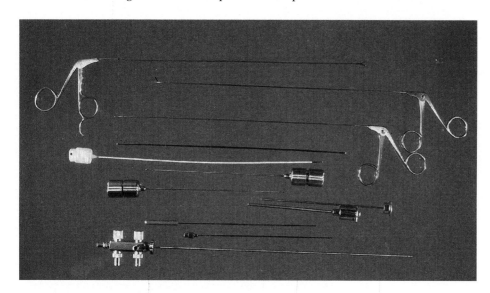

FIGURE 14–2. Surgical instruments used in operative fetoscopy. Most instruments are 5 Fr in diameter, or approximately 1.6 mm. Larger instruments (e.g., 3 mm) can also be used through the current trocars. The thinness of the instruments requires that the trocar through which they are inserted be manipulated with another hand, to avoid bending of the shaft.

series with fetoscopy in ongoing pregnancies. Hobbins and Mahoney reported 2 losses among 65 patients (3%) in continuing pregnancies.[9] They used an endoscope of 1.7 mm in diameter inserted transabdominally through a 2.2 × 2.7-mm cannula in patients at risk for hemoglobinopathies and other genetic disorders. Rodeck, using a similar endoscope, had a 3.7% pregnancy loss rate among 108 patients who underwent transabdominal fetoscopy for fetal blood sampling, skin biopsy, or evaluation for suspected anomalies.[10] An additional 37 patients underwent pregnancy termination based on the results of the examination. From these data a 3.0 to 3.7% corrected pregnancy loss rate is quoted for transabdominal fetoscopy.

Approximately 5 to 7% of patients in the above-mentioned series experienced amniotic fluid leakage, though the majority had a successful outcome. By comparison, second-trimester amniocentesis is associated with a 0.5 to 1% risk of pregnancy loss, probably reflective of the use of a smaller bore instrument. Within amniocenteses series, a statistically significant difference in the pregnancy loss rate occurs when an 18-gauge or wider needle is used. It is relatively safe to conclude that wider instruments are more likely to be associated with an increased rate of pregnancy loss. Therefore, we have not insisted on using trocars beyond 3 mm in diameter.

Concern about the possibility of injury to the visual pathways has existed since the inception of fetoscopy. We have shown in both chick and rat embryos that the use of endoscopic white light does not affect the developing retina or alter neurotransmission to the colliculi.[11] In addition, behavioral studies in the chick embryo also suggest lack of visual impairment after intense exposure during embryonic life. On the other hand, there are data to suggest that prolonged exposure to light may indeed be harmful.[12, 13] We conclude, therefore, that exposure to endoscopic white light, under the current working conditions, is unlikely to harm the developing visual pathways.

Tocolysis

In contrast to the experience with open fetal surgery, tocolysis is not a major issue in operative fetoscopy. Uterine contractions may occur during surgery despite general anesthesia, and become more organized within 1 to 3 hours after surgery. However, these are usually mild in character and are typically not uncomfortable. Nonetheless, we institute intravenous tocolysis with magnesium sulfate with a loading dose of 4 g followed by 2 g/hr. Indomethacin may also be used except in cases associated with poor fetal renal perfusion. Tocolysis is usually discontinued within 12 to 16 hours. Double intravenous tocolytic agents, central line placement, or more aggressive tocolytic therapy is not required. Patients are discharged home with oral tocolytics for 1 week prophylactically. Readmission for uterine contractions has not occurred.

Antibiotic Therapy

As infection may complicate any invasive intrauterine procedure, we cover all cases with antibiotics. Coverage is aimed at skin pathogens, mainly *Staphylococcus aureus*. However, gram-negative coverage is also added. Our typical regimen involves the use of a cephalosporin and an aminoglycoside. The antibiotics are begun prior to incision and continued for 24 hours. Patients are discharged on prophylactic oral antibiotic therapy for 1 week. Readmission for chorioamnionitis has not been a common complication. In our series, only 4 of 97 cases have had chorioamnionitis within 3 weeks of the procedure.

Anesthesia

Given the small diameter of the instruments used, the procedures can be performed under local or regional anesthesia with intravenous sedation. In these cases, paralysis of the fetus(es) may be necessary to avoid interference with the procedure or potential harm to the fetus(es). This can be accomplished by an intramuscular percutaneous injection of a muscle-blocking agent such as pancuronium bromide under ultrasound guidance. Extensive diaphragmatic excursion during spontaneous maternal breathing can be disruptive during the procedure. This will typically occur during sedation. Because of this and to avoid the need to paralyze the fetus(es), we prefer to do our procedures under general anesthesia. The level of anesthesia used is gauged by maternal response as well as by our monitoring of fetal movements. In cases where intubation is considered difficult, surgery is done under regional or local anesthesia. In 97 cases we have only had one mild complication from general anesthesia in a patient with unknown acetylcholinesterase deficiency, which delayed extubation for another hour after surgery.

Complications

Bleeding

Bleeding may complicate surgery at any time. The bleeding may originate from the uterine wall or the placenta. Bleeding from the uterine wall is identified with ultrasound as streaming into the amniotic cavity. The initial trocar insertion is the moment of highest risk and dictates the course of the surgery. If bleeding occurs at this point the degree of difficulty of the procedure is increased severalfold. If the source of bleeding is the uterine wall we increase the left lateral tilt on the table to decrease venous stasis within the myometrium. This usually solves the problem. In some instances, however, the trocar needs to be removed and either reinserted elsewhere or the surgical strategy changed. Rarely, a laparotomy is required to place a suture on the myometrium.

During the initial insertion the placenta is always avoided. This is done because, even if bleeding does not occur when initially traversing it, movement of the trocar during surgery will usually bring about this complication. Therefore, a placenta-free area is always sought. However, even in cases with a posterior placenta, bleeding from the uterine wall may occur.

Bleeding may also occur from placental vessels during laser photocoagulation. In these cases photocoagulation in front and behind the vessel defect may control the problem. However, visualization may be quickly obscured and the surgery may need to be interrupted.

Bleeding from the uterine wall may also result in membrane dissection. This is the most dreaded complication of this type of surgery as it can result in rupture of membranes and pregnancy loss. When the bleeding is confined to the amniotic cavity, the fluid clears within 2 to 4 weeks.

In our series, bleeding has been significant enough to interrupt the surgery in 4 of 97 cases. In three of them, bleeding was from the uterine wall and minilaparotomy was required. The bleeding stopped spontaneously in 2 cases and a suture on the myometrium was not required, whereas in the other the bleeding stopped with a stitch of 0-chromic. In one case, bleeding occurred during laser photocoagulation of communicating vessels for twin–twin transfusion syndrome, and the surgery was stopped. The patient was brought back to surgery a week later to complete the procedure, and the pregnancy progressed well thereafter.

Rupture of Membranes

Rupture of membranes within 3 weeks of the procedure is usually ascribed to the surgery. This may present in the form of gross rupture or insidious amniotic fluid leakage. The etiology of the rupture may be apparent in some cases, particularly if membrane dissection has occurred. In other cases, chorioamnionitis may also be present and explain the complication. In other cases, other than the surgery the explanation is not apparent. We have had 10 of 97 patients with rupture of membranes within 3 weeks of surgery.

There are a number of potential risk factors for the occurrence of premature rupture of membranes (PROM). The size of the trocars, the number of trocars used, the duration of surgery, and any intraoperative complications may all be risk factors. In our series, uterine contractions with or without cervical changes prior to surgery has been the most important risk factor for this complication.

Clinical Applications

Acardiac Twins

Twin reverse arterial perfusion (TRAP) sequence affects 1% of monozygotic twins or 1 in 35,000 births or 1 in 30 triplets. The proposed pathophysiology for this condition is that in the presence of artery-to-artery and vein-to-vein anastomoses in a monozygotic placenta, a hemodynamically advantaged twin (pump twin) perfuses the other twin (perfused twin) via retrograde flow. Inadequate perfusion of the recipient twin is responsible for the development of a characteristic and invariably lethal set of anomalies including acardia and acephalus. The diagnosis of acardiac twin is made by pulsed and color Doppler by demonstrating arterial blood flow perfusing the acardiac twin in a retrograde fashion. Typically, the pump twin is structurally normal, but it is at risk for developing in utero cardiac failure, and without treatment dies in 50 to 75% of cases, particularly if the acardiac/pump twin size ratio is greater than 50%. Subtle signs of hemodynamic decompensation in the pump twin include enlarged right atrium, increased reverse flow in the inferior vena cava, reverse flow in the ductus venosus, or pulsatile flow in the umbilical vein, all of which may occur prior to the appearance of ascites and edema.

The therapeutic goal of interrupting the vascular communication between the two twins, although simple in concept, had been difficult to accomplish. Methods previously employed have included removal of the anomalous twin, or sectio parva, whereby the abnormal fetus is selectively delivered. Sectio parva requires a hysterotomy and a subsequent cesarean section, and has been associated with abruptio placentae, preterm labor, preterm birth, and prolonged maternal hospitalization. Ultrasound-directed percutaneous thrombosis of the umbilical cord of the acardiac twin by the intra-arterial injection of either thrombogenic coils or fibrin superglue in the umbilical cord of the perfused twin circulation has also been tried. Unfortunately, although technically easier, these techniques have been associated with death of both twins and recanalization of the umbilical arterial flow after the procedure.

We have developed a minimally invasive operative technique to tie off the umbilical cord of the acardiac twin, or umbilical-cord ligation (UCL).[5] One or two 2- to 3-mm ports are introduced percutaneously into the amniotic cavity under ultrasound guidance. The use of ultrasound is essential in identifying the correct cord to ligate, as well as placental-free areas through which the trocars can be placed. An endoscope is delivered intra-amniotically to monitor the surgical procedure. Through the other port, a 3-0 Vicryl suture is passed with a small grasper beneath the umbilical cord (Fig. 14–3). The suture is grasped on the opposite side of the cord and retrieved outside of the maternal abdomen through the same operating port. Thus, a loop has been created around the cord with a single instrument. A simple extracorporeal knot is tied and delivered intra-amniotically with a custom-designed knot pusher to occlude the cord. The procedure is repeated for safety, and the suture is cut with small scissors inside the amniotic cavity. In selected cases, the procedure can be performed under ultrasound guidance alone, which limits the number of ports to one. As the acardiac twin usually lacks any amniotic fluid, access to the umbilical cord may be hindered by the dividing membrane. An amni-

oinfusion or amniorrhexis of this sac needs to be performed in order to reach the umbilical cord.

As of May 1998, we have performed umbilical-cord ligation in 25 patients with an acardiac twin in previable pregnancies. The technical success rate (i.e., the ability to ligate the cord) is 76%. The overall fetal survival rate is 60%. No adverse effects of the ligation have been seen in the pump twin, as gauged clinically and with Doppler studies.[15] The average gestational age at delivery is 33 weeks, with 75% of patients having delivered beyond 30 weeks.

Thirty-six percent of successfully ligated cases of acardiac twins have been complicated by remote intrauterine demise of the pump twin approximately 3 to 10 weeks after the procedure. In at least half of these cases cord entanglement was identified as the probable cause of death. Because of this, we have recently modified our ligation technique by placing two or three knots in the umbilical cord and transecting the cord between two knots (umbilical cord ligation and transection) (UCL&T).[16] Using this modification, eight of nine fetuses have survived, with an average gestational age of 34 weeks, and all but one case delivering after 30 weeks. The transected umbilical cord avoids the possibility of cord entanglement and demise of the pump twin from this cause.

Endoscopic umbilical cord ligation is the first endoscopic surgical procedure to be performed in a human pregnancy using more than one port. It exemplifies many of the concepts developed by us to perform operative fetoscopy, including the combined use of ultrasound, videomixer, amnioinfusion, suture material, and specialized instruments as previously described.

Twin–Twin Transfusion Syndrome (TTTS)

TTTS appears to result from a net unbalanced flow of blood between two fetuses in a monochorionic gestation. In the classic model, an artery from one twin supplies a placental cotyledon, which in turn is drained by a vein to the co-twin. Thus, blood is shunted from one twin (the donor) and transfused to the co-twin (the recipient) through placental vascular anastomoses. Vascular anastomoses are almost universally present in monochorionic placentas. These anastomoses are commonly of the arterioarterial type, but sometimes venous anastomoses can also be found. The anastomoses can be superficial, deep, or both superficial and deep. The most common superficial types are artery-to-artery (28%) in conjunction with vein-to-vein anastomoses (28%), followed by arteriovenous anastomoses (11%). An average of 3.1 anastomosis per placenta are present in each twin pair.[17] Despite the high frequency of occurrence of vascular anastomoses in monochorionic placentation, TTTS occurs only in 5.5 to 17.5% of monochorionic gestations.

Expectant or medical management of TTTS has been associated with a virtually 100% perinatal mortality.[18] Invasive treatment options include serial amniocentesis, coagulation of surface placental vessels, selective feticide, or selective fetectomy. Serial amniocentesis of the sac of the recipient twin (polyhydramnios) has been

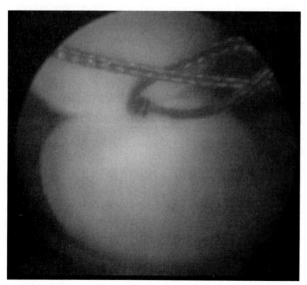

FIGURE 14–3. Umbilical-cord ligation under endoscopic guidance. The suture has been passed beneath the umbilical cord and is being grasped around it. The suture is retrieved outside the maternal abdomen where an extracorporeal knot is tied. The knot is delivered to the umbilical cord with a custom-designed knot pusher.

associated with an overall 50 to 60% survival rate. However, despite initial enthusiasm, support for this approach has dwindled somewhat. Additional risks reported with this technique include infection, rupture of membranes, and extra-amniotic fluid collections with disruption of the membranes. More significantly, death of one of the twins has been associated with significant morbidity of the surviving twin, including the appearance of porencephalic cysts and other major neurologic complications in approximately 15 to 36% of cases.[19, 20] Originally, these complications were thought to result from the release of thromboplastic substances from the dead twin into the surviving twin. More recently, however, acute anemia has been documented in the surviving twin, suggesting that perhaps hypotension from acute bleeding into the dead twin may be responsible for the observed complications.

Laser photocoagulation (LPC) of the vascular anastomoses has been advocated by several authors. In this technique, the purported culprit vessels are photocoagulated using yttrium-aluminum-garnet (YAG) laser via a fiber passed through an operating endoscope (Fig. 14–4). As arteries cross over veins on the surface of the placenta, the nature of the vessels can be determined endoscopically. In addition, vessels identified as crossing from one placental territory to the other beneath the dividing membrane may correspond to abnormal sharing of a cotyledon. Outcomes using LPC for TTTS have been slightly better than those reported with serial amniocentesis, with an overall success rate from 52 to 70% of at least one surviving fetus. Most importantly, the reported incidence of neurologic complications is only 4% compared to 25% for serial amniocentesis.[21]

We have had 32 patients referred for TTTS of which 24 underwent LPC. The remaining eight patients underwent umbilical-cord ligation for severe fetal hydrops.

Table 14–2 shows our clinical data. In the first 17 cases, LPC was performed using the technique described by Ville et al. (group I). In the last seven cases, we have modified the technique to include only a selective number of vessels. The vessels are identified endoscopically through a systematic evaluation of their placental course while using the dividing membrane as a reference point only. We have named this technique "selective laser photocoagulation of communicating vessels" (S-LPC) (group II).

The mean gestational age at the time of surgery was no different between the two groups (21.38 vs. 21.85, $p = 0.6$). The mean gestational age at delivery was 28.4 weeks for group I, and 30.7 weeks for group II, a difference that was not statistically significant ($p = 0.24$). Although the survival rates between the two groups is not yet statistically different, there is a trend for a better outcome with S-LPC, both in the total number of successful pregnancies (chi square = 4.1, DF = 2, $p = 0.063$, one-tailed test) as well as in the total number of fetuses (chi square = 4.3, DF = 2, $p = 0.059$, one-tailed test). Approximately 54 pregnancies would be necessary to show a significant difference in the number of successful pregnancies, with a power of 0.80. Only 19 pregnancies would be required to show an improved outcome in total number of fetuses.

Evidence of the effectiveness of S-LPC can be seen shortly following surgery. On the first postoperative day, it is possible to see the bladder of the donor twin and accumulation of a small amount of amniotic fluid within its sac. By postoperative days 5 to 7, the amniotic fluid volume is normal in the donor twin's sac. It is important to point out that normalization of the amniotic fluid volume without bladder filling in the donor twin cannot be interpreted as evidence of surgical success, as unintentional breaching of the dividing membrane

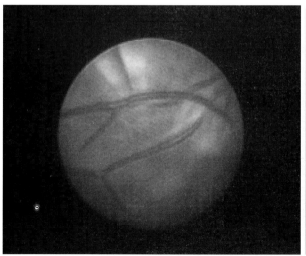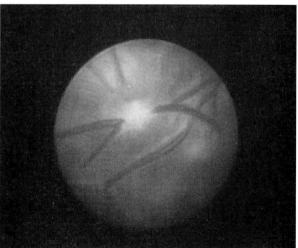

FIGURE 14–4. Laser photocoagulation of placental anastomoses in twin–twin transfusion syndrome. The communicating vessels are first identified with the diagnostic endoscope. The operating endoscope is used to deliver a 400-μm fiber with which the vessels are coagulated using 20 to 40 w.

TABLE 14–2. CLINICAL CHARACTERISTICS OF PATIENTS TREATED WITH LASER PHOTOCOAGULATION FOR TWIN–TWIN TRANSFUSION SYNDROME

CASE	GA DX	GA DEL	ALIVE D	ALIVE R	WEIGHT D	WEIGHT R	HYDROPS	PLACENTA
1	16	35	iufd	y		1,882	n/n	a
2	24	28	iufd	iufd			n/y	a
3	23	30	y	y	1,021	1,191	n/y	a
4	21	37	y	y	2,382	2,948	n/n	p
5	25	27	nnd	nnd	750	920	y/y	f
6	26	30	nnd	y	907	1,673	n/y	p
7	21	26	iufd	nnd	750	900	n/y	f
8	15.5	29	iufd*	y		652	n/n	p
9	24	26	iufd	iufd			n/y	a
10	22	36	y	y	2,268	2,336	n/n	p
11	27	29	y	y	962	1,164	n/n	a
12	20	23	iufd	iufd			n/n	a
13	17	33	y†	y‡			n/n	a/f
14	19	19	iufd	iufd			n/n	a
15	20	20	iufd	iufd			n/n	f
16	23	23	iufd	iufd			n/n	p
17	20	32	y	y	544	1,275	n/n	a
18	24	28	nnd	y	560	1,160	n/n	f
19	17	31	y	y	508	1,769	n/n	p
20	22	36	iufd	y		3,090	n/n	p
21	23	27	y	nnd	667	1,097	n/n	p
22	20	24	nnd	iufd§			n/n	a
23	23	32	y	y	1,644	1,644	n/n	p
24	24	37	y	iufd	2,637	388	n/n	p

* Intrauterine fetal demise from cord entanglement due to involuntary membrane disruption.
† Cerebral palsy.
‡ Hydrocephalus.
§ Intrauterine fetal demise from tight double-knot in the umbilical cord.
GA dx, gestational age at diagnosis; GA del, gestational age at delivery; Alive D, donor alive; Alive R, recipient alive; Weight D, weight of the donor; Weight R, weight of the recipient; Hydrops, hydrops of donor/recipient; Placenta, placental location; a, anterior; f, fundal; p, posterior; iufd, intrauterine fetal demise; nnd, neonatal demise; shaded cells, cases done with S-LPC.

may equilibrate the amniotic fluid volumes without affecting the appearance of the bladder of the fetus.

Figure 14–5 shows our survival data over the study period. The improved survival data, as well as the lack of untoward effect of a single fetal demise, provide preliminary clinical evidence of the effect of S-LPC in treating TTTS.

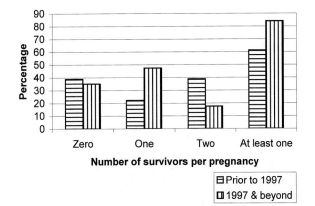

FIGURE 14–5. Survival data over time. The technique used after 1997 involved ablation of selected vessels while using the dividing membrane as an anatomic landmark (S-LPC).

Umbilical Cord Ligation in Twin–Twin Transfusion Syndrome

Selective feticide has also been proposed in severe TTTS. This procedure is only considered when one of the fetuses is deemed nonviable. Criteria for nonviability are based both on gross appearance of the fetus with severe hydrops and extremely poor cardiac contractility, as well as on severely abnormal Doppler findings including pulsatile umbilical-venous flow or absent/reverse flow in the umbilical artery. In this subset of patients, the overall survival rate with LPC is only 37.5% versus 62.5% in the less severe cases. Because of the presence of placental vascular communications, injection of potassium chloride into the cord of this twin may result in the death of both twins. Cardiac tamponade has been successful in one report, but it is unreliable and may carry similar risks as those of potassium chloride injection. In our opinion, umbilical cord ligation represents the best alternative method for selective feticide in this context.

We have performed UCL in eight patients with severe TTTS. Seven of eight fetuses have survived. The same signs of recovery seen after S-LPC are seen with UCL in TTTS. If the cord of the recipient fetus has been ligated, the bladder of the donor fetus can be seen within the next 24 hours, and normalization of the amniotic fluid volume occurs by approximately 5 to 7 days. If the cord of the donor fetus has been ligated, the bladder of the recipient fetus returns to normal size and polyhydramnios does not recur. One fetus died in the newborn period from extreme prematurity. That patient had undergone seven amniodrainage procedures prior to UCL at the referring institution, with gross bloody contamination of the amniotic cavity. All other patients did well and were delivered without complications.

UCL for severe TTTS is not only therapeutic, as it effectively interrupts all possible communications between the fetuses, but it is also of pathophysiologic importance. First, it demonstrates that by eliminating all possible communications between the fetuses, the syndrome disappears. Indeed, by tying off the umbilical cord of one fetus, all possible vascular anastomoses between the fetuses have been closed. As a corollary, there are probably no "beneficial" communications present between monochorionic fetuses that need to be preserved. This observation is at odds with reports suggesting that placental anastomoses may play a compensating role in TTTS, and that elimination of these anastomoses may be deleterious. Our observations with UCL in TTTS do not support this theory. Second, UCL avoids neurologic complications in the surviving fetus. Pathophysiologically, this may be due to the fact that the surviving fetus cannot bleed into the demised co-twin, as blood would only flow to the level of the knot. Therefore, acute fetofetal hemorrhage and hypotension are avoided. Finally, survival rates associated with UCL for severe TTTS may represent the ceiling of the best possible outcome in the surgical management of this disease, with nonsuccessful pregnancies being lost to surgical complications.

Amniotic Band Syndrome

Amniotic band syndrome (ABS) is a sporadic condition that occurs in approximately 1 per 1,200 to 1 per 15,000 live births. Although the exact cause of the syndrome is not known, early rupture of the amnion resulting in bands that insert on the body of the fetus is the most accepted view. The bands may lead to amputations, constrictions, and other deformities of the fetus.

Although some cases of ABS show congenital anomalies beyond surgical repair at the time of diagnosis (e.g., amputations, eccentric encephaloceles), some fetuses may show an isolated constriction of an extremity without amputation. In these cases, it has been speculated that the limb constriction can lead to subsequent amputation or significant functional impairment. Experimental work in sheep has shown that release of the constriction can restore the anatomy and functionality of the limb. However, surgical release of the band has not been previously undertaken in human fetuses. We have recently performed lysis of amniotic bands in two fetuses with constricting bands whose limbs were at risk of becoming amputated.[22] These cases represent the first antenatal experience of surgical treatment of amniotic bands. They also represent the first surgical treatment of a nonlethal birth defect in utero.

Case 1

The patient was a 30-year-old, gravida 2 para 0 at 21 weeks' gestation. The fetus had amniotic bands attached to the face and the left arm. Bilateral cleft lip was present. The left forearm was markedly edematous, with a circumference of 60.1 mm just distal to the elbow, versus 54.5 mm in the right forearm. The left hand was ulnarly deviated and the fingers were abnormally flexed. Arterial blood flow distal to the obstruction was documented with color and pulsed Doppler. Chromosome analysis showed a normal 46,XY complement.

After informed consent, a diagnostic fetoscopy was performed at 22 weeks' gestation under general anesthesia with a 2.7-mm 5-degree diagnostic endoscope (Richard Wolf, Inc, Vernon Hills, IL). Visualization of the left arm showed bands attached to the lower portion of the arm.

Scissors were applied at the level of the constriction and advanced gently into the skin (Fig. 14–6). Closure of the jaws resulted in snapping of the band, with immediate change in the contour of the skin. Follow-up ultrasound showed resolution of the edema within 6 days, with only a minimal indentation of the skin remaining posteriorly. Growth of the ulna and radius was concordant in both arms. The ulnar deviation of the hand and the abnormal flexion also appeared to improve on follow-up ultrasound.

The patient was electively delivered at 39 weeks. Physical exam showed bilateral cleft lip and a type 4 Tessier craniofacial cleft. There was right microphthalmia. The left arm had only minimal scarring posteriorly where the band had been attached. The baby has a functional left arm today.

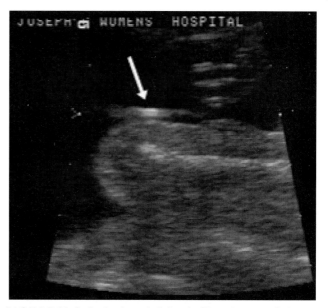

FIGURE 14–6. Lysis of amniotic bands. The scissors are being applied at the lower third of the left arm of the fetus. Closure of the jaws of the scissors produced an immediate release of the constriction evidenced by the change in the contour of the arm. Only one incision on the band was required.

Case 2

The patient was a 29-year-old gravida 2, para 1, referred at 23 weeks' gestation with a thick band constricting the left ankle of the fetus. Marked edema of the ankle and foot was present distal to the constriction (Fig. 14–7). Minimal blood flow in the pedal artery was shown with color and pulsed Doppler. Flexion or extension of the ankle were never documented.

Fetoscopy was performed at 23 weeks' gestation after informed consent. Under general anesthesia, a 2.7-mm 5-degree endoscope was introduced percutaneously into the amniotic cavity under ultrasound guidance. All anatomic landmarks of the left foot were lost due to edema. The foot did not appear necrotic, but was pale. The constriction around the left ankle was such that the bottom of the groove was not visible unless the endoscope was advanced within the groove. The constricting band was lysed using a 400-μm contact YAG-laser fiber. Follow-up ultrasounds showed marked resolution of the ankle edema. Flexion and extension of the ankle were now present and the foot continued to grow normally. The edema of the foot decreased, and the distal arterial blood flow was improved. The patient delivered spontaneously at 34.5 weeks. The baby underwent successful repair of the amniotic band with Z-plasties. The baby has a fully functional left foot.

Fetal Lower Obstructive Uropathy

Fetal lower obstructive uropathy (LOU) occurs sporadically in 1 per 5,000 to 8,000 males. Untreated, the obstruction may lead to hydronephrosis, renal dysplasia, pulmonary hypoplasia, and perinatal death.[23] Most cases of LOU represent severe forms of posterior urethral valves (PUVs), but other conditions such as urethral atresia, prune belly syndrome, may also be responsible for the

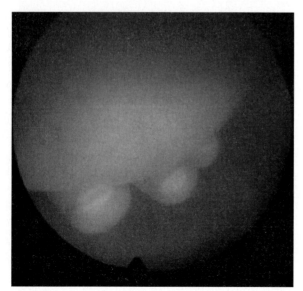

FIGURE 14–7. Marked edema on the dorsal aspect of the foot in a fetus with a constricting ring around the left ankle. Lysis of the band was accomplished endoscopically with YAG laser.

sonographic findings. Ultrasound and fetal vesicocenteses identify those fetuses most likely to benefit from in utero treatment of the urinary tract obstruction. Treatment of fetuses with LOU had thus far been performed with vesicoamniotic shunts or fetal vesicostomy. The goal of deriving the fetal urine from the bladder into the amniotic cavity is to avert the damage to the fetal kidneys that may result from the obstruction, and to prevent pulmonary hypoplasia.

Current surgical procedures for fetuses with LOU have significant limitations. First, they are palliative in nature, deferring the final treatment of the obstruction until after the birth of the child. Second, the incidence of complications of vesicoamniotic shunts—including obstruction, displacement, malfunction, or urinary ascites—is as high as to 40%. This requires replacement of the shunt and increases maternal and fetal morbidity. Third, fetal vesicostomy via open fetal surgery has not gained acceptance due to significant maternal and fetal morbidity (i.e., preterm labor, premature rupture of membranes, in utero fetal demise).

We have recently introduced fetal cystoscopy as part of the evaluation of fetuses with LOU. We have shown that fetal cystoscopy may help establish the correct diagnosis, overcoming the limitations of ultrasound in distinguishing among various possible conditions. In addition to its diagnostic potential, fetal cystoscopy may also allow the introduction of new treatment options for these fetuses. We have placed a urethral catheter in three fetuses with LOU in which PUVs were not thought to be present. The catheter was advanced antegradely from within the fetal bladder. One baby survived and has done well. One baby had megacystis-microcolon and died from the disease. The other pregnancy was voluntarily terminated despite adequate catheter function.

In cases where PUVs are apparent, direct ablation of the valves can be performed[24] (Fig. 14–8). We have performed this surgery in nine patients thought to have PUVs. PUVs were present in six of these nine patients. The urethra was made permeable in five of six patients. Two fetuses survived the neonatal period but died of unrelated complications (necrotizing enterocolitis, pneumonia). Chorioamnionitis was responsible for two losses, and one patient had voluntary interruption of pregnancy due to worsening renal changes. Despite these complications, we are encouraged to know that the obstruction can be eliminated in utero. Improvement in our current techniques should result in successful outcomes.

Chorioangiomas

Chorioangiomas occur in approximately 1% of all microscopically examined placentas. Most tumors are asymptomatic, but large tumors have been associated with polyhydramnios (18 to 35%), oligohydramnios, nonimmune fetal hydrops, cardiomegaly, growth retardation, premature labor (10%), fetal thrombocytopenia, microangiopathic hemolytic anemia, and intrauterine fetal death (16%). Maternal complications include thrombo-

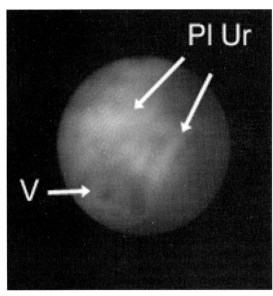

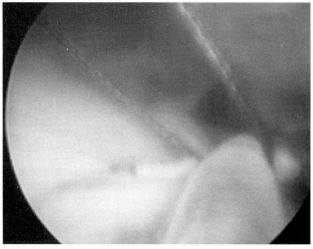

FIGURE 14-8. Endoscopic ablation of posterior urethral valves. The valves are identified anterior to the verumontanum. The plicae urethralis and the verumontanum serve as anatomic landmarks. The valves are ablated with short pulses of YAG laser energy.

FIGURE 14-9. Endoscopic devascularization of a large placental chorioangioma. The arterial blood supply has been identified. The artery has been dissected off the surface of the placenta. A suture has been passed beneath the vessel and is being retrieved outside the amniotic cavity to deliver an extracorporeal knot.

cytopenia, coagulopathy, toxemia, abruptio placentae, fetomaternal transfusion, hemolysis, and hemoglobinuria. Chorioangiomas can be diagnosed with ultrasound as uniform and nonuniform echogenic, multicystic masses, or as complex masses. Color Doppler can be used to confirm the vascular nature of the mass.

Management of patients with chorioangiomas is individualized. Since maternal and fetal complications may lead to premature termination of the pregnancy or to premature birth, serial ultrasound examinations including fetal echocardiography are suggested to determine the optimal time of delivery. Premature labor and acute onset of polyhydramnios may require hospitalization, and the use of tocolytic agents.

Large chorioangiomas are associated with a 30% fetal mortality rate, half of which are due to intrauterine fetal demises.[25] These figures are undoubtedly biased, as bad outcomes are less likely to be reported. Of the available reports, the most frequent cause of death was prematurity, followed by evidence of fetal heart failure or hydrops. Specific risk factors associated with a higher risk of fetal or neonatal death have not been identified, particularly since many diagnoses have been made retrospectively, and standard parameters of evaluation have not been established. Nonetheless, it is fair to say that fetuses with overt signs of failure diagnosed prior to viability constitute the highest risk group, and in whom in utero intervention is more clearly indicated. To date, cordocentesis has been used to manage three patients with chorioangiomas. Two fetuses were transfused and delivered within 24 hours for fetal distress. A third case was managed with serial intrauterine transfusions.

We have had the opportunity to evaluate a patient with a large chorioangioma (9 cm) and a hydropic fetus at 24 weeks' gestation.[26] Color Doppler disclosed a large

artery and vein located subchorionically. Hemodynamic evaluation of the fetus revealed signs of overt heart failure with pulsatile umbilical venous blood flow, enlarged right atrium, and tricuspid regurgitation. Cordocentesis revealed moderate fetal anemia and hypoalbuminemia. The vessels feeding the tumor were too large to be photocoagulated with YAG laser. Fetoscopy was performed at 24 weeks' gestation. Endoscopically, the artery was dissected off of the surface of the placenta, and a suture was placed around this vessel (Fig. 14-9). Remaining vessels were obliterated with bipolar electrocautery. Unfortunately, the fetus died 3 days later from hydrops. We speculate that perhaps with earlier intervention the fetus may have survived. Additionally, these fetuses may require pre- or postsurgical intravascular transfusions to correct the hematologic derangements associated with the disease.

Limitations of Operative Fetoscopy

Table 14-3 shows the limitations that we have identified in performing operative fetoscopy. The need for better instrumentation cannot be overemphasized. As no specific instruments are available for operative fetoscopy, this statement is even more relevant, and should stress

TABLE 14-3. LIMITATIONS OF OPERATIVE FETOSCOPY

Placental location
Access
Visualization
Instruments
Fetal position
Premature rupture of membranes

the need to continue to develop the necessary tools for this type of surgery.

Fetal position may be particularly limiting, and techniques to correct it are not available. Occasionally, external maneuvers may change the position of the fetus in the uterus, but these may not be effective or reliable. We have attempted to correct the fetal position from within the amniotic cavity with limited success. Further efforts to address this issue are being pursued.

The location of the placenta may also hinder the performance of operative fetoscopy. In open fetal surgery, if the placenta is anterior, the uterus is entered posteriorly. Although this technique is significantly more involved, it could be considered for operative fetoscopy in selected cases as well. Thus far, we have been able to avoid entering the placenta in most cases; however, we have had one instance in which no space free of placenta could be found, and in which bleeding from transplacental insertion of the trocars, though not resulting in fetal morbidity, forced us to abandon the procedure.

Some conditions may never become amenable to an endoscopic approach. Such may be the case for cystic adenomatoid malformation of the lung, pulmonary sequestrations, large fetal tumors, or other complex fetal anomalies. These cases should probably continue to be managed by teams with significant expertise in open fetal surgery.

Future of Operative Fetoscopy

A great deal of interest in the management of fetuses with diaphragmatic hernia has been generated recently. Wilson[27] and others have shown that tracheal ligation in fetal lambs with iatrogenic diaphragmatic hernias reverses the pathophysiologic effects of pulmonary hypoplasia. The net accumulation of fluid in the tracheobronchial tree resulted in expanded lungs. Histologic, molecular, and functional analysis of these lungs demonstrated cell proliferation and lack of arrest of pulmonary development. Based on these findings, Harrison and others have performed tracheal occlusion through open fetal surgery in three fetuses with diaphragmatic hernia. One fetus survived, requiring minimal ventilatory support at birth and intubation for a few weeks after birth due to tracheal instability. The other two fetuses died from postoperative complications. These animal and clinical experiences are extremely encouraging, and may completely change our approach to fetuses with diaphragmatic hernias. If an endoscopic procedure could be devised to obstruct the fetal trachea, it is likely that better results with lesser morbidity would be achieved.

Other conditions for which endoscopic fetal surgery could be potentially used are listed in Table 14–4. While much research is still needed to understand how these disorders could be addressed endoscopically in utero, it is clear that the list of conditions potentially amenable to in utero surgery is expanding as a result of the lesser morbidity associated with this technique. Further development of operative fetoscopy should make the fetus become a true endoscopic surgical patient.

TABLE 14–4. POSSIBLE FURTHER APPLICATIONS OF OPERATIVE FETOSCOPY

Diaphragmatic hernia
Sacrococcygeal teratoma and other fetal tumors
Laryngeal atresia
Aqueductal stenosis
Spina bifida
GI obstruction

REFERENCES

1. Johnson M, Bukowski T, Reitleman C, et al: In utero surgical treatment of fetal obstructive uropathy: A new comprehensive approach to identify candidates for vesicoamniotic shunt therapy. Am J Obstet Gynecol 170:1770–1776, 1994.
2. Harrison M, Adzick N, Flake A, et al: Correction of congenital diaphragmatic hernia in utero: VI. Hard-earned lessons. J Pediatr Surg 28:1411, 1993.
3. Krummel T, Longaker M: Fetal wound healing. In Harrison MR, Golbus MS, Filly RA (eds): The Unknown Patient. Philadelphia: W.B. Saunders Company, 1991, p 526.
4. Quintero R, Reich H, Puder K, et al: Operative fetoscopy: A new frontier in fetal medicine [abstract]. Am J Obstet Gynecol 179(1, part 2):297, 1994.
5. Quintero R, Reich H, Puder K, et al: Brief Report: Umbilical-cord ligation of an acardiac twin by fetoscopy at 19 weeks of gestation. N Engl J Med 330:469–471, 1994.
6. Quintero RA, Romero R, Reich H, et al: In utero percutaneous umbilical cord ligation in the management of complicated monochorionic multiple gestations. Ultrasound Obstet Gynecol 8:16–22, 1996.
7. Luks F, Deprest J, Marcus M, et al: Carbon dioxide pneumoamnios causes acidosis in fetal lamb. Fetal Diagn Ther 9:105, 1994.
8. Fisk NM, Giussani DA, Parkes MJ, et al: Amniofusion increases amniotic pressure in pregnant sheep but does not alter fetal acid-base status. Am J Obstet Gynecol 165:1459–1463, 1991.
9. Hobbins J, Mahoney M: Clinical experience with fetoscopy and fetal blood sampling. In Kaback MM, Valenti (eds): Intrauterine Fetal Visualization, A Multidisciplinary Approach. Amsterdam: Excerpta Medica 1976, pp 164–170.
10. Rodeck C: Fetoscopy guided by real-time ultrasound for pure fetal blood samples, fetal skin samples, and examination of the fetus in utero. Br J Obstet Gynecol 87:449, 1980.
11. Quintero R, Crossland W, Cotton D: Effect of endoscopic white light on the developing visual pathway: A histologic, histochemical, and behavioral study. Am J Obstet Gynecol 171:1142, 1994.
12. Aige-Gil V, Murilli-Ferrol N: Effects of white light on the pineal gland of the chick embryo. Histol Histopathol 7:1, 1992.
13. Sanchez del Campo F, Puchades A, Panchon A, et al: Action of laser light on the ocular development of chick embryos. Anat Anz 169:253, 1989.
14. Moore T, Gale S, Benirschke K: Perinatal outcome of forty-nine pregnancies complicated by acardiac twinning. Am J Obstet Gynecol 163:907–912, 1990.
15. Martinez-Poyer J, Quintero R, Carreño C, et al: Assessment of the effect of umbilical-cord ligation of acardiac twins [abstract]. Am J Obstet Gynecol 176:S152, 1997.
16. Quintero R, Lanouette J, Carreño C, et al: Percutaneous ligation and transection of the umbilical cord in complicated monoamniotic twin gestations via operative fetoscopy [abstract]. Am J Obstet Gynecol 176:S19, 1997.
17. Benirschke K, Driscoll S: The Pathology of the Human Placenta. New York: Springer-Verlag, 1967.
18. Saunders NJ, Snijders RJM, Nicolaides KH: Therapeutic amniocentesis in twin-twin transfusion syndrome appearing in the second trimester of pregnancy. Am J Obstet Gynecol 166:820–824, 1992.
19. Pinnette M, Pan Y, Pinnette S, Stubblefield P: Treatment of twin-twin transfusion syndrome. Obstet Gynecol 163:1513–1522, 1993.
20. Bajoria R, Wibblesworth J, Fisk N: Angioarchitecture of monocho-

rionic placentas in relation to the twin-twin transfusion syndrome. Am J Obstet Gynecol 172:856–863, 1995.

21. Ville Y: Monochorionic twin pregnancies: 'les liaisons dangereuses'. Ultrasound Obstet Gynecol 10:82–85, 1997.

22. Quintero R, Morales W, Phillips J, et al: In utero lysis of amniotic bands. Ultrasound Obstet Gynecol 10:316–320, 1997.

23. Crombleholme TM, Harrison MR, Golbus MS, et al: Fetal intervention in obstructive uropathy: Prognostic indicators and efficacy of intervention. Obstet Gynecol 162:1239–1244, 1990.

24. Quintero R, Johnson M, Muñoz H, et al: In utero endoscopic treatment of posterior urethral valves. Prenat Neonat Med 3:208–216, 1998.

25. Engel K, Haln T, Karschnia R: Sonographic diagnosis of a placental tumour with high-grade intrauterine foetal development deficiency, increasing anhydramnia and subsequent foetal death. Geburtsh Frauenheilk 41, 1981.

26. Quintero R, Reich R, Romero R, et al: In utero endoscopic devascularization of a large chorioangioma. Ultrasound Obstet Gynecol 8:48–52, 1996.

27. DiFiore JW, Fauza DO, Slavin R, Wilson JM: Experimental fetal tracheal ligation and congenital diaphragmatic hernia: A pulmonary vascular morphometric analysis (see comments). J Pediatr Surg 30:917–923, 1995 (discussion 923–924).

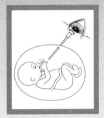

CHAPTER 15

Obstetric Endoscopy

JAN A. M. DEPREST and YVES VILLE

In the 1970s, direct fetal visualization through endoscopy was introduced into obstetrics. Various names were given to this technique: amnioscopy, fetoscopy, and embryoscopy,[1] the latter referring to its application in the first trimester. Fetoscopy was performed for diagnostic purposes (e.g., to obtain fetal blood in the diagnosis of hemoglobinopathies, to demonstrate pathognomic malformations, or to biopsy fetal skin or liver under direct vision). Fetoscopy was also used for therapeutic purposes, such as intravascular transfusion under direct visual control. The technique never became widely implemented because of its required skills, instruments, and invasiveness. In a report of the International Fetoscopy Group (1984),[2] data on about 3,000 procedures in 24 fetoscopy programs were pooled. The overall abortion rate, defined as any fetal loss prior to 28 weeks, was 4%. Abortions were more frequent following skin biopsy (16%) and fetal visualization (7.9%). The relatively large diameter of the instruments used may have played a role: rod lens telescopes of 3 mm or more were the minimum for sufficient illumination and appropriate image resolution. Some complications were also attributed to the "blind" introduction technique (i.e., without ultrasound [US] guidance). But fetoscopy soon became nearly completely abandoned, because of advances in high-resolution US used for diagnostic purposes or to guide invasive procedures.

Rapid advances of videoendoscopic technology and miniaturization of lightweight cameras boosted laparoscopy and hysteroscopy in the 1980s. Simultaneously, diameters of the endoscopes decreased dramatically, particularly fiber endoscopes; these had a high number of pixels that offered better image quality at a very small diameter. This renewed interest in direct visual access to the fetus, both for diagnostic and therapeutic procedures: the "new" fetoscopy came back in fetal medicine.[3–5] Since fetoscopy as such has not been very popular for about 20 years, we first introduce the reader to instrumental requirements for and surgical or technical aspects of fetoscopy. We then summarize the status of diagnostic embryofetoscopy, mostly used to rule out morphologic anomalies in early gestation, in patients at high risk or when US may not be able to detect them yet. Subsequently, we will review how fetoscopy is now being used to guide in utero operations on the placenta,

umbilical cord, and fetal membranes. To make the difference with fetoscopic interventions directed to the fetus, these fetoscopic manipulations on the fetal adnexae are usually called "obstetric endoscopy."[6] In addition, it must be remembered that fetoscopy is a surgical intervention, subject to complications. This will be dealt with in the last paragraph.

Instrumentation and Technique for Operative Fetoscopy

Fetoscopes and Image Display

Today, most clinicians use endoscopes of diameters of approximately 2 mm or less. Key elements of the scope are the diameter, length, field and angle of vision, as well as the technology of the image and light transmission within the scope, which determine the depth of vision. Image and light transmission can be either through fiberoptic bundles or through a conventional rod lens system. In general, the diameter of fiberoptic scopes determines the number of individual fibers of the scope, although the newer generation accomodates more fibers for the same diameter, providing a clearer image and better resolution for the same diameter. Fiberscopes have, in theory, a larger opening angle, and therefore a panoramic view, in spite of having no real lens at their tip. Current technology does not offer the possibility yet to look through the scope at a certain angle as, for instance, standard (rod lens) hysteroscopes do, where a 30-degree angle is typical. Such developments are under way. In our current clinical practice we use fiber-endoscopes with diameters ranging from 1.0 to 2.3 mm (Karl Storz, Tuttlingen, Germany) (Figs. 15–1 and 15–2). These continue to improve in resolution, having up to 50,000 pixels at the time of writing this chapter. The fibers in the scope are flexible and these optics can therefore be curved to a certain degree, which helps to overcome the current limitation of a 0-degree angle of view. This may be particularly helpful for operating on the anterior side of the uterus, without the need to enter the uterus posteriorly. We also have used steerable endoscopes in experimentation, as well as in cases of laser coagulation on an anteriorly located placenta.[7, 8] There

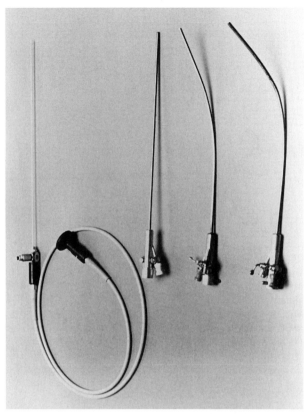

FIGURE 15–1. (From left to right) A 2.0-mm 0-degree fiber scope with deported eyepiece, rendering the weight of the scope during manipulation very light and comfortable. Straight and curved sheaths are at the right of the image.

is a tendency to manufacture fetoscopes with deported or remote eyepieces, making manipulation more elegant.

Rod lens endoscopes also contain fibers for illuminational light transmission, but the image itself is focused by a lens system. Rod lens scopes usually have a relatively large opening angle and offer a panoramic view, thanks to their lens design. However, these features may be limited by the diameter of the scope. With current technology there is a critical level of approximately 2-mm diameter, under which it is difficult to obtain enough light to work clinically, at least for longer fetoscopes. The smallest rod lens fetoscope we have been using is a pediatric cystoscope with a diameter of 1.9 mm (Olympus, Hamburg, Germany). This scope is, however, very short; a 25-cm or longer fetoscope seems more appropriate to meet the depth of a polyhydramniotic cavity or to bridge maternal adiposity in some cases.

Embryoscopes have a smaller diameter, but light instillation requirements are obviously much lower. Dumez initially used rod lens equipment of 1.7 mm, but smaller fiberoptics of 0.5 to 1.0 mm are available today. These semiflexible optics contain 10,000 pixels or more, and have a 70-degree field of vision.[9] When the scope has a deported eyepiece, manipulation is facilitated, as the instrument in the surgeon's hands is much lighter. Introduction is done through a single 18-gauge or larger double needle for operative manipulations. The second needle lumen acts as a side port for the introduction of an aspiration needle (24 gauge) or instruments to be used during the procedure (Fig. 15–2). Because of the limited view, the endoscope must be directed to the area to be visualized under US guidance.

The fetoscope is connected to a good-quality light fountain and a videocamera. We use a xenon light

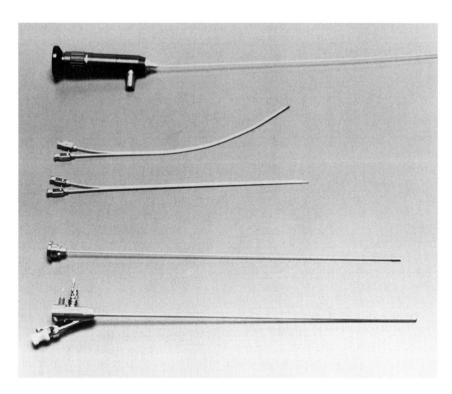

FIGURE 15–2. (From top to bottom) A 1.2-mm fiber endoscope, double needle (curved and straight), and operative sheath.

During the procedure, the sheath will inevitably be advanced or withdrawn to some extent, which causes some friction and possibly membrane disruption. In lengthy or complex procedures, so many manipulations or reinsertions of instruments are needed, that a real endoscopic port or cannula is preferable, just as in laparoscopy. The diameter of the cannula is chosen according to the largest instrument to be used through the port. We have been using cannulas designed for vascular access, which come in any diameter between 4 and 15 Fr (1.6 to 5 mm; Performa, Cook, Belgium). They are inserted either with the Seldinger technique,[10] which gradually expands the myometrial and membrane stab wound up to the desired diameter, or directly with purpose-designed pyramidal trocars (Karl Storz). The cannulas offer a leakproof seal and a side channel for infusion or removal of fluid; they are made of flexible material allowing for the use of curved instruments. Others have used different types of cannulas, particularly during (experimental) fetal surgical procedures, and we expect more from these as they become available clinically.[11, 12] Balloon-tipped cannulas are a need in that respect, but are not yet commercially available in the small range.

Uterine Entry Point

The exact point of entry into the amniotic cavity is a compromise between the theoretical optimal cannula position towards the target area, and the limitations imposed by the actual position of the fetus and placenta. The majority of obstetric endoscopic procedures are performed percutaneously with local anesthesia of the abdominal wall down to the myometrium, as earlier mentioned, without a formal cannula. The sheath can be easily inserted through an area free of placenta (Figs. 15–4 and 15–5). When an anterior placenta hampers entry through the anterior uterine wall, we suggest a

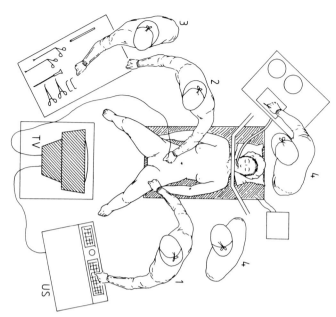

FIGURE 15–3. Organization of the operation room for operative fetoscopy. In this case cord ligation of the left-sided twin is performed with a target area above the cervix. US operator (1) and equipment (US) are on the left side, while the surgeon and his assisting nursing (2, 3) are on the right side. Videomonitor and endoscopic hardware (TV) are at the feet of the patient. Anesthesiologist (4) is at the head of the patient. (From Deprest JA, Evrard VA, Van Ballaer PP, et al: Experience with fetoscopic cord ligation. Eur J Obstet Gynaecol Reprod Biol 81:157–164, 1998. Copyright 1998, Elsevier Science, with permission.)

source, and a one- or three-chip digital image processing camera, as used in conventional laparoscopy. The camera projects the fetoscopic images on a videoscreen, but as US back-up is crucial, both images should be available to the operator. We therefore use a so-called Twin-video system (Karl Storz) to project both endoscopic and US images simultaneously; the relative size of each of those images on the screen can be decided upon by the operator. In very complex interventions, several monitors can be used. The monitor(s) is (are) set according to the rules applying in any endoscopic procedure: the operator, the target area, and the screen should be in one line, to allow comfortable manipulation of instruments by both the surgeon and his assistants (Fig. 15–3).

Techniques to Access the Pregnant Uterus and Distention Media

Sheaths and Cannulas

The endoscope is normally used with a sheath around it, its diameter and shape being dependent on the purpose of the endoscopic procedure. The sheath can be used for irrigation of the operative field and/or instrument insertion. To penetrate the abdominal and uterine wall, the sheath is loaded with a sharp trocar and inserted under US guidance. The trocar is then withdrawn and the sheath accommodates the scope, and eventually a laser fiber, forceps, scissors, or irrigation as required. During laser procedures an oval-shaped sheath is handy as it prevents the fiber from moving within the sheath.

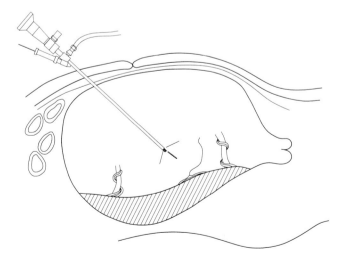

FIGURE 15–4. Schematic drawing of fetoscopic Nd:YAG laser coagulation of chorionic plate vessels, in case of a posterior placenta. The scope is inserted percutaneously. (From Deprest J, Van Schoubroeck D, Van Ballaer P, et al: Alternative access for fetoscopic Nd:YAG laser in TTS with anterior placenta. Ultrasound Obstet Gynecol 12:347–352, 1998, with permission.)

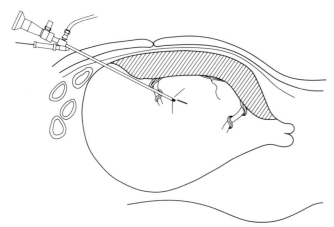

FIGURE 15–5. Schematic drawing of fetoscopic Nd:YAG laser co-agulation of chorionic plate vessels, in case of an anterior placenta. A percutaneous approach is being used. The inclination angle towards the targeted vessels is not optimal. (From Deprest J, Van Schoubroeck D, Van Ballaer P, et al: Alternative access for fetoscopic Nd:YAG laser in TTS with anterior placenta. Ultrasound Obstet Gynecol 12:347–352, 1998, with permission.)

transfundal insertion and the use of a flexible cannula and curved instruments. To do this safely, we make a 2- to 3-cm minilaparotomy to avoid bowel injury (Fig. 15–6).[10] However, this approach requires locoregional or general anesthesia, and is certainly more invasive than the percutaneous approach. As an alternative in case of an anteriorly located placenta, Ville used a very lateral uterine insertion with previous identification of uterine vessels using Doppler, and a steerable endoscope.[8, 13]

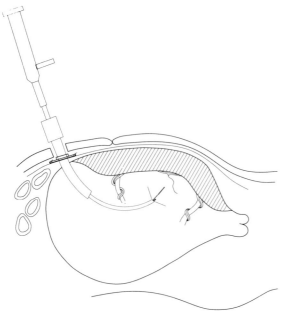

FIGURE 15–6. Fetoscopy for laser coagulation through minilaparotomy, extraplacental fundal insertion. Bowels have been retracted, and a trocar has been introduced. A bent fetoscope is used, allowing full visualization of the intertwin membrane and the intertwin vessels. (From Deprest J, Van Schoubroeck D, Van Ballaer P, et al: Alternative access for fetoscopic Nd:YAG laser in TTS with anterior placenta. Ultrasound Obstet Gynecol 12:347–352, 1998, with permission.)

However, in complex operative procedures, such as two-port fetoscopic cord ligation or fetal surgery, multiple cannulas are simply a necessity, and varying degrees of uterine distention may occur during the operation. Such operations are usually carried out through (a) formal abdominal incision(s) so that the uterine cannulas can move freely in relation to the maternal wall and uterine tearing is thus prevented. Although many obstetricians would try to perform all interventions percutaneously at any price, we feel that the maternal incision and morbidity should be considered separately from the invasiveness of the procedure to the uterus and fetus. Maternal abdominal wall incision may obviously be justified and even technically necessary in selected circumstances, certainly for fetal surgery.

Distention Media

Although fetoscopy can be performed in a natural amniotic fluid environment, the use of a distention medium can improve visualization and/or create more working space. We always have normal saline or Hartmann's solution available; during longer operations a blood warmer may be used. Care should be taken to avoid a rise in intra-amniotic pressure, and (intermittent) drainage may be needed. So far its clinical use has been safe in normal working conditions, as was reported earlier in experimental conditions.[14–16] A purpose-designed amniotic distention device controlling for all important parameters such as pressure and temperature is not commercially available yet, but research and product development are ongoing.

In one report on fetoscopic covering of a myelomeningocele, uterine distention was achieved with CO_2. No experience with this medium for "obstetric" interventions has been reported so far. The use of a gas distention medium probably facilitates complex endoscopic procedures because of a better depth of vision, more working space, and the ability to work in conditions with limited bleeding.[12] We have been hesitant to use CO_2, as it causes fetal acidosis.[17] However, other investigators have demonstrated in sheep that maternal hyperventilation could correct for this,[18] an observation which we could not confirm in physiologic conditions.[18a] In theory inert gases such as helium could also be used.[19] However, none of these distention techniques have been tested more formally in experimental conditions nor widely used clinically to date.

Additional Instrumentation

The choice of instruments, whenever needed, is dependent on the purpose of the procedure. For most obstetric interventions, a laser with coagulation abilities is helpful. For this purpose, a neodymium: yttrium-aluminum-garnet (Nd:YAG) laser has been mostly used, with a power output of 60 to 100 w (Dornier Medilas, Germany). The sheath of the endoscope should allow for the insertion of a laser fiber, usually with a diameter of 400 to 600 μm. Miniaturized forceps or scissors can be inserted through the same operative sheath, although this may be easier through an additional port. The length of the instruments should be sufficient, and they should not be too small in diameter, in order to resist bending.[10] The use of bipolar energy and forceps will be addressed later.

Diagnostic Embryoscopy and Fetoscopy in the First Trimester of Pregnancy

Early diagnosis or suspicion of fetal abnormalities at 10 to 14 weeks' gestation calls for immediate confirmation or reassurance, which cannot always be given by early second-trimester US examination. Microendoscopy allows for a sonoendoscopic approach by intra-amniotic fetoscopy at the same time amniocentesis is performed.[9, 20] Several congenital malformations have been diagnosed in the first trimester using embryoscopy (Table 15–1).

Embryoscopy is likely to remain confined to the early investigation of the pregnancy in a few families at high risk of recurrence of genetic conditions showing external fetal abnormalities. Detailed US examination of fetal anatomy at 10 to 14 weeks is increasingly being used, mainly under the influence of screening programs for fetal aneuploidy by the measurement of nuchal translucency (NT).[21] An increased NT above 4.5 mm often overlaps with cystic hygromata of the neck and may reveal genetic syndromes with normal karyotype, some of which could show external abnormalities or facial dysmorphy in the first trimester of pregnancy.[22] In those cases it is important to conduct a detailed morphologic examination of the fetus with both transabdominal and transvaginal US examination. However, complete fetal assessment is still unlikely at this early stage. One option is to wait for another detailed scan in the second trimester, but this is rarely welcomed by the parents whose anxiety calls for rapid fetal evaluation, especially when karyotyping is requested and when termination of pregnancy is an option. In any case, fetoscopy allows for in vivo fetal examination, which can be different from postmortem findings. Visualization of the fetal anatomy can only be partial; therefore, the needle must be directed towards the fetal part most likely to be affected. The success rate of such procedures is also influenced by the possibility of intra-amniotic bleeding from the placenta or the uterine wall, which in our experience is around 10% (unpublished data). An 18-gauge needle is an acceptable sampling device in the late first trimester of pregnancy; however, the safety of this procedure is still in evaluation, since there are no data allowing an estimation of the fetal loss rate. It seems reasonable to assume that this should remain below the risk of miscarriage in operative fetoscopy in the second trimester (10 to 12%).[13, 23] Although clinical experience with embryoscopy is very reassuring in terms of remote effects of light instillation on the developing retina, its risks are still not well documented in experimental conditions and are not known for clinical applications.[24, 25]

Embryoscopy

Embryoscopy aims at introducing an optical device in the exocoelomic space in contact with the intact amnion, after penetration of the chorion. Optimally this can be done at 9 weeks' gestation and, by definition, before 12 weeks, at which stage the chorion fuses with the amnion. Two routes are clinically used.

Transcervical Embryoscopy

For transcervical embryoscopy, a rigid endoscope is advanced through the cervical canal. The diameter of the transcervical embryoscope has gone down over the years, from a 10-mm hysteroscope[26] to a 1.7-mm fetoscope.[1] Dumez et al. reported their experience with diagnostic embryoscopy in 42 patients (all but a few done transcervically) at high risk for mainly autosomal dominant genetic conditions involving limb and/or facial abnormalities at 8 to 13 weeks' gestation.[1] They obtained a 97% rate of successful visualization of the fetus. Six patients underwent termination of pregnancy for facial or limb anomalies as part of a genetic syndrome (Table 15–1). They reported five cases (12.8%) of spontaneous

TABLE 15–1. ABNORMALITIES DIAGNOSED BY EMBRYOFETOSCOPY

INVESTIGATOR	GESTATIONAL AGE (WEEKS)	APPROACH	FETAL STRUCTURAL ABNORMALITIES	SYNDROME
Hobbins 1994	11 +5	TA	Polydactyly	Smith-Lemli-Opitz
Dommergues 1995	11	TC	Unilateral cleft lip	Van der Woude
Dumez 1992	9–10	TA	Limb and facial anomalies,	Ellis-van Creveld, Smith-Lemli-Opitz,
		TC	ectrodactyly, cleft palate	Baller-Gerold, Apert, Rothmund-Thomson, DOOR
Dumez 1994	10 +4	TC	Polydactyly	Meckel-Gruber
Quintero 1993	11	TA	Polydactyly, occipital, encephalocele	Meckel-Gruber
Ville 1996	12	TA	Club hands, hypoplasia of forearm	Trisomy 18
Ville 1996	11	TA	Frontal encephalocele	
	12		Facial cleft	
Quintero 1993	12 +2	TA	Cystic hygroma	
	11 +6		Omphalocele	
	11 +2		Neural tube defect	

TA, transabdominal; TC, transcervical.

abortion between 11 and 23 weeks, when the procedure was done after 10 weeks, and two cases of spontaneous rupture of membranes at 25 weeks, which delivered after 34 weeks. Another 31 babies were born alive and well at a mean gestational age of 39 weeks, all developing normally.

Transabdominal Embryoscopy

Before termination of pregnancy, a transabdominal procedure was performed on a total of 40 patients at 7 to 20 weeks using a 0.7- to 0.8-mm-diameter microendoscope passed transabdominally through a 16- to 19-gauge needle.[4, 28] A failure rate as high as 35% was reported. As these studies were performed on patients seeking termination of pregnancy, no fetal loss rate can be quoted.

Intra-amniotic Transabdominal Fetoscopy

From 11 weeks' gestation onward, the amnion and the chorion are usually fused, making exocoelomic embryofetoscopy impossible. Transabdominal fetoscopy in the first trimester of pregnancy is indicated when fetal abnormality is suspected during first-trimester US examination. This is becoming routine practice in many countries as part of the US screening for fetal aneuploidies at 10 to 14 weeks' gestation.[21] Several fetal abnormalities have thus been confirmed or ruled out. Pennehouat et al. examined 15 embryos/fetuses before termination of pregnancy.[28] They used a flexible fiberoptic endoscope of 0.5 mm in its outer diameter with a 55-degree field of vision. The scope was introduced into the amniotic cavity through a 21-gauge needle. The procedure was performed under continuous US control, directing the needle towards selected fetal parts, mainly the face, hands, feet, and genitalia. They noticed that only either the ventral face or the dorsal part of the fetal anatomy could be visualized at a time without manipulating the embryo with the needle.

Hobbins et al.[29] were able to diagnose a Smith-Lemli-Opitz syndrome at 10 weeks in one case and rule it out in another. The latter baby was born at 35 weeks and is reportedly developing normally. In another case, a 0.5-mm angioscope was used through a 20-gauge spinal needle to rule out Carpenter syndrome at 11 weeks' gestation.[30] Although the patient had immediate leakage of amniotic fluid and went into preterm labor at 21 weeks, she delivered a normal baby at 36 weeks. Reece et al.[31] reported on using intra-amniotic needle fetoscopy to rule out a neural tube defect that was suspected by US examination at 15 weeks' gestation. No complications were reported and a normal baby was delivered at term. Ville et al.[8, 9] used a specially designed 0-degree microendoscope and double needle as described above. Several abnormalities could be confirmed, including the association of frontal encephalocele and midline facial cleft in two cases at 11 and 12 weeks, the association of club hand and hypoplasia of the forearm at 12 weeks, confirmation of facial dysmorphy including one case of Pierre Robin syndrome, and one case with cutaneous angiomas. In one case where a presumed diagnosis of

meningocele was ruled out, the pregnancy was continued and a normal baby was delivered at term.

"Obstetric Endoscopy": Fetoscopic Surgery on the Placenta, Cord, and Membranes

Apart from case reports on ligation of the major vessels in a placental chorioangioma[32] and section of amniotic membranes or webs, laser coagulation of the chorionic plate vessels and cord obliteration account for the majority of present obstetric indications for operative fetoscopy.

Nd:YAG Laser Coagulation of Chorionic Plate Vessels for Fetofetal Transfusion Syndrome

Pathophysiology

Monochorionic (MC) twins have a three- to tenfold increased perinatal morbidity and mortality in comparison to dichorionic twins. This is thought to be related to the presence of certain patterns of vascular anastomoses between both fetal circulations. Anastomoses exist in virtually all monochorionic placentas, and in most cases fetofetal transfusion is a balanced phenomenon. In about 10 to 15% (range, 4 to 35%) of MC twins, a chronic imbalance in the net flow of blood across these communications may occur, resulting in a clinically relevant fetofetal transfusion syndrome (FFTS). Typically, the "donor" suffers from hypovolemia and hypoxia, and occasionally growth retardation. The recipient becomes hypervolemic, compensates with polyuria leading to polyhydramnios, and eventually develops hydrops due to cardiac failure. When occurring before 28 weeks' gestation, FFTS is associated with more than 80% fetal or perinatal loss.[33] A much more detailed review on the pathophysiology of this condition can be found elsewhere in the book.

Main problems are preterm labor and premature birth, as well as preterm premature rupture of membranes (PPROM) and its consequences, mainly as a consequence of extreme polyhydramnios. Intrauterine fetal death (IUFD) is another complication, but death of one twin does not arrest the transfusion process or improve the prognosis for the remainder. On the contrary, the survivor may acutely exsanguinate in the circulation of the dying fetus in up to 30% with a high risk of severe neurologic damage.[34, 35] The indication for active therapy is therefore obvious, and for years consisted of serial amnioreductions. Potential mechanisms explaining the benefit of this therapy are also detailed in the earlier mentioned section. Despite improving fetal survival rates (usually around 60%), significant neurologic morbidity in about 20% of survivors continues to be present.[33, 36] Furthermore, amniodrainage does not alter the cause of this condition, nor does it prevent the risk of neurologic damage in case of intrauterine death of one fetus.

Rationale for Surgical Therapy

More recently, laser coagulation of chorionic plate vessels has been introduced as a new and probably more cause-oriented approach. As mentioned earlier, the best pathophysiologic explanation for FFTS continues to be the chronic imbalance in blood flow between the fetuses across vascular communications in their shared placenta.[37, 38] FFTS is related to the presence of one (or few) arteriovenous (A-V) anastomoses in combination with a paucity (or absence) of arterioarterious (AA) or venovenous (VV) anastomoses, which normally compensate for the hemodynamic effects of A-V communications. For clarity, an arteriovenous anastomosis is not a real "anatomic" anastomosis, but a cotyledon that is fed by an artery from one fetus, and drained by a vein from the other. The afferent and efferent branches of this shared cotyledon run over the placental surface and plunge into the chorionic plate almost at the same point, and anastomose functionally in the villous capillaries of that "shared" cotyledon (Fig. 15–7).[39]

Provided that the "vascular" hypothesis is correct, and that anastomosing vessels could be identified, their interruption will result in the elimination of the shared

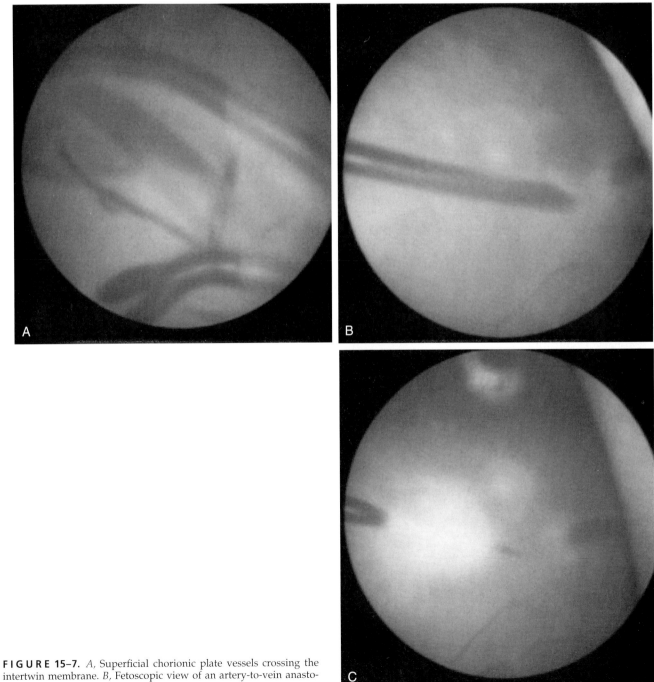

FIGURE 15–7. *A,* Superficial chorionic plate vessels crossing the intertwin membrane. *B,* Fetoscopic view of an artery-to-vein anastomosis prior to and, *C,* after coagulation.

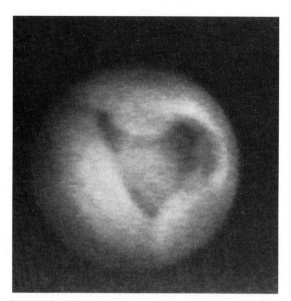

FIGURE 15–8. Embryoscopy, demonstrating cleft palate.

circulation, and therefore in the resolution of the abnormal intertwin blood transfer. It has been demonstrated in experimental conditions and by placental perfusion studies that the obliteration of the superficially located feeding vessels indeed eliminates the deeply located circulation or, in other words, the "shared" cotyledon.[40–42] That idea was already suggested by Benirschke in 1973,[43] and de Vore[44] proposed to use laser energy for this purpose. Julian De Lia et al. should be credited for introducing the clinical technique,[45, 46] but the procedure became more widely implemented, at least in Europe, after Ville et al. reported a modified and elegant percutaneous technique.[47]

Operative Technique

De Lia proposed an open approach with maternal laparotomy and purse-string hysterotomy for fetoscope insertion. In Europe, Nd:YAG laser coagulation is usually performed by percutaneous approach and under local[47] or epidural anesthesia. The sheath, loaded with a trocar, is inserted under US guidance into the polyhydramniotic sac. The trocar is then removed and a fetoscope and a 400- to 600-μm Nd:YAG laser fiber are inserted into the sheath. The laser tip is directed as close as possible to a 90-degree angle towards the target vessels. Coagulation is done using a nontouch technique with power settings of 40 to 100 w at about 1 cm distance or less. Selection of the vessels to be targeted is discussed below. Sections of approximately 1 cm are coagulated. Amnioinfusion may be needed to improve visualization or to clear the operative field in case of stained fluid, or to prevent suspended amniotic debris to become stuck to the tip of the fiber, making laser energy inefficacious and finally burn the fiber tip. The procedure is completed by amniodrainage till normal amniotic fluid pockets are seen on US.

The trocar is obviously inserted in an area free of placenta. In case of a posterior placenta, this can easily be done percutaneously. When the placenta is anterior, two problems arise. An anterior insertion may make it difficult to achieve a close to 90-degree angle with the target area, reducing efficacy of laser coagulation. It may also be difficult to avoid for sure the placenta, even with a lateral insertion. Therefore, we recently proposed a transfundal technique, described above (Fig. 15–6).[10, 48] However, it has not been proven that the results are improved by this additional invasiveness.

Selection of Vessels

The chorionic plate is inspected and the course of the vessels determined. Fetoscopic laser occlusion (FLOC) of the chorioangiopagus vessels, as proposed by DeLia,[42] is the identification and coagulation of anastomosing vessels along the vascular equator (Fig. 15–9). It is not clear whether that is always possible. In a more pragmatic approach, Ville et al.[47] described the surgical division of the vascular territory by coagulating all the vessels crossing the intertwin membrane (Fig. 15–9). Although overtreating, the latter is reproducible and may be faster because of its readily identifiable landmarks. However, as experience grows, we as well as

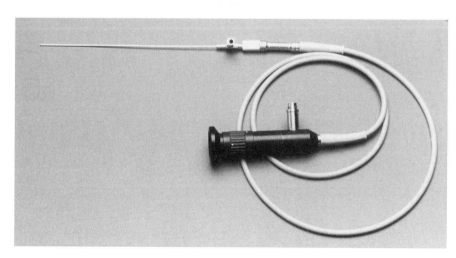

FIGURE 15–9. Embryofetoscope with deported eyepiece. (Courtesy Karl Storz.)

TABLE 15–2. FETOSCOPIC ND:YAG LASER COAGULATION FOR FFTS GROUPED BY REPORTS, INCLUDING INITIAL EXPERIENCE AND REPORTS WHERE THE LEARNING CURVE WAS EXCLUDED

AUTHOR, YEAR	NUMBER OF CASES	FETAL SURVIVAL	SURVIVAL OF AT LEAST ONE FETUS	NEUROLOGIC MORBIDITY
Series including first cases				
DeLia et al., 1990	31	53%	69%	4%
Ville et al., 1995	45	53%	71%	2%
Ville et al., 1998	132	55%	73%	5%
After the learning curve				
Hecher et al., 1999	69	61%	79%	6%
De Lia et al., 1999	100	69%	82%	4.3%

Nd:YAG, neodymium:yttrium-aluminum-garnet; FFTS, fetofetal transfusion syndrome.

others are using a "mixed" selection technique, namely, coagulating all obviously anastomosing vessels as well as those vessels that cannot be demonstrated to be part of the normal vascularization of the placenta. In other words, when vessels originating from the recipient cannot be followed completely, because they disappear on the other side of the membrane or under the fetus, and could in theory anastomose, they will be coagulated too. Coagulating more sparingly makes sense, as unnecessary coagulation of vessels not involved in the shunting will lead to the elimination of normal cotyledons and may impair fetomaternal blood-gas interchange for an already critically distressed fetus.

Results

Fetal survival following laser coagulation has been consistently reported to be around 55 to 68%, with a risk of about 5% of neurologic handicap in survivors (Tables 15–2 and 15–3).[13, 23, 42, 46, 47, 49] The technique has been shown to be reproducible in the hands of different surgeons. These results also appear to be better than those reported for amniodrainage, at least in respect to the occurrence of neurologic damage. Both a retrospective compilation of amniodrainage series published in 1997[8]

and a recently reported prospective multicenter study[50] yielded a 60% survival rate with about 19% risk for neurologic impairment. In a recent prospective (but not randomized) comparative study of laser versus amniodrainage conducted in Germany, the results of laser ($n = 73$) at one institution were prospectively compared with those of amniodrainages ($n = 43$) at another.[23] The inclusion criteria for both groups were the same, all cases being severe previable FFTS of comparable gestational age at diagnosis. The survival rate and neurologic morbidity for the laser group were 61% and 6%, respectively, and those of amniodrainage 51% and 19% (Table 15–3). This study probably represents the best available comparison at present, but still has the drawback of not being a randomized study.

A serious disadvantage of laser coagulation for FFTS is the procedure-associated risk of IUFD (25%) within hours after the procedure.[47] This may be due to the difficult differentiation by fetoscopy of those vessels involved from others not contributing to the pathologic shunting process, and, in case of coagulation of these, leading to IUFD. This argument is often used in emotional debates in favor of or against this therapeutic modality. However, it should be remembered that, when patients are treated with serial amnioreductions, the risk for a not directly procedure-related double IUFD

TABLE 15–3. PROSPECTIVE, COMPARATIVE STUDY OF FFTS PATIENTS TREATED WITH FETOSCOPIC LASER COAGULATION OR SERIAL AMNIODRAINAGE*

	LASER ($n = 73$)	SERIAL AMNIODRAINAGE ($n = 43$)	p VALUE
GA at diagnosis	20.7 (17–25)	20.4 (17.6–25)	0.438
Fluid drained (mL)	2,500 (650–7,500)	1,900 (350–3,000)	<0.001
GA at delivery	33.7 (25–40)	30.7 (28–37)	0.438
Survival	61%	51%	0.239
2 survivors	42%	42%	1.0
1 survivor	37%	19%	0.058
No survivors	21%	40%	0.033
Neonatal deaths	6%	14%	0.221
Neurologic morbidity†	6%	18%	0.030
Birthweight (g)			
Donor	1,750 g	1,145 g	0.034
Recipient	2,000 g	1,560 g	0.076

* From Hecher K, Plath H, Bregenzer T, et al: Endoscopic laser surgery versus serial amniocenteses in the treatment of severe twin-twin transfusion syndrome. Am J Obstet Gynecol 180:717–724, 1999, with permission.
† Defined as periventricular leukomalacia, grade III and IV intraventricular hemorrhage, parenchymal defects, and microcephaly.
FFTS, fetofetal transfusion syndrome; GA, gestational age.

is at least as high. This argument is all too often forgotten, because the event does not immediately follow the procedure.[23]

The comparable fetal survival rates, but the substantially reduced risk for neurologic damage, justify a randomized trial designed to confirm or reject the existence of differences between laser and amniodrainage in FFTS. A randomized multicenter trial comparing laser versus amniodrainage in the management of FFTS has recently been set up in the context of the Eurofoetus Programme, a research project supported by the European Commission. Participation in the trial is open to all centers throughout the world and all information is available via the Internet (www.eurofoetus.org). Inclusion criteria for the study are:

1. diagnosis of FFTS established at less than 25 weeks of gestation,
2. confirmed monochorionicity, and
3. polyhydramnios/oligohydramnios sequence as defined by well-described US criteria, varying with gestational age.

The randomization and the use of strict inclusion criteria aim at evaluating only severe and previable cases of FFTS, overcoming the limited comparability of most available data in the literature. In parallel, centers not participating or patients with FFTS not willing to be randomized could enter an observational study recording data from patients having undergone laser or amniodrainage therapy. Again, both initiatives are not limited to Europe, but are open to all fetal medicine units (consult www.eurofoetus.org).

Fetoscopic Cord Obliteration

Next to FFTS, MC twinning may be complicated by a number of rare conditions, such as twin reversed arterial perfusion (TRAP) sequence, or twins may be discordant for structural or genetic anomalies, for which they are at higher risk than singletons.[51, 52] In all these circumstances selective feticide may be contemplated for selected cases. In *dichorionic* multiple pregnancies, selective feticide with intracardiac or intrathoracic injection of potassium chloride is a well-established modality. The loss rate for the other twin is approximately 7% and may be independent of gestation.[53] The cause of this remains unknown. In *monochorionic* twins, vascular communications between the two fetuses are virtually always present and feticide by intracardiac KCl is not suitable, as the product may embolize to the other fetus. Also, following IUFD, blood may be "dumped" from the surviving twin into the dead fetus, since intertwin vessels remain patent. Such acute, agonal fetofetal transfusion may lead to hypovolemic shock in the survivor, causing either central nervous system (CNS) damage or IUFD of the survivor. Accordingly, techniques for selective feticide in monochorionic twins must include a method for arresting flow in the cord of the target fetus completely and permanently.[48]

Indications for Selective Termination in MC Twins

Twin Reversed Arterial Perfusion Sequence

TRAP sequence is a condition encountered in 1% of MZ pregnancies, where one twin is acardiac and survives only on the blood flow provided by the other twin. Blood flows from an umbilical artery of the pump twin in a reversed direction into the umbilical artery of the acardiac fetus, via an arterioarterial anastomosis. The umbilical vein of the parasitic fetus returns blood into the placenta and back to the pump twin. The condition places the pump twin at risk for in utero high-output cardiac failure and hydrops, potentially leading to IUFD and/or to polyhydramnios and its complications.[54] According to the largest available review by Healey, TRAP sequence is complicated by polyhydramnios in 51% of cases and by preterm labor in 75%.[55] In utero congestive heart failure occurs in 28% and intrauterine demise of both twins in 25%. Perinatal mortality is estimated to be about 30%. The proportional size of the acardiac fetus to the pump twin seems to be a useful predictive factor, and a twin weight ratio of above 50% (acardiac/pump twin) has a 71% predictive value for preterm delivery and a 45% predictive value for the death of the pump twin.[56] In this series by Moore et al., all 13 pregnancies with a size ratio above 80% developed cardiac failure in the pump twin. Although some pregnancies complicated by acardiac twinning will progress uneventfully into the viable period, allowing treatment by timed delivery, the complications described above may develop in other cases as early as the second trimester. In these cases, selective feticide of the acardiac fetus by interruption of blood flow may offer the best hope for intact survival for the pump twin. Moreover, in high-risk cases (generally those with a large acardiac twin at previable gestation), selective feticide should be considered before the development of hydrops in the pump twin.

Selected Cases of Fetofetal Transfusion Syndrome

In most cases of FFTS, therapy aimes at improving the survival for *both* twins. Unfortunately, in some cases of FFTS one of the twins may have already developed irreversible damage, particularly cerebral ventriculomegaly or hydrocephalus at the time of presentation. Additional cases may present with or develop signs of impending fetal death, including severe cardiac failure. As mentioned earlier, spontaneous IUFD does not improve the prognosis for the co-twin, but rather puts it at a higher risk for severe cerebral damage or IUFD. In these severe cases, or circumstances where standard therapies of amnioreduction and/or laser to chorionic vessels have failed, therapy may be rationally redirected toward selective feticide, where the aim is to improve the chance of intact survival of a healthy singleton pregnancy.

Twins Discordant for Structural Anomaly

Structural abnormalities are more common in MC twins. A large range of major and minor structural anomalies

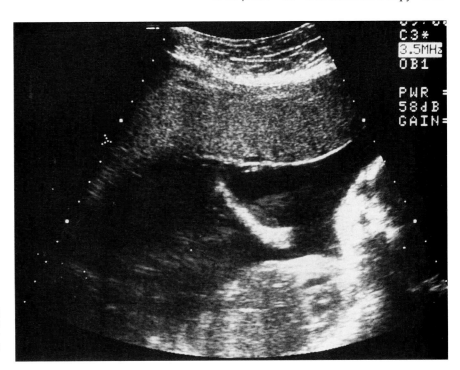

FIGURE 15–10. Cord embolization using enbucrilate gel. The thrombogenic material is visible within one of the umbilical cord vessels. In the second image the material is also visible in the fetal heart.

has been reported in association with twin pregnancies, including anencephaly, sirenomelia, neural tube defects, and holoprosencephaly.[57, 58] It has been observed that many of these anomalies occur in the midline, and are particularly prevalent in MC pregnancies.[59] In only about 15% of cases both twins are affected by the anomaly (so-called concordant twins), whilst in the majority of cases only one twin is affected (so-called discordant twins).[60] When the twins are discordant for the anomaly, selective feticide using any of the available techniques may be contemplated, but will also threaten the survival of the structurally normal fetus. Accordingly, making the decision to perform a selective feticide is never straightforward.

Techniques for Cord Occlusion in Monochorionic Twins

Fetoscopy may play a role in selective feticide in MC twins, but should be positioned in between currently available alternatives. It is unclear today which technique for selective termination in MC twins is the most effective and puts the co-twin at the lowest risk.

Embolization of the Umbilical Cord

One of the first techniques described for interruption of flow within the umbilical cord was embolization of cord vessels. This technique is based on well-established embolization techniques in interventional radiology, and cordocentesis under US guidance (Fig. 15–10). Fetal medicine specialists are very familiar with the latter, and any restrictions or complications should be the same as for funipuncture, using a 20-gauge needle. For instance, the incidence of PPROM, which is a major concern for the techniques described below, should be comparable to that of fetal transfusions. Different agents have been suggested to embolize the fetal circulation, such as absolute alcohol,[61, 62] coils,[63–65] and enbucrilate gel (Table 15–4).[66, 67] The procedure is relatively noninvasive and anecdotal successes have been reported. Unfortu-

TABLE 15–4. PUBLISHED DATA ON CORD EMBOLIZATION

AUTHOR, YEAR	NUMBER OF PROCEDURES	FAILURE OF EMBOLIZATION	IUFD	PPROM (≤32 wk)	PPROM (>32 wk)	NEONATAL SURVIVAL RATE
Hamada, 1989	1	0	0	0	0	1
Porreco, 1991	1	0	0	0	0	1
Dommergues, 1995	4	0	0	1	1	3
Bebbington, 1995	1	1	1	0	0	0
Denbow, 1999	6	4	3	0	0	3
Deprest, 1999	4	3*	2	0	0	2*
Total	17	8/17	6/17	1/17	1/17	10/17

* Failed embolization in one case was followed by a successful endoscopic cord ligation.
IUFD, intrauterine fetal death; PPROM, preterm premature rupture of membranes.

TABLE 15–5. FETOSCOPIC CORD LIGATIONS*

AUTHOR, YEAR	NUMBER OF CASES	FAILURE OF LIGATION	IUFD	PPROM (≤32 wk)	PPROM (>32 wk)†
McCurdy, 1993	1	0	1	—	—
Willcourt, 1996	1	0	0	0/1	0/1
Lémery, 1994	2	0	0	NA	NA
Quintero, 1996b	14‡	2	3	3/14	1/14
Deprest, 1996	4	0	0	2/4	0/4
Crombleholme, 1996	1	0	0	1/1	0/1
Totals	23	2/23	4/21	6/17	2/17

* Modified from Deprest JA, Evrard VA, Van Ballaer PP, et al: Experience with fetoscopic cord ligation. Eur J Obstet Gynaecol Reprod Biol 81:157–164, 1998. Copyright 1998, Elsevier Science, with permission.
† Calculation only for the successfully performed procedures, and with in utero surviving co-twin.
‡ 13 pregnancies, of which one was a quadruplet pregnancy, with two cord ligations.
IUFD, intrauterine fetal death; PPROM, preterm premature rupture of membranes; NA, not applicable.

nately, IUFD of both twins has also been observed, probably due to incomplete vascular obliteration or migration of the sclerosants or thrombogens to the co-twin.[68, 69] In a recent report, Denbow et al.[66] reported 12 attempts of umbilical vessel occlusion with absolute alcohol or enbucrilate gel and observed an overall success rate of 33% in six MC twins. In the conclusions of this series the authors discouraged any further use of this technique (Table 15–5).

Nd:YAG Laser Coagulation

For laser coagulation of the umbilical cord, the same instrumentation as for chorionic plate vessel coagulation is being used. As early as 16 weeks, a double-lumen needle can be used, accommodating a 1.0-mm fetoscope and a 400-μm laser fiber.[70] Coagulation of the umbilical cord is a fairly easy and straightforward procedure; the cord root of the target fetus is visualized and the vessels are then coagulated using a "no-touch" technique (Fig. 15–11). The successful use of laser cord coagulation has

been reported for an acardiac twin as late as 24 weeks.[71] Unfortunately, cord coagulation has been shown to have a high failure rate beyond 20 to 22 weeks of gestation. In our institution, where we attempt laser cord coagulation nearly always prior to any other technique, an overall success rate of 27% was noted (n = 11; unpublished data). When considering only cases prior to 20 weeks, three out of four cases were successful. The failure at advanced gestational age is probably due to the larger diameter of the cord vessels or the presence of hydropic perivascular tissue, absorbing the coagulation energy.[72, 73] At that gestational age, the procedure may also be impaired by floating vernix particles and/or stained amniotic fluid, causing poor transmission of light and laser energy absorption. Along with preterm labor and rupture of the membranes, risks of this procedure theoretically include vessel perforation.[16] This is so far an unpublished complication, but when it occurs it may result in almost certain fatal fetal hemorrhage, and death of both twins is then likely.

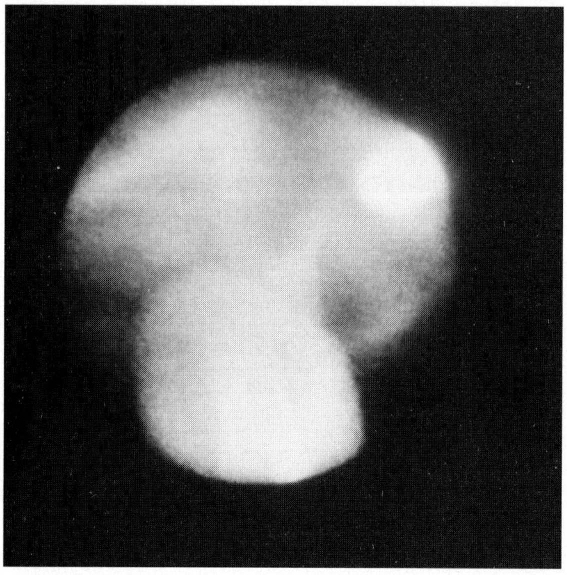

Fetoscopic Cord Ligation

Surgical ligation of the umbilical cord causes immediate, complete, and permanent interruption of both arterial and venous flow in the umbilical cord, irrespective of its diameter. The procedure has become clinically acceptable, since it was demonstrated to be feasible endoscopically. One or two ports are inserted as described above and a nonabsorbable suture is guided around the cord. Then it is tied with an extracorporeal knot, which is slipped in through the cannula by a purpose-designed knot pusher, using another instrument to act as a backstop relieving tension of the cord (Figs. 15–12 and 15–13). The first report was published by McCurdy et al.[74]; however, in that case, the pump twin also died in utero. A first successful case was published by Quintero et al.[75, 76] We recently reviewed the experience with the 23 procedures published to date (Table 15–5).[48] Cord ligation failed in two cases and IUFD of the co-twin occurred in four cases. The mean prolongation of pregnancy following the procedure was 8.5 weeks; preterm labor was not a clinical problem. The major limitation, however, was the risk for PPROM as high as 30%; the problem of PPROM will be dealt with below. These 23

FIGURE 15–11. Nd:YAG laser coagulation of cord vessels. A 400-μm fiber is used.

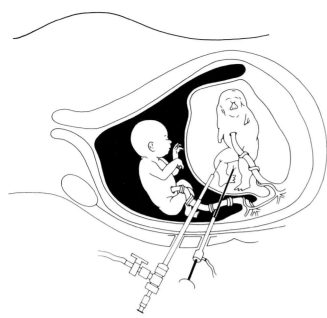

FIGURE 15–12. Technique of two-port fetoscopic cord ligation. The amniotic sac of the acardiac fetus, lying under the placenta, has been opened. Instruments are inserted into that sac to perform the actual procedure. Ports were attached to the fascia with a retention disc. Amnioinfusion goes in by the scope, and drainage is done through the ports. (From Deprest JA, Lerut TE, Vandenberghe K: Operative fetoscopy: New perspective in fetal therapy? Prenat Diagn 17:1247–1260, 1997, with permission.)

cases resulted in 17 live births, but three babies died in the neonatal period, one of them due to an unrelated cause (undiagnosed cystic fibrosis). This brings the total survival rate following successful cord ligation to 71% (n = 15/21). One baby was also born with the features of an amniotic band syndrome, likely caused by the procedure,[77] although it theoretically may have been related to prior amnioreduction procedures.[78]

Bipolar Cord Coagulation

We recently described an alternative technique to occlude the umbilical cord using bipolar coagulation for-

ceps and thus conventional, nonlaser equipment.[79] Initially we used fetoscopic back-up; however, this is not essential (Fig. 15–14). The procedure can indeed be carried out using US guidance through a single port, which may reduce access-related complications. If the cannula cannot be directly inserted into the target amniotic sac, the cord can even be grasped through the intertwin membranes. The key instrument in the procedure is a small-diameter bipolar coagulation forceps. Over time we have used different commercially available instruments, most with a disposable 3.0-mm forceps (Everest Medical, Minneapolis, MN). At this moment we are testing even smaller diameter instruments in experimental conditions.

In a collaborative experience of ten cases, there were no failed procedures and the operating time was usually limited to about 15 minutes. Unfortunately, two cases were complicated by rupture of the membranes shortly after the procedure, prompting termination of the pregnancy. In the eight other cases, healthy babies were born at a mean gestation of 35 weeks (i.e., > 15 weeks after the procedure). Two additional amniotic leaks, also PPROM cases, occurred, but they were transient and did not pose any clinical problem. In our series the indication for cord obliteration was a TRAP sequence in one half of the patients, the others presented with FFTS and either CNS abnormalities or impending fetal demise. Bipolar coagulation was effective in arresting umbilical blood flow in *all* cases. In the two cases where the procedure exceeded 30 minutes, the cord was very thick and hydropic. Postoperative IUFD of the co-twin did not occur. Maternal morbidity was minimal, even when a minilaparotomy was made.

Bipolar coagulation has a number of theoretical and practical advantages. First, it obliterates simultaneously both the umbilical arteries and veins, causing immediate cessation of flow, thus preventing agonal interfetal hemorrhage when a vessel remains patent. Second, the procedure can be performed through a single port. Moreover, the technique relies on existing standard and relatively inexpensive instrumentation. Fetal medicine specialists are familiar with performing invasive pro-

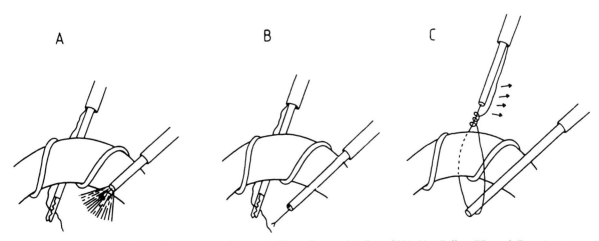

FIGURE 15–13. Steps in fetoscopic cord ligation. (From Deprest JA, Evrard VA, Van Ballaer PP, et al: Experience with fetoscopic cord ligation. Eur J Obstet Gynaecol Reprod Biol 81:157–164, 1998. Copyright 1998, Elsevier Science, with permission.)

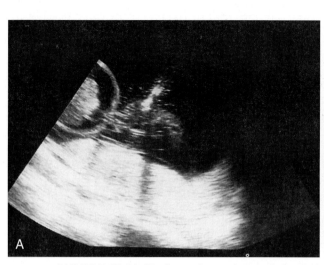

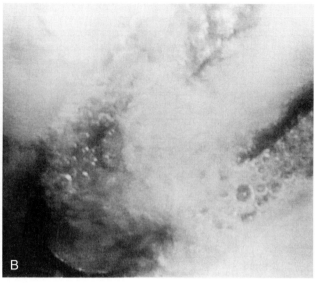

FIGURE 15–14. Bipolar cord coagulation. *A,* Same phase of the procedure, as visualized by US. *B,* Fetoscopic image of bipolar umbilical cord coagulation. Local heat production is visible as steam bubbles.

cedures under real-time ultrasound guidance. This also permits procedures in conditions where fetoscopy would be difficult, such as amniotic fluid stained with particles or blood. It also has the theoretical advantage that the electrical current does not travel through the umbilical cord, placenta, and/or other twin, since bipolar current passes only between the two blades of the instrument. As compared to cord ligation, the duration of the procedure has also been markedly reduced.

Monopolar Coagulation of the Cord and Other Fetal Vessels

Rodeck et al.[80] have described the use of monopolar thermocoagulation to arrest blood flow using conventional US-guided needling techniques. Their published experience includes so far four cases of TRAP sequence. In their first case, an attempt was made to coagulate the cord at 24 weeks. Although this was the surgical goal of the intervention, coagulation did not completely arrest flow in the umbilical cord. Nonetheless, the outcome of pregnancy was favorable. In the three following cases, the needle was directed to the acardiac aorta, successfully arresting flow in the fetal circulation. These latter three cases were all treated prior to 20 weeks and ended in uneventful term births. This elegant needle-based ultrasound-guided technique is certainly less complex and invasive than fetoscopic ligation. However, it remains to be demonstrated whether (1) arresting flow in the aorta precludes internal fetal hemorrhage or (2) fetofetal hemorrhage, and (3) if the technique would also work in other hemodynamic conditions and/or at a later gestational age. For instance, flow within a TRAP sequence fetus is clearly different than that in FFTS and/or discordant MC twins. Moreover, it was only successful at gestational ages where Nd:YAG laser of the cord has already proven effective; the upper gestational limit at which this procedure is successful remains to be established.

Assessment Before Selective Reduction

Thorough US fetal evaluation, including assessment of chorionicity, is obviously essential prior to embarking upon any of these procedures. The correct US identification of chorionicity may be difficult but is vital in planning therapy, and reviewing the images obtained at earlier US studies is essential. The specific criteria for case selection have not been established, and the optimal timing of procedures for each of the indications is unknown. The procedures discussed above are all associated with a variable but significant risk of complications and fetal death of the normal twin, and theoretically they should only be considered when the risks of not treating clearly outweigh those associated with the intervention.[81] The clinician will have to balance a number of factors in deciding whether to embark upon feticide. These include maternal risks, prognosis for both the normal as well as the abnormal fetus, risks for preterm delivery, risk of PPROM and other procedure-related complications, gestational age, availability of instrumentation, and operator experience.

Unfortunately the balance between risks and benefits remains unclear, as good data are not available for many of these factors. Decisions will therefore be based primarily on parental wish and local experience. Although the risk for preterm delivery of the normal twin is increased when carrying out selective termination, it should, however, also be noted that there is also an increased background preterm delivery rate for twins discordant for structural anomalies, reported to be as high as 79% when managed conservatively.[82]

Timing of the intervention may be even more difficult. For instance, the diagnosis of acardiac twin pregnancy can be easily made before 20 weeks, and at that time Nd:YAG laser coagulation is effective and of limited invasiveness. But as accurate criteria to predict IUFD of the pump twin are lacking, many would wait, thereby

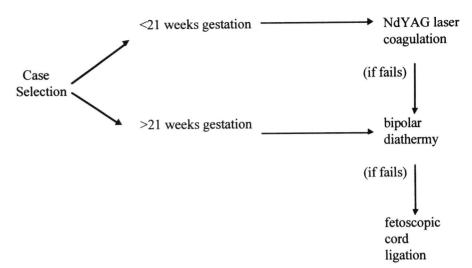

FIGURE 15–15. Suggested clinical flow chart of techniques for cord occlusion.

rendering conditions for a later intervention technically more challenging, and probably increasing the risk of procedure-related complications. The same issues apply to selective termination in cases of FFTS with poor prognosis or refractory to other therapy. The timing of the procedure is often difficult, as a judgment must be made between an early and perhaps unnecessary intervention, or leaving the procedure to a later point in time, making it more difficult and increasing the risk for in utero damage or cardiac decompensation of the normal twin.

Which is the Optimal Technique for Cord Occlusion?

There is no objective way to evaluate which is the optimal method of selective feticide in MC pregnancies today. Given the rarity of the indications, it is unlikely that this judgment will soon (or ever?) be possible. Based on the data presented above and our own experience, we suggest the simplest procedure with the fewest ports is likely to have the best outcome and fewest complications. Accordingly, we apply today the following clinical algorithm (Fig. 15–15). Prior to about 21 weeks, we prefer Nd:YAG laser coagulation, as this is a single-port technique with proven efficacy and technically not very demanding. If this technique is unsuccessful or for gestations beyond 21 weeks, bipolar cord coagulation is currently our method of choice. Sonoendoscopic cord ligation is reserved as a backup procedure if none of the above techniques are successful. If needle-based monopolar coagulation proves to be effective in more advanced gestations and in a wide range of hemodynamic situations, this would certainly affect the decision-making process.

Amniotic Band Syndrome

To date, the pathogenesis of amniotic bands and even their existence as a cause for some congenital anomalies have remained controversial. Amniotic band syndrome (ABSd) refers to amputation of fingers and/or limbs, and a wide spectrum of associated anomalies involving trunk and craniofacial anomalies. Two theories have been proposed to explain the pathogenesis. One is based on a developmental anomaly of the embryonic germinal disc,[83] and the amniotic band would be a by-product rather than the cause of fetal anomalies. The second theory claims that the primary problem is rupture of the amniotic membrane, and its detachment from the chorion.[84] In that scenario, the fetus would exit the amniotic cavity, and the outer amnion and naked chorion produce mesodermic fibrous strings that entangle and entrap different fetal organs like a "guillotine," leading to constriction and amputation. This theory became widely accepted, despite the small number of cases and inconsistent findings.[85]

The etiology has remained the source of much debate. It has so far been difficult to visualize an amnion at the precise place of amputation, or in most instances no amniotic sheet at all. The full sequence of a normal fetus, followed by the occurrence of amniotic rupture then by adhesion to the limbs and finally by amputation has not been described. Brohnstein therefore doubts this etiology. It is, for instance, difficult to explain why bands always cause transverse amputations and not diagonal constriction rings. The adhesion and constriction theory of Torpin, for instance, explains neither the associated anomalies nor the damage to internal organs. Brohnstein concludes therefore that the underlying reason must be an embryonic or teratogenic factor.

Moerman et al.[86] have reconciled both theories, and accept that both entities exist, and are just of different origin. We recently investigated a case of ABSd at 12 weeks' gestation in which the fetus appeared to be trapped in a "cob web" of bands[87] (Fig. 15–16). These bands were examined by transmission electron microscopy, and appeared to be cell-free tubules, carrying hooks acting like "Velcro" and constricting fetal elements. The case demonstrates early and increasing constriction as the fetus grows and moves. In addition, this fetus had grade 3 intraventricular hemorrhage, suggesting that bands could cause internal damage by redistrib-

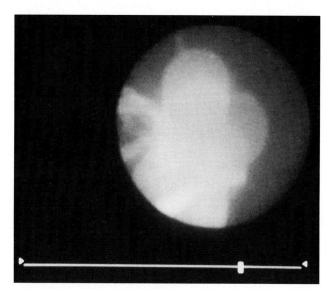

FIGURE 15-16. Fetoscopic image of the "cobweb" syndrome. (From Schwartzler P, Moscoso G, Senat M, Ville Y: The cobweb syndrome: 1st trimester sonographic diagnosis of multiple amniotic bands confirmed by fetoscopy and pathological examination. Hum Reprod 13:2966–2969, 1998, with permission.)

uting blood flow under external pressure. Also at later gestational age, modern ultrasound allows the detection of limb or finger amputations. In a recent report, Tadmor et al.[88] observed the progressive constriction of the lower limbs from 21 weeks onwards.

Though the consequences of ABSd are dramatic, they are not life threatening. Despite that, it would seem logical to try to arrest this process, particularly when the diagnosis of bands is made early and the amputation process has just started, moreover, as a causal relationship between the bands and the amputation is plausible.

In an ovine model, Crombleholme et al.[89] reproduced severe limb edema and dysfunction by limb constriction, caused by the extra-amniotic fixation of the lamb legs, which could be averted by the release of the constriction. The in utero release of amniotic bands in humans was therefore only a logical step pioneered by Quintero et al.[90] His group treated two cases of ABSd, at 22 and 23 weeks, lysing the band under sonoendoscopic control. The procedure restored adequate blood flow distal to the obstruction, and the limb could be preserved. In both cases, only mild or minimal limb dysfunction was present at birth. The assumption that human amniotic bands are amenable to a similar form of surgical release as in the animal model remains indeed speculative, and the success of surgery is based on the mechanistic etiologic mechanism.

Complications of Fetoscopic Procedures

The Risk for Rupture of the Fetal Membranes ("Iatrogenic" PPROM) and its Potential Therapy

The most important side effect of operative fetoscopy is the high risk of PPROM. Since this event is obvi-

ously related to the invasiveness of the procedure, and thus has causes other than spontaneous (idiopathic) PPROM, we would call this event "iatrogenic" PPROM (iPPROM). The exact incidence of iPPROM is difficult to define, given the limited experience with operative fetoscopy. In the pooled series of 17 successful cord ligations with surviving pump twin, there was frank rupture of the membranes in eight cases (47%), and in an additional two patients there was temporary amniotic fluid leakage prior to 32 weeks.[48] This remained as high even when considering only a single surgeon experience. For a much more common procedure such as Nd:YAG laser of chorionic plate vessels, Ville et al. reported an iPPROM rate of 10%.[13] Even after the "learning curve" of the procedure, iPPROM remains significant. In the more recent data from Hecher a risk of 12% of fetal loss was reported, most but not all related to iPPROM. As this operation is always carried out through a single port and its iPPROM rate is lower, we speculated that the number of ports used may be a risk factor for iPPROM.[49] However, other factors, such as operating time, complexity of the procedure, diameter of the port, use of and volume of amnioinfusion, previous invasive procedures, hemorrhage, underlying condition, or preexisting contractions may be as important.

Although further experience may reduce its incidence, iPPROM will certainly remain a limitation to the widespread application of operative fetoscopy. Therefore, innovative techniques to seal traumatic membrane defect have been proposed. Quintero reported the successful use of a cryoprecipitate plug after a fetoscopic cord ligation; however, it did not work in cases with spontaneous rupture of the membranes.[76, 90] In an in vitro study, adherence of platelets to the extracellular matrix at the place of the membrane defect was demonstrated, but its efficacy in vivo awaits further evidence. We have investigated in animal models whether sealing of the membrane defect at the end of the procedure would prevent iPPROM; this was so when using collagen plugs.[91–93] However, we have not applied it in clinical procedures yet; nevertheless, as it has been shown to be effective in primates this can be considered.[93] It is also hoped that any knowledge on this topic may be beneficial for patients with spontaneous PPROM, but that remains to be seen.[90]

Amniotic fluid leak after withdrawal of the fetoscope without surgical closure of the access site, causing anhydramnios, has been observed in 3 of 132 (2.3%) cases of laser coagulation for FFTS. However, leaking stopped spontaneously in all cases and amniotic fluid volume was restored.[13]

Other Complications and Considerations in Operative Fetoscopy

The exact nature and incidence of other, less frequent complications are not yet known. Access to the gestational sac is a critical step in any fetoscopy. Particularly hemorrhage from the trocar insertion site was already a problem in the earlier days of fetoscopy, and may still occur, even when using ultrasound guidance and the use of smaller diameter instruments.[13, 23, 42, 46] Bleeding may be intra-amniotic, intraperitoneal, or retroperitoneal. Intra-amniotic bleeding hampers fetoscopic view and may cause abortion of the fetoscopic procedure. In Ville's series with fetoscopic laser for FFTS, intra-abdominal bleeding prompted the need for transfusion of 7 units of blood in one patient, which was complicated by pulmonary edema. In his earlier experience, clinically symptomatic hemorrhage occurred in 2 of 44 cases.[8] Closing the uterine access site with a purse-string may prevent postoperative bleeding, but whether that would justify a minilaparotomy to expose the uterine wall is uncertain.[46, 49] It may as well only prevent intraperitoneal bleeding, not intra-amniotic hemorrhage.

Just as with serial amnioreductions, chorioamnionitis and abruptio placentae are possible. Amniotic fluid embolism is a theoretical complication of operative fetoscopy, but has not been reported so far. Maternal "hydrops" associated with severe hydrops fetoplacentalis has been described once by Ville, and we have seen this once following a laser procedure for FFTS.[8, 94] In another case, however, this was mildly present prior to the operation, but resolved completely after the laser procedure.[95] This reflects that this complication may as well be due to the primary condition as well. Amniotic bands developed probably as a result of (iatrogenic) disruption of the fetal membranes in one case of fetoscopic cord ligation.[77] These uncommon but serious complications demonstrate that operative fetoscopy remains an invasive procedure with its inherent risks. Patients should be counseled accordingly and monitored closely for any of these complications.

Theoretically, all known side effects of invasive in utero procedures might eventually be expected. This is one of the reasons driving the set-up of a registry of fetoscopic procedures, irrespective of their purpose. We have been able to do so with the support of the European Commission in its "Biomed Programme."[96] Data can be entered via the Internet, and the registry is open to all centers worldwide (http://www.eurofoetus.org). Maternal safety is the primary objective, but registration of large numbers may help to learn about fetal safety and outcome.

REFERENCES

1. Dumez Y, Mandelbort L, Dommergues M: Embryoscopy in continuing pregnancies. *In* Proceedings of the Annual Meeting of the International Fetal Medicine Society, Evian, France, May 1992.
2. International Fetoscopy Group: The status of fetoscopy and fetal tissue sampling. Prenat Diagn 4:79–81, 1984.
3. Estes JM, MacGillivray TE, Hedrick MH, et al: Fetoscopic surgery for the treatment of congenital anomalies. J Pediatr Surgr 27:950–954, 1992.
4. Quintero RA, Abuhamad A, Hobbins JC, Mahoney MJ: Transabdominal thin gauge embryofetoscopy: A technique for early prenatal diagnosis and its use in the diagnosis of a case of Meckel Gruber syndrome. Am J Obstet Gynecol 168:1552–1557, 1993.
5. Luks FI, Deprest JA: Endoscopic fetal surgery: A new alternative? [editorial]. Eur J Obstet Gynecol Reprod Biol 52:1–3, 1993.
6. Deprest JA, Gratacos E: Obstetrical endoscopy. Curr Opin Obstet Gynecol 11(2):195–203, 1999.
7. Luks FI, Deprest JA, Vandenberghe K, et al: Fetoscopy-guided fetal endoscopy in a sheep model. J Am Coll Surg 178:609–612, 1994.
8. Ville Y, Van Peborgh P, Gagnon A, et al: Traitement chirurgical du syndrome transfuseur-transfusé: Coagulation des anastomoses par un laser Nd:YAG sous contrôle écho-endoscopique. J Gynecol Obstet Biol Reprod 26:175–181, 1997.
9. Ville Y, Bernard JP, Doumerc S, et al: Transabdominal fetoscopy in fetal anomalies diagnosed by ultrasound in the first trimester of pregnancy. Ultrasound Obstet Gynecol 8:11–15, 1996.
10. Deprest J, Van Schoubroeck D, Van Ballaer P, et al: Alternative access for fetoscopic Nd:YAG laser in TTS with anterior placenta. Ultrasound Obstet Gynecol 12:347–352, 1998.
11. Luks FI, Deprest JA, Gilchrist BF, et al: Access techniques in endoscopic fetal surgery. Eur J Pediatr Surg 7:131–134, 1997.
12. Bruner JP, Richards WO, Tulipan NB, et al: Endoscopic coverage of fetal myelomeningocele in utero. Am J Obstet Gynecol 180:153–158, 1999.
13. Ville Y, Hecher K, Gagnon A, et al: Endoscopic laser coagulation in the management of severe twin transfusion syndrome. Br J Obstet Gynecol 105:446–445, 1998.
14. Fisk NM, Ronderos-Dumit D, Soliani A, et al: Diagnostic and therapeutic transabdominal amnio-infusion in oligohydramnios. Obstet Gynecol 78:270–278, 1991.
15. Skarsgard ED, Bealer JF, Meuli M, et al: Fetal endoscopic surgery: The relationship between insufflation pressure and the fetoplacental circulation. J Pediatr Surg 30:1165–1168, 1995.
16. Evrard V, Deprest J, Luks F, et al: Amnio-infusion with Hartmann's solution: A safe distension medium for endoscopic fetal surgery in the ovine model. Fetal Diagn Ther 12:188–192, 1997.
17. Luks FI, Deprest JA, Marcus M, et al: Carbon dioxide pneumamnios causes acidosis in the fetal lamb. Fetal Diagn Ther 9:101–104, 1994.
18. Saiki Y, Litwin DEM, Bigras JL, et al: Reducing the deleterious effects of intrauterine CO_2 during fetoscopic surgery. J Surg Res 69:51–54, 1997.
18a. Gratacós E, Wu J, Devlieger R, et al: Effects on fetal acid-base status of carbon dioxide (Co_2) amniodistension with and without maternal hyperventilation in a sheep model for fetal surgery. Am J Obstet Gynecol 182:S184 (Abstract 603), 2000.
19. Pelletier GJ, Srinathan SK, Langer JC: Effects of intraamniotic helium, carbon dioxide, and water on fetal lambs. J Pediatr Surg 30:1155–1158, 1995.
20. Ville Y: Diagnostic embryoscopy and fetoscopy in the first trimester of pregnancy. Prenat Diag 17:1237–1246, 1997.
21. Sebire NJ, Snijders RJ, Hughes K, et al: Screening for trisomy 21 in twin pregnancies by maternal age and fetal nuchal translucency thickness at 10–14 weeks of gestation. Br J Obstet Gynecol 103:999–1003, 1996.
22. Ville Y, Lalondrelle C, Doumerc S, et al: First trimester diagnosis of nuchal anomalies: Significance and fetal outcome. Ultrasound Obstet Gynecol 4:396–398, 1992.
23. Hecher K, Plath H, Bregenzer T, et al: Endoscopic laser surgery versus serial amniocenteses in the treatment of severe twin-twin transfusion syndrome. Am J Obstet Gynecol 180:717–724, 1999.
24. Quintero RA, Crossland WJ, Cotton DB: Effect of endoscopic white light on the developing visual pathway: A histologic, histochemical, and behavioral study. Am J Obstet Gynecol 171:1142–1148, 1994.
25. Deprest JA, Luks FI, Peers KHE, et al: Natural protection mechanisms of the fetal eye against endoscopic white light injury. Obstet Gynecol 94:124–127, 1999.
26. Westin J: Hysteroscopy in early pregnancy. Lancet 2:872, 1954.
27. Reece EA, Goldstein I, Chatwani A, et al: Transabdominal needle embryofetoscopy: A new technique paving the way for early fetal therapy. Obstet Gynecol 84:634–636, 1994.
28. Pennehouat GH, Thebault Y, Ville Y, et al: First trimester transabdominal fetoscopy. Lancet 340:429, 1992.
29. Hobbins JC, Jones OW, Gottesfeld S, Persutte W: Transvaginal ultrasonography and transabdominal embryoscopy in the first-trimester diagnosis of Smith-Lemli-Opitz syndrome, type II. Am J Obstet Gynecol 171:546–549, 1994.
30. Ginsberg NA, Zbarz D, Trom C: Transabdominal embryoscopy for the detection of Carpenter syndrome during the first trimester. J Assist Reprod Genet 11:373–375, 1994.
31. Reece EA, Homko CJ, Wiznitzer A, Goldstein I: Needle embryofetoscopy and early prenatal diagnosis. Fetal Diagn Ther 10:81–82, 1995.
32. Quintero R, Morales WJ, Kalter CS, Angel JL: In utero lysis of amniotic bands. Ultrasound Obstet Gynecol 10:316–320, 1997.

33. Ville Y: Monochorionic twin pregnancies: "Les liasons dangereuses". Ultrasound Obstet Gynecol 10:82–85, 1997.
34. Fusi L, McParland P, Fisk N, et al: Acute twin-twin transfusion: A possible mechanism for brain-damaged surviors after intrauterine death of a monochorionic twin. Obstet Gynecol 78:517–520, 1991.
35. Nicolini U, Pisoni MP, Cele E, Roberts A: Fetal blood sampling immediately before and within 24 hours of death in MC twin pregnancies complicated by single in utero fetal death. Am J Obstet Gynecol 179:800–803, 1998.
36. Deprest JA: Endoscopic feto-placental surgery: From animal experience to early clinical applications. Leuven University Press, Acta Biomedica Lovaniensia 199:1–179, 1999 (doctoral thesis).
37. Bajoria R, Wigglesworth J, Fisk N: Angioarchitecture of monochorionic placentas in relation to the twin-twin transfusion syndrome. Am J Obstet Gynecol 172:865–863, 1995.
38. Machin G, Still K, Lalani T: Correlations of placental vascular anatomy and clinical outcomes in 69 monochorionic twin pregnancies. Am J Med Genet 61:229–236, 1996.
39. De Lia JE, Cruikshank DP: Feticide versus laser surgery for twin-twin transfusion syndrome [letter]. Am J Obstet Gynecol 170:1480–1481, 1994.
40. Dumitrascu-Branisteanu I, Deprest J, Evrard V, et al: Time-related cotyledonary effects of laser coagulation of superficial chorionic vessels in an ovine model. Prenat Diagn 19:205–210, 1999.
41. Van Peborgh P, Rambaud C, Ville Y: Effect of laser coagulation on placental vessels: Histological aspects. Fetal Diagn Ther 12:32–35, 1997.
42. De Lia JE, Kuhlmann RS, Lopez KP: Treating previable twin-twin transfusion syndrome with fetoscopic laser surgery: Outcomes following the learning curve. J Perinat Med (in press) 1999.
43. Benirschke K, Kim CK: Multiple pregnancy. N Engl J Med 288:1276–1284, 1973.
44. De Vore G, Dixon J, Hobbins JC: Fetoscope-directed Nd:YAG laser: A potential tool for fetal surgery. Am J Obstet Gynecol 143:379–380, 1983.
45. De Lia JE, Cruikshank DP, Keye WR: Fetoscopic neodymium:YAG laser occlusion of placental vessels in severe twin-twin transfusion syndrome. Obstet Gynecol 75:1046–1053, 1990.
46. De Lia JE, Kuhlmann RS, Harstad TW, Cruikshank DP: Fetoscopic laser ablation of placental vessels in severe previable twin-twin transfusion syndrome. Am J Obstet Gynecol 172:1202–1211, 1995.
47. Ville Y, Hyett J, Hecher K, Nicolaides K: Preliminary experience with endoscopic laser surgery for severe twin twin transfusion syndrome. N Engl J Med 332:224–227, 1995.
48. Deprest JA, Evrard VA, Van Ballaer PP, et al: Experience with fetoscopic cord ligation. Eur J Obstet Gynaecol Reprod Biol 81:157–164, 1998.
49. Deprest JA, Lerut TE, Vandenberghe K: Operative fetoscopy: New perspective in fetal therapy? Prenat Diagn 17:1247–1260, 1997.
50. Mari G: Amnioreduction in twin-twin transfusion syndrome—a multicenter registry, evaluation of 579 procedures [abstract]. Am J Obstet Gynecol 177:S28, 1998.
51. MacGillivray I: Epidemiology of twin pregnancy. Semin Perinatol 10:4, 1984.
52. Van Allen MI, Smith DW, Shepard TH: Twin reversed arterial perfusion (TRAP) sequence: Study of 14 twin pregnancies with acardius. Semin Perinatol 7:285–293, 1983.
53. Evans MI: Selective termination for structural, chromosomal, and mendelian abnormalities: International experience. Am J Obstet Gynecol 180:S31, 1999.
54. Gilliam DL, Hendricks CH: Holoacardius; review of the literature and case report. Obstet Gynecol 2:647–653, 1953.
55. Healey MG: Acardia: Predictive risk factors for the co-twin's survival. Teratology 50:205, 1994.
56. Moore TR, Gale S, Bernischke K: Perinatal outcome of forty-nine pregnancies complicated by acardiac twinning. Am J Obstet Gynecol 163:907–912, 1990.
57. Adams D, Chervenak F: Multifetal pregnancies: Epidemiology, clinical characteristics and management. In Reece E, et al (eds): Medicine of the Fetus and Mother. Philadelphia: JB Lippincott Company, 1993, p 269.
58. Evans MI, Goldberg JD, Dommergues M, et al: Efficacy of second trimester selective termination for fetal abnormalities: International collaborative experience amongst the worlds largest centres. Am J Obstet Gynecol 171:90–94, 1994.
59. Nance W: Malformations unique to the twinning process. Prog Clin Biol Res 69:123, 1981.
60. Onyskowova A, Dolezal A, Jedlica V: The frequency and the character of malformations in multiple births. Acta Univ Carol 16:333, 1970.
61. Holzgreve W, Tercanli S, Krings W, Schuierer G: A simpler technique for umbilical cord blockade of an acardiac twin. N Engl J Med 331:57–58, 1995.
62. Sepulveda W, Bower S, Hassan J, Fisk N: Ablation of acardiac twin by alcohol injection into the intra-abdominal umbilical artery. Obstet Gynecol 86:680–681, 1995.
63. Hamada H, Okana M, Koresawa M, et al: Fetal therapy in utero by blockage of the umbilical blood flow of acardiac monster in twin pregnancy. Acta Obstet Gynecol Jpn 41:1803–1809, 1989.
64. Porreco R, Barton SM, Haverkamp AD: Occlusion of umbilical artery in acardiac, acephalic twin. Lancet 337:326–327, 1991.
65. Bebbington MW, Wilson RD, Machan L, Wittmann BK: Selective feticide in twin transfusion syndrome using ultrasound guided insertion of thrombogenic coils. Fetal Diagn Ther 10:32–41, 1995.
66. Denbow ML, Overton TG, Duncan KR, et al: High failure rate of umbilical vessel occlusion by ultrasound guided injection of absolute alcohol or enbucrilate gel. Prenat Diagn 19:527–532, 1999.
67. Dommergues M, Mandelbrot L, Delzoide A, et al: Twin-to-twin transfusion syndrome: Selective feticide by embolization of the hydropic fetus. Fetal Diagn Ther 10:26–31, 1995.
68. Roberts RM, Shah DM, Jeanty P, Beattie JF: Twin, acardiac, ultrasound guided embolization. Fetus 1(3):5–10, 1991.
69. Mahone PR, Sherer DM, Abramowicz JS, Woods JR: Twin-twin transfusion syndrome: Rapid development of severe hydrops of the donor following selective feticide of the hydropic recipient. Am J Obstet Gynecol 169:166–168, 1993.
70. Hecher K, Hackeloër BJ, Ville Y: Umbilical cord coagulation by operative microendoscopy at 16 weeks gestation in an acardiac twin. Ultrasound Obstet Gynecol 10:130, 1997.
71. Arias F, Sunderji S, Gimpelson R, Colton E: Treatment of acardiac twinning. Obstet Gynecol 91:818, 1998.
72. Ville Y, Hyett JA, Vandenbussche F, Nicolaides KH: Endoscopic laser coagulation of umbilical cord vessels in twin reversed arterial perfusion sequence. Ultrasound Obstet Gynecol 4:396–398, 1994.
73. Hecher K, Reinhold U, Gbur K, Hackelöer B-J: Interruption of umbilical blood flow in an acardiac twin by endoscopic laser coagulation. Geburtsh Frauenheilk 56:97–100, 1996.
74. McCurdy CM, Childers JM, Seeds JW: Ligation of the umbilical cord of an acardiac-acephalus twin with an endoscopic intrauterine technique. Obstet Gynecol 82:708–711, 1993.
75. Quintero RA, Romero R, Reich H, et al: In utero percutaneous umbilical cord ligation in the management of complicated monochorionic multiple gestations. Ultrasound Obstet Gynecol 8:16–22, 1996.
76. Quintero RA, Romero R, Dziecskowski J, et al: Sealing of ruptured amniotic membranes with intra-amniotic platelet cryoprecipitate plug [letter]. Lancet 347:1117, 1996.
77. Deprest J, Evrard V, Van Schoubroeck D, Vandenberghe K: Fetoscopic cord ligation. Lancet 348:890–891, 1996.
78. Von Eckardstein S, Reihs T, Crombach G: Constriction of an extremity after amnioreduction in a TRAP-like sequence. Fetal Diagn Ther 12:50–53, 1997.
79. Deprest J, Audibert F, Van Schoubroeck D, et al: Bipolar cord coagulation of the umbilical cord in complicated monochorionic twin pregnancy [abstract]. Am J Obstet Gynecol 180:S186, 1999.
80. Rodeck C, Deans A, Jauniaux E: Thermocoagulation for the early treatment of pregnancy with an acardiac twin. N Engl J Med 339:1293–1294, 1998.
81. Harrison MR: Professional considerations in fetal treatment. In Harrison MR, Golbus MS, Filly RA (eds): The Unborn Patient. Philadelphia: WB Saunders Company, 1991, pp 8–13.
82. Malone F, D'Alton ME: Management of multiple gestations complicated by a single anomalous fetus. Curr Opin Obstet Gynecol 9:213, 1997.
83. Streeter GL: Focal deficiencies in fetal tissues and their relation to intrauterine amputation. Contrib Embryol 22:1, 1930.
84. Torpin R: Amniochorionic mesoblastic fibrous strings and amniotic bands. Associated constricting fetal anomalies or fetal death. Am J Obstet Gynecol 91:65–75, 1965.

85. Brohnstein M, Zimmer EZ: Do amniotic bands amputate fetal organs? Ultrasound Obstet Gynecol 10:309–311, 1997.

86. Moerman P, Fryns JP, Vandenberghe K, Lauweryns JM: Constrictive amniotic bands, amniotic adhesions, and limb-body wall complex: Discrete disruption sequences with pathogenetic overlap. Am J Med Genet 42:470–479, 1992.

87. Schwartzler P, Moscoso G, Senat M, Ville Y: The cobweb syndrome: 1st trimester sonographic diagnosis of multiple amniotic bands confirmed by fetoscopy and pathological examination. Hum Reprod 13:2966–2969, 1998.

88. Tadmor O, Kreisberg G, Achiron R, et al: Limb amputation in amniotic band syndrome: Serial ultrasonographic and Doppler observations. Ultrasound Obstet Gynecol 10:312–315, 1997.

89. Crombleholme TM, Robertson F, Marx G, et al: Fetoscopic cord ligation to prevent neurological injury in monozygous twins. Lancet 348:191, 1996.

90. Quintero RA, Morales WJ, Kalter CS, et al: Transabdominal intra-amniotic endoscopic assessment of previable premature rupture of membranes. Am J Obstet Gynecol 179:71–76, 1998.

91. Deprest J, Papadopulos NA, Dumitrascu I, et al: Closure techniques for fetoscopic access sites in the midgestational rabbit model. Hum Reprod 14:1730–1734, 1999.

92. Gratacós E, Wu J, Yesildaglar, et al: Successful sealing of fetoscopic access sites with collagen plugs in the rabbit model. Am J Obstet Gynecol 182:142–146, 1999.

93. Luks FI, Deprest JA, Peers KHE, et al: Gelatin spongeplug to seal fetoscopy port sites: Technique in ovine and primate models. Ann J Obstet Gynecol 181:995–996, 1999.

94. Demeyere T, Van Schoubroeck D, Deprest J, Spitz B: Maternal hydrops after laser surgery in twin-to-twin transfusion syndrome. Fetal Diagn Ther 17:S124, 1998.

95. Claerhout F, Deprest J, Van Schoubroeck D, et al: In utero recovery of fetal hydrops and maternal hydrops in twin-twin transfusion syndrome. Fetal Diagn Ther 17:S125, 1998.

96. Eurofetus: Endoscopic Feto-Placental Surgery: From animal experimentation to early human experimentation. Programme funded by the European Commission, within the Biomed 2 Programme, PL 962383.

97. Willcourt RJ, Naughton MJ, Knutzen VK: Ligation of an umblical cord of an acardiac fetus; laparoscopic technique. J Am Assoc Gynecol Laparosc 2:319–321, 1995.

98. Lémery DJ, Vanlieferinghen P, Gasq M, et al: Umbilical cord ligation under US guidance. Ultrasound Obstet Gynecol 4:399–401, 1994.

ADDITIONAL READINGS

Bargy F, Sapin E: La chirurgie foetale: Pour quoi faire? Pediatrie 47:347–350, 1992.

Bealer JF, Raisanen J, Skarsgard E, et al: The incidence and spectrum of neurological injury after open fetal surgery. J Pediatr Surg 30:1150–1154, 1995.

Deprest JA, Luks FI, Peers KHE, et al: Intrauterine endoscopic creation of urinary tract obstruction in the fetal lamb: A model for fetal surgery. Am J Obstet Gynecol 172:1422–1426, 1995.

Harrison MR, Mychaliska GB, Albanese CT, et al: Correction of congenital diaphragmatic hernia in utero IX: Fetuses with poor prognosis (liver herniation and low lung-to-head ratio) can be saved by fetoscopic temporary tracheal occlusion. J Pediatr Surg 33:1017–1022, 1998.

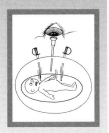

Operative Fetoscopy: FETENDO

MICHAEL R. HARRISON and CRAIG T. ALBANESE

Although open fetal surgery has successfully treated a limited number of fetal malformations, its effectiveness is limited by the occurrence of preterm labor and altered fetal homeostasis. These problems were the impetus for the development of minimally invasive fetal surgery. The theoretical benefits of fetoscopic surgery appear promising. The unique requirements of fetoscopic surgery necessitated modifications of existing endoscopic techniques, development of novel fetoscopic instruments, and multidisciplinary team approach. The technical and operative strategies led to the use of radially expanding and balloon tip trocars, miniaturized instruments, a fetoscopic irrigating pump and heat exchanger for working in a fluid medium, transuterine fetal fixation techniques, and new fetal monitoring methods. The constellation of techniques that allow real surgical procedures inside the uterus without hysterotomy we call FETENDO.

Many disorders are potentially amenable to correction in utero. Severe congenital diaphragmatic hernia, obstructive uropathy, and severe twin–twin transfusion syndrome have already been successfully treated using fetoscopic surgical techniques. Other life-threatening candidate disorders include cystic adenomatoid malformation of the lung, sacrococcygeal teratoma, hydrocephalus, and congenital high airway obstruction syndrome. But the most interesting application of minimally invasive surgical techniques will be the extension of surgical treatment to fetal diseases that are disabling but not life threatening: myelomeningocele, amniotic band syndrome, cleft lip, and other craniofacial defects. Although technically feasible, fetoscopic correction of many of these non–life-threatening anomalies is not currently warranted until potential maternal and fetal morbidity is dramatically lower. The future of fetoscopic surgical intervention depends on the continued evolution of fetoscopic techniques, the elucidation of the pathophysiology of fetal disorders, and a better understanding of preterm labor and fetal homeostasis.

The Rationale for Fetendo

Open fetal surgery has been successfully performed to treat a variety of life-threatening congenital anomalies.

However, preterm labor resulting from the hysterotomy is the predominant limiting factor preventing the broad application of open fetal surgery. Furthermore, open fetal surgery requires partial exteriorization of the fetus, which predisposes to fetal hypothermia and related secondary physiologic perturbations that may cause fetal morbidity.

We hypothesized that minimally invasive fetal surgery (FETENDO), by inducing less uterine trauma, would ameliorate preterm labor and maintain fetal homeostasis by protecting the intrinsic physiologic fetal milieu. Unfortunately, the existing equipment and techniques used for postnatal endoscopic surgery required significant modifications to meet the unique requirements of fetoscopic surgery. Among the novel challenges of fetoscopic surgery were: variable placental location, a thick vascular uterine wall with layers of membranes tenuously attached to the inner surface, a variable uterine wall compliance, a mobile fetus, the necessity of operating within a fluid medium, a cramped operative field, and suboptimal monitoring of the fetus with no intravenous access. These obstacles have been largely overcome experimentally and recently applied clinically.

This chapter chronicles the evolution of minimally invasive fetal surgery. The potential advantages of FETENDO, compared to open fetal surgery, are discussed in the context of experimental and clinical work. The technical details of fetoscopic surgery and monitoring techniques are presented. Lastly, specific disorders potentially amenable to fetoscopic intervention are discussed.

Experimental Background

The concept that uterine irritability (preterm labor) was directly related to the magnitude of uterine trauma (i.e., from simple needle puncture to full hysterotomy incision) was derived intuitively from early attempts at human fetal intervention (i.e., from fetal transfusions by percutaneous intraperitoneal injection to hysterotomy for exchange transfusions). In the early 1980s, this concept was first documented from our experimental fetal surgery work in the nonhuman primate (Fig. 16–1).[1]

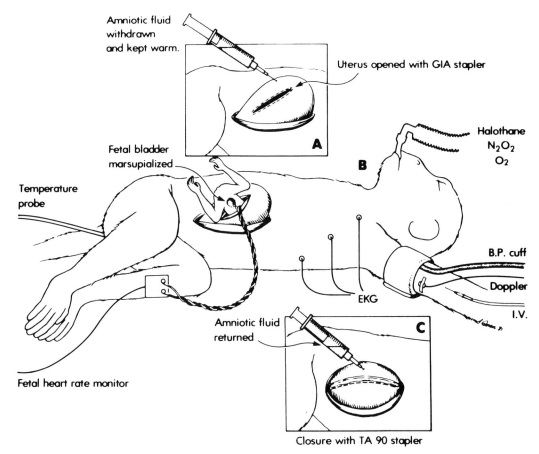

Amniotic fluid
withdrawn
and kept warm.

Uterus opened with GIA stapler

A

B

Halothane
N₂O₂
O₂

Fetal bladder
marsupialized

Temperature
probe

B.P. cuff

Doppler

EKG

I.V.

Amniotic fluid
returned

C

Fetal heart rate monitor

Closure with TA 90 stapler

F I G U R E 16–1. Techniques for open fetal surgery in the nonhuman primate.

Subsequently, we used the sheep model to develop the techniques for fetoscopic intervention (Fig. 16–2).[2, 3] More recently, fetoscopic techniques and their effect on fetal homeostasis and preterm labor have been systematically studied by a number of laboratories around the world.

The experimental effect of minimally invasive fetal surgery on preterm labor is inconclusive. Van der Wildt et al.[4] studied the effect of fetoscopic access in midtrimester rhesus monkeys and the resulting uterine contractions. Twenty-four hours postoperatively, no significant premature contractions were noted. Of the five monkeys, two died on the second and sixth postoperative days, respectively. Of the remaining three monkeys, recordings of myometrial activity were repeated during the third trimester and no premature contractions were noted.

In contrast, Luks and colleagues performed a study in third-trimester sheep to assess uterine contractions after open hysterotomy versus fetoscopic access.[5] The effects on the uterus were recorded based solely on access; no fetal manipulation was performed. Surprisingly, they found that uterine contractions were present 52% of the time (range, 34 to 72%), and there was no significant difference between control, hysterotomy, and endoscopic access. Furthermore, the rate, pattern, and amplitude of myometrial contractions were not significantly different between the groups. These findings are particu-

larly surprising because clinically significant preterm labor has been more prominent in the monkey compared to the sheep model.

In the same study, Luks assessed uteroplacental oxygen delivery after open hysterotomy versus fetoscopic access in third-trimester sheep.[5] Open hysterotomy caused a reduction in uterine blood flow and uteroplacental oxygen delivery to 73% of its initial value. The uteroplacental flow remained unchanged after the endoscopic approach. The 27% reduction in uteroplacental oxygen delivery seen in the hysterotomy group is probably higher during a surgical procedure given uterine and fetal manipulations. Experimental studies have demonstrated decreased fetal pH, increased serum lactate concentrations, and redistribution of fetal blood flow when uteroplacental oxygen delivery was reduced to 70% of control. Furthermore, during an operative procedure, the fetal oxygen demand could be increased resulting in more severe fetal hypoxemia. Therefore, fetoscopic access to the uterus may result in more stable fetal homeostasis.

Our initial clinical experience with human fetoscopic surgery has in general reflected the experimental work. Fetoscopic intervention is strikingly better than open fetal surgery for fetal homeostasis and produces less preterm labor with less use of tocolytics, decreased maternal hospital stay, and decreased maternal complications related to tocolysis.[6] But there has not yet been a

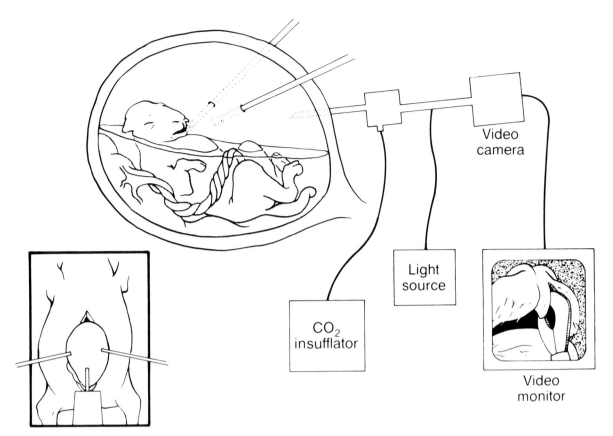

FIGURE 16–2. The operating set-up for fetoscopic surgery on the fetal sheep. The *inset* depicts the orientation of the equipment on the anesthetized ewe. The video monitor demonstrates the creation of a fetal cleft lip.

demonstrable prolongation of time in utero, since most fetuses still deliver early.

Operative Fetoscopic Techniques

Procedure

The anesthetic techniques, intraoperative monitoring, and tocolytic therapy developed from two decades of intensive experimental and clinical fetal intervention have been previously described.[7] Briefly, the mother and fetus are anesthetized with halogenated agents, which also provide profound uterine relaxation. Intraoperatively, nitroglycerin and occasionally terbutaline are administered as needed to achieve uterine relaxation.

The mother is placed in a modified lithotomy position with the knees low so the surgeons can work from three sides. The surgeon is usually between the legs with the assistants positioned on either side of the patient and the ultrasonographer is on the patient's right. The monitors (one for endoscopic imaging, one for sonographic imaging) are side by side opposite the surgical team. The intraoperative set-up is pictured in Figure 16–3.

The position of the placenta and the fetus determines whether a procedure can be performed percutaneously or requires maternal laparotomy and manipulation of the uterus (Fig. 16–4). When the placenta is anterior and blocks access through the maternal abdominal wall, the uterus is exposed through a low transverse abdominal incision. Intraoperative ultrasonography is used to map the placental edge. Thus far, placental position has never precluded access to the fetus, but intraoperative decisions about trocar placement must allow for both placental position and the uterine vessels in both uterine horns. In the case of an anterior placenta, and uterus is manipulated forward for posterior/superior insertion of the trocars.

The Crucial Role of Intraoperative Sonography

Operative manipulation of the fetus without hysterotomy depends on a close working relationship between surgical endoscopists and sonologists. The FETENDO procedure requires two simultaneous real-time views of the fetus in utero—a sonographic view on one video monitor and an endoscopic view on the same screen (window) or on a second side-by-side monitor so that all participants can see both views simultaneously. The evolution of the role of sonography is best illustrated by comparing Figure 16–5, which describes the initial and now outdated set-up, to the newer and better set-up outlined in Figure 16–3. In the outdated set-up, the sonographic image is displayed only on the monitor of the portable sonogram device, so the sonographer and surgical team must turn around to see it. The newer set-

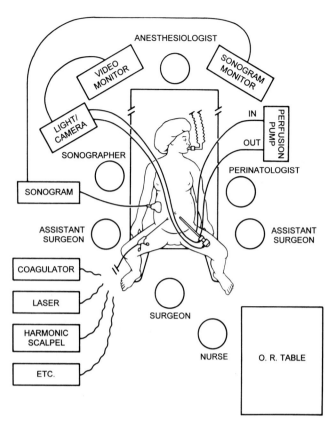

FIGURE 16–3. Drawing of the operating room set-up. Note two monitors at the head of the table; one for the fetoscopic picture and the other for the real-time ultrasound image.

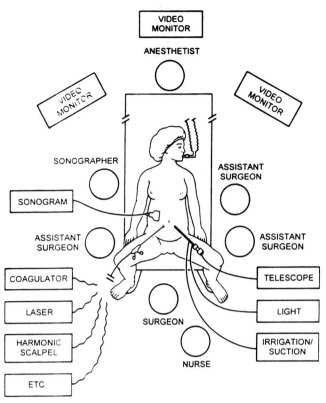

FIGURE 16–5. Before appreciating the necessity of having real-time ultrasound image available to all, only the fetoscopic images were displayed at the head of the table and the ultrasound image was displayed on the portable machine to the patient's right, out of the surgeon's view.

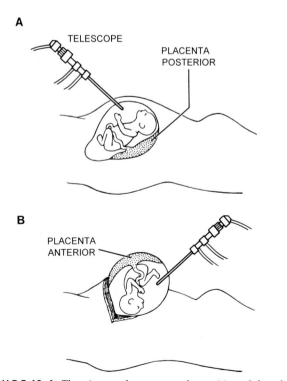

FIGURE 16–4. The pictures demonstrate the position of the telescope with respect to placental position. An anterior placenta necessitates forward displacement of the uterus.

up puts the sonographic and endoscopic images side-by-side for simultaneous viewing by the whole team.

The sonologist not only determines the trocar sites by mapping the position of placenta and fetus, but also helps guide insertion of the trocars in order to avoid inadvertent trauma to the fetus and/or umbilical cord. Because the operative field is quite "cramped," the sonologist is often required to guide the camera and instruments to the endoscopic "working area" in the uterus. In addition, many maneuvers are performed better under sonographic than endoscopic guidance (e.g., placing a T-bar through the trachea during the FETENDO clip procedure). FETENDO is thus a carefully orchestrated dance between endoscopic surgeon and sonologist. The "lead" changes depending on what is required for that sequence of the dance, but the cooperation and coordination must be maintained throughout for successful completion of this complex ensemble.

Trocars

The limiting factor in the success of fetoscopic surgery has proven to be the delicate handling of the uterus, hemostasis, and membrane separation. The membranes can be "tented" and pushed away from the myometrium by incorrectly placed trocars. In our early work, we used relatively large trocars with balloons that proved crucial

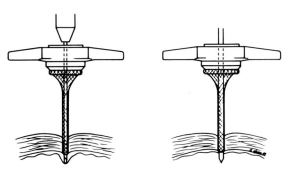

FIGURE 16–6. Two methods of deploying the radial expansion access system are depicted. On the left, a Veress needle (which comes in the kit) is used. This is not acceptable, since the blunt safety mechanism deploys once the muscle is completely pierced, allowing the membranes to be "tented" and pushed away. On the right, the system was modified by replacing the Veress needle with an extremely sharp diamond cut needle that sharply pierces the membranes, making only a small opening without pushing them off the undersurface of the myometrium.

for controlling bleeding from the myometrium and preventing membrane separation at the insertion sites. The trocars were placed with ultrasound guidance after placing a full-thickness U stitch that allowed us to pull up on the uterus and membranes as the trocar was advanced. Two sizes were used: 5 mm, which has an 8-mL balloon (Entec Corp., Madison, CT), and 10 mm, which as a 25-mL balloon (Origin Medsystems, Inc., Menlo Park, CA). In closing the uterine trocar sites, we strove to incorporate all membrane layers. The previously placed U stitches were tied over pledgets and fibrin glue was instilled into the insertion sites before tightening the sutures.

More recently, we have used a specially modified radially expanding access system (InnerDyne, Inc., Sunnyvale, CA), which is introduced with a small, very sharp needle and then expanded to accommodate 3-, 5-, or 7-mm trocars (Figs. 16–6 and 16–7). They control bleeding by outward pressure, and membrane separation is minimized using a swift insertion technique with the sharp needle. Newer radial expanding access sys-

tems with balloon tamponade capabilities are now being tested. Luks and colleagues also found that using a Seldinger technique for insertion of radially expanding trocars allowed safe access without membrane separation in experimental animals.[8]

Membrane Separation: The Achilles' Heel of Fetoscopic Surgery

Membrane rupture and separation with exposure of the biologically active space between membrane and myometrium to amniotic fluid is a powerful stimulus to preterm labor and is probably more harmful than myometrial disruption. The ideal closure of the trocar access sites would seal the membranes, prevent amniotic fluid extravasation, and later membrane separation, and also provide hemostasis and reinforcement for the myometrium. This closure is not yet available.

Many techniques have been tried experimentally and clinically. The work of Deprest et al.[9–11] first suggested that closure of the myometrium was superior to suturing of membranes, and later that a gelatin sponge plug may help. Our experience in humans confirms this experimental work. Initially, we used fibrin glue and myometrial/membrane sutures (Fig. 16–8). This proved inadequate to prevent membrane separation and preterm labor. More recently, we have developed a technique in which a plug is constructed by wrapping Dexon mesh around Gelfoam soaked in liquid thrombin and Toradol (Fig. 16–9), termed the uterine SEAL (seal entry, avoid labor) procedure. The components of the uterine seal plug are aimed at providing "bulk," promoting hemostasis, interrupting the prostaglandin pathway implicated in myometrial contractions, and occluding the hole in the membranes, while pulling the membranes up against the endometrium. An absorbable suture is tied to the mesh and is cut long. The plug is deployed

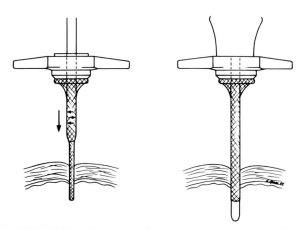

FIGURE 16–7. A 5-mm cannula/obturator is used to radially expand the sheath. This mechanism stabilizes the access system, controls myometrial bleeding by virtue of its outward expansion, and keeps the membranes from separating and tearing.

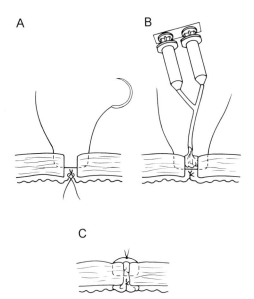

FIGURE 16–8. The membranes and myometrium are sutured separately (A). Fibrin glue is instilled before the myometrial suture is tied (B). The site is closed (C).

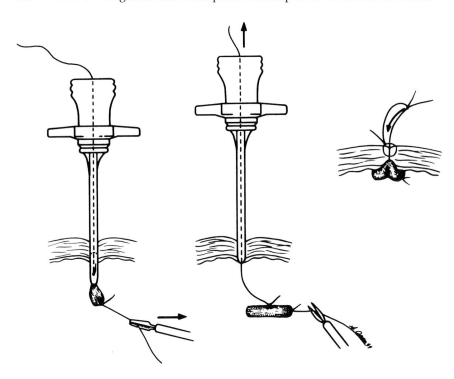

FIGURE 16–9. Steps required to perform the uterine "seal" procedure. The plug is first pulled down the 5-mm cannula, leaving the long centrally placed suture intact and hanging free from the top of the cannula. The polar "pull" suture is cut, and the cannula withdrawn (*center*). The plug is gently pulled up to the entry site, a myometrial suture is placed and tied, and the plug's suture is tied to the end of one of the myometrial sutures, which keeps the plug from migrating.

through the trocar and the trocar is removed. Because the tract was made by radial expansion it becomes smaller once the access system is removed, allowing one to snugly pull the plug against the membranes. The tract is closed with a simple partial thickness figure-of-eight Maxon stitch, incorporating the plug suture that is placed on moderate tension. Before tying the myometrial suture, fibrin glue is placed in the tract.

The Working Medium: Fluid Versus Gas

Most operative endoscopy is performed in a gas medium, commonly with CO_2. This makes visualization and surgical manipulation (cutting, catheterization, etc.) easy and familiar. However, it is not ideal for the normally aquatic fetal environment. Most problematic are the potential complications of CO_2 insufflation (air embolism or fetal acidosis). Luks et al.[12] demonstrated in six anesthetized ewes that CO_2 insufflation of the amniotic cavity produced severe fetal hypercapnia (57.6 ± 1.6 to 87.0 ± 7.0 mm Hg) and acidosis (from 7.22 ± 0.03 to 7.11 ± 0.8) despite normal maternal CO_2 pressure and pH. CO_2 was insufflated at low pressure (3 mm Hg) and rate (1.01/min). In the pilot experiment, CO_2 was insufflated for 1 hour and caused irreversible fetal acidosis, bradycardia, and death. The subsequent experiments lasted only 30 minutes and caused marked fetal hypercapnia and acidosis. Furthermore, an elevated Pa_{CO_2} may decrease cerebral blood flow. In addition, high CO_2 pressure has led to placental insufficiency in a lamb model.[13] Perhaps most important for fetal endoscopic manipulation, a gas medium would make ultrasonography, a crucial component of visualization, impossible.

Working in a fluid medium has many physiologic advantages but is technically difficult. By bathing the fetus in warm saline or lactated Ringer's solution throughout the case, the physiologic milieu of the fetus is maintained. Even with high volumes of fluid perfused into the uterus, less than 3% is systematically absorbed and maternal hypervolemia or altered maternal electrolytes have not been noted in our experience. The safest medium for endoscopic work in the uterus is an isotonic solution. Experimentally, Evrard et al.[14] demonstrated that amnioinfusion with Hartmann solution is a safe medium for endoscopic fetal surgery in the ovine model. The Hartmann solution was warmed to 38°C and radiolabeled with ^{99m}Tc red blood cells. They detected no absorption or diffusion of radioactivity in the fetus or membranes.

The major problem with a fluid medium is visibility. Amniotic fluid is normally filled with debris, and surgical dissection and bleeding further obscure the field of view. Continuous flow of clear fluid directly into the field with simultaneous retrieval is necessary. A specially designed fetoscopic irrigation system was developed that would deliver high flows at constant physiologic temperatures (37°C) within 10 minutes.[15] The high flows were necessary for effective visualization when working in a fluid medium obscured by cloudy amniotic fluid and bleeding. A heat exchanger was necessary to keep the fluid at 37°C. Once the uterus is distended with an adequate amount of fluid as judged by manual palpation, the fetoscopic irrigation system maintains this balance. However, given the changing uterine compliance during this procedure, volume controls are used to infuse or suction fluid as needed. The irrigating pump was connected to a 12-degree, 5-mm hysteroscope that is ideally suited to fetoscopic surgery. The telescope is inserted into two concentric sheaths. Fluid is pumped through the inner sheath, which exits at the tip of the telescope providing excellent end-on visualization. If the operative field is obscured by bleeding, increasing the flow effectively clears the field. Multiple perforations at the tip of the external sheath allows for effective fluid withdrawal (Fig. 16–10).

A problem with saline amnioinfusion is the difficulty of coagulating blood vessels because the current between the bipolar tips disseminates into the electrolyte-rich solution. Solutions such as glycine or sorbitol would allow for excellent bipolar coagulation, but may be toxic to the fetus. Luks et al. found that a specially designed bipolar cutting probe with a needle tip and a broad-based ring allowed a moderate amount of electrical cutting (personal communication). Perhaps the best solution to in utero coagulation is the harmonic scalpel, which we have adapted from the postnatal laparoscopy experience and have demonstrated it to work (cut and coagulate) in a saline medium. We have used it to dissect the fetal neck for temporary tracheal occlusion and to divide the umbilical cord in situ for twin–twin transfusion syndrome.

Fetal Orientation, Fixation, and Dissection

One of the most difficult and often frustrating aspects of FETENDO is manipulating the fetus into the correct position and maintaining that position while trocars are placed and the procedure performed. Maternal laparotomy is often necessary when the fetus or placenta are not aligned correctly as determined by sonography under anesthesia. This potential problem was best elucidated during the development of the technique to temporarily occlude the fetal trachea. Dissection of a delicate structure like the trachea is impossible when the fetal neck is normally flexed. To overcome this, a transuterine suture is placed through the center of the fetal chin and back out of the uterus under sonographic guidance (Fig.

16–11). Upward tension is placed and it is secured to a malleable retractor arm that is fixed to the operating table. The operative field is now exposed and can then be triangulated by the chin stitch and the two graspers. As in all endoscopic surgery, the camera and operative instruments must be carefully positioned to triangulate the operative field and the operator's orientation.

For difficult dissections like the midline neck, endoscopic visual localization may not be adequate, since the telescope visualizes only a very small portion of the fetal neck without the ability for a large panoramic view that would allow orientation and assessment of the midline of the fetal neck. Therefore, sonographic visualization of the midline and sonographic placement of "guides" for subsequent endoscopic dissection are crucial. For example, for the FETENDO clip procedure, ultrasound-guided placement of a transuterine T-fastener (Meditech, Boston Scientific Corp., Watertown, MA) within the lumen of the trachea allows rapid and reliable endoscopic dissection along the T-fastener for exposure of the anterior wall of the trachea (Fig. 16–11).[15]

Monitoring the Uterus and Fetus

Luks et al. performed a study of the predictive value of various monitoring methods in fetoscopic surgery.[16] Using a fetal lamb model, a balloon occluder was placed around the umbilical cord and inflated to reproduce fetal ischemia. Although intravascular oximetry and blood pressure provided a prompt and reliable response to fetal stress, these modalities are invasive and technically challenging. Bradycardia was found to be an insensitive and late sign of fetal distress. The most promising noninvasive modality was transcutaneous pulse oximetry, which was shown to have a rapid response time, high sensitivity, and negative predictive value. Although there was variability in the absolute oxygen saturation value, desaturation was predictive of acute fetal distress.

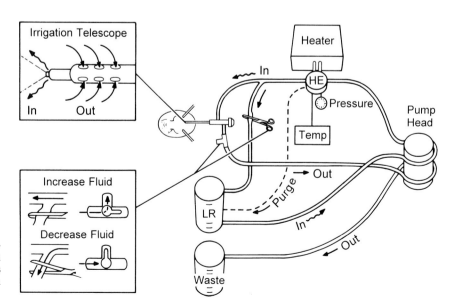

F I G U R E 16–10. The high-flow irrigating system consists of an extracorporeal pump and a heat exchanger that continuously circulates warmed lactated Ringer's solution via a sheath through which the telescope is placed (*inset*).

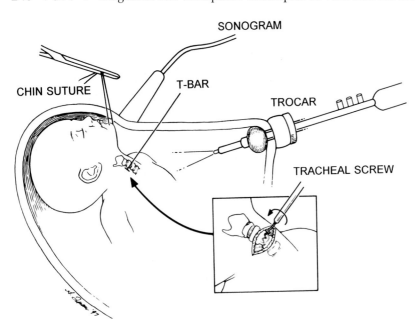

SONOGRAM

CHIN SUTURE

T-BAR

TROCAR

TRACHEAL SCREW

F I G U R E 16–11. Under sonographic guidance, the fetus' neck is exposed and the head stabilized by placing a temporary transuterine chin suture, and a T-fastener is placed in the fetal trachea to aid in localizing the midline fetal neck. After anterior tracheal dissection, a tracheal "screw" can be placed in the anterior tracheal wall to facilitate safe posterolateral dissection, if necessary.

Luks et al. have demonstrated the feasibility of fetoscopically placed temperature, amniotic pressure, and pulse oximetry sensors. These technical advances will aid in fetal monitoring and help to elucidate the fetal response during fetoscopic surgery. Furthermore, fetoscopically placed amniotic pressure monitoring will be essential when fetoscopic procedures are performed percutaneously, since direct palpation of the uterus to assess distention will be impossible.

We have used a variety of monitoring parameters during human fetoscopic surgery. Periodic sonography monitors heart rate and contractility. Direct uterine palpation is required to assess the degree of uterine distention, and intrauterine fluid balance is adjusted accordingly. The irrigating solution is warmed and maintained at 37° to 38°C. During open fetal surgery, a radiotelemeter is implanted under the fetal chest wall that transmits continuous electrocardiogram and intrauterine pressure.[7] Currently, we are working with the National Aeronautics and Space Administration (NASA) Sensors 2000 Program on developing a miniaturized radiotelemeter that can be inserted through a 5-mm trocar that could potentially be left in the amniotic space or inside the fetus. This device is presently being tested in animals.

Disorders Potentially Amenable to Fetoscopic Correction In Utero

Congenital Diaphragmatic Hernia

Fetuses with congenital diaphragmatic hernia (CDH) who have a poor prognosis with postnatal treatment can now be selected on the basis of liver herniation and a low lung/head ratio (LHR).[17,18] In this subset of fetuses, open in utero hernia reduction and complete repair proved unsuccessful because of umbilical vein occlusion while reducing the liver into the abdomen. Fortunately,

a serendipitous observation that fetuses with congenital high airway obstruction syndrome had abnormally large and well-developed lungs led to the idea that temporary tracheal occlusion might successfully be used to gradually enlarge the hypoplastic fetal lung. Temporary tracheal occlusion or the PLUG (*p*lug the *l*ung *u*ntil it *g*rows) technique has worked experimentally and clinically to reverse the pulmonary hypoplasia associated with CDH.[19,20] It increases lung mass, improves gas exchange, and reduces the viscera. Initial clinical experience showed that the PLUG strategy works in human fetuses, but complications from open fetal surgery limited survival.[6] After a decade of experimental work, we have now developed techniques for fetoscopic tracheal occlusion.[15]

Since the evolution of operative fetoscopy (FETENDO) was driven by the need to develop a minimally invasive fetal temporary tracheal occlusion, the technical developments of the FETENDO clip procedure will be described in detail. As usual, the techniques were first perfected in the fetal sheep model[21] (Fig. 16–12) and then applied clinically.

The procedures have been performed between 23 and 30 weeks' gestation. The mother and fetus are anesthetized with a halogenated inhaled anesthetic agent, which also provide profound uterine relaxation. General endotracheal anesthesia is coupled with narcotics administered via an epidural catheter. The uterus is exposed through a low transverse abdominal incision. Intraoperative ultrasonography delineates the margins of the placenta. No patient is excluded on the basis of placental position; an anterior placenta requires tipping the uterus forward and placement of the trocars superiorly and/or posteriorly.

The mother is placed in lithotomy position with the knees low enough to allow the surgeon to work between the abducted legs (Fig. 16–3). The surgical assistants are positioned on either side of the patient. The sonographer is on the patient's right. The perfusionist is back a few

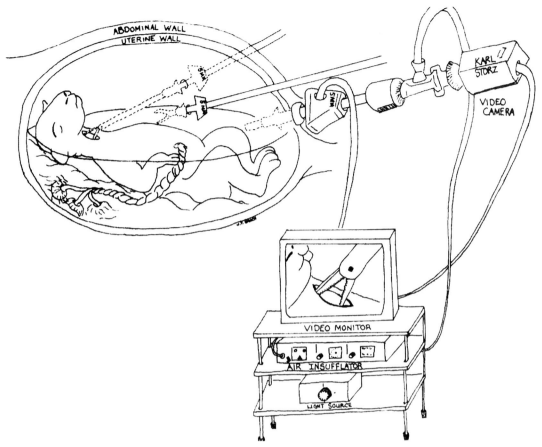

FIGURE 16–12. Fetal sheep model for external fetoscopic tracheal occlusion.

feet from the table on the patient's left. Two video monitors are placed at the head of the bed on either side of the patient. One displays the videoscopic image; the other, the real-time ultrasound image.

Initially, four trocars were inserted: one 10-mm port for the 6.5-mm (O.D.), 4.5-mm lens; a 12-degree hysteroscope placed through the irrigating sheath; two 5-mm ports for graspers placed on both ends of the neck incision; and one 10-mm working port for dissection and placement of the tracheal clips. Now the procedure requires only three 5-mm radially expanding trocars. Fetal orientation, fixation, and tracheal dissection are performed as described above (Fig. 16–11). The trachea was initially occluded with two standard, large titanium hemoclips placed with a reusable 10-mm clip applier (Karl Storz, Tuttlingen, Germany). A Prolene suture was tied in the crotch of the clips and left long to facilitate clip identification and removal at the time of delivery. More recently, the clip applier developed by US Surgical Corporation allows placement of an 8-mm long clip through a 5-mm port. To ensure complete occlusion, we place clips from both sides through both 5-mm ports. The skin incision is left open. An adequate volume of warmed lactated Ringer's solution remains in the uterus at the time of trocar removal and insertion site closure. Antibiotics are instilled into the amniotic cavity.

Thus far, the results achieved with the FETENDO clip procedure appear to justify the long and difficult evolution of techniques. In the last 3 years, 32 of 86 fetuses with CDH diagnosed before 25 weeks' gestation had both herniated liver and a low LHR. Because of the poor prognosis of these fetuses, fetal tracheal occlusion was offered. Thirteen had the trachea occluded by open fetal surgery; only one survived (8%). Eight had the trachea occluded fetoscopically (FETENDO clip); six survived (75%). Thirteen families chose postnatal treatment at an extracorporeal membrane oxygenation (ECMO) center; ten babies required ECMO and only five survived (38%). Although not statistically significant given the small number of cases, maternal morbidity, preterm labor, hospital stay, and time to delivery were better in the FETENDO clip group than in the open clip group. CDH fetuses with herniated liver and low LHR are at high risk of neonatal demise (62%) and appear to benefit from temporary tracheal occlusion when performed fetoscopically but not when performed by open fetal surgery.[6]

FETENDO clip may not be the final best technical solution to achieving minimally invasive temporary tracheal occlusion. An internal occlusion device like a balloon could be placed through the larynx using fetal bronchoscopy. We have developed in a sheep model videofetoscopic tracheal occlusion using an intratracheal plug (Fig. 16–13).[22] Others have developed detachable balloon techniques for achieving tracheal occlusion.[23, 24] These promising techniques are still being developed and tested experimentally.

Fetal Obstructive Uropathy

Prenatal intervention is possible for select fetuses with urinary tract obstruction whose renal and pulmonary development is threatened but potentially salvageable. Methods of fetal urinary tract decompression continue to be refined: open fetal surgery is no longer necessary, since the development of vesicoamniotic shunts that can be placed percutaneously under sonographic guidance and, more recently, endoscopic intervention. Catheter shunts are not always successful in decompressing the obstructed bladder, and carry a complication rate of approximately 25% due largely to displacement and obstruction.[25]

Open fetal surgery can relieve bladder outlet obstruction, but it carries the attendant risk of open surgery for the mother and fetus. Percutaneous methods carry less risk but are unreliable for long-term bladder decompression due to catheter migration or occlusion. However, there is a fetoscopic technique that holds a great deal of promise for improving the treatment of congenital urinary tract obstruction in utero. There are two possible approaches. Catheters or other shunt devices can be placed under direct vision, thereby ensuring proper positioning and minimizing the risks to the fetus. Estes et al. developed a fetoscopic approach to relieving urinary obstruction in fetal lambs.[26] A model of congenital obstructive uropathy was created by ligation of the urethra and urachus at 80 days' gestation in the fetal lamb. Seven days later the uterus was exposed by laparotomy and two 5-mm trocars were placed through the uterus and a vesicocutaneous fistula was created using a Wallstent, which is placed in a 7-Fr catheter that expands to 8 mm (21-Fr) in diameter when deployed. Examination 7 days later demonstrated that the stent was effective in relieving obstruction in all cases, while severe megacystis and hydroureter were noted in the controls. This fetoscopic technique should provide more reliable bladder drainage than catheter shunts due to the large caliber and

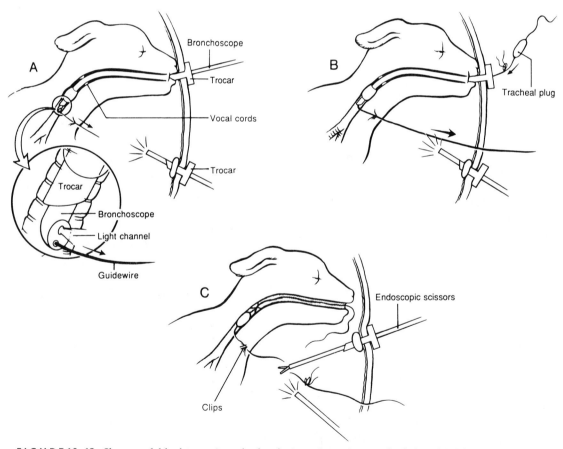

F I G U R E 16–13. Sheep model for fetoscopic tracheal occlusion using an intratracheal plug. *A,* With secure subglottic endotracheal trocar access, the sharp guidewire is advanced through the working channel of the bronchoscope, across the anterior trachea and cervical soft tissue, and into the uterine cavity under direct endoamniotic visualization. *B,* Once the bronchoscope has been withdrawn over the transtracheal guidewire, the compressed foam plug (attached via suture to the guidewire) is drawn into the trachea through the trocar. *C,* With the foam plug positioned inside the trachea, the endotracheal trocar is removed and replaced with a short endoamniotic trocar through which endoscopic clips are applied to the suture at its exit from the lamb's neck. The suture is divided with scissors.

wire mesh design of the stent, and direct visualization should decrease fetal morbidity. The problem with this approach to date is that the Wallstent incites granulation tissue ingrowth. Newer coated stents may circumvent this problem. The second approach utilizes endoscopic visualization within the obstructed urinary tract. This may allow direct repair by ablation of urethral valves or surgical shunting (vesicostomy). Quintero and colleagues have described a promising experience with in utero percutaneous cystoscopy in the management of fetal lower obstructive uropathy.[27] A trocar was placed through the maternal abdomen, uterus, and into the fetal bladder. Fetal cystoscopy was then performed through the trocar with a fiberoptic endoscope to allow visualization of the bladder, urethra, and ureteral orifices. In a report of 13 patients, fetal cystoscopy was possible in 11 patients, and the ureteral orifices were seen in 9 of 11 fetuses. In some patients, urethral vesicoamniotic shunts with a 5-Fr double-pigtail catheter could be passed over a guidewire. This group has also reported cystoscopically diagnosed posterior urethral valves and subsequent endoscopic fulguration of the valves in utero.[28] Although this experience is limited, in utero cystoscopy may aid in confirming ultrasound diagnosis, enhance our prognostic abilities, and facilitate the introduction of novel techniques such as urethral vesicoamniotic stents, which may have a lower incidence of dislodgement. Fetoscopic techniques may also allow the creation of a fetal vesicostomy without the need for a shunt.

Clinical Applications for Complicated Monochorionic Twin Pregnancies

In some monochorionic twin pregnancies abnormal chorionic blood vessels in the placenta connect the circulation of the two fetuses. Perinatal mortality is high for twin–twin transfusion syndrome (TTTS). Although serial amniocentesis has worked in many instances, fetoscopic ablation of placental vessels may improve outcome in severe cases. De Lia et al.[29] and Ville et al.[30] demonstrated the feasibility of fetoscopic placental vessel occlusion in severe TTTS in previable fetuses using a dual-channel fetoscope and neodymium:yttrium-aluminum-garnet (Nd:YAG) laser light. Fetoscopic laser ablation of placental vessels has been used extensively in Europe and is being compared to amniodrainage in a prospective trial in fetuses less than 25 weeks' gestation. The technique is described in Chapter 15. Newer methods to disrupt abnormal placental vascular connections (e.g., radiofrequency ablation) are being developed experimentally.

For some discordant monochorionic twins and for acardiac-acephalic or twin reversed arterial perfusion (TRAP) syndrome, obliteration of the umbilical cord of the abnormal twin is preferable because the demise of one twin threatens the other by embolization, hemodynamic change, or cord entanglement. Laser obliteration of the umbilical cord circulation is effective for small cords (< 21 weeks' gestation).[31] Thereafter, fetoscopic cord ligation is the preferred method, using a suture

tied either intra- or extracorporeally.[32] Division of the umbilical cord is believed preferable in order to prevent cord entanglement and demise of the normal fetus. However, this is difficult to achieve. The cord has been pulled out through a small hysterotomy, divided, and returned. Using fetoscopic techniques, the cord has been ligated in two places and divided within the uterus, but this is time consuming and difficult depending on placenta position, etc. We have adapted FETENDO techniques to place occluding clips and divide the cord. More recently, we have used the 5-mm harmonic scalpel to both coagulate the umbilical vessels and divide the cord completely using ultrasound guidance alone (unpublished data). Cases of late gestation ultrasound-guided monopolar and bipolar coagulation have been reported (J.A. Deprest, unpublished data).

Amniotic Band Syndrome

Amniotic band syndrome is a frequent cause of fetal deformations involving the limbs, craniofacial region, and trunk. The spectrum of morbidity ranges from the formation of syndactyly to limb amputation. This syndrome may be fatal if umbilical cord constriction is present. Cromblehome et al.[33] created an experimental model of amniotic band syndrome by banding the extremities of eight fetal lambs at 100 days' gestation with fetoscopic release at 125 days' gestation. In this model, there were no differences between fetoscopically released limbs and control limbs in terms of segmental limb length, circumference, joint range of motion, and histology. If amniotic band syndrome is causing umbilical cord constriction, fetoscopic release is warranted. Severe forms of this syndrome are good candidates for early release if this can be accomplished fetoscopically with acceptable fetal and maternal morbidity. Recently, Quintero et al.[34] treated two fetuses using endoscopic techniques. Lysis of bands at 22 weeks and 23 weeks, respectively, restored adequate blood flow distal to the obstruction, and only mild or minimal limb dysfunction was present at birth.

Sacrococcygeal Teratoma

Although most fetuses diagnosed with sacrococcygeal teratoma have an uneventful intrauterine course, a small subset (<20%) with large tumors develop hydrops from high-output failure, which leads rapidly to fetal demise. Excision of the tumor with open fetal surgery reverses the pathophysiologic process, but is fraught with the usual limitations of open fetal surgery.[35] Techniques are being developed that may be able to occlude the feeding vessels (e.g., injection of sclerorizing agents such as alcohol, or occluding feeding vessels with coils or embolic material). All these techniques risk embolization to the fetus. We have explored and abandoned shoring the neck of the tumor because the rectum and sphincter would be damaged. Hecher reduced the blood flow of a midtrimester fetus with the Nd:YAG laser. The procedure had to be repeated twice and was associated with intrauterine blood transfusion. We have recently successfully coagulated the feeding vessels at the base of the tumor to slow the vascular steal and reverse hydrops using a radiofrequency ablation probe under ultrasound guidance (unpublished data). We are also exploring the possibility of direct fetoscopic dissection using FET-ENDO techniques and the harmonic scalpel.

Cleft Lip Repair

Estes et al. created a fetal lip wound in midgestational fetal lambs and immediately repaired the wound fetoscopically. The full-thickness lip incision was created with hooked scissors and closed immediately with 6-0 nylon sutures. At harvest 14 days later, the fetuses were healthy, the sutures were intact, and there was no visible scar on the lip.[36]

Prior to clinical application, the natural history of cleft lip must be better defined and several technical hurdles regarding fetal cleft lip repair must be overcome. Specifically, the current Millard rotation-advancement repair commonly performed in many institutions will be very difficult to perform fetoscopically. It is likely that a new operation that is an amalgam of Millard's repair but simplified for the particular requirements of fetoscopic surgery will be required. Smaller specialized instruments will be required for precise handling of the tissues.

Congenital High Airway Obstruction Syndrome

Congenital high airway obstruction syndrome (CHAOS) is usually caused by laryngeal atresia and rarely by isolated tracheal stenosis. The constellation of findings include large echogenic lungs, flattened or inverted diaphragms, dilated airways distal to the obstruction, and fetal ascites and/or hydrops.[37] If hydrops does not develop in utero, these babies may be treated using the ex utero intrapartum treatment (EXIT) procedure, which maintains the baby on placental support while an airway is established by orotracheal intubation or tracheostomy (see Chapter 20). However, for selected fetuses who develop hydrops from lung overdistention caused by increased fluid accumulation, in utero fetoscopic tracheostomy would relieve the obstruction and possibly reverse the hydrops. The technique is similar to FETENDO clip for CDH.

Myelomeningocele

Myelomeningocele is a nonlethal defect that results in paraplegia, hydrocephalus, incontinence, sexual dysfunction, skeletal deformities, and often impaired mental development. Although it has been assumed that the spinal cord is intrinsically defective, recent studies suggest that neurologic impairment after birth may be due to exposure of the spinal cord in utero. We have shown in fetal lambs that exposure of the spinal cord causes neurologic damage that can be prevented or ameliorated by covering the defect in utero.[38, 39] More recently, we have shown in the fetal lamb model that Chiari malformation may be prevented by early repair of myelomeningocele.

Early attempts to repair myelomeningocele fetoscopically in human fetuses by placing a maternal skin graft on the lesion were unsuccessful (J. Bruneer, personal communication). This attempt was based on the questionable concept of maternal skin grafting. Indeed, after the first human cases have proven unsuccessful, Bruner has abandoned fetoscopic in utero repair of myelomeningocele in favor of open surgical repair.[40] The first cases done late in gestation to minimize the consequences of preterm labor were likewise unsuccessful. Early repair before 24 weeks by open surgery is being pursued.

The crucial unanswered question in the prenatal natural history of myelomeningocele is whether there is neurologic function to be salvaged by in utero repair. Currently, it is not possible to accurately distinguish active from passive leg movement early in gestation. If the fetus has active leg movement early in gestation and then progressively loses this function, in utero coverage of the spinal cord defect may salvage lower extremity neurologic function and may even ameliorate the consequences of the Chiari malformation including development of hydrocephalus. Further elucidation of the prenatal natural history of myelomeningocele will be necessary before the effect of intervention can be determined. The risks of open fetal surgery may not be justified for a nonlethal disease, making fetal repair of myelomeningocele an ideal candidate for FETENDO.

Chronic Fetal Vascular Access

One general limiting problem for fetal surgery is the lack of intravenous access to the fetus in the intraoperative and postoperative periods. A "fetal IV" and/or arterial line would allow fetal blood sampling, pressure monitoring, administration of blood products, intravenous fluids, and pharmacologic agents.

Although percutaneous umbilical blood sampling (PUBS) has proven very useful and safe for one-time vascular access, chronic access via the umbilical cord has proven difficult. Lemery et al.[41] tested the feasibility of ultrasound-guided umbilical vein catheterization in a baboon model. Although it was technically possible to cannulate all four fetuses studied, there was a high intraoperative complication rate secondary to fetal intraamniotic hemorrhage. Bleeding within the chorionic plate was noted and believed to be due to a transverse communicating artery, which is seen in 85% of preterm and 70% of term baboon placentas. In a surviving fetus, the catheter was used to withdraw blood daily, and when the fetus was harvested, the catheter and umbilical vessels remained patent.

An ideal technique for fetal vascular access should be safe for the mother, minimize the risk of infection, have a completely extra-amniotic course in order to avoid fetal or umbilical cord entanglement, remain patent throughout gestation, and have minimal risk of vasospasm to the umbilical cord. We have performed successful endoscopic catheterization of placental vessels for chronic fetal vascular access in six third-trimester pregnant rhesus monkeys.[42] Briefly, after the uterus was exposed through a midline maternal laparotomy, a 5-mm port was placed into the amniotic space and a 5-mm endoscope was used to locate chorionic villus for cannulation. A 17-gauge thin-walled trocar was passed through the myometrium adjacent to the placental edge and into the plane between the amnion and the chorion. The stylet was replaced by a 22-gauge 60-cm Centremark catheter (Menlo Care, Menlo Park, CA), which was used to cannulate the vessels. The catheter tip was then advanced within the lumen to the base of the umbilical cord. The catheter end was attached to a vascular access port (Model SLA-48, 18; Access Technologies, Skokie, IL), the system flushed with heparinized saline (10 U/mL), and the port placed in a subcutaneous pocket on the maternal anterior abdominal wall. Successful vascular access was obtained in all six third-trimester monkeys. Arterial and/or venous chorionic vessels were cannulated with equal success. We were able to transduce fetal arterial pressure, sample fetal blood, and infuse medication until the fetus was delivered. There was no intraoperative maternal or fetal morbidity or mortality. One fetus died 72 hours after the procedure, whereas the other five fetuses tolerated the procedure without complication. All catheters remained patent until planned delivery 1 to 14 days later. This technique demonstrated that chronic access to the fetal circulation is safe for the fetus and mother in a primate model. Chronic vascular access improves the ability to monitor and treat the postoperative fetal surgery patient. In addition, chronic vascular access in the fetus may have important applications in the treatment of intrauterine growth retardation, in utero hematopoietic stem cell transplantation, and other prenatal interventional therapies.

Conclusion

The elucidation of the natural history of several fetal disorders has paved the way for the development of fetal surgical intervention. Although open fetal surgery was successful in treating specific fetal pathophysiologic processes, preterm labor and altered fetal homeostasis resulting from the hysterotomy and fetal exposure and manipulation has limited its broad application. These limitations of open fetal surgery have stimulated the development of minimally invasive fetal surgery. The experimental and clinical experience suggests a diminution in the severity of postoperative preterm labor and less impaired fetal homeostasis. Despite these improvements, it must be emphasized that preterm labor remains the nemesis of fetal surgical intervention, whether open or fetoscopic. We have relied on the regimen used for spontaneus preterm labor, including external monitoring with a tocodynamometer, bedrest, intravenous magnesium sulfate, intravenous or subcutaneous β-mimetics, and oral prostaglandin synthetase inhibitors. Our experience suggests that this regimen is inadequate for fetal surgery. There has been limited success in iden-

tifying new tocolytic agents such as nitric oxide.[43] Future work in this area will need to address the unique contribution of uterine injury and particularly membrane disruption and separation during fetoscopic surgery in causing the cascade of events leading to preterm labor.

The improved outcomes seen with FETENDO versus open fetal surgery have become possible through the evolution of techniques that minimize uterine trauma, maintain fetal homeostasis, and allow for an expeditious surgical procedure. It is important to stress that fetoscopic surgery has only been made possible using multidisciplinary imaging and surgical techniques. Integration of sonographic and endoscopic visualization is crucial to success. Currently, life-threatening anomalies such as severe CDH are treated with fetoscopic surgical intervention. Other lethal defects may soon be converted from open fetal surgery to FETENDO repair. Some nonlethal disorders such as myelomeningocele, amniotic band syndrome, and cleft lip may soon be treated fetoscopically, but the specific techniques must have demonstrably low fetal and maternal morbidity to justify in utero intervention. The future of fetoscopic surgical intervention will necessitate progress in elucidating the natural history of fetal disorders, improving diagnostic and imaging techniques, instrumentation refinements, creation of novel disease-specific fetal surgical procedures, and a better understanding of preterm labor and fetal homeostasis. But the direction of the fetal treatment enterprise is already clear: minimally invasive surgical fetoscopy (FETENDO) is the future.

REFERENCES

1. Harrison MR, Anderson J, Rosen MA, et al: Fetal surgery in the primate I. Anesthetic, surgical, and tocolytic management to maximize fetal-neonatal survival. J Pediatr Surg 17:115–122, 1982.
2. Estes JM, Szabo Z, Harrison MR: Techniques for in utero endoscopic surgery. A new approach for fetal intervention. Surg Endosc 6:215–218, 1992.
3. Estes JM, MacGillivray TE, Hedrick MH, et al: Fetoscopic surgery for the treatment of congenital anomalies. J Pediatr Surg 27:950–954, 1992.
4. van der Wildt B, Luks FI, Steegers EAP, et al: Absence of electrical uterine activity after endoscopic access for fetal surgery in the rhesus monkey. Eur J Obstet Gynecol Reprod Biol 58:213–214, 1995.
5. Luks FI, Peers KH, Deprest JA, et al: The effect of open and endoscopic fetal surgery on uteroplacental oxygen delivery in the sheep. J Pediatr Surg 31:310–314, 1996.
6. Harrison MR, Mychaliska GB, Albanese CT, et al: Correction of congenital diaphragmatic hernia in utero IX: Fetuses with poor prognosis (liver herniation and low lung-to-head ratio) can be saved by fetoscopic temporary tracheal occlusion. J Pediatr Surg 33:1017–1023, 1998.
7. Albanese CT, Harrison MR: Surgical treatment for fetal disease: State of the art. Ann N Y Acad Sci 847:74–85, 1998.
8. Luks FI, Deprest JA, Gillchrist BE, et al: Access techniques in endoscopic fetal surgery. Eur J Pediatr Surg 6:1–4, 1996.
9. Deprest J, Papadopulos NA, Decaluw H, et al: Closure techniques for fetoscopic access sites in the rabbit at mid-gestation. Hum Reprod 14:1730–1734, 1999.
10. Luks FI, Deprest JA, Peers KH, et al: Gelatin spongeplug to seal fetoscopy port sites: Technique in ovine and primate models. Am J Obstet Gynecol 181:995–996, 1999.
11. Luks FI, Deprest JA, Gilchrist BF, et al: Access techniques in endoscopic fetal surgery. Eur J Pediatr Surg 7:131–134, 1997.
12. Luks F, Deprest JA, Marcus M, et al: Carbon dioxide pneumamnios causes acidosis in the fetal lamb. Fetal Diagn Ther 9:101–104, 1994.

13. Skarsgard ED, Bealer JF, Meuli M, et al: Fetal endoscopic (Fetendo) surgery: The relationship between insufflating pressure and the fetoplacental circulation. J Pediatr Surg 30:1165–1168, 1995.

14. Evrard VA, Verbeke K, Peers KH, et al: Amnioinfusion with Hartmann's solution: A safe distention medium for endoscopic fetal surgery in the ovine model. Fetal Diagn Ther 12:188–192, 1997.

15. Albanese CT, Jennings RW, Filly RA, et al: Endoscopic fetal tracheal occlusion procedure: Evolution of techniques. Pediatr Endosurg Innov Tech 2(2):47–53, 1998.

16. Luks FI, Johnson BD, Papadakis K, et al: Predictive value of monitoring parameters in fetal surgery. J Pediatr Surg 33:1297–1301, 1998.

17. Lipshutz GS, Albanese CT, Feldstein VA, et al: Prospective analysis of lung-to-head ratio predicts survival for patients with prenatally diagnosed congenital diaphragmatic hernia. J Pediatr Surg 32:1634–1636, 1997.

18. Albanese CT, Lopoo J, Goldstein RB, et al: Fetal liver position and perinatal outcome for congenital diaphragmatic hernia. Prenat Diagn 18:1138–1142, 1998.

19. DiFiore JW, Fauza DO, Slavin R, et al: Experimental fetal tracheal ligation reverses the structural and physiological effects of pulmonary hypoplasia in congenital diaphragmatic hernia. J Pediatr Surg 29:248–257, 1994.

20. Hedrick MH, Estes JM, Sullivan KM, et al: Plug the lung until it grows (PLUG): A new method to treat congenital diaphragmatic hernia in utero. J Pediatr Surg 29:612–617, 1994.

21. VanderWall KJ, Bruch SW, Meuli M, et al: Fetal endoscopic ('Fetendo') tracheal clip. J Pediatr Surg 31:1101–1104, 1996.

22. Bealer JF, Skarsgard ED, Hedrick MH, et al: The 'PLUG' odyssey: Adventures in experimental fetal tracheal occlusion. J Pediatr Surg 30:361–365, 1995.

23. Luks FI, Gilchrist BF, Jackson BT, Piasecki GJ: Endoscopic tracheal obstruction with an expanding device in a fetal lamb model: Preliminary considerations. Fetal Diagn Ther 11:67–71, 1996.

24. Flageole H, Evrard V, Deprest J, et al: The Plug-Unplug sequence: An important step to achieve type II pneumocyte maturation in the fetal lamb model. J Pediatr Surg 33:299–303, 1998.

25. Estes JM, Harrison MR: Fetal obstructive uropathy. Semin Pediatr Surg 2:129–135, 1993.

26. Estes JM, MacGillivray TE, Hedrick MH, et al: Fetoscopic surgery for the treatment of congenital anomalies. J Pediatr Surg 27:950–954, 1992.

27. Quintero RA, Hume R, Smith C, et al: Percutaneous fetal cystoscopy and endoscopic fulguration of posterior urethral valves. Am J Obstet Gynecol 172:206–209, 1995.

28. Quintero R, Johnson M, Munoz H, et al: In utero endoscopic treatment of posterior urethral valves. Prenat Neonat Med 3:208–216, 1998.

29. De Lia JE, Kuhlmann RS, Lopez KP: Treating previable twin-twin transfusion syndrome with fetoscopic laser surgery: Outcomes following the learning curve. J Perinat Med 27:61–67, 1999.

30. Ville Y, Hecher K, Gagnon A, et al: Endoscopic laser coagulation in the management of severe twin transfusion syndrome. Br J Obstet Gynaecol 105:446–453, 1998.

31. Hecher K, Hackerloer BJ, Ville Y: Umbilical cord coagulation by operative microendoscopy at 16 weeks gestation in an acardiac twin. Ultrasound Obstet Gynecol 10:130–132, 1997.

32. Deprest JA, Evrard VA, VanBallaer PP, et al: Fetoscopic cord ligation. Eur J Obstet Gynecol Reprod Biol 81:157–164, 1998.

33. Crombleholme TM, Dirkes K, Withney TM, et al: Amniotic band syndrome in fetal lambs. I. Fetoscopic release and morphometric outcome. J Pediatr Surg 30:974–978, 1995.

34. Quintero RA, Morales WJ, Phillips J, et al: In utero lysis of amniotic bands. Ultrasound Obstet Gynecol 10:316–320, 1997.

35. Langer JC, Harrison MR, Schmidt KG, et al: Fetal hydrops and death from sacrococcygeal teratoma: Rationale for fetal surgery. Am J Obstet Gynecol 160:1145–1150, 1989.

36. Estes JM, Whitby DJ, Lorenz HP, et al: Endoscopic creation and repair of fetal cleft lip. Plast Reconstr Surg 90:743–746, 1992.

37. Hedrick MH, Ferro MM, Filly RA, et al: Congenital high airway obstruction syndrome (CHAOS): A potential for perinatal intervention. J Pediatr Surg 29:271–274, 1994.

38. Meuli M, Meuli-Simmen C, Yingling CD, et al: A new model of myelomeningocele: Studies in the fetal lamb. J Pediatr Surg 30:1034–1037, 1995.

39. Meuli M, Meuli-Simmen C, Hutchins GM, et al: In utero surgery rescues neurologic function at birth in sheep with spina bifida. Nat Med 1:342–347, 1995.

40. Bruner JP, Richards WO, Tulipan NB, Arney TL: Endoscopic coverage of fetal myelomeningocele in utero. Am J Obstet Gynecol 180:153–158, 1999.

41. Lemery DJ, Santolaya-Forgas J, Wilson L Jr, et al: A non-human primate model for the in utero chronic catheterization of the umbilical vein. A preliminary report. Fetal Diagn Ther 10:326–332, 1995.

42. Hedrick MH, Jennings RW, MacGillivray TE, et al: Chronic fetal vascular access. Lancet 342:1086–1087, 1993.

43. Jennings RW, MacGillivray TE, Harrison MR: Nitric oxide inhibits preterm labor in the rhesus monkey. J Matern Fet Med 2:170–175, 1993.

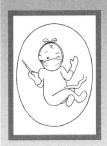

CHAPTER 17

Open Fetal Surgical Techniques

MICHAEL R. HARRISON and N. SCOTT ADZICK

Although most prenatally diagnosed malformations are best managed by appropriate medical and surgical therapy after maternal transport and planned delivery near term, a few simple anatomic abnormalities with predictable devastating developmental consequences may require correction before birth. In the 1980s, the pathophysiologic development of several potentially correctable lesions was worked out in animal models; the natural history was determined by serial observation of human fetuses; selection criteria for intervention were developed; and anesthetic, tocolytic, and surgical techniques for hysterotomy and fetal surgery were refined.[1–3] In the 1990s this investment in basic and clinical research has benefited an increasing number of fetal patients.

Clinical fetal surgical principles are based directly on experimental studies in over 2,000 operations on fetal lambs and over 400 operations on fetal rhesus monkeys during the past 20 years.[2, 4] These techniques have now been used in more than 120 open fetal surgical cases in humans. Since open fetal surgery poses obvious risks to the mother, fetal surgery should not be attempted until (1) the natural history of the fetal disease is established by following up untreated cases; (2) selection criteria for cases requiring intervention are developed; (3) the pathophysiology of the fetal disorder and its correction are defined in fetal animal models; and (4) hysterotomy and fetal surgery can be performed without undue risk to the mother and her reproductive potential.[5–7]

Fetal surgery is a team effort requiring a variety of input from the different team members. The operative team consists of two pediatric surgeons, a perinatologist, and a sonographer. The operative steps are performed by the pediatric surgeon with the assistance of others. It is important to stress that fetal surgery cannot develop and succeed unless a few surgeons are willing to devote considerable time and effort to developing, practicing, and perfecting all aspects of these new procedures: hysterotomy, fetal exposure, and correction; closure of the pregnant uterus; and maternal-fetal perioperative care and control of preterm labor.

Management of Mother and Fetus at Surgery

Breaching the uterus, whether by puncture or by incision, incites uterine contractions. In spite of technical advances, preterm labor is the Achilles' heel of fetal therapy. The regimen of preoperative indomethacin; intraoperative deep halogenated inhalation anesthesia; and postoperative indomethacin, magnesium sulfate, and β-sympathomimetics that was worked out in monkeys[4, 5] has proved inadequate for extensive procedures in humans. Although halogenated inhalation agents provide satisfactory anesthesia for mother and fetus, the depth of anesthesia necessary to achieve intraoperative uterine relaxation can produce fetal and maternal myocardial depression and affect placental perfusion.[8] Indomethacin can constrict the fetal ductus arteriosus, and the combination of magnesium sulfate and β-sympathomimetics can produce maternal pulmonary edema. Fluid restriction to avoid this complication can compromise maternal-placental-fetal circulation and contribute to recalcitrant preterm labor. The search for a more effective and less toxic tocolytic regimen led to the demonstration in monkeys that exogenous nitric oxide ablates preterm labor induced by hysterotomy.[9] For the last 2 years, we have used intravenous nitroglycerin intraoperatively and postoperatively; it is a potent tocolytic but requires careful control to avoid serious complications.[10, 11]

An epidural catheter is placed preoperatively to help manage postoperative pain. The use of "preemptive analgesia" beginning in the operative room also seems to have a salutary effect on postoperative uterine contractions. Indomethacin and antibiotics are given preoperatively, and isoflurane provides anesthesia for both mother and fetus.[12] The mother is positioned supine with towels placed under one side to lift her uterus off of the inferior cava to avoid compromise of venous return (Fig. 17–1). Maternal perioperative monitoring includes a radial arterial catheter, blood pressure cuff, large-bore intravenous catheters, bladder catheter,

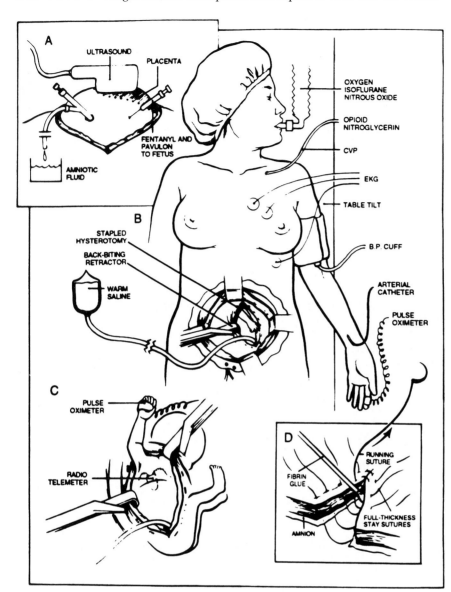

FIGURE 17–1. Fetal surgery techniques. *A,* The uterus is exposed through a low transverse abdominal incision. Ultrasonography is used to localize the placenta, inject the fetus with narcotic and muscle relaxant, and aspirate amniotic fetal fluid. *B,* The uterus is opened with staples that provide hemostasis and seal the membranes. Warm saline solution is continuously infused around the fetus. Maternal anesthesia, tocolysis, and monitoring are shown. *C,* Absorbable staples and back-biting clamps facilitate hysterotomy exposure of the pertinent fetal part. A miniaturized pulse oximeter records pulse rate and oxygen saturation intraoperatively. A radiotelemeter monitors fetal electrocardiogram and amniotic pressure during and after operation. *D,* After fetal repair the uterine incision is closed with absorbable sutures and fibrin glue. Amniotic fluid is restored with warm lactated Ringer's solution. (A videotape library of fetal surgery techniques is available.)

electrocardiogram (ECG) leads, and a transcutaneous pulse oximeter.

Opening and Closing the Gravid Uterus

The technical aspects of fetal surgery that have evolved over 20 years of experimental and clinical work are summarized in Figure 17–1. A videotape library of techniques to correct specific fetal defects and an atlas of fetal surgery are available.

The uterus is exposed through a low transverse abdominal incision. If a posterior placenta is present, superior and inferior subcutaneous flaps are raised and a vertical midline fascial incision is made to expose the uterus for a convenient anterior hysterotomy with the uterus remaining in the abdomen. Conversely, the presence of an anterior placenta necessitates division of the rectus muscles so that the uterus can be tilted out of the abdomen for a posterior hysterotomy. A large abdominal ring retractor (Turner-Warwick) is utilized to maintain exposure and prevent lateral compression of the uterine vessels. Sterile intraoperative ultrasound is used to delineate the fetal position and placental location. The edge of the placenta is marked under sonographic guidance using the electrocautery or a marking pen. The position and orientation of the hysterotomy is planned to stay parallel to and at least 6 cm from the placental edge and still allow exposure of the appropriate part of the fetus.

The hysterotomy is facilitated by the placement of two large monofilament sutures parallel to the intended incision site and through the full thickness of the uterine wall under sonographic guidance (Fig. 17–2). The electrocautery is used to incise the myometrium between the two stay sutures down to the level of the amniotic membranes. A uterine stapler (U S Surgical Corporation, Norwalk, CT) with absorbable Lactomer staples is then directly introduced through this point of fixation and

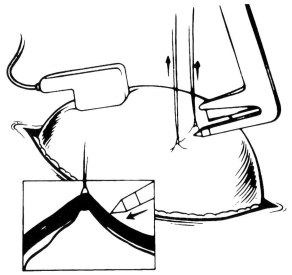

FIGURE 17–2. A large abdominal ring retractor is used for exposure. The placental edge is marked with the electrocautery or a marking pen, and the planned hysterotomy is made parallel to and away from the placental edge. We avoid a hysterotomy that is too close to the cervix due to the risk of amniotic fluid dissection beneath the membranes and consequent premature membrane rupture. Two large monofilament sutures are placed through the full-thickness wall under sonographic guidance. These stay sutures are lifted up as the uterine stapler is introduced through the uterine wall and membranes using a piercing attachment on the lower limb of the stapler.

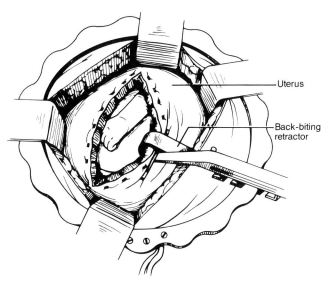

FIGURE 17–3. The hysterotomy is extended with a uterine stapling device. Back-biting uterine retractors gently compress the uterine edges and are attached to the abdominal ring retractor to facilitate exposure.

into the amniotic cavity by use of a piercing attachment on the lower limb of the stapler.[13, 14] The stapler is then fired, therby anchoring the amniotic membranes to the uterine wall and creating a hemostatic hysterotomy. Occlusive clamps are not placed on the hysterotomy edges because they cause tissue ischemia. Instead, a total of four specially designed gentle reverse-biting compression clamps are placed at the corners and lateral edges of the uterine incision to prevent venous bleeding at these unstapled sites as well as to keep the hysterotomy open (Fig. 17–3). The fetus and uterus are continually bathed in warm saline at 38° to 40°C using a level I warming device connected to a red rubber catheter that is placed in the uterine cavity.

For the fetal portion of the procedure, a surgical head lamp and 3.5X optical loupe magnification are helpful. The appropriate fetal part is exposed and intraoperative fetal monitoring is first provided by a miniaturized pulse oximeter that is wrapped around the fetal palm and protected with Tegaderm (3M, St. Paul, MN). We no longer place ECG electrodes but instead place a subcutaneously implanted radiotelemetry device that reliably measures the fetal ECG and temperature both intraoperatively and postoperatively.[15, 16] For instance, during a fetal lobectomy for a lung mass, a suture tied to each of the two telemeter leads is passed out from the inside of the thoracotomy wound through the muscles and skin of the chest wall and tied, one posterior and one anterior, so that the leads are fixed in an orientation that provides the best ECG signal (Fig. 17–4). The telemeter is then sutured into the chest wall pocket.

After repair of the defect, the fetus is returned to the uterus, and full-thickness 0 Maxon (Davis and Geck,

Danbury, CT) stay sutures are placed (Fig. 17–5). A watertight two-layer uterine closure is performed with running 2-0 Maxon and approximately 400 to 500 mL of warmed saline containing 500 mg of nafcillin is instilled into the amniotic cavity via the level I device just prior to completing the first layer. Fibrin glue can be added to help seal the uterine incision, and then the stay sutures are tied. The omentum usually is placed over the hysterotomy closure to help seal the closure with vascularized tissue and to prevent bowel adher-

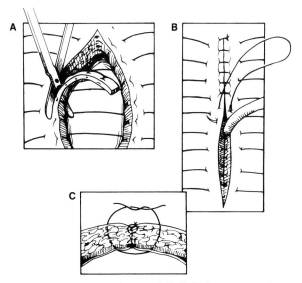

FIGURE 17–4. Uterine closure. *A,* Full-thickness stay sutures are placed first, then the staple line can be excised to allow muscle-to-muscle apposition. An assistant should hold up on the stay sutures to minimize bleeding during and after the staple removal. *B,* The uterus is closed in two layers of running sutures, and a soft rubber catheter is inserted prior to completing the first layer in order to place warm saline and antibiotics in the amniotic space. *C,* The stay sutures are tied last.

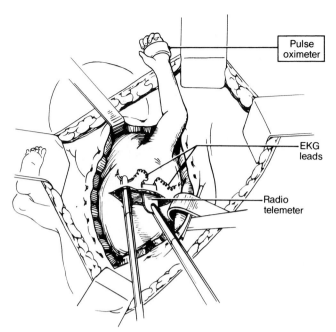

FIGURE 17–5. A transverse incision is made through the muscle (but not chest wall) and ECG leads sutured as far apart as possible to maximize the signal pickup across the fetal heart. The radiotelemeter device is placed in a pocket deep to the muscle on the chest wall.

ence to the site especially when a posterior hysterotomy is performed. The maternal laparotomy incision is closed in layers. It is important to use a subcuticular maternal skin closure covered with a transparent dressing so that monitoring devices can be placed on the maternal abdomen postoperatively.

Tocolysis begins as the patient emerges from anesthesia, and continues as the mother is transferred to the intensive care unit. Postoperative management takes place in the fetal intensive care unit. Maternal arterial pressure, central venous pressure, urine output, and oxygen saturation are continuously monitored. Fetal well-being and uterine activity are recorded externally by tocodynamometer and by a radiotelemeter implanted at surgery, which continuously records the fetal electrocardiogram and intra-amniotic pressure.[15] Patient-controlled analgesia and/or continuous epidural analgesics ease maternal stress and aid tocolysis. Vigilant fetal and uterine monitoring is crucial to control of preterm labor in the first week. Use of indomethacin requires daily echocardiographic monitoring of the fetus for ductal constriction and tricuspid regurgitation. All fetal surgery mothers have delivery by subsequent cesarean section.

When labor is controlled and the fetus stable (usually several days), the patient is transferred to the obstetric ward where radiotelemetric monitoring continues until discharge (usually 1 week). Outpatient monitoring and tocolysis continue and fetal sonograms are obtained at least weekly. Cesarean delivery is performed when membranes rupture or labor cannot be controlled, usually before 36 weeks.

Beyond these technical points, we have learned that, as a general principle, fetal surgery should be "all or none"; that is, the fetal repair should be complete and adequate to ensure a good chance for fetal survival, or else the otherwise doomed fetus should be removed. A partial or inadequate repair presents an ongoing threat to the mother with little potential benefit.

Techniques for Specific Fetal Defects

The only anatomic malformations that warrant consideration are those that interfere with fetal organ development and that, if alleviated, would allow normal development to proceed (Table 17–1). At present, only a small number of life-threatening malformations have been successfully corrected (the first six conditions listed). A few others should be successfully treated as their pathophysiologic characteristics are unraveled. When less invasive interventional techniques are developed and proved safe, a few nonlethal anomalies may be considered.

Fetal Vesicostomy for Urethral Obstruction

Fetal urethral obstruction produces pulmonary hypoplasia and renal dysplasia, and these often fatal consequences can be ameliorated by urinary tract decompression before birth. The natural history of untreated fetal urinary tract obstruction is well documented, and selection criteria that are based on fetal urine electrolyte and β_2-microglobulin levels and the ultrasonographic appearance of the fetal kidneys have proven reliable.[17, 18] Of all fetuses with urinary tract dilatation, as many as 90% do not require intervention. However, in fetuses with bilateral hydronephrosis caused by urethral obstruction, development of oligohydramnios necessitates treatment. If the lungs are mature, the fetus can be delivered early for postnatal decompression. If the lungs are immature, the bladder can be decompressed in utero by a catheter shunt placed percutaneously under ultrasonographic guidance,[19] by fetoscopic vesicostomy,[20] by placement of an improved wire mesh stent that may solve the technical problems encountered with shunts (malfunction, dislodgement, abdominal wall disruption),[21] or by open fetal vesicostomy.[22]

For open vesicostomy to relieve high-grade urethral obstruction in the setting of oligohydramnios, the lower extremities of the fetus are exteriorized and a transcutaneous pulse oximeter is placed around the fetal thigh.[22] A midline suprapubic incision is made through the fetal abdominal wall exposing the thick-walled and distended bladder. The bladder is then opened and marsupialized to the abdominal wall using interrupted 4-0 Maxon sutures (Fig. 17–6).

Open surgery is seldom necessary now that percutaneous placement of shunts and direct ablation of the obstructing tissue can be accomplished under sonographic or fetoscopic guidance.

Fetal Thoracotomy and Lobectomy for Cystic Adenomatoid Malformation of the Lung

Although congenital cystic adenomatoid malformation (CCAM) often presents as a benign pulmonary mass in

TABLE 17–1. MALFORMATIONS THAT MAY BENEFIT FROM TREATMENT BEFORE BIRTH

DEFECTS	EFFECT ON DEVELOPMENT (RATIONALE FOR TREATMENT)			TECHNIQUE
Life-Threatening Defects				
Urinary obstruction (urethral valves)	Hydronephrosis Lung hypoplasia	→ →	Renal failure Pulmonary failure	Percutaneous catheter Fetoscopic vesicostomy Open vesicostomy
Cystic adenomatoid malformation	Lung hypoplasia/hydrops	→	Fetal hydrops/demise	Open pulmonary lobectomy
Diaphragmatic hernia	Lung hypoplasia	→	Pulmonary failure	Open complete repair Bowel exteriorization Temporary tracheal occlusion
Sacrococcygeal teratoma	High output failure	→	Fetal hydrops/demise	Resect tumor Fetoscopic vascular occlusion*
Twin-twin transfusion syndrome	Vascular steal through placenta	→	Fetal hydrops/demise	Open fetectomy Fetoscopic division of placenta
Aqueductal stenosis	Hydrocephalus	→	Brain damage	Ventriculoamniotic shunt Open ventriculoperitoneal shunt*
Complete heart block	Low output failure	→	Fetal hydrops/demise	Percutaneous pacemaker Open pacemaker
Pulmonary/aortic obstruction	Ventricular hypertrophy	→	Heart failure	Percutaneous valvuloplasty Open valvuloplasty*
Tracheal atresia/stenosis/ obstruction by tumor	Overdistention by lung fluid	→	Hydrops/demise	Fetoscopic tracheostomy* Open tracheostomy* Ex utero intrapartum treatment (EXIT)
Nonlethal Defects				
Myelomeningocele	Spinal cord damage	→	Paralysis, neurogenic bladder, etc.	Fetoscopic coverage* Open repair*
Clefting/lip and palate	Facial defect	→	Persistent deformity	Fetoscopic repair* Open repair*
Metabolic/Cellular Defects				
Stem cell/enzyme defects	Hemoglobinopathy Immunodeficiency Storage diseases	→ → →	Anemia, hydrops Infection Retardation	Fetal stem cell transplant or gene therapy using fetal stem cells (autologous/allogeneic)*
Predictable organ failure	Hypoplastic heart/kidney/lung	→	Neonatal heart/kidney/lung failure	Induce tolerance for postnatal organ transplant*

* Not yet attempted in human fetuses.

infancy or childhood, some fetuses with large lesions die in utero or at birth from hydrops and pulmonary hypoplasia.[23] The pathophysiologic characteristics of hydrops and the feasibility of resecting the fetal lung have been studied in animals.[24, 25] Experience managing more than 80 cases suggests that most lesions can be success-fully treated after birth and that some lesions resolve before birth.[26] Although only a few fetuses with very large lesions will develop hydrops before 26 weeks, almost all have rapid progression and die in utero. Careful ultrasonographic surveillance of large lesions is necessary to detect the first signs of hydrops, because fetuses in whom hydrops develops (<10% of all fetuses with congenital cystic adenomatoid malformations) can be successfully treated by emergency resection of the cystic lobe in utero.

For resection of a large CCAM causing hydrops, the fetal chest is entered by a very generous fifth intercostal space thoracotomy. The lobe containing the CCAM lesion is deliverable out through the thoracotomy wound. Using techniques developed in experimental animals, the appropriate pulmonary lobe containing the lesion is resected.[27, 28] The pulmonary hilar structures that supply the mass can either be individually ligated and divided or else transected using a TA-30 vascular stapling device (U S Surgical Corporation, Norwalk, CT). The fetal thoracotomy is then closed in layers.

Nine fetuses have undergone open fetal surgical resection of the massively enlarged pulmonary lobe. Five of these had rapid resolution of hydrops, impressive bilateral in utero lung growth, and normal postnatal growth and development with a follow-up of 12 to 45

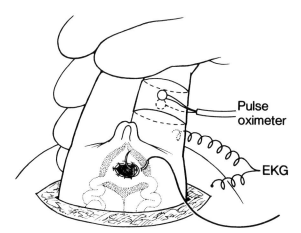

FIGURE 17–6. Diagram of intraoperative appearance of bladder marsupialization to the fetal abdominal wall to create a vesicoamniotic fistula.

months.[27, 28] Fetal pulmonary lobectomy has proved to be surprisingly simple and quite successful. For lesions with single large cysts, thoracoamniotic shunting has also been successful.[29]

Tracheal Occlusion for Fetal Diaphragmatic Hernia

Repair of fetal congenital diaphragmatic hernia (CDH) has proven technically difficult, especially when the left lobe of the fetal liver is incarcerated in the fetal chest.[14–17] Although success has been achieved in fetuses without liver herniation, these fetuses are selected for relatively good outcome and are more likely to do well with conventional postnatal therapy.[34]

Extensive animal studies have shown that obstructing egress of lung fluid by fetal tracheal occlusion results in large, fluid-filled lungs.[35, 36] The poor prognosis fetal CDH patient with massive liver herniation and low lung-to-head circumference ratio (LHR) might be helped by in utero tracheal occlusion. Before attempting clinical tracheal occlusion, a number of important technical issues had to be addressed. A reliable method of internal, endoscopically deployed, reversible, and atraumatic tracheal occlusion would be ideal. Unfortunately, to achieve the physiologic effect, complete tracheal occlusion is necessary. It has been our animal model and clinical experience that even small leaks result in minimal or no lung growth. The technical problem of complete occlusion by an internal device without ischemic or mechanical injury to the trachea has been difficult to solve. Attempts at occlusion with balloon devices or expansile foam plugs have failed either due to leak and no effect, or tracheal dilatation and tracheomalacia.[37] Surprisingly, tracheal occlusion in the fetal lamb by external application of completely occlusive vascular clips has been associated with minimal tracheal injury and is readily reversible at the ex utero intrapartum treatment (EXIT) procedure.

Through the hysterotomy, both fetal arms are delivered and a pulse oximeter is placed on one hand. The arms are gently pulled down to permit extension of the neck. Through a small transverse anterior neck wound, the trachea is dissected and the recurrent laryngeal nerves are identified. The trachea is occluded with two large titanium clips. A suture is first tied in the crotch of each clip and left long to facilitate identification and removal at the time of the EXIT delivery.

Fetal Sacrococcygeal Teratoma Resection

Most neonates with sacrococcygeal teratoma survive and malignant invasion is unusual. However, the outcome for sacrococcygeal teratoma diagnosed prenatally (by sonogram or elevated α-fetoprotein) is less favorable. In a subset of fetuses (<20%) with large masses, hydrops develops from high-output failure caused by extremely high blood flow through the tumor. Because hydrops progresses very rapidly to fetal death, frequent ultrasonographic follow-up is mandatory. Attempts to interrupt the vascular "steal" by ultrasonographically guided or fetoscopic techniques have not yet been successful. Excision of the tumor reverses the pathophysiologic process.

Through the hysterotomy, the caudal end of the fetus is delivered, including the tumor.[38, 39] The fetal radiotelemetry monitoring device is placed on the fetal upper back. The tumor resection is initiated by dissecting the base of the tumor in a circumferential plane away from the anorectum. If the base of the tumor is sufficiently narrow, then it is transected with the uterine stapling device that we had crafted initially for the hysterotomy incision (Fig. 17–7). This stapler contains large polyglycolic acid staples designed for compression of vascular tissues and permits amputation of the tumor and compression of its blood supply in a single maneuver with minimal blood loss. If the tumor has a broad base, then the stapler is ineffective, so an umbilical tape is applied at the base and the tape is tightened with a pump tourniquet for compression. The tumor is then resected across its base by direct dissection and suture ligation of vessels. Any residual tumor can be resected in the newborn period once the hydrops is resolved and the baby is clinically stable.

More recently, radiofrequency ablation of the vascular base of the tumor has been successful. The probe is deployed under ultrasonographic guidance and the power applied until the majority of the blood flow is stopped.

Fetectomy for Discordant Monochorionic Twins

In some twin pregnancies, abnormal chorionic blood vessels in the placenta connect the circulation of the two fetuses. These placental abnormalities are associated with very high perinatal mortality for discordant twins (e.g., acardiac-acephalus twin syndrome). Interrupting the abnormal placental vascular connections may improve outcome in severe cases. This has been accomplished by occluding the umbilical circulation percutaneously, by dividing the abnormal placental vessels endoscopically, and by removing the abnormal fetus by hysterotomy.[40, 41] All of these techniques have been successful in small series, and the optimal approach has not yet been determined.

Fetal Pacemaker Placement for Heart Block

Most fetuses who have structurally normal hearts but development of complete heart block associated with maternal collagen-vascular disease will survive without intervention. In a few with very slow rates (<50 bpm) hydrops may develop and death may occur in utero. If low-output failure cannot be reversed by increasing the heart rate with β-adrenergic receptor agonists or by treatment with steroids, a pacemaker can be placed.

Selected fetuses with complete heart block, which frequently causes hydrops and demise in utero, may be salvaged by open fetal surgery and pacemaker place-

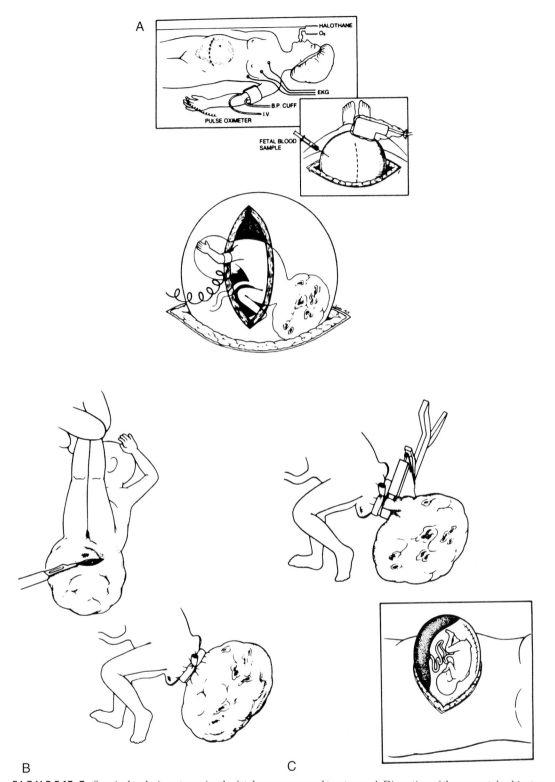

F I G U R E 17–7. Surgical technique to excise the fetal sacrococcygeal teratoma. *A,* Dissection of the anorectal sphincter mechanism from tumor. *B,* Application of a latex tourniquet around the base of the tumor. *C,* Application of stapling device to base of tumor.

ment.[42, 43] The fetal left chest is exposed and a left anterolateral thoracotomy is performed. The pericardium is opened, and a specially designed Medtronic model 4951 unipolar "fishhook" myocardial lead is placed on the apical surface of the left ventricle. The lead is attached to a Siemens-Pacesetter Dialog II model 2038T pacemaker (Siemens-Elema, Solna, Sweden), which is implanted posterolaterally in a subcutaneous pocket. This device is used because it is tiny, it transmits an ECG signal, and it is programmable by telemetry to a distance of 12 inches. The ventricular rate is gradually increased, and the myocardial performance is followed by sterile intraoperative fetal echocardiography. Placement of fetal pacemakers is only necessary when medical management of arrhythmias fails, but the techniques may prove useful as an adjunct to cardiac surgical procedures now being developed experimentally.

Fetal Myelomeningocele Repair

Myelomeningocele (MMC) is becoming less common because it can be detected early in gestation by α-fetoprotein screening or ultrasonography and may be prevented by vitamin supplementation. Although it has been assumed that the spinal cord is intrinsically defective, recent studies suggest that neurologic impairment after birth may be due to exposure of the spinal cord in utero. We have shown in fetal lambs that exposure of the spinal cord causes neurologic damage that can be prevented or ameliorated by repairing the anatomic defect in utero.[44, 45] The natural history of myelomeningocele in human fetuses must be elucidated, particularly the gestational age at which the lower extremity neurologic damage occurs.

There is limited experience with repair of human MMC. Early attempts at endoscopic covering with maternal skin were unsuccessful. Direct repair by open fetal surgery has proven feasible in a few cases.

The myelomeningocele lesion is positioned directly under the hysterotomy and the fetus remains entirely within the uterus. The cystic membrane is excised. Using techniques developed in fetal sheep, the exposed unprotected spinal cord is closed and covered either with mobilized skin flaps and/or AlloDerm.[45]

Lessons From the Fetal Surgery Enterprise

The steep learning curve derived from our experimental and clinical experience with fetal surgery has provided invaluable lessons regarding optimal maternal anesthesia and uterine relaxation, hysterotomy and fetal exposure techniques, intraoperative fetal monitoring, and reliable methods for amniotic membrane and uterine closure. However, many challenges remain. New issues include the need for better postoperative maternal-fetal monitoring,[10] reliable long-term fetal intravascular access for fetal blood sampling and infusions,[46] noninvasive maternal-fetal hemodynamic assessment,[47] less invasive methods of intervention including fetoscopy,[48] and effective detection and treatment of preterm labor.

The great promise of fetal therapy is that for some diseases the earliest possible intervention (i.e., before birth) will produce the best possible outcome (i.e., the best quality of life for the resources expanded). However, the promise of cost-effective, preventative fetal therapy can be subverted by misguided clinical applications (e.g., a complex in utero procedure that "half-saves" an otherwise doomed fetus for a life of intensive [and expensive] care). Enthusiasm for fetal intervention

must be tempered by reverence for the interests of the mother and her family, by careful study of the disease in experimental fetal animals and untreated human fetuses, and by a willingness to abandon therapy that does not prove effective and cost-effective in properly controlled trials.

REFERENCES

1. Harrison MR, Golbus MS, Filly RA (eds): The Unborn Patient: Prenatal Diagnosis and Treatment, 2nd ed. Philadelphia: WB Saunders Company, 1990.
2. Harrison MR, Adzick NS: The fetus as a patient: Surgical considerations. Ann Surg 213:279–291, 1990.
3. Harrison MR: Fetal surgery. West J Med 159:341–349, 1993.
4. Adzick NS, Harrison MR: Fetal surgical therapy. Lancet 343:897–902, 1994.
5. Harrison MR, Anderson J, Rosen MA, et al: Fetal surgery in the primate I. Anesthetic, surgical and tocolytic management to maximize fetal-neonateal survival. J Pediatr Surg 17:115–122, 1982.
6. Nakayama DK, Harrison MR, Seron-Ferre M, et al: Fetal surgery in the primate II. Uterine electromyographic response to operative procedure and pharmacologic agents. J Pediatr Surg 19:333–339, 1984.
7. Adzick NS, Harrison MR, Glick PL, et al: Fetal surgery in the primate III. Maternal outcome after fetal surgery. J Pediatr Surg 21:477–480, 1986.
8. Sabik JF, Assad RS, Hanley FL: Halothane as an anesthetic for fetal surgery. J Pediatr Surg 28:542–546, 1993.
9. Jennings RW, MacGillivray TE, Harrison MR: Nitric oxide inhibits preterm labor in the rhesus monkey. J Matern Fetal Med 2:170–175, 1993.
10. Bealer JF, Rice HE, Adzick NS, Harrison MR: Acute non-cardiac pulmonary edema complicating nitroglycerin tocolysis following open fetal surgery. (Submitted for publication.)
11. Harrison MR, VanderWall KJ, Bealer JF, et al: Nitroglycerin suppresses preterm labor after hysterotomy and fetal surgery. (Submitted for publication.)
12. Longaker MT, Golbus MS, Filly RA, et al: Maternal outcome after open fetal surgery: A review of the first 17 human cases. JAMA 265:737–741, 1991.
13. Adzick NS, Harrison MR, Flake AW, et al: Automatic uterine stapling devices in fetal operation: Experience in a primate model. Surg Forum 36:479–480, 1985.
14. Bond SJ, Harrison MR, Slotnick RN, et al: Cesarean delivery and hysterotomy using an absorbable stapling device. Obstet Gynecol 74:25–28, 1989.
15. Jennings RW, Adzick NS, Longaker MT, et al: Radio-telemetric fetal monitoring during and after open fetal surgery. Surg Gynecol Obstet 176:59–64, 1993.
16. Jennings RW, Adzick NS, Longaker MT, et al: New techniques in fetal surgery. J Pediatr Surg 27:1329–1333, 1992.
17. Nicolaides KH, Cheng HH, Snijders RJM, Moniz CF: Fetal urine biochemistry in the assessment of obstructive uropathy. Am J Obstet Gynecol 166:932–937, 1992.
18. Johnson MP, Bukowski TP, Reitleman C, et al: In utero surgical treatment of fetal obstructive uropathy: A new comprehensive approach to identify appropriate candidates for vesicoamniotic shunt therapy. Am J Obstet Gynecol 170:1770–1779, 1994.
19. Manning FA, Harrison MR, Rodeck CH, et al: Special report: Catheter shunts for fetal hydronephrosis and hydrocephalus. N Engl J Med 315:336–340, 1986.
20. MacMahan RA, Renou PM, Shekelton PA, Paterson RJ: In utero cystostomy. Lancet 340:1234, 1992.
21. Estes JM, Harrison MR: Fetal obstructive uropathy. Semin Pediatr Surg 2:129–135, 1993.
22. Crombleholme TM, Harrison MR, Langer JC, et al: Early experience with open fetal surgery for congenital hydronephrosis. J Pediatr Surg 23:1114–1121, 1988.
23. Adzick NS, Harrison MR, Glick PL, et al: Fetal cystic adenomatoid malformation: Prenatal diagnosis and natural history. J Pediatr Surg 20:483–488, 1985.

24. Rice HE, Estes JM, Hedrick MH, et al: Congenital cystic adenomatoid malformation: A sheep model of fetal hydrops. J Pediatr Surg 29:692–696, 1994.
25. Adzick NS, Hu LM, Davies P, et al: Compensatory lung growth after pneumonectomy in the fetus. Surg Forum 37:648, 1986.
26. MacGillivray TE, Harrison MR, Goldstein RB, Adzick NS: Disappearing fetal lung lesions. J Pediatr Surg 28:1321–1325, 1993.
27. Harrison MR, Adzick NS, Jennings RW, et al: Antenatal intervention for congenital cystic adenomatoid malformation. Lancet 336:965–967, 1990.
28. Adzick NS, Harrison MR, Flake AW, et al: Fetal surgery for congenital cystic adenomatoid malformation of the lung. J Pediatr Surg 28:806–812, 1993.
29. Adzick NS, Harrison MR: Fetal surgical techniques. Semin Pediatr Surg 2:136–142, 1993.
30. Harrison MR, Langer JC, Adzick NS, et al: Correction of congenital diaphragmatic hernia in utero V. Initial clinical experience. J Pediatr Surg 25:47–57, 1990.
31. Harrison MR, Adzick NS, Longaker MT, et al: Successful repair in utero of a fetal diaphragmatic hernia after removal of herniated viscera from the left thorax. N Engl J Med 322:1582–1584, 1990.
32. Harrison MR, Adzick NS, Flake AW, et al: Correction of congenital diaphragmatic hernia in utero VI. Hard-earned lessons. J Pediatr Surg 28:1227–1231, 1993.
33. Harrison MR, Adzick NS, Flake AW: The CDH two-step: A dance of necessity. J Pediatr Surg 28:813–816, 1993.
34. Harrison MR, Adzick NS, Bullard KM, et al: In utero repair of congenital diaphragmatic hernia: A prospective trial. J Pediatr Surg 32:1637–1642, 1997.
35. DiFiore JW, Fauza DO, Slavin R, et al: Experimental fetal tracheal ligation reverses the structural and physiological effects of pulmonary hypoplasia in congenital diaphragmatic hernia. J Pediatr Surg 28:1433–1439, 1993.
36. Hedrick MH, Estes JM, Sullivan KM, et al: Plug the lung until it grows (PLUG): A new method to treat congenital diaphragmatic hernia in utero. J Pediatr Surg 29:248–256, 1994.
37. Bealer JF, Skarsgard ED, Hedrick MH, et al: The PLUG odyssey: Adventures in experimental fetal tracheal occlusion. J Pediatr Surg 30:362–365, 1995.
38. Langer JC, Harrison MR, Schmidt KG, et al: Fetal hydrops and death from sacrococcygeal teratoma: Rationale for fetal surgery. Am J Obstet Gynecol 160:1145–1150, 1989.
39. Adzick NS, Crombleholme TM, Morgan MA, Quinn TM: A rapidly growing fetal teratoma. Lancet 349:538, 1997.
40. De Lia JE, Cruikshank DP, Keye WR: Fetoscopic neodymium: YAG laser occlusion of placental vessels in severe twin-twin fusion syndrome. Obstet Gynecol 75:1046–1053, 1990.
41. Fries MH, Goldberg JD, Golbus MS: Treatment of acardiac-acephalic twin gestations by hysterotomy and selective delivery. Obstet Gynecol 79:601–604, 1992.
42. Schmidt KG, Ulmer HE, Silverman NH, et al: Perinatal outcome of fetal complete atrioventricular block: A multicenter experience. J Am Coll Cardiol 17:360–366, 1991.
43. Crombleholme TM, Harrison MR, Longaker MT, et al: Complete heart block in fetal lambs I. Technique and acute physiologic response. J Pediatr Surg 25:587–593, 1990.
44. Meuli M, Meuli-Simmen C, Yingling CD, et al: A new model of myelomeningocele: Studies in the fetal lamb. J Pediatr Surg 30:1034–1037, 1995.
45. Meuli M, Meuli-Simmen C, Hutchins GM, et al: In utero surgery rescues neurologic function at birth in sheep with spina bifida. Nat Med 1:342–347, 1995.
46. Hedrick MH, Jennings RW, MacGillivray TE, et al: Endoscopic catheterization of placental vessels for chronic fetal venous access. Surg Forum 43:504–505, 1992.
47. Kleinman CS, Donnerstein RL, DeVore GR, et al: Fetal echocardiography for evaluation of in utero congestive heart failure: A technique for study of nonimmune hydrops. N Engl J Med 306:568–575, 1982.
48. Estes JM, MacGillivray TM, Hedrick MH, et al: Fetoscopic surgery for the treatment of congenital anomalies. J Pediatr Surg 27:950–954, 1992.

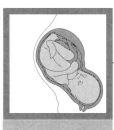

P A R T   III

Fetal Anatomic Defects Amenable to Treatment: The Craft of Fetal Treatment

18

Fetal Obstructive Uropathy

MARK PAUL JOHNSON

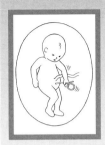

The field of fetal medicine has changed rapidly over the past two decades. The late 1970s witnessed the introduction of mid-gestational prenatal diagnosis, which began to be applied in the late first trimester during the 1980s. The 1990s has seen continued improvement in our prenatal diagnosis capabilities, and the development of a number of interventive approaches in which prenatally diagnosed disorders have been treated in utero. Thus, the fetus has now achieved the recognition as "potential patient," and numerous anomalies, previously associated with little hope of survival, are being reevaluated for possible treatment in utero.

Prenatal ultrasonography can detect most significant fetal malformations, and current diagnostic capabilities can identify urinary tract anomalies as early as 12 to 14 weeks' gestation. Obstructive abnormalities of the urinary tract are common and observed in about 1% of pregnancies. Fortunately, the majority of these have little clinical significance and only about 1 in 500 pregnancies are complicated by significant urologic malformations. The key, however, is prenatal identification and development of a coordinated prenatal and postnatal management plan directed at optimizing clinical outcomes in such cases. This chapter will review the diagnosis, evaluation, and management of the more commonly encountered prenatally detected urologic malformations.

Early Experimental Models

Embryology

Development of the genitourinary tract begins during the fourth week of gestation with a condensation of mesoderm that gives rise to the pronephros. This rudimentary structure regresses at 5 weeks' gestation as the mesonephros begins development. This second stage of development involves the caudal descent of the mesonephros until it comes in contact with the urogenital sinus. Development of the genital duct system results from interaction between the mesonephros and urogenital sinus, as well as induces the evagination of the ureteral bud. The third phase of development occurs from

11 to 32 weeks' gestation, and involves interaction between the ureteric bud and primitive mesoderm, known as nephrogenic blastema, to form the kidney, as well as the migration of the developing kidney cephalad. The ureteric bud undergoes extensive branching giving rise to the renal pelvis and calices and later contributing to the formation of glomeruli and functional nephrons from the nephrogenic blastema. The most rapid period of growth of the kidneys occurs between 18 and 32 weeks' gestation. It is during this period that the kidney may be most susceptible to damage from obstructive dilation that can interfere with normal developmental and differentiation processes.[1]

The ureter develops independently from the ureteral bud. Although initially patent until around day 35 of gestation, it subsequently loses its lumen due to the rapid growth and elongation associated with the ascent of the kidney from a sacral to thoracic position. The ureter begins recanalization at the midportion and progresses both cranially and caudally. The last segments to canalize are at the ureterovesical and ureteropelvic junctions. This may explain the frequency of obstructive abnormalities found at each end of the ureter.[2]

The bladder develops mostly from the vesical portion of the urogenital sinus, while the trigone region develops from the caudal ends of the mesonephric ducts. Bladder epithelium derives from urogenital sinus endoderm, while the muscular component arises from adjacent splanchnic mesenchyme. From 10 to 12 weeks' gestation, the bladder is continuous with the allantois via the urachus. This attachment later constricts and involutes, becoming the umbilical ligament. As the bladder enlarges, distal elements of the mesonephric ducts are incorporated as connective tissue elements in the trigone of the bladder. As the kidneys ascend in the pelvis, the ureters come to open separately into the bladder, entering obliquely through its base. Anomalous entrance of the ureters into the bladder are another common source of obstruction in the urinary tract.[1]

The majority of the urethra is derived from endoderm of the urogenital sinus. In the male, the distal part of the urethra forms from surface ectoderm of the glandular plate which grows from the tip of the penis to meet the penile urethra which has formed from the phallic part of the urogenital sinus. The smooth muscle and connective tissue components are derived from adjacent splanchnic mesenchyme.

Natural History of Obstructive Uropathy

The natural history of obstructive uropathy is highly variable and dependent on the severity, duration, and age of onset of the obstruction. Complete obstruction early in gestation of the urethra can lead to massive distention of the bladder, hydroureteronephrosis, and renal dysplasia. Inability of the urine to enter the amniotic space and replenish the amniotic fluid volume results in oligohydramnios that leads to pulmonary insufficiency and compression deformations of the face and extremities[3] (Fig. 18–1). Outcomes are measured in terms of postnatal survival and are dependent on two factors: pulmonary maturity and renal function. Of these, pulmonary development may be the more critical for neonatal survival.

Pulmonary hypoplasia is the leading cause of mortality in obstructive uropathy. Nakayama et al.[4] demonstrated that in cases of posterior urethral valves there is a 45% mortality rate that can be directly attributed to pulmonary insufficiency. This high mortality rate is generally not reflected in postnatal urologic series of lower urinary tract obstruction, as it represents the "hidden mortality" of this disorder due to the fact that these infants do not survive postnatally and die before transfer to a pediatric specialty center for treatment. Early midgestation oligohydramnios carries a poor prognosis for the fetus, and when associated with urethral obstruction, the mortality rate has been estimated to be as high as 95%.[5] Therefore, fetuses with oligohydramnios and lower urinary tract obstruction represent the most severe end of the obstructive uropathy spectrum, and are those fetuses that one would expect to identify earliest in gestation, and be at highest risk for pulmonary hypoplasia and renal dysplasia.

In order to better understand the natural progression of developmental abnormalities occurring in obstructive uropathy, an animal model was needed to study the process in greater detail. Such a model would require the following: (1) simulate congenital obstruction in humans, with high-grade obstruction causing subsequent pulmonary, renal, and skeletal deformities; (2) quantitatively assess the effect of obstruction on pulmonary and renal parenchymal development, and overall survival; and (3) allow correction of the obstruction in utero to evaluate whether such prenatal intervention improved survivals and decreased pulmonary and renal tissue damage.[6]

In the early 1980s, Dr. Michael Harrison's group in San Francisco developed a sheep model for surgically created urinary tract obstruction that was reasonably easy to study and reflected the pathophysiology observed in human fetuses.[7] Ureteral ligation and contralateral nephrectomy were performed in fetal lambs at 62 to 84 days' gestation (total sheep gestation = 144 days). The effects of ureteral ligation on renal histology were found to be dependent on when in gestation the obstruction occurred. Early obstruction in the second trimester resulted in renal dysplasia, while obstruction in the third trimester led to hydronephrosis alone. However, this surgical approach proved difficult, with a high rate of fetal loss and no postnatal survival because of pulmonary hypoplasia. Numerous other approaches were attempted without success. Finally, using a combination of urachal ligation and gradual occlusion of the urethra with an ameroid constrictor, they were able to consistently produce pulmonary hypoplasia, bladder dilation, hydroureters, and hydronephrosis. This model produced histologic changes in the kidneys similar to those seen in humans with increased fibrosis throughout the kidney, although interestingly, no cysts or parenchymal disorganization was observed, which are frequent findings in the human.

Having successfully developed an approach that reproduced the pathophysiologic changes found in humans, the next step was to determine if in utero decompression was beneficial.[8] After they had established urethral obstruction at 95 days, half of the fetal lambs underwent suprapubic cystostomy after 15 to 27 days of obstruction, to allow urine to flow freely from the fetal bladder. After birth, all of the lambs that had undergone cystostomy survived with minimal respiratory support, in contrast to those that had not undergone decompression who all required maximal respiratory support and died within the first 24 hours after birth. Lung weights were greater in lambs who had undergone cystostomy, although still less than normal control animals. These studies demonstrated that restoration of amniotic fluid volume resulted in improved lung growth and pulmonary survival. All lambs that had undergone cystostomy had mildly dilated urinary tracts and minimal histologic renal parenchymal damage. Fibrosis was prominent throughout the kidneys of nondecompressed lambs; however, no evidence of cystic dysplasia was observed.

To create renal dysplasia reflective of that seen in humans, Harrison's group found they needed to establish obstruction earlier in gestation. Using a unilateral ureteral obstruction model created at days 58 to 66 of gestation, they found obstructed kidneys demonstrated cystic changes and disorganized architecture. Fibrosis and parenchymal disorganization were present, and the medullary region contained a few abnormal appearing

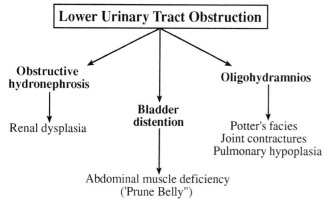

FIGURE 18–1. Malformations and deformations associated with lower urinary tract obstruction.

ducts buried by primitive epithelium, but no tubular-like structures were identified.[9] To determine whether in utero relief of obstruction would prevent renal dysplasia, they performed unilateral ureteral obstruction at days 58 to 66 followed by end ureterostomy to relieve obstruction at 20, 40, and 60 days' postobstruction. All decompressed kidneys had mildly dilated ureters and were overall smaller and weighed less than normal controls. Renal function was found to decrease as duration of obstruction increased. Histologic changes and abnormalities also increased as duration of obstruction increased. However, decompression, regardless of timing, improved both histology and function compared to non-decompressed controls. These studies provided evidence that in utero decompression of early ureteral obstruction could arrest histologic changes in the kidney, preventing severe dysplastic damage, and potentially preserve renal function (Fig. 18–2).

Experimental Studies for Evaluating Fetal Renal Function

Clinical assessment of renal function in obstructive uropathy has been difficult to do. Subjective tests such as rate of bladder refilling after bladder aspiration or urine output following Lasix stimulation have proven unreliable.[10–12] Several studies have looked at the predictive value of the sonographic appearance of the fetal kidneys as an indicator of damage; however, such observational impressions lack the sensitivity for correlating with renal function.[13–15] As renal function deteriorates, urine production falls, which should be reflected in amniotic fluid volume (AFV). However, quantitative analysis of AFV alone is a poor measure of renal function, because by the time oligohydramnios is sonographically observed, renal dysplasia and pulmonary hypoplasia may already be irreversibly established.[11, 16]

As the metanephric kidneys begin to function at 10 to 12 weeks' gestation, an ultrafiltrate of fetal serum is produced that is somewhat hypotonic because of tubular reabsorption of sodium and chloride. Between 16 and 21 weeks' gestation further maturation within the nephrons occurs, resulting in production of fetal urine that is progressively more hypotonic.[17, 18] Early clinical studies were able to correlate the observation that fetuses with urinary obstruction that were found postnatally to have normal renal function produce hypotonic urine in utero, while those with poor postnatal function produced isotonic or somewhat hypertonic urine.[19] Investigators next began to analyze the substances within the urine for predictive markers that might correlate with damage to the fetal kidneys.

In an elaborate set of experiments, again using a fetal sheep model of unilateral ureteral ligation in the mid-gestation, the San Francisco group investigated late-gestation comparative renal function in the obstructed and unobstructed kidney by serial selective urine samplings from catheters placed in the fetal bladder and proximal ureter of the obstructed kidney, and blood sampling using lines placed into the femoral artery and vein.[20] They found that, compared to the control side, the obstructed fetal kidney had a markedly decreased glomerular filtration rate (GFR) as well as abnormal proximal tubular function with increased sodium and chloride loss. The obstructed kidney was consistently smaller and weighed less than the contralateral control. Also, urine production as measured by an iothalamate clearance and creatine clearance was significantly less in the obstructed kidney compared to the unobstructed kidney. These experiments successfully demonstrated that upper urinary tract obstruction can result in altered growth, function, and histologic damage reflective of that observed in human clinical studies.

Appropriate prenatal management in human fetuses would depend on our ability to reliably determine the presence and extent of functional damage in the kidneys, and select those that might benefit from intervention and prevention of further progressive damage. Severe

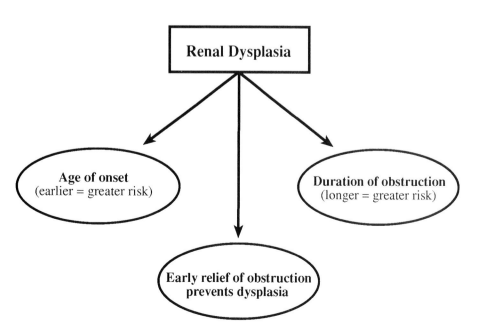

FIGURE 18–2. Concepts of renal dysplasia derived from fetal sheep model of ureteral obstruction. (From Glick PL, Harrison MR, Noall RA, Villa RL: Correction of congenital hydronephrosis in utero. III. Early mid-trimester ureteral obstruction produces renal dysplasia. J Pediatr Surg 18:681, 1983, with permission.)

oligohydramnios early in gestation and increased echo-genicity and presence of discrete parenchymal cysts are certainly consistent with advanced renal damage.[14, 19] However, minimal to moderate amniotic fluid volume changes and more subtle parenchymal changes on ultrasound are less reliable in predicting renal function and damage. Therefore, a simple and safe method of reliably determining renal damage was needed. The first useful approach came from observations based on the review of electrolyte patterns from fetal urine obtained during clinical evaluations of obstructive uropathies. The San Francisco group reviewed data from 20 human fetuses and categorized outcomes as "poor function" ($n = 10$) or "good function" ($n = 10$) based on renal histology at autopsy or biopsy, and/or renal and pulmonary function at birth.[19] Groups were compared for (1) amniotic fluid status at initial presentation, (2) ultrasound appearance of kidneys, (3) fetal urine composition, and (4) fetal urine output. Fetuses categorized with poor function were found to have moderate to severely decreased amniotic fluid volume, very echogenic and/or cystic kidneys on ultrasound, urine outputs of less than 2 mL/hr, and sodium concentrations greater than 100 mEq/L, chloride greater than 90 mEq/L, and osmolality levels greater than 210 mOsm/L. Those grouped as good function had normal to moderately decreased amniotic fluid, normal to mildly echogenic renal parenchyma, urine output greater than 2 mL/hr, and sodium concentrations less than 100 mEq/L, chloride less than 90 mEq/L, and osmolality values less than 210 mOsm/L. Numerous subsequent clinical series have supported these predictive criteria, and evaluation of urinary components has continued to evolve, as will be discussed later, with the addition of other markers such as calcium, β_2-microglobulin, and total protein. Lastly, use of multiple urine aspirations to document increasing or decreasing hypotonicity following repeated bladder drainage has helped select fetuses who would benefit from in utero treatment.

Pulmonary Hypoplasia Resulting from Early Bilateral Obstruction

Oligohydramnios secondary to fetal urinary tract obstruction, renal agenesis, or a prolonged amniotic fluid leak results in pulmonary hypoplasia and neonatal death.[21–24] Pulmonary changes include decreases in lung volume, alveolar size, airway generations, and radial alveolar count, as well as increased pulmonary arteriolar muscularization.[24, 25] To study the morphologic changes that occur within these lungs, investigators developed an animal model using fetal sheep, creating complete urinary tract obstruction in the early mid-gestation and examining the lungs and kidneys after term delivery. Bilateral ureteral obstruction was performed at 60 days' gestation (term, 145 days) during the pseudoglandular stage (40 to 80 days) of fetal lung development.[26] After bilateral obstruction, severe oligohydramnios resulted and the kidneys developed histologic changes consistent with dysplasia. To standardize lung volumes for differences in body weight, lung volume/body weight ratios

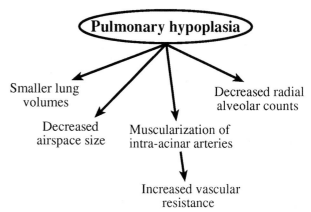

F I G U R E 18–3. Lung changes associated with oligohydramnios observed in a sheep model of bilateral ureteral obstruction. (From Adzick NS, Harrison MR, Hu LM, et al: Pulmonary hypoplasia and renal dysplasia in a fetal lamb urinary tract obstruction model. Surg Forum 38:666, 1987, with permission.)

were calculated. Lambs with ureteral obstruction were found to have significantly smaller lung volumes compared to controls. Radial alveolar counts paralleled lung volume results such that the smaller the lung volume, the lower the observed radial alveolar count. Airspace size within the term lungs was also smaller in the bilateral ureteral obstruction group. Muscularization of intra-acinar arteries was also greater in the obstruction group, and increased muscularization of peripheral pulmonary arterioles correlates with increased vascular resistance in these hypoplastic lungs (Fig. 18–3).

The mechanism by which oligohydramnios affects lung growth may have several components.[21, 22] The diminished size of the uterine cavity in the presence of oligohydramnios may limit intrathoracic space and restrict fetal breathing movements, both of which appear necessary for normal lung growth. Oligohydramnios may result in increased pressure on the fetal chest with increased fetal lung fluid loss and associated diminished lung volume within the airways and potential airspace. Also, loss of a potential pulmonary growth factor produced by the kidneys may interfere with normal lung growth and maturation. However, experimental pulmonary hypoplasia due to obstructive uropathy was also shown to be preventable with early reversal of obstruction or urinary diversion from the obstructed bladder into the amniotic space resulting in restoration of amniotic fluid volume within the uterine cavity.[21] This observation was an important piece of evidence to justify and support early in utero treatment of human obstructive uropathy.

Common Urinary Tract Anomalies

Differential Diagnosis

Urinary tract abnormalities continue to constitute a large portion of prenatally diagnosed congenital abnormalities, making up almost 50% of those abnormalities diagnosed with ultrasound.[27] The ability to reliably identify urinary tract structures allows diagnosis early in pregnancy. Between 14 and 18 weeks' gestation, 0.33% of fetuses will be identified as having renal abnormalities on ultrasound.[28] This percentage becomes higher as gestation progresses, as some abnormalities do not manifest until later in gestation. There is a familial influence, as 14% of parents of a fetus diagnosed with a urinary tract abnormality will themselves have an anomaly of the urinary tract. In 24% of sonographically detected urinary tract abnormalities, associated abnormalities will be detected and may provide evidence for an underlying genetic syndrome. Dilation of the urinary tract can be secondary to obstructive or nonobstructive causes. Obstructive causes include ureteropelvic junction (UPJ) obstruction (44% of cases), ureterovesical junction (UVJ) obstruction (21% incidence), multicystic dysplastic kidney, ureterocele/ectopic ureter, duplication of collecting system (12%), posterior urethral valves (PUV) (9%), urethral atresia, and pelvic tumors.[29] Nonobstructive causes include physiologic dilatation, vesicoureteral reflux (14%), prune belly syndrome, renal cysts, and megacalycosis[29] (Table 18–1).

Upper Tract Obstruction— Ureteropelvic Junction

The prenatal detection and management of upper tract disease remains controversial. Thomas[31] showed the estimated incidence of urinary tract dilatation in utero to be 1 in every 100 pregnancies, but only 1 in 500 were caused by clinically significant urologic problems. Approximately half of prenatally detected upper tract dilatations are caused by UPJ obstructions, with bilateral obstruction occurring in 21 to 36% of cases.[31] UPJ obstruction is also the most common cause of postnatal hydronephrosis followed by reflux (33%), UVJ obstruction (9 to 14%), and PUV (2 to 9%).[32]

Two forms of UPJ obstruction occur: *type I* obstruction is due to an anatomic or functional abnormality of the UPJ, while *type II* obstruction occurs secondary to vesicoureteral reflux leading to elongation of the ureter and kinking of the UPJ where it is fixed to the kidney. The most common cause of UPJ obstruction is an intrinsic

stenosis of the proximal portion of the ureter, often associated with an abnormally high insertion of the ureter into the renal pelvis. Occasionally, anatomic variation can result in the proximal ureter being trapped behind a band of tissue or blood vessels that are supplying the lower segment of the kidneys. Obstruction can also occur in the absence of anatomic stenosis or distortion due to an aperistaltic segment of the proximal ureter at the UPJ. Anatomic changes in the muscular and collagen components may prevent the normal propagation of peristaltic activity initiated by the pacemaker in the pelvocalyceal region.[33, 34]

Sonographic diagnosis is generally based on measurement of the diameter at the renal pelvis. Anderson et al.[35] found upper tract obstruction was not reliably detected before 24 weeks using a cut-off measurement of over 10 mm, and that the degree of renal pelvis dilation greater than 10 mm in the third trimester was not predictive and did not correlate with postnatal renal function. Fasolato et al.[36] found that 18% of infants with prenatally detected upper tract dilatation had confirmed abnormalities after birth, and this group all had renal pelvis diameters greater than 15 mm prenatally. They also found that all infants diagnosed with renal pelvis diameters of less than 10 mm had resolution of their upper tract dilatation in the first year of life.

Prenatal detection of upper tract diseases is important to improve postnatal management. Unilateral neonatal hydronephrosis has been shown to be associated with a 3.5 to 20% risk of renal deterioration in the postnatal period.[37] Also, while prenatally detected isolated renal pelvis dilatation has been shown to be a weak predictor of vesicoureteral reflux, it may prenatally identify infants for close postnatal surveillance and allow the earlier documentation and treatment of vesicoureteral reflux with improved outcomes.[38]

An algorithm for management of prenatally detected upper tract abnormalities has been suggested.[7, 32, 36, 39] Postnatal ultrasound should be performed at 3 to 7 days of age, and if normal should be repeated after 1 month of age to confirm normal status. If the initial scan is abnormal, antibiotics should be initiated and full radiologic evaluation undertaken including voiding cystourethrogram, intravenous pyelogram, and renal scintigram. Therapy should be based on test results, but surgical intervention has been recommended when there is less than 40% renal function and an obstructed pattern on renography, breakthrough infection or renal colic, marked hydronephrosis, and an anteroposterior diameter of more than 2 cm on ultrasound.

TABLE 18–1. SONOGRAPHIC DIFFERENTIAL DIAGNOSIS OF HYDRONEPHROSIS

Obstructive
Ureteropelvic junction obstruction
Ureterovesicle junction obstruction
Multicystic dysplastic kidney
Ureterocele/ectopic ureter
Duplication of the collecting system
Posterior urethral valves
Pelvic tumors

Nonobstructive
Physiologic dilatation
Vesicoureteral reflux
Prune belly syndrome
Megacalycosis
Renal cysts

Ureteral Obstruction

Ureterovesical junction abnormalities are recognized by megaureter in the absence of an enlarged bladder. Characteristic ultrasound findings are dilatation of the distal ureter more so than the upper collecting system (Fig. 18–4). Hyperperistalsis of the lower ureter and adynamic segments of the distal portion have been described.[40] Prenatal diagnosis may allow earlier identification, which prompts earlier postnatal evaluation and

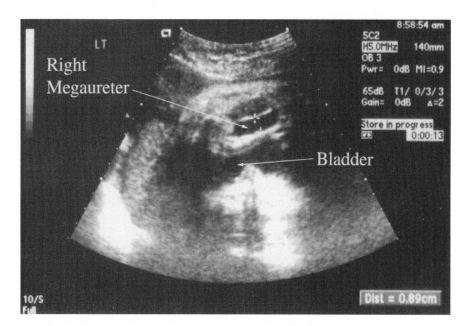

FIGURE 18–4. Isolated megaureter from ureterovesicle junction obstruction.

intervention, ideally before severe renal parenchymal damage occurs. This condition is more common in males and, although usually sporadic, may be familial with 32% of asymptomatic siblings of patients with reflux also exhibiting reflux.[41] Causes of megaureter other than reflux include bladder dysfunction or obstruction, primary megaureter from stenosis or fibrosis of the ureterovesical valves,[42] or benign primary megaureter that is congenital.[43] Congenital megaureter requires no prenatal intervention to protect renal function, and ultrasound findings include identification of a dilated peristaltic ureter with or without dilated renal pelvis.[43] Duplicated collecting systems may also give rise to megaureters and are a common urinary tract abnormality[44] (Fig. 18–5). Ectopic ureteroceles may occur with duplication, and if present occur bilaterally in 15% of cases. The normal

ureter opens into the lateral angle of the trigone. When complete ureteral duplication exists, the ureter draining the upper renal pole usually opens caudal and medial to the ureter draining the lower renal pole. Duplex ureters may open into the trigone, but commonly can enter at a number of abnormal positions, including one of the genital ductal systems or the urethra. The ureter draining the upper pole commonly ends in an ectopic ureterocele, which represents an expansion of the ureter within the bladder wall between the muscle and mucosal layers (Fig. 18–6). When a duplex system is present on one side, contralateral duplication can be found in 50% of cases. Ureteral duplication is seen more often in females and, if the ureterocele(s) is very large, can result in bladder outlet or contralateral UVJ obstruction. The opening of the ureterocele is usually obstructed by a

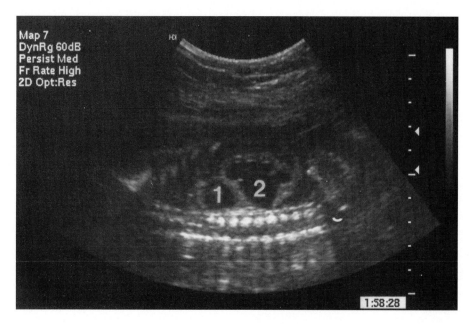

FIGURE 18–5. Duplication of renal collecting systems. (1 = upper pole; 2 = lower pole with pyelocaliectasis.)

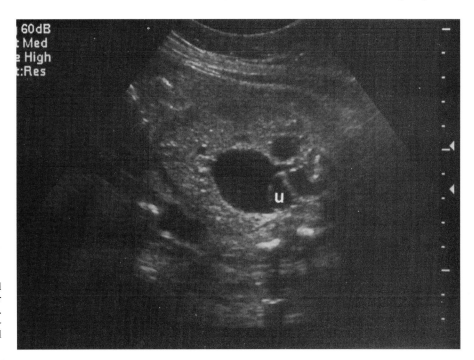

FIGURE 18–6. Ureterocele within fetal bladder associated with an ectopic ureter from a duplicated collecting system (Fig. 18–5). Dilated structures anterior to bladder represent the hydroureter associated with the ureterocele.

stenosis, or because it opens into the bladder at the level of the urogenital diaphragm and is obstructed by the closed bladder neck.

Hydronephrosis, and potentially cystic dysplasia, is common in the upper renal pole when the ureter is obstructed by an ectopic ureterocele. If the hydronephrosis is mild to moderate, careful renal evaluation can usually identify the normal or mildly dilated lower pole and collecting system. When hydronephrosis is severe,

or if the upper pole pelvis is markedly dilated, then identification of the lower pole system may not be apparent (Fig. 18–7). Therefore, when identification of a megaureter with an ectopic ureterocele is made, consideration should be given to the presence of a duplication system and an appropriate search made to identify the lower pole and collecting system if possible. Prenatal management of such patients revolves around amniotic fluid volume and evidence of bladder outlet obstruction,

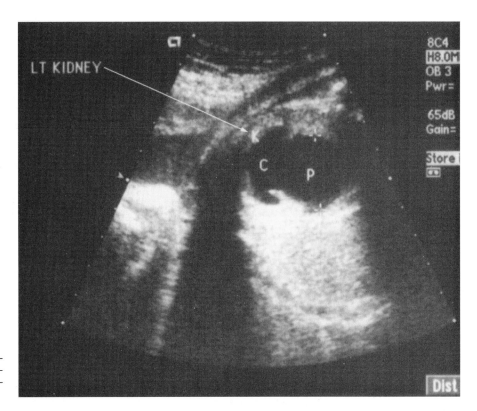

FIGURE 18–7. Ureteropelvic junction obstruction. (p = dilated renal pelvis; c = distended renal calyces; k = compressed renal parenchyma.)

and expectant management is appropriate if normal fluid is present. Early onset oligohydramnios due to bladder outlet obstruction arising from bladder distortion from a large ureterocele can potentially place the fetus at risk for pulmonary hypoplasia and contralateral ureteral obstruction and hydronephrosis.

In 1997, we reported[45] a case of an ectopic megaureter associated with a ureterocele that caused significant distortion and compression of the fetal bladder resulting in contralateral ureteral and bladder outlet obstruction. Progressive contralateral hydronephrosis and oligohydramnios developed in midgestation. Percutaneous ultrasound-guided drainage of the ureterocele allowed transient drainage and decreased hydronephrosis in the contralateral side until the ureterocele again enlarged. In this case, we were able to successfully place a vesicoamniotic diverting shunt catheter into the ureterocele leading to persistent drainage, restoration of bladder anatomy, resolution of contralateral UVJ obstruction, and preservation of contralateral renal function. Postnatally, this infant was found to have a distal ureteral duplication with one segment entering ectopically into the bladder associated with ureterocele formation and the other entering ectopically into the proximal penile urethra. More recently, we observed progressive growth of a right ureterocele within the fetal bladder until bladder outlet obstruction occurred. The ureterocele was percutaneously drained on two occasions, but recurred within days leading to progressive contralateral hydronephrosis and bladder distention at 25 weeks' gestation. Using a 1-mm microendoscope and a fetal transabdominal cystoscopic approach, we were able to directly visualize the long, tubular ureterocele sac extending into and obstructing the proximal urethra. Utilizing a yttrium-aluminum-garnet (YAG) laser, we were able to drain the ureterocele sac by placing a linear incision through the cyst wall, allowing collapse of the obstructing sac

and subsequent bladder drainage for the remainder of the pregnancy. Postnatally, the infant was confirmed to have duplication of the right collecting system, and ectopic insertion of the ureter associated with the ureterocele.

Urinary Extravasation in Obstructive Uropathy

Urinary extravasation resulting in an isolated perirenal urinoma or urinary ascites has been described primarily in the neonatal period and is presumed to result from increased pressure within an obstructed fetal urinary tract.[46–49] Both clinical and experimental studies have shown that fetal urinary tract obstruction can result in severe renal parenchymal injury. The degree of dysplasia varies with timing of onset, degree of obstruction, and in utero duration of obstruction. If urinary leakage into the fetal peritoneal cavity or perinephric space occurs from the high-pressure obstructed urinary tract before irreversible renal damage occurs, then a "safety valve" phenomenon may occur that may protect the fetal kidneys from additional damage[50] (Fig. 18–8).

In the fetus, the renal collecting tubules are short and straight. When the urinary tract becomes obstructed and hydronephrosis develops, pressure may increase within the kidney and be exerted directly on the tubules causing eventual renal parenchymal damage. The mechanism of "renal protection" by extravasation is most likely related to relief of intrarenal pressure from obstructive hydronephrosis. The degree of renal preservation likely depends on the time during gestation the leak occurs and the degree of histologic damage present at the time. Fetal lamb experiments have shown that subsequent renal function is inversely proportional to the duration

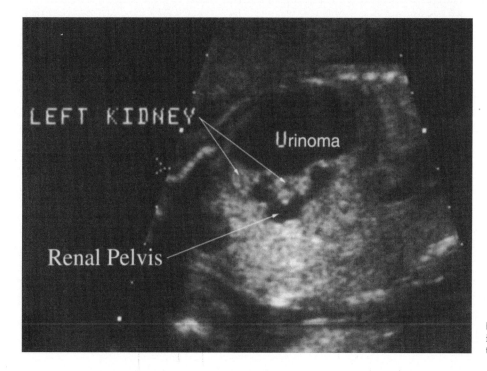

FIGURE 18–8. Subcapsular versus perinephric urinoma associated with a ureteropelvic junction obstruction.

of urinary tract obstruction and is directly proportional to the duration of in utero decompensation.[8]

In most cases, the precise location of extravasation is unclear, and it has been proposed that urinary ascites occurs by transudation across the renal capsule or Gerota's fascia. Some reports have demonstrated either calyceal or renal parenchymal tears, with subsequent ascites occurring from transudation or a peritoneal defect. However, extravasated urine may remain contained in a urinoma without subsequent drainage and development of ascites.[48, 51]

Some investigators hypothesize that the failure of contained urinomas to communicate with the peritoneal cavity results in inadequate decompression and progression of renal parenchymal damage.[48] Certainly there are exceptions to this concept, and the type of obstruction may play a role in the pathophysiologic outcome. Neonates have been reported with isolated perirenal urinomas and adequate renal function after postnatal urinary tract drainage.[46–49] Such cases appear to be associated with lower urinary tract obstruction, while isolated urinomas occurring with UPJ obstruction seem to be associated with nonfunctioning, severely damaged renal parenchyma and may represent an end-stage renal event.[8]

The contributions of urinary extravasation or bladder distention to the development of the "prune belly" phenotype remains controversial. The triad of abdominal muscular deficiency, obstructive uropathy, and failure of testicular descent was first described by Parker in 1985. However, there remains no consensus regarding the etiology and developmental pathogenesis of this group of findings. Disagreement continues in regards to whether abdominal muscular deficiency and laxity is an intrinsic malformation or simple deformation resulting from abdominal distention. Traditional opinion regards the prune belly triad as being a primary mesodermal defect.[52, 53] Recent experience supports the belief that deficiency and laxity of abdominal muscles in prune belly is a deformation secondary to abdominal distention at a critical time in early gestation. Based on accumulated experience with cases of babies born with abdominal muscular deficiencies from three different prenatal abnormalities—obstructive uropathy, nonimmune fetal ascites, and small bowel duplication—the most classic appearance of the prune belly phenotype occurred in early gestational ascites that subsequently resolved leaving the typical redundant, "stretched" prune belly abdominal wall.[54] The severity of abdominal wall laxity associated with bladder distention and/or urinary ascites may well be determined by how early in gestation as well as the severity and duration of distention that is present. The degree to which such potential secondary deformations can be prevented by in utero bladder decompression before birth is still unknown. However, many fetuses that we have successfully salvaged with prenatal vesicoamniotic shunt interventions have been born with minimal to no deficiency of abdominal wall musculature and its associated prune belly phenotype.

Urethral Obstruction

Lower urinary tract obstructions (LUTOs) generally involve developmental abnormalities of the penile urethra in male fetuses, with PUV and urethral atresia being the most common causes for early onset LUTO. Other urethral anomalies such as anterior urethral valves (Fig. 18–9), meatal stenosis (Fig. 18–10), epispadias, and hypospadias have also been associated with LUTO. As noted previously, the presence of a large ureterocele within the bladder can also obstruct the bladder neck and proximal urethra. The typical prenatal sonographic features of LUTO include an enlarged fetal bladder, bilateral hydronephrosis, and decreased amniotic fluid volume. A normal amniotic fluid volume would indicate the absence of complete urethral obstruction, and is more consistent with the diagnosis of urethral stricture, hypoplasia, or "incomplete" PUV. LUTO in female fetuses, generally associated with cloacal developmental abnormalities, is normally a component of syndromic abnormalities for which prenatal therapy has not been shown to be beneficial. Cases of congenital bladder atony in female fetuses have been reported that were caused by a neurologic deficit in the bladder, which may have benefited by vesicoamniotic shunt placement in the second trimester.[55] Finally, there are a number of genetic causes, such as megacystis-microcolon syndrome, as well as chromosomal aneuploidies, such as trisomies 21 and 18, which can be associated with LUTOs. It is the tremendous heterogeneity of underlying etiologies that has made the prenatal evaluation and treatment of LUTO a challenge, and has resulted in the highly variable success rates reported for prenatal treatment of these disorders. It has not been until recently that a stepwise algorithm for the prenatal evaluation and selection of fetuses for treatment was established. Following these guidelines, however, patient selection has improved and predictive precision increased in the evaluation of fetal function.

The contemporary history of treatment of fetal obstructive uropathy began with the work of Harrison and colleagues, who were able in the fetal sheep model to show the pathophysiologic link between obstructive uropathy, renal dysplasia, and pulmonary hypoplasia. They further demonstrated that relief of obstruction and restoration of amniotic fluid volume allowed normal lung growth, providing the first rationale for vesicoamniotic shunting as a means to prevent pulmonary hypoplasia, the leading cause of neonatal death in LUTO. Their research also indicated that early relief of obstruction may prevent severe renal dysplasia, adding additional support for prenatal intervention.

Histologic Changes Associated with LUTO

Complete urethral obstruction or significant restriction of urethral flow results in accumulation of urine within the fetal bladder, leading to marked distention. Prolonged obstruction results in smooth muscle hypertrophy and hyperplasia within the bladder wall, and eventual impairment of contractile capacity as well as compliance and elasticity. Bladder distention results in elevated pressures within the bladder, which may overcome the delicate physiologic valve mechanism at the ureterovesical junctions. Bladder wall distortion–associated hypertrophy may contribute to loss of the

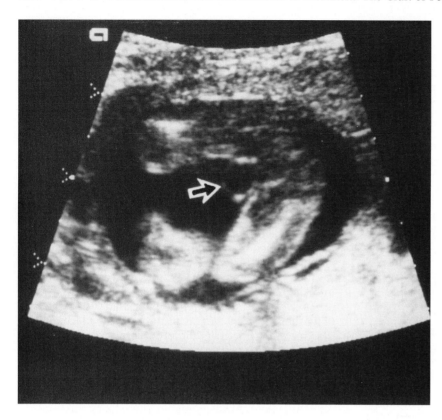

FIGURE 18–9. Megaurethra associated with anterior urethral valves. *Arrow* points to marked dilated penile urethra due to distal obstruction.

physiologic valve mechanism resulting in reflux and the development of hydroureters and progression of hydronephrosis. Ureteral distention also seems to elicit smooth muscle hypertrophy, particularly in the distal ureter where smooth muscle is more prevalent. This may

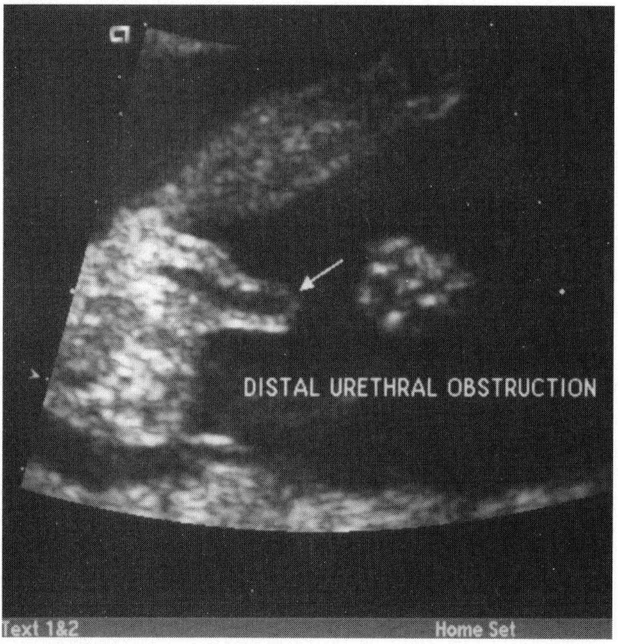

FIGURE 18–10. Dilated penile urethra from distal urethral stenosis. Note normal amniotic fluid volume, as fetal urine can still pass through the urethra and enter the amniotic space.

further distort the ureterovesical junctions, diminishing elasticity in ureteral wall, and contribute to worsening reflux and associated renal damage.

Our ongoing clinical studies indicate there is a subset of male fetuses in which no anatomic urethral obstruction can be demonstrated on fetal autopsy, although these fetuses appear sonographically identical to those in which complete obstruction is confirmed postnatally. Histologically, these fetuses may have a defect in the development and response of smooth muscle throughout the upper and lower urinary tract, resulting in dilatation of the bladder and subsequent reflux hydronephrosis. In such cases, we have found little to no change in the smooth muscle component of the urinary tract when compared to age-matched controls. This is in contrast to cases with confirmed urethral obstruction, where the typical hypertrophic and hyperplastic response in the smooth muscle component is observed in the walls of the bladder and distal ureters in response to obstruction, which is progressive and reflective of duration of obstruction[56] (Figs. 18–11 and 18–12).

Long-term prognosis in cases without anatomic urethral obstruction following shunt intervention appears to be better than outcomes in cases of anatomic obstruction such as posterior urethral valves, and it would therefore be helpful to reliably differentiate these two groups prenatally.[57] We have recently begun using fine-needle fetoscopy to perform in utero fetal cystoscopy during the prenatal evaluation of obstructive uropathy to directly examine the bladder mucosa, ureteral orifices, and proximal urethra.[58] In cases of true urethral obstruction, the proximal urethra has been markedly dilated,

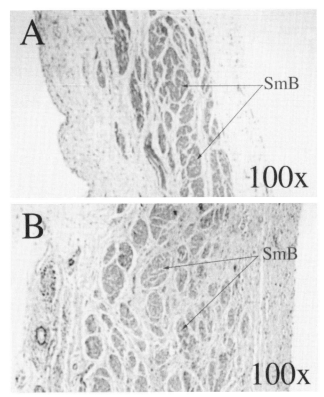

FIGURE 18–11. H&E stain of upper bladder dome (*A*) and lower bladder (*B*) regions from a fetus with urethra-patent obstructive uropathy. Note prominence of connective tissue component (SmB = smooth muscle bundles). Magnification listed in lower right corners.

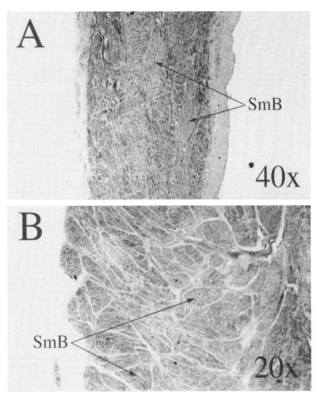

FIGURE 18–12. H&E stain of upper bladder dome (*A*) and lower bladder (*B*) regions from a fetus with complete urethral obstruction from posterior urethral valves. Note hypertrophic and hyperplastic response of smooth muscle component with minimal increase in connective tissue component. (SmB = smooth muscle bundles). Magnification listed in lower right corners.

with muscular trabeculations noted in the trigone of the bladder (Fig. 18–13). In cases of urethra patent uropathy, the proximal urethra and bladder neck was much less distended and the trigone was without trabeculation (Fig. 18–14). However, sonographically both groups demonstrated characteristic features of the "keyhole sign" of bladder and proximal urethral distention (Fig. 18–15). The capability to differentiate these two groups prenatally may direct future changes and refinements in our interventive approaches in an effort to optimize long-term outcomes.

Hydronephrosis develops from continued urine production in the face of obstructed drainage as well as reflux from the distended bladder. The renal pelvises and calices of the upper collecting system become progressively distended and compress the renal parenchyma against the distended renal capsule. Histologic studies indicate a progressive dilation of the distal to proximal renal tubules associated with development of peritubular and interstitial fibrosis. Sonographically, the degree of compression and associated fibrosis is reflected by the echogenic appearance of the parenchyma. Eventually, these processes may trigger cystic degeneration of the kidneys, heralded by the appearance of discrete cysts in the renal cortex on ultrasound, and renal insufficiency at birth.

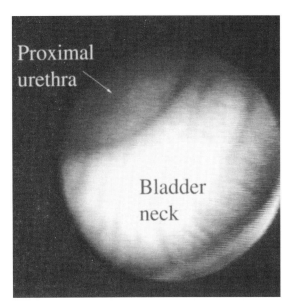

FIGURE 18–13. In utero fetal cystoscopic image of bladder neck and proximal urethra in a fetus with complete urethral obstruction from posterior urethral valves. Note tense distention of both structures. Mucosa was noted to be quite pale in appearance.

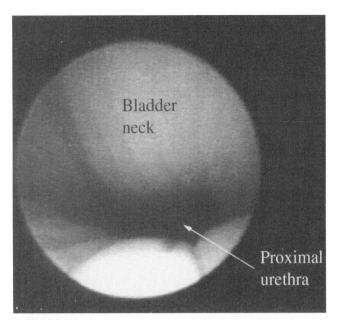

FIGURE 18–14. In utero fetal cystoscopic image of bladder neck and proximal urethra in a fetus with urethral-patent obstructive uropathy. Bladder neck and proximal urethra only mildly distended. Mucosa was pink and more normal in appearance than that observed in complete obstructive cases such as in Figure 18–13.

Mechanisms of Histologic Damage

Harrison's group was able to demonstrate that early urinary tract obstruction resulted in more histologic damage to the kidney than obstruction later in gestation.[8] Carr et al.[59] have shown, through analysis of gene-specific and nonspecific mRNA expression in the fetal kidney, that mid-gestation is the period of greatest renal growth and development. They suggest that obstruction and hydronephrosis in early mid-gestation would have

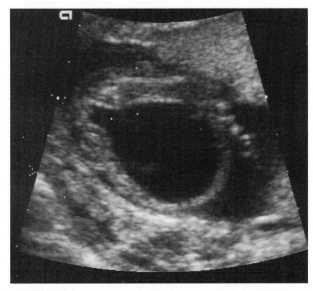

FIGURE 18–15. Sonographic image of a typical bladder seen in lower urinary tract obstruction. Note the "keyhole" appearance that is used to describe the combination of dilated bladder and proximal urethra.

its greatest impact on renal development if present during this maximal growth phase of renal development. Changes in mRNA expression indicate that significant intrarenal physiologic changes occur secondary to obstruction, which may change mechanisms of cell proliferation and differentiation, potentially irreversibly, if obstructive hydronephrosis is present in the early stages of the mid-gestation. Such alterations may predispose the kidney to or promote the dysplastic process.

Utilizing a mid-gestational sheep model of unilateral ureteral ligation, Attar et al.[60] found a characteristic pattern after 10 days' obstruction of absent normal nephron precursors and cortical architecture dominated by cyst-like structures containing abnormal glomerular tufts. They observed prominent vascular-like spaces that they felt represented dilated venules or lymphatics as well as increased interstitial edema. Increased numbers of pyknotic nuclei were observed in the interstitial tissues and dilated lumens of the cystic structures, reflecting increased cell apoptosis. They also noted increased expression of both proliferating cell nuclear antigen (PCNA; a marker for cycling cells) and PAX2 (a growth-stimulating transcription factor that is usually down-regulated during normal renal maturation) after 10 days' obstruction, indicating cellular gene deregulation as well as increased cell turnover and death. In kidneys evaluated after only 1 day of obstruction, they found a pattern of dilatation of proximal nephron precursors and increased expression of PAX2 and PCNA in cells lining these primitive tubules. Such findings imply that early obstructed urine flow and hydronephrosis results in morphologic abnormalities of the developing proximal nephron rather than in elements that will develop into collecting ducts. Attar postulates that early increases in intrarenal pressure may cause stretch within the primitive epithelia that triggers an initial growth response.

Nguyen and Kogan,[33] using a similar model, found that prolonged obstruction resulted in renal parenchymal disorganization, fibrosis, and the reappearance of primitive epithelial structures. They demonstrated elevated renin levels present in the obstructed kidney only, and proposed that obstruction may activate the renin-angiotensin system and alter the expression of growth factors that promote fibrosis. They suggest that increased angiotensin II expression, which regulates growth factors such as transforming growth factor-$\beta 1$ (TGF-$\beta 1$), platelet-derived growth factors, and clusterin, may activate pathways that lead to interstitial fibrosis. TGF-$\beta 1$ stimulates extracellular matrix production, and its expression in obstructed kidneys was shown to be increased. They found a cell-aggregating glycoprotein, clusterin, to be transiently increased early in obstruction, and suggested it may temporarily protect against cell death. Angiotensin II, however, suppresses clusterin expression, and as angiotensin II levels increase with prolonged obstruction, clusterin levels were found to fall and cell apoptosis increased. They also noted that expression of epithelial growth factor (EGF) was decreased in obstructed kidneys, but not in the contralateral unobstructed kidney. Normal EGF expression in the unobstructed kidney may potentiate the observed compensatory growth seen in the unobstructed side, because EGF has a strong mitogenic effect on renal tissues that is potentiated by angiotensin II.

Preliminary studies[61] in our laboratory in urine obtained at the time of vesicocentesis during the prenatal evaluation of human fetuses with LUTO have found increased levels of EGF in cases of good-prognosis fetuses with less renal damage than cases in which more advanced renal impairment and histologic damage is present. In human fetuses, it may be that EGF levels increase early in obstruction as the kidney tries to respond to cell damage and death, but expression later falls as progressive cell death and focal hypoxia diminish the number of cells that can contribute to this response, and the expression of other cellular regulators is altered. This seems consistent with other reports of an observed brief proliferative response of renal tissues to decreased blood flow, followed by increased epithelial apoptosis and tubular atrophy, interstitial fibrosis, and increased TGF-β1 expression.[62, 63]

Contemporary Approach to Prenatal Intervention

The early use of a double-pigtail catheter placed into the fetal bladder to allow obstructed urine to flow into the amniotic space met with highly variable success. The criteria for intervention were highly variable, and evaluation of the fetus before treatment was minimal in most cases. Therefore, fetuses with underlying chromosomal abnormalities, other significant structural anomalies, and advanced renal dysplasia were treated unnecessarily with a predictable poor outcome. In 1994, we proposed an algorithm for the prenatal evaluation and selection of fetal candidates for the prenatal intervention that has improved the ability to predict which fetuses might benefit from intervention and those in whom intervention would not improve the clinical outcome.[64] The three major components of this evaluation algorithm include obtaining (1) a fetal karyotype, (2) a detailed sonographic evaluation to rule out other structural anomalies that might impact on the prognosis for the fetus, and (3) serial urine evaluations to determine the extent of the underlying renal damage present (Fig. 18–16). To be considered a candidate for prenatal evaluation and potential treatment, the fetus must have a normal male karyotype, and ultrasound must demonstrate oligo-/anhydramnios or document decreasing amniotic fluid volume, as well as absence of other fetal anomalies that would adversely affect the prognosis and clinical outcome for the infant.

Given that oligohydramnios is one of the criteria, amniocentesis for fetal karyotyping is generally not possible. We therefore use transabdominal chorionic villus sampling (TA-CVS) or cordocentesis to obtain a fetal karyotype. Fetal blood sampling provides a rapid banded fetal karyotype in around 72 hours, but carries a slightly higher complication risk than TA-CVS, which can provide a preliminary aneuploid screen using fluorescent in-situ hybridization (FISH) technology within 48 hours and a full, banded karyotype within 5 to 7 days. Documentation of a normal male karyotype is important, as female fetuses are usually not found to have simple urethral obstructions and typically have more complex developmental abnormalities of the cloaca. Past attempts at in utero shunt therapy have proven unsuccessful in improving the prognosis for these fetuses; therefore, in utero shunt therapy is not indicated. We have also encountered fetuses with trisomy 21, trisomy 18, and Klinefelter syndrome with apparent isolated bladder distention, hydronephrosis, and decreased amniotic fluid volume in the absence of other major sonographic markers, and an overall aneuploid rate in our LUTO database of 7%.

Role of Ultrasound in Evaluation

Detailed anatomic survey is necessary to rule out the presence of other anomalies such as neural tube or cardiac defects that seem to occur in higher frequency with LUTO, and certainly would dramatically impact on the prognosis for that infant. Certainly, in utero intervention would not be warranted when the fetus is afflicted by another life-threatening anomaly. One must look carefully for other, more subtle phenotypic signs, such as limb-shortening or facial abnormalities that may indicate the presence of an underlying genetic syndrome that might alter the underlying long-term prognosis.

Detailed evaluation of the fetus in the presence of severe oligo-/anhydramnios can be extremely difficult and frustrating. We therefore use amnioinfusion to reestablish the fluid-tissue interface, allowing better sonographic evaluation of the fetus. Early experience using normal saline or 5% dextrose in lactated Ringer's solution showed an associated increased risk of premature rupture of membranes, preterm labor, and chorioamnionitis. We have subsequently found that these risks can be significantly reduced, or eliminated, by using plain lactated Ringer's solution, warmed to 37°C, and infused through a closed, sterile intravenous tubing system to restore amniotic fluid volumes to a low normal level.[65] In addition, the patient is started on a 14-day course of oral antibiotics with an initial 1-g oral or intravenous loading dose, followed by a 500-mg dose given four times daily of a broad-spectrum cephalosporin or penicillin. Since we began the use of warmed lactated Ringer's solution and antibiotics, the incidence of obstetric complications following invasive prenatal testing and vesicoamniotic shunt placement has decreased dramatically.

The urinary tract must be carefully evaluated from the kidneys to the distal urethra, for clues as to the underlying etiology and renal status. Long axis measurement of the kidney is useful in evaluating the underlying hydronephrosis and, in general, kidneys that measure large for gestational age and are less hyperechogenic are associated with a better prognosis. Kidneys that are hyperechogenic and measure appropriate or small for gestational age are generally found to have poor underlying function due to renal fibrosis. The finding of small kidneys in such cases likely reflects the

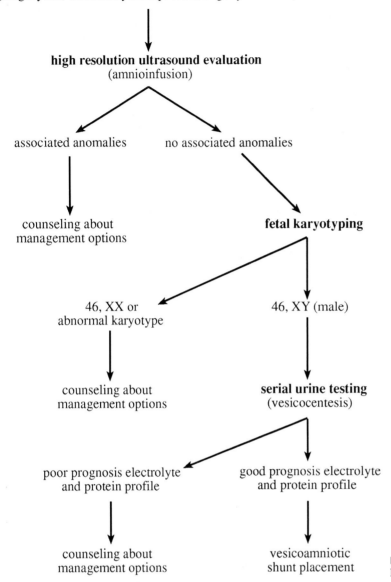

FIGURE 18–16. Algorithm for the evaluation of fetal lower urinary tract obstruction.

underlying contraction phase of fibrosis and scarring in these severely damaged tissues.

The renal parenchyma is then examined for the degree of echogenicity, parenchymal compression, and absence of discrete cortical cysts (Fig. 18–17). Care must be taken when possible microcystic changes are found to ensure that what the sonographer is seeing is not dilated calices. The presence of cortical cysts is associated with advanced, irreversible parenchymal damage, which renders the fetus not amenable to interventive therapy (Fig. 18–18). Occasionally, a large unilocular cystic structure can be found adjacent to the renal capsule. In many cases this represents a subcapsular urinoma that can usually be differentiated from a large dilated renal pelvis or cortical macrocyst. Such urinomas can result from increased intrarenal pressure from obstructive hydronephrosis, with rupture and extravasation of urine through the parenchyma to beneath the renal capsule (Fig. 18–8).

This may transiently decrease intrarenal pressure and associated damage, serving a temporary protective function for the kidney. Early in our investigative experience, we drained several such urinomas for diagnostic purposes and to allow evaluation of underlying renal parenchyma, and consistently found much better than expected renal function in these kidneys. Also, following placement of vesicoamniotic shunts and diminished hydronephrosis, we have not found the urinomas to recur, supporting the role of increased renal pressure in their etiology.

Next, the ureters should be evaluated for abnormalities. The presence of significant pyelectasis in the absence of hydroureters may indicate the presence of a UPJ obstruction. Successful vesicoamniotic shunting of a urethral obstruction in the presence of a concurrent UPJ obstruction would not be expected to be of benefit to that kidney and therefore fail to prevent further dam-

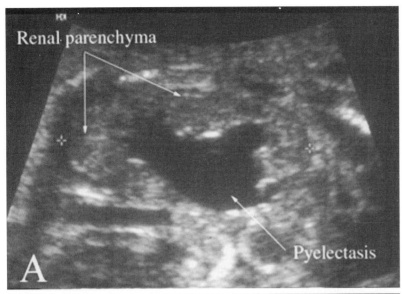

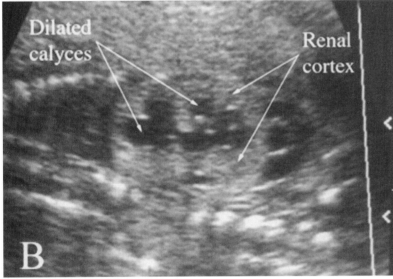

FIGURE 18–17. Hydronephrosis in obstructive uropathy. *A*, Pyelocaliectasis and compression of the renal parenchyma. *B*, Distended calices that extend into the echogenic renal cortex. Such dilated calices are often mistaken for cortical cysts.

age to that kidney. Megaureters and obvious distortion of the ureterovesicle junctions indicate severe reflux, which is generally associated with more advanced renal damage and a poorer prognosis (Fig. 18–19). Megaureters may also be present in megacystis-megaureter and pseudo–prune belly syndromes, which are associated with highly variable outcomes.

The bladder is carefully evaluated prior to and following complete drainage by fine-needle vesicocentesis. Prior to drainage, overall size is assessed as well as degree of apparent proximal urethral dilation (i.e., "keyhole sign") as an indicator of level and etiology of apparent obstruction. The presence of an abnormal bladder shape or urachal abnormalities may indicate the presence of an underlying developmental abnormality of cloacal differentiation, which represents more complex anomalies that have not benefited from simple shunt-diverting procedures.

We have observed that the shape of the bladder before and after urine drainage may provide a clue to the un-derlying source of obstruction in these cases (Fig. 18–20). Early observations suggest that after drainage of the bladder by vesicocentesis, fetuses with urethral atresia or complete obstructing posterior urethral valves demonstrate bladders that are symmetrically round and very thick walled with a bagel or donut-like appearance. Bladders that are symmetrically thick walled but elongated and somewhat tubular in appearance after drainage seem to occur in fetuses with incomplete urethral obstruction such as incomplete posterior urethral valves, urethral strictures, or urethral meatus abnormalities. Fetuses with patent but hypoplastic urethras demonstrate a more unusual appearance to the bladder, being somewhat elongated and segmented in appearance, giving rise to what we refer to as a "snowman" bladder. These bladders seem to demonstrate the typical thickening caused by hypertrophy and hyperplastic changes in the lower bladder neck region, but have minimal thickening in the bladder dome, making them more susceptible to bladder rupture. This group of fetuses seem to have the

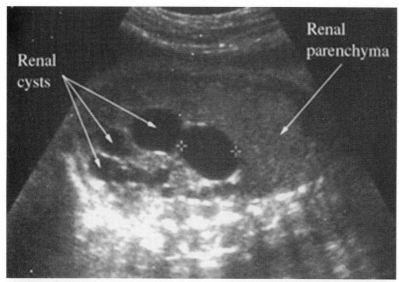

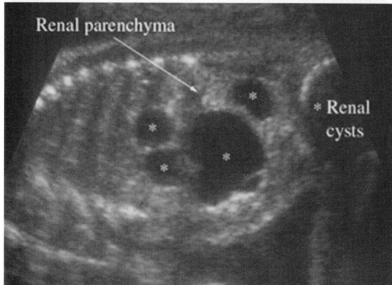

FIGURE 18–18. Renal cysts. Careful sonographic evaluation can usually differentiate these discrete structures from dilated components of the renal collecting system. Cortical cysts carry a poor prognosis and are reflective of significant, irreversible renal dysplasia.

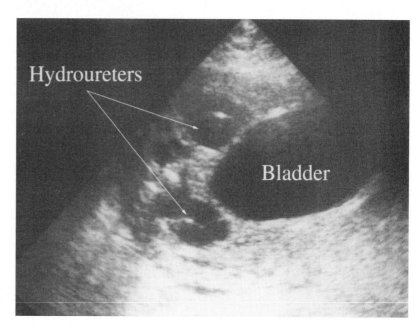

FIGURE 18–19. Oligohydramnios, distended bladder, and bilateral hydroureters in mid-gestation obstructive uropathy.

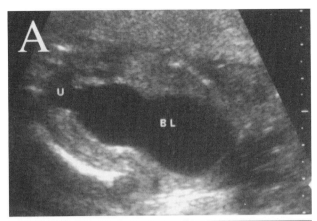

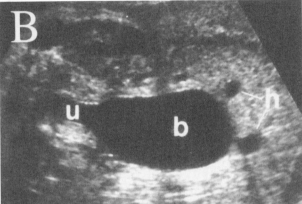

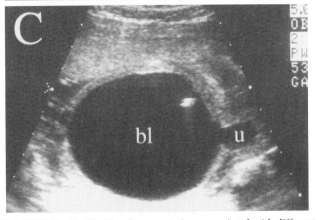

FIGURE 18–20. Bladder shape variations associated with different underlying etiologies of obstruction. In *A*, note the segmented, "snowman" shape with a very thin bladder dome observed in cases of urethral-patent obstructive uropathy. In *B*, note the elongated, tubular appearing bladder and bilateral hydroureters commonly seen in incomplete urethral obstructions. In *C*, note the round, symmetrically thickened appearance of the bladder wall associated with complete urethral obstruction.

finding has been shown to be associated with anterior urethral valves, or abnormalities of the tip of the penis such as meatal stenosis, epispadias, or hypospadias (Fig. 18–10).

Evaluation of Fetal Renal Function

The last and perhaps most important component of the prenatal evaluation is the serial analysis of fetal urine, obtained by ultrasound-guided fine-needle bladder drainage (vesicocentesis). The importance of serial sampling has been well described,[66] and must be performed at set intervals for the information to retain its predictive value. We recommend complete bladder drainage at 48- to 72-hour intervals, and the analysis of fetal urine for sodium, chloride, osmolality, calcium, β_2-microglobulin, and total protein (Table 18–2). A minimum of three bladder aspirations is usually necessary to provide optimal predictive value; however, additional vesicocentesis may be necessary to establish a clear pattern of decreasing or increasing hypertonicity. Reflux and urinary stasis likely cause increased intrarenal pressure, progressive dilatation of the renal tubules and collecting systems, and probable altered blood flow to the delicate proximal renal tubules, resulting in altered physiologic function. Decreased solute reabsorption and catabolism and subsequent increased loss of substances in the fetal urine results, and the degree of urine hypertonicity present has been positively correlated with the extent of underlying histologic renal damage.[67]

The initial bladder drainage collects urine that has been present in the fetal bladder for an undetermined period of time and does not reflect present renal function. The second bladder drainage represents urine from the upper tracts that has drained into the bladder and again does not represent recent renal urine production. The third bladder drainage, however, represents urine that has recently been formed by the kidneys, and is most reflective of the degree of underlying renal function and damage. In cases of severe renal damage, a decrease in hypertonicity is not observed, and increasing values reflective of progressive and more advanced renal disease may be observed. In select cases, however, a pattern of progressively decreasing hypertonicity and improving values that fall below established thresholds can be observed, which indicates potential renal salvage and identifies fetuses that hold the greatest potential to benefit from in utero intervention (Fig. 18–21).

best prognosis for long-term survival, and have been shown to have an underlying smooth muscle and connective tissue abnormality.[61]

Lastly, the penile urethra should be evaluated for clues to the etiology of obstruction. Occasionally, the degree of proximal urethral dilation (keyhole sign) will be mild to moderate, and a dilated membranous penile urethra can be traced to its distal end. Such a

TABLE 18–2. URINE VALUES FOR SELECTING FETUSES FOR PRENATAL THERAPY

Sodium	<100 mmol/L
Chloride	<90 mmol/L
Osmolality	<200 mOsm/L
Calcium	<8 mg/dL
β_2-Microglobulin	<6 mg/L
Total protein	<20 mg/dL

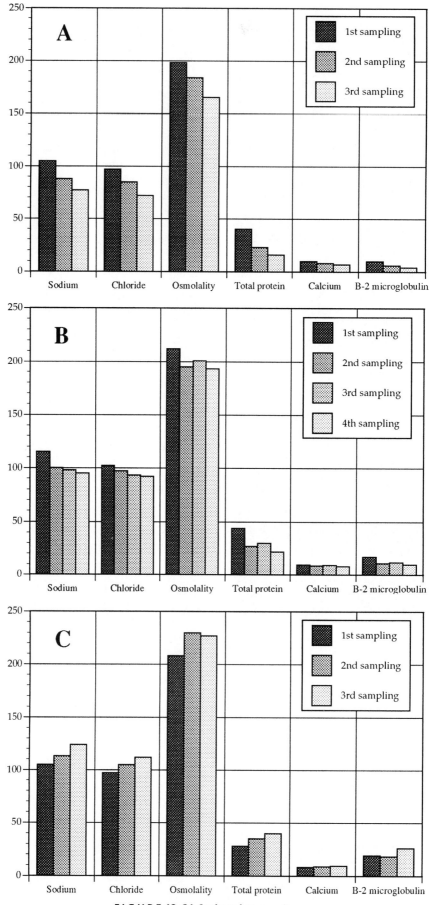

F I G U R E 18–21 *See legend on opposite page*

Patient Selection for Intervention

Fetuses with isolated bladder dilatation, bilateral hydronephrosis, decreased amniotic fluid volume, absent associated congenital anomalies, a 46,XY (male) karyotype, and serially decreasing urinary hypertonicity with electrolyte and protein values below recommended thresholds (Fig. 18–21A), would be considered potential candidates for vesicoamniotic shunt placement. Fetuses who meet all other criteria, but have urine values demonstrating minimal improvement and cluster around the threshold cutoffs (Fig. 18–21B), can be counseled that placement of a vesicoamniotic shunt may help ensure a live birth and reduce the risk of lethal pulmonary hypoplasia, but the infant would be expected to have renal insufficiency, likely require early dialysis, and may need early replacement if it survives the neonatal period. As with any invasive prenatal procedure, the patient must have a clear understanding of the potential risks of the procedure itself to the mother and fetus, the level of experience of the operator, as well as the possible complications that can occur later in the pregnancy.

Vesicoamniotic Shunting

The success of intervention for LUTO remains controversial. In a review of the evaluation and treatment of LUTO, Coplen looked at successful shunt interventions in the five largest reported series in the literature.[68] In this combined series, overall survival after intervention was 47%, and shunt-related complications occurred in 45% if cases. While not all pregnancies had oligohydramnios present, of those that did, 56% died despite intervention. Failure to restore amniotic fluid volume was associated with 100% mortality. Vesicoamniotic shunting in cases of poor urinary prognosis was associated with postnatal renal insufficiency in 87.5% of cases, but while intervention did not alter renal outcomes, it did improve neonatal chances of pulmonary survival.

Technical Considerations and Surgical Approach

Vesicoamniotic shunting represents a temporary therapeutic intervention allowing simple diversion of fetal urine from the obstructed bladder into the amniotic space (Fig. 18–22). It is essential that patients understand that such therapy is not curative, but is in essence preventative in nature, and that the infant will require further evaluation and treatment for the obstruction follow-

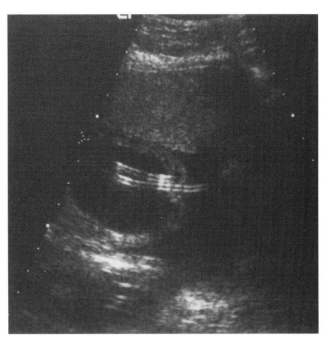

FIGURE 18–22. Vesicoamniotic shunt within fetal bladder immediately after placement. Note the proximal segment coiling within the bladder, and the straight midsegment traversing the abdominal wall. The distal segment is disappearing into the amniotic space created by amnioinfusion performed at time of shunt placement.

ing birth. Pregnancies complicated by anhydramnios present a technical challenge when placing a vesicoamniotic shunt, both from a visualization perspective and also because the distal end of the shunt catheter needs to be placed into a pocket of amniotic fluid. As noted earlier, we utilize amnioinfusion at time of initial evaluation to assist sonographic evaluation, but in most cases the amniotic space must be reexpanded with fluid for successful shunt placement. Again, because of the associated risks of subsequent obstetric complications, prophylactic antibiotics are recommended. Amnioinfusion is performed under continuous ultrasound guidance, using warmed lactated Ringer solution and a 20-gauge spinal needle inserted as high in the fundus as possible to decrease the risk of fluid leakage. One must be exceedingly careful and utilize color Doppler to identify and avoid umbilical cord vessels, which always seem to be present in the small apparent fluid pockets present in these cases. We use a closed, sterile system consisting of a warmed IV bag of lactated Ringer's solution connected by a sterile set of IV tubing to a three-way stopcock valve with a 30-mL syringe attached, and IV exten-

---

FIGURE 18–21. Graphic representation of fetal urine analysis based on serial vesicocenteses in the evaluation of renal damage. A, Good-prognosis profile: stepwise improvement (decreasing hypertonicity) noted for each urinary marker with each of three bladder aspirations. Final values are below screening thresholds, representing absence of severe histologic renal damage. B, Intermediate-prognosis profile: minimal improvement in urine markers with serial samplings that has been shown to be associated with the presence of moderate fibrocystic damage within the kidney and high likelihood of moderate renal insufficiency following successful prenatal vesicoamniotic shunt placement. C, Poor-prognosis profile: progressive worsening hypertonicity noted on serial urine samplings with values above screening thresholds. This pattern is associated with severe fibrocystic damage within the kidneys, and such cases do not demonstrate a renal benefit from in utero vesicoamniotic shunt placement.

sion tubing connected to the infusion needle. The syringe and stopcock are used to intermittently draw fluid from the IV bag and then infuse fluid into the developing amniotic space to restore volume levels to low normal and create an adequate pocket of fluid to place the distal end of the shunt catheter into.

Prior to selecting a fetus for shunting, evaluation of renal function is necessary using serial bladder aspirations (vesicocentesis). These procedures are also carried out under continuous ultrasound guidance to ensure appropriate needle position and placement throughout the procedure (Fig. 18–23). Using a 22-gauge needle, the fetal abdomen is carefully approached just above the pubic rami and lateral to midline. Before entering the abdomen and distended bladder, color Doppler is used to ensure that the potential needle track does not pass through and traumatize the umbilical arteries that course laterally around the bladder. The needle is then passed into the lower aspect of the bladder and the urine completely drained while constantly maintaining needle-tip placement within the cavity of the shrinking bladder. Needle placement into the upper bladder will not allow complete drainage as the bladder shrinks downward into the fetal pelvis.

We do not paralyze the fetus with intramuscular pancuronium prior to either vesicocentesis or vesicoamniotic shunt placement procedure. For shunt placement procedures, we do utilize local anesthesia with 1% lidocaine, and IV maternal and fetal sedation using a combination of morphine (4 to 10 mg) and Valium (4 to 10 mg) usually in two doses with total dose dependent on initial maternal response and level of fetal and maternal sedation and pain relief required. For cases that are likely to be particularly challenging, we have used epidural anesthesia and light IV fetal-maternal sedation with good success.

Careful sonographic evaluation prior to attempted shunt placement is important to identify the position of the placenta and fetus. If possible, one should always try to approach the fetus without having to pass the shunt trocar needle through the placenta, although we have done so without problems in most cases. If a transplacental approach is unavoidable, care should be taken to try and traverse the placenta in a single smooth motion, keeping lateral motion of the trocar to a minimum, and utilizing color Doppler prior to passage through the chorionic plate to identify surface vessels along the plate that must be avoided. If possible, the fetus should be in back-down, vertex position, allowing a straight approach as high in the uterine fundus as possible. If the fetus proves uncooperative, we have ambulated the patient for several minutes or had the mother lie in a variety of positions to encourage position changes, postponed the procedure until the following day, or externally manipulated the fetus into a better, vertex position. If these measures fail and the only approach is through the lower uterine segment, then strict bed rest for at least 72 hours is recommended, as our experience indicates the risk of amniotic fluid leakage is quite high.

Once the appropriate approach is chosen, IV sedation is given and the maternal skin is anesthetized with 1% lidocaine. A small 3- to 5-mm stab wound is made through the skin to allow easy passage of the shunt trocar, which is then introduced under continuous ultrasound guidance into the amniotic space near the lower fetal abdomen. An adequate pocket of amniotic fluid needs to be present in which to drop the distal end of the shunt catheter on exiting the fetal abdomen. If insufficient fluid space is present, then an additional amnioinfusion can be performed through the shunt trocar after removing the sharp stylet. We have routinely used the shunt apparatus offered by Rocket of London, as well as their Rodeck vesicoamniotic shunt catheters (Fig. 18–24). The tip of the trocar is positioned in the same manner as the vesicocentesis needle and color Doppler used to confirm the trocar will not pass near

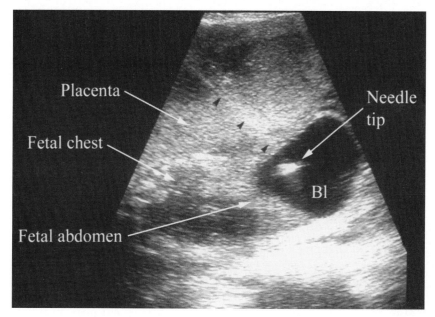

FIGURE 18–23. Sonographic image of fetal urine sampling by vesicocentesis. Note needle tip within enlarged, obstructed fetal bladder (*Bl*), and absence of amniotic fluid (anhydramnios) around fetus at time of initial evaluation.

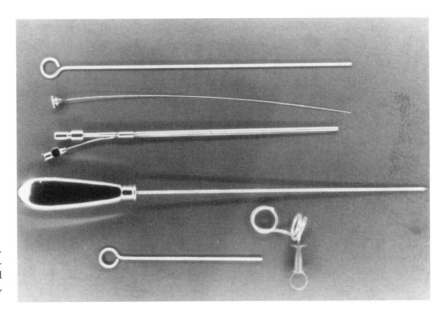

FIGURE 18–24. Vesicoamniotic shunt apparatus. Note shunt trocar with sampling sideport, introducing stylet, long and short push rods, and double-pigtail shunt (Rocket of London, London, UK).

to and damage the umbilical arteries on passage through the bladder wall. The trocar is then quickly inserted into the bladder and positioned into a central location. At this point, the operative assistant should have carefully and gently uncurled and straightened the vesicoamniotic catheter. The catheter is then completely threaded into the trocar sheath prior to removal of the internal wire stylet. If the wire is removed prior to threading the catheter, difficulty with kinking and directing the catheter down the trocar sheath may be experienced. Once in place, a short push rod is introduced and used to push the proximal coiled segment of the catheter into the bladder. This is then removed and a long push rod gently introduced until it comes in contact with the distal tip of the shunt catheter within the trocar sheath. The push rod is then held in place while the shaft of the trocar sheath is slowly pulled back approximately 1 cm. At this point, the trocar sheath should lie just outside of the fetal abdomen, with the straight segment of the shunt catheter (Fig. 18–25) traversing the region of abdomen between the bladder and amniotic space. Failure to perform this part of the maneuver may result in partial displacement of the proximal end of the catheter and increased risk for shunt displacement.

The trocar sheath is now slowly directed slightly away from the insertion site and the long push rod advanced to displace the distal end of the catheter into the amniotic space. Position of the proximal and distal coiled segments of the catheter, as well as initiation of bladder drainage is confirmed sonographically. The patient is then placed on external fetal/uterine monitoring for 2 to 4 hours, and any evidence of uterine contractions aggressively managed with tocolytic therapy.

Complications

Counseling of the patient prior to initiation of a course of prenatal evaluation includes discussion of potential complications of any invasive procedure such as chorioamnionitis, premature rupture of fetal membranes, direct trauma to the fetus, and intraplacental bleeding and possible associated onset of preterm labor if a transplacental approach is necessary.

Following vesicocentesis, transient vesicoperitoneal fistulas can occur that result in urinary ascites (Fig. 18–26). Such fistulas spontaneously close in 10 to 14 days followed by reenlargement of the bladder. In some cases, massive urinary ascites can develop, resulting in extreme distention of the fetal abdomen, which may potentiate abdominal wall changes characteristic of the prune belly phenotype.

Vesicoamniotic shunt displacement is also a common complication, occurring in approximately 40% of cases in our clinical series.[69] Despite the fact that the Rodeck catheter is designed such that the distal end curls to lie flat against the fetal abdomen, it may become entangled in fetal extremities or more directly dislodged (Fig. 18–27), necessitating replacement with recurrence of bladder distention. As noted earlier, if the shunt catheter is placed too high within the distended bladder, it may be placed under tension as the bladder shrinks with drainage, and eventually displaced and drawn within the fetal abdomen (Fig. 18–28), resulting in massive urinary ascites and loss of optimal diverting function.

We have also had several cases in our series of successful shunt placements at 19 to 21 weeks' gestation in which catheter placement and function was considered optimal with observed decreasing hydronephrosis and maintenance of reasonable amniotic fluid volumes. However, at 27 to 29 weeks' gestation, amniotic fluid volumes fell, renal parenchyma became increasingly echodense, and renal growth stopped and actually regressed over time. All such fetuses died near or shortly after birth. On autopsy, all demonstrated severe fibrocystic renal dysplasia, and all were found to have appropriately placed, patent shunt catheters. The etiology of

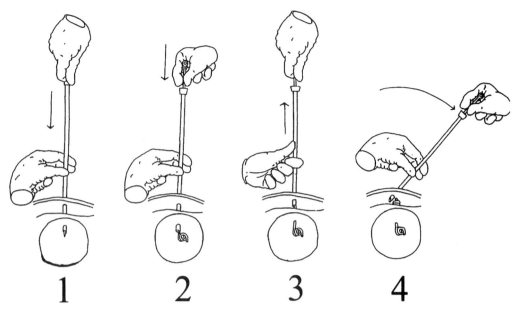

FIGURE 18–25. Graphic illustration of the four-step technique for placing a vesicoamniotic shunt. (From Johnson MP, et al: Fetal shunt procedures. *In* Evans MI, et al [eds]: Invasive Outpatient Procedures in Reproductive Medicine. Philadelphia: Lippincott-Raven Publishers, 1997, with permission.)

this late-onset renal dysplasia despite resolution of obstructive hydronephrosis remains unclear.

Follow-up

After a fetal vesicoamniotic shunt procedure, a follow-up sonographic evaluation should be performed 24 to 48 hours later to confirm catheter placement and function. Weekly exams are suggested for at least 6 to 8 weeks to confirm catheter placement and function, progressive

resolution of the hydronephrosis, and maintenance of amniotic fluid volume. At that point, usually around 28 weeks' gestation, evaluation can be spaced to every 2 weeks, depending on maintenance of amniotic fluid volume.

Prenatal consultation with the pediatric urologist and neonatologist who will care for the infant after birth is recommended so that issues of postnatal evaluation, management, and treatment options can be discussed; a tentative plan formulated; and a professional relationship established between the family and postnatal medi-

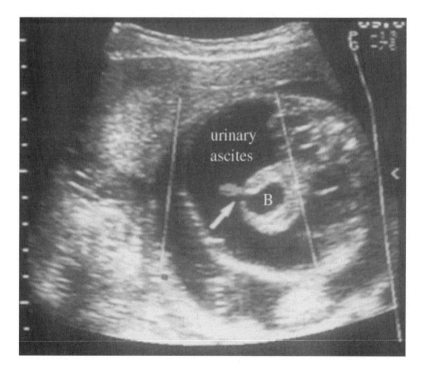

FIGURE 18–26. Sonographic image of a transient bladder fistula and urinary ascites following vesicoamniotic shunt displacement from a fetal bladder with urethral obstruction. *Arrow* points to streaming of fetal urine through the bladder wall defect using color Doppler. (B = bladder lumen.) Note the thickening of the bladder wall from smooth muscle hypertrophy resulting from longstanding urethral obstruction.

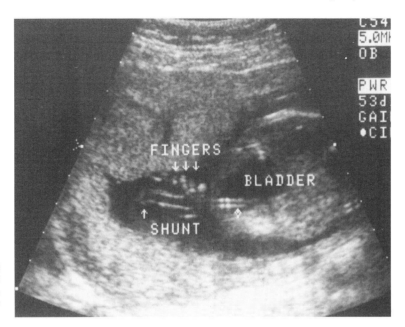

FIGURE 18–27. Sonographic image of a fetus grasping the distal, intra-amniotic segment of a vesicoamniotic shunt catheter just prior to pulling it out of the bladder, and into the amniotic space. This is postulated to be the leading cause of catheter displacement.

cal team. This greatly facilitates communications and understanding of postnatal management issues that may arise, reduces family anxiety, and fosters a trusting relationship between the family and medical team.

Route of delivery should be dictated by routine obstetric indications and not influenced by the presence of an indwelling catheter. Pregnancies that have undergone shunting in our experience have experienced spontaneous rupture of fetal membranes and onset of labor with vaginal delivery at 33 to 36 weeks' gestation. This gestational age for delivery has not been found to be different than occurred in an age-matched cohort of unshunted fetuses with LUTO, but the family should be counseled

about this tendency for early delivery in pregnancies complicated by LUTO.

Outcomes After Prenatal Intervention

Perhaps the most difficult question still confronting us is whether the contemporary approach to fetal evaluation and intervention actually improves postnatal renal outcomes. Unfortunately, there have been no randomized trials or large multicenter studies to address this issue. Present data represent outcomes reported by the first international registry, or individual investigative groups.[70–73] Unfortunately, the international registry data predate the contemporary era, and the majority of single center reports are quite small.

Short-Term Outcomes

In 1996, we reported our experience with 55 sequential fetuses evaluated in a single center for sonographically diagnosed obstructive uropathy.[62] Of the 55 cases, 13 (24%) had posterior urethral valves, 11 (20%) had urethral atresia, nine (16%) had urethra patent prune belly syndrome, and the remainder had a variety of other anatomic causes for their urinary tract obstructions. Of the 55 fetuses, 33 were found to have a good prognosis by urine electrolyte and protein analysis, and 22 of these underwent vesicoamniotic shunting. Fourteen of the 22 shunted fetuses survived, and 5 of the 11 nonshunted fetuses survived the postnatal period. Many of the nonshunted fetuses were, however, not considered candidates for intervention because of the presence of adequate amniotic fluid volumes at the time of evaluation. Twenty-two fetuses were found to have a poor prognosis on the basis of urinary profile. Six of these fetuses underwent shunt placement at parental request despite

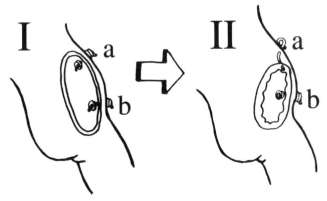

FIGURE 18–28. Importance of insertion site in shunt placement for obstructive uropathy. In I, shunt catheter *a* has been placed into the dome and *b* into the lower segment of the distended fetal bladder. With subsequent bladder drainage and return of the previously distended dome of the bladder into the fetal pelvis (II), the proximal tip of catheter *a* becomes displaced from the shrinking bladder dome, while catheter *b* remains in good functional position. (From Johnson MP, et al: Fetal shunt procedures. *In* Evans MI, et al [eds]: Invasive Outpatient Procedures in Reproductive Medicine. Philadelphia: Lippincott-Raven Publishers, 1997, with permission.)

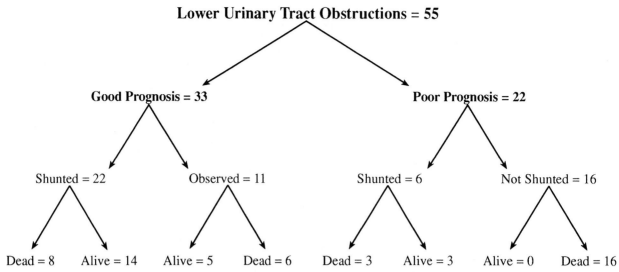

FIGURE 18–29. Prenatal urinary prognosis and postnatal outcomes in a series of prenatally diagnosed lower urinary tract obstructions evaluated at a single center.

the poor predicted prognosis. Three of the six fetuses shunted survived, and none of those without shunting survived, although 11 of the remaining 16 unshunted fetuses were terminated on the basis of poor renal prognosis (Fig. 18–29).

The overall gross survival rate was 40%, postnatal survival was 61%, and shunted survival was 61%. A nadir creatinine greater than 1 mg/dL in the first year of life occurred in 23% of surviving infants. When evaluated by diagnosis group, those with posterior urethral valves had a 46% gross survival, 60% postnatal survival, and 67% shunted survival with 33% having a nadir creatinine greater than 1 mg/dL. Urethra patent prune belly patients faired better with a 67% gross survival, 86% postnatal survival, and 100% shunted survival with only 17% having an elevated nadir creatinine. In contrast, none of the original 11 fetuses with urethral atresia survived; however, only four underwent shunt placement (Table 18–3). Since that report, however, we have two additional patients with urethral atresia who have survived after shunting, and have good postnatal renal function with nadir creatinines of less than 1 mg/dL at over 1 year of age.

Long-Term Outcomes

In 1999, we evaluated outcomes of 14 children who underwent vesicoamniotic shunt placement and had survived beyond 2 years of age.[74] The children's ages range from 25 to 114 months (mean, 54.3 months). Of the 14 children, seven (50%) had urethra-patent prune belly syndrome; four (29%) had posterior urethral valves; and one each had urethral atresia, megacystis, and bilateral reflux–megaureters. Growth during the first year was impaired, with seven below the fifth percentile and 12 below the 25th percentile. Weight was also decreased with five below the fifth percentile, and eight below the 25th percentile. Four children required postnatal ventilatory support, two of whom required prolonged support up to 1 month. Two infants have been diagnosed with mild asthma, and four have recurrent bronchitis or frequent respiratory infections. No child, however, has any respiratory restrictions to its physical activities. Eight children void spontaneously, four children are catheterized in addition to voiding, and two children are catheterized only. Three of the four children with posterior urethral valves have undergone surgical bladder augmentation. Current renal function is normal in six (46%) children with a creatinine clearance greater than 70 mL/min, three (21%) children have renal insufficiency, and five (36%) have developed end-stage renal disease (ESRD) and have undergone successful renal transplantation with normally functioning grafts (Table 18–4). Nadir creatinine was less than 0.8 mg/dL in eight infants of whom six have normal function, one has insufficiency, and one had developed ESRD as an adolescent. Nadir creatinine was between 0.8 and 1.0 mg/dL in two children, and both have gone on to develop renal insufficiency. Four children had nadir

TABLE 18–3. FETAL OUTCOMES BASED ON DIAGNOSIS-SPECIFIC GROUPS

DIAGNOSIS	N	GROSS SURVIVAL	POSTNATAL SURVIVAL	SHUNTED SURVIVAL	RENAL FAILURE
Posterior urethral valves	13	46%	60%	67%	33%
Urethral patent prune belly	9	67%	86%	100%	17%
Urethral atresia	11	0%	0%	0%	NA

TABLE 18–4. LONG-TERM OUTCOMES FOLLOWING VESICOAMNIOTIC SHUNTING

Growth	<5th percentile, 7/14 (50%)	<25th percentile, 12/14 (86%)	
Weight	<5th percentile, 5/14 (36%)	<25th percentile, 8/14 (57%)	
Renal function	Normal, 6/14 (46%)	Renal insufficiency, 3/4 (21%)	ESRD, 5/14 (36%)
Bladder control	Void spontaneously, 8/14 (57%)	Void and catheterize, 4/14 (29%)	Catheterize only, 2/14 (14%)

ESRD, end-stage renal disease.

creatinine greater than 1.0 mg/dL, and all progressed to ESRD.

Future Directions

In Utero Cystoscopic Treatment

Among the challenges for the future, we must focus our efforts to further refine the approach to intervention in LUTO, and develop techniques to decrease the greatest technical complication, that of shunt displacement and migration. One technique currently under development is the cystoscopic disruption of posterior urethral valves.[75] In this approach, a tiny endoscope is passed through the shunt cannula and directed into the proximal urethra under direct visualization and ultrasound guidance (Figs. 18–30 and 18–31). If the source of obstruction can be visualized, then it can be evaluated to determine whether it represents posterior urethral

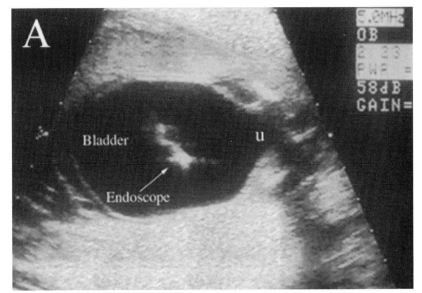

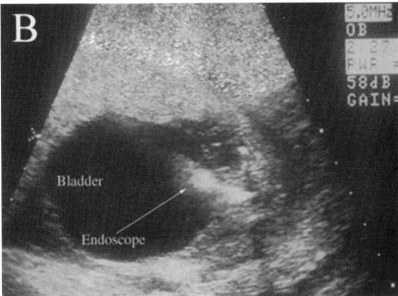

FIGURE 18–30. Sonographic images of mid-gestational fetal cystoscopy. *A,* Microendoscope within fetal bladder during process of evaluating bladder mucosa, musculature, and ureteral openings (u = proximal urethra.) *B,* The microendoscope has been directed into the proximal urethra in an attempt to visualize the origin of obstruction.

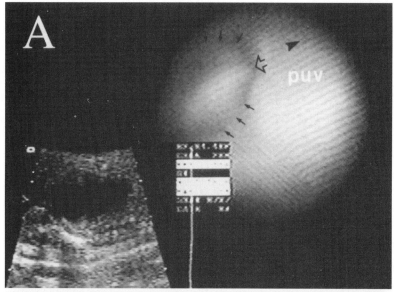

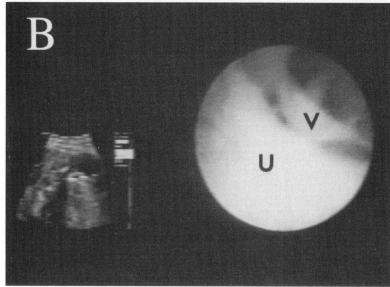

F I G U R E   18–31. Upper panel (*A*) demonstrates the appearance of posterior urethral valves (puv) as seen by antegrade in utero fetal cystourethroscopy. *Solid arrowhead* points to tiny urethral aperture, *open arrowhead* and *small arrows* outline the ventral aspect of the penile urethra. Lower panel (*B*) shows remnants of posterior valves following laser resection. (u = urethra; v = valve.)

valves or an atresia. If valves can be confirmed, then laser ablation or mechanical disruption may be technically possible. This approach has been used investigatively with mixed results, but may hold great promise for the future by relieving the obstruction without the need for a diverting catheter. Perhaps more importantly, it may allow for a more normal physiologic state of bladder cycling with storage and voiding, which has been suggested to play an important role in long-term bladder function.[76] As experience and instrumentation improve, this may become the treatment of choice for fetuses with posterior urethral valves. For cases of LUTO due to other etiologies, diverting shunt therapy will likely remain the intervention of choice.

Understanding Mechanisms of Renal Damage

Continuing investigation of the mechanisms of tissue response to obstruction will expand our understanding of underlying pathologic processes, and the role that growth factors and immunoproteins play in this process may provide us with the opportunity to modulate renal tissue response. Nguyen and Kogan[33] demonstrated that injection of insulin-like growth factor type I (IGF-1) to neonatal opossums with complete ureteric surgical obstruction resulted in decreased caliectasis and interstitial fibrosis in the injected obstructed kidney compared to its contralateral noninjected obstructed kidney. Steinhardt et al.[77] studied the effects of an intradermal IGF-1 injection on renal damage, also using a fetal opossum model with unilateral surgical ureteric obstruction of 1 week duration. In the obstructed kidneys, it appeared that IGF-1 prevented the development of cortical and medullary fibrosis and caliceal dilatation. They also observed a decrease in tubular cystic change, and suggested IGF-1 may serve a protective role on the renal architecture in the setting of urinary tract obstruction.

Investigators need to continue to search for better markers of underlying renal damage to identify fetuses with salvageable renal function. Cellular growth factors and immunoproteins are presently under investigation as indicators of renal response to obstruction and focal hypoxia. Preliminary studies indicate that elevated urinary levels of epidermal growth factor may identify fetuses in the early stages of renal damage from obstruction, whereas other growth factors such as transforming growth factor, a potent modulator of collagen, may reflect changes associated with more advanced fibrocystic renal damage.[61] Bussieres et al.[78] found that fetal urinary levels of IGF-1 and its binding protein-3 were elevated in cases of bilateral obstructive uropathy in the human fetus, and levels positively correlated with postnatal plasma creatinine values. They found that both IGF-1 and IGF-binding protein-3 were sensitive (0.90, 0.80) and specific (0.88, 0.88) for predicting postnatal renal insufficiency. Although they conclude that this probably represents proximal tubular dysfunction in reabsorption and catabolism of these substances, it might also represent altered IGF-1 gene expression in response to injury that could influence the histologic progression to dysplasia, considering IGF plays a role in early nephrogenesis.

Conclusion

Although tremendous improvements in patient selection have resulted in more consistent success in fetal intervention for LUTO, short-term outcomes remain highly variable between centers, and long-term outcomes into the adolescent and young adult years remain to be determined. With careful prenatal evaluation and case selection, vesicoamniotic shunt placement has been shown to be successful in preventing the mortality associated with pulmonary hypoplasia, and appears to result in improved postnatal renal function. Whereas shunt displacement will remain an ongoing problem, fetal cystoscopy and endoscopic surgery holds great promise for the future. Also, further understanding of the role of specific growth factors and immunoproteins, such as EGF and IGF-1, may provide the pharmacologic means to prevent significant renal damage associated with obstruction, and improve renal outcomes. Although the time for randomized trials has passed, it is hoped that the use of multicenter cooperation and international registries will provide enough well-structured clinical data to determine and define finally and accurately the proper role for in utero surgery for the treatment of LUTO.

REFERENCES

1. Moore KL, Persaud TVN: The urogential system. *In* The Developing Human: Clinically Oriented Embryology, 5th ed. Philadelphia: WB Saunders Company, 1993, p 265.
2. Ruano-Gil D, Coca-Payeras A, Tejedo-Mateu A: Obstruction and normal recanalization of the ureter in the human embryo. Its relation to congenital ureteric obstruction. Eur Urol 1:278, 1975.
3. Jones KL: *In* Smith's Recognizable Patterns of Human Malformation, 4th ed. Philadelphia: WB Saunders Company, 1988, pp 562 and 572.
4. Nakayama DK, Harrison MR, deLorimier AA: Prognosis of posterior urethral valves presenting at birth. J Pediatr Surg 21:43, 1986.
5. Mahony BS, Callen PW, Filly RA: Fetal urethral obstruction: Ultrasound evaluation. Radiology 157:221, 1985.
6. Housley HT, Harrison MR: Fetal urinary tract abnormalities. Natural history, pathophysiology, and treatment. Urol Clin North Am 25:63, 1998.
7. Harrison MR, Filly RA: The fetus with obstructive uropathy: Pathophysiology, natural history, selection, and treatment. *In* Harrison MR, Golbus MS, Filly RA (eds): The Unborn Patient: Prenatal Diagnosis and Treatment, 2nd ed. Philadelphia: WB Saunders Company, 1991, p 328.
8. Harrison MR, Ross NA, Noall R, deLorimier AA: Correction of urogenital hydronephrosis in utero. The model: Fetal urethral obstruction produces hydronephrosis and pulmonary hypoplasia in fetal lambs. J Pediatr Surg 18:247, 1983.
9. Glick PL, Harrison MR, Noall RA, Villa RL: Correction of congenital hydronephrosis in utero. III. Early mid-trimester ureteral obstruction produces renal dysplasia. J Pediatr Surg 18:681, 1983.
10. Kramer SA: Current status of fetal intervention for congenital hydronephrosis. J Urol 130:641, 1983.
11. Bellinger MF, Comstock CH, Grosso D, Zaino R: Fetal posterior urethral valves and renal dysplasia at 15 weeks gestational age. J Urol 129:1238, 1983.
12. Wladimiroff JW: Effect of furosemide on fetal urine production. Br J Obstet Gynecol 82:221, 1975.
13. Chinn DH, Filly RA: Ultrasound diagnosis of fetal genitourinary tract anomalies. Urol Radiol 4:115, 1982.
14. Mahony BS, Filly RA, Callen PW, et al: Fetal renal dysplasia: Sonographic evaluation. Radiology 152:143, 1984.
15. Glazer GM, Filly RA, Callen PW: The varied sonographic appearance of urinary tract in the fetus and newborn with urethral obstruction. Radiology 144:563, 1982.
16. Crombleholme TM, Harrison MR, Longaker MT, Langer JC: Prenatal diagnosis and management of bilateral hydronephrosis. Pediatr Nephrol 2:334, 1988.
17. Lumbers ER, Hill KJ, Bennett VJ: Proximal and distal tubular activity in chronically catheterized fetal sheep compared with the adult. Can J Physiol Pharmacol 66:697, 1988.
18. Lipitz S, Ryan G, Samuell C, et al: Fetal urine analysis for the assessment of renal function in obstructive uropathy. Am J Obstet Gynecol 168:174, 1993.
19. Glick PL, Harrison MR, Golbus MS, et al: Management of the fetus with congenital hydronephrosis. II. Prognostic criteria and selection for treatment. J Pediatr Surg 20:376, 1985.
20. Adzick NS, Harrison MR, Flake AW, Laberge JM: Development of a fetal renal function test using endogenous creatinine clearance. J Pediatr Surg 20:602, 1985.
21. Nakayama DK, Glick PL, Harrison MR, et al: Experimental pulmonary hypoplasia due to oligohydramnios and its reversal by relieving thoracic compression. J Pediatr Surg 18:347, 1983.
22. Adzick NS, Harrison MR, Glick PL, et al: Experimental pulmonary hypoplasia and oligohydramnios: Relative contributions of lung fluid and fetal breathing movements. J Pediatr Surg 19:658, 1984.
23. Wigglesworth JS, Dejai R, Guerrini P: Fetal lung hypoplasia: Biochemical and structural variations and their possible significance. Arch Dis Child 56:606, 1981.
24. Inselman LS, Mellins RB: Growth and development of the lung. J Pediatr 98:1, 1981.
25. Hislop A, Hey E, Reid L: The lungs in congenital bilateral renal agenesis and dysplasia. Arch Dis Child 54:32, 1979.
26. Adzick NS, Harrison MR, Hu LM, et al: Pulmonary hypoplasia and renal dysplasia in a fetal lamb urinary tract obstruction model. Surg Forum 38:666, 1987.
27. Helin I, Personn PH: Prenatal diagnosis of urinary tract abnormalities by ultrasound. Pediatrics 78:879, 1986.
28. Brumfield CG, Guinn D, Davis R, et al: The significance of nonvisualization of the fetal bladder during an ultrasound examination to evaluate second trimester oligohydramnios. Ultrasound Obstet Gynecol 8:186, 1996.
29. Merguerian P: The evaluation of prenatally detected hydronephrosis. Monogr Urol 16:1, 1995.
30. Thomas DF: Fetal uropathy. Br J Urol 66:225, 1990.
31. Reddy PP, Mandell J: Prenatal diagnosis: Therapeutic implications. Urol Clin North Am 25:171, 1998.

32. Nguyen HT, Kogan BA: Upper urinary tract obstruction: Experimental and clinical aspects. Br J Urol 81(Suppl 2):13–21, 1998.

33. Anderson KR, Weiss RM: Physiology and evaluation of ureteropelvic junction obstruction. J Endourol 10:87, 1996.

34. Starr NT, Maizzels M, Chou P, et al: Microanatomy and morphometry of the hydronephrotic "obstructed" renal pelvis in asymptomatic infants. J Urol 148:519, 1992.

35. Anderson N, Clautice-Engle T, Allan R, et al: Detection of obstructive uropathy in the fetus; Predictive value of sonographic measurements of renal pelvic diameter at various gestational ages. AJR Am J Roentgenol 164:719, 1995.

36. Fasolato V, Poloniato A, Bianchi C, et al: Feto-neonatal ultrasonography to detect renal abnormalities: Evaluation of 1-year screening program. Am J Perinatol 15:161, 1998.

37. Freedman ER, Rickwood AMK: Prenatally diagnosed pelviureteric junction obstruction: A benign condition? J Pediatr Surg 29:769, 1994.

38. Walsh G, Dubbins PA: Antenatal renal pelvis dilatation: A predictor of vesicoureteral reflux? AJR Am J Roentgenol 167:899, 1996.

39. Valentin L, Marsal K: Does the prenatal diagnosis of fetal urinary tract anomalies affect perinatal outcome? Am N Y Acad Sci 847:59, 1998.

40. Wood BP, Ben-Ami T, Teele RL, Rabinowitz R: Ureterovesical obstruction and megaloureter: Diagnosis by real-time US. Radiology 156:79, 1985.

41. Jerkins GR, Noe HN: Familial vesicoureteral reflux: A prospective study. J Urol 128:774, 1982.

42. Tokunaka S, Koyanagi T: Morphologic study of primary nonreflux megaureters with particular emphasis on the role of ureteral sheath and ureteral dysplasia. J Urol 128:399, 1981.

43. Dunn V, Glasier CM: Ultrasonographic antenatal demonstration of primary megaureters. J Ultrasound Med 4:101, 1985.

44. Jeffrey RB, Laing FC, Wing VW, Haddick W: Sonography of the fetal duplex kidney. Radiology 153:123, 1984.

45. Johnson MP, Schroeder E, Quintero RA, et al: In utero treatment of obstruction ureterocele [abstract]. Am J Obstet Gynecol 176(1 pt 2):84, 1997.

46. Mitchell ME, Garrett RA: Perirenal urinary extravasation associated with urethral valves in infants. J Urol 124:688, 1980.

47. Greenfield SP, Hensle TW, Berdon WE, Geringer AM: Urinary extravasation in the newborn male with posterior urethral valves. J Pediatr Surg 17:751, 1982.

48. Kay R, Brereton RJ, Johnston JH: Urinary ascites in the newborn. Br J Urol 52:451, 1980.

49. Cass AS, Khan AU, Smith S, Godec C: Neonatal perirenal urinary extravasation with posterior urethral valves. Urology 18:258, 1981.

50. Parker RM: Neonatal urinary ascites: A potentially favorable sign in bladder outlet obstruction. Urology 3:589, 1974.

51. Moncada R, Wang JJ, Love L, Bush I: Neonatal ascites associated with urinary outlet obstruction (urinary ascites). Radiology 90:1165, 1968.

52. Burton OC: Agenesis of abdominal musculature associated with genitourinary and gastrointestinal anomalies. J Urol 656:607, 1951.

53. Ives EJ: The abdominal muscle deficiency triad syndrome—experience with ten cases. Birth Defects 10:127, 1974.

54. Nakayama DK, Harrison MR, Chinn DH, deLorimier AA: The pathogenesis of prune belly. Am J Dis Child 138:834, 1984.

55. Tomlinson M, Johnson MP, Goncalves L, et al: Correction of hemodynamic abnormalities by vesicoamniotic shunting in familial congenital megacystis. Fetal Diagn Ther 11:46, 1996.

56. Freedman AL, Qureshi F, Shapiro E, et al: Smooth muscle development in the obstructed fetal bladder. Urology 49:104, 1997.

57. Freedman AL, Bukowski TP, Smith CA, et al: Fetal therapy for obstructive uropathy: Diagnosis-specific outcomes. J Urol 156:720, 1996.

58. Quintero RA, Johnson MP, Romero R, et al: In utero percutaneous cystoscopy in the management of fetal lower obstructive uropathy. Lancet 346:537, 1995.

59. Carr MC, Schlessel RN, Peters CA, et al: Expression of cell growth regulated genes in the fetal kidney: Relevance to in utero obstruction. J Urol 154:242, 1995.

60. Attar R, Quinn F, Winyard PJD, et al: Short-term urinary flow impairment deregulates PAX2 and PCNA expression and cell survival in fetal sheep kidneys. Am J Pathol 152:1225, 1998.

61. Johnson MP, Romero R, Edwin S, et al: Evidence for differential expression of growth factors and cytokines in the urine of fetuses with obstructive uropathy [abstract]. Am J Obstet Gynecol 180 (1 part 2):24, 1999.

62. Truong LP, Petrusevska G, Yang G, et al: Cell apoptosis and proliferation in experimental chronic obstructive uropathy. Kidney Int 50:200, 1996.

63. Kaneto H, Morrisey J, Klahr S: Increased expression of TGF-β1 mRNA in the obstructed kidney of rats with unilateral ligation. Kidney Int 44:313, 1993.

64. Johnson MP, Bukowski TP, Reitleman C, et al: In utero surgical treatment of fetal obstructive uropathy: A new comprehensive approach to identify appropriate candidates for vesicoamniotic shunt therapy. Am J Obstet Gynecol 170:1770, 1994.

65. Feldman B, Hassan S, Kramer RL, et al: Amnioinfusion in the evaluation of fetal obstructive uropathy: The effect of antibiotic prophylaxis on complication rates. Fetal Diagn Ther 14:172, 1999.

66. Johnson MP, Corsi P, Bradfield W, et al: Sequential urinalysis improves evaluation of fetal renal function in obstructive uropathy. Am J Obstet Gynecol 173:59, 1995.

67. Qureshi F, Jacques SM, Seifman B, et al: In utero fetal urine analysis and renal histology do correlate with the outcome in fetal obstructive uropathies. Fetal Diag Ther 11:306, 1996.

68. Coplen DE: Prenatal intervention for hydronephrosis. J Urol 157:2270, 1997.

69. Hassan S, Mariona L, Kasperski S, et al: Complications of vesicoamniotic shunting [abstract]. Am J Obstet Gynecol 176:583, 1997.

70. Manning FA, Harrison MR, Rodeck C: Catheter shunts for fetal hydronephrosis and hydrocephalus: Report of the international Fetal Surgery Registry. N Engl J Med 315:336, 1986.

71. Crombleholme TM, Harrison MR, Golbus MS, et al: Fetal intervention in obstructive uropathy: Prognostic indicators and efficacy of intervention. Am J Obstet Gynecol 162:1239, 1990.

72. Sholder AJ, Maizels M, Depp B, et al: Caution in antenatal intervention. J Urol 139:1026, 1998.

73. Coplen DE, Hare JY, Zderic SA, et al: 10-year experience with prenatal intervention for hydronephrosis. J Urol 156:1142, 1996.

74. Freedman AL, Johnson MP, Smith CA, et al: Long-term outcome in children after antenatal intervention for obstructive uropathies. Lancet 345:374, 1999.

75. Quintero RA, Hume R, Smith C, et al: Percutaneous fetal cystoscopy and endoscopic fulguration of posterior urethral valves. Am J Obstet Gynecol 172:206, 1995.

76. Close CE, Carr MC, Burns MW, Mitchell ME: Lower urinary tract changes after early valve ablation in neonates and infants: Is early diversion warranted? J Urol 157:984, 1997.

77. Steinhardt GF, Liapis H, Phillips B, et al: Insulin-like growth factor improves renal architecture in fetal kidneys with complete ureteral obstruction. J Urol 154:690, 1995.

78. Bussieres C, Laborde K, Souberbielle JC, et al: Fetal urinary insulin-like growth factor I and binding protein 3 in bilateral obstructive uropathies. Prenat Diagn 15:1047, 1995.

CHAPTER 19

The Fetus with a Lung Mass

N. SCOTT ADZICK

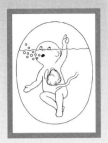

Prenatal diagnosis provides insights into the in utero evolution of fetal lung lesions such as congenital cystic adenomatoid malformation (CCAM) and extralobar pulmonary sequestration (EPS). Serial sonographic study of fetuses with lung lesions has helped define the natural history of these lesions, determine the pathophysiologic features that affect clinical outcome, and formulate management based on prognosis.[1–6] In a series of more than 175 prenatally diagnosed cases, we have found that the overall prognosis depends on the size of the lung mass and the secondary physiologic derangement: a large mass causes mediastinal shift, hypoplasia of normal lung tissue, polyhydramnios, and cardiovascular compromise leading to fetal hydrops and death.[7] Hydrops is a harbinger of fetal or neonatal demise, and manifests itself as fetal ascites, pleural and pericardial effusions, and skin and scalp edema.

Smaller thoracic lesions can cause respiratory distress in the newborn period, and the smallest masses may be asymptomatic until later in childhood when infection, pneumothorax, or malignant degeneration may occur. Large fetal lung tumors may partially disappear on serial prenatal sonography, illustrating that improvement can occasionally occur during fetal life.[8–10] In particular, many EPSs dramatically decrease in size before birth and may not need treatment after birth.[7]

The finding that fetuses with hydrops are at very high risk for fetal or neonatal demise led us to perform fetal surgical resection of the massively enlarged pulmonary lobe (fetal lobectomy) for cystic/solid lesions or thoracoamniotic shunting for unilocular cystic lesions.[7, 11–13] When this fetal lung lesion topic was reviewed in the last (1991) edition of this book, it was predicted that fetal therapy would be a future option for CCAM, and indeed fetal therapy is now performed successfully for lung lesions associated with nonimmune hydrops. The fetus with a lung mass but without hydrops has an excellent chance for survival with maternal transport, planned delivery, and neonatal evaluation and surgery.

Prenatal Diagnosis and Natural History

CCAM is characterized by an overgrowth of terminal respiratory bronchioles that form cysts of various sizes.

Cha has identified two histologic patterns of fetal CCAM, pseudoglandular and canalicular.[14] Stocker defined three types of CCAM (types I to III) based primarily on cyst size.[15] We have classified prenatally diagnosed CCAM into two categories based on gross anatomy and ultrasound findings.[1] Macrocystic lesions contain single or multiple cysts that are 5 mm in diameter or larger on prenatal ultrasound, whereas microcystic lesions appear echogenic on sonography. CCAM usually arises from one lobe of the lung and bilateral lung involvement is rare. We have learned that the overall prognosis depends primarily on the *size* of the CCAM rather than on the lesion type, and the underlying growth characteristics are likely to be important.

Resected large fetal CCAM specimens demonstrate increased cell proliferation and markedly decreased apoptosis compared to normal fetal lung tissue.[16] Examination of factors that enhance cell proliferation or down-regulate apoptosis in CCAM may provide further insights into the pathogenesis of this tumor and may suggest new therapeutic approaches. With regard to cell proliferation, we examined the role of pneumocyte mitogens like keratinocyte growth factor (KGF) and platelet-derived growth factor (PDGF) in rapidly growing fetal CCAMs. CCAM-like lesions occur in transgenic mice that overexpress KGF,[17] but we found no differences in the expression of KGF protein or KGF mRNA in CCAM and normal lung. In contrast, fetal CCAMs that grew rapidly, progressed to hydrops, and required in utero resection showed increased PDGF-B gene expression and PDGF-BB protein production compared to either normal fetal lung or term CCAM specimens.

Extralobar pulmonary sequestrations are masses of nonfunctioning lung tissue that are supplied by an anomalous systemic artery and do not have a bronchial connection to the native tracheobronchial tree. On prenatal ultrasonography, an EPS appears as a well-defined echodense, homogeneous mass. Detection by color flow Doppler of a systemic artery from the aorta to the fetal lung lesion is a pathognomonic feature of fetal EPS[18] (Fig. 19–1). However, if this Doppler finding is not detected, then an echodense microcystic CCAM and an EPS can have an identical prenatal sonographic appearance. Ultrafast fetal magnetic resonance imaging (MRI) may help differentiate CCAM from EPS.[19] Furthermore,

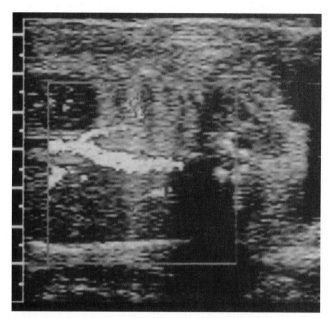

F I G U R E 19–1. By Doppler studies, a systemic artery (*curved arrow*) from the descending aorta (Ao) is seen supplying the mass (*) consistent with the diagnosis of pulmonary sequestration.

we and others have also described prenatally diagnosed lung masses that display clinicopathologic features of both CCAM and sequestration, which suggests a shared embryologic basis for some of these lung lesions. The ability to differentiate intralobar and extralobar sequestration before birth is limited unless an extralobar sequestration is highlighted by a pleural effusion or is located in the abdomen. There are no diagnostic hallmarks for the specific prenatal diagnosis of an intralobar sequestration.

Huge fetal lung lesions have reproducible pathophysiologic effects on the developing fetus. Esophageal compression by the thoracic mass causes interference with fetal swallowing of amniotic fluid and results in polyhydramnios. Polyhydramnios is a common obstetric indication for ultrasonography, so a prenatal diagnostic marker exists for many large fetal lung tumors. Support for this concept comes from the absence of fluid in the fetal stomach in some of these cases, and the alleviation of polyhydramnios after effective fetal treatment.[2] The hydrops is secondary to vena caval obstruction and cardiac compression from large tumors causing an extreme mediastinal shift.[20] Like CCAMs, a fetal EPS can also cause fetal hydrops, either from the mass effect or from a tension hydrothorax that is the result of fluid or lymph secretion from the EPS.[7] Although there is some association of both polyhydramnios and hydrops with fetal lung lesions, our experience indicates that either can occur independently of the other.

Although sonographic prenatal diagnosis is becoming increasingly sophisticated, diagnostic errors are possible. Diaphragmatic hernia can be distinguished by careful sonographic assessment, an amniogram with or without a computed tomography (CT) scan, or by ultrafast MRI.[19] We and others have experience with other fetal thoracic masses including bronchogenic and enteric cysts, mediastinal cystic teratoma, congenital lobar emphysema, hemangioma, and bronchial atresia.[20, 21] We have described two cases of intrathoracic gastric duplication cyst associated with hydrops that were treated with placement of a thoracoamniotic shunt.[22] Several years ago, we had an unusual case of unilateral pulmonary agenesis in which the prenatal sonographic findings included a densely echogenic left lung mass with flattening of the left hemidiaphragm and a marked mediastinal shift to the right. A chest x-ray after birth revealed right-sided pulmonary agenesis and hyperinflation of the remaining left lung. A bronchoscopic evaluation demonstrated a long area of tracheobronchial stenosis to the solitary left lung. Retention of fetal lung fluid with overdistention of the left lung secondary to the high-grade airway obstruction during fetal life resulted in sonographic findings similar to those of a large microcystic CCAM.

Associated anomalies in our series were extremely uncommon compared to some other reports.[2] This difference may reflect a referral bias of cases to our centers for possible fetal or postnatal treatment, such that fetuses with associated anatomic anomalies may not be referred.

Although a large pulmonary lesion diagnosed in utero is an ominous finding, the natural history of prenatally diagnosed pulmonary lesions is variable. Approximately 15% of our CCAM lesions decreased in size during gestation, and the majority (68%) of EPS lesions shrank dramatically before birth. Several other groups have also reported the involution of some pulmonary lesions,[4, 5, 8–10] although the mass is invariably detectable by chest CT scan after birth.[23] Although regression of a lung lesion and associated hydrops has been reported, this is a very rare circumstance.[6, 24]

The exact mechanism by which these lesions shrink is unclear. The masses that shrank in our experience and in other reported cases were usually echodense lesions. The echogenic appearance on ultrasonography is due to the large number of tissue/fluid interfaces. As the lung lesions decreased in size, they also became less echogenic implying that they were losing fluid/tissue interfaces. CCAMs and sequestrations usually do not communicate directly with the tracheobronchial tree, although abnormal channels to the airway and the gastrointestinal tract have been reported. Perhaps the lesions shrink due to decompression of fetal lung fluid through these abnormal channels. Another possible explanation is that the pulmonary lesions outgrow their vascular supply and involute. Initial impressions concerning the prognosis of large pulmonary lesions should be tempered with the understanding that they can shrink in size or even "disappear."

Recently, we have determined CCAM volume by sonographic measurement using the formula for a prolate ellipse. A cystic adenomatoid malformation volume ratio (CVR) was obtained by dividing the CCAM volume by head circumference to correct for fetal size. We found that a CVR greater than 2 is predictive of hydrops for CCAM fetuses. The CVR may be useful in selecting fetuses at risk for hydrops and thus need close ultrasound observation and possible fetal intervention.

Experimental Studies: Rationale for Fetal Surgery

Experimental studies have elucidated the pathophysiologic consequences of fetal intrathoracic masses and have demonstrated that fetal pulmonary resection is straightforward. Simulation of the thoracic mass effect with an intrathoracic balloon in the third-trimester fetal lamb resulted in pulmonary hypoplasia and death at term due to respiratory insufficiency, whereas lambs that underwent simulated resection of the mass by balloon deflation in the middle of the third trimester had sufficient lung growth to permit survival at birth.[25, 26] In addition, we have shown that intrauterine pneumonectomy in fetal lambs is technically feasible at early and mid-gestation and can induce compensatory growth of the remaining lung by term.[27]

Hydrops caused by large CCAM lesions has been attributed to direct mediastinal compression, obstruction of venous return, protein loss from the tumor, or unspecified humoral factors that increase capillary permeability. In order to study the etiology of hydrops associated with huge fetal lung masses, we created a fetal sheep model in which a surgically implanted intrathoracic tissue expander was gradually inflated over several days while monitoring fetal arterial, venous, intrathoracic, and intra-amniotic pressures and while monitoring for sonographic indications of hydrops.[28] We found that balloon inflation resulted in hydrops as a result of cardiac venous obstruction and increasing central venous pressure (Figs. 19–2 and 19–3). Simulation of prenatal resection of the fetal thoracic mass by deflating the expander resulted in complete resolution of the hydrops and return of pressures to normal. This model may be used to further evaluate the pathophysiologic and sonographic features of large fetal chest masses.

Experiments in nonhuman primates led to the development of the necessary surgical, anesthetic, and tocolytic techniques prior to clinical use and have shown that fetal intervention is safe for the mother and her future reproductive potential.[29–31] The salvage of human fetuses with severe diaphragmatic hernia or obstructive

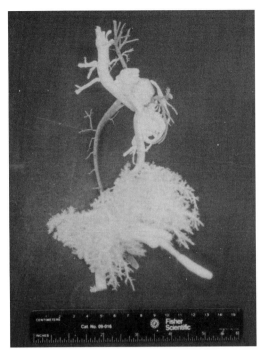

FIGURE 19–3. Silicone vascular digestion cast of a postmortem sheep, constructed while the tissue expander was fully inflated. The white silicone fills the venous system via the umbilical vein, and the black silicone fills the arterial system via the aorta. Note the dramatic lateral displacement and compression of the venae cavae by the tissue expander. The aortic position is unchanged.

uropathy by in utero repair established a sound basis for open fetal surgery based on extensive animal studies.[32]

Clinical Experience

Methods

Case study review was performed for 175 fetal lung lesion patients (134 CCAMs and 41 EPSs) referred to the University of California at San Francisco (UCSF) Fetal Treatment Center from July 1, 1983, to June 30, 1995, and referred to the Center for Fetal Diagnosis and Treatment at the Children's Hospital of Philadelphia (CHOP) from July 1, 1995, to December 31, 1997. All patients had evaluation of their sonographic findings at UCSF or CHOP and patient management was subsequently performed either in San Francisco, Philadelphia, or at the referring institution. Details of care and outcome at the referring institution were tracked by a written protocol and telephone follow-up. The following data were compiled: gestational age at the time of diagnosis and delivery; size and location of the lesion; presence of hydrops (defined as an abnormal fluid accumulation in one or more serous cavities and/or soft tissue edema); presence of other anomalies; fetal therapy; and postnatal course including diagnostic studies, need for respiratory support, surgery, pathology, and outcome.

In the absence of nonimmune hydrops, serial sonography was done to monitor the size of the lesion and to look for signs of hydrops. In any fetus where interven-

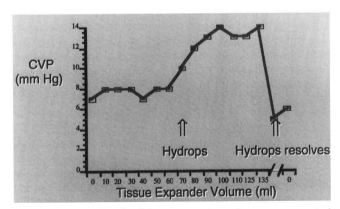

FIGURE 19–2. Graph of tissue expander volume versus central venous pressure (CVP) for a fetal sheep. This animal began to show evidence of hydrops and had an increase in CVP at the expander volume of 75 mL. After expander deflation, all evidence of hydrops disappeared, and the CVP returned to baseline.

tion was considered, fetal echocardiography was used to rule out cardiac defects, and karyotyping was performed after amniocentesis or cordocentesis. Prenatal and postnatal imaging studies as well as operative and pathologic criteria were used to differentiate CCAM from EPS.

Thirteen cases of CCAM associated with fetal hydrops underwent open fetal surgery. For fetal surgery candidates, each family underwent extensive discussion of the risks and benefits of fetal therapy for a lung tumor associated with hydrops. The first six cases were performed under a protocol approved by the institutional review board (IRB) of UCSF, and subsequent cases were not considered experimental by the IRB.

Fetal surgery candidates had a normal karyotype by amniocentesis or percutaneous umbilical blood sampling, and no other anatomic abnormalities were present on detailed sonographic survey. Fetal surgical techniques have been previously described in detail[33] and in Chapter 11. In brief, indomethacin and antibiotics were given preoperatively, isoflurane provided the necessary uterine relaxation and anesthesia for both mother and fetus, and a low transverse maternal laparotomy was performed. Sterile intraoperative sonography delineated both the fetal and placental position. The hysterotomy was facilitated by the placement of two large absorbable monofilament sutures parallel to the intended incision site and through the full thickness of the uterine wall. A uterine stapler (US Surgical Corporation, Norwalk, CT) with absorbable Lactomer staples[34] was then directly introduced through this point of fixation and into the amniotic cavity using a piercing attachment on the lower limb of the stapler. The stapler was then fired, thereby anchoring the amniotic membranes to the uterine wall and creating a hemostatic hysterotomy. The fetal chest was entered by a fifth intercostal space thoracotomy. Invariably, the lesion readily decompressed out through the thoracotomy wound consistent with increased intrathoracic pressure from the mass. Using techniques developed in experimental animals, the appropriate pulmonary lobe containing the lesion was resected.[27] The fetal thoracotomy was closed, the fetus was returned to the uterus, warmed saline containing 500 mg of nafcillin was instilled into the amniotic cavity, and the uterine and abdominal incisions were closed in layers. Tocolysis with intravenous magnesium sulfate and β-mimetics began as the mother emerged from anesthesia. All fetal surgery mothers had subsequent cesarean delivery.

Results

Congenital Cystic Adenomatoid Malformation

There were 134 cases of CCAM diagnosed between 17 weeks' and 38 weeks' gestation. Fourteen women underwent pregnancy termination: 12 fetuses had nonimmune hydrops, one had multiple structural abnormalities and hydrops, and one was otherwise normal. One hundred twenty women elected to continue their pregnancies after the diagnosis was made: 101 women were man-

aged expectantly, 13 women carrying hydropic fetuses underwent open fetal surgery, and 6 women carrying fetuses with a large unilocular pulmonary cyst had percutaneous placement of a thoracoamniotic shunt.

In the expectant management group, there were 76 fetuses with CCAM lesions that were not associated with nonimmune hydrops; all survived. These cases were usually managed with maternal transport, planned delivery near or at term, and resection of the mass during the neonatal period (66 cases have undergone resection; ten others are being followed). Many of the babies with large lesions required substantial ventilatory support and four needed treatment with extracorporeal membrane oxygenation (ECMO). Only one had a karyotype abnormality (Down syndrome). Twenty-five hydropic fetuses were followed expectantly and all died either before or after preterm labor and delivery at 25 to 36 weeks' gestation; nine mothers had associated placentomegaly and preeclampsia. One hydropic fetus had another serious anomaly (tetralogy of Fallot), and one hydropic fetus had bilateral CCAMs.

Fifteen CCAM lesions appeared large at 20 to 26 weeks' gestation with an associated contralateral mediastinal shift, but then clearly decreased in size during the third trimester with return of the heart back toward the midline. Although four of these shrinking lesions were associated with polyhydramnios including one case with fetal ascites, these phenomena resolved as the masses decreased in size.

Seven cystic lesions proved to have a previously unrecognized systemic arterial blood supply present at the time of operation consistent with a pulmonary sequestration (five intralobar and two extralobar pulmonary sequestrations). Histologic sections revealed CCAM pathology, so these are "hybrid" lesions as previously described.[35, 36]

Open Fetal Surgery for CCAM

The knowledge that hydrops is highly predictive of fetal or neonatal demise led to fetal surgical resection of a massive multicystic or predominantly solid CCAM (fetal lobectomy) in 13 cases at 21 to 29 weeks' gestation, with eight healthy survivors at 1 to 7 years' follow-up (Table 19–1). All cases had histologic confirmation of the diagnosis of CCAM. In one multicystic case (case 3), a thoracoamniotic shunt failed to adequately decompress the mass effect prior to open fetal surgery. In the eight fetuses that survived, fetal CCAM resection led to hydrops resolution in 1 to 2 weeks, return of the mediastinum to the midline within 3 weeks, and impressive in utero lung growth (Fig. 19–4). Mean postoperative pregnancy duration was 8 weeks (range, 2 to 13 weeks). Developmental testing every 6 to 12 months has been normal in all eight survivors.

There were five fetal deaths in the fetal surgery resection cases. In case 1, the mother had already developed the maternal "mirror" syndrome.[37] The fetal operation was successful, the hydrops improved, but the placentomegaly and maternal hyperdynamic state remained, and the fetus was delivered 1 week later. In case 6, a 21-week-gestation fetus became bradycardic and died 8

T A B L E 19–1. FETAL CCAM RESECTIONS

CASE NO.	FETAL HYDROPS	AGE	PARITY	SURGERY WEEKS	PRENATAL COURSE	DELIVERY WEEKS	NEONATAL OUTCOME	LESION LOCATION
1	Yes	24	G2P1	27	Preterm labor and "mirror syndrome" necessitated delivery 1 wk postoperatively	28	Died from lung hypoplasia at 40 hr	RML
2	Yes	25	G4P1	23	Hydrops resolved 1 wk after surgery	30	Ventilated for 2 d, discharge DOL 24; left pneumothorax, alive & well at 7 yr	LLL
3	Yes	30	G5P0	26	Failed shunt at 25 wk hydrops resolved 2 wk after surgery	34	Ventilated for 6 d, discharge DOL 36; alive & well at 6 yr	LLL
4	Yes	30	G2P1	26	Hydrops resolved 1 wk after surgery	33	Ventilated for 2 d, discharge DOL 73; alive & well at 6 yr	LLL
5	Yes	25	G4P2	24	Postoperative indocin-induced ductus arteriosus constriction, preterm labor/delivery 2 wk postoperative	26	Ventilated for 4 wk, right pneumothorax; PDA ligation; discharge DOL 73; alive & well at 5 yr	RML
6	Yes	30	G7P2	21	Fetal demise 8 hours postoperative autopsy: no apparent cause of death	21	—	RML, RLL
7	Yes	24	G1P0	25	Intraoperative fetal demise 2 hr to uterine contractions	—	—	RUL
8	Yes	30	G4P3	24	Minimal uterine activity on nitroglycerin, hydrops resolved 1 wk after surgery	30	Ventilated for 10 d, discharge DOL 27; alive & well at 5 yr	RML, RLL
9	Yes	24	G3P1	24	Intraoperative fetal demise after induction of maternal anesthesia	—	—	LUL
10	Yes	25	G2P1	22	Intraoperative 10 mL fetal blood transfusion, hydrops resolved 10 d after surgery	35	Discharge DOL 5; alive & well at 18 mo	LLL
11	Yes	24	G1P0	21	Intraoperative fetal demise; arrest immediately after fetal thoracotomy	—	—	RUL
12	Yes	38	G3P1	22	Hydrops resolved 1 wk after surgery	35	Discharge DOL 5; alive & well at 12 mo	LLL
13	Yes	19	G1P0	29	Intraoperative 10 mL fetal blood transfusion; hydrops resolved 2 wk after surgery	37	Discharge DOL 9; alive & well at 6 mo	RUL

CCAM, congenital cystic adenomatoid malformation; DOL, day of life, PDA, patent ductus arteriosus; RML, right middle lobe; LLL, left lower lobe; RLL, right lower lobe; RUL, right upper lobe.

hours postoperatively; postmortem did not elucidate the cause of death. In case 7, fetal death was due to uncontrolled intraoperative uterine contractions, which hallmarks this limitation of fetal surgery. Finally, in cases 9 and 11 massive hydrops was present at 21 weeks' gestation and both fetuses died intraoperatively—one died during induction of maternal anesthesia and the other died immediately after the fetal thoracotomy was made.

With regard to maternal morbidity, there was one wound seroma and one wound infection that developed after cesarean delivery and each required drainage. There were two maternal blood transfusions of 1 U of packed red blood cells in cases 1 and 11. Two cases of mild postoperative interstitial pulmonary edema responded to furosemide diuresis. In case 1, a uterine wound dehiscence was evident at the time of cesarean delivery in each of her two subsequent pregnancies.

Six mothers have delivered normal babies by planned cesarean delivery subsequent to the fetal surgery pregnancy.[32]

Catheter Shunt Placement for CCAM

Six fetuses with a single large predominant cyst underwent thoracoamniotic shunt placement using a Rocket catheter (Rocket Ltd, London, England). Fetal thoracentesis alone was ineffective, since fetal lung fluid rapidly filled the aspirated cyst. Three nonhydropic fetuses with large cystic lesions had shunts placed at 25, 28, and 30 weeks' gestation that functioned for 11, 10, and 2 weeks, respectively. All three patients survived, although one case required ECMO support for 4 days and another required high-frequency ventilation for 2 weeks. Of the three hydropic fetuses with a large solitary cyst, two survived after shunt placement at 24 and 30 weeks'

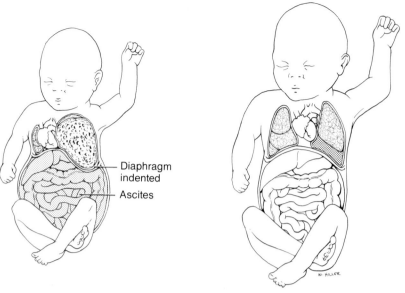

Pre-op

6 weeks post-op

FIGURE 19–4. Fetal anatomy preoperatively and 6 weeks after fetal surgery.

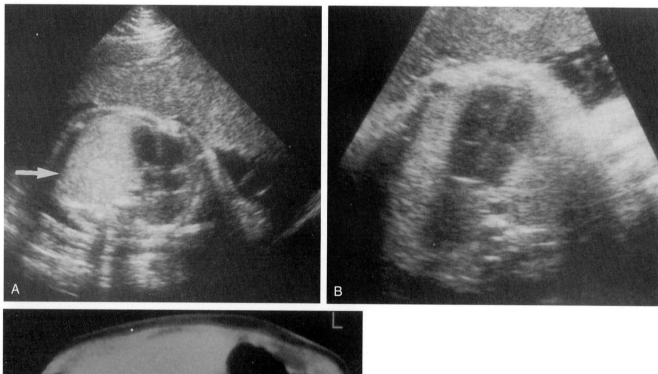

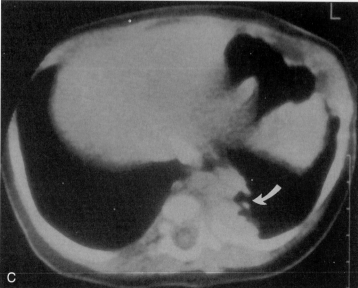

FIGURE 19–5. *A,* Prenatal ultrasound at 22 weeks' gestation demonstrating a large, echogenic mass in the left chest shifting the heart and mediastinum to the right. *B,* By 37 weeks, the heart is in the midline with normal appearing lungs. The mass is no longer visible by ultrasound. *C,* Postnatal chest CT scan shows a small mass in the left inferoposterior chest.

gestation and the shunt functioned for 10 and 4 weeks, respectively, prior to delivery, and high-frequency oscillation was required in one and ECMO was used in the other. The third hydropic fetus died after premature rupture of membranes 3 days following shunt placement at 22 weeks' gestation.

Pulmonary Sequestration

Extralobar pulmonary sequestrations are echodense lesions that have a systemic arterial blood supply arising from the aorta that is usually detectable by prenatal color flow Doppler. There were 41 EPS cases with the age of diagnosis varying between 18 and 36 weeks' gestation. There were two twin pregnancies in which one fetus was affected. There were no other associated significant anatomic or karyotypic anomalies. There were two terminations of pregnancy. Of the 39 pregnancies that continued, 28 lesions regressed and completely or nearly completely disappeared on serial prenatal ultrasound (Fig. 19–5). One lesion had associated ascites at 24 weeks' gestation that disappeared as the lesion regressed during the third trimester. All of these infants were asymptomatic after birth. The lesion was often undetectable on postnatal chest x-ray but could invariably be detected by postnatal CT or MRI. All of these babies have been followed without resection.

Eleven fetuses with larger EPSs were treated before and/or after birth. Seven nonhydropic babies underwent postnatal resection because of respiratory symptoms and all survived; one required ECMO. Three fetuses presented with an EPS and hydrops at 27, 29, and 30 weeks' gestation. The hydrops appeared to be a consequence of a tension hydrothorax from fluid or lymph secretion by the mass (Fig. 19–6). The hydrops

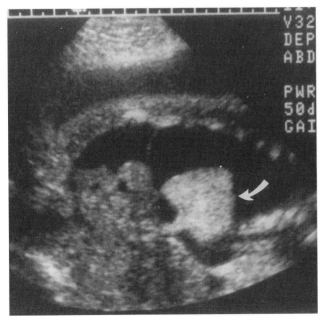

FIGURE 19–6. Longitudinal scan of a fetus with an EPS and associated tension hydrothorax and hydrops. The EPS and vascular stalk are seen in the chest outlined by the pleural effusion, and ascites and body wall edema are present.

resolved after weekly fetal thoracenteses in one case and thoracoamniotic shunt placement in the two other cases. All three survived after delivery at 33 to 35 weeks' gestation, required ventilatory support, and subsequently underwent EPS resection. Another fetus with sequestration, hydrops, and preterm labor diagnosed at 34 weeks' gestation was not treated prenatally and this baby died from pulmonary hypoplasia despite postnatal resection and the use of ECMO for 3 weeks.

The Fetal Surgery Experience

Fetuses with life-threatening lung lesions were selected for prenatal treatment according to predetermined guidelines, including the gestational age of the fetus, the size of the intrathoracic lesion, maternal health, and the development of fetal hydrops. The finding that fetuses with large tumors and hydrops are at high risk for fetal or neonatal demise led to several therapeutic maneuvers. Fetal thoracentesis alone was ineffective for treatment because of rapid reaccumulation of cyst fluid.[38] At best, thoracentesis may serve as a temporizing maneuver prior to shunt placement or resection. Thoracoamniotic shunting was performed in several cases that had a large predominant cyst as long as there was not a large solid component to the CCAM. Ten years ago, Clark documented resolution of hydrops after 3 weeks of catheter drainage,[39] and successful shunt placement has been reported in several other cases of unilocular CCAM lesions.[2, 5, 40] However, many of these shunts dislodged or clogged after relatively short periods of time. Multicystic or predominantly solid CCAM lesions do not lend themselves to catheter decompression and require resection.

Fetal surgical resection of the massively enlarged pulmonary lobe (fetal lobectomy) was performed at 21 to 29 weeks' gestation in 13 cases with eight survivors. These encouraging results demonstrate that fetal CCAM resection is reasonably safe and technically feasible, reverses hydrops over 1 to 2 weeks, and allows sufficient lung growth to permit survival and normal postnatal development. We have used serial ultrafast fetal MRI examinations to measure lung growth after fetal surgical CCAM resection (Table 19–2). The steep learning curve derived from our experience with more than 100 open fetal surgery cases for a variety of life-threatening fetal anomalies has provided invaluable lessons regarding optimal maternal anesthesia and uterine relaxation, hysterotomy and fetal exposure techniques, intraoperative fetal monitoring, and reliable methods for amniotic membrane and uterine closure.[41]

In contrast, the five unsuccessful fetal CCAM resection cases highlight other challenges. We learned in case 1 that the maternal hyperdynamic state referred to as the "mirror syndrome" cannot be reversed solely by treatment of the underlying fetal condition. This preeclamptic state is associated with molar pregnancies and fetal conditions that cause placentomegaly, and may be caused by a factor released by poorly perfused placental tissue that leads to endothelial cell injury.[19, 42] Until the pathophysiology of the maternal mirror syndrome is

T A B L E 19–2. FETAL CCAM: POSTOPERATIVE LUNG VOLUMES BY ULTRAFAST MRI

GESTATIONAL AGE	EVENT	R LUNG VOLUME	L LUNG VOLUME
22 wk	Hydrops/lobectomy	—	—
24 wk		8.5	5.0
26 wk		14.7	10.4
30 wk		27.6	15.2
33 wk		34.6	23.5
35 wk	Delivery/no ventilator required	—	—

CCAM, congenital cystic adenomatoid malformation; MRI, magnetic resonance imaging; R, right; L, left.

understood, earlier intervention before the onset of placentomegaly and the related maternal preeclamptic state may be the only approach to salvage these doomed fetuses. Case 13 illustrates that placentomegaly can regress after fetal surgical CCAM resection if clinical signs of the maternal "mirror syndrome" are not present preoperatively.

As illustrated in unsuccessful cases 6, 7, 9, and 11, our clinical focus has shifted from the technical details of the fetal surgical procedure to the crucial need for better postoperative maternal–fetal monitoring[43] reliable long-term fetal intravascular access for fetal blood sampling and infusions,[44] and noninvasive maternal–fetal hemodynamic assessment.[45] The detection and treatment of preterm labor remains the "Achilles' heel" of fetal surgery. As a result of ongoing work in fetal animal models, the concept of a fetal intensive care unit with a specially trained cadre of physicians and nurses has become a clinical reality.

In the future, minimally invasive approaches to fetal lung lesions associated with hydrops may be possible. Laser therapy to fulgurate a fetal CCAM has been reported,[46] but we believe that this approach is not clinically warranted at the current time. For example, a mother carrying a 28-week-gestation fetus with a large right-sided CCAM and hydrops was turned down for open fetal surgery by our group because of maternal psychosocial difficulties, and she decided to seek yttrium-aluminum-garnet (YAG) laser therapy at another medical center. Using a percutaneous technique under ultrasound guidance, a laser fiber was deployed in the fetal right chest, and the procedure was repeated twice during the next 4 weeks. After birth, the baby died from pulmonary hypoplasia and had a severely caved-in right chest with multiple rib fractures as a result of the prenatally applied laser energy (Fig. 19–7). It is possible that laser therapy or techniques such as radiofrequency thermal ablation will be clinically useful for fetal lung lesions associated with fetal hydrops if the result is a decrease in mass effect, but experimental studies in animal models to rigorously test these techniques should be mandatory prior to clinical trials.

We have learned from prenatal diagnosis that there is a wide spectrum of clinical severity for the fetus with a lung mass. Accurate prognostic information is necessary for providing appropriate management and parental counseling (Fig. 19–8). If an associated life-threatening anomaly is present or if the mother is sick with the mirror syndrome, then the family may choose to terminate the pregnancy. If the fetus is not hydropic and an isolated fetal lung lesion is present, then the mother is followed by serial ultrasound, and arrangements are made for the best possible care after birth. Some CCAMs and many EPSs will shrink in size, so it is important to try to differentiate these lesions using prenatal diagnostic criteria, although this is not always possible.[7] All fetuses with fetal thoracic masses and without hydrops in our series survived in the setting of maternal transport, planned delivery, and immediate postnatal evaluation at a facility with ECMO capability. Interestingly, our impression is that these nonhydropic fetuses with lung masses have a much better prognosis than those with diaphragmatic hernia despite a similar degree of mediastinal shift as judged by sonography. In asymptomatic neonates with a cystic lung lesion, we recommend elective resection because of the risks of infection and occult malignant transformation.[47-51] In contrast, we have simply followed patients with asymptomatic noncystic EPS if we are confident of the diagnosis based on postnatal imaging studies.

If the fetus is hydropic at presentation or if hydrops develops during serial follow-up, then management depends upon the gestational age. For those hydropic fetuses greater than 32 weeks' gestation, early delivery should be considered so that the lesion can be resected ex utero, but the neonatal outcome is dismal. For those hydropic fetuses less than 32 weeks' gestation, there is now a new therapeutic option, which is to treat the lesion before birth.

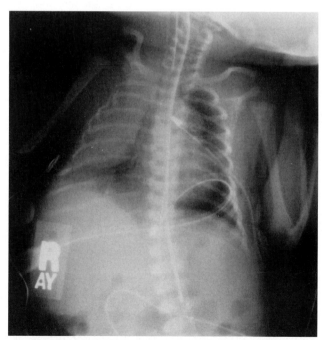

F I G U R E 19–7. Chest x-ray appearance of a neonate with a right CCAM who underwent attempted laser ablation during fetal life. The laser energy caused a thoracoplasty-like collapse of the right chest wall with distortion and fracture of all of the ribs. This baby died shortly after birth due to respiratory insufficiency.

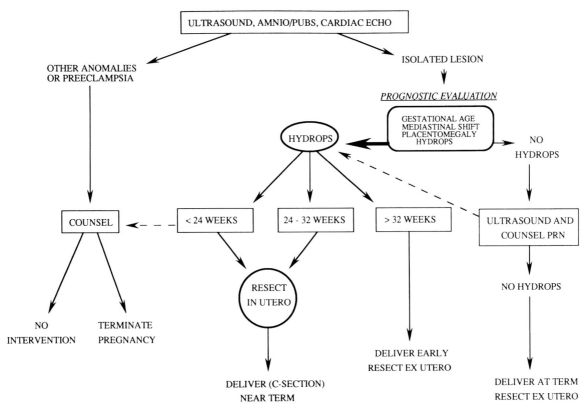

FIGURE 19–8. Algorithm for management of the fetus with a CCAM.

REFERENCES

1. Adzick NS, Harrison MR, Glick PL, et al: Fetal cystic adenomatoid malformation: Prenatal diagnosis and natural history. J Pediatr Surg 20:483–488, 1985.
2. Thorpe-Veeston JG, Nicolaides KH: Cystic adenomatoid malformation of the lung: Prenatal diagnosis and outcome. Prenatal Diagn 14:677–688, 1994.
3. Sakala EP, Perrott WS, Grube GL: Sonographic characteristics of antenatally diagnosed extralobar pulmonary sequestration and congenital cystic adenomatoid malformation. Obstet Gynecol Surv 49:647–655, 1994.
4. Miller JA, Corteville JE, Langer JC: Congenital cystic adenomatoid malformation in the fetus: Natural history and predictors of outcome. J Pediatr Surg 31:805–808, 1996.
5. Dommergues M, Louis-Sylvestre C, Mandelbrot L, et al: Congenital adenomatoid malformation of the lung: When is active fetal therapy indicated? Am J Obstet Gynecol 177:953–958, 1997.
6. Taguchi T, Suita S, Yamanouchi T, et al: Antenatal diagnosis and surgical management of congenital cystic adenomatoid malformation of the lung. Fetal Diagn Ther 10:400–407, 1995.
7. Adzick NS, Harrison MR, Crombleholme TM, et al: Fetal lung lesions: Management and outcome. Am J Obstet Gynecol 179:884–889, 1998.
8. Saltzman DH, Adzick NS, Benacerraf BR: Fetal cystic adenomatoid malformation of the lung: Apparent improvement in utero. Obstet Gynecol 71:1000–1003, 1988.
9. MacGillivray TE, Harrison MR, Goldstein RB, Adzick NS: Disappearing fetal lung lesions. J Pediatr Surg 28:1321–1325, 1993.
10. Budorick NE, Pretorius DH, Leopold GR, Stamm ER: Spontaneous improvement of intrathoracic masses diagnosed in utero. J Ultrasound Med 11:653–662, 1992.
11. Harrison MR, Adzick NS, Jennings RW, et al: Antenatal intervention for congenital cystic adenomatoid malformation. Lancet 336:965–967, 1990.
12. Kuller JA, Yankowitz J, Goldberg JD, et al: Outcome of antenatally diagnosed cystic adenomatoid malformation. Am J Obstet Gynecol 167:1038–1041, 1992.
13. Adzick NS, Harrison MR, Flake AW, et al: Fetal surgery for cystic adenomatoid malformation of the lung. J Pediatr Surg 28:806–812, 1993.
14. Cha I, Adzick NS, Harrison MR, Finkbeiner WE: Fetal congenital cystic adenomatoid malformations of the lung: A clinicopathologic study of eleven cases. Am J Surg Pathol 21:537–544, 1997.
15. Stocker TJ, Manewell JE, Drake RM: Congenital cystic adenomatoid malformation of the lung: Classification and morphologic spectrum. Hum Pathol 8:155–171, 1977.
16. Cass DL, Yang EY, Liechty KW, et al: Increased cell proliferation and decreased apoptosis in congenital cystic adenomatoid malformation: Insights into pathogenesis. Surg Forum 47:659–661, 1997.
17. Simonet WS, DeRose ML, Bucay N, et al: Pulmonary malformation in transgenic mice expressing keratinocyte growth factor in the lung. Proc Natl Acad Sci USA 92:12461–12465, 1995.
18. Hernanz-Schulman M, Stein SM, Neblett WW, et al: Pulmonary sequestration: Diagnosis with color Doppler sonography and a new theory of associated hydrothorax. Radiology 180:817–821, 1991.
19. Quinn TM, Hubbard AM, Adzick NS: Prenatal magnetic resonance imaging enhances prenatal diagnosis. J Pediatr Surg 33:312–316, 1998.
20. Albright EB, Crane JP, Shackelford GD: Prenatal diagnosis of a bronchogenic cyst. J Ultrasound Med 7:91–95, 1988.
21. Richards DS, Langham MR, Dolson LH: Antenatal presentation of a child with congenital lobar emphysema. J Ultrasound Med 11:165–168, 1992.
22. Ferro MM, Milner R, Cannizzaro C, et al: Intrathoracic alimentary tract duplication cysts treated in utero by thoracoamniotic shunting. Fetal Diagn Treat 13:343–347, 1998.
23. Winters WD, Effmann EL, Nghiem HV, Nyberg DA: Disappearing fetal lung massses: Importance of postnatal imaging studies. Pediatr Radiol 27:535–539, 1997.
24. daSilva OP, Ramanan R, Romano W, Evans M: Nonimmune hydrops fetalis, pulmonary sequestration, and favorable neonatal outcome. Obstet Gynecol 88:681–683, 1996.
25. Harrison MR, Jester JA, Ross NA: Correction of congenital diaphragmatic hernia in utero I. The model: Intrathoracic balloon produces fatal pulmonary hypoplasia. Surgery 88:174–180, 1980.

26. Harrison MR, Bressack MA, Churg AM, et al: Correction of congenital diaphragmatic hernia in utero II. Simulated correction permits fetal lung growth with survival at birth. Surgery 88:260–268, 1980.

27. Adzick NS, Harrison MR, Hu LM, et al: Compensatory growth after pneumonectomy in fetal lambs: A morphologic study. Surg Forum 37:309–311, 1986.

28. Rice HE, Estes JM, Hedrick MH, et al: Congenital cystic adenomatoid malformation: A sheep model. J Pediatr Surg 29:692–696, 1994.

29. Harrison MR, Anderson J, Rosen MA, et al: Fetal surgery in the primate I. Anesthetic, surgical, and tocolytic management to maximize fetal-neonatal survival. J Pediatr Surg 17:115–122, 1982.

30. Nakayama DK, Harrison MR, Seron-Ferre M, et al: Fetal surgery in the primate II. Uterine electromyographic response to operative procedure and pharmacologic agents. J Pediatr Surg 19:333-339, 1984.

31. Adzick NS, Harrison MR, Glick PL, et al: Fetal surgery in the primate III. Maternal outcome after fetal surgery. J Pediatr Surg 21:477–480, 1986.

32. Longaker MT, Golbus MS, Filly RA, et al: Maternal outcome after open fetal surgery: A review of the first 17 human cases. JAMA 265:737–741, 1991.

33. Adzick NS, Harrison MR: Fetal surgical techniques. Semin Pediatr Surg 2:136–142, 1993.

34. Adzick NS, Harrison MR, Flake AW: Automatic uterine stapling devices in fetal operation: Experience in a primate model. Surg Forum 36:479–480, 1985.

35. Cass DL, Crombleholme TM, Howell LJ, et al: Cystic lung lesions with systemic arterial blood supply: A hybrid of congenital cystic adenomatoid malformation and bronchopulmonary sequestration. J Pediatr Surg 32:986–990, 1997.

36. Hirose R, Suita S, Taguchi T, et al: Extralobar pulmonary sequestration mimicking cystic adenomatoid malformation in prenatal sonographic appearance and histologic findings. J Pediatr Surg 30:1390–1393, 1995.

37. Creasy R: Mirror syndromes. In Goodlin RC (ed): Care of the Fetus. New York: Masson, 1979, pp 48–50.

38. Chao A, Monoson RF: Neonatal death despite fetal therapy for cystic adenomatoid malformation. J Reprod Med 35:655–657, 1990.

39. Clark SL, Vitale DJ, Minton SD, et al: Successful fetal therapy for cystic adenomatoid malformation associated with second trimester hydrops. Am J Obstet Gynecol 157:294–297, 1987.

40. Bernaschek G, Deutinger J, Hansmann M, et al: Feto-amniotic shunting: Report of the experience of four European centres. Prenat Diagn 14:821–833, 1994.

41. Adzick NS, Harrison MR: Fetal surgical therapy. Lancet 343:897–902, 1994.

42. Langer JC, Harrison MR, Schmidt KG, et al: Fetal hydrops and death from sacrococcygeal teratoma: Rationale for fetal surgery. Am J Obstet Gynecol 160:1145–1150, 1989.

43. Jennings RW, Adzick NS, Longaker MT, et al: New techniques in fetal surgery. J Pediatr Surg 27:1329–1333, 1992.

44. Hedrick MH, Jennings RW, MacGillivray TE, et al: Endoscopic catheterization of placental vessels for chronic fetal venous access. Surg Forum 43:504–505, 1992.

45. Kleinman CS, Donnerstein RL, DeVore GR, et al: Fetal echocardiography for evaluation of in utero congestive heart failure: A technique for study of nonimmune hydrops. N Engl J Med 306:568–575, 1982.

46. Fortunato S, Lombardo S, Dantrell J, Ismael S: Intrauterine laser ablation of a fetal cystic adenomatoid malformation with hydrops: The application of minimally invasive surgical techniques to fetal surgery. Am J Obstet Gynecol 177:S84, 1997.

47. Ueda K, Gruppo R, Martin L, Bove K: Rhabdomyosarcoma arising in a congenital cystic adenomatoid malformation. Cancer 40:383–388, 1977.

48. Benjamin DR, Cahill JL: Bronchoalveolar carcinoma of the lung and congenital cystic adenomatoid malformation. Am J Clin Pathol 95:889–892, 1991.

49. Murphy JJ, Blair GK, Fraser GC, et al: Rhabdomyosarcoma arising within congenital pulmonary cysts: Report of three cases. J Pediatr Surg 27:1364–1367, 1992.

50. d'Agnostino S, Bonoldi E, Dante S, et al: Embryonal rhabdomyosarcoma of the lung arising in cystic adenomatoid malformation. J Pediatr Surg 32:1381–1383, 1997.

51. Ribet ME, Copin MC, Soots JG, Gosselin BH: Bronchioloalveolar carcinoma and congenital cystic adenomatoid malformation. Ann Thorac Surg 60:1126–1128, 1995.

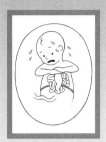

CHAPTER *20*

The Fetus with a Diaphragmatic Hernia

MICHAEL R. HARRISON

Congenital diaphragmatic hernia (CDH) is an anatomically simple defect that can be easily corrected by removing the herniated viscera from the chest and closing the diaphragm.[1, 2] However, most infants with CDH die of pulmonary insufficiency despite optimal postnatal care because their lungs are too hypoplastic to support extrauterine life. The pulmonary hypoplasia, universally seen with CDH, has been well documented clinically and experimentally; it appears to be caused by compression of the developing fetal lung by herniated bowel.

The clinical spectrum of CDH ranges from minimally affected infants who do well with modern neonatal care to severely affected infants who die despite all interventions. Two decades of research have led to advances in prenatal diagnosis of CDH and have better defined the natural history of CDH. Fetuses with CDH now can be stratified into low- and high-risk groups based on gestational age at diagnosis, presence or absence of liver herniation, and an estimation of lung size: the lung-to-head ratio (LHR). Low-risk fetuses have an excellent chance of survival with postnatal therapy. High-risk fetuses have a terrible prognosis without intervention to increase lung size before birth. For fetuses without liver herniation, complete repair of the defect by open surgery works, but is not necessary because this group does equally well without fetal surgery. Fetuses with liver herniated into the chest and low LHR most need in utero treatment, but complete repair has proved technically impossible. Temporary tracheal occlusion is a new strategy to achieve fetal lung growth before birth that appears promising experimentally and clinically, and can now be accomplished without open surgery using newly developed fetoscopic techniques (FET-ENDO clip).

Natural History of Congenital Diaphragmatic Hernia

CDH occurs in approximately 1 in 2,400 births.[3] Neonates with CDH often die soon after birth because lung tissue compressed by the herniated viscera is inadequately developed, and hypoplasia of the pulmonary vascular bed leads to pulmonary hypotension or persistent fetal circulation syndrome. As a result of advances in ultrasonography, CDH is now diagnosed before birth with increasing frequency. Because the family can choose to terminate the pregnancy, carry to term for postnatal management, or attempt fetal intervention,[4] accurate counseling regarding the expected outcome is crucial.

The outcome reported for infants with CDH (and other life-threatening defects that can now be diagnosed before birth) varies widely, depending on whether the disease is studied before or after birth. Tertiary neonatal referral centers with extracorporeal membrane oxygenation (ECMO) available report that 70 to 76% of neonates with CDH can be saved. In contrast, data on 150 fetuses with this condition show that only 20 to 27% survive.[5, 6] This discrepancy between the "visible" mortality reported for neonates with CDH and the mortality based on all prenatally diagnosed (i.e., unselected) cases has been called the "hidden mortality" of CDH.[2] The magnitude of the hidden mortality for CDH (and other life-threatening fetal diseases) is not known and cannot be accurately determined retrospectively or from birth defects monitoring programs because many cases go unrecognized unless there is an autopsy.[7, 8] On the other hand, the reports that CDH mortality exceeds 75%[5, 6] reflect the outcome of fetuses with life-threatening chromosomal and anatomic anomalies as well as those with isolated CDH.

A Prospective Study of Outcome

To accurately determine the outcome for potentially salvageable fetuses with isolated CDH diagnosed before 24 weeks' gestation, we identified 83 such fetuses and followed them prospectively.

There were 83 fetuses with well-documented CDH diagnosed before 24 weeks' gestation who did not have associated chromosomal or anatomic abnormalities and were delivered at a teritiary neonatal center.[9] Typically, most hernias were on the left side (75 of 83, 90%). Forty-eight of these 83 patients died, a mortality of 58% (95% confidence interval [CI], 41 to 75%). Of the 48 patients

297

who did not survive, seven died in utero. This unexpectedly high rate of fetal demise included four fetuses who died spontaneously near term, one who died after attempted version, and two who died after percutaneous umbilical sampling. Four nonsurvivors delivered prematurely because of polyhydramnios secondary to the fetal CDH. Sixteen nonsurvivors had severe respiratory distress at birth and could not be resuscitated sufficiently prior to ECMO therapy. Thirty-one neonates died despite resuscitation and urgent ECMO support that lasted from 2 to 30 days.

Of the 35 surviving patients, 22 received ECMO. Nine of these infants have severe chronic illness attributable to the intensity of their management; two have chronic lung disease that requires home oxygen; two have severe developmental delay secondary to intracranial hemorrhage sustained while on ECMO; and four are fed by gastrostomy. Another survivor has Simpson-Golabi syndrome. Neonatal outcome in this small sample did not correlate with hernia side (four neonates with right-sided hernias died) or demographic variables such as maternal age, indication for sonography, maternal health, or socioeconomic status.

Not unexpectedly, cost was related to the intensity and duration of neonatal care. Fetal and early neonatal demise were relatively inexpensive, generally less than $10,000. The median hospitalization expenditures for four nonsurvivors who received ECMO was $107,000 (range, $105,000 to $305,000), for seven survivors who received ECMO was $170,000 (range, $128,000 to $244,000), and for three survivors who did not receive ECMO was $171,000 (range, $28,000 to $194,000). The nine infants with severe long-term sequelae have ongoing costs.

The cumulative survival plot shown in Figure 20–1 shows that 34% of these infants died in utero or soon after birth. Without prenatal diagnosis or autopsy, many of these deaths would not be attributed to CDH. These cases represent a substantial hidden mortality.[9]

Hidden Mortality

This study documents for the first time the magnitude of the hidden mortality and explains how a disease diagnosed before birth can appear to have a different outcome than the same disease diagnosed after birth. When cumulative survival is plotted both before and after birth (Fig. 20–1), we begin to understand why previous studies from tertiary neonatal centers underestimated the hidden mortality of CDH. Patients reported from tertiary neonatal centers have already been selected by their ability to survive birth, resuscitation, and transport. The most severely affected do not make it to the neonatal centers. In our study, seven fetuses were stillborn, four others died soon after premature delivery, and six neonates died immediately after birth before ECMO could be started. If not diagnosed before birth, CDH would not be recognized as the cause of death in most of these stillborns unless an autopsy was performed. Even some of those correctly diagnosed after birth would not be reported as deaths in an ECMO registry. For example, three families in this series delivered at an ECMO center that has reported 70% survival for diaphragmatic hernia: two died immediately after birth and the third after ECMO; only the last patient would be reported as an ECMO failure. The inset of the Figure 20–1 demonstrates how survival based on postnatal cases appears to be approximately 63%, but when prenatally diagnosed cases are considered, survival is actually 42%. Of further concern is the finding that 9 of the 35 survivors have severe long-term sequelae attributable to their intensive support. One of these died after a year of repeated hospitalizations and multiple procedures for hydrocephalus,

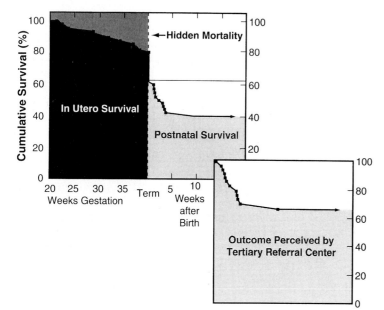

F I G U R E 20–1. A cumulative survival plot for 83 fetuses with isolated congenital diaphragmatic hernia diagnosed before 24 weeks' gestation. Seven fetuses died in utero, four died soon after premature delivery, and 16 died immediately after birth; most of these would not be recognized as having congenital diaphragmatic hernia unless an autopsy was performed. These deaths represent a significant hidden mortality that is not perceived when only infants seen at tertiary neonatal referral centers are considered (*inset*).

gastroesophageal reflux, and recurrent diaphragmatic hernia.

This study does not address the outcome for all fetuses with CDH diagnosed prenatally. We excluded from analysis 24 elective terminations and 11 fetuses with associated life-threatening anomalies who died soon after birth. Such associated anomalies may occur even more frequently than observed in our study because fetuses with obvious associated anomalies would not be referred.[10, 11] We also excluded 10 fetuses because they were diagnosed after 24 weeks' gestation; all of those survived.

CDH is now frequently diagnosed prior to 24 weeks' gestation, when the family can choose between termination or attempted treatment. This difficult choice has rested on widely discrepant estimates of outcome based on retrospective studies. This study establishes the mortality for isolated CDH in a referred sample of patients diagnosed before 24 weeks' gestation and followed prospectively. This information should assist families in making decisions about management. As new modes of therapy become available, including repair before birth, their effectiveness can be measured against the natural history and expected outcome of CDH.

Natural History: Timing of Herniation Determines Severity of Pulmonary Hypoplasia

Prenatal diagnosis has provided a new perspective on the important pathophysiologic features of fetal CDH. Fetal CDH appears to have a dynamic variation in the timing and amount of herniated viscera, and this accounts for the spectrum of severity seen postnatally (Fig. 20–2). Fetuses who have a relatively small volume of viscera (no dilated stomach) or herniate late in gestation generally do well with conventional treatment after birth, as demonstrated by the survival of most fetuses diagnosed later than 24 weeks' gestation. On the other hand, most fetuses with CDH are identifiable early in gestation, when a large volume of viscera has already herniated into the thorax. Most of these infants will die soon after birth from pulmonary hypoplasia, despite our most sophisticated (and expensive) neonatal intensive care.

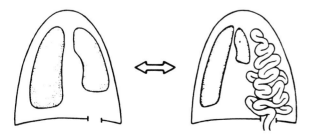

F I G U R E 20–2. Fetal CDH appears to be a dynamic process, and early herniation of a large volume of viscera through a large defect leads to severe lung hypoplasia and neonatal death.

Prenatal Sonographic Characteristics of CDH

Once CDH is suspected, either due to the presence of oligohydramnios, the presence of a mediastinal shift, or inability to demonstrate the normal fetal upper abdominal anatomy, a specific search for herniated abdominal contents within the thorax can be made. The herniated abdominal contents associated with left-sided CDH are the easiest to detect. The echo-free, fluid-filled stomach and small bowel contrast dramatically compared with the more echogenic fetal lung. Herniated abdominal contents associated with right-sided CDH are more difficult to identify because of the subtle intrinsic difference in echogenicity between the fetal liver and the lung.

To increase certainty that apparently herniated abdominal organs truly lie within the thorax rather than high in the abdomen, one must image the chest in a true transverse plane and use thoracic bony landmarks (e.g., the number of ribs from the thoracic apex, and inferior margin of the scapula). We believe that if the abdominal organs are at the same level as the four-chamber view of the heart, then the abdominal organs lie within the thorax and a CDH is present. Similarly, abdominal organs extending to the inferior margin of the scapula are probably herniated. Clearly, this aspect of the examination of CDH requires the greatest care in technique and interpretation. In a normal fetus, the slightest angulation off the true transverse plane may cause the heart and stomach, or heart and gallbladder, to lie in the same plane and lead to a false suspicion of CDH. If one can observe the diaphragm, then the delineation of the thorax from abdomen is defined, and the location of the herniated abdominal contents is easily confirmed. The actual delineation of the diaphragm is not always possible. The ability to identify a portion of the diaphragm itself is not helpful in excluding CDH, because most defects involve only a portion of the entire diaphragm.

When intervention is being considered, accuracy of diagnosis becomes crucial. Fortunately, in our experience, no false-positive diagnoses of CDH were made by ultrasound. However, it is quite possible that false-positive interpretations could arise in cases of cystic lung disease (e.g., congenital lobar emphysema, cystic adenomatoid malformation) or with mediastinal cystic processes (e.g., neurenteric cysts, bronchogenic cysts, thymic cysts). Although a fluid-filled structure may be present within the chest and may even cause a mediastinal shift, the fetal upper abdominal anatomy would be normal and, thus, would exclude a large CDH. It is particularly important to exclude large cystic adenomatoid malformations, which may actually decrease in size (and disappear) with increasing gestational age. In cases in which doubt exists, computed tomography (CT) or magnetic resonance imaging (MRI) may clarify the situation. Echocardiography will exclude cardiac malformations, and MRI may detect subtle associated malformations. However, Fryn's syndrome and multiple pterygium syndrome are very difficult to recognize and must specifically be sought to avoid inappropriate intervention.

Assessing Severity: Liver Herniation and Lung/Head Ratio

The most important factor in a family's decision about treatment is where their fetus is on the spectrum of severity (i.e., what are the chances of survival). Initial clinical experience suggested that fetuses with prenatally diagnosed CDH could be stratified into those with relatively "good" prognosis, presumably amenable to aggressive postnatal care, and those with "poor" prognosis who would potentially benefit from in utero intervention. A number of potential prognostic indicators have been suggested. A prospective study in 1994 suggested that detection of CDH prior to 25 weeks' gestation predicted up to 58% mortality.[9] In addition, polyhydramnios,[12] presence of an intrathoracic stomach,[13, 14] small lung/thorax transverse area ratio,[15, 16] and underdevelopment of the left heart[17] have been associated with poor prognosis. However, none of these parameters has been universally accepted or applied.

More recently, it has become clear that the two best prognostic indicators are the presence or absence of liver herniation into the chest across the diaphragmatic defect ("liver-up" versus "liver-down" CDH) and sonographic measurement of the LHR. When liver herniation was first recognized as a problem (because it made surgical repair difficult), accurate measurement of liver herniation was difficult because sonography could not distinguish liver from other herniated viscera. Then, color flow Doppler of the course of the umbilical vein and hepatic vessels was shown to accurately identify herniated liver. Liver substance can now be accurately distinguished by high-resolution ultrasound and by new ultrafast magnetic resonance scanners. In our prospective study, the absence of liver herniation (liver-down) predicted 75 to 80% survival with either fetal intervention or standard postnatal treatment.[18] A retrospective review of 48 patients with prenatally diagnosed CDH found 93% survival in the liver-down group versus 43% survival in the liver-up group.[19] These data suggest that the absence of liver herniation predicts a favorable prognosis and that most of these infants do well with postnatal therapy. Conversely, liver-up CDH has a poor prognosis without intervention.

The sonographically determined LHR has emerged as a good prognostic indicator for prenatally diagnosed CDH. The LHR is determined by obtaining a transverse axial image through the chest at the level of the four-chamber view of the heart at gestational age 24 to 26 weeks. Two measurements of the right lung are made— the longest length (in millimeters), then the length perpendicular to this initial measurement (in millimeters). The lung measurements are multiplied, then divided by head circumference (in millimeters). Thus, the LHR describes the relative size of the right lung at a given gestational age. LHR less than 1.0 is associated with mortality approaching 100%, whereas LHR greater than 1.4 is associated with no mortality. For LHR between 1.0 and 1.4, mortality is approximately 60%. Both retrospective and prospective studies have confirmed the usefulness of LHR in predicting postnatal survival.[20, 21]

When combined with sonographic information about the presence or absence of liver herniation, the LHR is very useful in counseling families about their choices in managing the fetus with a CDH (Fig. 20–3). For fetuses with liver-down CDH with a favorable LHR ($\geq$1.4), postnatal treatment is the best option because outcome is very favorable. For fetuses with liver-up CDH and a more ambiguous LHR (1.0 to 1.4), postnatal treatment may be suboptimal because the majority of these infants require very intensive care including ECMO and many will not survive.[20] For fetuses with liver-up and low LHR (<1.0), survival is very unlikely unless the severe pulmonary hypoplasia can be reversed before birth.

Experimental Pathophysiology: Pulmonary Hypoplasia is Reversible

Initial studies in the fetal lan.b were undertaken to unravel the pathophysiology and the reversibility of pulmonary hypoplasia in CDH. Fetal lambs had a silicone rubber balloon progressively inflated in their left hemithorax during the last trimester to simulate compression by herniated viscera.[22] Lambs with inflated intrathoracic balloons deteriorated rapidly at delivery despite maximal resuscitation, and soon died of severe respiratory failure. At autopsy, the lungs were severely hypoplastic. To determine if pulmonary hypoplasia was reversible, the balloon was deflated at 120 days' gestation (simulated correction).[23] All lambs with simulated correction of CDH were easily resuscitated and had normal pulmonary function. Simulated correction produced increased lung weight, air capacity, compliance, and area of the pulmonary vascular bed (Fig. 20–4). Because the fetal lung maintains remarkable plasticity even late in gestation, in utero repair may allow the hypoplastic lung in fetuses with CDH to grow and develop.

Although the sheep model demonstrated that in utero correction of CDH allowed the lung to grow and develop enough to ensure survival at birth, it differed from human CDH in several respects. The human diaphragmatic defect is present much earlier in gestation (the first trimester), although the viscera may not herniate until later. Also, although the high mortality of infants with CDH has been attributed to respiratory insufficiency from pulmonary parenchymal hypoplasia, other major physiologic abnormalities, such as pulmonary hypertension and persistent fetal circulation, inevitably contribute to poor outcome in these cases.

To address these vascular physiologic differences, CDH was created in fetal lambs early in gestation (60 days; term = 145 days), and morphometric analysis of the pulmonary vascular bed was subsequently performed.[24] The CDH was repaired in experimental lambs at 100 days' gestation, and an unrepaired group served as controls. The unrepaired CDH group demonstrated decreased cross-sectional area of the pulmonary vascular bed, decreased number of vessels per unit of area of the lung, and increased muscularization of the arterial tree, similar to findings in human CDH. In utero repair of CDH at 100 days ameliorated this abnormal pulmonary arteriolar muscle hyperplasia, allowed impressive

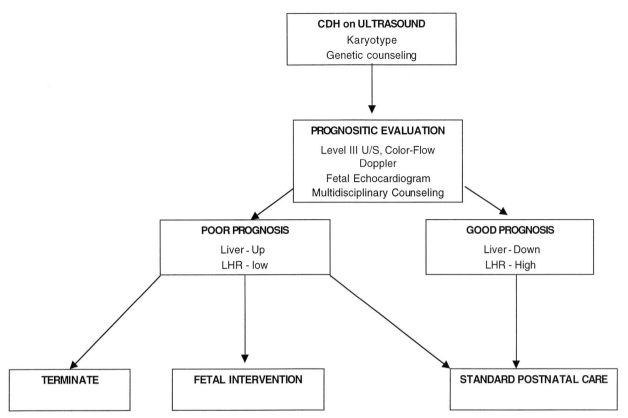

FIGURE 20–3. Diagnostic and treatment algorithm for a fetus with a congenital diaphragmatic hernia. The prognostic evaluation allows families to potentially have three choices: terminate, standard postnatal care, and fetal intervention. Termination is a choice of the family based on their understanding of the prognosis and their personal beliefs. If the fetus is in the good-prognosis group (liver in the abdomen, LHR favorable), postnatal care at a tertiary center with extracorporeal membrane oxygenation support capability is recommended. If the fetus is in the poor-prognosis group (liver in the hemithorax, LHR low), postnatal care at a center with extracorporeal membrane oxygenation support capability is recommended if the fetus is greater than 30 weeks' gestation, and fetal intervention if less than 30 weeks' gestation.

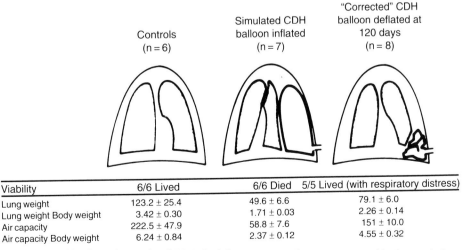

Viability	6/6 Lived	6/6 Died	5/5 Lived (with respiratory distress)
Lung weight	123.2 ± 25.4	49.6 ± 6.6	79.1 ± 6.0
Lung weight Body weight	3.42 ± 0.30	1.71 ± 0.03	2.26 ± 0.14
Air capacity	222.5 ± 47.9	58.8 ± 7.6	151 ± 10.0
Air capacity Body weight	6.24 ± 0.84	2.37 ± 0.12	4.55 ± 0.32

FIGURE 20–4. Fetal lambs with simulated CDH died despite maximal resuscitation and had severely hypoplastic lungs. Lambs "corrected" by balloon deflation in the middle of the last trimester had sufficient lung growth and development to permit survival at birth. Lung weight and air capacity were greater than for lambs with CDH but less than controls. (CDH = congenital diaphragmatic hernia.)

restoration of lung volume, and restored the pulmonary arterial tree almost to normal.[24]

After the experimental rationale for in utero treatment of CDH was established, surgical techniques for in utero repair were developed in a fetal lamb model. The diaphragmatic defect was created in the fetal lamb by making a hole in the left diaphragm at 100 days' gestation, allowing herniation of abdominal viscera and reliably producing pulmonary hypoplasia. At a second operation at day 120, the diaphragmatic hernia was repaired.[25] Initial attempts at repair were unsuccessful because reduction of viscera increased intra-abdominal pressure, causing decreased umbilical blood flow and subsequent fetal demise. A Silastic (Dow Corning Corp., Midland, MI) abdominal silo overcame this problem. In addition, intrathoracic volume displacement also affected umbilical flow by shifting the mediastinum and impeding venous return. To stabilize the mediastinum and to minimize the pressure-volume changes in the chest, the air in the partially empty left side of the chest was replaced by warm Ringer's lactate solution before the diaphragm was closed. When these changes were used for repair of the diaphragmatic hernia, six of ten lambs were viable after term delivery. At autopsy, the lungs were well expanded, histologically mature, and much larger than those of the controls. These studies showed that correction of diaphragmatic hernia is technically feasible when an appropriate procedure is used. This observation has been confirmed by several investigators.[26]

Experimental Pathophysiology of Tracheal Occlusion

The technique of complete repair developed in the lamb model worked in human fetuses only when the liver was not herniated. Complete repair failed when the liver was up in the chest because reducing the liver back into the abdomen resulted in acute obstruction of umbilical venous return.[27, 28] All attempts to salvage these fetuses (e.g., leaving the abdomen open, resecting herniated liver, placing a loose diaphragmatic patch over the liver) failed. For these severe cases with liver herniation, we continued to explore, in the fetal lamb model, other approaches to improving lung growth before birth.

Experimental work in our laboratory and others[29–34] has shown that fetal tracheal obstruction can correct the pulmonary hypoplasia associated with CDH. Normally, the fetal lung produces a continuous flow of lung fluid that exits through the trachea into the amniotic fluid. Experimentally, external drainage of fetal lung fluid retards lung growth, resulting in pulmonary hypoplasia,[35, 36] whereas tracheal obstruction markedly accelerates lung growth, resulting in pulmonary hyperplasia.[29–39] In fetal lambs with surgically created diaphragmatic hernias, tracheal obstruction expands the fetal lung, which not only pushes the viscera back into the abdomen but produces lungs that at birth are larger and functionally better than untreated controls (Fig. 20–5). Thus, fetal tracheal obstruction does more than passively distend the fetal lung; it appears to accelerate growth and improve function.[29–34] However, tracheal ob-

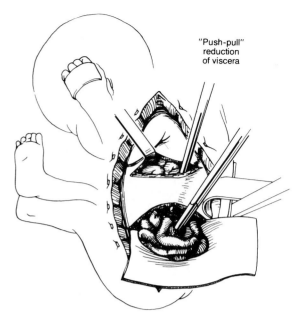

FIGURE 20–5. The viscera (stomach, bowel, spleen) are reduced through the defect and out onto the abdominal patch in the "two-step" repair of a diaphragmatic hernia.

struction may also delay or depress pulmonary maturation as measured by surfactant production.[40, 41]

To apply this strategy of tracheal obstruction to the treatment of human CDH, we had to develop techniques to achieve temporary tracheal occlusion that did not damage the fetal trachea and could be easily reversed at birth. Using the fetal lamb model, we developed and tested a variety of techniques including an internal occlusion device ("plug") made of water-permeable, expandable, polymeric foam that can be placed through the larynx, and external occlusion devices such as metal clips.[32] Translaryngeal placement of a foam plug appeared to be simple and easy to reverse at birth, but produced tracheomalacia. External metal clips were used in subsequent cases. The techniques for temporarily occluding the fetal trachea and reversing the obstruction at the time of birth were developed and tested in the lamb model prior to human application.

Prenatal Treatment of CDH in Human Fetuses: The Saga

Salvage of severely affected fetuses who have isolated diaphragmatic hernia has remained an unsolved problem for several decades. Although in mild to moderate cases, pulmonary hypoplasia may be reversible with aggressive postnatal surgical care (including ECMO), affected neonates often require weeks or months of treatment.[23–25, 42] ECMO is generally limited to 1 to 2 weeks, and although useful for marginal babies, it clearly cannot salvage severely affected neonates. Long-term support or replacement of lung function after birth will require either an artificial placenta or neonatal lung transplantation. Repair before birth with continued support on "placental ECMO" while the fetal lung grows and recovers would be ideal.[4, 25, 43] Unfortunately, application to human fetuses has proven difficult and the history of this enterprise over the last two decades (outlined in the series of papers titled "Correction of CDH in Utero," I–IX) epitomizes the saga of fetal surgery itself.

A Prospective Trial of Open Repair

In fetal sheep, in utero repair of CDH allows the fetal lung to grow and decreases both morbidity and mortality.[23] Early experience with repair in human fetuses showed that fetal correction is technically feasible in selected cases.[4, 27, 44] The problem of liver herniation into the chest, however, was particularly challenging. Attempts to reduce the incarcerated liver kinked the umbilical vein, resulting in fetal death.[43] Clearly, an open repair is not a viable option for these fetuses.

In fetuses with evidence of liver herniation, in utero repair proved to be technically possible (Fig. 20–5). Although in utero repair has the potential to improve lung growth and development, whether repair would improve pulmonary growth and function enough to improve outcome could not be determined without a proper trial. To critically assess the role of fetal surgery in the treatment of CDH without liver herniation, a prospective trial was designed and conducted. This study examined the safety and efficacy of open fetal surgery for selected cases of CDH.[18]

Four fetuses in whom CDH without liver herniation was diagnosed underwent open fetal surgery for repair of the CDH. Seven comparison fetuses were treated conventionally. Neonatal mortality was the principal outcome variable. Secondary outcome variables included death of all causes until 2 years of age, number of days of ventilatory support, length of hospital stay, requirement for ECMO, and total hospital charges.

There was no difference in survival between the fetal surgery group and the postnatally treated comparison group (75% vs. 86%). Fetal surgery patients were born more prematurely than the comparison group (32 weeks' vs. 38 weeks' gestation). Length of ventilatory support and requirement for ECMO were equivalent in the fetal surgery group and the postnatally treated comparison group. Length of hospital stay and hospital charges did not differ between the groups.

This study demonstrated that open fetal surgery is physiologically sound and technically feasible, but does not improve survival over standard postnatal treatment in the subgroup of CDH fetuses without liver herniation, primarily because overall survival in this subgroup is favorable with or without intervention.

Fetuses with CDH without liver herniation, liver-down CDH, can undergo repair successfully in utero, but this may not offer a significant advantage compared with postnatal care. In our series, in utero correction of these selected cases of CDH did not improve survival. However, despite greater prematurity in the fetal surgery group (32 weeks' gestation at birth vs. 38 weeks' gestation in the comparison group), these infants had comparable pulmonary function as measured by ventilator and ECMO requirements. Two of the fetal surgery patients required far less ventilatory support than comparison infants. In the comparison group, a number of

the patients also had characteristics that we now recognize as good prognostic indicators: diagnosis of fetal CDH after 24 weeks' gestation and minimal mediastinal shift.[21] The comparable pulmonary function in the more premature fetal surgery group may be the result of improved lung growth after fetal repair, suggesting that the rationale for in utero correction of CDH is physiologically sound.

Total hospital charges were higher in the fetal surgery group than in the comparison group, but this difference did not reach statistical significance. Both groups had costs comparable to previously published average cost for postnatally treated CDH survivors ($177,000).[45] The financial data, however, have a number of shortcomings. First, a set fee was negotiated for fetal evaluation and surgery as part of the trial ($17,449), so cost estimate for the fetal surgery group may not accurately represent the cost of performing this procedure outside the trial. Second, two patients in the fetal surgery group and three in the comparison group received care at referring institutions. Hospital charges inevitably vary from site to site. Still, we can conclude that although fetal intervention provided no significant savings, it incurred no significantly excess cost when compared with postnatal treatment.

The overall mortality rate in our study was low. Both treatment and comparison groups had survival much greater than is reported for CDH in general (75% and 86%, respectively, in our groups vs. up to 60% in all cases of CDH). Moreover, neither of the deaths (one neonatal death in the treated group, one in utero death in the comparison group) was attributable to pulmonary hypopolasia. These results are consistent with previous data showing 100% survival in ten fetuses with prenatally diagnosed liver-down CDH.[21] Pulmonary hypoplasia appears to be less severe in these cases, predicting a good chance of survival regardless of treatment modality. Indeed, the most significant advances to come from two decades of experimental and clinical work on fetal CDH have been the development of sonographic predictors of outcome (liver herniation, LHR[21, 46]) and development of anesthetic and surgical techniques that have allowed correction of other fetal defects (urinary tract obstruction, cystic adenomatoid malformation, sacrococcygeal teratoma).[47]

Despite the favorable response of the fetal lungs after in utero repair, this approach did not improve survival compared with postnatal care. In fact, the one death in the fetal survival group was directly attributable to the fetal intervention (maternal hypotension and/or perioperative indomethacin administration). Clearly, CDH without liver herniation usually has a more benign course and better prognosis than CDH with liver herniation regardless of treatment modality. Given the potential risks of fetal surgery to both mother and fetus, we abandoned in utero repair for CDH without liver herniation.

Dilemma: The High-Risk Fetus Proves Unfixable

By the mid-1990s, much of the uncertainty about the natural history and prognosis for a fetus with CDH had been resolved by two decades of experimental work and clinical observation. Fetuses with liver herniation into the hemithorax and a low LHR have a very poor prognosis with conventional treatment after birth. The only CDH fetuses who are now candidates for intervention in our program are those with poor prognosis by virtue of liver herniation, low LHR, and early diagnosis.

The high-risk CDH fetus could now be identified, but attempts to salvage those fetuses by complete repair proved unsuccessful. For fetuses with liver-up CDH and an unfavorable LHR, prognosis is grim and in utero intervention may offer the only hope for survival. Attempts at open repair of CDH in these fetuses proved impossible because of obstruction of umbilical venous return when the liver was reduced in the abdomen.[27] In the most frustrating and agonizing part of the CDH saga, liver-up fetuses proved unfixable despite extensive efforts to solve this problem of umbilical vein kinking using a variety of techniques.

A New Approach: Temporary Tracheal Occlusion or "PLUG" (Plug the Lung Until It Grows)

In the course of exploring the pathophysiology of CDH, experimental work has shown that fetal tracheal obstruction can improve the pulmonary hypoplasia associated with CDH. Throughout gestation, the fetal lung produces lung fluid that exits through the trachea into the amniotic fluid. External drainage of lung fluid in experimental animals retards lung growth, resulting in pulmonary hypoplasia, whereas prevention of lung fluid efflux by tracheal occlusion accelerates lung growth, resulting in pulmonary hyperplasia. In fetal lambs with surgically created diaphragmatic hernia, tracheal obstruction expands the fetal lung, reduces the herniated viscera back into the abdomen, and produces lungs that are larger and functionally better at birth than untreated controls.[29-34]

The optimal method of temporary tracheal occlusion is still evolving. Because of concern that tracheal occlusion could produce fetal lung overdistention requiring reversal before delivery, we initially developed and tested in fetal lambs a cuffed endotracheal tube or tracheostomy tube connected to a magnetically activated valve. However, these more complicated devices frequently malfunctioned in animals and did not appear necessary because we did not see lung overdistention in our initial cases. We tested both internal occlusive devices and external clips, and tried to assess the efficacy in producing complete occlusion, their potential for tracheal damage, and their ease of reversibility at birth. In case 1, an internal foam plug performed well experimentally and achieved a good result, but produced enough tracheomalacia that the baby required prolonged stenting of the affected cervical tracheal segment. When the internal foam plug was made smaller (in case 2), we saw no lung enlargement, presumably because the plug leaked. External clips also performed well experimentally. Although theoretically attractive, the spring-loaded aneurysm clip did not work clinically, presum-

ably because it allowed some leakage of lung fluid. The external metal hemoclip worked best; it produced complete, easily reversible occlusion without tracheal damage in four cases. We continue to explore experimentally newer materials and other methods of temporarily obstructing the fetal trachea, including devices that may allow the occluding device to be turned on or off noninvasively to modulate lung growth.

The Ex Utero Intrapartum Treatment (EXIT) Procedure

Because delivery in anything other than an optimal controlled environment would lead to rapid demise from airway obstruction, we modified the anesthetic and surgical technique of cesarean delivery to maintain fetoplacental circulation while the fetal airway is secured (Fig. 20-6). The mother is anesthetized using high doses of inhaled halogenated agents supplemented with single doses of nitroglycerin or terbutaline as necessary to ensure complete uterine relaxation throughout the procedure. The fetal head and shoulders are delivered through the previous hysterotomy, but the lower torso

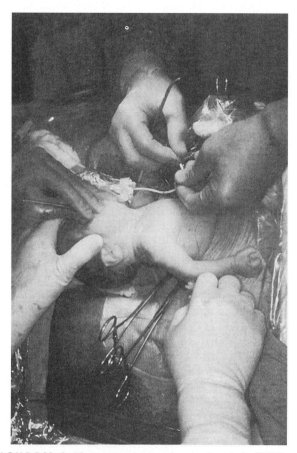

FIGURE 20-6. The ex utero intrapartum tracheoplasty (EXIT) procedure is a modification of cesarean delivery that allows time to correct the fetal tracheal obstruction and secure the airway while the fetus remains on placental support. The upper torso is brought out of the uterus, and a bronchoscope is passed to observe the tracheal lumen while the external clip is removed.

and umbilical cord remain within the uterus. Because the umbilical circulation provides gas exchange, there is adequate time to expose the fetal neck, pass a bronchoscope, remove an internal plug or external clip, repair the trachea (if necessary), secure the airway with an endotracheal or tracheostomy tube, suction lung fluid, administer surfactant, and begin ventilation—all before the umbilical cord is divided and the baby delivered.

This technique evolved with experience.[48] Initially we delivered the entire fetus and worked on the maternal abdomen, but found that the torso and umbilical cord could be left inside while the head and neck were exposed. In the first cases, we opened the trachea to remove the internal plug, and closed it surgically. In the first two cases with external clips, we opened the neck incision to remove the clip. Finally, we learned that the clip could be pulled off the trachea without reopening the neck incision. Intraoperative bronchoscopy allowed us to monitor the "unplugging," visualize the trachea at the area of previous occlusion by the clip, and examine the distal trachea before intubation. In several cases, the EXIT procedure proved to be lifesaving because removing the clip proved difficult and the baby could be maintained on the umbilical circulation when establishing an airway.

Initial Experience with Open "PLUG"

The initial clinical experience suggested that impeding the normal egress of fetal lung fluid by controlled tracheal obstruction can enlarge the hypoplastic lungs, partially reduce the viscera back into the abdomen, and improve lung function at birth.[49] Although plagued by a variety of frustrating problems and complications, this early experience showed that the strategy of occluding the fetal trachea to induce growth and development of the fetal lung works in human fetuses as it did in the experimental fetal lamb model. In the five cases in which the lungs enlarged in utero (noted on serial sonograms), beginning about 1 week after the trachea was occluded, lung function after birth and/or lung size at autopsy suggested that the lungs were no longer hypoplastic. Some of the herniated viscera had been reduced by the time of birth, as evidenced by a nonscaphoid abdomen and by the anatomic findings at the time of postnatal repair. In contrast, when the fetal lung did not enlarge before birth, probably because the trachea was not completely occluded by the small internal foam plug (case 2) or the springy aneurysm clip (case 6), the lungs remained hypoplastic. We have noted in fetal lambs that even a small leak of fetal lung fluid appears to abrogate the effect on lung development (Figs. 20–7 and 20–8; Table 20–1).

This initial clinical experience illustrates the agonizing and frustrating process of attempting to develop techniques to salvage human fetuses based on physiologic observations made in fetal animals. Most of the complications that limited success and contributed to morbidity and cost in this series, especially preterm labor and delivery, were related to the hysterotomy, not the fetal problem. Achieving fetal tracheal occlusion without hys-

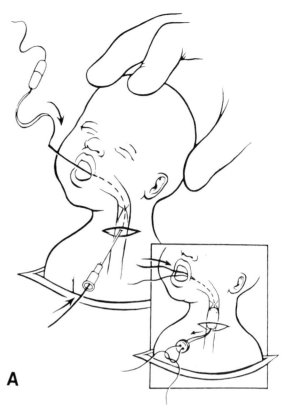

A

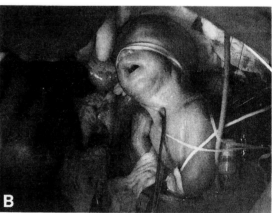

B

FIGURE 20–7. *A,* The procedure used (in cases 1 and 2) to place an internal foam "plug" in the trachea of a fetus with diaphragmatic hernia. A flexible guidewire is passed retrograde up the trachea and out of the mouth. A suture attached to the leading end of the plug is fixed to the wire and pulled through the larynx. The plug is secured in the upper trachea by tying the suture to a button. *B,* The plug being pulled into the trachea of the fetus's mouth.

terotomy should improve the risk/benefit calculus and would allow this promising physiologic strategy to be applied successfully. Clearly, the techniques for fetal surgery in general and for temporary tracheal occlusion and its reversal in particular were still evolving.

The Evolution of Fetoscopic Tracheal Occlusion

Occluding the trachea to accelerate lung growth in fetuses with congenital diaphragmatic hernia is a novel

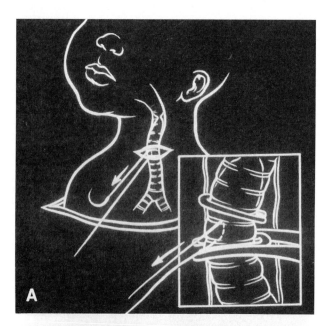

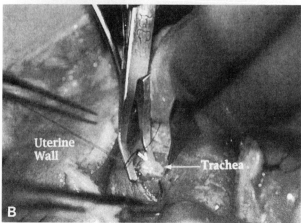

FIGURE 20–8. *A,* The procedure used (in cases 3 and 8) to place an external clip on the trachea of a fetus with diaphragmatic hernia. The technique and type of clip evolved with experimental and clinical experience. *B,* The clip being applied. The fetal trachea is exposed and the clip is about to be applied. In subsequent cases, we learned to do this without bringing the fetal head out of the uterus.

strategy supported by extensive experimental work.[29, 30] One method of occlusion, opening the uterus and directly occluding the fetal trachea using a metal clip, is limited in part by complications of the large uterine incision.[50] Preterm labor after a large uterine incision is inevitable. By using fetoscopy to perform fetal surgery, the uterine incision is smaller and hopefully the risk of preterm labor is reduced as well. Building on fetoscopic techniques (FETENDO), we have been refining strategies of tracheal occlusion[4–6] and have now applied these strategies clinically.

When we first attempted this strategy of temporary tracheal occlusion, the technique of tracheal occlusion evolved from an internal plug to an external clip, and the EXIT procedure was developed for unplugging the trachea at the time of birth.[51] We learned that temporary occlusion of the fetal trachea accelerates fetal lung growth and ameliorates the often fatal pulmonary hypo-

plasia associated with severe CDH. Although the strategy proved physiologically sound and technically feasible, complications encountered during the evolution of these techniques, related principally to open fetal surgery, limited survival.[49, 50]

Recently, several technical advances have made it possible to occlude the fetal trachea endoscopically.[48, 52–54] Fetoscopic tracheal occlusion has been successfully performed in fetal lambs using miniaturized instruments and a variety of new techniques.[54] Fetal endoscopic surgery presented a host of new challenges not encountered in laparoscopic surgery. These include variable placental location, a uterine wall with layers of membranes tenuously attached to the anterior surface and a variable wall compliance, a mobile fetus, the necessity of operating within a fluid medium impairing vision and the ability to coagulate, a cramped operative field, and suboptimal monitoring of the fetus with no intravenous access. These obstacles have been largely overcome (Fig. 20–9). An experienced sonographer is crucial for identifying the placenta and fetal position for the safe introduction of trocars. Although the prevention of membrane separation remains a formidable challenge, we have found that balloon-tip trocars work well. Currently, we place two 5-mm trocars and one 10-mm trocar (Fig. 20–10). The development of miniaturized instruments and telescopes has also allowed significant advances. We use continuous warm saline irrigation to avoid the potential complications of carbon dioxide insufflation (air embolism or fetal acidosis) (Fig. 20–11). When closing the uterine trocar sites, it is essential to be certain that all membranes are incorporated into the closure. Given the multiple new challenges, initial human cases begin with a maternal laparotomy and subsequent insertion of trocars into the uterus. This approach allows the safest introduction of trocars, manual fetal manipulation, and palpation of the uterus to ensure adequate relaxation and the appropriate volume of infused saline. We secure the fetal position with a temporary transuterine suture through the fetal chin, and place a T-bar (using sonographic guidance) into the fetal trachea to aid in the neck dissection (Fig. 20–12). By bathing the fetus in warm saline throughout the case, the physiologic milieu of the fetus was maintained. Despite a high volume of fluid perfused into the uterus (up to 40 L), less than 3% was systematically absorbed and never caused hypervolemia or altered maternal electrolytes.

This procedure is the culmination of years of experimental work on the use of trachea occlusion for the prenatal treatment of congenital diaphragmatic hernia. The evolution from an open procedure to a fetoscopic procedure was an obvious progression. Because it is minimally invasive, a fetoscopic procedure is advantageous for both mother and fetus. Small holes lessen the uterine insult and may decrease preterm labor. Allowing the fetus to remain in its "natural environment" may require less fetal manipulation, attenuate temperature changes in the amniotic fluid, and ultimately decrease the fetal stress response. In this case, the mother and fetus did remarkable well postoperatively and did not suffer any major morbidity.

T A B L E 20–1. PROCEDURES AND LUNG RESPONSE

PATIENT NO.	MATERNAL AGE (YR)/PARITY	GESTATIONAL AGE (WK) AT TIME OF			Enlargement Before Birth*	RESPONSE OF THE LUNG			COMMENTS
		Fetal Procedure	Fetal Surgery	Fetal Delivery		Function After Birth†	Lung/Body‡	Pulmonary Hypoplasia	
1	24/G1,P0	Foam plug	26.5	30	3	3		No	Good pulmonary function at 20 mo
2	24/G2,P1	Foam plug	26.5	30.5	0	0	0.0058	Yes	Plug not occlusive (?); pulmonary death at birth
3	34/G4,P3	Hemoclip (3)	25	29	3	—	0.016	No	Umbilical cord accident
4	41/G3,P2	Hemoclip (1)	24.9	28	3	3	0.021	No	Intracranial hemorrhage; support withdrawn
5	19/G1,P0	Aneurysm clip (11 mm)	27	27	—	—	0.0078	Yes	Tocolytic failure (aborted)
6	35/G2,P0	Aneurysm clip (15 mm)	27.3	33.7	1	1	0.032	§	Clip not occlusive (?); pulmonary death at 4 mo
7	23/G1,P0	Hemoclip (2)	26	29.3	3	4	0.024	No	Discharged home, unrelated bowel necrosis at 4 mo
8	23/G1,P0	Hemoclip (2)	26.9	32	2	1	0.018	No	CNS damage at 4 mo; support withdrawn

* Lung enlargement before birth was determined by serial sonographic assessment of the size of both lungs (right always greater than left), and the degree to which rightward mediastinal shift was corrected and viscera were reduced from the chest: 0, none; 1, minimal; 2, moderate; 3, good; 4, excessive.
† Lung function after birth was determined by clinical assessment and the need for respiratory support: 0, unable to resuscitate; 1, intensive support + ECMO; 2, intensive support; 3, moderate support; 4, minimal support.
‡ The ratio of combined lung weight (right and left) to body weight at the time of autopsy. Pulmonary hypoplasia is likely if the ratio is <0.015 before 28 weeks' gestation <0.012 after 28 weeks' gestation.
§ In case 6, the lung was traumatized and edematous owing to months of intensive support.

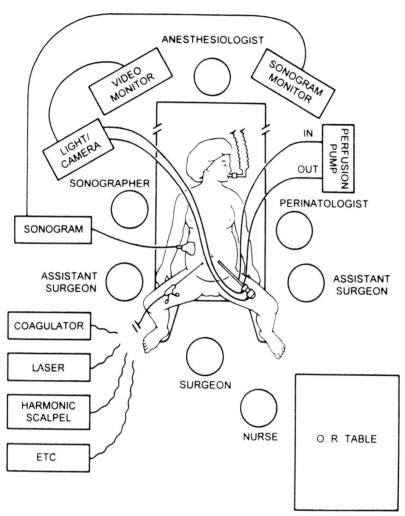

F I G U R E 20–9. Bird's eye view of the operating room setup for the fetoscopic tracheal occlusion procedure. Only two of the four ports are pictured.

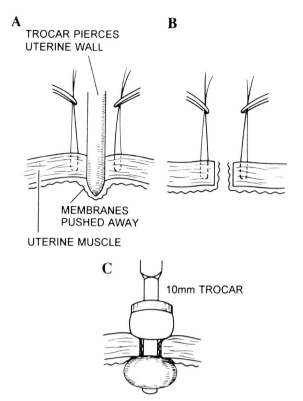

A

TROCAR PIERCES
UTERINE WALL

MEMBRANES
PUSHED AWAY

UTERINE MUSCLE

B

C

10mm TROCAR

FIGURE 20-10. Sutures are placed and the myometrium is pierced with the trocar (*A*). The membranes are pulled into the tract, facilitating separate closure (*B*). A 10-mm trocar has been inserted and the 25-cc balloon inflated (*C*). The compressible foam flange and the balloon together seal the membranes, prevent amniotic fluid leak during the procedure, and control myometrial bleeding.

Initial Experience with FETENDO Clip

Initial experience with tracheal occlusion by open fetal surgery demonstrated that the strategy of tracheal occlusion works to reverse pulmonary hypoplasia in human fetuses with CDH, as it did in sheep, and that the tech-

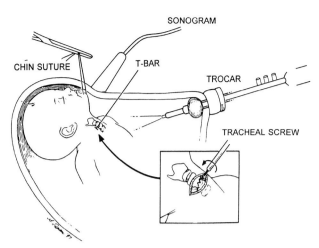

FIGURE 20-12. Under sonographic guidance, the fetus neck is exposed and the head stabilized by placement of a transuterine chin suture, and a T-bar is placed in the fetal trachea to aid in localizing the midline fetal neck. After anterior trachea dissection, a tracheal "screw" is placed in the tracheal wall and anterior traction is applied, allowing safe posterolateral tracheal dissection.

nique of an external clip is superior to an internal plug. However, complications associated with the hysterotomy and open surgery severely compromised survival.[49] We then developed video-fetoscopic techniques (FETENDO) that allow dissection of the fetal trachea and placement of an occluding clip without hysterotomy. We then applied the FETENDO clip procedure in eight human fetuses and compared this with 13 similar cases who were offered the procedure but elected postnatal treatment and 13 cases who underwent tracheal occlusion by open fetal surgery.

Over a 3-year period at the UCSF Fetal Treatment Center, 34 of 86 fetuses with an isolated left CDH met criteria for the poor-prognosis group. Thirteen families chose postnatal treatment at an ECMO center, 13 underwent open fetal tracheal occlusion, and eight underwent fetoscopic tracheal occlusion.[50]

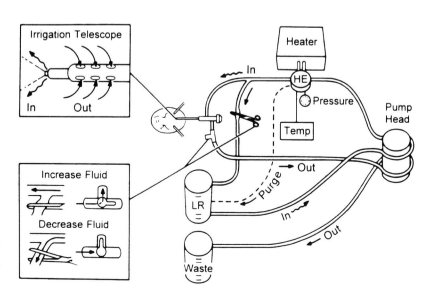

FIGURE 20-11. The high-flow irrigating system consists of an extracorporeal pump and a heat exchanger that continually circulate warmed lactated Ringer's solution via a sheath through which the telescope is placed (*inset*.)

Survival was 38% in the group treated by standard postnatal therapy, 15% in the open trachael occlusion group, and 75% in the FETENDO group. There were less postoperative pulmonary complications noted in mothers who underwent the FETENDO procedure versus the open tracheal occlusion procedure. All but one FETENDO clip patient had a striking physiologic response demonstrated by sonographic enlargement of the small left lung and documented postnatally by plain radiographs and its subjective appearance during repair of the CDH. In contrast, only 5 of the 13 open tracheal occlusion patients demonstrated lung growth.

The mothers tolerated the FETENDO surgery much better than open fetal surgery. Although not statistically significant at this stage, preterm labor, tocolysis, hospital stay, and discomfort were less with FETENDO surgery. The noncardiogenic pulmonary edema seen usually 24 to 36 hours after open fetal surgery was infrequently observed after FETENDO and, when present, was clinically mild. Premature rupture of membranes remains an unsolved problem. This complication may be associated with trocar insertion or may be related to the trocar site closure. The avoidance of a long hysterotomy appears to decrease the incidence of preterm labor by decreasing uterine injury. Future work in this area will need to address the unique contribution of uterine injury and manipulation during fetal surgery in causing the cascade of events leading to preterm labor.

The most striking finding was the positive effect of the FETENDO clip on growth of the fetal lung. Evidence of lung growth and correction of mediastinal shift by sonogram was subtle and slow to appear, usually requiring several weeks. The lungs, however, were strikingly enlarged on imaging studies after birth and at the time of surgical repair. Most importantly, lung function was surprisingly good despite premature delivery (Table 20–2).

For the subset of CDH fetuses with the worst prognosis (liver-up, low LHR), temporary occlusion of the fetal trachea accomplished without hysterotomy (FETENDO clip) appears to improve because another problem (multiple pterygium syndrome) became apparent after birth.[7] One other fetus had no lung response for unknown reasons (possibly not completely occluded). The other six showed good lung enlargement and good function after birth. Most importantly, a similar group of 13 patients who did not have fetal intervention but optimal postnatal care had strikingly worse outcomes (38% survival), emphasizing the very poor prognosis of this subset of fetal CDH. Finally, survival with tracheal occlusion by FETENDO appears to be superior to occlusion by open fetal surgery.

We are continuing to refine prenatal selection for CDH fetuses with the worst prognosis, and to develop better fetoscopic techniques to achieve temporary tracheal occlusion without hysterotomy. The strategy of tracheal occlusion to enlarge hypoplastic lungs appears sound, and the evolution of FETENDO surgery makes it technically feasible and perhaps applicable to other fetal diseases. The development of FETENDO surgery opens up new vistas in fetal treatment.

This initial experience suggests that fetuses with a left CDH who have liver herniation and a low LHR are at high risk of neonatal demise and appear to benefit from temporary tracheal occlusion when performed fetoscopically, but not when performed by open fetal surgery.

As with any promising but unproved therapy, the efficacy and safety of the FETENDO clip procedure must be established in a proper prospective trial. We have proposed a randomized trial comparing FETENDO clip to postnatal management for high-risk CDH fetuses.

Postnatal Treatment of CDH

Survival of a neonate with CDH requires intensive care nursery with ECMO capability. At birth, the infant should be intubated and a nasogastric tube placed to decompress the intrathoracic stomach. Ventilatory support (either conventional or high-frequency ventilation) can be then initiated. Ideally, prenatal diagnosis allows both the time and place of birth to be planned so that the infant can be delivered at a site with neonatal intensive care capabilities. In the absence of a prenatal diagnosis, an infant with CDH who is born at a facility without these capabilities should be transferred to a tertiary care nursery immediately after initial resuscitation. Timing of surgical correction remains controversial. Delayed repair has been widely advocated and has improved survival in some series. At present, it is generally agreed that urgent repair does not improve outcome for neonates with CDH. Decisions about the timing of repair are based on an individual infant's hemodynamic and respiratory stability.

ECMO has increasingly been used to rescue infants with CDH and respiratory failure that is unresponsive to maximal medical therapy, yet the safety and efficacy of ECMO in this setting remain controversial. In a number of series, ECMO has been reported to improve survival when compared with historical controls. Recently published retrospective studies from two major tertiary care centers suggest that high-frequency ventilation may be equivalent to ECMO in salvaging these critically ill neonates. Most centers currently reserve ECMO for those infants with severe respiratory failure in whom all other treatment modalities have been exhausted.

A number of innovative therapies have been developed that target the lung immaturity and vascular changes associated with CDH. One of the functional defects in these small, immature lungs is a relative deficiency of surfactant. Replacing surfactant by exogenous administration immediately after birth appears to improve lung compliance and pulmonary function in both preterm and term infants born with CDH. Inhaled nitric oxide (NO) is a potent vasodilator that has been shown to decrease vascular resistance in infants with persistent pulmonary hypertension. Because pulmonary hypertension exacerbates the respiratory failure seen in neonates with CDH, inhaled NO has been suggested as an adjunct to ventilatory support in these infants. A recent randomized, prospective trial, however, concluded that inhaled NO therapy did not improve mortality or reduce the need for ECMO in infants with CDH and respiratory

TABLE 20-2. THE FETAL, NEONATAL, AND MATERNAL CLINICAL CHARACTERISTICS AND OUTCOME FOR STANDARD POSTNATAL CARE, OPEN FETAL TRACHEAL OCCLUSION, AND FETENDO CLIP IN FETUSES WITH POOR PROGNOSTIC FACTORS*

PATIENT NO.	MATERNAL AGE/PARITY	GA AT DIAGNOSIS (WK)	LUNG TO HEAD RATIO	GA AT SURGERY	MATERNAL OUTCOME			FETAL/NEONATAL OUTCOME			
					Tocolytic Rx at Discharge	Maternal Hospital Stay (d)	Delivery GA (wk)/POD (d)	Fio₂†	ECMO	Complications/ Comment	Survival‡
Standard Postnatal Care											
1	22/G5,P0	19	0.6		—		33	1.0	No	Too small for ECMO	No
2	35/G1,P0	20	1.2		—		39		Yes		Yes
3	37/G2,P1	20	1.1		—		38		Yes		Yes
4	22/G3,P2	21	1.0		—		37		Yes		No
5	32/G5,P2	24	1.4		—		40		Yes		No
6	29/G1,P0	18	1.4		—		36		Yes		No
7	29/G4,P2	21	0.7		—		39		Yes		Yes
8	31/G2,P1	20	1.4		—		39		Yes		No
9	30/G2,P0	22	1.0		—		35		Yes		Yes
10	41/G8,P2	18	1.0		—		38	0.60	No	Death at 90 min of age	No
11	30/G2,P1	19	1.2		—		36	1.0	No		Yes
12	21/G2,P1	23	1.3		—		38		Yes		No
13	17/G1,P0	19	1.0		—		37		Yes		No
Mean	29 ± 2	20 ± 0.5	1.1 ± 0.1				37 ± 0.5				38%
Open Tracheal Occlusion											
1	24/G1,P0	23	—	27	N, T	16	30/21	0.48	No	Good pulmonary function	Yes
2	24/G2,P1	18	—	27	N	30	31/25	—	No	Plug not occlusive, death at birth	No
3	34/G4,P3	18	—	25	TP	6	29/30	—	No	Umbilical cord accident, IUFD	No
4	41/G3,P2	20	—	25	N, TP	12	28/22	0.40	No	Intracranial hemorrhage, support withdrawn	No
5	19/G1,P0	20	—	27	VA	10	27wk	—	No	Tocolytic failure, IUFD	No
6	35/G2,P0	20	—	27	TP		34/45	1.0	Yes	Plug not occlusive, death at 4 mo of age	No
7	23/G1,P0	19	—	26	TP	9	29/23	0.21	No	Discharged home, death from bowel necrosis at 4 mo	Yes
8	23/G1,P0	18	—	27	TP	8	32/36	—	Yes	CNS damage at 4 mo, support withdrawn	No

TABLE 20–2. THE FETAL, NEONATAL, AND MATERNAL CLINICAL CHARACTERISTICS AND OUTCOME FOR STANDARD POSTNATAL CARE, OPEN FETAL TRACHEAL OCCLUSION, AND FETENDO CLIP IN FETUSES WITH POOR PROGNOSTIC FACTORS* (Continued)

PATIENT NO.	MATERNAL AGE/PARITY	GA AT DIAGNOSIS (WK)	LUNG TO HEAD RATIO	GA AT SURGERY	MATERNAL OUTCOME			FETAL/NEONATAL OUTCOME			
					Tocolytic Rx at Discharge	Maternal Hospital Stay (d)	Delivery GA (wk)/POD (d)	Fio2†	ECMO	Complications/ Comment	Survival‡
9	31/G3,P2	23	1.4	26	NA	13	27/9	0.35	No	Hydrops from rapid, excessive lung growth	No
10	23/G2,P1	21	0.5	29	T	9	30/9	0.81	No	Ipsilateral sequestration	No
11	30/G3,P2	20	—	30	N, TP	12	33/16	—	No	Trisomy 12p, death at 4 hr of age	No
12	30/G3,P1	21	0.9	30	NA	11	31/8	—	No	Death at 1 hr of age	No
13	30/G1,P0	26	1.4	30	NA	26	33/19	1.0	No	Death at 30 hr of age	No
Mean*	**28 ± 1.7**	**21 ± 0.6**	**1.1 ± 0.2**	**27 ± 0.5**		**13.5 ± 2**	**30 ± 0.6/ 22 ± 3.2**				**15%**
FETENDO Clip											
1	24/G1,P0	23	1.4	30	N	11	33/21	0.21	No	Multiple pterygium syndrome, support withdrawn	No
2	34/G6,P3	16	1.1	30	NA	15	31/12	0.34	No	Normal at 16 mo of age	Yes
3	28/G3,P1	21	1.1	30	TP	9	33/21	0.45	No	Lung function good (1 L nasal prong O2), vocal cord paresis	Yes
4	30/G3,P0	19	1.2	28	TP	9	35/46	0.75	Yes	Lung function normal, vocal cord paresis	Yes
5	32/G11,P1 *	20	0.7	29	T	6	35/40	—	Yes	No biologic response	No
6	30/G3,P2	19	0.7	27	N	6	31/24	0.30	No	Moderate VSD	Yes
7	21/G2,P1	18	0.8	28	N	5	29/10	0.25	No	Large VSD	Yes
8	32/G4,P0	19	1.0	27	N	12	32/33	0.35	No	Lung function normal	Yes
Mean*	**29 ± 1.6**	**19 ± 0.7**	**1.0 ± 0.1**	**29 ± 0.5**		**9 ± 1.2**	**32 ± 0.7/ 26 ± 4.5**				**75%**

* Summary statistics (bold) presented as mean±standard error.
† Fio2 at 48 hours of age.
‡ Survival = discharged from hospital.
G, gravida; P, para; GA, gestational age; POD, postoperative day; IUFD, intrauterine fetal demise; NA, not applicable; T, terbutaline; N, nifedipine; TP, terbutaline pump; VSD, ventriculoseptal defect; Fio2, frequency of inspired oxygen.

failure, although the transient improvement in oxygenation seen in the NO-treated infants might allow stabilization, transport, and initiation of ECMO. Finally, partial liquid ventilation (PLV) has been explored as a way of improving gas exchange in a number of animal models, in adults with respiratory distress syndrome, and in a small number of neonates with infant respiratory distress syndrome. These studies have shown improvements in both oxygenation and lung compliance with PLV. While these preliminary data are intriguing, the safety and efficacy of PLV in neonates with CDH remains to be proven.

Fetal CDH: The Sequel

Despite intensive clinical and experimental efforts, mortality from CDH remains high. However, over two decades of research in multiple centers has led to a better understanding of the pathophysiology, prognosis, and treatment options for fetuses with CDH. It now appears that fetuses with prenatally diagnosed CDH can be stratified into high- and low-risk groups based on sonographic parameters. Fetuses with liver herniation into the chest and with favorable LHR have an excellent chance of survival with postnatal therapy. Prenatal diagnosis allows the timing and place of delivery to be planned in advance so that these infants can be treated in a tertiary care nursery with ECMO capability. Innovations such as inhaled NO and partial liquid ventilation hold promise for further improving the outcome in these neonates. Fetuses with liver herniation into the chest and an unfavorable LHR have a grim prognosis, and it is these fetuses who may benefit from in utero intervention. Recent advances such as fetoscopic temporary tracheal occlusion (FETENDO clip) may improve lung growth and development and may decrease mortality in these infants. FETENDO clip appears to work and, for the first time, offers hope to the fetus with high-risk CDH, but efficacy must be proven in a proper, randomized trial.

With many technical difficulties overcome, the final barriers to successful fetal repair—including proper patient selection and an effective strategy to reverse pulmonary hypoplasia—are beginning to yield. There may yet be an end to the long, often frustrating, frequently discouraging saga of fetal treatment for CDH.

REFERENCES

1. Harrison MR, deLorimier AA. Congenital diaphragmatic hernia. Surg Clin North Am 61:1023–1035, 1981.
2. Harrison MR, Bjordal RI, Langmark E, Knutrud O: Congenital diaphragmatic hernia: The hidden mortality. J Pediatr Surg 13:227–230, 1978.
3. Butler N, Claireaux AE: Congenital diaphragmatic hernia as a cause of perinatal mortality. Lancet 1:659–661, 1962.
4. Harrison MR, Adzick NS, Longaker MT, et al: Successful repair in utero of a fetal diaphragmatic hernia after removal of herniated viscera from the left thorax. N Engl J Med 322:1582–1584, 1990.
5. Adzick NS, Harrison MR, Glick PL, et al: Diaphragmatic hernia in the fetus: Prenatal diagnosis and outcome in 94 cases. J Pediatr Surg 20:357–361, 1985.
6. Sharland GK, Lockhart SM, Howard AJ, Allen LD: Prognosis in fetal diaphragmatic hernia. Am J Obstet Gynecol 166:9–13, 1992.
7. Wenstorn KD, Welner CP, Hanson JW: A five-year statewide experience with congenital diaphragmatic hernia. Am J Obstet Gynecol 165:838–842, 1991.
8. Torfs CP, Curry CJ, Bateson TF, Honore LK: A population-based study of congenital diaphragmatic hernia. Teratology 46:555–565, 1992.
9. Harrison MR, Adzick NS, Estes JM, Howell LJ: A prospective study of the outcome of fetuses with congenital diaphragmatic hernia. JAMA 271:382–384, 1994.
10. Benjamin DR, Juul S, Siebert JR: Congenital posterolateral diaphragmatic hernia: Associated malformations. J Pediatr Surg 23:899–903, 1988.
11. Thorpe-Beeston JG, Gordan CM, Nicolaides KH: Prenatal diagnosis of congenital diaphragmatic hernia: Associated malformations and chromosomal defects. Fetal Ther 4:21–28, 1989.
12. Stringer MD, Goldstein RB, Filly RA, et al: Fetal diaphragmatic hernia without visceral herniation. J Pediatr Surg 30:1264–1266, 1995.
13. Hatch E, Kendall J, Blumhagen J: Stomach position as an in utero predictor of neonatal outcome in left-sided diaphragmatic hernia. J Pediatr Surg 27:778–779, 1992.
14. Burge DM, Atwell JD, Freman NV: Could the stomach site help predict outcome in babies with left-sided congenital diaphragmatic hernia diagnosed antenatally? J Pediatr Surg 24:567, 1989.
15. Teixeira J, Sepulveda W, Hassan J, et al: Abdominal circumference in fetuses with congenital diaphragmatic hernia: Correlation with hernia content and pregnancy outcome. J Ultrasound Med 16:407, 1997.
16. Hasegawa T, Kamata SK, Imura K: Use of lung-thorax transverse area ratio in the antenatal evaluation of lung hypoplasia in congenital diaphragmatic hernia. J Clin Ultrasound 18:705, 1990.
17. Crawford DC, Wright VM, Drake DP, Allan LD: Fetal diaphragmatic hernia: The value of fetal echocardiography in the prediction of postnatal outcome. Br J Obset Gynecol 96:705, 1989.
18. Harrison MR, Adzick NS, Bullard KM, et al: Correction of congenital diaphragmatic hernia in utero VII: A prospective trial. J Pediatr Surg 32:1637–1642, 1997.
19. Albanese CT, Lopoo J, Goldstein RB, et al: Fetal liver position and perinatal outcome for congenital diaphragmatic hernia. Prenatal Diagn 18:1138–1142, 1998.
20. Lipshutz GS, Albanese CT, Feldstein VA, et al: Lung-to-head ratio predicts survival in prenatally diagnosed congenital diaphragmatic hernia. J Pediatr Surg 32:1634–1636, 1997.
21. Metkus AP, Filly RA, Stringer MD, et al: Sonographic predictors of survival in fetal diaphragmatic hernia. J Pediatr Surg 31:148–151, 1996.
22. Harrison MR, Jester JA, Ross NA: Correction of congenital diaphragmatic hernia in utero I. The model: Intrathoracic balloon produces fatal pulmonary hypoplasia. Surgery 88:174–182, 1980.
23. Harrison MR, Bressack MA, Churg AM, deLorimier AA: Correction of congenital diaphragmatic hernia in utero II. Simulated correction permits fetal lung growth with survival at birth. Surgery 88:260–268, 1980.
24. Adzick NS, Outwater KM, Harrison MR, et al: Correction of congenital diaphragmatic hernia in utero IV. An early gestational fetal lamb model for pulmonary vascular morphometric analysis. J Pediatr Surg 20:673–680, 1985.
25. Harrison MR, Ross NA, deLorimier AA: Correction of congenital diaphragmatic hernia in utero III. Development of a successful surgical technique using abdominoplasty to avoid compromise of umbilical blood flow. J Pediatr Surg 16:934–942, 1981.
26. Soper RT, Pringle KC, Scofield JC: Creation and repair of diaphragmatic hernia in the fetal lamb: Techniques and survival. J Pediatr Surg 19:33, 1984.
27. Harrison MR, Adzick NS, Flake AW, et al: Correction of diaphragmatic hernia in utero: VI. Hard-earned lessons. J Pediatr Surg 28:1411–1418, 1993.
28. MacGillivray TE, Jennings RW, Rudolph AM, et al: Vascular changes with in utero correction of diaphragmatic hernia. J Pediatr Surg 29:992–996, 1994.
29. Wilson JM, DiFiore JW, Peters CA: Experimental fetal tracheal ligation prevents the pulmonary hypoplasia associated with fetal nephrectomy: Possible application for CDH. J Pediatr Surg 28:1433–1440, 1993.
30. Hedrick MH, Estes JM, Sullivan KM, et al: Plug the lung until it grows (PLUG): A new method to treat congenital diaphragmatic hernia in utero. J Pediatr Surg 29:612–617, 1994.

31. DiFiore JW, Fauza DO, Slavin R, et al: Experimental fetal tracheal ligation reverses the structural and physiological effects of pulmonary hypoplasia in congenital diaphragmatic hernia. J Pediatr Surg 29:248–257, 1994.
32. Bealer JF, Skarsgard ED, Hedrick MH, et al: The "PLUG" odyssey: Adventures in experimental fetal tracheal occlusion. J Pediatr Surg 30:361–365, 1995.
33. Beierle EA, Langham MR, Cassin S: In utero lung growth in fetal sheep with diaphragmatic hernia and tracheal stenosis. J Pediatr Surg 31:141–146, 1996.
34. Luks FI, Gilchrist BF, Jackson BT, Piasiecki GJ: Endoscopic tracheal obstruction with an expanding device in the fetal lamb model. Fetal Diagn Ther 11:67–71, 1996.
35. Carmel J, Friedman F, Adams F: Fetal tracheal ligation and tracheal development. Am J Dis Child 109:452–456, 1965.
36. Alcorn D, Adamson T, Lambert T, et al: Morphologic effects of chronic tracheal ligation and drainage in the fetal lamb lung. J Anat 22:649–660, 1976.
37. Moessinger AC, Harding R, Adamson TM, et al: Role of lung fluid in growth and maturation of the fetal sheep lung. J Clin Invest 86:1270–1277, 1990.
38. Hooper SB, Man VKM, Harding K: Changes in lung expansion after pulmonary DNA synthesis and IGFII gene expression in fetal sheep. Am J Physiol 265:L403–L409, 1993.
39. Hooper SB, Harding R: Fetal lung liquid: A major determinant of the growth and functional development of the fetal lung. Clin Exp Pharmacol Physiol 22:235–247, 1995.
40. O'Toole S, Sharma A, Karamanoukian H, et al: Tracheal ligation does not correct the surfactant deficiency associated with CDH. J Pediatr Surg 31:1–16, 1996.
41. Bullard KM, Sonne J, Hawgood SB, et al: Tracheal ligation increases cell proliferation but decreases surfactant protein in fetal murine lungs in vitro. J Pediatr Surg 32:207–213, 1997.
42. Beals DA, Schlou BL, Vacanti JP, et al: Pulmonary growth and remodeling in infants with high risk congenital diaphragmatic hernia. J Pediatr Surg 27:997–1002, 1987.
43. Harrison MR, Langer JC, Adzick NS, et al: Correction of congenital diaphragmatic hernia in utero. V. Initial clinical experience. J Pediatr Surg 5:47–57, 1990.
44. Harrison MR, Adzick NS, Flake AW, et al: The CDH two-step: A dance of necessity. J Pediatr Surg 28:813–816, 1993.
45. Metkus AP, Esserman L, Sola A, et al: Cost per anomaly: What does a diaphragmatic hernia cost? J Pediatr Surg 30:226–230, 1996.
46. Bootstaylor BS, Filly RA, Harrison MR, et al: Prenatal sonographic predictors of liver herniation in congenital diaphragmatic hernia. J Ultrasound Med 14:515–520, 1995.
47. Harrison MR: Fetal surgery. Am J Obstet Gynecol 174:1255–1264, 1996.
48. Albanese CT, Jennings RW, Filly RA, et al: Endoscopic fetal tracheal occlusion: Evolution of techniques. Lancet 2:47–53, 1998.
49. Harrison MR, Adzick NS, Flake AW, et al: Correction of congenital diaphragmatic hernia in utero VIII: Response of the hypoplastic lung to trachael occlusion. J Pediatr Surg 31:1339–1348, 1996.
50. Harrison MR, Mychaliska GB, Albanese CT, et al: Correction of congenital diaphragmatic hernia in utero IX: Fetuses with poor prognosis (liver herniation and low lung-to-head ratio) can be saved by fetoscopic temporary tracheal occlusions. J Pediatr Surg 33:1017–1023, 1998.
51. Mychaliska GB, Bealer JF, Graf JL, et al: Operating on placental support: The ex utero intrapartum treatment procedure. J Pediatr Surg 32:227–231, 1997.
52. Estes JM, MacGillivary TE, Hedrick MH, et al: Fetoscopic surgery for treatment of congenital anomalies. J Pediatr Surg 27:950–954, 1992.
53. Skarsgard ED, Meuli M, VanderWall KJ, et al: Fetal endoscopic tracheal occlusion ("FETENDO-PLUG") for congenital diaphragmatic hernia. J Pediatr Surg 31:1335–1338, 1996.
54. VanderWall KJ, Bruch SW, Kohl T, et al: Fetoscopic tracheal clip occlusion for the treatment of congenital diaphragmatic hernia. J Pediatr Surg 31:1101–1104, 1996.

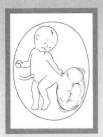

CHAPTER 21

The Fetus with Sacrococcygeal Teratoma

ALAN W. FLAKE

Sacrococcygeal teratoma (SCT) remains a relatively rare diagnosis, but is the most common tumor of the newborn, with an incidence of 1 in 35,000 to 40,000 live births.[1-4] In the past two decades, prenatal diagnosis of SCT has had a major impact on pre-, peri-, and postnatal management of fetuses effected by this tumor. It has become increasingly apparent that survival and optimal outcome of fetal SCT depend upon anticipation and recognition of pathophysiologic events in utero, which dictate specific obstetric and surgical management. The purpose of this chapter is to review our current understanding of fetal SCT and provide guidelines for optimal management.

Definition, Origin, and Pathology

SCT has been defined as either a neoplasm composed of tissues from all three germ layers[5, 6] or a neoplasm formed from multiple tissues foreign to the part and lacking organ specificity.[7] In either case the presence of multiple tissues suggests origin from a pluripotent cell, which is the basis for speculation about the embryogenesis of SCT. Evidence argues against SCT either having a germ cell origin or representing a form of fetus in fetu.[8] Rather, SCT is thought to arise from totipotent somatic cells[9] that originate from the primitive knot (Hensen's node) or caudal cell mass and escape normal inductive influences. Neverthelesss, a number of cases of fetus in fetu with remarkable resemblance to SCT have been described,[10-13] and there may be circumstances in which such etiologic distinctions are unclear. Although rare, familial cases of SCT have been described, suggesting a possible genetic predisposition. Familial tumors have all been predominantly presacral (American Academy of Pediatrics Surgical Section [AAPSS] classification type IV), and eight kindreds have been described.[14, 15]

Descriptions of the pathology of SCT are as diverse as the tissues themselves. From a clinical perspective, however, the histology of SCT fits into one of three categories[1, 16-18]: (1) tumor elements are all mature with little or no mitotic activity; (2) immature elements (embryonal) are present in varying amounts, particularly primitive neuroepithelium; or (3) vitelline differentiation (yolk sac) is present. It is important to emphasize that all three histologic groups have the potential for malignant or metastatic recurrence as endodermal sinus tumor.[19, 20] Children with SCT should be closely followed for at least 3 years for recurrence regardless of the initial histologic classification. Although once nearly uniformly fatal, prognosis for recurrent disease has improved significantly with modern chemotherapy.[19, 21]

Postnatal SCT

Presentation of SCT after birth can vary from appreciation of a massive external tumor at birth to delayed diagnosis of an entirely presacral tumor. SCT is uniformly intimately attached to the coccyx and has been classified by the relative amounts of presacral (or pelvic) and external tumor present (AAPSS classification).[22] AAPSS type I is completely external with no significant presacral component. At the other extreme, AAPSS type IV is completely internal with no visible external component. The value of this classification system relates to the ease of surgical resection, the timing of diagnosis, and the likelihood of malignancy. Type I SCTs are recognized at birth, are generally easily resectable, and have a very low incidence of malignancy. Type IV tumors, in contrast, are recognized only when they become symptomatic at a later age, and are frequently malignant at the time of diagnosis. Fortunately, the majority of tumors are type I or II. The clinical classification relates to histology with the relative likelihood of embryonal or malignant histology increasing with increasing AAPSS classification. Treatment consists of en bloc resection of the tumor and coccyx at the time of diagnosis. Outcome is dependent primarily upon whether the patient develops a malignant recurrence. In addition, there have been a number of disturbing reports of a surprisingly high rate of long-term functional abnormalities in children and adults following neonatal resection of benign SCT.[23-27] These include neurogenic bladder and other urologic functional abnormalities, issues with fecal incontinence, hypergonadotropic hypogonadism and sperm abnormalities in males, and vertebral anomalies.

Many of these may be related to surgical trauma during resection, rather than the tumor itself.

Prenatal SCT

With the widespread application and improved sophistication of obstetric sonography, the majority of SCTs are now detected in utero. Diagnosis depends upon the recognition of a characteristic caudal and/or intra-abdominal mass by a skilled sonographer. Diagnosis can routinely be accomplished during the second trimester[28] and has been reported as early as 13 weeks' gestation.[29]

Widespread application of screening sonography has resulted in an increased number of SCTs being detected in asymptomatic mothers. The most-common obstetric indication for sonography is a uterus too large for gestational dates that may be due to either rapid enlargement of tumor mass or the onset of associated polyhydramnios.[30] Other less common presentations include maternal preeclampsia, spotting, or rapid weight gain. Maternal serum screening is not useful in pregnancies complicated by SCT,[31] and amniotic fluid levels of α-fetoprotein or other markers have been inconsistent.[32-35]

Fetal SCT may be either cystic, solid, or mixed in sonographic appearance and may have bizarre echogenic patterns secondary to areas of tumor necrosis, cystic degeneration, internal hemorrhage, or calcification.[28, 36-39] Important sonographic observations include abdominal or pelvic extension, bowel or urinary obstruction, integrity of the fetal spine, and documentation of lower extremity function. The differential diagnosis (Fig. 21–1) of a cystic pelvic or sacral mass[28] includes myelomeningocele,[40] neuroectodermal cyst,[41] meconium pseudocyst,[42] and obstructive uropathy. The absence of spinal dysraphic features, presence of solid components and calcification, lack of meconium appearance to the contained fluid, and presence of normal kidneys will essentially exclude these possibilities. The presence of vertebral anomalies does not rule out SCT,[23] and SCT frquently causes secondary obstructive uropathy in utero.

Recently, ultrafast magnetic resonance imaging (MRI) using sequences requiring less that 0.5 second per image has allowed fetal imaging without the necessity for fetal sedation or paralysis.[43] We have found fetal MRI helpful in the assessment of atypical SCT or primarily cystic SCT where doubt may exist following ultrasound assessment (Fig. 21–2). However, MRI adds little to the ultrasound evaluation in most cases.

Natural History of Fetal SCT

To define the prenatal natural history of SCT we reviewed the literature and our experience with fetal SCT.[30] A total of 27 cases of prenatally diagnosed SCT were analyzed. Five cases were electively terminated, and 15 of the 22 remaining fetuses died in utero or soon after birth. The majority of cases in this series presented at 22 to 34 weeks' gestation with a uterus large for gestational dates or with symptoms of acute polyhydramnios. The presence of placentomegaly and/or hydrops in association with fetal SCT was predictive of fetal death in utero in seven of seven cases. A subsequent analysis of our experience and survey data from the

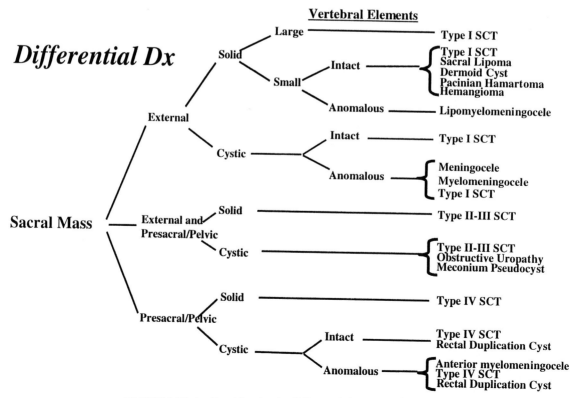

F I G U R E 21–1. Algorithm for the differential diagnosis of fetal SCT.

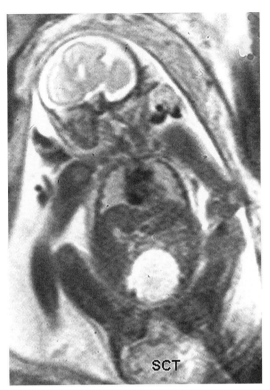

FIGURE 21–2. HASTE MRI of fetal SCT.

International Fetal Medical and Surgical Society[44] confirmed the high mortality of fetal SCT. In this analysis, 22 of 42 cases died in utero, or at birth. When placentomegaly or hydrops occurred, 15 of 15 fetuses died precipitously. A maternal indication for sonography was also a bad prognostic factor. Twenty-two of 32 fetuses died when there was an obstetric reason to scan the mother, whereas nine of ten fetuses detected by routine screening ultrasound survived. Although diagnosis prior to 30 weeks' gestation was associated with poor outcome, the incidental finding of SCT was favorable at any gestational age.

Other published series of prenatally diagnosed cases generally confirm our experience. Sheth published a series of 15 cases with only six survivors.[39] The presence of fetal hydrops resulted in rapid fetal death in three of four cases. The lone survivor presented acutely at 35 weeks and was salvaged by emergency cesarean section. Of interest, there were three cases of severe obstructive uropathy with secondary renal dysplasia, which had previously been considered to be an extremely rare complication of SCT. A more favorable series was reported by Gross[45] with ten prenatally diagnosed SCTs including one set of twins. The twins diagnosed at 19 weeks were aborted, and the remaining eight fetuses survived the perinatal period. However, four of the survivors presented at birth between 37 and 40 weeks' gestation, only three had polyhydramnios, and no fetus had findings of placentomegaly or hydrops. Nakayama has reported survival of two fetuses presenting with hydrops at 27 and 30 weeks' gestation.[46] Both premature babies were critically ill but survived with intensive care and tumor resection.

Although AAPSS classification may be a major determinant of ultimate survival and morbidity it does not appear to predict fetal survival. Most SCTs that induce high-output physiology are predominantly solid and large in size; however, absolute predictions of physiologic behavior or malignant potential cannot be made on the basis of findings such as tumor size, solid or cystic composition, or presence or absence of calcifications. An exception may be the unilocular cystic variety of SCT, which has a relatively favorable prognosis because of its benign pathology and relatively limited vasculature and metabolic demand.[37, 47] Serial sonography has documented variable growth rates of SCT in utero. The relative size of the SCT compared to the fetus may increase, decrease, or stay the same as gestation proceeds. In our experience, a rapid phase of tumor growth frequently precedes the development of placentomegaly and hydrops.

Although understanding of the natural history of fetal SCT is undoubtedly still evolving, some important observations have been made (Table 21–1). It is clear that the prognosis of fetal SCT is worse than neonatal SCT and that a particularly poor prognostic finding is the association of placentomegaly and/or hydrops. Although a few exceptions have been reported, the association of an immature fetus with SCT and placentomegaly/hydrops is generally fatal. In addition, SCTs discovered following the development of a maternal indication for ultrasonography should be considered to be high risk and have a relatively poor prognosis. Finally, fetal survival may in many cases depend upon appropriate obstetric and perinatal management.

Pathophysiology and Rationale for Fetal Surgery

As documented above, SCT frequently causes fetal death, but not by the mechanism usually responsible for death in postnatal series (i.e., malignant degeneration). Instead, death appears to result from a variety of mechanisms that are secondary effects of the SCT. These can be divided into complications related to either the tumor mass or the tumor physiology (Fig. 21–3). Mass effects include dystocia secondary to tumor bulk and premature delivery secondary to increased intrauterine volume with or without polyhydramnios. Dystocia may result in traumatic tumor rupture and hemorrhage during vaginal or cesarean delivery. Dystocia has been reported as an obstetric problem in 6 to 13% of postnatal series of SCT,[45, 48, 49] but this is probably an underestimation of the true incidence of the problem. The unexpected presence of a large SCT is an obstetrician's nightmare and a classic cause of arrested delivery.[50, 51]

TABLE 21–1. FETAL SCT—NATURAL HISTORY

Fetal SCT worse than newborn SCT
Different pathophysiology
Placentomegaly ± hydrops predicts fetal death

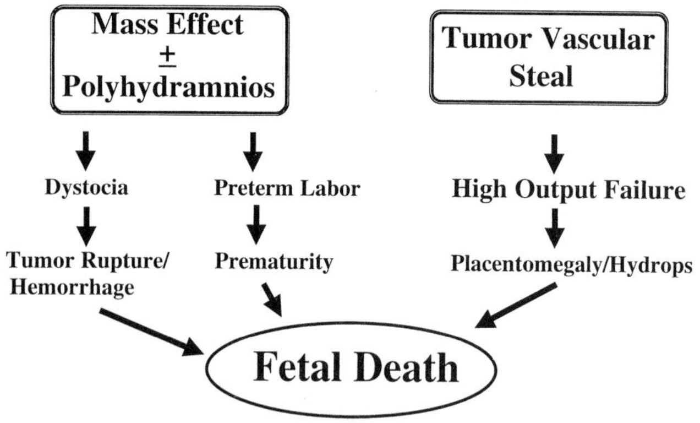

```
┌─────────────────────┐        ┌─────────────────────┐
│    Mass Effect      │        │  Tumor Vascular     │
│        ±            │        │      Steal          │
│  Polyhydramnios     │        │                     │
└─────────────────────┘        └─────────────────────┘
     ↓           ↓                        ↓
  Dystocia   Preterm Labor        High Output Failure
     ↓           ↓                        ↓
Tumor Rupture/ Prematurity        Placentomegaly/Hydrops
Hemorrhage
        ↘         ↓        ↙
          ┌───────────────┐
          │  Fetal Death  │
          └───────────────┘
```

FIGURE 21–3. Pathophysiology of SCT.

Typically, the fetus is delivered in a normal fashion until tumor bulk stops progress. Attempts to deliver the tumor have included vaginal incisional drainage,[52] vaginal delivery after abdominal debulking or drainage,[50, 53] and blind dissection of the tumor.[54] The best option is probably emergency abdominal delivery after partial vaginal delivery, with intubation and ventilation of the partially delivered fetus on the perineum.[49, 55] As expected in these desperate circumstances, fetal morbidity and mortality have been high. Probably the greatest contribution of prenatal diagnosis of SCT is prevention of dystocia by elective or emergent cesarean delivery. Tumor mass effect with or without polyhydramnios may also result in preterm delivery induced by uterine distention. A large proportion of prenatally diagnosed SCTs are delivered prematurely,[30, 44] resulting in perinatal mortality and morbidity from lung immaturity. Massive polyhydramnios is a frequent finding with large fetal SCTs, but the underlying pathophysiology of polyhydramnios is unclear in this circumstance.

The physiologic consequences of fetal SCT are dependent upon the metabolic demands and secondary blood flow of the tumor and the presence or absence of hemorrhage and secondary anemia. The metabolic requirements of the tumor vary dramatically and depend upon tumor size, rate of growth, ratio of cystic to solid composition, and probably the tissue components of the tumor. Blood flow has been attributed to the middle sacral artery, which may vary from minimally enlarged to the size of the common iliac artery.[56, 57] However, in reality, these tumors can usually be documented by power Doppler to derive blood supply from one or both internal iliac circulations (Fig. 21–4). Thus SCT has the potential to "steal" blood flow from the fetus and placenta. A second potential mechanism for increased metabolic demand is spontaneous internal or external hemorrhage from SCT resulting in fetal anemia.[58] This may be related to minor trauma, or necrotic or cystic degeneration of the tumor as it outgrows its blood supply. Since both of these mechanisms are potential etiologies of high-output failure, delineation of the pathophysiology in individual cases is essential because management will differ. The anemic, hydropic fetus with SCT might be treated by in utero transfusion, whereas the only hope for a fetus with vascular steal from the tumor would be early delivery or prenatal tumor resection. Evidence supporting high-output failure due to vascular steal is convincing. Other large vascular tumors such as hemangiomas and chorioangiomas have been documented to cause similar physiologic derangement.[59] The physiology seen in acardiac twins is analogous to a large SCT, since one twin is the "pump" and the acardiac twin is perfused by reversed umbilical flow. In acardiac twins the development of heart failure and hydrops of the pump twin is directly proportional to the ratio of acardiac to pump twin size. If the ratio is greater than 70%, all pump twins die of heart failure and hydrops, whereas

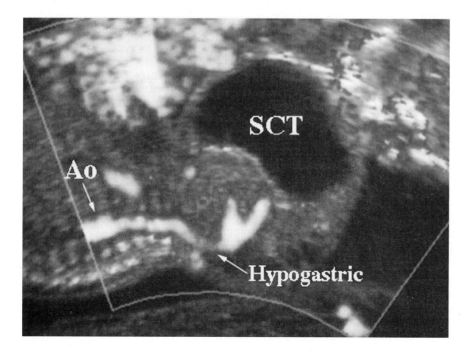

FIGURE 21–4. Power Doppler examination of fetal SCT demonstrating vascular supply arising from the internal iliac artery. *See Color Plate 1*

death is unlikely if the ratio is less than 25%.[60] Open surgery to remove the acardiac twin or interruption of the acardiac twin's umbilical cord has reversed heart failure and hydrops in the normal twin.[61, 62] The strongest evidence supporting high-output failure secondary to tumor vascular steal comes from echocardiographic and Doppler ultrasound measurements on three fetuses we have managed.[44, 63, 64] When hydrops was present, all fetuses had dilated ventricles that maintained a normal fractional shortening index, a dilated inferior vena cava that reflected increased venous return from the lower body, pericardial and pleural effusions as a manifestation of fetal hydrops, and marked placentomegaly. Serial examinations in one fetus documented dramatic increases in combined ventricular output, descending aortic flow, and umbilical venous flow. In these cases, high-velocity blood flow could be seen in noncystic areas of the tumor. Although placental flow was increased, placental flow as a percentage of descending aortic flow was decreased, thereby confirming a tumor steal of descending aortic blood flow. Anemia was not the etiology of hydrops, since the fetal hematocrit was near normal in each case. Although congestive heart failure has been attributed to fetal anemia in SCT,[58] the evidence is inconclusive. Other reports have found normal cardiac output and no cardiac failure in hydropic fetuses with severe anemia secondary to erythroblastosis.[65] In our experience, the presence of high-output physiology has always been related to tumor blood flow with minimal, if any, contribution from anemia. Finally, postnatal measurements of umbilical arterial blood gases before and after removal of a large SCT demonstrate that the tumor acts as a large arteriovenous shunt.[66]

Clear documentation of high-output failure secondary to tumor vascular steal, combined with our observation of the uniformly fatal outcome of immature fetuses who develop placentomegaly and hydrops, suggested to us that resection of the tumor in utero might reverse hydrops and prevent fetal demise.

The Maternal "Mirror Syndrome"

Prior to considering fetal surgery for SCT, we had experience with six cases of fetal SCT and hydrops. In each case serial sonography demonstrated the development of progressive placentomegaly and hydrops fetalis. In all six cases, the pregnancy culminated in premature labor with fetal death from either hydrops or immaturity. The development of placentomegaly and hydrops was also associated with potentially devastating maternal complications. This condition appeared to be similar to the maternal "mirror syndrome" previously described in association with erythroblastosis fetalis in which the maternal condition begins to mirror that of the fetus.[67] All of the mothers experienced progressive symtoms suggestive of preeclampsia including vomiting, hypertension, peripheral edema, proteinuria, and pulmonary edema. The pathophysiology of this condition remains unclear. A maternal hyperdynamic state is seen in molar pregnancies and a variety of fetal conditions associated with placentomegaly. This state may result from the release of a placental substance[68] such as human chorionic gonadotropin,[69] which is known to stimulate thyroxine production. An important question with regard to fetal intervention for SCT was whether reversal of the fetal high-output state might also reverse the placentomegaly and secondary preeclampsia and allow continuation of pregnancy.

Fetal Surgery for SCT

There have now been seven open fetal procedures performed for SCT with associated high-output physiology, five at the University of California at San Francisco (UCSF), and two at Children's Hospital of Philadelphia. Only two fetuses have survived, one from each institution, but much has been learned about the feasibility of SCT resection in utero and the requirements for success.

Selection of Patients

The primary positive selective criteria for consideration of fetal intervention has been the presence of associated placentomegaly/hydrops or the clear evolution of high-output physiology in an AAPSS type I or II SCT at less than 30 weeks' gestation (Table 21-2). It has become clear, however, that there are also negative selective criteria. First, the presence of maternal eclampsia (mirror syndrome) is a contraindication for fetal intervention. Our first patient developed mild hypertension, peripheral edema, and proteinuria during the evolution of hydrops in the fetus. Prior to planned fetal surgery, the mother progressed to preterm labor that was controlled over the next 2 days with aggressive tocolytic therapy. We then proceeded with fetal surgery with the hope that resection of the tumor would reverse the fetal and maternal pathophysiology. The fetal hydrops did resolve over the next 2 weeks; however, the placentomegaly and maternal preeclampsia did not. Control of preterm labor was difficult because the mother's illness precluded effective tocolytic therapy, and her illness progressed to pulmonary edema despite fetal improvement. On the 12th postoperative day, active labor began and a 26-week fetus was delivered by cesarean section and subsequently died of pulmonary immaturity at 6 hours of age. No evidence of hydrops was present at delivery or autopsy. The mother's illness resolved within 2 days after delivery.

TABLE 21-2. SELECTION CRITERIA FOR FETAL SURGERY FOR SCT

POSITIVE	NEGATIVE
AAPSS Type I or II	AAPSS III or IV
High-output physiology	Maternal "mirror" syndrome
Placentomegaly/hydrops	Fetal dilated cardiomyopathy (advanced)
	Evidence of tumor hemorrhage* (fetal anemia)

* May improve with fetal transfusion.

A second contraindication for fetal intervention is advanced fetal pathophysiology. We operated on a fetus that had severe hydrops with marked chamber dilation and intermittent bradycardia on preoperative scans. During the procedure the fetus became bradycardic and died with application of a tourniquet around the base of the tumor. A severely ill fetus with far-advanced high-output cardiac failure is unlikely to survive the operative procedure, presumably because of the inability to compensate for the increase in afterload incurred with removal of the low-resistance tumor vascular bed. The ideal patient for consideration of fetal intervention appears to be one in which high-output physiology evolves during serial Doppler observation, so that the fetus can be referred prior to maternal or severe fetal compromise. In our experience, the pathophysiology can progress rapidly, and early referral can be the limiting factor in our ability to salvage the fetus.

The Operative Procedure

The object of SCT resection in utero is to occlude the tumor vascular supply and remove the low-resistance tumor vascular bed from the fetal circulation. This differs from the postnatal procedure, where every effort is made to remove the entire tumor en bloc with the coccyx. Following hysterotomy, the lower extremities and tumor mass are exteriorized (Fig. 21–5). Care is taken to keep the remainder of the fetus in the amniotic space to avoid uterine volume contraction. A dilator is placed in the fetal rectum to allow palpation of the rectum and

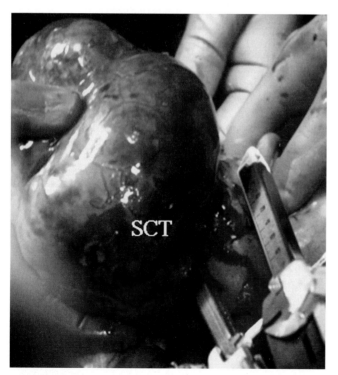

FIGURE 21–5. Photograph of open fetal surgical procedure for SCT. The GIA stapler is being applied across the pedicle of the tumor. *See Color Plate 1*

avoid injury during the resection. An incision is made around the base of the tumor avoiding the anal sphincter complex. The incision is carried deeply enough to allow placement of a tourniquet around the base of the tumor and prevent slippage. Depending upon the width of the base, either a uterine stapling device is deployed across the base, or the tumor is cut across and vessels are individually suture ligated. The entire fetal portion of the procedure takes approximately 10 to 15 mintues. A cord blood specimen is then obtained for the fetal hematocrit, and warmed blood is transfused if necessary. With this approach, fetal blood loss and operative time are minimized, improving the likelihood of a successful outcome.

Other "less invasive" approaches have been suggested for management of fetal SCT such as tumor embolization or radiofrequency or laser ablation. These approaches remain clinically unproven and need investigation in animal models. Although no animal model exists for fetal SCT, many of the physical and thermal effects of the ablation techniques should be investigated in normal fetal models prior to clinical application.

Results of Open Fetal Surgery for SCT

There have been seven open fetal procedures performed for SCT. Two of the deaths are described above and, we now know, were the result of ill-advised patient selection (one maternal mirror syndrome, one fetal bradycardia and cardiomyopathy). Another fetus experienced premature closure of the ductus arteriosus related to indomethacin tocolysis, with secondary right ventricular dysfunction and hypertrophic cardiomyopathy. This ultimately led to premature delivery and fetal demise. Finally, there have been four cases in which resection of the SCT reversed the fetal pathophysiology and resulted in delivery of a nonhydropic neonate. In one case the tumor was resected at 28 weeks' gestation and the nonhydropic fetus delivered 8 days later following onset of preterm labor. Following delivery, despite prematurity, the fetus did surprisingly well and required only minimal ventilatory support. There was clinical evidence of obstructive uropathy with an enlarged bladder, mild hydronephrosis, and the early development of azotemia. However, the hydronephrosis and azotemia improved with urethral catheter drainage. Residual tumor resection was attempted on the 13th day of life when her cardiopulmonary and renal status were stable. A combined abdominal-perineal approach resulted in straightforward resection of the tumor. While performing the perineal portion of the procedure, during the dissection of the presacral space, the baby experienced complete cardiovascular collapse and electromechanical dissociation with acute elevation of ST segments on electrocardiogram. She could not be resuscitated and expired secondary to a presumed paradoxical air embolus via the presacral veins. Autopsy confirmed air in the coronary circulation. In another interesting case, operated on at UCSF, a hydropic fetus with extensive intrapelvic extension of SCT and associated obstructive uropathy and rectal atresia secondary to tumor underwent bilateral loop ureterostomies and complete resection with rectal reconstruction in utero. The fetus was delivered 3 weeks later and was reportedly doing well for 3 days when it suddenly died due to an atrial perforation from a femoral catheter. Although unsuccessful, these two cases document reversal of fetal pathophysiology following resection of the tumor. In two subsequent cases the fetuses have survived their neonatal courses.[70] One has done well to date; the other initially did well but returned with lung metastases and local recurrence of endodermal sinus tumor at 1 year of age. This patient has undergone re-resection and intensive chemotherapy and currently has no evidence of disease at 27 months of age.

The histopathology of tumors resected in utero with either subsequent definitive resection after birth or autopsy follow-up are of interest.[71] These cases represent a preselected subset of rapidly growing, predominantly solid, highly vascularized tumors. From our small experience it appears that tumors resected in utero are more immature, and have a higher likelihood of malignant elements than SCTs resected in the postnatal period. In addition, in four of six cases in which only debulking was performed in utero, no residual tumor could be found at reoperation (with coccygectomy) or autopsy, suggesting that many of these tumors involute after occlusion of their blood supply. However, the local recurrence of germ cell tumor with distant metastases seen in one fetal surgery survivor, with no residual tumor found at neonatal coccygectomy, is disconcerting and documents that even prenatal resection of SCT with no apparent residual disease does not avoid the risk of malignancy.

Management of the Fetus with SCT

The pathophysiologic rationale for fetal surgical intervention in selected cases of SCT is sound. Our opinion is that once high-output physiology is documented in the immature fetus, early fetal intervention offers the best hope for fetal survival. Our current recommendations are shown in the algorithm in Figure 21–6. Briefly, all fetuses diagnosed with SCT should undergo detailed sonographic evaluation to confirm the diagnosis and

rule out associated anomalies. An assessment of placental size, type of SCT, and the presence or absence of hydrops should be made. Doppler echocardiography should be performed with a detailed evaluation for high-output physiology. Recommendations then depend on tumor size, gestational age, and the presence or absence of documented high-output physiology secondary to tumor vascular steal. If the tumor is small (smaller than the diameter of the fetus) and asymptomatic, a relatively optimistic outlook can be given, particularly late in gestation. These fetuses can be followed by serial sonography to term vaginal delivery. If the tumor is large, or obstetric indications for sonography are present, a guarded prognosis should be given and the pregnancy followed by frequent sonography. If no placentomegaly or hydrops evolves, the fetus should be delivered by elective cesarean section after pulmonary maturity is established, to avoid dystocia and/or tumor rupture and hemorrhage. If placentomegaly and hydrops evolve after pulmonary maturity is established, the fetus should be delivered by emergent cesarean section and treated ex utero. If high-output failure develops prior to 30 weeks' gestation, and the tumor is anatomically amenable to resection (AAPSS type I or II), then fetal surgery should be considered. The gestational limit for early delivery versus fetal intervention is in evolution. Our bias is that, in general, the severely hydropic fetus has a better chance of recovery with placental support. We are therefore leaning toward fetal intervention in cases with severe hydrops as late as 32 weeks' gestation.

Summary

We have learned a great deal about the pathophysiology and natural history of SCT. The pathophysiologic rationale for fetal intervention in appropriately selected cases is sound. The feasibility of resection of SCT by open fetal surgery has been established and survival has been achieved. The challenge in the future will be to improve on our current results, and this can best be accomplished by early referral of these cases to experienced centers that can offer informed counseling and timely intervention for this anomaly. In addition, less invasive approaches to fetal SCT need to be developed and experimentally validated prior to clinical application.

REFERENCES

1. Bale P: Sacrococcygeal developmental abnormalities and tumors in children. Perspect Pediatr Pathol 1:9–56, 1984.
2. Berry C, Keeling J, Hilton C: Teratomata in infancy and childhood: A review of 91 cases. J Pathol 98:241–250, 1969.
3. Grosfeld J, Ballantine T, Lowe D, et al: Benign and malignant teratomas in children: Analysis of 85 patients. Surgery 80:297–305, 1976.
4. Mahour G, Woolley M, Trivedi S, et al: Teratomas in infancy and childhood: Experience with 81 cases. Surgery 76:309–319, 1974.
5. Gross R, Clatworthy H, Meeker I: Sacrococcygeal teratomas in infants and children. Surg Gynecol Obstet 92:341–354, 1951.
6. Mahour GH, Wolley MM, Trivedi SN, Landing BH: Sacrococcygeal teratoma: A 33-year experience. J Pediatr Surg 10:183–188, 1975.
7. Willis R: The Borderland of Embryology and Pathology. London: Butterworth and Co., 1958.

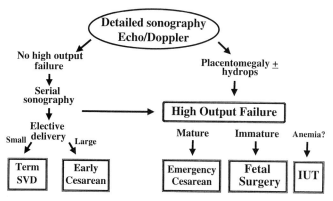

FIGURE 21–6. Algorithm for the management of a fetus with SCT.

8. Linder D, Hecht F, McCaw B, et al: Origin of extragonadal teratomas and endodermal sinus tumours. Nature 254:597–600, 1975.

9. Mintz B, Cronmiller C, Custer R: Somatic cell origin of teratocarcinomas. Proc Natl Acad Sci U S A 75:2839–2846, 1978.

10. Ouimet A, Russo P: Fetus in fetu or not? [see comments]. J Pediatr Surg 24:926–927, 1989.

11. de Lagausie P, de Napoli Cocci S, Stempfle N, et al: Highly differentiated teratoma and fetus-in-fetu: A single pathology? [see comments]. J Pediatr Surg 32:115–116, 1997.

12. Sanal M, Kucukcelebi A, Abasiyanik F, et al: Fetus in fetu and cystic rectal duplication in a newborn. Eur J Pediatr Surg 7:120–121, 1997.

13. Montgomery ML, Lillehei C, Acker D, Benacerraf BR: Intra-abdominal sacrococcygeal mature teratoma or fetus in fetu in a third-trimester fetus. Ultrasound Obstet Gynecol 11:219–221, 1998.

14. Ashcraft KW, Holder TM, Harris DJ: Familial presacral teratomas. Birth Defects 11:143–146, 1975.

15. Goto T, Aoyama K: [Familiar sacrococcygeal teratoma]. Nippon Rinsho 53:2779–2785, 1995.

16. Carney J, Thompson D, Johnson C, et al: Teratomas in children: Clinical and pathologic aspects. J Pediatr Surg 7:271–282, 1972.

17. Gonzalez-Crussi F, Winkler R, Mirkin D: Sacrococcygeal teratoma in infants and children. Relationship of histology and prognosis in 40 cases. Arch Pathol Lab Med 102:420–425, 1978.

18. Noseworthy J, Lack E, Kozakewich H, et al: Sacrococcygeal germ cell tumors in childhood: An updated experience with 118 patients. J Pediatr Surg 16:358–364, 1981.

19. Rescorla FJ, Sawin RS, Coran AG, et al: Long-term outcome for infants and children with sacrococcygeal teratoma: A report from the Childrens Cancer Group. J Pediatr Surg 33:171–176, 1998.

20. Bilik R, Shandling B, Pope M, et al: Malignant benign neonatal sacrococcygeal teratoma. J Pediatr Surg 28:1158–1160, 1993.

21. Ein SH, Mancer K, Adeyemi SD: Malignant sacrococcygeal teratoma—endodermal sinus, yolk sac tumor—in infants and children: A 32-year review [review]. J Pediatr Surg 20:473–477, 1985.

22. Altman RP, Randolph JG, Lilly JR: Sacrococcygeal teratoma: American Academy of Pediatrics Surgical Section Survey-1973. J Pediatr Surg 9:389–398, 1974.

23. Lahdenne P, Heikinheimo M, Jaaskelainen J, et al: Vertebral abnormalities associated with congenital sacrococcygeal teratomas. J Pediatr Orthop 11:603–607, 1991.

24. Lahdenne P, Dunkel L, Heikinheimo M, et al: Hypergonadotropic hypogonadism and sperm abnormalities in men born with benign sacrococcygeal teratoma. J Androl 12:226–230, 1991.

25. Rintala R, Lahdenne P, Lindahl H, et al: Anorectal function in adults operated for a benign sacrococcygeal teratoma. J Pediatr Surg 28:1165–1167, 1993.

26. Milam DF, Cartwright PC, Snow BW: Urological manifestations of sacrococcygeal teratoma. J Urol 149:574–576, 1993.

27. Boemers TM, van Gool JD, de Jong TP, Bax KM: Lower urinary tract dysfunction in children with benign sacrococcygeal teratoma. J Urol 151:174–176, 1994.

28. Holzgreve W, Mahony BS, Glick PL, et al: Sonographic demonstration of fetal sacrococcygeal teratoma. Prenat Diagn 5:245–257, 1985.

29. Kuhlmann RS, Warsof SL, Levy DL, et al: Fetal sacrococcygeal teratoma [review]. Fetal Ther 2:95–100, 1987.

30. Flake AW, Harrison MR, Adzick NS, et al: Fetal sacrococcygeal teratoma. J Pediatr Surg 21:563–566, 1986.

31. Kirkinen P, Heinonen S, Vanamo K, Ryynanen M: Maternal serum alpha-fetoprotein and epithelial tumour marker concentrations are not increased by fetal sacrococcygeal teratoma [see comments]. Prenat Diagn 17:47–50, 1997.

32. Szabo M, Varga P, Zalatnai A, et al: Sacrococcygeal teratoma and normal alphafetoprotein concentration in amniotic fluid. J Med Genet 22:405–408, 1985.

33. Brock DJ, Richmond DH, Liston WA: Normal second-trimester amniotic fluid alphafetoprotein and acetylcholinesterase associated with fetal sacrococcygeal teratoma. Prenat Diagn 3:343–345, 1983.

34. Hecht F, Hecht BK, O'Keeffe D: Sacrococcygeal teratoma: Prenatal diagnosis with elevated alphafetoprotein and acetylcholinesterase in amniotic fluid. Prenat Diagn 2:229–231, 1982.

35. Dupont M, Boulot P: Faint-positive amniotic fluid acetylcholinesterase in a case of sacrococcygeal teratoma. Biol Neonate 63:397–398, 1993.

36. Horger EOD, McCarter LM: Prenatal diagnosis of sacrococcygeal teratoma. Am J Obstet Gynecol 134:228–229, 1979.

37. Hogge WA, Thiagarajah S, Barber VG, et al: Cystic sacrococcygeal teratoma: Ultrasound diagnosis and perinatal management. J Ultrasound Med 6:707–710, 1987.

38. Morrow RJ, Whittle MJ, McNay MB, et al: Prenatal diagnosis of an intra-abdominal sacrococcygeal teratoma. Prenat Diagn 10:753–756, 1990.

39. Sheth S, Nussbaum AR, Sanders RC, et al: Prenatal diagnosis of sacrococcygeal teratoma: Sonographic-pathologic correlation. Radiology 169:131–136, 1988.

40. Evans MJ, Danielian PJ, Gray ES: Sacrococcygeal teratoma: A case of mistaken identity. Pediatr Radiol 24:52–53, 1994.

41. Bloechle M, Bollmann R, Wit J, et al: Neuroectodermal cyst may be a rare differential diagnosis of fetal sacrococcygeal teratoma: First case report of a prenatally observed neuroectodermal cyst. Ultrasound Obstet Gynecol 7:64–67, 1996.

42. Lockwood C, Ghidini A, Romero R, Hobbins JC: Fetal bowel perforation simulating sacrococcygeal teratoma. J Ultrasound Med 7:227–229, 1988.

43. Kirkinen P, Partanen K, Merikanto J, et al: Ultrasonic and magnetic resonance imaging of fetal sacrococcygeal teratoma. Acta Obstet Gynecol Scand 76:917–922, 1997.

44. Bond SJ, Harrison MR, Schmidt KG, et al: Death due to high-output cardiac failure in fetal sacrococcygeal teratoma [review]. J Pediatr Surg 25:1287–1291, 1990.

45. Gross SJ, Benzie RJ, Sermer M, et al: Sacrococcygeal teratoma: Prenatal diagnosis and management. Am J Obstet Gynecol 156:393–396, 1987.

46. Nakayama DK, Killian A, Hill LM, et al: The newborn with hydrops and sacrococcygeal teratoma. J Pediatr Surg 26:1435–1438, 1991.

47. Mintz MC, Mennuti M, Fishman M: Prenatal aspiration of sacrococcygeal teratoma. AJR Am J Roentgenol 141:367–368, 1983.

48. Giugiaro A, Boario U, Di Francesco G, et al: Considerazioni su tre casi di rottura intraparto di teratoma sacro-coccigeo. Minerva Pediatr 29:1517–1524, 1977.

49. Musci MN Jr, Clark MJ, Ayres RE, Finkel MA: Management of dystocia caused by a large sacrococcygeal teratoma. Obstet Gynecol 62:10s–12s, 1983.

50. Tanaree P: Delivery obstructed by sacrococcygeal teratoma. Am J Obstet Gynecol 142:239, 1982.

51. Foruhan B, Jennings P: Unusual presacral tumours obstructing delivery. Br J Obstet Gynecol 85:231–233, 1978.

52. Weiss D, Wajntraub G, Abulafia Y, et al: Vaginal surgical intervention for sacrococcygeal teratoma obstructing labor. Acta Obstet Gynecol Scand 55:183–188, 1976.

53. Edwards W: A fetal sacrococcygeal tumor obstructing labor after attempted home confinement. Obstet Gynecol 61:19s–21s, 1983.

54. Abbott PD, Bowman A, Kantor HI: Dystocia caused by sacrococcygeal teratoma. Obstet Gynecol 27:571–574, 1966.

55. Johnson JW, Porter J Jr, Kellner KR, et al: Abdominal rescue after incomplete delivery secondary to large fetal sacrococcygeal teratoma. Obstet Gynecol 71:981–984, 1988.

56. Smith B, Passaro E, Clatworthy H: The vascular anatomy of sacrococcygeal teratomas: Its significance in surgical management. Surgery 49:534–539, 1961.

57. Smith WL, Stokka C, Franken EA Jr: Arteriography of sacrococcygeal teratomas. Radiology 137:653–655, 1980.

58. Alter DN, Reed KL, Marx GR, et al: Prenatal diagnosis of congestive heart failure in a fetus with a sacrococcygeal teratoma. Obstet Gynecol 71:978–981, 1988.

59. Dum R: Hemangioma of placenta (chorio-angioma). J Obstet Gynecol Br Emp 66:51–57, 1959.

60. Moore T, Gale S, Benirschke K: Perinatal outcome of forty-nine pregnancies complicated by acardiac twinning. Am J Obstet Gynecol 167:33–37, 1990.

61. Ginsberg N, Applebaum M, Rabin S, et al: Term birth after midtrimester hysterotomy and selective delivery of an acardiac twin. Am J Obstet Gynecol 167:33–37, 1992.

62. Quintero RA, Romero R, Reich H, et al: In utero percutaneous umbilical cord ligation in the management of complicated monochorionic multiple gestations. Ultrasound Obstet Gynecol 8(1):16–22, 1996.

63. Langer JC, Harrison MR, Schmidt KG, et al: Fetal hydrops and death from sacrococcygeal teratoma: Rationale for fetal surgery [see comments]. Am J Obstet Gynecol 160:1145–1150, 1989.

64. Schmidt KG, Silverman NH, Harison MR, Callen PW: High-output cardiac failure in fetuses with large sacrococcygeal teratoma: Diagnosis by echocardiography and Doppler ultrasound. J Pediatr 114:1023–1028, 1989.

65. Phibbs R, Johnson P, Tooley W: Cardiorespiratory status of erythroblastosis newborn infants. II. Blood volume, hematocrit, and serum albumin concentration in relation to hydrops. Pediatrics 53:13–23, 1974.

66. Calenda E, Bachy B, Guyard MF: Sacrococcygeal teratoma and venous shunting through a tumor: Biological evidence [letter]. Anesth Analg 74:165–166, 1992.

67. Nicolaides K, Gainey H: Pseudotoxemic state associated with severe Rh isoimunization. Am J Obstet Gynecol 89:41–45, 1964.

68. Jeffcoate T, Scott J: Some observations on the placental factor in pregnancy toxemia. Am J Obstet Gynecol 77:475–489, 1959.

69. Nisula B, Taliadouros G: Thyroid function in gestational trophoblastic neoplasia: Evidence that the thyrotropic activity of chorionic gonadotropin mediates the thyrotoxicosis of choriocarcinoma. Am J Obstet Gynecol 138:77–85, 1980.

70. Adzick NS, Crombleholme TM, Morgan MA, Quinn TM: A rapidly growing fetal teratoma. Lancet 349:538–540, 1997.

71. Graf JL, Housely HT, Albanese CT, et al: A surprising histological evolution of preterm sacrococcygeal teratoma. J Pediatr Surg 33:177–179, 1998.

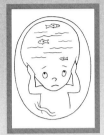

CHAPTER 22

The Fetus with Hydrocephalus

PETER P. SUN and LESLIE N. SUTTON

Congenital internal hydrocephalus develops in utero, and may cause such enlargement of the head as to prevent birth until the fluid is let out, or may be moderate at the time of birth, and afterward rapidly increase. The causes and pathological mechanisms are practically unknown. It has been ascribed to maternal grief or other emotion, but on no reasonable ground.

Gowers, 1888

Neonatal hydrocephalus is one of the most common congenital anomalies affecting the nervous system, occurring with an incidence of 0.3 to 2.5 per 1,000 live births.[1] Traditionally, the signs of a large head, a bulging fontanel, and distended scalp veins led to a radiographic imaging study showing enlargement of the ventricular system, and a ventriculoperitoneal shunt was performd in the early neonatal period. The result, in terms of intellectual outcome as the child matured, has remained somewhat unpredictable. Some infants with extreme hydrocephalus and virtually no cortical mantle visible on the initial imaging studies have grown up to be remarkably normal adults, prompting John Lorber to question, "Is the brain really necessary?"[2] Numerous attempts have been made to correlate the thickness of cortical mantle with ultimate IQ, with variable results. Serial imaging studies of shunted hydrocephalic infants often show dramatic reconstitution of the brain over time, and the mechanism of this process remains a topic of active investigation.

With the routine use of high-quality ultrasonography, ventricular enlargement is now routinely diagnosed in utero. This knowledge has facilitated obstetric care, but presents a challenge for the team counseling parents regarding their fetus. There are clearly four options: (1) termination of the pregnancy; (2) completion of the pregnancy to term, delivery by the most appropriate route, probably cesarean section, and neonatal shunting; (3) early induced delivery to hasten insertion of the shunt and presumably prevent further irreversible damage to the brain; and (4) some form of fetal intervention, such as serial cephalocentesis, fetal ventriculoperitoneal shunt, or ventriculoamniotic shunt.

It is clear that fetal ventriculomegaly associated with other brain or chromosomal abnormalities carries a poor prognosis. However, the prenatal management of those cases of isolated congenital hydrocephalus diagnosed in utero remains undefined. Fetal shunting was performed in the early 1980s with the hope that in utero intervention would improve outcome.[3, 4] At that time, however, knowledge was limited regarding the natural history and outcome of fetal hydrocephalus. Imaging was suboptimal, and significant brain anomalies were not appreciated. As a result, patient selection was spotty, and the outcomes were mixed.[5, 6] Furthermore, the techniques of fetal surgery were crude by today's standard, and the morbidity was high. A de facto moratorium has been in place for over a decade. Recent refinements in fetal imaging, surgical techniques, and drugs to hasten fetal lung maturity and to prevent premature labor have again raised the possibility that some unborn children with isolated hydrocephalus might now be candidates for fetal intervention. The selection of suitable candidates will depend on a firm grasp of embryology, radiology, and the natural history of fetal hydrocephalus. The selection of the optimal surgical procedure will depend on preliminary work in the animal laboratory.

Embryology

The central nervous system (CNS) from its earliest form as the neural plate is bathed by fluid, at first by the amniotic fluid and after neurulation has occurred, by cerebrospinal fluid (CSF).[7] The ventricular system is formed as the caudal neuropore closes during the fourth week of gestation.[8] At this stage, the ventricular system matches the tubular shape of the brain, but it is already demarcated into the cavities of the prosencephalon (the future lateral ventricles), mesencephalon (the future aqueduct of Sylvius), and the rhombencephalon (the future fourth ventricle), and is continuous with the central canal of the spinal cord. The subsequent morphologic evolution of the ventricular system is caused by evaginations, flexures, and differential growth of parts of the brain. The fourth ventricle becomes apparent as a large cavity of the rhombencephalon at 4.5 weeks. At the same time, bilateral vesicular evaginations develop in the anterior prosencephalon as the telencephalon. The mantles of these telencephalic vesicles grow immensely to become the cerebral hemispheres, while the cavities become the lateral ventricles. The posterior prosencephalon becomes the diencephalon, and its cavity becomes the third ventricle. A persistent connection between the telencephalic vesicles and diencephalon remains as the interventricular foramen of Monroe. The cavity of the mesencephalon becomes the aqueduct, which connects the third and fourth ventricles (Fig. 22–1).

As the cerebral hemispheres develop, they expand caudally in a curved direction to form the temporal lobes. The lateral ventricles develop into a C-shaped structure with an anterior and inferior horn at 7 weeks. By 13 weeks, a posterior horn can be seen in the occipital region of the lateral ventricle. The corpus callosum begins as a thickening in the midline region between the two telencephalic vesicles known as the commissure plate at 8 weeks.[8] It grows with the cerebral hemispheres in a curved caudal direction so that the caudal end of the corpus callosum sits over the third ventricle by 20 weeks. In doing so, a double layer of pia-arachnoid is formed (velum interpositum) over the roof of the third ventricle. The inferior portion of the corpus callosum becomes thinned to form the septum pellucidum that separates the anterior portion of the two lateral ventricles.

The choroid plexus appears in the fourth ventricle at the sixth week, and in the lateral ventricles at the seventh week.[9] One third of the lateral ventricle is filled by choroid plexus at 8 weeks, and by 11 weeks it fills the atria.[10, 11] The proportion of the lateral ventricles filled by the choroid plexus diminishes by the end of the second trimester. The enormous size of the early choroid plexus suggests a function in nourishing the embryonic brain in addition to CSF formation.[12, 13]

In the neonate, approximately 300 to 600 mL of CSF is produced per day. About 80 to 90% of CSF is produced from the choroid plexus by an active pump[14] and the rest originates from the brain parenchyma. CSF production is influenced by chronic changes in intracranial pressure, but production continues despite high-pressure states such as hydrocephalus.[15] Aided by arterial pulsations of the brain and choroid plexus, CSF flows from the lateral ventricles through the foramen of Monroe to the third ventricle and then through the aqueduct of Sylvius, which has become the narrowest section of the pathway to the fourth ventricle. From the fourth ventricle, CSF leaves the ventricular system into the subarachnoid space via the outlets developed in the fourth ventricle: the midline foramen of Magendie and the lateral, paired foramina of Luschka. CSF then flows passively into the venous system via the arachnoid granulations.

The embryonic and fetal development of CSF circulation is a dynamic process intimately related to brain development. Anencephaly results from failure of the anterior neuropore to close properly to form the ventricular system. As the choroid plexus begins to appear, the roof of the rhombencephalon becomes very thin and is

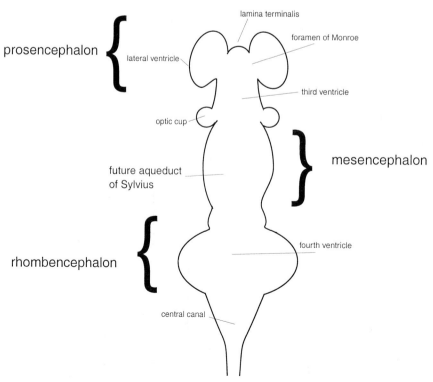

F I G U R E 22–1. Embryonic human brain.

thought to allow some passage of fluid and macromolecules into the subarachnoid space.[16] The actual perforation of the roof to form the fourth ventricular outlets does not occur until later.[17, 18] During this time, adequate ventricular distention by CSF plays a critical role in brain development.[19-21] Cannulation and drainage of the ventricles in early chick embryos results in small, disorganized brains.[22] Growth of the surrounding cranial mesenchyme is also affected by lack of ventricular distention. Failure to maintain distention of the primitive ventricular system from open myelomeningoceles has been theorized to cause hindbrain anomalies (the Chiari malformations).[23]

The subarachnoid space develops independently of CSF circulation as a loose mesenchymal condensation around the neural tube as early as the fifth week.[24] As the fourth ventricular outlets mature, CSF fills the subarachnoid spaces. The subarachnoid space becomes most prominent during the second trimester and gradually diminishes to the neonatal size during the third trimester.[25, 26] Arachnoid villi begin to develop as depressions in the sagittal sinus filled with arachnoid tissue at 26 weeks. Well-developed arachnoid villi are not seen until the 35th week and are not fully mature until term.[27] This morphologic sequence indicates that embryonic CSF reabsorption is not carried out by arachnoid villi or granulations. It is thought that fenestrations in embryonic perineural vessels are capable of CSF reabsorption, analogous to that of lower animals that do not have arachnoid granulations.[28] Some degree of pressure exists in the subarachnoid space prior to the formation of arachnoid villi, which may be necessary for arachnoid granulation development.

Etiology and Differential Diagnosis

Ventricular enlargement must be distinguished from hydrocephalus. Ventriculomegaly can be caused by brain destruction, morphologic maldevelopment, or increased pressure from altered CSF dynamics. Only the latter can be properly termed hydrocephalus. The distinction can be difficult to make by imaging criteria, but it is critical for parental counseling and treatment because fetal ventriculomegaly from a destructive process or morphologic maldevelopment carries a poor prognosis. In these cases the ventricles are not only relatively enlarged but are often distorted due to overlying parenchymal abnormalities. While alterations of CSF dynamics and hydrocephalus may be present in some cases, it is secondary.

True fetal hydrocephalus may arise from a variety of processes, including dysembryogenesis, congenital infection, vascular injury, and tumors. If obstruction arises within the ventricular system, the hydrocephalus is considered obstructive. If there is open communication between the ventricular system and subarachnoid space and there is failure of absorption arising within the subarachnoid space or arachnoid granulations, the hydrocephalus is considered communicating. Rarely, excessive CSF production is seen with choroid plexus tumors. The resultant CSF accumulation produces increased pressure and subsequent dilatation of the ventricles with thinning and stretching of the cerebral mantle. In the acute phase, the ependymal cells lining the ventricles become flattened and the white matter becomes edematous.[29] To some extent, brain compliance can accommodate the ventricular dilatation without significant brain damage. As the process continues, axonal degeneration occurs with associated focal neuronal loss, and the edema is replaced by gliosis.[30-32] Cortical neurons then demonstrate a loss of synaptic connections and dendritic richness.[33]

The most common form of isolated, obstructive hydrocephalus is so-called aqueductal stenosis, which accounts for up to 20% of cases of fetal hydrocephalus.[34] In fact, the aqueduct is not truly stenotic, but occluded by gliosis, forking, or septum formation.[35, 36] Blockage at the aqueduct is inferred from enlargement of the lateral and third ventricles proximal to the obstruction with a small fourth ventricle distally. The prenatal diagnosis of isolated aqueductal stenosis, however, is one of exclusion. It is confirmed only by a thorough evaluation of the neuraxis to exclude other causes of hydrocephalus. The prognosis can be favorable, and many patients with postnatally treated isolated aqueductal stenosis will have normal neurodevelopmental outcome. Much less common than aqueductal stenosis is isolated atresia or stenosis of the foramen of Monroe.[37] It typically involves only one foramen and gives rise to unilateral hydrocephalus.

In utero infections can cause hydrocephalus by inflammation and scarring of the CSF pathways. Toxoplasmosis produces a secondary aqueductal stenosis and also affects the subarachnoid spaces.[38, 39] Cytomegalovirus induces a basal arachnoiditis that impairs CSF flow. Rubella, mumps, varicella, and parainfluenza have been implicated in the development of hydrocephalus as well. In utero hemorrhagic or ischemic lesions can obliterate CSF pathways and cause hydrocephalus. Infections and vascular lesions often produce extensive parenchymal damage that ultimately determines the outcome, which is often poor. Obstruction of CSF pathways by strategically placed mass lesions can also occur. Prenatal CNS tumors are rare. Vein of Galen aneurysms cause hydrocephalus by obstruction of the aqueduct of Sylvius or intracranial venous hypertension from the associated heart failure. Arachnoid cysts in the velum interpositum, suprasellar region, or quadragerminal plate can enlarge to compress the adjacent third ventricle or aqueduct.

Hydrocephalus can have a genetic basis. Classic X-linked recessive hydrocephalus (Bickers-Adam syndrome) accounts for approximately 7% of male hydrocephalus cases.[40] The condition is characterized by aqueductal stenosis and severe mental retardation. Half of the children have an adduction thumb deformity. The disease is genetically heterogeneous and has been mapped to chromosome Xq28 and Xq27.3, which encode the neural cell adhesion molecule L1.[41, 42] Hydrocephalus may also be present in a number of major and minor chromosomal aberrations affecting chromosomes 8, 9, 13, 15, 18, and 21.[43-49]

Hydrocephalus is often associated with congenital malformation syndromes, and it is vital to define associated anomalies prior to recommending specific treatment. The Chiari II malformation accounts for approximately 30% of fetuses identified with ventriculomegaly.[50, 51] It accompanies myelomeningocele, and is defined as herniation of the hindbrain structures (cerebellar vermis and tonsils) into the cervical spinal canal with a shallow posterior fossa and vertically oriented tentorium, which have distinct sonographic appearances (the so-called lemon and banana signs). Affected children will have a variable level of paralysis of the legs and perhaps brain stem malfunction as well. Intelligence may be affected, particularly in patients with higher spinal levels, in whom magnetic resonance imaging (MRI) may show brain parenchymal abnormalities such as agenesis of the corpus callosum and polymicrogyria. The hydrocephalus is thought to be a result of an increase in CSF flow resistance at the fourth ventricular outlets secondary to the posterior fossa abnormalities. At birth, 15% of neonates with the Chiari II malformation will have hydrocephalus and 80 to 90% will eventually develop hydrocephalus after closure of the myelomeningocele.[52, 53] The *Dandy-Walker malformation* accounts for 2 to 10% of children with hydrocephalus.[54–56] It is defined by hypoplasia of the cerebellar vermis, cystic dilatation of the fourth ventricle, and hydrocephalus. Most fetuses with Dandy-Walker malformations have ventriculomegaly on sonography, but the hydrocephalus may not be overt at birth. The Dandy-Walker malformation is believed to arise from failure of the fourth ventricular outlet to open, accounting for the dilatation of the fourth ventricle and hydrocephalus. The two compartments may not communicate and a dual-shunt system is often required. In its most severe form, the syndrome is often associated with other CNS, cardiac, genitourinary, ocular, and facial anomalies, and is often accompanied by mental retardation of variable degree despite successful shunting. So-called Dandy-Walker variants are common, however, and are characterized by a lesser degree of vermian hypoplasia. These individuals often do not develop hydrocephalus, and may be mentally normal, having none of the associated cerebral abnormalities.

It is also important to distinguish the Dandy-Walker syndrome from arachnoid cysts of the posterior fossa, and from the "mega cisterna magna," which carry a good prognosis.

The most severe destructive prenatal brain disorder that leads to fetal ventriculomegaly is hydranencephaly. The cerebral hemispheres are absent or nearly absent secondary to massive bilateral internal carotid artery occlusion or other intrauterine catastrophe.[57] Most of the forebrain is replaced by CSF within a thin gliotic membrane. Variable amounts of medial occipital lobe are spared due to collateral blood supply. The cerebellum, midbrain, thalamus, basal ganglia, and choroid plexus are preserved. The head is usually normal sized or small. A careful search for compressed cortical mantle should be made to distinguish hydrancephaly from massive hydrocephalus. A more limited in utero injury may lead to a localized cystic cavitation, termed a *porencephaly.* The cause can be vascular, traumatic, degenerative, or inflammatory. These cavitations may be in communication with the ventricular system and resemble asymmetric ventriculomegaly (Fig. 22–2). Other cystic abnormalities in the brain can also mimic hydrocephalus. Large arachnoid cysts near the ventricular system may resemble asymmetric hydrocephalus. Arachnoid cysts usually occur in isolation and are uncommonly associated with other brain anomalies. Choroid plexus cysts are very commonly seen between 15 and 26 weeks. They rarely become large enough to be mistaken for hydrocephalus, and most resolve by 24 weeks. Isolated choroid plexus cysts are benign.[58–60]

Holoprosencephaly refers to a spectrum of disorders due to absent or incomplete partition of telencephalic vesicles into cerebral hemispheres and lateral ventricles. It is not uncommon, and the frequency is estimated to be as high as 1 in 250 pregnancies and to represent 16% or more of all cases of prenatal ventriculomegaly.[61, 62] Approximately 50% have chromosomal abnormalities.[63–66] Maternal diabetes, fetal alcohol, or other toxin exposure are possible etiologies.[67] In the alobar and sem-

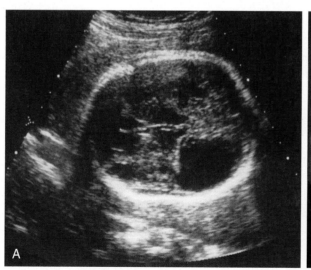
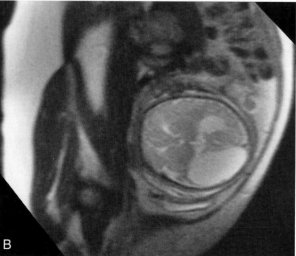

FIGURE 22–2. *A,* Fetal sonogram at 30 weeks resembling a unilaterally dilated atrium. *B,* MRI at 36 weeks with axial brain image reveals the occipital porencephalic cyst in communication with the ventricular system.

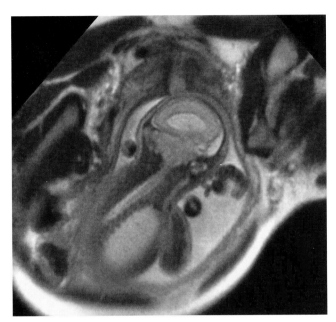

FIGURE 22–3. MRI at 29 weeks with coronal brain image demonstrates an alobar holoprosencephaly with a distorted monoventricle and absent midline structures.

ilobar forms, the lateral ventricles assume a variety of relatively enlarged and distorted "monoventricular" shapes while the head size ultimately becomes microcephalic due to loss of brain mass[68] (Fig. 22–3). The midline structures are variably absent or fused. The fused thalami serves as a key sonographic feature to distinguish the ventriculomegaly in alobar and semilobar prosencephaly from isolated hydrocephalus. Facial anomalies and extracranial malformations are common. In lobar holoprosencephaly, there is cleavage of the ventricular system and thalamus, but other midline structures such as the septum pellucidum, corpus callosum, and olfactory tracts are absent. Infants with alobar and semilobar holoprosencephaly usually die. Rare survivors are profoundly retarded.

Relative ventricular enlargement and distortion also occur in neuronal migration disorders. *Schizencephaly* defines a full-thickness cleft in the cerebral hemispheres caused by abnormal neuronal migration. The absence of a portion of the brain mantle distorts and enlarges portions of the ventricular anatomy. In *lissencephaly* there is a paucity of gyri and sulci from interruption of neuronal migration from the germinal matrix to the brain surface, mimicking the early fetus. The ventricles also appear relatively enlarged.

More subtle distortions of ventricular anatomy are seen in *agenesis of the corpus callosum* (ACC). ACC may be complete or partial. Axons that would have formed the corpus callosum gather into two aberrant bundles of fibers that run longitudinally along the medial walls of the lateral ventricles. These bundles displace the lateral ventricles superolaterally and make them appear more parallel than normal (Fig. 22–4A). The absence of the corpus callosum gives the atria and occipital horns a disproportionally enlarged appearance, termed culpocephaly, which may easily be confused with hydrocephalus (Fig. 22–4B). Additionally, in the absence of the corpus callosum, the third ventricle can dilate and displace superiorly into the interhemispheric fissure. The septum pellucidum is absent with complete ACC. The diagnosis can be made with MRI after 20 weeks when normal development of the corpus callosum is complete, but can be missed with sonography.[69, 70] Up to 85% of patients with ACC have other associated CNS malformations including various forms of hydrocephalus.[71] ACC is also a component of the Aicardi, Apert, and other syndromes. The high rate of mental retardation and epilepsy of ACC in postnatal series is likely due to the associated abnormalities and syndromes rather than the specific abnormality of the corpus callosum itself. As an isolated prenatal finding, the prognosis appears quite good with an 85% chance of normal outcome in a recent series.[72] Fetal hydrocephalus in isolated association with agenesis of corpus callosum has a variable outcome, as 4 of 13 patients derived from four series were normal at 12 months.[73–76]

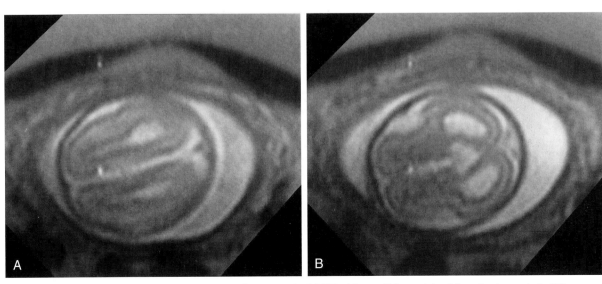

FIGURE 22–4. Agenesis of the corpus callosum on fetal MRI with parallel ventricles (*A*) and culpocephaly (*B*).

Radiology

The radiographic diagnosis of hydrocephalus has traditionally relied on sonographic measurements of ventricular enlargement. Several criteria have been proposed, the most useful of which is the transverse atrial width. Due to the lack of constraints from the striatum and Laplace's law (larger spheres require less pressure than the smaller to dilate when interconnected), the atrium is the first portion of the ventricular system to dilate with hydrocephalus. Each atrium as measured perpendicular to the ventricular axis is normally between 4 and 8 mm, with an upper limit of normal at 10 mm.[77, 78] The utility of the measurement is based on the fact that the atria are easily identified and the measurement is nearly constant between 15 and 35 weeks of gestation. The smallest measurement is considered the most accurate, as errors tend to occur when the measurement is not truly axial, or when the vein of Galen is misidentified as the medial wall, which tend to give a larger measurement.[79] The upper limit of 10 mm has been criticized as too sensitive, since some fetuses with measurement of 10 to 12 mm are normal.[80] There is clearly an increased rate of associated malformations with atrial widths greater than 10 mm, however.[77, 81] The second objective measurement is the lateral ventricular ratio (LVR), which is the ratio of the lateral ventricle width (from the parietal lateral ventricular wall to the midline echo) to the hemispheric width (from the midline echo to the inner table of the skull in the same transverse plane).[82, 83] The ratio is normally 70% during early pregnancy and decreases to 33% at 24 weeks. It then remains stable until term. The wide variation limits the usefulness of the LVR. The cranial size may remain normal in the setting of ventriculomegaly, but if it is enlarged it provides additional evidence for active hydrocephalus rather than a purely destructive process. The choroid plexus normally fills the ventricular atrium by the end of the first trimester and continues to do so during the second trimester. As the ventricles dilate, the posterior portion of the choroid plexus settles dependently into the enlarged atrium and becomes separated from the medial wall of the atrium, forming the basis of the "dangling choroid plexus" sign.[84] A separation of more than 3 mm between the choroid plexus and the medial wall is considered abnormal.[85] Isolated dilatation of the lateral ventricles and third ventricle suggests aqueductal stenosis. The size of the third ventricle changes with gestational age. The mean width of the third ventricle is approximately 1 mm during the second trimester, but after 32 weeks it can be up to 2 mm. An upper limit of 3.5 mm is proposed.[86]

Recently, fetal MRI has been developed as a more anatomically precise modality for prenatal neuroimaging.[70, 87–90] There is no apparent risk to the mother or fetus from the radiofrequency pulses or the magnetic field.[91] The technique is now being used in several centers. Fetal MRI is able to image the cerebral cortex well, and is also more sensitive than ultrasound in evaluating the subarachnoid space and ventricular morphology.[87] In a series of 18 fetuses with ultrasound-diagnosed CNS abnormalities, MRI revealed additional abnormalities in ten.[70] These included agenesis of the corpus callosum, polymicrogyria, porencephaly, agenesis of the septum pellucidi, and cerebellar hypoplasia. Undoubtedly, fetal MRI will facilitate accurate diagnosis of brain anomalies and prove valuable in selecting among the therapeutic options.

Natural History

A thorough understanding of the natural history of fetal hydrocephalus should form the basis for rational treatment and parental counseling. Unfortunately, understanding of the natural history is presently insufficient to definitively provide an exact prognosis. Current knowledge derives from outcome data obtained from untreated and treated postnatal hydrocephalus patients and studies of hydrocephalus diagnosed in utero since the initial experience with fetal shunting.

Before shunts were widely available, the prognosis of untreated hydrocephalus was dismal. The mortality rate was up to 50% in infancy, and the long-term survival was less than 30%.[92, 93] Of those who survived with compensated hydrocephalus, most were disabled and over half were mentally retarded.[94] The ability to effectively treat hydrocephalus came with the introduction of silicone ventricular shunts in the mid 1950s and the subsequent development of noninvasive neuroimaging in the 1970s. The CSF is typically diverted to the peritoneum. The mortality of shunted hydrocephalus dropped to less than 15% and almost half of the patients have an IQ greater than 80 and are able to work.[95] In Lorber's series, 84% reached normal intelligence.[96] The prognosis of children with hydrocephalus became more dependent on the etiology than on the hydrocephalus itself. Patients with Chiari II malformations consistently have the best long-term cognitive outcomes after shunting: over 70% have an IQ above 80 and the mean IQ is reported to be between 84 and 94.[95, 97–99] In aqueductal stenosis, approximately 50 to 65% are considered normal.[100–102] The outcome with Dandy-Walker malformations is less favorable; only 30 to 50% have normal IQs despite a generally later onset in infancy.[54, 103, 104] Hydrocephalic patients with additional CNS disorders such as porencephalic cavities or seizures have much worse outcomes.[105, 106] Prognostic variables relating to the hydrocephalus itself have been reported. A young age at diagnosis, delayed treatment, and infectious treatment complications are associated with a worse outcome.[107] The degree of ventriculomegaly has also been reported to be a significant variable. A preshunt cortical mantle of less than 20 mm and failure of the postshunting mantle to achieve 30 mm are poor prognostic signs,[108, 109] but this has not been a consistent observation.[110, 111] Shunting halts the hydrocephalus and usually results in reexpansion of the cerebral mantle on imaging. However, once axonal degeneration and neuronal loss have taken place in adult animal models, the reexpansion of the cerebral mantle does not result in restoration of lost elements but rather the formation of a glial scar.[112, 113] Clinical experience points to a critical age limit of 2 to 6 months in neonatal hydrocephalus, after which irreversible functional loss occurs if the hydrocephalus persists.[96, 114] Early intervention is clearly beneficial in neonatal hydrocephalus if there is clinical and radiographic evidence of increased intracranial pressure.

The outcome of pediatric and neonatal hydrocephalus cannot be extrapolated to fetal hydrocephalus. The fetal brain is different from the postnatal brain. The predominate neurodevelopmental process is cellular proliferation and migration before 32 weeks, versus dendritic formation and myelination in the postnatal period. At the same time, CSF dynamics in the fetus within a uterine environment are presumed to be different from those in the postnatal infant.

Attempts to describe the outcome of fetal hydrocephalus are complicated by diverse etiologies and difficulties distinguishing ex vacuo ventriculomegaly from hydrocephalus. Severe CNS abnormalities such as hydrancephaly, holoprosencephaly, and migration abnormalities are common causes of ventriculomegaly. Cochran reported a 36% incidence of these anomalies in a series of 41 fetuses with ventriculomegaly.[115] Extracranial malformations involving facial, cardiac, gastrointestinal, genitourinary, and skeletal structures are also frequently present in association with ventriculomegaly. Nyberg reported 61 fetuses with ventriculomegaly on sonogram, of whom 27 had multiple extra-CNS anomalies, and all ultimately died.[50] Up to 36% of cases with fetal ventriculomegaly with associated multisystem malformations have chromosomal defects.[116] The accurate detection of these abnormalities is critical, yet a false-negative rate of 20 to 60% has been reported.[115, 117, 118] Additionally, many destructive or genetic etiologies of true hydrocephalus such as toxoplasmosis-induced obstructive hydrocephalus and X-linked hydrocephalus can produce a poor outcome independent of the elevated CSF pressure. Many of these fetuses who are diagnosed before the legal limit are aborted, particularly if the ventriculomegaly is severe or associated anomalies are suspected. Overall, major series of fetal ventriculomegaly report a 54 to 84% incidence of associated abnormalities and a mortality of 50 to 91%.[1, 50, 51, 74, 115, 117–121] Of the survivors, between 16 and 68% have a normal cognitive outcome (Table 22–1).

Isolated fetal hydrocephalus from common etiologies (aqueductal stenosis, Chiari II, Dandy-Walker malformations) and communicating hydrocephalus without associated abnormalities account for approximately 50% of all cases of fetal ventriculomegaly. The outcome is variable in this group. One may obtain 184 cases from 11 published series that were not terminated, fully treated, and followed for outcome (Table 22–2).[1, 51, 73–75, 115–117, 119, 122] The overall mortality rate was 27%, with most deaths occurring in the immediate postpartum period. Only 48% of the survivors had a normal cognitive outcome. Many with isolated ventriculomegaly did not develop postnatal hydrocephalus and 70% required postnatal shunting. As with postnatal hydrocephalus, the outcome of fetal hydrocephalus is influenced by the etiology. The literature provides 110 cases of hydrocephalus from confirmed Chiari II malformations, aqueductal stenosis, and Dandy-Walker malformations with their respective outcome data (Table 22–3). Fetal hydrocephalus from Chiari II malformations (myelomeningocele) had the best cognitive outcome. The mortality was 23%, and 67% of survivors were cognitively normal in 43 cases.[1, 51, 115–117, 119, 121–124] Leakage of CSF from the open myelomeningocele may allow ventricular decompression and explain the relatively good cognitive outcome. Of 51 cases of fetal aqueductal stenosis, the mortality was 16% and only 40% of the survivors had a normal cognitive outcome.[1, 51, 110, 115, 119, 122, 125] Fetal Dandy-Walker malformations had the worst outcome, with only 31% of 16 survived cases considered normal.[1, 51, 73, 122, 124]

These results do not accurately portray the natural history of fetal hydrocephalus due to the selection bias from terminated cases. Most myelomeningoceles detected before the legal limit are terminated. In a large series from the United Kingdom, 172 of 267 cases of fetal ventriculomegaly had Chiari II malformations associated with myelodysplasia, and 153 before the legal limit of 28 weeks were terminated.[116] In a separate series of isolated fetal ventriculomegaly of diverse etiologies, Gupta found that 12% are terminated.[126] Presumably, most severely affected fetuses were more likely to be aborted, and the survivors fared better than the group as a whole. Nevertheless, the outcome of the three common etiologies of congenital hydrocephalus in the fetus paral-

TABLE 22–1. FETAL VENTRICULOMEGALY

	N	N ASSOCIATED ABNORMALITIES	N DIED (N TERMINATED)	N SURVIVOR NL (%)
Chervenak et al.[118]	50	42	36 (13)	6 (42%)
Glick et al.[74]	24	13	13 (8)	7 (64%)
Pretorius et al.[34]	40	28	34 (9)	3 (50%)
Cochrane et al.[115]	40	30	21 (0)	3 (16%)
Serlo et al.[1]	38	32	28 (4)	6 (60%)
Vintzileos et al.[51]	20	14	11 (4)	—
Nyberg et al.[62]	61	51	41 —	—
Hudgins et al.[117]	47	35	28 (15)	13 (68%)
Drugan et al.[119]	43	31	19 (17)	8 (33%)
Rousseau et al.[121]	40	26	12 (3)	16 (57%)
Holzgreve et al.[120]	118	90	72 (27)	—

NL, normal.

T A B L E 22–2. FETAL HYDROCEPHALUS (INCLUDING ISOLATED AQUEDUCTAL STENOSIS, CHIARI II, DANDY-WALKER) WITHOUT OTHER SEVERE ABNORMALITY

						DEVELOPMENTAL OUTCOME			
SERIES	N* APPARENT	N† CONFIRMED	N SURVIVED	S/P/R‡	Shunt	NI	Mild	Mod	Severe
Glick et al.[135]	14	14	11	9/1/1	6	7	1	3	0
Cochrane et al.[115]	19	18	7	—	8	2	—	—	—
Serlo et al.[1]	11	10	9	—	9	6	2	1	0
Vintzileos et al.[51]	9	7	7	2/5/0	7	3	3	0	1
Hudgins et al.[117]	17	14	13	11/2/1	9	10	2	0	1
Drugan et al.[119]	16	15	15	11/3/—	9	8	5	2	0
Oi et al.[122]	12	12	6	—	7	3	0	3	0
Nicolaides et al.[116]	230§	49	25	—	5	12	1	3	2
Amato et al.[73]	13	13	13	—	13	3	7	—	2
Twining et al.[75]	25	9	9	6/0/3	1	5	3	1	0
Levitsky et al.[125]	37	23	18	—/8/—	19	3	3	10	5
Total		184	133 (73%)		93 (70%)	64 (48%)	27	23	11

* Apparent in utero diagnosis.
† Not terminated.
‡ s/p/r: stable/progression/resolution.
§ 153 of 172 Chiari II malformations electively terminated.

lels their neonatal counterpart, but appears to be worse in each case. Studies of overt hydrocephalus at birth (head circumference 2 to 3 SD above normal) provide additional insight. Patients born with such large heads would presumably have had fetal hydrocephalus and yet survived pregnancy and delivery. In Fernell's series, the mortality at age 2 was 20% and normal development was seen in 44% of patients without other severe anomalies.[127] Renier reported a series of 47 patients that excluded those with Chiari II malformations.[128] The mortality was 34%, and only 28% had normal intelligence. Of those with aqueductal stenosis in the series, 46% had normal IQs and the mortality at 10 years was 20%. Those with Dandy-Walker malformations did worse. Only 20% had normal IQs and 40% mortality at 10 years. McCullough reported a mortality rate of 14% and normal intelligence in 53% in a series of 37 patients with different etiologies.[98] Collectively, these studies suggest a somewhat worse developmental prognosis for prenatal hydrocephalus than for postnatal hydrocephalus (Table 22–4).

Other prognostic variables in fetal hydrocephalus have been examined. Fetuses with mild ventriculomegaly have a better outcome than those with severe ventriculomegaly. Mild isolated fetal ventriculomegaly (10 to 12 mm of atrial diameter) carries an excellent prognosis. Resolution of the ventriculomegaly occurs in one third of cases, and the rest remain stable and mild. Development delay occurs in 3%, which is indistinguishable from the 2.5% risk in the general population.[129] The incidence of abnormal outcome increases to 23% in isolated ventriculomegaly with an atrial width between 12 and 15 mm, but this is mostly related to metabolic or intrinsic brain disorders.[129, 130] Static mild isolated ventriculomegaly between 10 and 12 mm atrial width may be a normal physiologic variation that does not usually lead to postnatal hydrocephalus. However, there should be a high level of suspicion for an underlying brain disorder when the ventricles measure 12 to 15 mm in the absence of any associated malformations.

With more severe ventriculomegaly, the relationship between residual cortical thickness in fetal hydrocephalus and cognitive outcome has not been consistently established. A series of 25 fetuses with hydrocephalus who survived at least 10 years was evaluated by Kirkinen.[124] Out of this group, 48% had a normal outcome, and they had a significantly smaller ventricular index on the last prenatal ultrasound than those with a poor outcome. In a series of 26 fetuses with myelodysplasia, none with in utero macrocephaly had a normal outcome.[131] Leviski's series of fetal aqueductal stenosis demonstrated a correlation between the fetal cerebral mantle width and outcome.[125] Postnatal measurements of prenatal hydrocephalus also support a relationship. McCul-

T A B L E 22–3. OUTCOME OF FETAL HYDROCEPHALUS BY ETIOLOGY

			DEVELOPMENTAL OUTCOME			
ETIOLOGY	REFERENCES	NO. OF PATIENTS	Normal (%)	Mild/Moderate	Severe	Dead
Aqueductal stenosis	1, 51, 110, 115, 119, 122, 123	51	17 (40%)	18	8	8
Dandy-Walker	1, 51, 73, 122, 125	16	5 (31%)	*	*	*
Spina bifida	1, 51, 115–117, 119, 121, 122, 124, 125	43	22 (67%)	7	4	10

* Data not provided.

TABLE 22–4. PERCENTAGE OF NORMAL DEVELOPMENTAL OUTCOME

	COMBINED	CHIARI II	AQUEDUCTAL STENOSIS	DANDY-WALKER
Fetal hydrocephalus*	48%	67%	40%	29%
Overt hydrocephalus at birth[98, 127, 128]	28–53%	—	46%	20%
Neonatal hydrocephalus[95, 96, 99, 100–104]	50–80%	70%	50–65%	30–50%

* See text.

lough reported that a brain mantle of less than 1 cm in neonates with overt hydrocephalus at birth predicted an IQ of less than 80.[98] Renier showed a correlation between the postshunt reexpansion of cerebral mantle and outcome in neonates with overt hydrocephalus. However, there was no correlation between preshunt head size and outcome.[128] Several other studies have also found no correlation between brain mantle, ventricular width, and other measures of fetal ventriculomegaly, and outcome.[110, 116, 117] There are also reports of neonates with very little cerebral mantle at birth who ultimately had excellent outcomes.[57, 96] The degree of ventriculomegaly in fetal hydrocephalus or neonatal hydrocephalus is not associated with outcome in a simple way, and other factors are clearly important.

Radiographic progression of fetal ventriculomegaly is variable and depends on the etiology (Fig. 22–5). Overall, most cases do not progress. The progression rate from the limited studies which were documented by serial ultrasound was 20%.[51, 74, 75, 119] Rousseau, in a study of 40 fetuses, noted no progression in any.[121] On the other hand, Vintzileos reported progression before 32 weeks in five of seven fetuses, including all four with aqueductal stenosis.[51] Most of Levitsky's patients with aqueductal stenosis also progressed.[125] The cognitive outcome in progressive isolated fetal hydrocephalus has been reported in 16 patients: six were normal, four were mildly delayed, three were moderately delayed, and three were severely delayed.[1, 51, 74, 117, 119] A final in utero cortical width of less than 1.5 cm was noted in 5 of these 16 patients, and all 5 had moderate to severe delay after shunting in the neonatal period.[1, 119] This small series does not give the complete story, since progression is not detected prior to the first imaging study and many of those detected before the legal limit underwent termination of pregnancy. It does suggest, however, that in utero progression is an unfavorable prognostic factor if the mantle thickness is less that 1.5 cm. Otherwise, it is not uniformly ruinous for the fetus. Prominent ventriculomegaly may also regress. Twinning reported a case diagnosed at 31 weeks with an atrial diameter of 30 whose ventriculomegaly decreased on subsequent im-

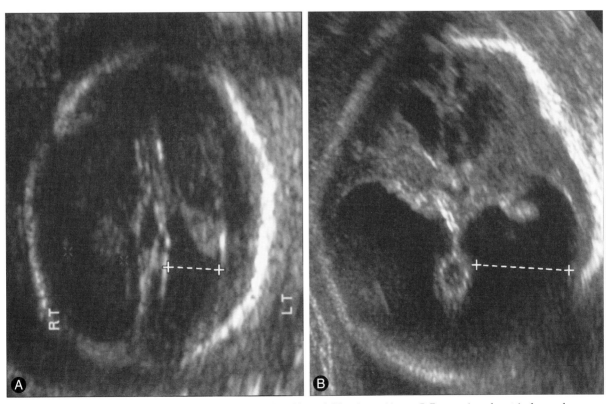

FIGURE 22–5. *A,* Fetal sonogram at 20 weeks with mild atrial dilatation at 11 mm. *B,* Progression of ventriculomegaly at 32 weeks to 39 mm.

aging, and the child was normal at 3 years of age without a shunt.[75]

The duration and time of onset of the fetal hydrocephalus affects outcome. In a series of 20 patients with fetal hydrocephalus diagnosed between 24 and 40 weeks, those who remained in utero for more than 1 month after diagnosis all had poor outcomes.[122] The analysis also included assessment of intracranial pressure. Three patients with marked ventriculomegaly and macrocephaly had further head enlargement immediately after birth. Therapeutic cephalocentesis was performed in two fetuses, with CSF pressure found to be 350 and 400 mm Hg, normal being 40 to 50 mm Hg. Intrauterine pressure was measured to be 160 mm Hg during a ventriculoamniotic shunting procedure.[4] The fetal brain is thus subjected to high pressures from both hydrocephalus and uterine constriction. Oi suggested that allowing this to persist for over a month puts the fetus at risk for irreversible brain damage. Another series, however, reported in utero hydrocephalus of more than 1-month duration that did well.[119] Oi has recently incorporated fetal MRI to provide more precise morphologic diagnosis.[132] Patients received IQ and developmental assessment at a mean of 1.8 years postnatally. In cases of aqueductal stenosis, communicating hydrocephalus, and Chiari II–associated hydrocephalus, the outcome was worse when the diagnosis was made before 32 weeks. This implies that neuronal maturation is affected by the development of hydrocephalus in the period before lung maturation.

Animal Models

Animal models of human hydrocephalus have been developed to determine the efficacy of in utero intervention and to explore various surgical options. Michejda and Hodgens successfully induced hydrocephalus in 90% of gravid rhesus monkeys with serial steroid injections.[133] The hydrocephalus, however, was accompanied by other malformations including porencephaly, cranium bifidum, and encephaloceles. A hysterotomy was performed to measure the fetal intracranial pressure, which was 45 to 55 mm Hg in controls and greater than 100 mm Hg in hydrocephalic fetal monkeys. A valved ventriculoamniotic shunt was developed for intrauterine treatment in this model. It allowed drainage of CSF at 60 mm Hg. The device was placed in the fetus at the end of the second trimester or the beginning of the third trimester. Treated animals were delivered by cesarean section at term. The untreated monkeys had severe and progressive ventricular enlargement with growth retardation and motor difficulties, and most died within 2 weeks. In contrast, most of the treated monkeys lived, showed progressive physical dexterity, and grew at a normal rate.

Harrison et al. developed a model of hydrocephalus in sheep by injecting kaolin into the cisterna magna.[134, 135] An inflammatory reaction was induced that fibrosed the subarachnoid space around the fourth ventricle and the animals developed obstructive hydrocephalus within a couple of weeks. Ventriculoamniotic, ventriculopleural, and ventriculojugular shunts were performed 20 days after kaolin injection. The shunted lambs had reduced head circumferences and more normal ventricular sizes, whereas the unshunted lambs had large heads, bulging fontanels, and marked ventriculomegaly. All specimens, however, demonstrated inflammatory arachnoiditis from the kaolin, making detailed histologic analysis of the autopsied brains difficult.

These experiments demonstrate that in utero shunts are technically possible and can be effective in animal models. Unfortunately, there is no large animal model of aqueductal stenosis to simulate isolated hydrocephalus without accompanying anomalies. The H-Tx rat strain have hydrocephalus at 18 to 19 days' gestation from a developmental aqueductal stenosis.[136, 137] However, fetal experimentation in a model would be technically challenging. Another limitation of animal models is the difficulty in assessing higher cortical function, which is the area of most concern in humans.

Treatment Options

The first interventions for human fetal hydrocephalus were performed to minimize maternal morbidity and mortality, without concern for the fetus. Prior to effective prenatal diagnosis with sonography, marked fetal hydrocephalus was not detected until labor arrest or uterine rupture occurred from dystocia. Trocar drainage of the fetal ventricle was performed to reduce the size of the fetal head in order to allow for safe vaginal delivery. The fetus rarely survived.

The development of routine real-time sonography made detection of ventriculomegaly during the second and third trimesters routine. This led to the hope that in utero treatment of fetal ventriculomegaly would improve outcome by preventing the detrimental effects of persistently elevated pressure on fetal brain development. The difficulty with these early efforts was patient selection. The first attempt to treat fetal hydrocephalus was by Birnholz and Frigoletto, who performed serial cephalocentesis to decompress the ventricles in a fetus with ventriculomegaly.[138] Ventricular punctures were performed under ultrasound guidance every 2 weeks from diagnosis at 25 weeks until delivery by cesarean section at 34 weeks. Postnatal CT revealed additional abnormalities not seen on ultrasound: asymmetric ventriculomegaly, a posterior cyst, and agenesis of the corpus callosum. The child was subsequently diagnosed with Becker's muscular dystrophy and remained impaired with a seizure disorder.

Intermittent drainage does not effectively address the constant production of CSF. Additionally, intermittent ventricular puncture can produce porencephaly in the immature brain. Clewell first described treating a human fetus with a ventriculoamniotic shunt in 1982.[4] A Silastic shunt with a one-way valve was inserted percutaneously through the posterior skull into the ventricle of a male fetus with a needle under ultrasound guidance. Serial ultrasounds demonstrated a decrease in ventricular size and an increase in thickness of the cerebral mantle. The shunt worked for 9 weeks, at which time the ventricles enlarged, and the infant was delivered at 34 weeks. The shunt catheter was found to be occluded by tissue that had grown into the lumen. The family had a known history of X-linked hydrocephalus and the infant had the characteristic bilateral hand deformity. In the same year, Frigoletto placed a ventriculoamniotic shunt in a 23-week fetus with a facial cleft.[140] Technical complications with inserting the shunt through the needle caused the valve to be lost, and the fetus had a valveless shunt. Serial ultrasounds showed a decrease in ventricular size. The infant was delivered at 28 weeks by cesarean section because of an amniotic fluid leak, but the shunt appeared to be working. The infant had diabetes insipidus, seizures, and possible sepsis, and died at age 5 weeks. Reflux of amniotic fluid may have caused chemical ventriculitis. A third ventriculoamniotic shunt was reported the following year by Depp on a fetus with Dandy-Walker malformation.[141] At follow-up, the child had developmental delay, spastic diplegia, and hemiparesis. Thus, fetal shunting had an inauspicious beginning, since these three patients all had poor functional outcomes that could have been foreseen: X-linked hydrocephalus, hydrocephalus with extra-CNS malformations, and Dandy-Walker malformation.

The burgeoning interest in fetal therapy, however, led to the Kroc Foundation Symposium in 1982 for workers in the field. The Fetal Surgery Registry was set up along with patient selection guidelines for in utero treatment of hydrocephalus[142]:

1. The presence of a multispecialty team with level III ultrasonography, high-risk obstetric unit, neonatal intensive care, and access to other subspecialties
2. A singleton pregnancy
3. Absence of any other significant anomalies
4. Progressive ventricular dilatation
5. A normal karyotype
6. Viral cultures
7. Adequate follow-up
8. Gestational age less than 32 weeks or lung immaturity
9. A consensus by the team to proceed

A total of 41 cases of fetal hydrocephalus treated up to 1987 by in utero decompression were reported by the Fetal Surgery Registry.[143] Of these, 39 cases were treated by ventriculoamniotic shunting and two by serial cephalocentesis. Hydrocephalus was defined as progressive ventriculomegaly determined by strict sonographic criteria. The etiology was mixed and did not strictly adhere to the guidelines, largely because of difficulty recognizing other anomalies. Thus, the series included five subjects with associated anomalies (including one holoprosencephaly, one Dandy-Walker syndrome, one prosencephaly, and one Chiari II malformation), along with 32 with aqueductal stenosis. The mean gestational age at diagnosis was 25 weeks and the mean age at treatment was 27 weeks. Seven treated fetuses died, one before birth and six after birth. The stillbirth was directly related to needle trauma to the brain stem. Three died as a result of premature labor within 48 hours of shunt placement. Chorioamnionitis was suspected on clinical grounds and coagulase-negative *Staphylococcus* infection confirmed in one. A gonococcal ventriculitis has also been reported from a ventriculoamniotic shunt.[144] The procedure-related mortality was 10% (4 of 39). The remaining three postnatal deaths were due to lethal anomalies not recognized prior to treatment. Twelve of the 34 survivors were normal at follow-up, all of whom had aqueductal stenosis. Outcome did not correlate with duration of treatment.

It is difficult to draw conclusions from this experience. Clearly, the treatment-related mortality was high. Patient selection was hampered by difficulty in recognizing associated malformations. Perhaps most importantly, there was no untreated concurrent control group. Given the selection bias, a comparable historic control group is difficult to gather from the literature. Vintzileos reported nine postnatally treated hydrocephalics who would have been candidates for in utero shunting. He compared the outcome to those who underwent fetal shunting for isolated aqueductal stenosis and noted no difference.[51] Table 22–5 compares the 51 patients with isolated fetal aqueductal stenosis and reported outcomes gleaned from the literature with the cases of aqueductal stenosis in the Fetal Surgery Registry. The rates of normal cognitive outcome and survival are remarkably similar. The fetal shunt group actually had more patients with severe impairments.

Soon after the reports of human fetal ventriculoamniotic shunts emerged, a voluntary moratorium was in-

TABLE 22–5. OUTCOME OF ISOLATED AQUEDUCTAL STENOSIS TREATED IN THE NEONATAL PERIOD COMPARED WITH PATIENTS WHO UNDERWENT FETAL SHUNTING

| | | DEVELOPMENTAL OUTCOME | | | |
	SERIES	Normal	Mild/Moderate	Severe	Dead
Neonatal shunts	Serlo et al.[1]	0	2	1	0
	Cochrane et al.[115]	1	0	1	1
	Amacher & Reid[110]	3	1	0	0
	Drugan et al.[119]	3	1	1	0
	Levitsky et al.[125]	3	10	4	5
	Twinning et al.[75]	2	1	0	1
	Oi et al.[122]	2	1	1	1
	Vintzileos et al.[51]	3	2	0	0
	Total 51 pts	17(40%)	18(42%)	8(18%)	8(16%)
Fetal registry[141]	32 pts	12(43%)	2(7%)	14(50%)	4(13%)

voked, pending further knowledge of the natural history of fetal hydrocephalus. Venes also noted that there was no conclusive correlation between ventricular size and cognitive outcome, and that since CSF flow may be required for the normal development of CSF pathways, in utero shunting might actually cause irreversible hydrocephalus.[145]

Although the de facto moratorium is still in place, advances in fetal surgery and prenatal diagnosis and further understanding of the natural history suggest the need for a reevaluation. The outcome of isolated fetal hydrocephalus is worse than neonatal and pediatric counterparts with the same etiologies (Table 22–4). This suggests an in utero component of neurodevelopmental impairment that is not reversible by postnatal treatment in a selected group of fetuses. The process occurs before 32 weeks, when lung immaturity precludes delivery and the damage may be irreversible after a duration of only 4 gestational weeks. Fetal MRI provides superior structural delineation to detect associated abnormalities. Ultrasound capabilities have also improved.[81] Along with other prenatal diagnostic advances such as rapid fetal blood sampling, chorionic villus sampling, and polymerase chain reaction (PCR) analysis for genetic disorders, reliable patient screening is now possible. Finally, the experience of fetal surgeons in the treatment of life-threatening diseases such as diaphragmatic hernia suggests open or endoscopic shunting procedures that would likely be safer and more effective than the percutaneous, ultrasound-guided technique. While we now have some indications of which fetuses with isolated hydrocephalus will likely do poorly, there is currently no definitive prognostic variable set with which to select patients who would benefit from in utero shunting. The fetus with isolated, rapidly progressive fetal hydrocephalus from non–X-linked aqueductal stenosis diagnosed before 28 weeks would be the ideal patient to be considered by selected centers with fetal surgery expertise. In the meantime, prospective analysis of the potential variables in the outcome of fetal hydrocephalus with MRI-based diagnosis is needed.

Present Status

The finding of fetal ventriculomegaly mandates a prompt, thorough work-up that begins with a concerted effort to rule out additional anomalies. Subsequent management decisions depend on the rate of progression, gestational age and, ultimately, the family's wishes (Fig. 22–6). A team that includes obstetricians, perinatologists, fetal surgeons, and pediatric neurosurgeons is necessary for optimal care.

The diagnosis of fetal hydrocephalus can be made as early as 15 weeks. At present, the average gestational age at diagnosis is around 30 weeks, but there is a trend toward earlier diagnosis as routine ultrasounds are performed during the early second trimester.[116] For those patients diagnosed before the legal limit of abortion, there is urgency to complete the work-up to allow an informed parental decision. The family gestational history is reviewed for previous outcomes, early drug exposures, and unexpected illnesses, and the family history is reviewed for X-linked hydrocephalus and neural tube malformations. A complete ultrasound examination is carried out to search for additional abnormalities, but there is a persistent false-negative rate with ultrasound evaluation alone. In a review of 318 cases of apparently isolated fetal ventriculomegaly detected by ultrasound, 25% were found to have additional associated anomalies after birth.[126] Ideally, an MRI scan is obtained and interpreted by an experienced pediatric neuroradiologist to evaluate the fetal brain for subtle abnormalities such as agenesis of the corpus callosum and cortical dysplasia. Amniocentesis is performed for viral cultures, chromosomal analysis, and α-fetoprotein levels. The dismal prognosis of ventriculomegaly associated with infections, chromosomal abnormalities, and severe CNS and extracranial abnormalities may influence the family's decision to continue the pregnancy. Isolated ventriculomegaly detected before the legal limit may be reason enough to terminate the pregnancy for some families who cannot accept the prospect of having a handicapped child.

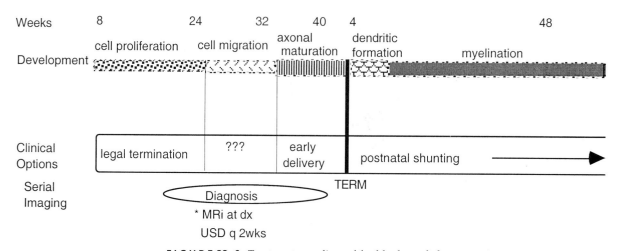

FIGURE 22–6. Treatment paradigm of fetal hydrocephalus.

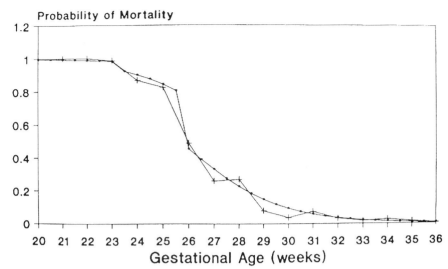

FIGURE 22–7. Actual (+) and predicted (•) mortality by gestational age at midpoint of each week from 20 through 36 completed weeks. (From Copper RL, Goldenberg RL, Creasy RK, et al: A multicenter study of preterm birth weight and gestational age-specific neonatal mortality [see comments]. Am J Obstet Gynecol 168:78–84, 1993, with permission.)

Isolated hydrocephalus is followed with serial ultrasounds. This affords additional opportunity to detect potentially missed abnormalities and to assess progression of ventriculomegaly. If the ventriculomegaly is stable, the fetus is carried to term. This does not deny the possibility of ongoing, irreversible damage in stable hydrocephalus, but concedes that at present there are no data to mandate preterm intervention. Cesarean section is performed when head size precludes vaginal delivery at the discretion of the obstetrician.[146] There is no clear indication to deliver by cesarean section in the absence of macrocephaly in the term fetus.[147]

A small group will show rapidly progressive ventricular enlargement on serial sonograms. This does not necessarily lead to devastating outcome, but it does appear to be an adverse predictor, prompting consideration of early delivery and early shunting. The morbidity and mortality from prematurity argue against early delivery and shunting before 32 weeks (Fig. 22–7). Beyond this point, there continues to be a small risk of complications from early delivery that diminishes as gestation progresses to term. Approximately 16% of infants delivered at 32 weeks will weigh less than 1,500 g and will have a 7.7% incidence of cerebral palsy.[148, 149] The gestational age-specific mortality at 32 weeks is 3.5% and decreases to 0.5% by 36 weeks.[150] The 3 to 4% incidence of necrotizing enterocolitis in infants with birth weights less than 2,000 g can seriously complicate the distal placement of the shunt.[151] Another significant source of morbidity from early delivery is the increased risk of shunt infection. The overall shunt infection rate is between 5 and 10% but is higher in preterm infants and may be as high as 20%.[152, 153] A shunt infection may be devastating in the neonate or premature infant, especially with gram-negative organisms. In Reiner's series, only 5% of patients with shunt infections from overt hydrocephalus at birth had normal IQs at a mean follow-up of 7 years and half died by age 10.[128] These risks are very real and must be weighed against the largely theoretical benefit of early delivery.

For the fetus with rapidly progressive hydrocephalus, early delivery and shunting may be considered after 32

weeks. Assessment of lung maturity is vital, since high intra-abdominal pressure translated from positive-pressure mechanical ventilation can interfere with shunt function. If the lungs are mature, delivery can be induced with the understanding that there is still a higher incidence of perinatal respiratory distress. A cesarean section is preferred, followed immediately by shunt insertion to eliminate vaginal and ICU flora exposure.

Those who develop progressive ventricular enlargement and cortical thinning before 28 weeks may have irreversible damage by 32 weeks.[122] Early delivery and shunting may not help these fetuses and is probably not worth the potential morbidity. It is in this group that fetal shunting could be considered, but only in the context of a clinical trial in the setting of a center with extensive experience in fetal surgery.

REFERENCES

1. Serlo W, Kirkinen P, Jouppila P, Herva R: Prognostic signs in fetal hydrocephalus. Childs Nerv Syst 2:93–97, 1986.
2. Lorber J: Is your brain really necessary? Nurs Mirror 152:29–30, 1981.
3. Clewell WH, Johnson ML, Meier PR, et al: Placement of ventriculo-amniotic shunt for hydrocephalus in a fetus [letter]. N Engl J Med 305:955, 1981.
4. Clewell WH, Johnson ML, Meier PR, et al: A surgical approach to the treatment of fetal hydrocephalus. N Engl J Med 306:1320–1325, 1982.
5. Bannister CM: Is the intrauterine treatment of fetal hydrocephalus helpful or harmful? Fetal Ther 1:146–149, 1986.
6. Clewell WH: Congenital hydrocephalus: Treatment in utero. Fetal Ther 3:89–97, 1988.
7. Lemire RJ (ed): Normal and Abnormal Development of the Human Nervous System. Hagerstown, MD: Harper & Row, 1975, p 95.
8. O'Rahilly R, Muller F: Human Embryology and Teratology. New York: Wiley-Liss, 1966, pp 362–366.
9. O'Rahilly R, Muller F: Ventricular system and choroid plexuses of the human brain during the embryonic period proper. Am J Anat 189:285–302, 1990.
10. Chinn DH, Callen PW, Filly RA: The lateral cerebral ventricle in early second trimester. Radiology 148:529–531, 1983.
11. Petrikovsky BM, Kaplan GP: Size disparity of the choroid plexuses of the lateral ventricles: Prenatal diagnosis and neonatal outcome. Prenat Diagn 16:670–672, 1996.

12. Duckett S: The choroid plexus of the lateral ventricles during early human fetal life. Anat Anz 129:77–83, 1971.
13. Spector R, Johanson CE: The mammalian choroid plexus. Sci Am 261:68–74, 1989.
14. Pollay M, Hisey B, Reynolds E, et al: Choroid plexus Na+/K+-activated adenosine triphosphatase and cerebrospinal fluid formation. Neurosurgery 17:768–772, 1985.
15. McComb JG: Cerebrospinal fluid physiology of the developing fetus. AJNR Am J Neuroradiol 13:595–599, 1992.
16. Jones HC: Intercellular pores between ependymal cells lining the roof of the fourth ventricle in mammalian fetuses. Z Kinderchir 37:130–133, 1980.
17. Wilson JT: On the nature and mode of origin of the foramen of Magendie. J Anat 71:423–426, 1936.
18. Gardner E, O'Rahilly R, Prolo P: The Dandy-Walker and Arnold-Chiari malformations. Arch Neurol 32:393–407, 1975.
19. Muller F, O'Rahilly R: The development of the human brain from a closed neural tube at stage 13. Anat Embryol 177:203–224, 1988.
20. O'Rahilly R, Gardner E: Initial development of the human brain. Bibl Anat 19:140–141, 1981.
21. Schoenwolf GC, Desmond ME: Neural tube occlusion precedes rapid brain enlargement. J Exp Zool 230:405–407, 1984.
22. Desmond ME, Jacobson AG: Embryonic brain enlargement requires cerebrospinal fluid pressure. Dev Biol 57:188–198, 1977.
23. Mclone DG, Nadich TP: Developmental morphology of the subarachnoid space, brain vasculature, and contiguous structures, and the cause of the Chiari II malformation. AJNR Am J Neuroradiol 13:463–482, 1992.
24. O'Rahilly R, Muller F: The meninges in human development. J Neuropathol Exp Neurol 45:588–608, 1986.
25. Dorovini-Zis K, Dolman CL: Gestational development of the brain. Arch Pathol Lab Med 101:192–180, 1977.
26. Pilu G, De Palma L, Romero R, et al: The fetal subarachnoid cisterns: An ultrasound study with report of a case of congenital communicating hydrocephalus. J Ultrasound Med 5:365–372, 1986.
27. Gomez DG, DiBenedetto AT, Pavese AM, et al: Development of arachnoid villi and granulations in man. Acta Anat 111:247–258, 1982.
28. Osaka K, Handa H, Matsumoto S, Yasuda M: Development of the cerebrospinal fluid pathway in the normal and abnormal human embryos. Childs Brain 6:26–38, 1980.
29. Rubin RC, Hochwald GM, Tiell M, et al: Hydrocephalus: I. Histological and ultrastructural changes in the pre-shunted cortical mantle. Surg Neurol 5:109–114, 1976.
30. Rubin RC, Hochwald GM, Tiell M, Liwnicz BH: Hydrocephalus: II. Cell number and size, and myelin content of the pre-shunted cerebral cortical mantle. Surg Neurol 5:115–118, 1976.
31. Del Bigio MR, Bruni JE, Fewer HD: Human neonatal hydrocephalus: An electron microscopic study of the periventricular tissue. J Neurosurg 63:56–64, 1985.
32. Weller RO, Shulman K: Infantile hydrocephalus: Clinical, histological, and ultrastructural study of brain damage. J Neurosurg 36:255–267, 1972.
33. McAllister JP II Chovan P: Neonatal hydrocephalus. Mechanisms and consequences. Neurosurg Clin North Am 9:73–93, 1998.
34. Pretorius DH, Davis K, Manco-Johnson ML, et al: Clinical course of fetal hydrocephalus: 40 cases. AJR Am J Roentgenol 144:827–831, 1985.
35. Shellshear I, Emery JL: Gliosis and aqueductal formation in the aqueduct of Sylvius. Dev Med Child Neurol 37(Suppl):22–29, 1976.
36. Russell DS: Observations on the pathology of hydrocephalus. Special Report Series Medical Research Council. Vol. No. 265. London: HM Stationery Office, 1949.
37. Pattern RM, Mack LA, Finberg HJ: Unilateral hydrocephalus: Prenatal sonographic diagnosis. AJR Am J Roentgenol 156:359–363, 1991.
38. Kaiser G: Hydrocephalus following toxoplasmosis. Z Kinderchir 40:10–11, 1985.
39. Hirsch JF, Hirsch E, Sainte Rose C, et al: Stenosis of the aqueduct of Sylvius. Etiology and treatment. J Neurosurg Sci 30:29–39, 1986.
40. Halliday J, Chow CW, Wallace D, Danks DM: X linked hydrocephalus: A survey of a 20 year period in Victoria, Australia. J Med Genet 23:23–31, 1986.
41. Strain L, Gosden CM, Brock DJ, Bonthron DT: Genetic heterogeneity in X-linked hydrocephalus: Linkage to markers within Xq27.3. Am J Hum Genet 54:236–243, 1994.
42. Lyonnet S, Pelet A, Royer G, et al: The gene for X-linked hydrocephalus maps to Xq28, distal to DXS52. Genomics 14:508–510, 1992.
43. Habib Z: Genetics and genetic counselling in neonatal hydrocephalus. Obstet Gynecol Surv 36:529–534, 1981.
44. Ribeiro MC, Brunoni D: Terminal deletion 1q43 in a newborn with hydrocephalus. Ann Genet 30:126–128, 1987.
45. Fahmi F, Schmerler S, Hutcheon RG: Hydrocephalus in an infant with trisomy 22. J Med Genet 31:141–144, 1994.
46. McDuffie RS Jr: Complete trisomy 9: Case report with ultrasound findings. Am J Perinatol 11:80–84, 1994.
47. Strain L, Brock DJ, Bonthron DT: Prenatal diagnosis of X-linked hydrocephalus [letter]. Prenat Diagn 14:415–416, 1994.
48. Walker ME, Lynch-Salamon DA, Milatovich A, Saal HM: Prenatal diagnosis of ring chromosome 6 in a fetus with hydrocephalus. Prenat Diagn 16:857–861, 1996.
49. Jouet M: The role of genetics in understanding hydrocephalus and spina bifida. An update. Eur J Pediatr Surg 6:35–36, 1996.
50. Nyberg DA, Mack LA, Hirsch J, et al: Fetal hydrocephalus: Sonographic detection and clinical significance of associated anomalies. Radiology 163:187–191, 1987.
51. Vintzileos AM, Campbell WA, Weinbaum PJ, Nochimson DJ: Perinatal management and outcome of fetal ventriculomegaly. Obstet Gynecol 69:5–11, 1987.
52. Rekate HL: Management of hydrocephalus and the erroneous concept of shunt independence in spina bifida patients. Barrows Neurol Inst Q 4:17–20, 1988.
53. Dias MS, McLone DG: Hydrocephalus in the child with dysraphism. Neurosurg Clin North Am 4:715–726, 1993.
54. Hirsch JF, Pierre-Kahn A, Renier D, et al: The Dandy-Walker malformation. A review of 40 cases. J Neurosurg 61:515–522, 1984.
55. Nyberg DA, Cyr DR, Mack LA, et al: The Dandy-Walker malformation prenatal sonographic diagnosis and its clinical significance. Ultrasound Med 7:65–71, 1988.
56. Cornford E, Twining P: The Dandy-Walker syndrome: The value of antenatal diagnosis. Clin Radiol 45:172–174, 1992.
57. Sutton LN, Bruce DA, Schut L: Hydranencephaly versus maximal hydrocephalus: An important clinical distinction. Neurosurgery 6:34–38, 1980.
58. Reinsch RC: Choroid plexus cysts—association with trisomy: Prospective review of 16,059 patients. Am J Obstet Gynecol 176:1381–1383, 1997.
59. Geary M, Patel S, Lamont R: Isolated choroid plexus cysts and association with fetal aneuploidy in an unselected population. Ultrasound Obstet Gynecol 10:171–173, 1997.
60. Diagiovanni LM, Quinlan MP, Verp MS: Choroid plexus cysts: Infant and early childhood developmental outcome. Obstet Gynecol 90:191–194, 1997.
61. Carrasco CR, Steirman ED, Harnsberger HR, et al: An algorithm for prenatal ultrasound diagnosis of congenital anomalies. J Ultrasound Med 4:163–165, 1985.
62. Nyberg D, Mack L, Bronstein A, et al: Holoprosencephaly: Prenatal sonographic diagnosis. AJR Am J Roentgenol 149:150–158, 1987.
63. Chervenak FA, Isaacson G, Hobbins JC, et al: Diagnosis and management of fetal holoprosencephaly. Obstet Gynecol 60:322–326, 1985.
64. Roach E, DeMyer W, Palmer K, et al: Holoprosencephaly: Birth data, genetic and demographic analysis of 30 families. Birth Defects 11:294, 1975.
65. Warkany J, Passarge E, Smith CB: Congenital malformations in autosomal trisomy syndromes. Am J Dis Child 112:502–517, 1966.
66. Frints SG, Schoenmakers EF, Smeets E, et al: De novo 7q36 deletion: Breakpoint analysis and types of holoprosencephaly. Am J Med Genet 75:153–158, 1998.
67. Barr M Jr, Hanson JW, Currey K, et al: Holoprosencephaly in infants of diabetic mothers. J Pediatr 102:565–568, 1983.
68. Demyer W: Classification of cerebral malformations. Birth Defects 7:78–93, 1971.
69. Bennett GL, Bromley B, Benacerraf BR: Agenesis of the corpus callosum: Prenatal detection usually is not possible before 22 weeks of gestation. Radiology 199:447–450, 1996.

70. Levine D, Barnes PD, Sher S, et al: Fetal fast MR imaging: Reproducibility, technical quality, and conspicuity of anatomy. Radiology 206:549–554, 1998.

71. Parrish M, Roessmann U, Levinsohn M: Agenesis of the corpus callosum: A study of frequency of associated malformations. Ann Neurol 6:349–354, 1979.

72. Gupta JK, Lilford RJ: Assessment and management of fetal agenesis of the corpus callosum. Prenat Diagn 15:301–312, 1995.

73. Amato M, Huppi P, Durig P, et al: Fetal ventriculomegaly due to isolated brain malformations. Neuropediatrics 21:130–132, 1990.

74. Glick PL, Harrison MR, Nakayama DK, et al: Management of ventriculomegaly in the fetus. J Pediatr 105:97–105, 1984.

75. Twining P, Jaspan T, Zuccollo J: The outcome of fetal ventriculomegaly. Br J Radiol 67:26–31, 1994.

76. Wilson RD, Hitchman D, Wittman BK: Clinical follow-up of prenatally diagnosed isolated ventriculomegaly, microcephaly and encephalocele. Fetal Ther 4:49–57, 1989.

77. Farrell TA, Hertzberg BS, Kliewer MA, et al: Fetal lateral ventricles: Reassessment of normal values for atrial diameter at US. Radiology 193:409–411, 1994.

78. Siedler DE, Filly RA: Relative growth of the higher fetal brain structures. J Ultrasound Med 6:573–576, 1987.

79. Filly RA, Goldstein RB: The fetal ventricular atrium: Fourth down and 10 mm to go [editorial; comment]. Radiology 193:315–317, 1994.

80. Hilbert PL, Hall BE, Kurtz AB: The atria of the fetal lateral ventricles: A sonographic study of normal atrial size and choroid plexus volume. Am J Radiol 164:731–734, 1994.

81. Filly RA, Goldstein RB, Callen PW: Fetal ventricle: Importance in routine obstetric sonography. Radiology 181:1–7, 1991.

82. Pretorius DH, Drose JA, Manco-Johnson ML: Fetal lateral ventricular ratio determination during the second trimester. J Ultrasound Med 5:121–124, 1986.

83. Denkhaus H, Winsberg F: Ultrasound measurements of the fetal ventricular system. Radiology 131:781–787, 1979.

84. Cardoza JD, Filly RA, Podrasky AE: The dangling choroid plexus: A sonographic observation of value in excluding ventriculomegaly. AJR Am J Roentgenol 151:767–770, 1988.

85. Hertzberg BS, Lile R, Foosaner DE, et al: Choroid plexus-ventricular wall separation in fetuses with normal-sized cerebral ventricles at sonography: Postnatal outcome. AJR Am J Roentgenol 163:405–410, 1994.

86. Hertzberg BS, Kliewer MA, Freed KS, et al: Third ventricle: Size and appearance in normal fetuses through gestation. Radiology 203:641–644, 1997.

87. Girard N, Raybaud C, Poncet M: In vivo MR study of brain maturation in normal fetuses. AJNR Am J Neuroradiol 16:407–413, 1995.

88. Revel MP, Pons JC, Lelaidier C, et al: Magnetic resonance imaging of the fetus: A study of 20 cases performed without curarization. Prenat Diagn 13:775–799, 1993.

89. Quinn TM, Hubbard AM, Adzick NS: Prenatal magnetic resonance imaging enhances fetal diagnosis. J Pediatr Surg 33:553–558, 1998.

90. Yuh WT, Nguyen HD, Fisher DJ, et al: MR of fetal central nervous system abnormalities. AJNR Am J Neuroradiol 15:459–464, 1994.

91. Elster AD: Does MR imaging have any known effects on the developing fetus? AJR Am J Roentgenol 162:1493, 1994.

92. Foltz EL, Shurtleff DB: Five year comparative study of hydrocephalus in children with and without operation (113 cases). J Neurosurg 20:1064–1070, 1963.

93. Yashon D, Jane JA, Sugar O: The course of severe untreated hydrocephalus; prognostic significance of the cerebral mantle. J Neurosurg 23:509, 1965.

94. Laurence KH, Coates S: The natural history of hydrocephalus. Detailed analysis of 182 unoperated cases. Arch Dis Child 37:345–362, 1962.

95. Hirsch JF: Consensus: Long-term outcome in hydrocephalus. Childs Nerv Syst 10:64–69, 1994.

96. Lorber J: The results of early treatment of extreme hydrocephalus. Dev Med Child Neurol 16(Suppl):21–29, 1968.

97. Hemmer R, Weissenfels E: [20 years of treatment of hydrocephalus. A catamnestic application (author's transl)]. Arch Psychiatr Nervenkrank 230:257–264, 1981.

98. McCullough DC, Balzer-Martin LA: Current prognosis in overt neonatal hydrocephalus. J Neurosurg 57:378–383, 1982.

99. Raimondi AJ, Soare P: Intellectual development in shunted hydrocephalic children. Am J Dis Child 127:664–671, 1974.

100. Villani RM, Gaini SM, Giovanelli M, et al: Treatment of non-neoplastic stenosis of the aqueduct of Sylvius with extrathecal CSF shunts. J Neurosurg Sci 30:55–60, 1986.

101. Giuffre R, Palma L, Fontana M: Infantile nontumoral aqueductal stenosis. J Neurosurg Sci 30:41–46, 1986.

102. Villani R, Tomei G, Gaini SM, et al: Long-term outcome in aqueductal stenosis. Childs Nerv Syst 11:180–185, 1995.

103. Sawaya R, McLaurin RL: Dandy-Walker syndrome. Clinical analysis of 23 cases. J Neurosurg 55:89–98, 1986.

104. Kalidasan V, Carroll T, Allcutt D, Fitzgerald RJ: The Dandy-Walker syndrome—a 10-year experience of its management and outcome. Eur J Pediatr Surg 5:16–18, 1995.

105. Fernell E, Hagberg B, Hagberg G, et al: Epidemiology of infantile hydrocephalus in Sweden: A clinical follow-up study in children born at term. Neuropediatrics 19:135–142, 1988.

106. Riva D, Milani N, Giorge C, et al: Intelligence outcome in children with shunted hydrocephalus of different etiology. Childs Nerv Syst 10:70–73, 1994.

107. Lumenta CB, Skotarczak U: Long-term follow-up in 233 patients with congenital hydrocephalus. Childs Nerv Syst 11:173–175, 1995.

108. Young HF, Nulsen F, Weiss M, et al: The relationship of intelligence and cerebral mantle in treated infantile hydrocephalus. IQ potential in hydrocephalic children. Pediatrics 52:38, 1973.

109. Nulsen FE, Rekate HL: Results of treatment for hydrocephalus as a guide to future management. In Neurosurgery AAoPNSoP (ed): Pediatric Neurosurgery. New York: Grune & Stratton, 1982, pp 229–241.

110. Amacher AL, Reid WD: Hydrocephalus diagnosed prenatally: Outcome of sugical therapy. Childs Brain 11:119–125, 1984.

111. Laurence KM: Neurological and intellectual sequelae of hydrocephalus. Arch Neurol 20:73–81, 1969.

112. Rubin RC, Hochwald G, Tiell M, et al: Reconstitution of the cerebral cortical mantle in shunt-corrected hydrocephalus. Dev Med Child Neurol 35(Suppl):151–156, 1975.

113. Rubin RC, Hochwald GM, Tiell M, et al: Hydrocephalus: III. Reconstitution of the cerebral cortical mantle following ventricular shunting. Surg Neurol 5:179–183, 1976.

114. Hagberg B, Naglo AS: The conservative management of infantile hydrocephalus. Acta Paediatr Scand 61:165–177, 1972.

115. Cochrane DD, Myles ST, Nimrod C, et al: Intrauterine hydrocephalus and ventriculomegaly: Associated anomalies and fetal outcome. Can J Neurol Sci 12:51–59, 1985.

116. Nicolaides KH, Berry S, Snijders RJ, et al: Fetal lateral cerebral ventriculomegaly: Associated malformations and chromosomal defects. Fetal Diagn Ther 5:5–14, 1990.

117. Hudgins RJ, Edwards MS, Goldstein R, et al: Natural history of fetal ventriculomegaly. Pediatrics 82:692–697, 1988.

118. Chervenak FA, Duncan C, Ment LR, et al: Outcome of fetal ventriculomegaly. Lancet 2:179–181, 1984.

119. Drugan A, Krause B, Canady A, et al: The natural history of prenatally diagnosed cerebral ventriculomegaly. JAMA 261:1785–1788, 1989.

120. Holzgreve W, Feil R, Louwen F, Miny P: Prenatal diagnosis and management of fetal hydrocephaly and lissencephaly. Childs Nerv Syst 9:408–412, 1993.

121. Rosseau GL, McCullough DC, Joseph AL: Current prognosis in fetal ventriculomegaly. J Neurosurg 77:551–555, 1992.

122. Oi S, Matsumoto S, Katayama K, Mochizuki M: Pathophysiology and postnatal outcome of fetal hydrocephalus. Childs Nerv Syst 6:338–345, 1990.

123. Chervenak FA, Hobbins JC, Wertheimer I, et al: The natural history of ventriculomegaly in a fetus without obstructive hydrocephalus. Am J Obstet Gynecol 152:574–575, 1985.

124. Kirkinen P, Serlo W, Jouppila P, et al: Long-term outcome of fetal hydrocephalus. J Child Neurol 11:189–191, 1996.

125. Levitsky DB, Mack LA, Nyberg DA, et al: Fetal aqueductal stenosis diagnosed sonographically: How grave is the prognosis? AJR Am J Roentgenol 164:725–730, 1995.

126. Gupta JK, Bryce FC, Lilford RJ: Management of apparently isolated fetal ventriculomegaly. Obstet Gynecol Surv 49:716–721, 1994.

127. Fernell E, Uvebrant P, von Wendt L: Overt hydrocephalus at birth—orgin and outcome. Childs Nerv Syst 3:350–353, 1987.

128. Renier D, Sainte-Rose C, Pierre-Kahn A, Hirsch JF: Prenatal hydrocephalus: Outcome and prognosis. Childs Nerv Syst 4:213–222, 1988.

129. Vergani P, Locatelli A, Strobelt N, et al: Clinical outcome of mild fetal ventriculomegaly. Am J Obstet Gynecol 178:218–222, 1998.

130. Patel MD, Filly AL, Hersh DR, Goldstein RB: Isolated mild, fetal cerebral ventriculomegaly: Clinical course and outcome. Radiology 192:759–764, 1994.

131. Brumfield CG, Acronin PA, Cloud GA, Davis RO: Fetal myelomingocele: Is antenatal ultrasound useful in predicting neonatal outcome? J Reprod Med 40:26–30, 1995.

132. Oi S, Honda Y, Hidaka M, et al: Intrauterine high-resolution magnetic resonance imaging in fetal hydrocephalus and prenatal estimation of postnatal outcomes with "perspective classification." J Neurosurg 88:685–694, 1998.

133. Michejda M, Hodgens GH: In utero diagnosis and treatment of non-human primate fetal skeletal abnormalities. I Hydrocephalus. JAMA 246:1093–1109, 1981.

134. Nakayama DK, Harrison MR, Berger MS, et al: Correction of congenital hydrocephalus in utero I. The model: Intracisternal kaolin produces hydrocephalus in fetal lambs and rhesus monkeys. J Pediatr Surg 18:331–338, 1983.

135. Glick PL, Harrision MR, Nakayama DK, et al: Correction of congenital hydrocephalus in utero: II. Efficacy of in utero shunting. J Pediatr Surg 19:870–881, 1984.

136. Jones HC, Bucknall RM: Inherited prenatal hydrocephalus in the H-Tx rat: A morphological study. Neuropathol Appl Neurobiol 14:263–274, 1988.

137. Jones HC, Bucknall RM: Changes in cerebrospinal fluid pressure and outflow from the lateral ventricles during development of congenital hydrocephalus in the H-Tx rat. Exp Neurol 98:573–583, 1987.

138. Birnholz JC, Frigoletto FD: Antenatal treatment of hydrocephalus. N Engl J Med 304:1021–1023, 1981.

139. Baumbach LL, Chamberlain JS, Ward PA, et al: Molecular and clinical correlations of deletions leading to Duchenne and Becker muscular dystrophies. Neurology 39:465–474, 1989.

140. Frigoletto FD, Birnhplz JC, Greene MF: Antenatal treatment of hydrocephalus by ventriculoamniotic shunting. N Engl J Med 248:2496–2497, 1982.

141. Depp R, Sabbagha RE, Brown JT, et al: Fetal surgery for hydrocephalus: Successful in utero ventriculoamniotic shunt for Dandy-Walker syndrome. Obstet Gynecol 61:710–714, 1983.

142. Harrison MR, Filly RA, Golbus MS, et al: Fetal treatment 1982. N Engl J Med 307:1651–1652, 1982.

143. Manning FA, Harrison MR, Rodeck C: Catheter shunts for fetal hydronephrosis and hydrocephalus. Report of the International Fetal Surgery Registry. N Engl J Med 315:336–340, 1986.

144. Bland RS, Nelson LH, Meis PJ, et al: Gonococcal ventriculitis associated with ventriculoamniotic shunt placement. Am J Obstet Gynecol 147:781–784, 1983.

145. Venes JL: Management of intrauterine hydrocephalus [letter]. J Neurosurg 58:793–794, 1983.

146. Chervenak FA, McCullough LB: Ethical analysis of the intrapartum management of pregnancy complicated by fetal hydrocephalus with macrocephaly. Obstet Gynecol 68:720–725, 1986.

147. Kuller JA, Katz VL, Wells SR, et al: Cesarean delivery for fetal malformations. Obstet Gynecol Surv 51:371–375, 1996.

148. Babson SG, Benda GI: Growth graphs for the clinical assessment of infants of varying gestational age. J Pediatr 89:815–818, 1976.

149. Escobar GJ, Littenberg B, Petitti DB: Outcome among surviving very low birthweight infants: A meta-analysis. Arch Dis Child 66:204–211, 1991.

150. Copper RL, Goldenberg RL, Creasy RK, et al: A multicenter study of preterm birth weight and gestational age-specific neonatal morality [see comments]. Am J Obstet Gynecol 168:78–84, 1993.

151. Engum SA, Grosfeld JL: Necrotizing enterocolitis. Curr Opin Pediatr 10:123–130, 1998.

152. Boynton BR, Boynton CA, Merritt TA, et al: Ventriculoperitoneal shunts in low birth weight infants with intracranial hemorrhage: Neurodevelopmental outcome. Neurosurgery 18:141–145, 1986.

153. James HE, Bejar R, Merritt A, et al: Management of hydrocephalus secondary to intracranial hemorrhage in the high risk newborn. Neurosurgery 14:612–618, 1984.

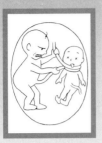

CHAPTER 23

The Fetus with Twin-Twin Transfusion Syndrome

NICHOLAS M. FISK and MYLES J. O. TAYLOR

T win-twin transfusion syndrome (TTTS) arguably presents the greatest challenge in modern day fetal therapy. First, two fetuses are involved. Second, the natural history of fetal loss or damage is extremely high compared to other correctable defects. Third, because the defect is in the placenta, these fetuses are structurally normal, and thus potentially completely salvageable. Finally, it is relatively common, occurring in 10 to 15% of monochorionic (MC) twins,[1] affecting about 1 in 3,200 pregnancies, or 1 in 1,600 fetuses.

TTTS makes a disproportionate contribution to perinatal morbidity and mortality. It accounts for 17% of perinatal deaths in twins overall,[2] which survivors are at risk of long-term neurologic sequelae.[3] Treatments that have been advocated include digoxin, serial amnioreduction, prostaglandin inhibitors, "give-and-take" transfusion, sectio parvae, selective fetocide, laser ablation, and septostomy. The length of this list demonstrates how elusive development of optimal therapy has proven. The chief obstacle has been lack of understanding of the underlying physiology.

Pathophysiology

The condition presents in MC twins usually in the second trimester with gross discordance in amniotic fluid volume. The net "recipient" develops polyhydramnios due to an atrial naturetic peptide (ANP)-mediated polyuria[4–6] and the net "donor" oligohydramnios/anhydramnios ("stuck twin" appearance) due to hypovolemic oliguria.[7, 8] The recipient may go on to develop cardiac dysfunction manifesting as cardiomegaly and tricuspid regurgitation, eventually leading to hydrops and fetal death.[9, 10] The donor is growth restricted, often with a velamentous cord insertion, small placental share, and absent end-diastolic frequencies in the umbilical artery.[10–13] TTTS is distinguished from discordant growth restriction, which complicates 40% of MC twin,[1] by the absence of polyhydramnios.

Intertwin Transfusion

Although TTTS is attributed to intertwin transfusion along placental vascular anastomoses, it is important to remember that anastomoses are present in almost all MC twins. Anastomoses were found in 83% of MC placentae in pooled historical studies,[7] this figure increasing in modern studies using rigorous injection techniques on fresh placentae to 95 to 100%.[13–15]

With anastomoses almost universal, intertwin transfusion is a normal event in MC twins. This concept is supported by injection studies, in which passage of marker substance injected into one twin is detected in the other. Agents used included adult red cells,[16, 17] pancuronium,[18] and Levovist.[19, 20] Further evidence for ubiquitous transfusion between MC twins comes from co-twin sequelae of single intrauterine death. When one MC twin dies in utero, there is a 25% risk of ischemic cerebral or renal lesions in the surviving twin,[21] and a similar risk of co-twin intrauterine death shortly afterwards. Fetal blood sampling data[22, 23] support the observation that these sequelae are due to acute intertwin transfusion from the initially healthy twin into the agonal co-twin.[24]

If intertwin transfusion is a normal event in MC twins, it must be relatively balanced to avoid clinical manifestation. It follows that TTTS is a consequence of unbalanced intertwin transfusion, as suggested more than a century ago by Schatz[25] and recently supported by computer modeling.[26] The pivotal question is how such dysequilibrium is mediated, in particular how the pattern of anastomoses differs in TTTS placentae compared to non-TTTS MC controls.

Vascular Anatomy

Anastomoses within the placenta are of two different anatomic and functional types. The *superficial* type connects a chorionic vessel of one twin with the same type of vessel in its co-twin; these are either arterioarterial (AA) or venovenous (VV) and allow bidirectional flow (Fig. 23–1). The *deep* type comprises a cotyledon sup-

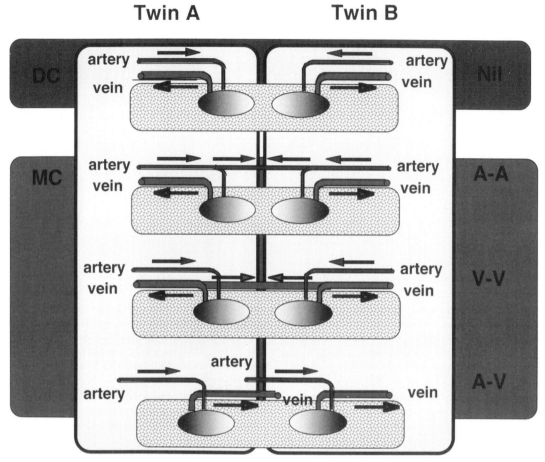

FIGURE 23–1. The three types of anastomoses in monochorionic placentae, the superficial, AA + VV, and the deeper AV.

plied by a chorionic artery of one twin, and drained by a chorionic vein of the co-twin. These are known as arteriovenous (AV) anastomoses and produce unidirectional flow. Strictly speaking, AVs are not anastomoses, as they do not bypass the normal capillary circulation, and instead represent a shared cotyledon. AAs and VVs are true anastomoses, although an anastomotic site cannot be defined, these vessels instead appearing as a seamless single connection between the two circulations (Fig. 23–2). AAs and AVs are found in the majority of MC placentae, whereas VVs are present in 25% or less.[13]

TTTS is associated with a paucity of superficial anastomoses. Using controlled injection studies, two groups have shown that superficial anastomoses are significantly less frequent in TTTS (10 to 17%) than in non-TTTS MC placentae (≥80%).[14, 15] The most common finding in TTTS was the presence of a small number of deep AV anastomoses together with absence of superficial anastomoses. These findings support Schatz's original hypothesis that bidirectional superficial anastomoses compensate for any hemodynamic imbalance built up by unidirectional AV connections.[25] In a more recent study comparing placental angioarchitecture in 21 TTTS with 49 non-TTTS MC pregnancies,[13] our group showed that only the frequency of AAs was different, but not

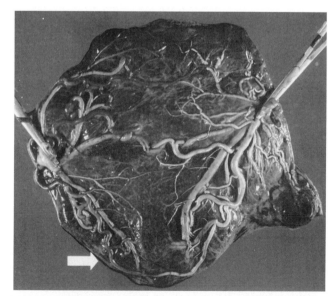

FIGURE 23–2. An injection study of a monochorionic placenta. Arteries from the left and right twins' placental cord insertions are shown in red and yellow with veins in blue and green, respectively. An AA anastomosis is seen (*arrow*). *See Color Plate 2*

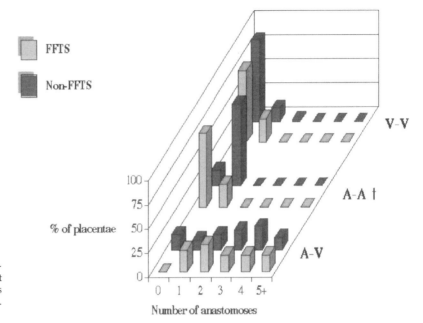

FIGURE 23–3. Placental injection studies in 82 consecutive monochorionic twins.[13] There is no significant difference in the number of VV and AV anastomoses but significantly fewer AAs in twins affected by TTTS. († $p = 0.001$.)

AVs or VVs (Fig. 23–3). Those affected by TTTS had fewer AA anastomoses, present in only 24% compared to 84% of MC controls. There was always at least one AV anastomosis in TTTS placentae, whereas there were no AVs in 16% of MC controls. Seventy-eight percent with 1 or more AV anastomoses and no AA anastomoses developed TTTS.

The protective role of AAs in equilibrating interfetal transfusion set up by deep AVs has recently been confirmed in vivo.[13, 27] Arterial vessels on the chorionic plate with a bidirectional spectral Doppler pattern (Fig. 23–4) are known to represent AA anastomoses based on (1) their correlation with postnatal anatomy,[27] (2) mathematical modeling showing that their periodicity is a function of the net difference in fetal heart rates,[28] and (3) transformation to a unidirectional arterial pattern during single intrauterine death.[13] In 76 MC pregnancies insonated at fortnightly intervals using color Doppler energy, we found functional AA anastomoses in only 14% with TTTS compared to 70% without TTTS.[13, 27]

Embryology

The vascular anastomotic patterns that characterize TTTS could arise secondary to asymmetric developmental or hemodynamic influences. Deficient placentation suggested by the high frequency in the donor of diminished placental share, velamentous insertion, and abnormal umbilical Dopplers implicates discordant trophoblast invasion and/or asymmetric splitting of the inner cell mass. Similarly, the rarity of TTTS in monoamniotic twins with anastomoses suggests that the timing of embryonic splitting may be important. Currently, the tools for studying early embryology and angiogenesis in MC twins remain crude.[29]

Hemodynamics

Understanding the pathophysiology behind TTTS has been limited by the relative inaccessibility of the human fetus, and the lack of a suitable animal model with MC placentation. Accordingly, our group developed a computer-based mathematical model of MC twins linking known fetal and placental physiologic variables in a dynamic real-time synthesis of hematologic, hydro-osmotic, and metabolic relationships. Transfusion along placental vascular anastomoses between twins with otherwise identical physiology reproduced the clinical features of TTTS.[26] In the model, the direction and symmetry of anastomoses determined the net hydrostatic and osmotic gradients and thus TTTS severity, with the more extreme findings occurring with increasing numbers of unidirectional anastomoses in the same direction only. These findings support the concept that TTTS is caused by net imbalance in flow between the twins set up by uncompensated deep AV anastomoses.

Unbalanced net intertwin transfusion can account for most of the hemodynamic changes in TTTS. Doppler studies of the recipient have shown venous waveform patterns consistent with raised central venous pressure.[10, 30] Typically, donor fetuses show little abnormality in cardiac function while recipient fetuses frequently develop cardiomegaly, tricuspid regurgitation, and ventricular hypertrophy.[9, 31] Right ventricular outflow obstruction (RVOT) may develop in recipients, of sufficient severity to warrant valvotomy in infancy.[9] RVOT obstruction could simply be attributed to transfusional volume overload, although recent work suggests in contrast that raised afterload may be present. Relative hypertension has been observed in recipient twins in the neonatal period.[30] Plasma levels of endothelin 1, a potent endothelially derived vasoconstrictor, are two- to threefold higher in recipient fetuses compared to donor and con-

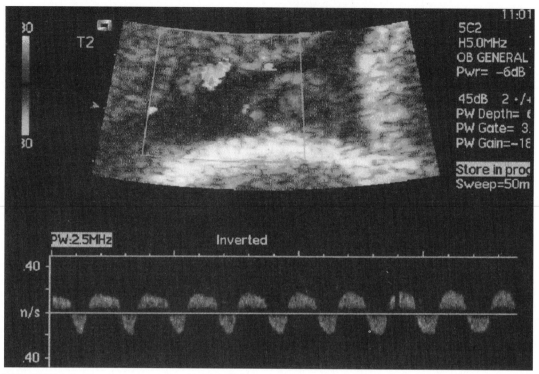

FIGURE 23–4. The characteristic interference pattern seen with pulsed wave Doppler insonation of an AA anastomosis.

trol fetuses.[32] This is consistent with anecdotal observations of reversal of flow in the ductus arteriosus in severely affected recipients.

Paired hematologic data obtained at fetal blood sampling in 36 TTTS pregnancies showed that only 25% had a greater than 5-g/dL difference in hemoglobin levels.[33] There was a wide range of discordancy (−1 to +14.6 g/dL), with the recipient's hemoglobin being a mean of 3.8 g/dL higher than the donor's. Thus, although there are significant differences in red cell mass between donor and recipient fetuses, only a minority have sufficient discordance to satisfy the now outmoded neonatal diagnostic criteria (>5 g/dL). The factors determining the degree of discordancy have yet to be determined but may include disease severity and anastomotic configuration.

Notwithstanding the above, many questions regarding the underlying pathophysiology remain unanswered. For instance, we know little of net transfusional flow rates and their determinants. Presumably, a minimal flow is required to maintain anastomotic patency; it is difficult to envisage how a flow rate even as low as 1 mL/hr though an uncompensated AV anastomosis would not over days lead to a lethal degree of volume overload in the recipient. On the other hand, preliminary calculations of flow down a single AV derived from AA waveforms referenced to anastomotic pattern at injection study suggest a figure as low as 5 mL/day, seemingly insufficient to prevent thrombosis.[13]

Natural History

Survival

Prognosis is poor in TTTS diagnosed in the second trimester. Survival with conservative management was only 20% in pooled series with TTTS diagnosed before 28 weeks (Table 23–1).[34–48] Neonatal deaths outnumber

T A B L E 23–1. PERINATAL SURVIVAL RATES AFTER CONSERVATIVE MANAGEMENT OF TTTS PRESENTING PRIOR TO 28 WEEKS

AUTHOR	PERIOD	SURVIVAL
Weir et al.[39]	1971–1978	0/16
Wittmann et al.[40]	1977–1978	0/4
Elejalde et al.[34]	Not stated	0/2
Chescheir & Seeds[35]	1982–1987	0/4
Pretorius et al.[38]	Not stated	1/14
Brown et al.[36]	1984–1986	1/8
Patten et al.[37]	1979–1987	3/48
Urig et al.[41]	1983–1987	0/10
Gonsoulin et al.[42]	1985–1989	6/15
Mahony et al.[43]	1986–1987	2/10
Radestad & Thomassen[44]	1980–1987	2/12
Bromley et al.[45]	Not stated	8/14
Pinette et al.[46]	1989–1992	4/6
Reisner[47]	1986–1992	4/10
Dennis et al.[48]	Not stated	6/10
Total	**1971–1992**	**37/183 (20%)**

fetal deaths by 2:1.[49] Although there was a trend to increasing survival in later studies, reflecting earlier diagnosis, case selection, and improved neonatal care, few would advocate conservative expectancy in any but the mildest of cases.

Morbidity

The natural history for short and long term morbidity cannot be meaningfully quantified from the small numbers in conservatively managed series. However, series overall attest to high rates of neonatal morbidity, in excess of that expected due to gestational age at delivery.[47, 50] The recipient is most at risk, being prone to circulatory complications as a result of hypertrophic cardiomyopathy and polycythemia. In addition to the usual neonatal complications of growth restriction, 12 to 30% of donors have renal failure and/or renal tubular dysgenesis,[47, 50, 51] presumably as a consequence of chronic hypoperfusion in utero, although this is rare in long-term survivors.

Antenatally Acquired Cerebral Lesions

Survivors of TTTS are at risk of neurologic injury, not just as a consequence of preterm delivery but also from antenatally acquired insults. Again, the natural history cannot be determined from conservatively managed series. Bejar reported that five of nine TTTS survivors undergoing neonatal intensive care had evidence of preexisting white matter lesions.[52] Our group recently reported evidence of antenatally acquired white matter lesions on Day 1 to 3 neonatal cranial scans in 35% (11 of 31) of double survivors delivered preterm. The frequency in donors and recipients was similar.[3]

Although clearly cause for concern, two issues warrant consideration. First, all but one of these lesions was minor, comprising mild ventriculomegaly, subependymal pseudocysts, small white matter cysts, basal ganglia echogenicity, or lenticulostriate vasculopathy[3] (Fig. 23–5); these are not uncommon in preterm infants and are not necessarily associated with long-term impairment. Indeed, 6% of 177 unselected, well, term neonates investigated in the same institution showed evidence on scan of some antenatally acquired brain insult.[53]

Second, although MC twins have a tenfold increased risk of antenatally acquired cerebral white matter lesions compared to dichorionic twins, these are not confined to pregnancies complicated by TTTS or single intrauterine death.[52] Bejar et al. found that 20% of double survivors undergoing neonatal intensive care from non-TTTS MC pregnancies delivered prior to 36 weeks also had evidence of antenatally acquired white matter lesions. Although it is tempting to postulate differing mechanisms in donor (anemia, hypotension) and recipient (polycythemia and intravascular sludging),[3] the high frequency in non-TTTS MC neonates suggests that a common mechanism may be perturbations in anastomotic blood flow affecting cerebral perfusion.

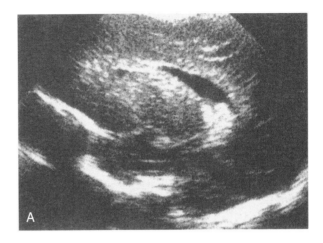

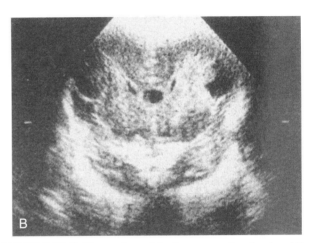

FIGURE 23–5. Neonatal cranial ultrasonographs showing (*A*) a minor lesion (subependymal cyst), and (*B*) a major lesion (porencephalic cyst). (From Denbow ML, et al: Neonatal cranial ultrasonographic findings in preterm twins complicated by severe fetofetal transfusion syndrome. Am J Obstet Gynecol 178:479–483, 1998, with permission.)

Long-Term Sequelae

Apart from survival, the other important outcome measure is handicap. There are, however, no formal studies of long-term outcome in cohorts of TTTS survivors. Interpreting published case series is problematic because these are small, use unstated or imprecise assessment methods, have variable and sometimes insufficient follow-up periods, and often confuse abnormalities on imaging with disability. In addition, handicap rates are further confounded by survival rates and the effects of treatment.

Published series with follow-up of more than ten survivors were reviewed for evidence of major neurodevelopmental sequelae. Those with abnormalities on imaging but not on clinical examination were not included, so that the following rates may be underestimates. Mahony et al.'s[43] series raised the initial concern with a figure of 23% (3 of 13). Pinette et al.'s[46] series showed 2 of 15 cases (13%), both following single intrauterine death. Reisner et al.[4] considered their rate of 15% (3 of 20) no different from that expected based on gestational age at delivery. More recent series show lower rates, De Lia et al.[54] having 1 in 28 (4%) at 1 to 68 months, Trespidi et al.[55] 2 in 26 (8%) at 3 to 24 months, Quintero et al.[56] 1 of 23 (4%) after an unspecified interval, and Ville et al.[57] 4 in 145 (3%) at 12 to 51 months.

Management Techniques

The choice of management technique for second-trimester TTTS is controversial. Most have been developed in the last 5 to 10 years, and none has yet been formally assessed by randomized trial. Comparison of methods is confounded by differing selection criteria (e.g., severity, gestational age), the evolving nature of each technique, multiple therapies, and use of historical rather than contemporaneous controls. Early studies emphasized survival as the primary outcome, whereas more recent studies are beginning also to address sequelae in survivors.

Amnioreduction

The principal aim of amnioreduction is to control polyhydramnios to allow prolongation of gestation. The risk of preterm labor and amniorrhexis associated with polyhydramnios is considered mediated through raised amniotic pressure.[58, 59] This rises linearly in relation to the degree of excess amniotic fluid,[58, 60] and exceeds the reference range when the amniotic fluid index rises above 40 to 45 or the deepest pool 12 cm. Accordingly, these thresholds are recommended as indications for intervention.[61] Amnioreduction restores normal amniotic pressure.[58, 62, 63] Small volumes of fluid (<1 L) were removed in initial series in view of concerns regarding precipitation of abruption or preterm labor.[64, 65] Although this is sufficient to restore amniotic pressure,[58, 66] it seems likely with rapid reaccumulation of fluid that pressure soon rises again. Then one group advocated removing all the excess amniotic fluid (up to 5 to 10 L).[41, 67] Their low 1.5% complication rate[68] and the clinical improvement reported after serial procedures[67] led to the widespread uptake in the 1990s of *serial aggressive amnioreduction* as first-line therapy for TTTS.

As a secondary aim, there is some evidence that amnioreduction in TTTS may ameliorate fetal condition and the disease process. Several groups have reported maintenance of normal amniotic volume, and/or resolution of hydrops after amnioreduction.[46, 67, 69] Rosen et al. reported less divergence in hourly fetal urine production rates following serial amnioreduction.[6] There are two possibilities. First, this apparent amelioration could simply be a gestational age effect, as severe polyhydramnios necessitating drainage is rare after 30 weeks. Alternatively, it could be a true treatment effect, although any mechanism remains speculative. Fetal blood gas status is inversely correlated with amniotic pressure in polyhydramnios,[70] suggesting that uteroplacental perfusion is impaired in severe polyhydramnios.[71] Consistent with this, amnioreduction has been shown acutely to increase uterine artery blood flow by 70%.[72]

The patient is wedged in the lateral position to avoid supine hypotension and should be comfortable, as the procedure may take up to 1 hour. Antibiotics and a prostaglandin synthase inhibitor may be given prophylactically. A large amniotic pocket is located by ultrasound slightly lateral and midway down the uterus, avoiding the placenta and donor twin. This site is chosen to allow maximal flexibility of the needle to minimize maternal discomfort and contractions, as the relationship between the overlying skin, uterus, and amniotic cavity changes greatly during drainage. An 18-gauge needle is inserted under ultrasound guidance, and extension tubing is attached to the hub. Amniotic pressure may be measured, as described elsewhere.[61] Fluid is aspirated as rapidly as possible via a 50-mL syringe and three-way tap until the amniotic fluid index (AFI) reaches the low-normal range, usually with a deepest pool 6 to 8 cm. Care is taken to avoid puncturing the septum, as this can rarely create pseudomonoamniotic twins predisposing to cord entanglement.[73] Approximately 1 L needs to be removed for every 10 cm the AFI is elevated.[74] Thereafter, amniotic fluid volume is monitored two to three times per week with repeat amnioreductions indicated in the presence of symptoms or an AFI greater than 40 cm. Chronic drainage catheters are not recommended because of a high incidence of infection and blockage, the latter due to kinking between the skin and uterine entry sites, which move apart as uterine volume diminishes.

Serial aggressive amnioreduction is associated with an overall perinatal survival rate in the region of 60% (Table 23–2), both from the available, albeit uncontrolled, published series,[41-44, 46, 48, 50, 55, 62, 67, 75-79] and from the interim international amnioreduction registry (http//:info.med.yale.edu/obgyn/mari).[80] Table 23–2 shows a 50% double survival and 20% single survival rate in published series of severe TTTS presenting prior to 28 weeks. Although some series comprise only five to ten pregnancies, their exclusion makes no difference to the overall survival rate. Note that the large series of Reisner et al.[47] is excluded because (1) it includes six dichorionic pregnancies and (2) cases earlier than 28 weeks cannot be distinguished.

Although amnioreduction appears to represent an improvement on conservative management, it does not work in at least one third of cases, and morbidity remains high among survivors. Indeed, as per Table 23–2, 50% of cases will still be complicated by one or more fetal or neonatal loss. Because of this and because amnioreduction does not seem to address the underlying disease process, a number of other treatments have been developed.

Septostomy

Amniotic septostomy creates an artificial hole within the septum[81, 82] to allow equilibration of amniotic fluid volume. Its rationale is based on the observation that TTTS is extremely rare in monoamniotic twins,[83] and on anecdotal improvement observed when septa are inadvertently ruptured at amnioreduction. Amniotic

T A B L E 23–2. PERINATAL SURVIVAL RATES AFTER SERIAL AGGRESSIVE AMNIOREDUCTION FOR TTTS PRESENTING PRIOR TO 28 WEEKS

		NUMBER OF SURVIVORS			
AUTHOR	NO. OF CASES	0	1	2	SURVIVAL
Urig et al.[41]	5	2	0	3	6/10(60%)
Mahony et al.[43]	7	2	1	4	9/14(64%)
Radestad & Thomassen[44]	9	6	0	3	6/18(33%)
Gonsoulin et al.[42]	11	NA	NA	NA	11/22(50%)
Elliot et al.[67]	16	3	1	12	25/32(78%)
Saunders et al.[77]	19	10	4	5	14/38(37%)
Pinette et al.[46]	9	0	3	6	15/18(83%)
Weiner & Ludomirski[62]	11	NA	NA	NA	11/22(50%)
Dickinson[78]	9	3	1	5	11/18(61%)
Cincotta et al.[50]	13	2	7	4	15/26(57%)
Trespidi et al.[55]	23	8	4	11	26/46(57%)
Dennis & Winkler[48]	11	1	2	8	18/22(82%)
Kilby et al.[76]	9	4	0	5	10/18(56%)
Bruner et al.[79]	6	0	4	2	8/12(67%)
Hecher et al.[75]	43	17	8	18	44/86(51%)
Mari et al.*	223	65	50	108	266/446(60%)
Total Survival	**424**				**495/848(58%)**
Breakdown of survivors	402	123(31%)	85(21%)	194(48%)	

* International Amnioreduction Registry (unpublished data).
NA, data not available.

pressure is raised in the recipient's sac and likely to be reduced in the donor's sac[58, 59] based on both experience with aberrant amniotic volumes in singleton gestations and physiologic principles related to diminished volume within a semidistensible membrane. This pressure gradient causes the septum to move towards the donor to minimize the gradient.[84] When it can no longer do so, as in stuck twins, the pressure gradient rises again. Disruption of the dividing membrane therefore causes fluid to move along a hydrostatic pressure gradient from the sac with polyhydramnios into the sac with oligohydramnios; indeed, fluid may be observed "spuming" from the larger into the smaller sac.[85]

Saade et al. used a 20- to 22-gauge needle in 12 pregnancies between 16 and 26 weeks gestation with severe TTTS and a mean fetal weight discordancy of 31%.[86] Septostomy was followed in all cases by rapid reaccumulation of amniotic fluid around the donor. Survival was 83% and mean prolongation of pregnancy was 8 weeks. Three of these pregnancies were treated with concomitant amnioreduction, so that it is difficult to separate the effects of the two treatments. However, the authors of this series instead suggested that therapeutic success with amnioreduction is attributable to inadvertent septostomy (Fig. 23–6).

Another group used laser to fenestrate the membrane, leading to equilibration of amniotic fluid volume, and improvement in fetal Dopplers and growth.[82] This technique presumably carries a greater risk of cord entanglement secondary to pseudomonoamniotic twins, something not yet observed with needle puncture in either the pilot, needle septostomy series,[86] or series of transseptal diagnostic amniocenteses.[87–89]

The mechanism by which this treatment might work is unclear, particularly in normalizing polyhydramnios, but by allowing oral rehydration, the donor fetus may be able to correct its hypovolemia and/or remove net fluid from the amniotic cavity. Although the results of the pilot study appear promising,[86] whether this treatment establishes a role in TTTS must await the results of the multicenter randomized trial underway comparing septostomy with amnioreduction (http://www.med.unc.edu/tts/).

Medical Treatment

Prostaglandin synthase inhibitors, like indomethacin and sulindac, act on the fetal kidney to reduce fetal urine output and have successfully been used to treat polyhydramnios in singleton and twin pregnancies.[90, 91] In TTTS, however, their use is contraindicated because of their concomitant but harmful effects on renal function in the already oliguric donor, which may manifest as renal failure in the neonatal period.[92]

An anecdotal case report describes resolution of hydrops after maternal digoxin administration,[93] although spontaneous resolution has certainly been reported in TTTS. There are no published series using this treatment.

It seems unlikely that drug therapy will play a major role in the treatment of TTTS, as the desirable effect of a drug in one twin may have deleterious effects on the other. Even if selective delivery systems to an individual fetus could be developed, the sharing of their circulation would render confinement of the drug effect to one twin problematic.

Another approach that has been tried is "give-and-take" transfusion. Weiner and Ludomirsky performed simple intravascular transfusion on the donor and isovolemic partial exchange transfusion in four cases of severe TTTS at 21 to 22 weeks.[62] Not only was survival poor at 25% but, not surprisingly, frequent procedures were

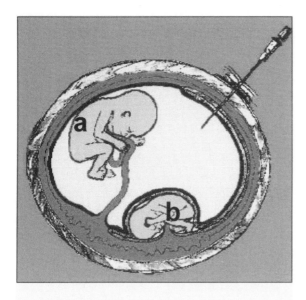

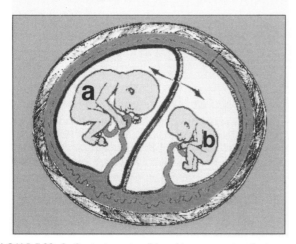

FIGURE 23–6. Septostomy is achieved by puncturing the intertwin membrane with a 20- to 22-gauge needle. Equal distribution of liquor volume is achieved. (From Saade G, Ludomirsky A, Fisk N: Feto-fetal transfusion. *In* Fisk N, Moise K [eds]: Fetal Therapy: Invasive and Transplacental. Cambridge: Cambridge University Press, 1997, pp 227–251, with permission.)

needed, every 1 to 2 days, to maintain normal hemoglobin concentrations.

Selective Termination

The rationale for selective fetocide is complete interruption of the transfusion process. One twin is terminated to allow survival of the other. Although suggested by many groups, its chief disadvantage is its inherent 50% perinatal mortality rate. Accordingly, most consider it only appropriate in the management of refractory or severe TTTS. It may be performed once intrauterine death of one twin appears imminent, or once other treatment options have failed. Indeed, this helps parents feel that the procedure is absolutely necessary to allow even a single twin to survive. However, timing is crucial; delay may result in death of one or both fetuses or damage in a survivor.

A variety of ultrasound-guided needle techniques have been described, including intracardiac potassium, saline pericardial tamponade, and intraluminal injection of thrombogenic coils and sclerosants. Case reports and one small case series attest to survival in 64% (7 of 11).[94-98] As with vessel occlusion for other complicated MC twins, it is likely that this is an overestimate, our group recently reporting a failure rate of 67% with absolute alcohol and enbucrilate gel.[20] Safe fetocide requires blockage of both umbilical arteries and the vein. Because TTTS is characterized by a lack of superficial anastomoses,[13-15] implicated in acute transfusional complications of single intrauterine death,[52] cord occlusion might seem less important in TTTS. Notwithstanding this, exsanguination has been reported after selective fetocide in TTTS.[20]

Accordingly, a definitive method of complete cord occlusion is required. As discussed in Chapter 9, fetoscopic cord ligation although effective,[99] is lengthy, and associated with up to a 30% risk of amniorrhexis.[100] In our opinion, the preferred procedure for all selective termination procedures in MC twins is now bipolar cord coagulation (Fig. 23–7).[101, 102] The limited published experience of complete cord occlusion in severe TTTS shows a perinatal survival rate in residual twins of 86% (12 of 14) by either fetoscopic (*n* = 7)[100, 103] or ultrasound-guided (*n* = 7) ligation/occlusion techniques.[101, 104]

Whether to terminate the donor or the recipient has been the subject of debate. The donor has until recently been preferred on theoretical grounds that (1) the recipient is then less likely to exsanguinate into the donor, as blood would have to flow in the reverse direction to the previous transfusional gradient and the commonest anastomotic configuration; and (2) the growth-restricted donor may not be able to overcome its deficient placentation to thrive for weeks in utero. However, increasing arguments suggest that selective termination of the recipient may instead be preferable. Polyhydramnios enables better visualization, and makes occlusion of the cord away from the uterine wall technically easier, thereby avoiding maternal injury. Further, recipients seem slightly more at risk of preexisting damage than donors.[3] Preliminary experience with ultrasound-guided bipolar cord occlusion in TTTS[101, 102] suggests that umbilical arterial end-diastolic frequencies and growth velocity return after termination of the recipient.

An alternative to selective fetocide is sectio parvae, where one fetus is delivered by hysterotomy to allow the other to continue in utero.[105] However, the risks of preterm labor and maternal morbidity mean that ultrasound-guided cord occlusion techniques are preferable. Although sectio parvae might be expected to have the advantage of allowing the delivered twin some chance of survival, it is effectively a form of selective termination in that the delivered twin is usually extremely preterm or previable and thus not expected to survive.

Laser Photocoagulation

Interruption of the vascular anastomoses between the fetuses is the most logical of therapeutic approaches to

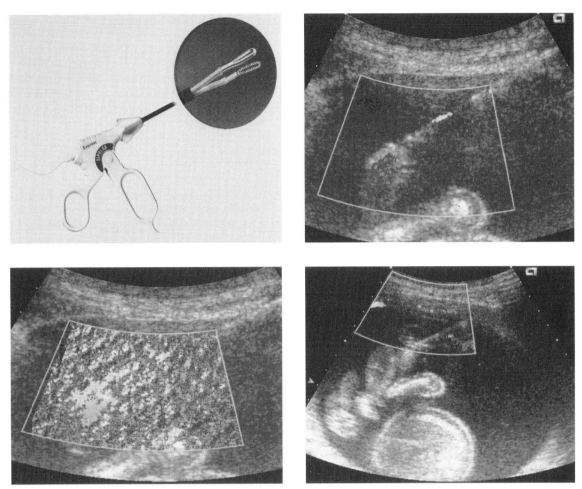

FIGURE 23–7. Cord occlusion with 3-mm bipolar diathermy forceps (*upper left;* Everest Medical, Minneapolis, MN). The cord is identified (*upper right*), diathermied (*lower left*), and cessation of flow achieved in the umbilical cord (*lower right*). *See Color Plate 2*

date. The technique of laser coagulation of placental vessels using a neodymium:yttrium-aluminium-garnet (Nd:YAG) laser was first developed in animals[106, 107] and later applied to humans.[108, 109] To date, five groups have reported experience in a total of 312 cases of TTTS.[56, 57, 75, 110] The overall survival rate for cases presenting prior to 28 weeks calculated in Table 23–3 is 58%.

The most common technique, the so-called *blitzkrieg* method of photocoagulating all surface chorionic vessels crossing the intertwin septum,[57, 109] has been associated with procedure-related fetal loss rates of between 15 and 50%.[75, 111] These can be explained by an understanding of the placental anatomy. Although none of the clinical series document the number of vessels ablated, both groups who developed the procedure describe photocoagulating six to ten communicating vessels crossing the intertwin septum.[108, 112] In contrast, we now know that there are a median of only three anastomoses in TTTS.[13]

TABLE 23–3. PERINATAL SURVIVAL RATES AFTER LASER ABLATION PLUS CONCOMITANT AMNIOREDUCTION FOR TTTS PRESENTING PRIOR TO 28 WEEKS

		NUMBER OF SURVIVORS			
AUTHOR	NO. OF CASES	0	1	2	SURVIVAL
De Lia et al.[110]	25	8	9	8	25/50(50%)
De Lia et al.*[54]	70	14	18	38	94/140(67%)
Ville et al.†[57]	132	35	50	47	144/264(55%)
Quintero et al.[56]	24	7	5	12	29/48(60%)
Deprest et al.[103]	6	2	0	4	8/12(67%)
Total Survival	**257**	**66(26%)**	**82(32%)**	**109(42%)**	**300/514(58%)**

* Adjusted for failed procedures as per http://www.tttsfoundation.org/handout.htm.
† Hecher et al.[75] not tabulated, as 18 cases also included in Ville et al.[57]

In addition, the site of the intertwin septum bears little geometric relation to the vascular equator, and often overlies the donor territory. This suggests that a number of normal chorionic plate vessels are also being ablated. Sheep studies confirm that laser ablation of a normal chorionic vessel leads to infarction of the entire cotyledon.[113] This explains the full-thickness placental necrosis seen after laser[114] and the high rate of intrauterine death within 24 hours of the procedure.

There are other variations to this technique. De Lia et al. photocoagulate vessels in the vascular equator rather than along the intertwin septum,[110, 115] and attribute their lower immediate procedure-related fetal death rate of 18% to less devitalization of normal donor cotyledons. Although they claim to ablate anastomoses rather than all connections in this region, review of their lased placental pathology (Fig. 23–8)[110] makes it clear that significant collateral damage to normal cotyledons still occurs, with the placenta transected in what is still essentially a *blitzkrieg* approach. Hecher et al.[75] describe coagulating superficial and arteriovenous anastomoses only rather than all vessels crossing the intertwin septum as per the Ville technique, yet 25% of their cases were included in Ville's latest series.[57] Notwithstanding this, both groups acknowledge ablating fewer vessels than previously.

There are two basic endoscopic approaches. The *open* method involves laparotomy under general anesthesia, with insertion of a 3.8 × 2.5 to 2.9 mm rigid operative scope.[54, 110] The *percutaneous* approach uses a *rigid* 1.9- to 2.0-mm pediatric cystoscope inserted under local anesthesia and continuous ultrasound guidance.[57, 75] The chief technical problem is access to the chorionic plate in anteriorly sited placentas. With the open technique, this has now been overcome by exteriorizing the uterus.[110] With the percutaneous technique a lateral approach may be used, but even then the placenta was transgressed in 9 of 57 (16%) cases.[57] Others have used

a minilaparotomy[116] or a flexible fetoscope to overcome this.[56]

Most workers use a 400-μm fiber 1 cm from the vessel to deliver 30 to 60 w until coagulation is achieved, estimated by blanching, shrinkage, and absent flow over a 1- to 2-cm segment. Studies in an underwater rat model show that the successful occlusion rate decreases with vessel diameter from 89% for vessels less than 1 mm diameter to 40% for vessels larger than 1.5 mm.[117] This is the reason why laser occlusion of the umbilical cord is not feasible after 20 weeks.[118] A minority of failures are perforations, essentially vessel rupture secondary to boiling of intravascular or interstitial fluid, which in the rat model were confined to larger vessels (>1 and especially >1.5 mm).[117] Notwithstanding this, in clinical series the perforation rate is low, between 1 and 7%,[57,75,110] and in many cases can be dealt with by lasering the vessel either side of the perforation.

Visualization may be impaired by intra-amniotic blood, either fresh from the uterine puncture site or the chorionic plate, or old from prior amnioreduction. In most cases this can be overcome by amniotic fluid replacement. As a result, few procedures are abandoned/not completed with the percutaneous approach (reported as <1%),[57, 75] although a much greater rate has been documented using the larger bore scope for the open procedure (22%).[110] On the other hand, the percutaneous approach may not always completely separate the two circulations,[119] additional procedures (repeat laser, amnioreduction, or rescue transfusion) being required in 18% in the largest series.[57]

In terms of maternal complications, there have been three cases of pulmonary edema, one following transfusion for massive intraperitoneal hemorrhage, and one with the maternal mirror syndrome. There was also one case of maternal death from disseminated intravascular coagulation 6 weeks later.

Apart from procedure-related intrauterine death, fetal complications are rare. Aplasia cutis, limb necrosis, amniotic bands, and microphthalmia/anopthalmia have been reported, although the relationship to endoscopic laser is not clear.[110, 116, 120, 121]

Some argue that laser reduces the chance of neurologic injury in survivors, Ville et al. concluding that their rate of neurologic handicap of less than 5% was much lower than after serial amnioreduction.[57] They base the latter on two outcome studies. The first by Pinette et al. they cite as showing a 36% cerebral palsy rate, whereas it actually shows no case of cerebral palsy in those treated by serial amnioreduction, the only cases of neurologic handicap occurring in pregnancies managed conservatively.[46] The second, by Trespidi et al., is cited as showing a 15% severe handicap rate in survivors; that paper in fact shows 3 of 26 survivors (11.5%) had handicap at follow-up, but in one of these the problem was pulmonary.[55] In Ville et al.'s study, the "handicap rate" after laser seems to have been assessed by postal or telephone contact, an approach well known to underestimate deficits. No mention is made of neonatal cranial ultrasound scans or pediatric assessment. Imaging studies may be used as an additional end point, but cannot be equated with handicap. Hecher et al. reported a 6%

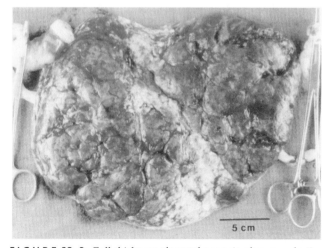

F I G U R E 23–8. Full-thickness placental necrosis after nonselective laser ablation of all surface chorionic vessels crossing the intertwin septum. (From De Lia JE, Cruikshank DP, Keye WR Jr: Fetoscopic neodymium: YAG laser occlusion of placental vessels in severe twin-twin transfusion syndrome. Obstet Gynecol 75:1046–1053, 1990, with permission. Courtesy of the American College of Obstetricians and Gynecologists.)

incidence of abnormal neonatal head scans after laser treatment compared to 18% after amnioreduction in pregnancies managed by amnioreduction in a different center a few years previously,[75] but the extent to which this may be attributed to earlier gestational age at delivery is not clear. The interpretation of neonatal ultrasound scans is notoriously variable, a recent study finding abnormalities in 20% of well term neonates.[53] Brain injury is clearly a problem in TTTS and it is important that cohort analyses compare like with like. Outcome studies reporting both neonatal imaging and long-term neurodevelopmental follow-up are urgently required.

Laser plus concomitant amnioreduction does not appear to have an obvious survival advantage over the conventional therapy of serial aggressive amnioreduction. Both from Tables 23–2 and 23–3, and from comparison of a single-center laser series with semihistorical controls from another center,[122] it is apparent that laser compared to amnioreduction increases the proportion of single survivors, by reducing the number of double deaths, albeit at the expense of also reducing the number of double survivors. Deaths after laser tend to be clustered around the time of the procedure,[57, 109] increasing gestational age at delivery by about 3 weeks in continuing "singleton" pregnancies.[75]

Selective Ablation of AV Anastomoses

Although an important technical and therapeutic advance, the results of nonselective laser separation remain disappointing for what theoretically should be a correctable defect. The chief problem appears to be cotyledonary loss from ablation of nonanastomotic vessels. Several groups have suggested that the therapeutic goal should instead be selective ablation of those few AV anastomoses involved in the disease process.[8, 56, 123] The question is how to identify them. There are three possible approaches in vivo: contrast angiography, endoscopic inspection, and Doppler.

The microbubble contrast agent Levovist can document intertwin transfusion in some, but not all, MC twins but provides insufficient enhancement to delineate shared cotyledons.[19, 20] This may be improved by development of newer generation contrast agents. Similarly, there are considerable technical barriers to magnetic resonance angiography, since ultrasound-guided fetal blood sampling would be required for contrast administration within the magnet.

Rigorous endoscopic inspection of the chorionic plate vasculature (Fig. 23–9) can also be used to allow selective identification of AV anastomoses.[100] Quintero et al. recently reported that perinatal survival improved from 44% to 57% in seven selectively, compared to 17 conventionally, ablated cases.[56] However, selective identification has then been followed by laser ablation, rendering it impossible to validate this scientifically. In pilot experiments using direct visualization ex vivo under optimal conditions compared with "gold standard" injection studies, we could only correctly identify two thirds of AV anastomoses. On the one hand, visualization in utero might be even worse due to a narrower field of view

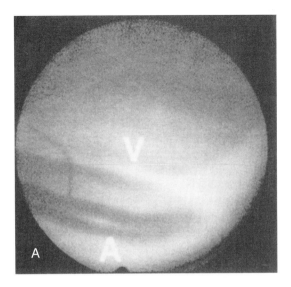

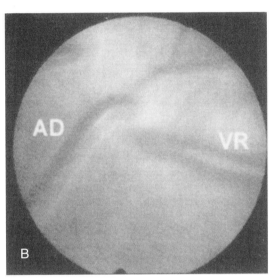

FIGURE 23–9. *A,* Endoscopic appearance of a paired artery and vein supplying a normal cotyledon. *B,* An arteriovenous anastomosis. An unpaired artery (AD) from the donor enters the shared cotyledon and an unpaired vein (VR) emerges to run to the recipient twin. (From Quintero RA, et al: Selective photocoagulation of placental vessels in twin-twin transfusion syndrome: Evolution of a surgical technique. Obstet Gynecol Surv 53:S97–S103, 1998, with permission.)

and smaller vessels at earlier gestations; on the other hand, visualization might be aided by the different color of arteries and veins in vivo. Although the unpaired artery from one twin is known invariably to terminate by entering the shared cotyledon within 5 mm of the origin of an exiting unpaired vein to the other twin,[13, 124, 125] there appears considerable variation in vessel direction, number, and tortuosity, which may complicate their identification (Fig. 23–10). Some AVs join at acute angles, may involve more than one artery or vein, or on one side involve a normal artery and vein pair. Furthermore, a normal cotyledon may be supplied by an artery and vein that run unpaired along the majority of their course. A prerequisite to this approach will be better characterization of the anatomic variation of AVs.

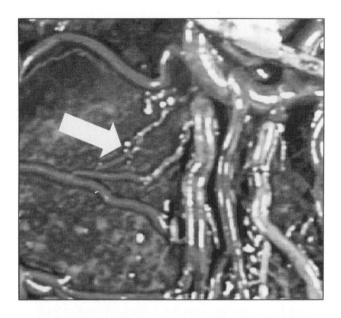

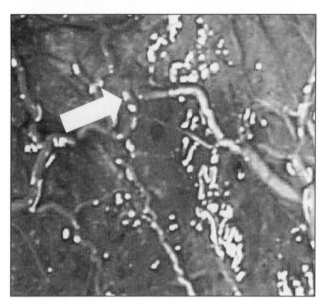

FIGURE 23–10. Placental injection study demonstrating variation in AV configurations. *A,* The vein emerges at approximately 180 degrees to the entering artery. *B,* In contrast, the angle between the artery and vein is only approximately 90 degrees. *See Color Plate 3*

Doppler can detect AA anastomoses but has not hitherto been considered capable of identifying AVs because of their lack of distinguishing spectral waveform. However, because the course and direction of small chorionic plate arteries and veins can be mapped with Doppler, AV anastomoses may be able to be distinguished by an unpaired artery entering a cotyledon from which a vein emerges towards the contralateral twin. In the future, preoperative localization of AV(s) for selective ablation may reduce procedure times and thus operative morbidity such as amniorrhexis. Indeed, accurate noninvasive localization may pave the way for minimally invasive ablative techniques such as interstitial laser and focused ultrasound surgery.[126, 127]

Delivery

At postviable gestations, delivery is a further option. However, this is rarely advisable prior to 28 weeks. This is both because of the high neonatal morbidity and mortality rates in TTTS and because the degree of severity needed to warrant intervention then is likely to be associated with severe growth restriction and renal impairment in the donor, and cardiac compromise and polycythemia in the recipient, further compromising neonatal outcome. For this reason, results of the various management strategies (Tables 23–1 through 23–3) above are compared for cases presenting prior to 28 weeks.

In contrast, delivery 32 weeks or later is relatively straightforward with a very high chance of intact survival. Further, it should reduce the chance of cerebral white matter lesions being acquired in the late third trimester.[52] In our view, the high morbidity rates warrant delivery of all MC pregnancies with complications at 32 weeks.

Our group has used fetal blood sampling in the remaining interval between 28 and 32 weeks to assist with timing of delivery.[33] Essentially, cases with major hematologic discordance are not considered candidates for conservative management. Further, preliminary analysis of the Amnioreduction Registry data suggest that the greater the hemoglobin discordancy, the greater the chance of an abnormal neonatal head scan (G. Mari, personal communication).

Management Strategy

With increasing uptake of routine chorionicity and serial fetal surveillance of MC twin pregnancies,[128] cases of TTTS should be diagnosed earlier, before the major complications of preterm labor, amniorrhexis, hydrops, and intrauterine death render the prognosis for treatment poor. In this regard, predictive tests, such as absent AA anastomoses on Doppler, positive nuchal translucency, and abnormal ductus venosus waveforms, may prove valuable.[27, 129]

For established disease, selection of the most appropriate treatment has to date been highly contentious, largely because these have not been subjected to controlled trials. Treatment preferences of various investigators have been an "all or nothing" phenomenon, with a single method advocated as primary treatment in all cases. However, the disease ranges widely in severity from mild disease, which may resolve spontaneously, to the most severe cases with extremely poor outcome. It seems logical to reserve more aggressive treatments for those who warrant it. There are two approaches.

With the *sequential* approach, amnioreduction is tried initially, proceeding to laser or selective fetocide if unsuccessful.[130] Theoretically, this should increase survival rates over those reported with either technique alone, both by minimizing procedure-related losses from laser in milder cases, and by terminating intertwin transfusion in severe cases refractory to amnioreduction. There is concern, however, that severe cases with discordant placental share may be more likely to succumb in utero from nonselective approaches to laser. Selective fetocide might arguably be preferable in this circumstance; indeed, if half the cases respond to amnioreduction, and the remainder undergo fetocide, survival rates could approach 75%, again considerably greater than with either technique alone.

With the *tailored* approach, aggressive treatments are used ab initio in severe cases.[123, 131] Most prognostic factors relate to parameters that develop during treatment such as hydrops and lack of bladder filling following amniocentesis.[76, 132] Recently we used multiple logistic regression analysis to determine poor prognostic factors identifiable at presentation: absent AA anastomoses, absent end-diastolic frequencies (EDFs) in the donor umbilical artery, and abnormal venous Doppler waveforms in the recipient.[131] The probability of one or more twins surviving was only 33% if there was absent EDFs in the donor or 37% with abnormal venous flow in the recipient. All babies survived when an AA anastomosis was detected, compared to a 45% chance of double death when absent.

Conclusion

The treatment of twin-twin transfusion remains controversial, although better understanding of the underlying physiology is leading to more rational approaches. Poor survival with conservative management has improved from 20% to around 60% with amnioreduction or nonselective laser ablation, while in severe cases elective fetocide by cord occlusion leads to an 85% single survival rate. As a result, prevention of neurodevelopmental sequelae in survivors is assuming greater importance. More rational treatment by selective identification and targeted ablation of the few AV anastomoses mediating the disease with minimal collateral damage is being developed. In addition, selecting treatments by sequential or tailored approaches may optimize survival and reduce handicap rates.

Acknowledgment

The authors acknowledge the long-term support from the Richard and Jack Wiseman Trust for work in this area.

R E F E R E N C E S

1. Sebire N, et al: The hidden mortality of monochorionic twin pregnancies. Br J Obstet Gynaecol 104:1203–1207, 1997.
2. Steinberg LH, et al: Acute polyhydramnios in twin pregnancies. Aust N Z J Obstet Gynaecol 30:196–200, 1990.
3. Denbow ML, et al: Neonatal cranial ultrasonographic findings in preterm twins complicated by severe fetofetal transfusion syndrome. Am J Obstet Gynecol 178:479–483, 1998.
4. Nageotte MP, et al: Atriopeptin in the twin transfusion syndrome. Obstet Gynecol 73:867, 1989.
5. Wieacker P, et al: Pathophysiology of polyhydramnios in twin transfusion syndrome. Fetal Diagn Ther 7:87–92, 1992.
6. Rosen DJ, et al: Fetal urine production in normal twins and in twins with acute polyhydramnios. Fetal Diagn Ther 5:57–60, 1990.
7. Fisk N: The scientific basis of feto-fetal transfusion syndrome and its treatment. *In* Ward H, Whittle M (eds): Proceedings of the RCOG Study Group on Multiple Pregnancy. London: RCOG Press, 1995, pp 235–250.
8. Duncan KR, Denbow M, Fisk NM: The aetiology and management of twin twin transfusion syndrome. Prenat Diagn 17:1227–1236, 1997.
9. Zosmer N, et al: Clinical and echographic features of in utero cardiac dysfunction in the recipient twin in twin-twin transfusion syndrome. Br Heart J 72:74–79, 1994.
10. Hecher K, et al: Doppler studies of the fetal circulation in twin-twin transfusion syndrome. Ultrasound Obstet Gynecol 5:318–324, 1995.
11. Machin GA: Velamentous cord insertion in monochorionic twin gestation—an added risk factor. J Reprod Med 42:785–789, 1997.
12. Fries MH, et al: The role of velamentous cord insertion in the etiology of twin-twin transfusion syndrome. Obstet Gynecol 81:569–574, 1993.
13. Denbow M, et al: Placental angioarchitecture in monochorionic twin pregnancies: Relationship to fetal growth, feto-fetal transfusion syndrome and pregnancy outcome. Am J Obstet Gynecol 182:417–426, 2000.
14. Machin G, Still K, Lalani T: Correlations of placental vascular anatomy and clinical outcomes in 69 monochorionic twin pregnancies. Am J Med Genet 61:229–236, 1996.
15. Bajoria R, Wigglesworth J, Fisk NM: Angioarchitecture of monochorionic placentas in relation to the twin-twin transfusion syndrome. Am J Obstet Gynecol 172:856–863, 1995.
16. Fisk NM, et al: Fetofetal transfusion syndrome: Do the neonatal criteria apply in utero? Arch Dis Child 65:57–61, 1990.
17. Bruner JP, Rosemond RL: Twin-to-twin transfusion syndrome: A subset of the twin oligohydramnios-polyhydramnios sequence. Am J Obstet Gynecol 169:925–930, 1993.
18. Tanaka M, et al: Intravascular pancuronium bromide infusion for prenatal diagnosis of twin-twin transfusion syndrome. Fetal Diagn Ther 7:36–40, 1992.
19. Denbow ML, et al: Ultrasound microbubble contrast angiography in monochorionic twin fetuses. Lancet 349:773, 1997.
20. Denbow M, et al: Intravascular microbubble contrast administration in twin fetuses: Early experience with Levovist. Radiology (in press) 2000.
21. Fusi L, Gordon H: Twin pregnancy complicated by single intrauterine death. Problems and outcome with conservative management. Br J Obstet Gynaecol 97:511–516, 1990.
22. Okamura K, et al: Funipuncture for evaluation of hematologic and coagulation indices in the surviving twin following co-twin's death. Obstet Gynecol 83:975–978, 1994.
23. Nicolini U, et al: Fetal blood sampling immediately before and within 24 hours of death in monochorionic twin pregnancies complicated by single intrauterine death. Am J Obstet Gynecol 179:800–803, 1998.
24. Fusi L, et al: Acute twin-twin transfusion: A possible mechanism for brain-damaged survivors after intrauterine death of a monochorionic twin. Obstet Gynecol 78:517–520, 1991.
25. Schatz F: Klinische Beiträge zur Physiologie des Fetus. Berlin: Hirschwald, 1900.
26. Talbert D, et al: Hydrostatic and osmotic pressure gradients produce manifestations of fetofetal transfusion syndrome in a computerised model of monochorionic twin pregnancy. Am J Obstet Gynecol 174:598–608, 1996.
27. Denbow ML, et al: Colour Doppler energy insonation of placental vasculature in monochorionic twins: Absent arterio-arterial anastomoses in association with twin-to-twin transfusion syndrome. Br J Obstet Gynaecol 105:760–765, 1998.
28. Hecher K, et al: Artery-to-artery anastomosis in monochorionic twins. Am J Obstet Gynecol 171:570–572, 1994.
29. Fisk N, et al: X-chromosome inactivation patterns do not implicate asymmetric splitting of the inner cell mass in the aetiology of twin-twin transfusion syndrome. Mol Hum Reprod 5:52–56, 1999.
30. Tolosa J, et al: Fetal hypertension and cardiac hypertrophy in the discordant twin syndrome. Proceedings of the SPO abstract. Am J Obstet Gynecol 168:292, 1993.
31. Simpson LL, et al: Cardiac dysfunction in twin-twin transfusion syndrome: A prospective, longitudinal study. Obstet Gynecol 92:557–562, 1998.

32. Bajoria R, Sullivan M, Fisk N: Endothelin levels in monochorionic twins with severe twin-twin transfusion syndrome. Hum Reprod 14:1614–1618, 1999.
33. Denbow M, et al: Haematological indices at fetal blood sampling in monochorionic pregnancies complicated by feto-fetal transfusion syndrome. Prenat Diagn 18:941–946, 1998.
34. Elejalde BR, et al: Diagnosis of twin to twin transfusion syndrome at 18 weeks of gestation. J Clin Ultrasound 11:442–446, 1983.
35. Chescheir NC, Seeds JW: Polyhydramnios and oligohydramnios in twin gestations. Obstet Gynecol 71:882–884, 1988.
36. Brown DL, et al: Twin-twin transfusion syndrome: Sonographic findings. Radiology 170:61–63, 1989.
37. Patten RM, et al: Disparity of amniotic fluid volume and fetal size: Problem of the stuck twin-US studies. Radiology 172:153–157, 1989.
38. Pretorius DH, et al: Doppler ultrasound of twin transfusion syndrome. J Ultrasound Med 7:117–124, 1988.
39. Weir PE, Ratten GJ, Beischer NA: Acute polyhydramnios—a complication of monozygous twin pregnancy. Br J Obstet Gynaecol 86:849–853, 1979.
40. Wittmann BK, Baldwin VJ, Nichol B: Antenatal diagnosis of twin transfusion syndrome by ultrasound. Obstet Gynecol 58:123–127, 1981.
41. Urig MA, Clewell WH, Elliott JP: Twin-twin transfusion syndrome. Am J Obstet Gynecol 163:1522–1526, 1990.
42. Gonsoulin W, et al: Outcome of twin-twin transfusion diagnosed before 28 weeks of gestation. Obstet Gynecol 75:214–216, 1990.
43. Mahony BS, et al: The "stuck twin" phenomenon: Ultrasonographic findings, pregnancy outcome, and management with serial amniocenteses. Am J Obstet Gynecol 163:1513–1522, 1990.
44. Radestad A, Thomassen PA: Acute polyhydramnios in twin pregnancy. A retrospective study with special reference to therapeutic amniocentesis. Acta Obstet Gynecol Scand 69:297–300, 1990.
45. Bromley B, et al: The natural history of oligohydramnios/polyhydramnios sequence in monochorionic diamniotic twins. Ultrasound Obstet Gynecol 2:317–320, 1992.
46. Pinette MG, et al: Treatment of twin-twin transfusion syndrome. Obstet Gynecol 82:841–846, 1993.
47. Reisner DP, et al: Stuck twin syndrome: Outcome in thirty-seven consecutive cases. Am J Obstet Gynecol 169:991–995, 1993.
48. Dennis LG, Winkler CL: Twin to twin transfusion syndrome: Aggressive therapeutic amniocentesis. Am J Obstet Gynecol 177:342–347, 1997.
49. Skupski D: Changes in survival of twins delivered after twin-twin transfusion syndrome versus preterm singletons over the calendar years 1970–1994. Fetal Diagn Ther 13:334–338, 1998.
50. Cincotta R, Oldham J, Sampson A: Antepartum and postpartum complications of twin transfusion. Aust N Z J Obstet Gynaecol 36:303–308, 1996.
51. Barr M, Sedman AB, Heidelberger KP: Renal tubular dysgenesis in twins. Pediatr Nephrol 12:408–413, 1998.
52. Bejar R, et al: Antenatal origin of neurologic damage in newborn infants. II. Multiple gestations. Am J Obstet Gynecol 162:1230–1236, 1990.
53. Mercuri E, et al: Incidence of cranial ultrasound abnormalities in apparently well neonates on a postnatal ward: Correlation with antenatal and perinatal factors and neurological status. Arch Dis Child Fetal Neonatal Ed 79:F185–F189, 1998.
54. De Lia JE, Kuhlmann RS, Lopez KP: Treating previable twin-twin transfusion syndrome with fetoscopic laser surgery: Outcomes following the learning curve. J Perinat Med 27:61–67, 1999.
55. Trespidi L, et al: Serial amniocenteses in the management of twin-twin transfusion syndrome: When is it valuable? Fetal Diagn Ther 12:15–20, 1997.
56. Quintero RA, et al: Selective photocoagulation of placental vessels in twin-twin transfusion syndrome: Evolution of a surgical technique. Obstet Gynecol Surv 53:S97–S103, 1998.
57. Ville Y, et al: Endoscopic laser coagulation in the management of severe twin-to-twin transfusion syndrome. Br J Obstet Gynaecol 105:446–453, 1998.
58. Fisk NM, et al: Amniotic pressure in disorders of amniotic fluid volume. Obstet Gynecol 76:210–214, 1990.
59. Weiner CP, et al: Normal values for human umbilical venous and amniotic fluid pressures and their alteration by fetal disease. Am J Obstet Gynecol 161:714–717, 1989.
60. Fisk NM, et al: Normal amniotic pressure throughout gestation. Br J Obstet Gynaecol 99:18–22, 1992.
61. Kyle P, Fisk N: Oligohydramnios and polyhydramnios. In Fisk N, Moise K (eds): Fetal Therapy: Invasive and Transplacental. Cambridge: Cambridge University Press, 1997, pp 203–226.
62. Weiner CP, Ludomirski A: Diagnosis, pathophysiology, and treatment of chronic twin-to-twin transfusion syndrome. Fetal Diagn Ther 9:283–290, 1994.
63. Garry D, et al: Intra-amniotic pressure reduction in twin-twin transfusion syndrome. J Perinatol 18:284–286, 1998.
64. Cabrera-Ramirez L, Harris RE: Controlled removal of amniotic fluid in hydramnios. South Med J 69:239–240, 1976.
65. Feingold M, et al: Serial amniocenteses in the treatment of twin to twin transfusion complicated with acute polyhydramnios. Acta Genet Med Gemellol Roma 35:107–113, 1986.
66. Fisk N: Amniotic pressure in disorders of amniotic fluid volume. PhD Thesis. London: University of London, 1992.
67. Elliott JP, Urig MA, Clewell WH: Aggressive therapeutic amniocentesis for treatment of twin-twin transfusion syndrome. Obstet Gynecol 77:537–540, 1991.
68. Elliott JP, et al: Large-volume therapeutic amniocentesis in the treatment of hydramnios. Obstet Gynecol 84:1025–1027, 1994.
69. Wax JR, et al: Stuck twin with cotwin nonimmune hydrops: Successful treatment by amniocentesis. Fetal Diagn Ther 6:126–131, 1991.
70. Fisk NM, Vaughan J, Talbert D: Impaired fetal blood gas status in polyhydramnios and its relation to raised amniotic pressure. Fetal Diagn Ther 9:7–13, 1994.
71. Tabor BL, Maier JA: Polyhydramnios and elevated intrauterine pressure during amnioinfusion. Am J Obstet Gynecol 156:130–131, 1987.
72. Bower SJ, et al: Uterine artery blood flow response to correction of amniotic fluid volume. Am J Obstet Gynecol 173:502–507, 1995.
73. Feldman DM, et al: Iatrogenic monoamniotic twins as a complication of therapeutic amniocentesis. Obstet Gynecol 91:815–816, 1998.
74. Denbow ML, et al: Relationship between change in amniotic fluid index and volume of fluid removed at amnioreduction. Obstet Gynecol 90:529–532, 1997.
75. Hecher K, et al: Endoscopic laser surgery versus serial amniocenteses in the treatment of severe twin-twin transfusion syndrome. Am J Obstet Gynecol 180:717–724, 1999.
76. Kilby MD, et al: Bladder visualisation as a prognostic sign in oligohydramnios polyhydramnios sequence in twin pregnancies treated using therapeutic amniocentesis. Br J Obstet Gynaecol 104:939–942, 1997.
77. Saunders NJ, Snijders RJ, Nicolaides KH: Therapeutic amniocentesis in twin-twin transfusion syndrome appearing in the second trimester of pregnancy. Am J Obstet Gynecol 166:820–824, 1992.
78. Dickinson J: Severe twin-twin transfusion syndrome: Current management concepts. Aust N Z J Obstet Gynaecol 35:16–21, 1995.
79. Bruner JP, Anderson TL, Rosemond RL: Placental pathophysiology of the twin oligohydramnios-polyhydramnios sequence and the twin-twin transfusion syndrome. Placenta 19:81–86, 1998.
80. Mari G: Amnioreduction in twin-twin transfusion syndrome—a multicenter registry, evaluation of 579 procedures. Am J Obstet Gynecol 178:S28, 1998.
81. Saade G, et al: Amniotomy: A new approach to the "stuck twin" syndrome. Am J Obstet Gynecol 172:429, 1995.
82. Hubinont C, et al: Nd:YAG laser and needle disruption of the interfetal septum: A possible therapy in severe twin to twin transfusion syndrome. J Gynecol Surg 12:183–189, 1996.
83. Bajoria R: Abundant vascular anastomoses in monoamniotic versus diamniotic monochorionic placentas. Am J Obstet Gynecol 179:788–793, 1998.
84. Quintero R, et al: Amniotic fluid pressures in severe twin-twin transfusion syndrome. Prenat Neonat Med 3:607–610, 1998.
85. Saade G, Ludomirsky A, Fisk N: Feto-fetal transfusion. In Fisk N, Moise K (eds): Fetal Therapy: Invasive and Transplacental. Cambridge: Cambridge University Press, 1997, pp 227–251.
86. Saade GR, et al: Amniotic septostomy for the treatment of twin oligohydramnios-polyhydramnios sequence. Fetal Diagn Ther 13:86–93, 1998.

87. Sebire NJ, et al: Single uterine entry for genetic amniocentesis in twin pregnancies. Ultrasound Obstet Gynecol 7:26–31, 1996.

88. Buscaglia M, et al: Genetic amniocentesis in diamniotic twin pregnancies by a single transabdominal insertion of the needle. Prenat Diagn 15:17–19, 1995.

89. van Vugt JM, Nieuwint A, van Geijn HP: Single-needle insertion: An alternative technique for early second-trimester genetic twin amniocentesis. Fetal Diagn Ther 10:178–181, 1995.

90. Kirshon B, Mari G, Moise K Jr: Indomethacin therapy in the treatment of symptomatic polyhydramnios. Obstet Gynecol 75:202–205, 1990.

91. Lange IR, et al: Twin with hydramnios: Treating premature labor at source. Am J Obstet Gynecol 160:552–557, 1989.

92. Buderus S, et al: Renal failure in two preterm infants: Toxic effect of prenatal maternal indomethacin treatment? Br J Obstet Gynaecol 100:97–98, 1993.

93. De Lia J, et al: Twin transfusion syndrome: Successful in utero treatment with digoxin. Int J Gynaecol Obstet 23:197–201, 1985.

94. Weiner CP: Diagnosis and treatment of twin to twin transfusion in the mid-second trimester of pregnancy. Fetal Ther 2:71–74, 1987.

95. Bebbington MW, et al: Selective feticide in twin transfusion syndrome using ultrasound-guided insertion of thrombogenic coils. Fetal Diagn Ther 10:32–36, 1995.

96. Dommergues M, et al: Twin-to-twin transfusion syndrome: Selective feticide by embolization of the hydropic fetus. Fetal Diagn Ther 10:26–31, 1995.

97. Wittmann BK, et al: The role of feticide in the management of severe twin transfusion syndrome. Am J Obstet Gynecol 155:1023–1026, 1986.

98. Chestnut DH: Epidural anesthesia and instrumental vaginal delivery [editorial; comment]. Anesthesiology 74:805–808, 1991.

99. Quintero RA, et al: Brief report: Umbilical-cord ligation of an acardiac twin by fetoscopy at 19 weeks of gestation. N Engl J Med 330:469–471, 1994.

100. Quintero RA, et al: In utero percutaneous umbilical cord ligation in the management of complicated monochorionic multiple gestations. Ultrasound Obstet Gynecol 8:16–22, 1996.

101. Deprest J, et al: Bipolar coagulation of the umbilical cord in complicated monochorionic twin pregnancy. Am J Obstet Gynecol 182:340–345, 2000.

102. Deprest J, Gratacos E: Obstetrical endoscopy. Curr Opin Obstet Gynecol 11:195–203, 1999.

103. Deprest JA, et al: Experience with fetoscopic cord ligation. Eur J Obstet Gynecol Reprod Biol 81:157–164, 1998.

104. Lemery D, et al: Fetal umbilical cord ligation under ultrasound guidance. Ultrasound Obstet Gynecol 4:399–401, 1994.

105. Urig MA, et al: Twin-twin transfusion syndrome: The surgical removal of one twin as a treatment option. Fetal Ther 3:185–188, 1988.

106. De Lia JE, Rogers JG, Dixon JA: Treatment of placental vasculature with a neodymium-yttrium-aluminium-garnet laser via fetoscopy. Am J Obstet Gynecol 151:1126–1127, 1985.

107. De-Lia JE, et al: Neodymium:yttrium-aluminum-garnet laser occlusion of rhesus placental vasculature via fetoscopy. Am J Obstet Gynecol 160:485–489, 1989.

108. De-Lia JE, Cruikshank DP, Keye W Jr: Fetoscopic neodymium:YAG laser occlusion of placental vessels in severe twin-twin transfusion syndrome. Obstet Gynecol 75:1046–1053, 1990.

109. Ville Y, et al: Preliminary experience with endoscopic laser surgery for severe twin-twin transfusion syndrome. N Engl J Med 332:224–227, 1995.

110. De Lia JE, et al: Fetoscopic laser ablation of placental vessels in severe previable twin-twin transfusion syndrome. Am J Obstet Gynecol 172:1202–1208, 1995.

111. Fisk NM, Bajoria R, Wigglesworth J: Twin-twin transfusion syndrome. N Engl J Med 333:388, 1995.

112. Ville Y, et al: Successful outcome after Nd: YAG laser separation of chorioangiopagus-twins under sonoendoscopic control. Ultrasound Obstet Gynecol 2:429–431, 1992.

113. Branisteanu-Dumitrascu I, et al: Time-related cotyledonary effects of laser coagulation of superficial chorionic vessels in an ovine model. Prenat Diagn 19:205–210, 1999.

114. De Lia JE, Cruikshank DP, Keye WR Jr: Fetoscopic neodymium:YAG laser occlusion of placental vessels in severe twin-twin transfusion syndrome. Obstet Gynecol 75:1046–1053, 1990.

115. De Lia J, Khulmann R, Clark S: Fetoscopic laser treatment of twin-twin transfusion syndrome: Expectations and results post learning curve. Fetal Diagn Ther 13:64, 1998.

116. Deprest JA, et al: Alternative technique for Nd:YAG laser coagulation in twin-to-twin transfusion syndrome with anterior placenta. Ultrasound Obstet Gynecol 11:347–352, 1998.

117. Evrard VA, et al: Underwater Nd:YAG laser coagulation of blood vessels in a rat model. Fetal Diagn Ther 11:422–426, 1996.

118. Ville Y, et al: Endoscopic laser coagulation of umbilical cord vessels in twin reversed arterial perfusion sequence. Ultrasound Obstet Gynecol 4:396–398, 1994.

119. Van Peborgh P, et al: Management of a case of twin-to-twin transfusion syndrome by a combined surgical approach. Fetal Diagn Ther 13:75–78, 1998.

120. Stone CA, Quinn MW, Saxby PJ: Congenital skin loss following Nd:YAG placental photocoagulation. Burns 24:275–277, 1998.

121. Lundvall L, et al: Limb necrosis associated with twin-twin transfusion syndrome treated with YAG-laser coagulation. Acta Obstet Gynecol Scand 78:349–350, 1999.

122. Hecher K, Campbell S: Characteristics of fetal venous blood flow under normal circumstances and during fetal disease. Ultrasound Obstet Gynecol 7:68–83, 1996.

123. van Gemert MJ, Major AL, Scherjon SA: Placental anatomy, fetal demise and therapeutic intervention in monochorionic twins and the transfusion syndrome: New hypotheses. Eur J Obstet Gynecol Reprod Biol 78:53–62, 1998.

124. Benirschke K, Kaufmann P: Pathology of the Human Placenta. New York: Springer-Verlag, 1995.

125. Baldwin V: The Pathology of Multiple Pregnancy. New York: Springer-Verlag, 1994.

126. Sohn C, et al: Treatment of the twin-twin transfusion syndrome: Initial experience using laser-induced interstitial thermotherapy. Fetal Diagn Ther 11:390–397, 1996.

127. Denbow M, Rivens IH, Rowland IJ, et al: Preclinical development of noninvasive occlusion with focussed ultrasonic surgery for fetal therapy. Am J Obstet Gynecol 182:387–392, 2000.

128. Fisk NM, Bryan E: Routine prenatal determination of chorionicity in multiple gestation: A plea to the obstetrician. Br J Obstet Gynaecol 100:975–977, 1993.

129. Sebire NJ, et al: Increased nuchal translucency thickness at 10–14 weeks of gestation as a predictor of severe twin to twin transfusion syndrome. Ultrasound Obstet Gynecol 10:86–89, 1997.

130. Machin GA, Keith LG: Can twin-to-twin transfusion syndrome be explained, and how is it treated? Clin Obstet Gynecol 41:105–113, 1998.

131. Taylor M, et al: Antenatal factors at diagnosis predictive of outcome in severe twin-twin transfusion syndrome. Am J Obstet Gynecol (in press) 2000.

132. Bebbington MW, Wittmann BK: Fetal transfusion syndrome: Antenatal factors predicting outcome. Am J Obstet Gynecol 160:913–915, 1989.

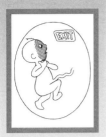

CHAPTER 24

The Fetus with Airway Obstruction

TIMOTHY M. CROMBLEHOLME and CRAIG T. ALBANESE

The widespread use of prenatal ultrasound has uncovered increasing numbers of fetal structural malformations that have a direct impact on perinatal management and fetal outcome. There is perhaps no more striking example of this than fetal airway obstruction. The causes of fetal airway obstruction may be either extrinsic to the airway caused by mass effect compressing it or intrinsic to the larynx or trachea. Extrinsic causes of fetal airway obstruction may be due to the mass effect of a giant cervical lymphangioma or teratoma, or less commonly by fetal goiter, hemangioma, choristoma, epignathus, neuroblastoma, mucocele, branchial cleft cyst, or laryngocele.[1-6] Intrinsic causes of fetal airway obstruction usually fall under the clinical syndrome of congenital high airway obstruction syndrome (CHAOS).[7] CHAOS is a prenatal clinical syndrome manifested by nonimmune hydrops that occurs as a result of complete, or near-complete, intrinsic obstruction of the fetal airway.[7]

This chapter focuses on the natural history, pathophysiology, key diagnostic prenatal sonographic and magnetic resonance imaging (MRI) findings, and the treatment and outcome of fetal airway obstruction.

The Pathogenesis of Fetal Airway Obstruction

Extrinsic Compression of the Fetal Airways

While a number of fetal neck masses have been anecdotally reported to compromise the fetal airway (Table 24–1), the vast majority of cases are either lymphangioma or teratoma. As the most is known about these two etiologies of extrinsic fetal airway obstruction, we will focus our discussion on them.

Cervical Lymphangioma

Lymphangioma is a benign malformation composed of dilated cystic lymphatics.[8] These malformations are often present at birth and are second only to hemangioma as a cause of a soft tissue mass in the newborn.[8-11] Lymphangiomas can occur in almost any location but are most commonly seen in the soft tissue of the neck, axilla, thorax, and lower extremities.[8] Isaacs reported a series of 97 consecutive lymphangiomas from the Children's Hospital of Los Angeles in which 45 occurred in the neck, 22 in the chest wall, 12 in the extremities, and four in the abdominal wall. Other less common sites included the omentum, mesentery, larynx, tongue, bowel, retroperitoneum, mediastinum, conjunctiva, and mouth.[10] These lesions can vary in size from tiny subepidermal skin blebs to large dilated cystic fluid-filled masses which, when located in the neck, are commonly referred to as cystic hygromas.

The lymphatic system develops at the end of the fifth week of gestation with sprouting from the six primary lymph sacs situated in the neck, iliac region, and retroperitoneum. Goetsch suggested that lymphangiomas are developmental defects secondary to sequestration of lymphatic tissue in early embryonic life.[12] Cervical lymphangiomas are believed to result from a failure of the jugular lymph sacs to join the lymphatic channels. The hygroma develops fibriller sprouts from the existing cystic spaces. These endothelial-lined cystic spaces secrete lymph-like fluid that causes local distention and gradual enlargement of cysts. Over time, the walls thicken, with connective tissue septae separating large cysts.[8, 13]

There is a disparity between isolated lymphangiomas that are diagnosed at birth in otherwise healthy infants, and those detected prenatally in the second trimester (Table 24–2). These two groups of fetuses appear to have lymphangiomas of differing origin, pathophysiology, natural history and, most importantly, outcome.[14-16] Early-diagnosed lymphangiomas are usually located in the posterior triangle, and have a 60% incidence of chromosomal abnormalities, other structural anomalies, hydrops fetalis, a high incidence of intrauterine demise; and rare postnatal survival (Table 24–3). Lymphangiomas diagnosed early in utero are commonly seen in association with Turner syndrome, hydrops, oligohydramnios, single-vessel umbilical cord, Noonan syndrome, fetal alcohol syndrome, Fryns syndrome, and trisomies 18 and 21.[13, 17-19] Chromosomal abnormalities are found in more than 60% of fetuses with cystic hy-

TABLE 24-1. DIFFERENTIAL DIAGNOSIS OF FETAL AIRWAY OBSTRUCTION

Causes of extrinsic obstruction
  Cervical teratoma
  Congenital goiter
  Solid thyroid tumors
  Thyroid cyst or thyroglossal duct cyst
  Branchial cleft cyst
  Neuroblastoma
  Hamartoma
  Hemangioma
  Lipoma
  Laryngocele
  Lymphangioma
  Nuchal edema
  Parotid tumor
  Choristoma
  Neural tube defects
    Occipital encephalocele
    Cervical myelomeningocele
  Twin sac of a blighted ovum

Causes of intrinsic obstruction
  Laryngeal atresia
  Laryngeal stenosis
  Laryngeal web
  Tracheal atresia
  Tracheal stenosis
  Laryngeal cyst

TABLE 24-3. ASSOCIATED ANOMALIES IN 27 FETUSES WITH CERVICAL LYMPHANGIOMA*

Structural anomalies	
Cardiac defects	6
Hydronephrosis	3
Neural tube defect	3
Cleft lip/palate	2
Multiple pterygium syndrome	2
Skeletal anomalies	1
Imperforate anus	1
Ambiguous genitalia	1

* Adapted from Langer JC, Fitzgerald PG, Desa D, et al: Cervical cystic hygroma in the fetus: Clinical spectrum and outcome. J Pediatr Surg 25:58–62, 1990, with permission.

that are characteristic features of Turner syndrome are believed to be the sequelae of fetal cystic hygromas that spontaneously resolved.

Precise estimates of the incidence of cystic hygroma and lymphangioma are difficult to ascertain and depend on whether prenatal or postnatal data are evaluated. Fonkalsrud estimated the incidence of cystic hygroma to be 1 in 12,000 births, with 50 to 65% of cases present at birth, and 80 to 90% present by the second year of life.[30, 31] A total of 52 confirmed diagnoses of cystic hygroma were reported to the South East Thames Regional Congenital Malformation Registry in a region with an annual birth rate of 52,000, yielding an incidence of 1 in 1,000 births. This series included terminations, intrauterine demise, stillbirths, and postnatal deaths, thus providing a more accurate account of the incidence of cystic hygroma.[32] However, the incidence of cystic hygroma was as high as 1 in 300 among spontaneous abortuses reported by Byrne et al.[33]

The natural history of prenatally diagnosed cystic hygroma appears to be dependent upon gestational age at diagnosis, location of the cystic hygroma and, most importantly, whether or not there are associated chromosomal or structural abnormalities.[14] The mortality of a posteriorly located cystic hygroma diagnosed prior to 30 weeks' gestation is extremely high because of the significant incidence of nonimmune hydrops and associated chromosomal defects. In the report by Langer et al. of 27 cases diagnosed prior to 30 weeks' gestation, only two fetuses survived. Of the 25 that did not survive, 21 developed nonimmune hydrops, four spontaneously aborted, and 21 had elective terminations. The only two survivors demonstrated spontaneous regression and were subsequently diagnosed with Noonan syndrome at birth.[14] Cystic hygroma associated with nonimmune hydrops is almost uniformly fatal, and approximately 80% of these cases have chromosomal abnormalities. In

groma (Table 24–4), with the majority being female 46,X karyotype,[17, 20, 21] although trisomy 13, trisomy 18, trisomy 21, and Kleinfelter syndrome have all been reported.[13, 22-24] Conversely, fetuses with normal karyotype appear to have a much higher incidence of consanguinity or a previous history of abnormal fetuses.[14] Cystic hygromas in karyotypically normal fetuses are more likely to be associated with familial conditions such as Noonan syndrome, multiple pterygium syndrome, polysplenia syndrome, Robert syndrome or an isolated autosomal recessive trait.[25-29] In contrast, isolated cystic hygroma usually presents in the third trimester, often with a previously normal sonogram earlier in gestation. These lymphangiomas are usually located anteriorly or anterolaterally, and are not generally associated with other anomalies or hydrops.[14-16] Langer et al. suggested that in these cases, the lymphangioma develops late in gestation, as one of his cases had a normal ultrasound at 17 weeks' gestation.[14] If this is true, it is unlikely that the embryologic mechanism in the late-presenting group of cystic hygromas is the same as the early-gestation group. Cystic hygromas may also regress in utero, presumably due to the development of collateral lymphatic and venous connections. Interestingly, the webbing of the neck and puffiness of the hands and feet

TABLE 24-2. CHARACTERISTICS OF EARLY VERSUS LATE-DIAGNOSED CERVICAL LYPHANGIOMA

	LOCATION	CHROMOSOMAL ANOMALIES	STRUCTURAL ANOMALIES	MORTALITY
Early (second trimester)	Posterior	Approximately 60%	Many	High
Late (third trimester or postnatal)	Anterior	Rare	Usually isolated	Low

TABLE 24–4. CHROMOSOMAL ABNORMALITIES ASSOCIATED WITH CERVICAL LYMPHANGIOMA

45,X
Trisomy 18
Trisomy 13
Trisomy 21
13q
18p
Partial 11q/22q trisomy
Trisomy 22 mosaicism

a review of 100 fetuses with nuchal thickening or cystic hygroma detected sonographically at 10 to 15 weeks' gestation, Nadel et al. found that a good prognosis could be expected if the karyotype was normal, there were no septae in the mass, and no hydrops.[34]

The major concern for fetuses with large cystic cervical masses later in gestation is airway compromise at birth. These fetuses may benefit by delivery using the ex utero intrapartum treatment (EXIT) strategy (see below).

Cervical Teratoma

Cervical teratoma is a rare tumor with only 150 congenital cases described. Since the first prenatal diagnosis of fetal cervical teratoma in 1978, there have been only 18 published reports of cervical masses detected in utero.[2, 3, 35–50] Teratomas are composed of tissues foreign to its anatomic site, with all three germ layers represented. Neural tissue is the most common histologic component, with cartilage and respiratory epithelium also observed.[35] Thirty to 40% contain thyroid tissue, but it is uncertain whether this represents actual involvement of the gland or ectopic thyroid tissue.[36] Cervical teratoma is theorized to originate from either totipotential germ cells or result from abnormal development of a conjoined twin.[40, 51] There is no apparent relationship to maternal age or parity.[40] Unlike other teratomas, males and females are equally affected[52, 53] and there is no racial predilection.[41] There has been one report of congenital cervical teratoma occurring in siblings, but no other familial cases have been described.[54]

Cervical teratomas are usually large and bulky, typically 5 to 12 cm in diameter.[52, 55] Tumor masses greater than the size of the fetal head have also been reported.[36, 52, 56] They can extend from the mastoid process and body of the mandible, superiorly displacing the ear, to the clavicle and sternal notch. Posteriorly, they can reach the anterior border of the trapezius. Involvement of the oral floor, protrusion into the oral cavity (epignathus), and extension into the superior mediastinum have also been noted.[36]

Polyhydramnios is present in up to 40% of the prenatally diagnosed cases and is more commonly observed in association with large tumors.[57–59] Polyhydramnios is believed to be due to esophageal obstruction, as has been demonstrated by contrast amniography.[60, 61] An empty stomach may be the first sonographic clue to esophageal obstruction from cervical teratoma.[41, 61] Other associated anomalies include chondrodystrophia fetalis and im-

perforate anus,[62] hypoplastic left ventricle and trisomy 13,[63, 64] and mandibular hypoplasia as a result of the mass effect on the developing mandible.[48, 50]

Lymphangioma is the most likely entity to be mistaken for cervical teratoma in cases detected prenatally. The similarities in size, sonographic findings, clinical characteristics, location, and gestational age at presentation make this ultrasonographic distinction difficult.[52] Cystic hygromas are typically multiloculated cystic masses with poorly defined borders that infiltrate the normal structures of the neck. This contrasts with the usually well-defined borders of cervical teratomas. Furthermore, cystic hygromas tend to be smaller than cervical teratomas, unilateral, and more frequently involve the posterior triangle.[45]

Amniotic fluid α-fetoprotein (AFP) has been suggested as an aid in the differential diagnosis of a fetal cervical neck mass. AFP may be either elevated or normal in cervical teratomas. Since fewer than 30% of cervical teratomas have an elevated AFP, this assay is not particularly helpful in the differential diagnosis of fetal cervical masses.[65] An elevated serum AFP in the newborn, however, may be helpful in following the patient for signs of teratoma recurrence following presumptive complete resection.

The natural history of fetal cervical teratomas is not well characterized. Although they are most often malignant in adults, the vast majority of cervical teratomas in fetuses and infants are benign.[60] Rare cases of malignancies in this age group have, however, been described.[42, 43, 65–68] The true malignant potential of cervical teratoma is uncertain.[47, 52, 56, 63, 69, 70] Despite the existence of primitive tissue types in the tumor and metastases to regional lymph nodes, many infants have remained free from recurrence following complete resection. These cases suggest that a malignant biologic behavior is uncommon in this population.[52, 63, 71] Immature tissue seen histologically may merely reflect the immaturity of the host; thus pathologic studies are not completely reliable in predicting prognosis.[52, 53]

Intrinsic Obstruction of the Fetal Airway

CHAOS is a prenatal clinical syndrome manifested by the presence of extremely large echogenic lungs, flattened or inverted diaphragms, a dilated tracheobronchial tree, ascites, and other manifestations of nonimmune hydrops due to complete or near-complete intrinsic obstruction of the fetal airway.[7] The fetal lungs normally produce fluid that leaves the trachea with fetal breathing movements at an estimated rate of 4 mL/kg/d under a positive pressure with respect to the amniotic fluid pressure. Complete obstruction of the upper trachea or larynx results in elevated intratracheal pressure and distention of the tracheobronchial tree due to accumulation of fetal lung fluid. The lungs become distended and the mediastinal structures compressed by the huge lungs, impeding venous return, leading to the development of hydrops. No fetus diagnosed prenatally with CHAOS associated with hydrops has survived without intervention.

The airway obstruction in CHAOS may be due to one of several etiologies, including laryngeal atresia, tracheal atresia, or laryngeal cyst (Table 24–1), but the fetal clinical presentation is the same. Three types of laryngeal atresia are recognized. Type I, in which the supraglottic and infraglottic parts of the larynx are atretic; type II, in which the atresia is infraglottic; and type III, which is glottic. Laryngeal atresia can only partially be accounted for by failure of epithelial recanalization. Abnormal cricoid development occurs with types I and II. Tracheal atresia occurs when the midportion of the foregut developed into esophagus only, with no endoderm left to form a trachea.

Most cases of CHAOS occur as sporadic, isolated malformations without known risk of recurrence. However, a wide range of anomalies can be seen in association with laryngeal atresia (Table 24–5). For example, CHAOS may be one fetal presentation of Fraser syndrome (cryptophthalmos-syndactyly syndrome). This inherited disorder is characterized by variable expression of cryptophthalmos, renal agenesis, syndactyly, abnormalities of ears and external genitalia, and laryngeal stenosis or atresia.[72, 73] Fraser syndrome has only been correctly diagnosed twice in the second trimester.[72, 74] Often, a previously affected pregnancy will prompt sonographic surveillance for Fraser syndrome, since this syndrome is believed to be inherited as an autosomal recessive disorder.[75] The sonographic features of cryptophthalmos, renal agenesis, and syndactyly in a fetus with CHAOS suggests the diagnosis of Fraser syndrome.[76]

The true incidence of CHAOS is unknown. Congenital obstruction of the fetal airway resulting in CHAOS was initially thought to be extremely rare.[7] However, 22 cases of this syndrome have been reported since 1989.[7, 72, 73, 77–90] This syndrome may be more common than generally appreciated because many of the affected fetuses die in utero or are stillborn.[72, 76, 80–82, 84, 86, 91]

The principal non-airway obstructing lesion that CHAOS is mistaken for on prenatal ultrasound is bilateral congenital cystic adenomatoid malformation (CCAM). Bilateral CCAM is an unusual finding, as CCAM is usually lobar, not involving the entire lung, and less than 2% of cases are bilateral.[92] An important distinguishing feature is the compressed rim of normal lung, which can usually be seen in CCAM but not in CHAOS. The uniformly echogenic lungs which are massively enlarged associated with flattened diaphragms, a midline compressed mediastinum, and often dilated trachea and mainstem bronchi allow CHAOS to be distinguished from CCAM.

Our understanding of the natural history of CHAOS is limited by the rarity of this entity. Only 52 cases of complete laryngeal atresia and CHAOS have ever been reported. In ten of these cases, the fetus was stillborn, suggesting that the fetus may be compromised in utero, not just at birth.[72,73,76,78,81,82,89–91,93] The fetus identified with sonographic features of CHAOS should be presumed to be at significant risk of intrauterine demise and a virtually 100% mortality should the pregnancy progress to delivery without intervention. Diagnosis in the mid second trimester appears to correlate with poor outcome. Survivors with laryngeal atresia have been rare. At least one case has been reported in which CHAOS presented at 23 weeks' gestation with polyhydramnios and fetal ascites, but no other manifestations of nonimmune hydrops. However, at 30 weeks' gestation, the amniotic fluid volume normalized and the ascites resolved. At birth, the infant was found to have a severe subglottic stenosis with a 1-mm hole that allowed the egress of lung fluid.[81] In contrast to the nonsurvivors, this patient had incomplete subglottic stenosis, which may have lessened the effects of airway occlusion and contributed to its survival.

Malformations of the esophagus and trachea including tracheoesophageal fistula, which are commonly associated with laryngeal atresia, allow decompression of the obstructed tracheobronchial tree. These fetuses do not become hydropic, do not develop CHAOS, and more commonly present at birth.

To date, there have been three survivors of prenatally diagnosed CHAOS.[73, 89, 90] Crombleholme et al. reported a case of CHAOS associated with massive ascites and other features of nonimmune hydrops at 20 weeks that was delivered 11 weeks later.[89] Similarly, DeCou et al. reported a case in which a hydropic fetus diagnosed with CHAOS at 18 weeks' gestation was delivered 17 weeks later.[73] Albanese et al., in an unpublished report, successfully delivered a 25-week-gestation hydropic fetus with laryngeal atresia that was first noted at 22 weeks' gestation.[90]

A fetus in the mid second trimester with isolated CHAOS presents a dilemma, as there is insufficient information known about the natural history of this syndrome to predict which fetuses will progress to hydrops and intrauterine demise versus premature delivery because of polyhydramnios. A fetus presenting in the third trimester with signs of fetal airway obstruction without associated anomalies or hydrops likely has incomplete obstruction and will do well until delivery. These fetuses need to be managed using the EXIT strategy in order to obtain and secure the airway while on placental support as laryngoscopy, bronchoscopy, and tracheostomy may be required (see EXIT procedure below).

In an attempt to replicate the pathophysiology of CHAOS in an animal model, Ferro and Hedrick ligated

T A B L E 24–5. ANOMALIES ASSOCIATED WITH CHAOS

Hydrocephalus
Vertebral anomalies
Absent radius
Bronchotracheal fistula
Esophageal atresia
Tracheoesophageal fistula
Syndactyly
Genitourinary anomalies
Uterine anomalies
Imperforate anus
Cardiac anomalies
Anophthalmia
Fraser syndrome

CHAOS, chronic high airway obstruction syndrome.

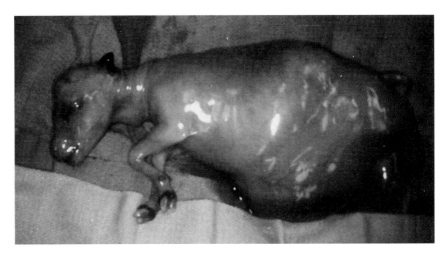

FIGURE 24–1. Fetal lamb that underwent tracheal ligation and subsequently developed massive ascites and other manifestations of CHAOS due to massive enlargement of the fetal lungs compromising venous return to the heart. (From Ferro M, Hedrick M, Harrison MR, Adzick NS: Unpublished observation.)

the trachea of a fetal lamb. The fetus became progressively more hydropic, with massive ascites and extremely large lungs that compressed the mediastinum. This model appeared to replicate all of the features of CHAOS observed clinically (Fig. 24–1). They were also able to demonstrate that in utero tracheostomy could reverse the hydrops associated with CHAOS (Fig. 24–2). It is uncertain, however, if fetal tracheostomy, while reversing the hydrops, would ultimately result in pulmonary hypoplasia as is seen in normal fetal lambs that undergo tracheostomy in utero.[49]

Diagnosis of Fetal Airway Obstruction

Distinguishing between the various causes of fetal airway obstruction poses a significant challenge to the sonographer. As previously noted, the main differential diagnosis is between extrinsic causes of airway obstruction such as lymphangioma or cervical teratoma and

intrinsic fetal airway obstruction and the CHAOS syndrome.

Ultrasound

The differential diagnosis of fetal airway obstruction due to extrinsic compression by a neck mass is extensive (Table 24–1). The management approach to each condition may differ significantly, highlighting the importance of accurate prenatal diagnosis. The presence of skull or vertebral column defects suggests the diagnosis of encephalocele, especially if associated with hydrocephalus. Congenital goiter is most commonly observed in mothers taking propylthiouracil for hyperthyroidism. A fetal goiter is homogeneous in its echotexture and is symmetric about the trachea. Neuroblastoma in the cervical region arises in the sympathetic chain and presents as a unilateral posterior neck mass. Branchial cleft cysts are unilateral and appear as unilocular anterolateral neck cysts.

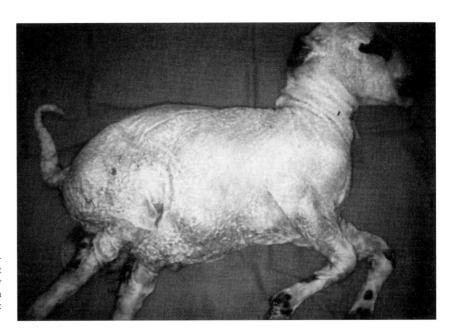

FIGURE 24–2. Another fetal lamb that underwent tracheal ligation developing CHAOS that subsequently underwent in utero tracheostomy with reversal of the hydropic changes. (From Ferro M, Hedrick M, Harrison MR, Adzick NS: Unpublished observation.)

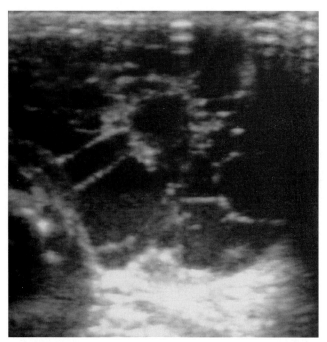

FIGURE 24–3. Prenatal ultrasound appearance of a cervical lymphangioma with its complex cystic spaces and absence of calcifications or solid components.

The sonographic features of lymphangioma include fluid-filled cystic spaces divided by fine septae located in the anterior and posterior triangles of the neck (Fig. 24–3). They often have a dense midline posterior septum, extending from the fetal neck across the full width of the hygroma. This septum is the sonographic equivalent of the nuchal ligament.[94] Cysts separated by septae are helpful in distinguishing nuchal edema from cystic hygroma. Solid components should be excluded to distinguish cystic hygroma from a cervical teratoma with cystic components. Once a cystic hygroma has been detected, one should search for signs of nonimmune hydrops such as fetal skin edema, ascites, pleural, or pericardial effusions. In addition, known structural anomalies should be searched for (Table 24–3).

In contrast to lymphangiomas, cervical teratomas are typically asymmetric, unilateral, and well demarcated (Fig. 24–4). Most are multiloculated, irregular masses with solid and cystic components. As many as 50% have calcifications.[3, 63] Calcifications may be difficult to appreciate on ultrasound and are more easily seen on plain radiographs.[41, 59, 95] Calcifications, when present in a partially cystic and solid neck mass, are virtually pathognomonic of cervical teratoma.[63]

The sonographic features of CHAOS are due to complete, or near-complete, obstruction of the upper airway. The lungs are distended and appear sonographically to be extremely echogenic and diffusely enlarged.[7, 73, 81, 83–85, 88–90] The diaphragm may be inverted and the mediastinal structures compressed (Fig. 24–5A). The heart may appear elongated with a shift in its axis, and the chambers are small and compressed by the large lungs (Fig. 24–5B). The dilation of the tracheobronchial tree can be traced up to the level of the tracheal obstruction. In order to meet criteria for CHAOS, signs of nonimmune hydrops must be seen. Polyhydramnios may also be observed secondary to esophageal compression. It has also been noted that the fetus with CHAOS may exhibit qualitatively abnormal breathing movements. Baarsma et al. observed that a fetus with complete laryngeal atresia exhibited large-amplitude vigorous jerky breathing movements as it tried in vain to move tracheal fluid through an atretic larynx.[96]

The etiology of CHAOS may vary from laryngeal or tracheal obstruction or stenosis, to an intraluminal web or cyst (Fig. 24–6). It may be difficult, however, if not impossible, to distinguish these conditions sonographically. Recently, the use of high-speed MRI has aided in the prenatal diagnosis of CHAOS, lymphangioma, and teratoma.[88, 89, 97]

Fetal MRI

Detection of a giant neck mass in the fetus permits the development of therapeutic strategies for dealing with

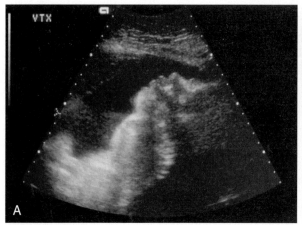

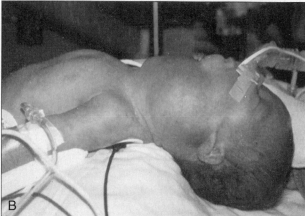

FIGURE 24–4. *A,* Panel on the left is a prenatal ultrasound of a fetus in sagittal section demonstrating a complex cervical mass resulting in hyperextension of the neck due to a cervical teratoma. This has been referred to as the "flying fetus" sign, as the head extension is similar to that observed in ski jumpers. *B,* Panel on the right shows the appearance of the same patient postnatally. *See Color Plate 2*

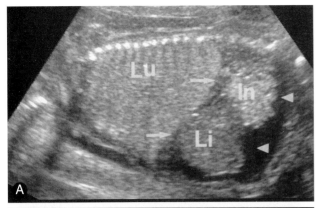

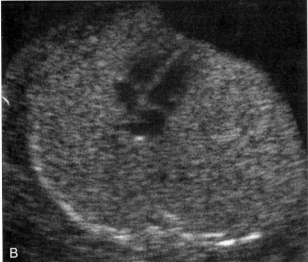

FIGURE 24–5. *A,* In the upper panel is a sonogram in sagittal view demonstrating CHAOS in a fetus at 20 weeks' gestation. There are extremely large homogeneously echogenic lungs with inversion of the diaphragm. *B,* In the lower panel is a cross-sectional view of the same fetus as shown in Figure 24–5*A,* again demonstrating extremely large echogenic lungs with a compressed mediastinum and heart.

expected airway compromise at birth. The two most common etiologies, lymphangioma and cervical teratoma, can often but not always be distinguished by prenatal ultrasound (Fig. 24–7). In addition, it is often difficult to evaluate the airway and surrounding tissues of the neck by ultrasound. Magnetic resonance imaging using fast scanning techniques has increased the potential usefulness of MRI for the prenatal evaluation of congenital abnormalities. Hubbard et al. described the first cases of giant fetal neck masses evaluated by fetal MRI.[97] These pregnant mothers were referred for prenatal MRI after a giant fetal neck mass was identified by ultrasound. MRI images were obtained in the transverse, sagittal, and coronal planes with fields of view large enough to include the entire maternal abdomen. Scans were performed in a Siemens 1.5-T (tesla) Vision Magnetom using a phased-array body coil. Sequences less than 20 seconds in length were performed with a breath hold to decrease motion during imaging. Neither maternal sedation nor fetal neuromuscular blockade was needed. The images of the neck mass in the first fetus were obtained using axial and sagittal T1-weighted spin-echo,

axial, and sagittal echo-planer imaging technique (EPI). In the second fetus, sagittal and coronal EPI and flash 2 images were obtained. In the third fetus axial, sagittal, and coronal half-Fourier single-shot turbo spin-echo (HASTE) images were obtained. Fetal movements and amniotic fluid created motion artifacts that distorted the traditional spin echo images, since these sequences require 1 to 3 minutes to acquire a set of images. The HASTE images provided the best anatomic definition of the fetus and neck mass.[97] The acquisition time with the HASTE sequence is less than 20 seconds per 19 slices, so there is little time for motion artifact. The sequence uses T2 weighting and provides good tissue contrast. Although good images could also be obtained with the EPI technique, all images were characterized by moderate susceptibility to artifacts caused by magnetic field inhomogeneities and differences in tissue interfaces. The EPI sequence is very fast, however, and can obtain an anatomic slice in less than 400 ms. Fetal MRI provided a correct diagnosis of the tumor in each case. In addition, MRI allowed more global imaging of the mass than ultrasound because of its larger field of view.

In our experience using both spin-echo and fast sequences, the HASTE and EPI sequences demonstrated excellent image quality because of decreased motion artifacts. In a report by Crombleholme et al., MRI provided better detail about the size and position of the mass and its relationship to the airway compared to ultrasound.[48, 50] Improved visualization of the relation-

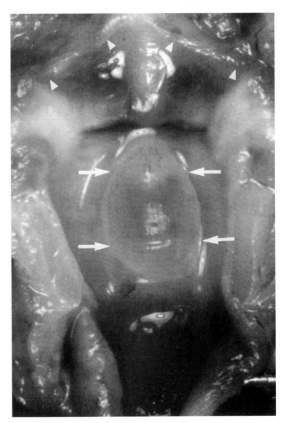

FIGURE 24–6. Autopsy of a fetus at 23 weeks' gestation with CHAOS. This is a posterior view of the trachea and larynx with the back wall completely opened to reveal the laryngeal cyst.

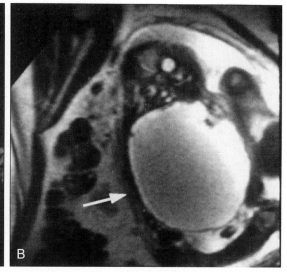

FIGURE 24–7. Panel *A* is a conventional ultrasound image and panel *B* is a high-speed MRI of the same fetus with a giant neck mass. The *curved arrows* indicate the location of the orbits and the *wide arrows* point to the cervical teratoma. As this direct comparison demonstrates, the MRI offers higher resolution, a larger field of view, and more anatomic details than the ultrasound. (From Liechty KW, Crombleholme TM, Weiner S, et al: The ex utero intrapartum treatment procedure for a large fetal neck mass in a twin gestation. Obstet Gynecol 93:824–825, 1999, with permission. Courtesy of the American College of Obstetricians and Gynecologists.)

ship of the mass to the entire airway may help predict which patients are at the highest risk for airway obstruction. Concern exists about performing MRI on the developing fetus, but follow-up studies of prenatal MRI have not demonstrated any deleterious effects in humans.[98]

Fetal MRI is also useful in evaluating causes of airway compromise other than fetal neck masses. Fetal MRI of two fetuses with CHAOS demonstrated all of the characteristic features of this syndrome[88, 89] (Fig. 24–8). However, there are limitations to the resolution of fetal MRI. In two cases, CHAOS was diagnosed but the occluding laryngeal cyst and complete subglottic atresia could not be precisely defined.

Ex Utero Intrapartum Treatment Procedure

There have been several anecdotal reports of intrapartum laryngoscopy or bronchoscopy for fetuses with neck masses in which the fetus was delivered (vaginally or by cesarean section) but the cord was not clamped.[1, 3, 6, 99–102] However, in these cases there was no attempt to prevent uterine contraction, and in most, the fetus was removed from the uterus resulting not only in uterine contraction but placental separation and nearly immediate cessation of uteroplacental gas exchange.[103] In contrast, the EXIT procedure can be viewed as a "half" delivery in which a hysterotomy is performed, only the head and shoulders are delivered, and uterine relaxation is maintained by high concentrations of an inhalational anesthetic and intravenous tocolytics, ensuring the maintenance of uteroplacental blood flow and gas exchange. This strategy began as a means to establish an airway after the fetal trachea was occluded to promote lung growth for fetuses with severe congenital diaphragmatic hernia (CDH).[104] In over 40 cases per-

formed for fetuses with an occluded trachea, this strategy provided time for neck dissection, clip removal, bronchoscopy, endotracheal intubation, surfactant administration, and placement of umbilical arterial and venous catheters. Unlike the EXIT procedure, a conven-

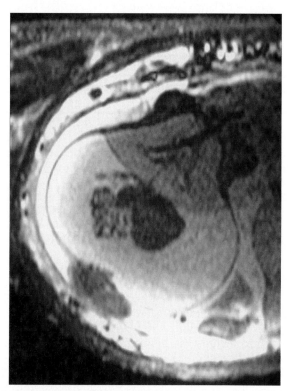

FIGURE 24–8. Fetal MRI demonstrating massively enlarged lungs, dilated tracheobronchial tree, inverted diaphragms, and massive ascites. (From Crombleholme TM, Sylvestri K, Flake AW, et al: Salvage of a fetus with congenital high airway obstruction syndrome [CHAOS]. Fetal Diagn Ther [in press].)

tional cesarean delivery makes no attempt to prevent bleeding from the hysterotomy, since hemostasis is achieved by return of uterine tone following the relatively rapid delivery of the fetus. Because of the potential for hemorrhage in a relaxed uterus with a conventional hysterotomy, in the EXIT procedure the uterus is opened using a hemostatic uterine stapling device.[105] Care is taken not to manipulate or unnecessarily expose the umbilical cord in order to avoid spasm of the vessels and compromise of blood flow. However, we have had one case in which there was a true knot in the nonvisualized portion of the umbilical cord within the uterus. Each time the fetus was repositioned the knot tightened and the fetal pulse oximeter reading dropped.

A successful EXIT procedure is a carefully orchestrated event in which all members have specific roles and responsibilities. The scrubbed personnel consist of two pediatric/fetal surgeons, a perinatologist/obstetrician, a neonatologist, and a nurse. After hysterotomy, the fetal head, neck, and shoulders are delivered (Fig. 24–9). A sterile pulse oximeter is placed on the fetal hand, covered with aluminum foil, and secured with a Tegaderm dressing, and a long oximeter cord is handed across the sterile field to the anesthesiologist. A variety of sterile instruments need to be available, such as a laryngoscope with at least two different sized blades, a bronchoscope, various endotracheal and tracheostomy tubes, an Ambubag with a manometer and sterile tubing that is passed off the field to an oxygen source, and a sterile syringe filled with surfactant (if necessary). A

cocktail of a narcotic and paralytic agent is administered intramuscularly to the fetus to supplement transplacental inhalational anesthetic agents before beginning any procedure. After the airway is obtained and secured, the umbilical cord is clamped and divided and the child taken to the resuscitation table by the neonatologist. Skarsgard et al. were the first to apply these principles of the EXIT procedure to the management of the fetus with a prenatally diagnosed tracheal obstruction.[106] Liechty et al. reported a series of five giant fetal neck masses managed by the EXIT procedure describing cord blood gas data for procedures lasting 8 to 54 minutes on placental support.[50] The ability of inhalational anesthetic agents to maintain uterine relaxation and uteroplacental gas exchange is apparent in the relatively normal cord blood gas values seen after up to 54 minutes on uteroplacental support (Table 24–6).

The most serious and immediate maternal risk during the EXIT procedure is intraoperative hemorrhage. This may result from uterine atony, and this risk can be minimized by decreasing the concentration of the inhalational anesthetic and administering oxytocin before umbilical cord ligation. This, in combination with the hemostatic uterine stapling device, has kept the average intraoperative maternal blood loss at 930 mL, well within the accepted range for traditional cesarean delivery.[50, 107] In addition, the placenta can be injured during hysterotomy, resulting in hemorrhage. This has occurred in the setting of polyhydramnios caused by an obstructing neck mass, in which the edge of the placenta was compressed, obscuring it from view by the sonographer. We now perform intraoperative amnioreduction in cases with severe polyhydramnios before performing an EXIT procedure to allow better placental visualization.

Although fetal neck masses can cause polyhydramnios and preterm labor, the most feared aspect of their management is treating a compromised airway at the time of delivery. The EXIT strategy allows a ''controlled'' approach to airway management for these babies. Airway compromise is a function of the location of the mass and distortion of the airway, not necessarily the absolute size of the neck mass. In each of our cases, conventional cesarean delivery and routine newborn airway management would have been difficult, if not impossible, and may have resulted in anoxic brain injury or death.

In addition to its use in giant fetal neck masses, the EXIT procedure has been successfully applied in the perinatal management of CHAOS. DeCou et al. reported the first case of CHAOS in which the EXIT strategy was used.[73] Crombleholme et al. reported the first long-term survivor of a fetus with CHAOS due to tracheal atresia who was salvaged by the EXIT procedure,[89] a 38-year-old female referred at 31 weeks' gestation for evaluation of a suspected bilateral CCAM with nonimmune hydrops. Although originally detected at 19 weeks' gestation, after 12 weeks of observation the fetus remained hydropic, but anticipated intrauterine fetal demise had not occurred. Ultrasound revealed a fetus with huge bilateral homogeneously echogenic lungs, a dilated proximal airway, and everted diaphragms. There was

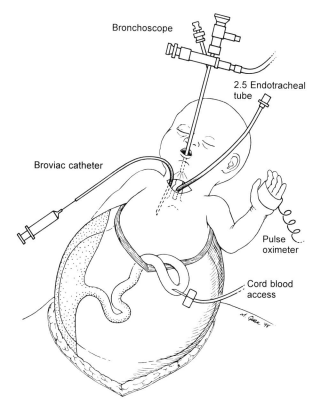

FIGURE 24–9. Schematic representation of a fetus with laryngeal atresia and CHAOS undergoing tracheostomy with a 2.5-Fr endotracheal tube using the EXIT strategy.

Labels in figure: Bronchoscope; 2.5 Endotracheal tube; Broviac catheter; Pulse oximeter; Cord blood access

T A B L E 24–6. EXIT PROCEDURE FOR FETAL NECK MASSES

CASE	DIAGNOSIS	EXIT DURATION	PROCEDURES PERFORMED	CORD GAS pH	Pco$_2$	Po$_2$	EBL	GESTATIONAL AGE AT BIRTH	OUTCOME
1	Lymphangioma	8 min	DL	n/a	n/a	n/a	1,000 mL	36 wk	Died in OR
2	Teratoma	54 min	DL, BR, TR	7.27	52	34	2,000 mL	34 wk	Died in NICU
3	Lymphangioma	21 min	DL	7.25	53	48	1,000 mL	38 wk	Resected Alive and well
4	Teratoma	8 min	DL, CD	7.22	62	36	150 mL	38 wk	Resected Alive and well
5	Teratoma	50 min	DL, BR, TR	7.15	75	48	500 mL	33 wk	Resected Alive and well
	Mean	28 + 22 min		7.22 + 0.05	61 + 11	42 + 8	930 + 698 mL	36 + 2 wk	

DL, direct laryngoscopy; BR, bronchoscopy; TR, tracheostomy; CD, cyst decompression; n/a, not applicable; NICU, neonatal intensive care unit; OR, operating room; EBL, estimated blood loss; EXIT, ex utero intrapartum treatment.

fetal anasarca, massive ascites, placentomegaly, and polyhydramnios. Fetal MRI confirmed the sonographic findings and localized the region of airway obstruction to the larynx or proximal trachea (Fig. 24–8). Forty-eight hours later at 31 weeks' gestation, after two doses of β-methasone, an EXIT procedure was performed. While on placental support, the fetal head and neck were exposed and laryngotracheoscopy was performed (Fig. 24–10A). A completely obstructing web was noted in the immediate subglottic trachea (Fig. 24–10B). A fetal tracheostomy was performed that resulted in a rush of cloudy fluid from the distal airways. Surfactant was administered via the tracheostomy and ventilation was established prior to clamping and dividing the umbilical cord. The infant required minimal ventilatory support and was weaned to room air within 24 hours. Because of diaphragmatic dysfunction, likely due to chronic stretch in utero caused by the massively enlarged lungs and tracheomalacia, the newborn required continued ventilatory support. The infant had resolution of the

tracheomalacia at 5 months of age and complete recovery of diaphragmatic function at 9 months of age, allowing him to be weaned from ventilatory support. He has had normal neurologic development and achieved all developmental milestones. A reconstructive laryngotracheoplasty was performed at 1 year of age.[89]

Previous experience had suggested that the development of nonimmune hydrops in CHAOS is uniformly fatal.[7] The survival of two fetuses with CHAOS for 12 and 17 weeks, despite massive ascites, placentomegaly, and anasarca, challenges our previous understanding of the natural history of CHAOS.[89, 93] These cases suggest that the prenatal natural history of CHAOS may be more favorable than previously thought. Furthermore, fetal intervention or delivery too early in gestation may lead to pulmonary hypoplasia since, in experimental animals, external drainage of lung fluid by fetal tracheostomy bypasses the necessary laryngeal stenting mechanism and equalizes fetal lung and amniotic fluid pressures.[49] CHAOS diagnosed prior to viability may

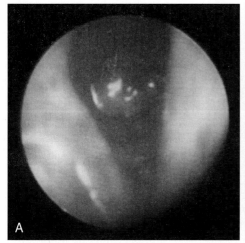
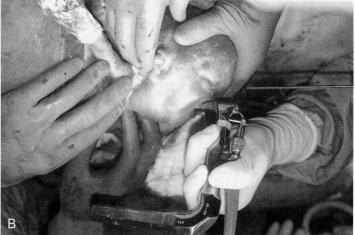

F I G U R E 24–10. EXIT procedure for a fetus with CHAOS at 31 weeks' gestation. *A,* Many of the essential elements involved in the EXIT procedure are demonstrated in this intraoperative photograph of a fetus with a large cervical teratoma undergoing bronchoscopy. Uterine volume is maintained by only delivering the fetal head, neck, and shoulders through the hysterotomy, as indicated by the *thin arrow.* The fetal pulse oximeter is indicated by the *black arrow* and monitors fetal heart rate and hemoglobin saturation. The bronchoscope is indicated by the *wide arrow* and is used to help define the airway anatomy and is essential in confirming the need for tracheostomy. *B,* The tracheoscopic view of the obstructing tracheal atresia.

warrant close observation until lung maturity unless there is progression in hydrops, development of preterm labor, or signs of cardiac compromise necessitating the EXIT procedure. Application of the EXIT procedure in cases of CHAOS offers the potential for salvage of these otherwise doomed fetuses. Before offering an EXIT procedure to the parents of a fetus with CHAOS, it is important that the family understands that, depending upon the nature of the malformation, perfect laryngeal reconstruction and adequate speech may not be possible and a lifelong tracheostomy may be necessary.

Historically, the risk of loss of a normal co-twin has precluded fetal intervention for twin gestations.[108] However, the EXIT has been applied to twin gestations discordant for an anomaly such as a large cervical lymphangioma in one co-twin.[109] However, if intervention can be accomplished without compromise of the normal co-twin, fetal therapy might be considered. Application of the EXIT procedure in twins must be based upon the assumption that the risks of decreased placental blood flow and compromised uteroplacental gas exchange must be borne by the anomalous twin and priority given for delivery of the normal twin first. Liechty et al. reported the successful use of the EXIT strategy in the management of a twin pregnancy in which one of the twins had a large cervical lymphangioma compromising the fetal airway.[109]

Lower uterine segment transverse hysterotomy is preferred for the EXIT procedure, as it allows the possibility of future vaginal delivery. However, a low anterior placenta or extremely large neck mass may make this incision impossible. In such cases, a classic hysterotomy is necessary, which would preclude future vaginal delivery because of the risk of uterine rupture during labor. Thus, all mothers should be counseled that cesarean delivery may be required for all future pregnancies.

Anesthetic Considerations During the Exit Procedure

The features that distinguish the EXIT procedure from a conventional cesarean delivery are, in large part, due to the anesthetic management. Of paramount importance is the uterine relaxation achieved with inhalational anesthetics, most notably isoflurane. Biehl et al. investigated the uptake of isoflurane by the fetal lamb in utero by anesthetizing eight pregnant ewes with 2% isoflurane in oxygen.[110] Isoflurane crossed the placenta rapidly, appearing in the fetal circulation 2 minutes after the initial exposure. However, the arterial levels of isoflurane rose more slowly in the fetus and remained at approximately two thirds of the maternal levels by 90 minutes. Dwyer et al. examined the uptake of isoflurane by the human fetus in mothers undergoing cesarean section.[111] Twelve parturients received 0.8% isoflurane in a 50% nitrous oxide in oxygen mixture. The umbilical venous partial pressure of isoflurane as a fraction of maternal arterial partial pressure was 0.71. The ratio of the maternal arterial partial pressure to inspired partial pressure was 0.44. Hence, isoflurane crossed the placenta, but fetal levels were less than maternal levels. Despite this rapid

placental transfer during anesthesia, we noted during one EXIT procedure that the first end-tidal concentration of isoflurane in the neonate was only 0.2%, much lower than expected, most likely due, in part, to the fact that isoflurane is more soluble in maternal than fetal blood.[112] The blood gas partition coefficient for maternal and fetal blood is 1.51 and 1.35, respectively. This lower fetal solubility is advantageous, as it favors more rapid elimination of isoflurane from the newborn after the EXIT procedure is completed.

Tunstall and Sheikh administered 1.25% isoflurane in 100% oxygen to 56 parturients undergoing elective cesarean delivery.[113] There were no cases of maternal awareness nor of apparent central nervous system depression of the newborn. Piggott et al. increased the concentration of isoflurane to 1.8% for 5 minutes, then decreased it to 1.2% without apparent neonatal depression.[114] We have administered isoflurane concentrations up to 2.5% to completely anesthetize the fetus in order to allow fetal laryngoscopy, bronchoscopy, tracheostomy, or tumor resection.[50]

Preservation of uteroplacental gas exchange with high concentrations of maternal isoflurane are well tolerated by the fetus for EXIT procedures lasting up to 75 minutes. Careful attention to maintenance of maternal systemic blood pressure, often with the use of α-adrenergic agents such as ephedrine, is essential in order to safely use the high concentration of isoflurane required for uterine relaxation. Occasionally, additional uterine relaxation is required, even when the end-tidal isoflurane concentration is over 2.5%. This suggests that extensive manipulation of the uterus (e.g., forward displacement of the uterus to make a posterior hysterotomy because of an anterior placenta) may stimulate the uterus to contract, even if high concentrations of isoflurane are used. We have found that intraoperative use of nitroglycerin is well-tolerated and provides excellent temporary uterine relaxation. Nitroglycerin has been used to provide uterine relaxation for removal of a retained placenta, for fetal version, for extraction of a second twin, for primary tocolysis following fetal surgery, and as an intraoperative adjunct to isoflurane to achieve uterine relaxation.[115, 116] Nitroglycerin is metabolized to nitric oxide, which activates guanyl cyclase, increases cGMP, and decreases intracellular calcium, resulting in uterine relaxation.[117] One concern with nitroglycerin as a tocolytic agent is the possibility of maternal pulmonary edema.[118] However, cases of pulmonary edema associated with the use of nitroglycerin in fetal surgery have occurred when continuous infusions of high doses were used for prolonged periods for postoperative tocolysis. Pulmonary edema does not appear to occur as a result of intraoperative intermittent dosing of nitroglycerin when it is used as an adjunct for temporary uterine relaxation.

Postnatal Management and Follow-up

Once an airway has been established, the care of the newborn should focus on underlying lung disease, exclude associated anomalies or chromosomal abnormalities, if this has not already been done. Once the newborn is able to be transported, a computed tomography (CT) scan and MRI scan with magnetic resonance angiography should be obtained of the infant's head and neck to confirm the diagnosis and define the lesion's extent.

Obstructing fetal neck masses can cause mortality in up to 80 to 100% of untreated infants.[52, 54, 55, 65, 95, 119] Delaying surgery can result in retention of secretions, atelectasis, and/or pneumonia due to interference with swallowing.[52, 120] In addition, precipitous airway obstruction may occur due to hemorrhage into the tumor,[52, 54, 55, 63] even in minimally symptomatic newborns. For this reason, endotracheal intubation is indicated in all patients regardless of the presence or absence of symptoms. Mortality decreases to between 9 and 17% in infants treated surgically.[52, 54, 55, 59, 95] It should be noted, however, that these tumors tend to be large, disfiguring masses that envelope vital structures in the neck. Extensive neck dissection and multiple procedures may be necessary to achieve the goals of complete extirpation of the tumor with acceptable functional and cosmetic results.

The infant with a large lymphangioma has an intrinsically unstable airway and should proceed to resection as soon as the evaluation is completed. Lymphangiomas of more modest size can be dealt with on a more elective basis if they do not pose a risk for airway compromise. Since this is a benign lesion, the surgical approach is focused on resection of as much of the mass as possible without sacrifice of vital structures. Some surgeons have recommended a conservative approach in asymptomatic lymphangiomas because of occasional spontaneous regression. More commonly, these lesions grow proportionately with the infant. There may also be acute increases in size of the cyst due to hemorrhage or infection. Since complete resection is possible in only 75% of cases and the recurrence rate is 10 to 27%,[121] alternative treatments have been tried with variable results. These include laser treatment and injection of sclerosing agents such as boiling water, sodium morrhuate, bleomycin, and OK-432.[122–124]

In a review of 18 cases of cervical and oral facial teratomas, Azizkhan et al. reported that life-threatening airway obstruction occurred in seven cases (39%), two of whom died without ever having a secure airway.[68] Two neonates with prenatally diagnosed tumors survived because tracheostomies were performed in the delivery room by a pediatric surgeon. The overall survival was 83% (15 of the 18 infants). Morbidity included two cases with recurrent laryngeal nerve injury, two with hypothyroidism, and two with developmental delay and mental retardation secondary to airway obstruction and asphyxia at birth. These infants are at risk for transient or permanent hypoparathyroidism and hypothyroidism. Cervical teratoma may completely replace the thyroid gland, and tumor resection may result in even permanent hypothyroidism. More commonly, thyroid tissue may be preserved but may not be adequately functioning, and an interval of thyroxine supplementation may be necessary. Due to the massive nature of these tumors and the difficulty of identifying parathyroid glands, transient or permanent hypoparathy-

roidism may be observed. Calcium and vitamin D supplementation may be needed postoperatively.

Cervical teratomas are functional tumors in approximately one third of the cases, producing markedly elevated levels of AFP. However, an elevated AFP level obtained immediately postoperatively must be interpreted with caution. AFP levels in normal newborns have an enormous range of values, with some as high as 200,000 U in the first month of life. The AFP values progressively fall during infancy until levels of less than 4 U are obtained at 1 year of age. While an elevated AFP may not necessarily be abnormal, the levels should decrease during infancy. A rising AFP should alert the clinician to the possibility of recurrence. While cervical teratoma is generally a benign tumor, there is the possibility of malignant transformation. We recommend following AFP levels at 3-month intervals in infancy and yearly thereafter, with CT or MRI scanning twice a year for the first 3 years of life in order to detect recurrent teratoma.

In the absence of a tracheoesophageal fistula, the surgical management of CHAOS is elective once an airway is established. The initial evaluation should be directed toward diagnosing the level of obstruction to allow planning of definitive surgical repair. The ideal timing of reconstruction in these extremely rare cases has not been established. However, bronchoscopy performed in the newborn period will exclude simple causes of laryngeal obstruction, such as laryngeal cyst or web. The majority of webs are located at the level of the glottis or immediately subglottic and are readily diagnosed at laryngoscopy or bronchoscopy. These webs can occasionally be cut endoscopically with a knife or laser. Although lasers can be used, the small airway of the newborn may make avoidance of thermal damage to surrounding tissues difficult. An infant urethral resectoscope with a narrow cutting loop can be used with brief bursts of cutting current. There are only anecdotal reports of successful reconstruction and long-term outcome in this condition.[81, 89, 91]

Conclusions

The keys to a successful outcome in managing a fetus with airway obstruction are early prenatal recognition, accurate prenatal diagnosis, and the controlled execution of the EXIT strategy to secure the fetal airway. Although multiple causes of fetal airway obstruction have been outlined above, the approach to their management in many respects is the same. However, a better characterization of the natural history of fetal airway obstruction, due to either extrinsic or intrinsic etiologies, will allow us to fine tune our management to fit the specific lesion. The use of high-resolution ultrasound and fetal MRI are providing ever more precise anatomic detail and essential information in planning the EXIT strategy. The early gestation diagnosis of CHAOS raises a therapeutic dilemma, as it is unknown if fetal tracheostomy is necessary, and if so, whether pulmonary hypoplasia will result. Only through experience will the natural history of CHAOS become more fully understood and the indications for fetal intervention better defined. At present, hydrops in fetuses with CHAOS appears to be better tolerated than other causes of hydrops. An expectant approach to CHAOS is recommended until a gestational age at which an EXIT procedure can be performed with acceptable risks of prematurity.

REFERENCES

1. Catalano PJ, Urken ML, Alcarez M, et al: New approach to the management of airway obstruction in "high risk" neonates. Arch Otolaryngol Head Neck Surg: 118:306–309, 1992.
2. Holinger LD, Birnholz JC: Management of infants with prenatal ultrasound diagnosis of airway obstruction by teratoma. Ann Otol Rhinol Laryngol 96:61–64, 1987.
3. Kelly MF, Berenholz L, Rizzo KA, et al: Approach for oxygenation of the newborn with airway obstruction due to a cervical mass. Ann Otol Rhinol Laryngol 99:179–182, 1990.
4. Ferlito A, Deveney KO: Developmental lesions of the head and neck: Terminology and biologic behavior. Ann Otolaryngol Head Neck Surg 120:444–448, 1994.
5. Shipp TD, Bromley B, Benacerraf B: The ultrasonographic appearance and outcome for fetuses with masses distorting the fetal face. J Ultrasound Med 14:673–678, 1995.
6. Schulman SR, Jones BR, Slotnick N, et al: Fetal tracheal intubation with intact uteroplacental circulation. Anesth Analg 76:197–199, 1993.
7. Hedrick MH, Martinez-Ferro, Filly RA, et al: Congenital high airway obstruction syndrome (CHAOS): A potential for perinatal intervention. J Pediatr Surg 29:271–274, 1994.
8. Isaacs H Jr: Tumors of the Fetus and Newborn. Philadelphia: WB Saunders Company, 1997, pp 69–72.
9. Potter EL, Craig JM: Pathology of the Fetus and Infant, 3rd ed. Chicago: Year Book Medical Publishers, 1941, p 177.
10. Isaacs H Jr: Tumors of the Newborn and Infant. St. Louis: Mosby-Year Book, 1991.
11. Isaacs H Jr: Neoplasms in infants: A report of 265 cases. Pathol Ann 18:165–171, 1983.
12. Goetsch E: Hygroma colli cysticum and hygroma axillae. Arch Surg 36:394–401, 1938.
13. Chervenak FA, Isaacson G, Blakemore KJ, et al: Fetal cystic hygroma: Cause and natural history. N Engl J Med 309:822–826, 1983.
14. Langer JC, Fitzgerald PG, Desa D, et al: Cervical cystic hygroma in the fetus: Clinical spectrum and outcome. J Pediatr Surg 25:58–62, 1990.
15. Lyngbye T, Haugaard L, Klebe JG: Antenatal sonographic diagnoses of giant cystic hygroma of the neck. Acta Obstet Gynecol Scand 65:873–875, 1986.
16. Benacerraf BR, Frigoletto FD: Prenatal sonographic diagnosis of isolated congenital cystic hygroma, unassociated with lymphedema or other morphologic abnormality. J Ultrasound Med 6:63–66, 1987.
17. Welborn JL, Timm NS: Trisomy 21 and cystic hygromas in early gestational age fetuses. Am J Perinatol 11:19–25, 1994.
18. Golden WL, Schneider BF, Gustashaw KM, et al: Prenatal diagnosis of Turner syndrome using cells cultured from cystic hygromas in two pregnancies with normal maternal serum alpha-fetoprotein. Prenat Diagn 9:683–689, 1989.
19. Pijpers L, Reuss A, Stewart PA, et al: Fetal cystic hygroma: Prenatal diagnosis and management. Obstet Gynecol 72:223–224, 1988.
20. Cohen MM, Schwartz S, Schwartz MF, et al: Antenatal detection of cystic hygroma. Obstet Gynecol Surv 44:481–485, 1989.
21. Romero R, Pilu G, Jeanty P, et al: Cystic hygroma in prenatal diagnosis of congenital anomilies. Norwalk, CT: Appleton & Lange, 1988, pp 115–118.
22. Marchese C, Savin E, Dragone E, et al: Cystic hygroma: Prenatal diagnosis and genetic counseling. Prenat Diagn 5:221–227, 1985.
23. Greenberg F, Carpenter RJ, Ledbetter DH: Cystic hygroma and hydrops fetalis in a fetus with trisomy 13. Clin Genet 24:389–391, 1983.
24. Stephens TD, Shepard TH: Down syndrome in the fetus. Teratology 22:37–41, 1980.
25. Zarabi M, Mieckowski GC, Maser J: Cystic hygroma associated with Noonan's syndrome. J Clin Ultrasound 11:398–404, 1983.
26. Chen H, Immken L, Blumberg B, et al: Lethal form of multiple pterygium syndrome. Presented at the 1982 March of Dimes Birth Defects Conference, Atlanta, Georgia, 1982.
27. Graham JM, Stephens TD, Shepard TH: Nuchal cystic hygroma in a fetus with presumed Robert's syndrome. Am J Med Genet 15:163–167, 1983.
28. Cowchock ES, Wapner RJ, Kurtz A, et al: Not all cystic hygromas occur in the Ullrich-Turner syndrome. Am J Med Genet 12:327–331, 1982.
29. Zelante L, Perla G, Villani G: Prenatal diagnosis of recurrence of cystic hygroma with normal chromosomes. Prenat Diagn 4:383–386, 1984.
30. Fonkalsrud EW: Malformations of the lymphatic system and hemangioma. In Ashcraft KW, Holder TM (ed): Pediatric Surgery. Philadelphia: WB Saunders Company, 1980, pp 1042–1061.
31. Bill AHJ, Sumner DS: A unified concept of lymphangioma and cystic hygroma. Surg Gynecol Obstet 120:79–86, 1965.
32. Fisher R, Partington A, Dykes E: Cystic hygroma. Comparison between prenatal and postnatal diagnosis. J Pediatr Surg 31:473–476, 1996.
33. Byrne J, Blanc WA, Warburton D, et al: The significance of cystic hygroma in fetuses. Hum Pathol 15:61–67, 1984.
34. Nadel A, Bromley B, Benacerraf BR: Nuchal thickening or cystic hygromas in the first- and early second-trimester fetuses: Prognosis and outcome. Obstet Gynecol 82:43–48, 1993.
35. Schoenfeld A, Edelstein T, Joel-Cohen SJ: Prenatal ultrasonic diagnosis of fetal teratoma of the neck. Br J Radiol 51:742–744, 1978.
36. Jordan RB, Gauderer MWL: Cervical teratomas. An analysis, literature review and proposed classification. J Pediatr Surg 23:583–591, 1988.
37. Patel RB, Gibson YU, D'Cruz CA, Burkhalter JL: Sonographic diagnosis of cervical teratoma in utero. AJR Am J Roentgenol 139:1220–1222, 1982.
38. Trecet JC, Claramunt V, Larraz J, et al: Prenatal ultrasound diagnosis of fetal teratoma of the neck. J Clin Ultrasound 12:509–511, 1984.
39. Zerella JT, Finberg FJ: Obstruction of the neonatal airway from teratomas. Surg Gynecol Obstet 170:126–131, 1990.
40. Hitchcock A, Sears RT, O'Neill T: Immature cervical teratoma arising in one fetus of a twin pregnancy. Acta Obstet Gynecol Scand 66:377–379, 1987.
41. Suita S, Ikeda K, Nakano H, et al: Teratoma of the neck in a newborn infant—a case report. Z Kinderchir 35:9–11, 1982.
42. Baumann FR, Nerlich A: Metastasizing cervical teratoma of the fetus. Pediatr Pathol 13:21–27, 1993.
43. Thurkow AL, Visser GHA, Oosterhuis JW, de Vries JA: Ultrasound observations of a malignant cervical teratoma of the fetus in a case of polyhydramnios: Case history and review. Eur J Obstet Gynecol Reprod Biol 14:375–384, 1983.
44. Kagan AR: Cervical mass in a fetus associated with maternal hydramnios. AJR Am J Roentgenol 140:507–509, 1983.
45. Pearl RM, Wisnicki J, Sinclair G: Metastatic cervical teratoma of infancy. Plast Reconstr Surg 77:469–473, 1986.
46. Roodhooft AM, Delbeke L, Vaneerdeweg W. Cervical teratoma: Prenatal detection and management in the neonate. Pediatr Surg Int 2:181–184, 1987.
47. Cunningham MJ, Myers EN, Bluestone CD: Malignant tumors of the head and neck in children. A twenty-year review. Int J Pediatr Otorhinolaryngol 13:279–292, 1987.
48. Crombleholme TM, Hubbard A, Howell L, et al: EXIT procedure (ex utero intrapartum treatment) for giant fetal neck masses. Am J Obstet Gynecol 272:584, 1997.
49. O'Callaghan SP, Walker P, Wohle C, et al: Perinatal care of a woman with the prenatal diagnosis of a massive fetal neck tumor (cervical teratoma). Br J Obstet Gynecol 104:261–263, 1997.
50. Liechty K, Crombleholme TM, Flake AW, et al: Intrapartum airway management for giant fetal neck masses: The exit procedure (ex utero intrapartum treatment). Am J Obstet Gynecol 177:870–874, 1997.
51. Ashley DJB: Origin of teratomas. Cancer 32:390–394, 1973.
52. Batsakis JG, Littler ER, Oberman HA: Teratomas of the neck. Arch Otolaryngol 79:619–624, 1964.

53. Tapper D, Lack EE: Teratomas in infancy and childhood. Ann Surg 198:398–410, 1983.
54. Hurlbut HJ, Webb HW, Moseley T: Cervical teratoma in infant siblings. J Pediatr Surg 2:424–426, 1967.
55. Silberman R, Mendelson IR: Teratoma of the neck. Arch Dis Child 35:159–170, 1960.
56. Owor R, Master SP: Cervical teratomas in the newborn. East Afr Med J 51:376–381, 1974.
57. Lloyd JR, Clatworthy HW: Hydramnios as an aid to the early diagnosis of congenital obstruction of the alimentary tract: A study of the maternal and fetal factors. Pediatrics 21:903–909, 1958.
58. Bale GF: Teratoma of the neck in the region of the thyroid gland. Am J Pathol 26:565–579, 1949.
59. Hajdu SI, Faruque AA, Hajdu E, Morgan WS: Teratoma of the neck in infants. Am J Dis Child 3:412–416, 1966.
60. Mochizuki Y, Noguchi S, Yokoyama S, et al: Cervical teratoma in a fetus and an adult. Acta Pathol Jpn 36:935–943, 1986.
61. Rosenfeld CR, Coln CD, Duenhoelter JH: Fetal cervical teratomas as a cause of polyhydramnios. Pediatrics 64:174–179, 1979.
62. McGoon DC: Teratomas of the neck. Surg Clin North Am 32:1389–1395, 1952.
63. Gundry SR, Wesley JR, Klein MD, et al: Cervical teratomas in the newborn. J Pediatr Surg 18:382–386, 1983.
64. Dische MR, Gardner HA: Mixed teratoid tumors of the liver and neck in trisomy 13. Am Soc Clin Pathol 69:631–637, 1987.
65. Schoenfeld A, Ovadia J, Edelstein T, Liban E: Malignant cervical teratoma of the fetus. Acta Obstet Gynecol Scand 61:7–12, 1982.
66. Touran T, Applebaum H, Frost DB, et al: Congenital metastatic cervical teratoma: Diagnostic and management considerations. J Pediatr Surg 24:21–23, 1989.
67. Heys RF, Murray CP, Kohler HG: Obstructed labour due to fetal tumours: Cervical and coccygeal teratoma. Gynaecologia 164:43–54, 1967.
68. Azizkhan RG, Haase GM, Applebaum H, et al: Diagnosis, management and outcome of cervicofacial teratomas in neonates: A children's cancer group study. J Pediatr Surg 30:312–316, 1995.
69. Watanatittan S, Othersen HB, Hughson MD: Cervical teratoma in children. Prog Pediatr Surg 14:225–239, 1981.
70. Pupovac D: Ein fall von teratoma colli mit veranderungen in den regionaren lymphdrusen. Arch Klin Chir 53:59–67, 1986. (Reviewed by Silberman and Mendelson)
71. Dunn CJ, Nguyen DL, Leonard JC: Ultrasound diagnosis of immature cervical teratoma: A case report. Am J Perinatol 9:445–447, 1992.
72. Schauer GM, Dunn LK, Godmilow L, et al: Prenatal diagnosis of Fraser syndrome at 18.5 weeks' gestation, with autopsy findings at 19 weeks. Am J Med Genet 37:583–591, 1990.
73. DeCou JM, Jones DC, Jacobs HD, Touloukian RJ: Successful ex utero intrapartum treatment (EXIT) procedure for congenital high airway obstruction syndrome (CHAOS) owing to laryngeal atresia. J Pediatr Surg 33:1563–1565, 1998.
74. Feldman E, Shalev E, Weiner E, et al: Microphthalmic-prenatal ultrasound diagnosis: A case report. Prenat Diagn 5:205–207, 1995.
75. Fraser GR: Our genetic load: A review of some aspects of genetic variation. Ann Hum Genet 25:387–415, 1962.
76. Fox H, Cocker J: Laryngeal atresia. Arch Dis Child 39:641–645, 1964.
77. Arizawa M, Imai S, Suchara N, et al: Prenatal diagnosis of pulmonary atresia. Cesta Obstet Gynecol 41:907–910, 1989.
78. Delechotte P, Lemery D, Vanlieferinghen P: Association atresie laryngee et agenesie renale bilaterale: Hyperplasie versus hypoplasie pulmonaire. Presented at Quaterereinae journee de la Societe Francaise de Foetopathologie, Paris-Bichat, France, 1988.
79. Didier F, Droulle P, Marchal C: A propos du depistage antenatal dis atresies tracheale at laryngee. Arch Fr Pediatr 47:396–397, 1990.
80. Fang SH, Ocejo R, Sin M, et al: Congenital laryngeal atresia. Arch J Dis Child 143:625–627, 1989.
81. Richards DS, Yancey MK, Duff P, et al: The perinatal management of severe laryngeal stenosis. Obstet Gynecol 80:537–540, 1992.
82. Scurry JP, Adamson TM, Cussen LJ: Fetal lung growth in laryngeal atresia and trachal agensis. Aust Paediatr J 25:47–51, 1989.
83. Tournier G, Goossens M, Bessis R, et al: Diagnostic antnatal et maladies gentiques pneumologiques. Rev Mal Respir 5:231–238, 1988.
84. Watson WJ, Thorp JM, Miller RC, et al: Prenatal diagnosis of laryngeal atresia. Am J Obstet Gynecol 163:1456–1457, 1990.
85. Weston MJ, Porter HJ, Berry PJ, et al: Ultrasonographic prenatal diagnosis of upper respiratory tract atresia. J Ultrasound Med 11:673–675, 1992.
86. Wigglesworth JS, Desai R, Hislap AA: Fetal lung growth in congenital laryngeal atresia. Pediatr Pathol 7:515–525, 1987.
87. Silver MM, Thurston WA, Patrick JE: Perinatal pulmonary hypoplasia due to laryngeal atresia. Hum Pathol 19:110–113, 1988.
88. Sylvester KG, Rosanen Y, Kitano Y, et al: Tracheal occlusion reverses the high impedance to flow in the fetal pulmonary circulation and normalizes its physiologic response to oxygenation at term. J Pediatr Surg 33:1071–1075, 1998.
89. Crombleholme TM, Sylvester K, Flake AW, et al: Salvage of a fetus with congenital high airway obstruction syndrome (CHAOS). Fetal Diagn Ther (in press).
90. Albanese CT, unpublished data, 1996.
91. Smith II, Bain AD: Congenital atresia of the larynx: A report of nine cases. Ann Otol 74:338–349, 1965.
92. Stocker JT, Madewell JER, Drake RM: Congenital adenomatoid malformation of the lung: Classification and morphologic spectrum. Hum Pathol 8:155–171, 1977.
93. Cohen SR: Congenital atresia of the larynx with endolaryngeal surgical correction: A case report. Laryngoscope 81:1607–1615, 1971.
94. Chervenak FA, Isaacson G, Tortora M: A sonographic study of fetal cystic hygromas. J Clin Ultrasound 13:311–315, 1985.
95. Goodwin BD, Gay BB: The roentgen diagnosis of teratoma of the thyroid region. Am J Roentgenol Radium Ther Nucl Med 95:25–31, 1965.
96. Baarsma R, Bekedam DJ, Visser GH: Qualitatively abnormal fetal breathing movements associated with tracheal atresia. Early Hum Dev 32:63–69, 1993.
97. Hubbard A, Crombleholme TM, Adzick NS: Prenatal MRI evaluation of giant neck masses in preparation for the fetal EXIT procedure. Am J Perinatol 15:253–257, 1998.
98. Baker PN, Johnson IR, Harvey PR, et al: A three year follow up of children imaged in utero with echo-planar magnetic resonance. Am J Obstet Gynecol 170:32–33, 1993.
99. Langer JC, Tabb T, Thompson P, et al: Management of prenatally diagnosed tracheal obstruction: Access to the airway in utero prior to delivery. Fetal Diagn Ther 7:12–16, 1992.
100. Tanaka M, Sato S, Naito H, Nakayama H: Anesthetic management of a neonate with prenatally diagnosed cervical tumour and upper airway obstruction. Can J Anaesth 41:236–240, 1994.
101. Schwartz MZ, Silver H, Schulman S: Maintenance of the placental circulation to evaluate and treat an infant with massive head and neck hemangioma. J Pediatr Surg 28:520–522, 1993.
102. Stocks RM, Egerman RS, Woodson GE, et al: Airway management of neonates with antenatally detected head and neck anomalies. Arch Otolaryngol Head Neck Surg 123:641–645, 1997.
103. McNamara H, Johnson N: The effect of uterine contractions on fetal oxygen saturation. Br J Obstet Gynaecol 102:644–647, 1995.
104. Mychalishka GB, Bealor JF, Graf JL, et al: Operating on placental support: The ex utero intrapartum treatment (EXIT) procedure. J Pediatr Surg 32:227–230, 1997.
105. Bond SJ, Harrison MR, Slotnick RN, et al: Cesarean delivery and hysterotomy using an absorbable stapling device. Obstet Gynecol 74:25–28, 1989.
106. Skarsgard ED, Chitkara U, Krane EJ, et al: The OOPS procedure (operation on placental support): In utero airway management of the fetus with prenatally diagnosed tracheal obstruction. J Pediatr Surg 31:826–828, 1996.
107. Hood DD, Holubec DM: Elective repeat cesarean section. Effect of anesthesia type on blood loss. J Reprod Med 35:368–372, 1990.
108. Harrison MR, Filly RA, Golbus MS, et al: Fetal Treatment 1982. N Engl J Med 307:1651–1652, 1982.
109. Liechty KW, Crombleholme TM, Weiner S, et al: The ex utero intrapartum treatment procedure for a large fetal neck mass in a twin gestation. Obstet Gynecol 93:824–825, 1999.
110. Biehl DR, Yarnell R, Wade JG, et al: The uptake of isoflurane by the foetal lamb in utero: Effect on regional blood flow. Can Anaesth Soc J 30:581–586, 1983.

111. Dwyer R, Fee JPH, Moore J: Uptake of halothane and isoflurane by mother and baby during caesarean section. Br J Anaesth 74:379–383, 1995.
112. Gaiser RR, Cheek TG, Kurth CD: Anesthetic management of caesarean delivery complicated by ex utero intrapartum treatment of the fetus. Anesth Analg 84:1150–1153, 1997.
113. Tunstall ME, Sheikh A: Comparison of 1.5% enflurane with 1.25% isoflurane in oxygen for caesarean section: Avoidance of awareness without nitrous oxide. Br J Anaesth 62:138–143, 1989.
114. Piggott SE, Bogod DG, Rosen M, et al: Isoflurane with either 100% oxygen or 50% nitrous oxide in oxygen for caesarean section. Br J Anaesth 65:325–329, 1990.
115. DeSimone CA, Norris MC, Leighton BL: Intravenous nitroglycerine aids manual extraction of the placenta. Anesthesiology 73:787, 1990.
116. Wesson A, Elowsson P, Axemo P, et al: The use of intravenous nitroglycerine for emergency cervico-uterine relaxation. Acta Anaesthesiol Scand 39:847–849, 1995.
117. Ignarro LJ: Biologic actions and properties of endothelium-derived nitric oxide formed and released from artery and vein. Circ Res 65:1–21, 1989.
118. DiFederco EM, Harrison MR, Matthey MA: Pulmonary edema in a woman following fetal surgery. Chest 109:1114–1117, 1996.
119. Garmel S, Crombleholme TM: The ultrasound diagnosis and management of fetal tumors. Postgrad Obstet Gynecol 15:1–8, 1985.
120. Gonzalez-Crussi F: Extragonadal Teratomas, Atlas of Tumor Pathology. Series 2. Fascicle 18, Bethesda, MD: Armed Forces Institute of Pathology, 1982, pp 118–127.
121. Hancock BJ, St-Vil D, Lebs FI, et al: Complications of lymphangiomas in children. J Pediatr Surg 27:220–225, 1982.
122. Ogita S, Tsuto T, Nakamura K, et al: OK-432 therapy for lymphangiomas in children: Why and how does it work? J Pediatr Surg 31:477–480, 1996.
123. Tanaka K, Inomata Y, Utsunomiya H, et al: Sclerosing therapy with bleomycin emulsion for lymphangioma in children. Pediatr Surg Int 5:270–275, 1990.
124. Tanigawa N, Shimomatsuya T, Takahashi K, et al: Treatment of cystic hygroma and lymphangioma with the use of bleomycin fat emulsion. Cancer 60:741–749, 1987.

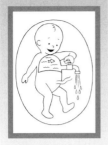

CHAPTER 25

Fetal Hydrothorax

DIANA LEE FARMER and CRAIG T. ALBANESE

The antenatal diagnosis of fetal pleural effusion was first reported by Carroll in 1977.[1] Hydrothorax (also referred to as fetal pleural effusion or fetal chylothorax) is an uncommon fetal lesion with an estimated incidence of 1 in 15,000 pregnancies.[2] However, with the improved resolution and widespread use of screening ultrasound, fetal pleural effusion is being diagnosed more frequently, and the true incidence is likely higher. Males are affected twice as often as females,[3,4] and 70% of cases are unilateral, predominately affecting the right side.[3]

The significance of fetal pleural effusion ranges from a transient, inconsequential finding to a life-threatening fetal diagnosis. The prognosis of small-volume, unilateral, isolated fetal pleural effusion is usually good, and spontaneous resolution is seen. However, the prognosis is poor when fetal pleural effusion is found in association with chromosomal abnormalities, multiple congenital malformations, or hydrops. Fetal hydrothorax has a perinatal mortality of 57 to 100%.[5] Mortality is higher when the fetal pleural effusion occurs in association with generalized hydrops than when it is an isolated finding.[6,7] As shown in other models, it is thought that intrathoracic compression of the developing lung produces pulmonary hypoplasia, which has been the main cause of perinatal death in fetuses with hydrothorax.[8,9] Large pleural effusions may cause hydramnios by interfering with fetal swallowing. Hydrops is the main cause of fetal death and is believed to be caused by mediastinal shift resulting in vena caval obstruction and/or direct cardiac compression.

Etiology and Natural History

The etiology of fetal pleural effusion is varied and associated with a wide spectrum of perinatal outcomes. Various causes include generalized fluid retention in association with immune and nonimmune hydrops and anatomic defects in chest or lung development. Fetal pleural effusion may be an isolated finding (primary), due to leakage of lymph (chylothorax) or may be secondary due to generalized hydrops or specific anatomic abnormalities.

In the neonate, isolated pleural effusion is most commonly a chylothorax, definitively diagnosed by identi-

fication of chylomicrons in the milky pleural fluid after feeding.[3] Prior to the advent of prenatal ultrasound, the newborn with chylothorax was identified by the development of respiratory distress. Neonatal mortality is reported to be between 15 and 20%.[3] While chylothorax is the most common cause of hydrothorax in neonates, the definitive diagnosis of this entity is difficult in the nonfed intrauterine fetus.[10] Some investigators have suggested that the diagnosis can be made in the fetus by demonstration of a high mononuclear cell count in the aspirated fetal pleural fluid.[11,12] However, this has not been confirmed by the finding of postnatal chylothorax. The cause of nonimmune hydrops that is not associated with fetal cardiac abnormalities or dysrhythmias remains unexplained in over 50% of cases,[13] despite detailed investigation with fetal blood sampling and ultrasound. Therefore, congenital chylothorax has been suggested as the primary cause of many cases of unexplained hydrops.[9] Because of the difficulty of documenting chylothorax in utero, the terms "fetal hydrothorax" and "primary fetal pleural effusion" are more appropriate.

Secondary fetal hydrothorax may be due to specific lesions such as congenital cystic adenomatoid malformation (CAM), bronchopulmonary sequestration, or congenital diaphragmatic hernia (CDH).[15,16] Fetal hydrothorax may also be part of a nonimmune hydrops fetalis (NIHF), which may be caused by cardiac defects, anemia, infection, or chromosomal abnormalities.[4] Fetal hydrothorax secondary to immune or nonimmune hydrops tends to be relatively unimpressive compared to the associated skin edema and ascites seen.

Prenatal series report aneuploidy in 1.8 to 5.8% of fetuses with hydrothorax.[17-19] It has been reported with Down, Turner, and Noonan syndromes. Fetal pleural effusion has been reported with diffuse congenital lymphangiomatosis, including chylopericardium, diffuse hemangioma, congenital lymphedema, and pulmonary lymphangiectasia.[20] Fetal hydrothorax with cervical hygroma without chromosomal abnormalities has also been reported. Primary fetal pleural effusions are rarely observed before 15 weeks' gestational age except in cases of Turner syndrome. Bilateral fetal hydrothorax has been reported as an isolated finding in first-trimester pregnancies complicated by Down and Turner syndromes.[21]

In unilateral pleural effusion, mediastinal shift and kinking of the great vessels impair venous return and lead to congestive heart failure and eventual hydrops.[22] In bilateral pleural effusion, congestive heart failure is a result of increased intrathoracic pressure (tamponade effect), cardiac compression, and low-output failure, rather that impaired venous return. This also eventually leads to hydrops. Abnormal reversed flow in the vena cava in bilateral fetal pleural effusions and its return to normal after drainage of the effusion (decreasing intrathoracic pressure) corroborates this mechanism.[23] Hydrops fetalis, on the other hand, whether immune or nonimmune, may present with fetal pleural effusions. In these cases, however, the pleural effusions are not as prominent as cervical hygroma, generalized skin edema, placental edema, or ascites. Large pleural effusion in early pregnancy may lead to pulmonary hypoplasia,[7] and in late pregnancy may lead to polyhydramnios and possible preterm delivery with consequent prematurity. Hydrops, pulmonary hypoplasia, and prematurity all increase fetal or perinatal death due to hydrothorax.

Natural history, first reported by Longaker et al.,[2] is complicated by a broad clinical spectrum, including variable gestational age at presentation, differing amounts and rates of fluid accumulation, and different causes as outlined above. Rarely, affected fetuses may undergo spontaneous resolution in utero or after a single aspiration in the prenatal period. In some cases, however, hydrothorax precipitates nonimmune fetal hydrops. When hydrothorax with hydrops is first noted near term, prompt delivery has resulted in survival of affected infants.

Clinical Experience and Intrauterine Therapy

Since first reported in 1977, many cases have been reported and a reasonable clinical experience has been gained. There remains no consensus in the literature on optimal management of fetal hydrothorax. Recommended options include elective abortion,[2, 6, 8, 24] observation with serial ultrasound,[25-27] or intrauterine fetal therapy. In 1982, fetal therapy was reported independently by several authors and included fetal thoracentesis,[11, 12, 28-34] shunt placement,[2, 5, 9, 35, 36] or both.[2, 37] Postnatal therapy, based on the neonate's respiratory status, may include the use of ventilatory support, tube thoracostomy, and surgery.[38-42]

The literature on fetal hydrothorax was reviewed extensively by Weber and Philipson[43]; 124 cases were identified from 38 reports. Maternal and fetal characteristics were identified, and eight potential prognostic indicators were evaluated by meta-analysis (Table 25–1). These included gestational age at diagnosis, gestational age at delivery, gender of the fetus, hydramnios, hydrops, extent of effusion (unilateral or bilateral), mode of delivery, and presence of other abnormalities. The types of management identified were abortion, observation, antenatal therapy by thoracentesis and/or shunt insertion, and postnatal therapy. Possible neonatal outcomes were good outcome including spontaneous resolution of fetal pleural effusion, and/or neonatal survival and poor outcome consisting of fetal or neonatal death.

Results of this meta-analysis revealed 54% surviving patients (including 11 cases of spontaneous resolution), and 46% deaths (9 fetal, 44 neonatal). Stepwise logistic regression analysis indicated the highest predicted probability (97%) of poor outcome when three statistically significant predictors of poor outcome were all present (Table 25–2). These identified predictors were delivery at less than 32 weeks, the presence of hydrops, and no fetal intervention. The chance of poor outcome (death) ranged from 30 to 36% when one risk factor was present and from 77 to 81% when two risk factors were present.

The most important finding of this review was that the outcome with fetal pleural effusion was found to be

T A B L E 25–1. VARIABLES ASSOCIATED WITH OUTCOME*

VARIABLE	DESCRIPTION	POOR OUTCOME	P
Gest age dx	≤31	59% (35 of 59)	.051
	≥32	38% (18 of 47)	
Gest age del	≤31	89% (16 of 18)	.0004
	≥32	39% (33 of 84)	
Hydrops	Yes	69% (29 of 42)	<.0001
	No	20% (8 of 40)	
Antenatal therapy	None	50% (35 of 70)	.06
	Thoracentesis	42% (5 of 12)	
	Shunt	22% (5 of 23)	
Gender of fetus	Male	53% (32 of 60)	.99 (NS)
	Female	52% (14 of 27)	
Hydramnios	Yes	40% (23 of 58)	.69 (NS)
	No	50% (7 of 14)	
Extent of effusion	Bilateral	52% (42 of 81)	.11 (NS)
	Unilateral	33% (11 of 33)	
Mode of delivery	Cesarean	47% (9 of 19)	.32 (NS)
	Vaginal	66% (21 of 32)	
Postnatal therapy	Yes	45% (18 of 40)	.99 (NS)
	No	47% (16 of 34)	
Other abnormalities	Yes	75% (12 of 16)	.08 (NS)
	No	42% (11 of 26)	

NS, not significant.
* From Weber A, Philipson EH. Fetal pleural effusion: A review and meta-analysis for prognostic indicators. Obstet Gynecol 79:281, 1992, with permission. Courtesy of the American College of Obstetricians and Gynecologists.

TABLE 25–2. STEPWISE LOGISTIC REGRESSION RESULTS*†

VARIABLE	IMPROVEMENT (*P*)	GOODNESS OF FIT (*P*)
Gest age del	<.001	.003
Antenatal therapy	.005	.021
Hydrops	.003	.173

* From Weber A, Philipson EH: Fetal pleural effusion: A review and meta-analysis for prognostic indicators. Obstet Gynecol 79:281, 1992, with permission. Courtesy of the American College of Obstetricians and Gynecologists.
† Independent variables considered: extent of effusion (bilateral, unilateral), gestational age at diagnosis (31 and 32 weeks), gestational age at delivery (31 and 32 weeks), antenatal therapy (some, none), hydrops (present, absent), and thoracentesis and shunt placement.
Gest age del, gestational age at delivery in weeks.

related to three variables: gestational age at delivery, presence or absence of hydrops, and antenatal therapy.

In a similar 1998 review by Aubard et al., 204 cases were identified and reviewed.[24] They found four factors that correlated with the course of primary fetal pleural effusion: the presence of hydrops, gestational age at time of birth, unilateral or bilateral nature of effusion (with unilateral having a better prognosis), and the occurrence of spontaneous resolution. With multivariate analysis, however, only fetal hydrops remained a prognostic factor.

The presence of hydrops predicts poor outcome. The pathophysiology of hydropic change associated with primary fetal pleural effusion includes vena caval obstruction with diminished venous return, cardiac compression, and low-output cardiac failure.[45] If hydrops is present at the time of initial diagnosis, it can be unclear whether the effusion is primary or secondary. The dilemma facing the clinician is that this distinction often cannot be made by antenatal ultrasound.

Pleural effusion may affect fetal lung development and hemodynamics as well as postnatal respiratory mechanics. The goals of antenatal therapy are to prevent lung compression and allow normal development, to prevent or reverse hydropic change, and to improve postnatal respiratory function.

As stated in the review by Weber and Philipson,[43] the number of cases was too small for statistical analysis comparing thoracentesis and shunt placement; however, for women considering prolongation of pregnancy, the shunt offers the advantage of continuous drainage. Experience with thoracentesis has shown that fluid may reaccumulate rapidly. Complications have been reported with both shunt placement and thoracentesis. In one case of thoracentesis, umbilical cord torsion and fetal death occurred; this result was believed to be procedure-related.[2] In one case of shunt placement, the shunt was noted to be under the neonate's chest wall at birth; no surgical intervention was considered necessary.[5] Other complications include significant catheter migration, infection, bleeding, damage to the fetus, initiation of premature rupture of membranes, and preterm labor.

Unilateral Hydrothorax

Wilkins-Haug and Doubilet[46] have proposed that unilateral and bilateral effusions may differ in both natural history and response to intervention, due to possible differences in the underlying lesions. Although unilateral and bilateral effusions have some causative factors in common, including chromosomal abnormalities, viral infections, and cardiac and thoracic structural anomalies, they suggest that bilateral effusions are more likely to be one of the manifestations of a global abnormality, such as arthrogryposis, skeletal dysplasia, or metabolic storage disease, which generally has a poor prognosis. In addition, when pleural effusions are due to lymphatic leak ("chylous" effusion), unilateral lesions usually result from an isolated abnormality in the integrity of the thoracic lymphatic system, where bilateral lesions may represent a more severe generalized lymph leak. Other series appear to support this hypothesis.[44]

In the reviews by Weber and Philipson and others, combining unilateral and bilateral collections, survival rates were found to be only 54 to 64%.[43, 44, 47] The prognosis was especially poor if the effusions were diagnosed prior to 32 weeks' gestation (survival rate, 40 to 45%) or if hydrops was present at any gestational age (survival rate, 30%). The survival rate appeared to be better for unilateral effusions (67%) than for bilateral effusions (48%), but the difference was not statistically significant, possibly because of insufficient sample size.[43]

In these reviews, when unilateral and bilateral effusions were considered together and thoracentesis and thoracoamniotic shunting are combined, intervention did not appear to influence outcome: survival rates were 69% and 63% with and without intervention, respectively.[47] Although survival after thoracoamniotic shunting alone appeared to be promising (78%, 18 of 23 cases), the rates could not be subdivided into unilateral versus bilateral or hydrops versus no hydrops owing to insufficient numbers of cases.[43, 44, 47]

Unilateral hydrothorax may remain stable, undergo spontaneous resolution, or progress to hydrops. Table 25–3 summarizes the current experience with untreated isolated unilateral effusion. With observational management alone, cases in which the infants survived are characterized by late third-trimester presentation with delivery within 2 weeks of diagnosis and a lack of hydrops. Three of these survivors had had normal second- and third-trimester ultrasonographic assessments at 7, 11, and 13 weeks prior to their documentation of a unilateral effusion.[40, 48, 49]

Thoracoamniotic shunting has been employed for unilateral effusion, both without and with hydrops (Table 25–4). The reported outcome in both groups appears to be good. In the nonhydropic group, whether shunting improves outcome is unclear, as survival may be high in cases of unilateral effusions without hydrops even if no intervention is undertaken. In the hydropic group, however, intervention may yield a clear-cut benefit, although cases with unilateral effusion and hydrops without intervention are few and historical.[2] Thoracoamniotic shunting appears to lead to a good outcome in the presence of hydrops and a unilateral effusion. This intervention even appears to be of value when the condition is diagnosed and treated well prior to term.

Although the numbers of treated infants remain small, a growing literature supports the use of thoracoamniotic shunting in fetuses with unilateral effusion and NIHF.

TABLE 25–3. LITERATURE REVIEW FOR NATURAL HISTORY OF UNTREATED UNILATERAL PLEURAL EFFUSIONS WITHOUT STRUCTURAL OR KARYOTYPIC ABNORMALITIES

	DIAGNOSIS (WK)	EDEMA	ASCITES	POLYHYDRAMNIOS	DELIVERY (WK)	NEONATAL OUTCOME
Bruno et al.[40]	33	—	—	—	36	Good
Schmit et al.[51]	34	+	+	+	34	Good
Parker and James[50]	35	—	—			Good
Calisti et al.[48]	36	—	—			Good
Longaker et al.[2]	36	?	?	?	36	Good
	27	?	?	?	37	Good
Meizner[39]	38	—	—	+	38	Good
Wilson et al.[20]	33	—	—	+	40	Neonatal death
Reece et al.[24]	31	?	?	+	?	Neonatal death
	36	?	?	?	?	Neonatal death
Lien et al.[53]	16	—	—	—	41	Good, effusion resolved in utero at 19 wk
Adams et al.[56]	16	—	—	—	40	Good, effusion resolved in utero at 28 wk
Longaker et al.[2]	30	?	?	?	40	Good, effusion not present at term

Shunt placement for unilateral effusions without hydrops remains speculative. After shunt placement, initial resolution of the effusion followed by decrease in the edema and polyhydramnios is anticipated during the following 2 to 4 weeks. Although shunt placement appears to be efficacious, further investigation in a larger series will be needed to assess outcome and evaluate complications.

Fetal Investigations

When fetal pleural effusion with NIHF is diagnosed and intervention is contemplated, the fetus should be evaluated carefully. It is essential to establish etiology as this will determine the management and affect the fetal outcome. Chromosomal anomalies as well as cardiac and thoracic structural anomalies, including pulmonary sequestration, cystic adenomatoid malformation, and diaphragmatic hernia must be looked for. Major cardiovascular defects are more commonly found early in gestation prior to 20 weeks. Fetal echocardiography may be indicated. Although other abnormalities do not inevitably predict a poor outcome, the specific nature of associated anomalies may guide management, particularly if they are incompatible with survival.

Chromosomal abnormalities are documented by karyotyping from amniocentesis and chorionic villus

TABLE 25–4. LITERATURE REVIEW OF THORACOAMNIOTIC SHUNT PLACEMENTS FOR UNILATERAL HYDROTHORAX

	GESTATIONAL AGE AT SHUNT (WK)	EDEMA	ASCITES	POLYHYDRAMNIOS	GESTATIONAL AGE AT DELIVERY (WK)	OUTCOME
No Other Body Cavity Fluid Collections						
Rodeck et al.[5]	25	–	–	+	39	Good
	27	–	–	+	39	Good
Nicolaides and Azar[57]	20	–	–	–	36	Good
	20	–	–	–	39	Good
	24	–	–	+	39	Good
	27	–	–	+	32	Good
	27	–	–	–	39	Good
	29	–	–	+	31	Good
	30	–	–	+	34	Good
	31	–	–	+	38	Good
	31	–	–	–	38	Good
	33	–	–	+	39	Good
Nonimmune Hydrops						
Nicolaides and Azar[57]	26	+	+	+	37	Good
	32	+	+	+	39	Good
	32	+	+	+	40	Good
	33	+	+	+	38	Good
	33	+	–	+	38	Good
	34	+	+	+	36	Good
Bernascheck et al.[51]	30	+	+	+	33	Good
Lasser and Timor-Tritsch et al.[58]	23	+	+	+	40	Good
Wilkins-Haug and Doubilet[46]	25	+	+	+	40	Good
	27				36	Good

sampling (CVS). CVS is the method of choice in cases of hydrops diagnosed before 15 weeks' gestation. CVS enables more rapid karyotyping, DNA analysis, and biochemical diagnosis. Fetal pulmonary maturity should also be evaluated in anticipation of antenatal therapy and possible preterm delivery.

Maternal Investigations

Immunologic and infectious causes have to be ruled out in cases of fetal hydothorax. Recommended laboratory studies on the mother include (1) compete blood cell count, (2) blood type and antibody screen, (3) hemoglobin electrophoresis, (4) TORCH titers (*toxoplasma*, *other* infections, *rubella*, *cytomegalovirus*, and *herpesvirus*), (5) Kleihauer-Betke test, and (6) serologic tests for syphilis (Venereal Disease Research Laboratories [VDRL]). In cases of unexplained nonimmune fetal hydrops in mothers with a previous history of pregnancies at risk, blood glucose, glucose-6-phosphate dehydrogenase (G6PD), or pyruvate kinase screening is recommended. Delta optical density of amniotic fluid may also be tested if hydrops is thought to be of immune etiology.

Current Guidelines for Antenatal Therapy

It is not unexpected that outcome is related to gestational age at delivery. Perinatal mortality is related to prematurity, the underlying condition resulting in pleural effusion, the effect of the effusion itself, or a combination of these factors. With careful patient selection, management may include attempts to prolong pregnancy to decrease the risk of prematurity-related morbidity and mortality, particularly at less than 32 weeks' gestation.

Management decisions will be influenced by gestational age and the risk of morbidity related to prematurity, and by the presence of other abnormalities. When fetal pleural effusion is diagnosed at less than 32 weeks' gestation and there is no evidence of hydrops, management may be conservative with serial ultrasound examinations for progression of effusion and development of hydrops. Conservative management may continue as long as the effusion is stable or decreasing, with the knowledge that even large pleural effusions may resolve spontaneously with no adverse effect on lung development. Survival after spontaneous resolution is 100%.[2, 9, 27, 41, 52–54]

With ascites or hydrops, antenatal therapy by thoracentesis for short-term drainage, or shunt placement for long-term drainage, should be considered. Close observation with serial ultrasound may be continued if hydrops resolves. If preterm labor occurs, tocolysis may be considered, particularly when the gestational age is less than 32 weeks. In cases complicated by hydramnios, indomethacin may be an appropriate choice for tocolysis because of its associated effect of decreasing amniotic fluid volume.[55] If the fetal condition deteriorates despite antenatal therapy, delivery should be considered regardless of gestational age.

After 32 weeks gestational age, if fetal hydrothorax is diagnosed without hydrops, serial ultrasound examination is indicated. Appearance of ascites or hydrops is an indication for delivery. If fetal hydrothorax with hydrops is diagnosed after 32 weeks then immediate delivery is indicated with consideration of thoracentesis just prior to delivery if significant respiratory compromise seems likely.

Because the mode of delivery does not appear to influence neonatal outcome, management should be guided by standard obstetric indications. In all cases, delivery should be planned at a center where appropriate neonatal services are available.

REFERENCES

1. Carroll B: Pulmonary hypoplasia and pleural effusions associated with fetal death in utero: Ultrasonic findings. AJR Am J Roengenol 129:749–750, 1977.
2. Longaker MT, Laberge JM, Dansereau J, et al: Primary fetal hydrothorax: Natural history and management. J Pediatr Surg 24:573–576, 1989.
3. Chemick V, Reed MH: Pneumothorax and chylothorax in the neonatal period. J Pediatr 76:624–632, 1970.
4. Brodmari RF: Congenital chylothorax: Recommendations for treatment. N Y State J Med 75:553–557, 1975.
5. Rodeck CH, Fisk NM, Fraser DL, Nicolini U: Long-term in utero drainage of fetal hydrothorax. N Engl J Med 319:1135–1138, 1988.
6. Castillo RA, Devoe LD, Hadi HA, et al: Nonimmune hydrops fetalis: Clinical experience and factors related to a poor outcome. Am J Obstet Gynecol 155:812–816, 1986.
7. Harrison MR, Bressach MA, Chung AM, deLorimier AA: Correction of congenital diaphragmatic hernia in utero. II. Simulated correction permits fetal lung growth with survival at birth. Surgery 88:260–268, 1980.
8. Castillo RA, Devoe LD, Falls C, et al: Pleural effusions and pulmonary hypoplasia. Am J Obstet Gynecol 157:1252–1255, 1987.
9. Roberts AB, Clarkson PM, Pattison NS, et al: Fetal hydrothorax in the second trimester of pregnancy: Successful intra-uterine treatment at 24 weeks gestation. Fetal Ther 1:203–209, 1986.
10. Eddleman KA, Levine AB, Chitkara U, et al: Reliability of pleural fluid lymphocyte counts in the antenatal diagnosis of congenital chylothorax. Obstet Gynecol 78:530, 1991.
11. Benacerraf BR, Frigoletto FD, Wilson M: Successful midtrimester thoracentesis with analysis of the lymphocyte population in the pleural effusion. Am J Obstet Gynecol 155:398–399, 1986.
12. Elser H, Borruto F, Schneider A, Schneider K: Chylothorax in a twin pregnancy of 34 weeks—sonographically diagnosed. Eur J Obstet Gynecol Reprod Biol 16:205–211, 1983.
13. Nicolaides KH, Rodeck CH, Lange I, et al: Fetoscopy in the assessment of unexplained fetal hydrops. Br J Obstet Gynaecol 92:671–679, 1985.
14. Meizner I, Bar-Ziv J, Insler V: Prenatal ultrasonic diagnosis of fetal thoracic and intrathoracic abnormalities. Isr J Med 22:350–354, 1986.
15. Shipley CF, Simmons CL, Nelson GH: Intrauterine diagnosis of hydrothorax in a fetus who had a combination chylothorax and pulmonary sequestration after delivery. J Perinatol 15:237–239, 1995.
16. Chan V, Greenough A, Nicolaides K: Antenatal and postnatal treatment of pleural effusion and extralobar pulmonary sequestration. J Perinat Med 24:335–338, 1996.
17. Achiron RA, Weissman A, et al: Fetal pleural effusion: The risk of fetal trisomy. Gynecol Obstet Invest 39:153–156, 1995.
18. Shimizu TK, Hashimoto, et al: Bilateral pleural effusion in the first trimester: A predictor of chromosomal abnormality and embryonic death? Am J Obstet Gynecol 177:470–471, 1997.
19. Nicholades KH, Rodeck CH, Gosden CM: Rapid karyotyping in nonlethal fetal malformations. Lancet i:283–286, 1986.
20. Wilson RH, Duncan A, Hume R, Bain AD: Prenatal pleural effusion associated with congenital pulmonary lymphangiectasia. Prenat Diagn 5:73–76, 1985.

21. Cademan A, Pergament E: Bilateral pleural effusion at 8.5 weeks gestation with Down syndrome and Turner syndrome [letter]. Prenat Diagn 13:659–660, 1993.

22. Romero R, Pilu G, Jeanty P, et al: Prenatal Diagnosis of Congenital Anomalies. Norwalk, CT: Appleton & Lange, 1989, pp 195–197.

23. Gonen R, Degani S, Shapiro I, et al: The effect of drainage of fetal chylothorax on cardiac and blood vessel hemodynamics. J Clin Ultrasound 21:265–268, 1993.

24. Reece EA, Lockwood CJ, Rizzo N, et al: Intrinsic intrathoracic malformations of the fetus: Sonographic detection and clinical presentation. Obstet Gynecol 70:627–632, 1987.

25. Thomas DB, Anderson JC: Antenatal detection of fetal pleural effusions and neonatal management. Med J Aust 2:435–436, 1979.

26. Jouppila P, Kirkinen P, Herva R, Koivisto M: Prenatal diagnosis of pleural effusions by ultrasound. J Clin Ultrasound 11:516–519, 1983.

27. Adams H, Jones A, Hayward C: The sonographic features and implications of fetal pleural effusions. Clin Radiol 39:398–401, 1988.

28. Petres RE, Redwine FO, Cruikshank OP: Congenital bilateral chylothorax—antepartum diagnosis and successful intrauterine surgical management. JAMA 248:1360–1361, 1982.

29. Schmidt W, Harms E, Wolf O: Successful prenatal treatment of non-immune hydrops fetalis due to congenital chylothorax—case report. Br J Obstet Gynaecol 92:685–687, 1985.

30. Benacerraf BR, Frigoletto FD: Mid-trimester fetal thoracentesis. J Clin Ultrasound 13:202–204, 1985.

31. Benacerraf BR, Frigoletto FD: In utero treatment of a fetus with diaphragmatic hernia complicated by hydrops. Am J Obstet Gynecol 155:817–818, 1986.

32. Whittle MJ, Gilmore OH, McNay MB, et al: Diaphragmatic hernia presenting in utero as a unilateral hydrothorax. Prenat Diagn 9:115–118, 1989.

33. Landy HJ, Daly V, Heyl PS, Khoury AN: Fetal thoracentesis with unsuccessful outcome. J Clin Ultrasound 18:50–53, 1990.

34. Gilsanz V, Emons O, Hansmann M, et al: Hydrothorax, ascites, and right diaphragmatic hernia. Radiology 158:243–246, 1986.

35. Booth P, Nicolaides KH, Greenough A, Gamsu HR: Pleuroamniotic shunting for fetal chylothorax. Early Hum Dev 15:365–367, 1987.

36. Blott M, Nicolaides KH, Greenough A: Pleuroamniotic shunting for decompression of fetal pleural effusions. Obstet Gynecol 71:798–800, 1988.

37. Seeds JW, Bowes WA: Results of treatment of severe fetal hydrothorax with bilateral pleuroamniotic catheters. Obstet Gynecol 68:577–580, 1986.

38. Lange IR, Manning FA: Antenatal diagnosis of congenital pleural effusions. Am J Obstet Gynecol 140:839–840, 1981.

39. Meizner I, Carmi R, BarZiv J: Congenital chylothorax—prenatal ultrasonic diagnosis and successful postpartum management. Prenat Diagn 6:217–221, 1986.

40. Bruno M, Iskra L, Dolfin C, Farina D: Congenital pleural effusion: Prenatal ultrasonic diagnosis and therapeutic management. Prenat Diagn 8:157–159, 1988.

41. Pijpers L, Reuss A, Stewart PA, Wladimiroff JW: Noninvasive management of isolated bilateral fetal hydrothorax. Am J Obstet Gynecol 161:330–332, 1989.

42. Peleg D, Golichowski AM, Ragan WD: Fetal hydrothorax and bilateral pulmonary hypoplasia. Acta Obstet Gynecol Scand 65:451–453, 1985.

43. Weber A, Philipson EH: Fetal pleural effusion: A review and meta-analysis for prognostic indicators. Obstet Gynecol 79:281, 1992.

44. Aubard Y, Derouineau I, et al: Primary fetal hydrothorax: A literature revue and proposed antenatal clinical strategy. Fetal Diagn Ther 13: 325–333, 1998.

45. Bessone IN, Ferguson TB, Burford TH: Chylothorax. Ann Thorac Surg 12:527–550, 1971.

46. Wilkins-Haug LE, Doubilet P: Successful thoracoamniotic shunting and review of the literature in unilateral pleural effusion with hydrops. J Ultrasound Med 16:153–160, 1997.

47. Hagay Z, Reece A, Roberts A, et al: Isolated fetal pleural effusion: A prenatal management dilemma. Obstet Gynecol 81:147, 1993.

48. Calisti A, Manzoni D, Pintus C, Perrilli L: Prenatal diagnosis and management of some fetal intrathoracic abnormalities. Eur J Obstet Gynecol Reprod Biol 22:61–68, 1986.

49. Lange IR, Harman CR, Ash KM, et al: Twin with hydramnios: Treating premature labor at source. Am J Obstet Gynecol 160:552–557, 1989.

50. Parker M, James D: Spontaneous variation in fetal pleural effusions: Case report. Br J Obstet Gynaecol 98:403, 1991.

51. Bernascheck G, Deutinger J, Hansmann M, et al: Fetoamniotic shunting—report of the experience of four European centres. Prenat Diagn 14:821, 1994.

52. Schmidt W, Harma E, Wolf D: Successful prenatal treatment of non-immune hydrops fetalis due to congenital chylothorax. Br J Obstet Gynaecol 92:685, 1985.

53. Lien JM, Colmorgen GHC, Gehret IF, Evantash AB: Spontaneous resolution of fetal pleural effusion diagnosed during the second trimester. J Clin Ultrasound 18:54–56, 1990.

54. Yaghoobian J, Comrie M: Transitory bilateral isolated fetal pleural effusions. J Ultrasound Med 7:231–232, 1988.

55. Jaffe R, DiSegni E, Altaras M, et al: Ultrasonic real-time diagnosis of transitory fetal pleural and pericardial effusion. Diagn Imag Clin Med 55:373–375, 1986.

56. Adam H, Jones A, Hayward C: The sonographic features and implications of fetal pleural effusions. Clin Radiol 39:398, 1988.

57. Nicolaides K, Azar G: Thoraco-amniotic shunting. Fetal Diagn Ther 5:153, 1990.

58. Lasser D, Timor-Tritsch I: In utero treatment of fetal hydrothorax with pleuroamniotic shunting at 23 weeks' gestation. Am J Obstet Gynecol 164:416, 1991.

26

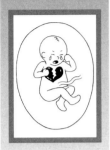

The Fetus with Congenital Heart Disease

NORMAN H. SILVERMAN and FRANK L. HANLEY

Although structural abnormalities of the heart and great vessels are fairly common congenital abnormalities, accounting for approximately 8 in 1,000 live newborns,[1, 2] fetal echocardiography (cardiac ultrasonography) has only recently attracted attention. Because the fetal heart is small and beats rapidly, it could be imaged clearly only after high-resolution real-time ultrasound scanners became available, allowing the image to be magnified. Since the advent of cross-sectional scanners, which provide real-time directed M-mode, pulsed Doppler echocardiography, and color-coded Doppler flow mapping, the assessment of fetal cardiac anatomy and function has enabled the perinatal ultrasonographer to recognize congenital heart defects,[3–11] arrhythmias,[12–17] and disturbed cardiac function in utero.[18–20] The information from fetal echocardiography may help choose a site and route of delivery when one has recognized a serious cardiac abnormality, has augmented the ability to provide genetic counseling, and has permitted sophisticated monitoring of cardiac arrhythmias during transplacental treatment. In the future, acquisition of such information may facilitate decisions about cardiac surgery in utero.[21, 22]

Clinical Indications for Fetal Echocardiography

Common indications for fetal echocardiography are most frequent when obstetric sonographers identify cardiac abnormalities. Other indications include previous congenital heart disease in siblings or parents; a maternal disease known to affect the fetus, such as diabetes mellitus or connective tissue disease; maternal use of drugs that might cause cardiac abnormalities in the fetus, such as lithium, alcohol, or progesterones[23]; and obstetric examinations indicating abnormal cardiac findings due to chromosomal abnormalities, diaphragmatic hernia, exomphalos, hydrops, polyhydramnios or oligohydramnios, or the presence of a very fast or slow fetal heart rate. A common indication is a positive family history of congenital heart disease. Although in our ex-

perience—and in that of others[24]—the rate of recurrence is low when there is one previously affected child, this rate might be increased when there is more than one previously affected child or when the mother has congenital heart disease.[24–26] Most of those women, who are referred because their disease is considered to be a risk to fetal cardiac development, have diabetes mellitus. Euglycemic control in diabetics at the time of conception and in early pregnancy may diminish the risk, and we have not found cardiac abnormalities in the offspring of such diabetic women. Structural cardiac defects are encountered more frequently when other fetal abnormalities have been detected previously on obstetric ultrasound examination, especially when there is nonimmune hydrops, exomphalos, or diaphragmatic hernia.

In the presence of a very slow fetal heart rate (<80 bpm), the fetus is at high risk for congenital heart block; fetal echocardiography should be performed not only to evaluate the arrhythmia but also to rule out the presence of a structural cardiac defect. The association of complete heart block with structural cardiac defects appears to have an extremely poor prognosis, presumably because of the adverse interaction of structural defects, bradycardia, and the additional atrioventricular valve regurgitation. In fetuses with complete heart block but without structural cardiac defect, the mother frequently suffers from a connective tissue disorder.[27, 28] This can be substantiated by obtaining maternal serum for anti-Ro and anti-La antibodies. Such antibodies have been recognized in a variety of collagen vascular diseases that produce congenital heart block. Other arrhythmias have, in our experience, no association with any structural abnormality of the heart.

We prefer to perform the initial study between 16 and 22 weeks of gestation, because the valves are well developed, the size of the heart is adequate for study, and the fetal size and position usually allow best access to the heart. If necessary, however, it is possible to display the fetal cardiac anatomy and to analyze cardiac rhythm and function from 14 weeks to term, although recent reports suggest that there is "continuing development" of malformations.[29]

Equipment

High-resolution ultrasound imaging is the cornerstone of fetal echocardiography. For studying the fetal heart, it is desirable to use ultrasound systems equipped with M-mode, pulsed Doppler, continuous wave, and color flow Doppler ultrasound. The transducer frequency for cardiac imaging should be as high as possible; we prefer 8-, 7.5-, or 5-MHz transducers, but have also used transducers with 3-MHz frequency when deeper penetration is required. Both linear array and sector scanners may be used to image the fetal heart. Image magnification and cine-loop facilities, which capture a few seconds of time in digital format, allow one to image the beating heart in real time, slow motion, or still image, and have augmented our ability to recognize structural abnormalities. Recording the studies on videotape for later playback and analysis or, with current systems, digital storage of cardiac motion in real time is essential for a fetal cardiac examination.

Investigational Technique

Cross-Sectional Imaging

In order to define the cardiac position and situs, it is necessary to orient the cross-sectional image to the fetal body by noting the position of the head, body, and limbs. It is also important to estimate fetal age using biparietal diameter or femur length measurements, because cardiac dimensions relate to gestational age and fetal weight.[5, 30–32] The best access to the heart is achieved through the fetal abdomen, but imaging is also possible through the rib cage and from the back because the fetal lungs, being filled with fluid, are not a barrier to the passage of ultrasound as they are postnatally. In later gestation, however, when the fetal back may be very close to the maternal abdominal wall, much of the ultrasonic energy is absorbed by the vertebral bodies, scapulae, and ribs, which become ossified, resulting in poorer imaging potential from this direction. To improve imaging it may be necessary to turn the mother onto one side or the other, or to elevate her chest or pelvis. We have occasionally found it helpful to have the mother walk around, empty a full bladder, or delay the examination for hours or even days. In the presence of polyhydramnios the fetus may lie at some distance from the transducer when the mother is recumbent; the fetus can be brought closer to the transducer by having the mother rest on her knees and elbows.

Once the fetal heart is located, only slight movements of the transducer are needed to display the cardiac structures because, with the fetal heart at some distance from the transducer, small movements subtend great angle changes. We consider that a complete cardiac examination must encompass scanning of the fetal heart from side to side and from top to bottom. Reference planes similar to those obtained postnatally are gathered, namely, four-chamber as well as long- and short-axis

cuts (Fig. 26–1). It should be noted that these terms are derived from traditional cardiac reference planes established postnatally.

Although the four-chamber plane (Fig. 26–1A) is very valuable for defining comparative sizes of the chambers, it allows the display of only the atrioventricular connections. It does not pass through a plane that allows recognition of the aorta and pulmonary arteries and, therefore, will not define the complexes of transposition of the great arteries, tetralogy of Fallot, truncus arteriosus, or double-outlet right ventricle. It also does not pass through the outlet part of the ventricular septum and will not define outlet ventricular septal defects and aortic override as found in tetralogy of Fallot, truncus arteriosus, or double-outlet right ventricle. It may not pass through a plane where most ventricular septal defects lie. The arterial valve anatomy is not defined in the

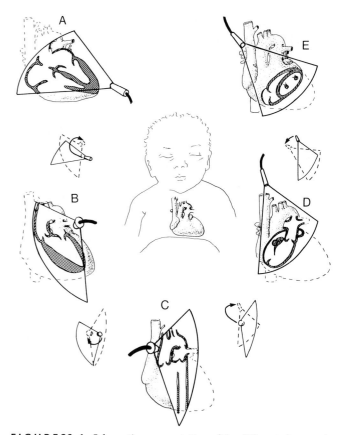

FIGURE 26–1. Schematic representation of the different views and approaches used to image the fetal heart and great vessels. The fetal heart has a more horizontal axis compared to its postnatal lie in the chest (*center*). Note that all the views are shown as being obtained from the chest or the abdominal wall; however, it is also possible to achieve all these imaging planes from the back. *A,* Four-chamber view, showing both atria and the foramen ovale within the atrial septum, both ventricles, and the atrioventricular valves. *B,* After slight clockwise rotation and tilt of the transducer toward the fetal left shoulder, the long axis comes into view. *C,* Further clockwise rotation and tilt of the transducer results in sagittally oriented planes, which are valuable for depicting the aortic arch and the "ductus-arch." *D,* Perpendicular to the long axis the short axis views are obtained. At the base of the heart the aorta lies centrally and is surrounded by the structures of the right ventricle and the pulmonary artery as postnatally. *E,* Further toward the apex, the left ventricular morphology with two papillary muscles can be seen.

four-chamber view, so that aortic and pulmonic stenosis cannot be detected from this plane. Abnormalities of the aortic arch such as interruption and coarctation will not be identified either. Therefore, the mere display of a four-chamber view is not adequate for a fetal cardiac examination. It should be appreciated that when the four-chamber view is obtained from a subcostal equivalent view, simply rotating the transducer along its axis by approximately 90 degrees brings the great veins and great arteries into view, allowing one to establish the venoatrial, atrioventricular, and ventriculoarterial connections.

The cardiac segments should be assessed sequentially in a manner similar to that performed postnatally.[33] These segments are the situs (or atrial arrangement), the atrioventricular connections, the ventricular morphology, and the ventricular arterial connections. In utero, left- and right-sided body orientation must be established to define the cardiac position within the chest. Inappropriate identification or assumption of levocardia and situs solitus can lead to serious errors. Although the echocardiographic views might be obtained from unusual transducer planes, the reference to cardiac position and situs (atrial arrangement) is facilitated by noting that the left atrium lies closer to the vertebral column, and the right ventricle lies closer to the anterior chest wall (Fig. 26–2). Furthermore, in situs solitus the fluid-filled stomach is left-sided, whereas the hepatic veins and the inferior vena cava as well as the superior vena cava drain into the right-sided atrium (Fig. 26–3). Magnifying the image aids in recognizing anatomic details considerably (Fig. 26–4).

Determining the atrial situs requires the identification of the venous connections and of the atrial morphology. The venous connections can be established in utero

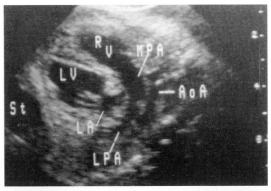

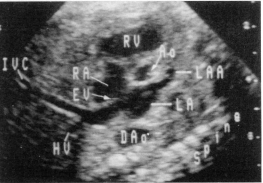

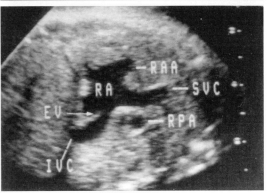

FIGURE 26–3. Series of magnified parasagittal views in the fetus, representing a sweep from the left to the right side. *Top,* The fluid-filled stomach (St) is seen inferior to the left ventricle (LV). The right ventricle (RV) lies anteriorly and is in continuation with the main pulmonary artery (MPA), which gives rise to the left pulmonary artery (LPA). A part of the aortic arch (AoA) can be seen above the pulmonary "arch." The left atrium (LA) lies between the left pulmonary artery and the left ventricle. *Middle,* In a sagittal view obtained to the right of the previous cut, the inferior vena cava (IVC) and a hepatic vein (HV) draining into the right atrium (RA) are demonstrated. The eustachian valve (EV) separates the inferior vena cava from the rest of the right atrium and is pointing towards the atrial septum. Note the narrow-based, finger-like left atrial appendage (LAA) lying behind the aortic root (Ao). The descending aorta (DAo) is seen lying between the left atrium (LA) and the spine. *Bottom,* This cut was obtained by directing the transducer further to the fetal right side in a sagittal orientation demonstrating the entry of the inferior (IVC) and of the superior vena cava (SVC) into the right atrium (RA). The right atrium is characterized by the presence of the eustachian valve (EV) and of a broad-based right atrial appendage (RAA). The right pulmonary artery (RPA) is visible in cross-section posterior to the superior vena cava. Note: the scale marker on the right shows centimeter marking and the depth from the transducer.

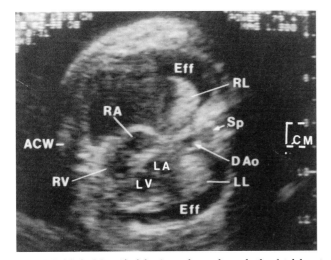

FIGURE 26–2. Magnified horizontal cut through the fetal heart (four-chamber view) and thorax. The right ventricle (RV) is seen close to the anterior chest wall (ACW), whereas the left atrium (LA) lies more posteriorly in front of the descending aorta (DAo) and the spine. The eustachian valve (EV) is noted within the right atrium (RA). In this and most subsequent echocardiographic images a centimeter (CM) scale marker is included on the right of the figure. (LV = left ventricle.) The CM scale marker in this and subsequent figures is shown on the right.

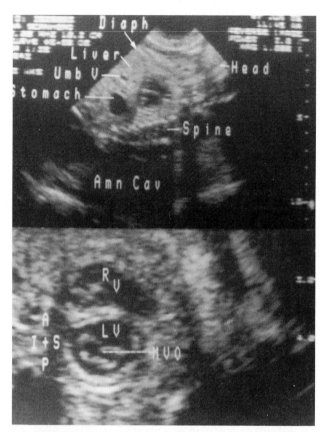

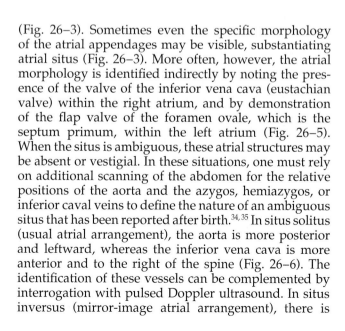

F I G U R E 26–4. Short-axis view of a fetal heart at 22 weeks' gestation. *Top,* This frame shows the position of the head, spine, and abdominal organs (stomach, liver) indicating the superior, inferior, anterior, and posterior directions. (Amn Cav = amniotic cavity; Diaph = diaphragm; Umb V = umbilical vein.) In this and the subsequent figures a scale marker in centimeters is included. The depth in the top panel is up to 11 cm. *Bottom,* After magnification (3×) this frame shows focus on the heart, which lies between 2.5 and 4.5 cm away from the transducer. The cardiac structures are better demonstrated than above; the left ventricle (LV), the mitral valve orifice (MVO), and the right ventricle (RV) can be identified. (A = anterior; I = inferior; P = posterior; S = superior.)

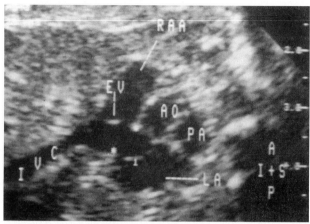

F I G U R E 26–5. Magnified fetal sagittal view at the site of entry of the inferior vena cava (IVC) into the right atrium with its broad-based right atrial appendage (RAA). The eustachian valve (EV) is seen within the right atrium, and the flap valve of the foramen ovale or septum primum (1) is seen within the left atrium (LA). The asterisks indicate the boundaries of the foramen ovale. (Ao = aorta; PA = pulmonary artery; A = anterior; I = inferior; P = posterior; S = superior.)

(Fig. 26–3). Sometimes even the specific morphology of the atrial appendages may be visible, substantiating atrial situs (Fig. 26–3). More often, however, the atrial morphology is identified indirectly by noting the presence of the valve of the inferior vena cava (eustachian valve) within the right atrium, and by demonstration of the flap valve of the foramen ovale, which is the septum primum, within the left atrium (Fig. 26–5). When the situs is ambiguous, these atrial structures may be absent or vestigial. In these situations, one must rely on additional scanning of the abdomen for the relative positions of the aorta and the azygos, hemiazygos, or inferior caval veins to define the nature of an ambiguous situs that has been reported after birth.[34, 35] In situs solitus (usual atrial arrangement), the aorta is more posterior and leftward, whereas the inferior vena cava is more anterior and to the right of the spine (Fig. 26–6). The identification of these vessels can be complemented by interrogation with pulsed Doppler ultrasound. In situs inversus (mirror-image atrial arrangement), there is

mirror-image arrangement of these vessels, with the aorta posterior and to the right, the inferior vena cava anterior and to the left, and the stomach noted on the right. When the situs is ambiguous, there is either left atrial isomerism (polysplenia syndrome or double left-sidedness) or right atrial isomerism (asplenia syndrome or double right-sidedness). In left atrial isomerism the inferior vena cava is usually interrupted above the renal veins, and lower body venous drainage is via an azygos or hemiazygos venous system. These veins are identified posteior to the aorta and on either the same or the opposite side of the spine. Doppler interrogation allows rapid differentiation of arterial and venous structures (Fig.

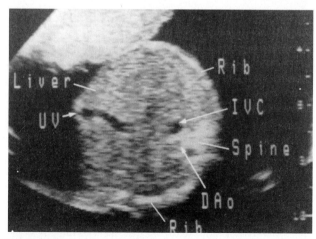

F I G U R E 26–6. Horizontal cut at the umbilical level in a fetus of 22 weeks' gestation demonstrating normal situs. Liver and umbilical vein (UV) lie anterior, the spine lies posterior. Note the inferior vena cava (IVC) more anterior and to the right of the spine, whereas the descending aorta (DAo) can be seen more posterior and to the left of the spine.

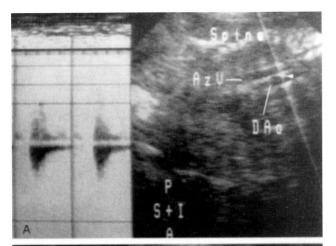

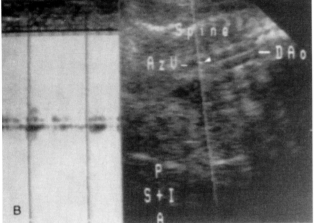

FIGURE 26–7. Abdominal sagittal view in a fetus of 23 weeks' gestation with left atrial isomerism (polysplenia syndrome) and complete heart block. *A,* In the right panel, two parallel vessels are recognized on the same side of the spine. The Doppler sample volume is placed in the anterior vessel (*arrowhead*). The Doppler display (*left*) shows an arterial flow signal at a rate of 57 bpm, thus identifying the descending aorta (DAo). *B,* In the right panel the Doppler sample volume is now seen in the posterior vessel (*arrowhead*). The Doppler display (*left*) demonstrates a low-velocity venous flow signal, thus indicating an azygous vein (AzV). This finding strongly suggests the presence of an interrupted inferior vena cava with azygous continuation of the lower body veins. (A = anterior; I = inferior; P = posterior; S = superior.)

noninflated lungs keep the diaphragm at a higher level within the chest, making the heart lie more horizontal than it does after birth. The four-chamber view usually allows identification of the prominent eustachian valve within the right atrium and the flap valve of the foramen ovale (septum primum) within the left atrium. In real time, the septum primum moves forward to the left atrial cavity and back toward the atrial septum twice during each cardiac cycle. The phasic movement of this interatrial valve appears to mirror the interatrial flow dynamics in the fetus. Both atrioventricular valves may be seen in the normal heart, and the tricuspid valve lies closer to the cardiac apex than does the mitral valve. The right ventricle often shows the septal attachment of the tricuspid valve leaflets, the moderator band, or the associated large anterior papillary muscle, and this right ventricle may appear slightly larger than the left ventricle.[5]

The four-chamber view allows definition of atrioventricular connections, evaluation of atrioventricular valve malformations, comparative assessment of chamber size, and identification of some positions of ventricular septal defects. Furthermore, more cranial scanning toward the outflow tracts in the four-chamber view may display the ventriculoarterial connections (Fig. 26–9), but this is not always possible, and other planes should be used to define these connections.

By rotating the transducer clockwise from the four-chamber view and tilting it slightly toward the fetal left shoulder, the scan plane is oriented in the long axis of the heart similar to long-axis views observed postnatally (Fig. 26–1*B*). These views often allow better definition of venoatrial, atrioventricular, and ventriculoarterial connections. The crossing of the right and the left ventricular outflow tract as well as the perpendicular relationship of the aorta (posterior) and of the pulmonary artery (anterior) can be defined (Fig. 26–10). This crossing of the great arteries will be absent when transposition of the great arteries occurs. Furthermore, long-axis

26–7). In right atrial isomerism there is almost invariably juxtaposition of the abdominal aorta and the inferior vena cava on the same side of the spine, either side by side, or in an anteroposterior relationship with the posterior vessel being the aorta. Again, in this situation it has been extremely valuable to confirm which vascular structure is which by pulsed Doppler interrogation of these vessels.

Having established the situs, the atrioventricular and ventriculoarterial connections are determined using a variety of examining planes. The four-chamber view (Fig. 26–1*A*) is easily obtained by tracing the inferior vena cava to the right atrium and then angling the transducer slightly cranially until the four chambers are visualized (Fig. 26–8). The relatively large fetal liver and the

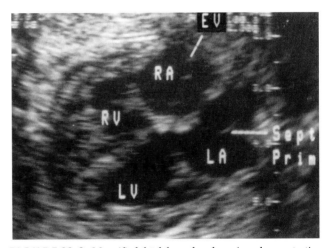

FIGURE 26–8. Magnified fetal four-chamber view demonstrating the eustachian valve (EV) within the right atrium (RA) and the flap valve of the foramen ovale, the septum primum, within the left atrium (LA). (LV = left ventricle; RV = right ventricle.)

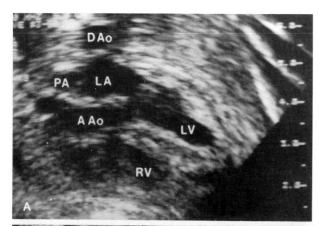

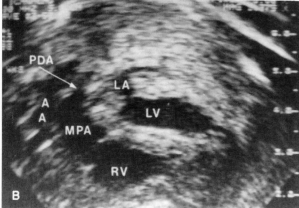

FIGURE 26–9. From the fetal four-chamber view, anterior angulation of the transducer displays the ventriculoarterial connections. *A,* The ascending aorta (AAo) is seen arising from the left ventricle (LV). The circular right pulmonary artery (PA) lies above the left atrium (LA) and behind the ascending aorta. (DAo = descending aorta.) *B,* With even further anterior angulation of the ultrasonic beam, the main pulmonary artery (MPA) is displayed arising from the right ventricle (RV) as it lies below the aortic arch (AA). The ductus arteriosus (PDA) is seen arising from the distal end of the main pulmonary artery.

planes demonstrate the left-sided structures of the heart similarly to views obtained postnatally (Fig. 26–10, *top*). With slight motion of the scan plane toward the fetal left side, the right ventricular outflow tract, the pulmonary valve, the main pulmonary artery, and the descending aorta also can be demonstrated (Fig. 26–10, *bottom*). From the long axis, slight clockwise rotation allows one to display the aortic root and the entire aortic arch (Fig. 26–1C), including the origin of the head and neck arteries, the aortic isthmus, the innominate vein, and the right pulmonary artery (Fig. 26–11). This plane is important because the origin of the head and neck vessels may help to identify the side of the aortic arch. Moving the plane slightly farther leftward shows the main pulmonary artery and its continuation into the descending aorta, where the ductus arteriosus is defined as that vessel connecting the pulmonary trunk at the site of origin of its branches to the descending aorta ("ductus-arch," Fig. 26–12). Aortic isthmus narrowing is a normal

feature in utero (Fig. 26–13), but may be distinguished from coarctation.

Short-axis views similar to those obtained postnatally can be acquired (Fig. 26–1D and E). This plane lies perpendicular to the long axis of the heart. Because of the horizontal lie of the fetal heart, the long-axis and short-axis views are often at right angles or parallel to the fetal spine, respectively. The short-axis views allows visualization of the fetal heart in cross-section from the level of the cardiac apex through the level of the ventricles, where the papillary muscle architecture in the left ventricle is best displayed, and more cranially where the mitral valve morphology is characteristic (Fig. 26–4, *bottom*), up to the level of the great arteries where the right ventricular outflow tract, the pulmonary trunk with its bifurcation into the branch pulmonary arteries (Fig. 26–14), and the ductus arteriosus can be seen. In this plane, obstructive lesions of the right ventricular outflow tract and of both semilunar valves can be dis-

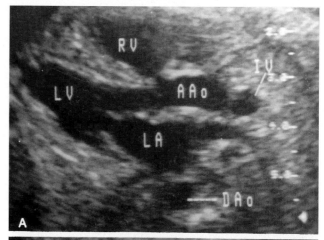

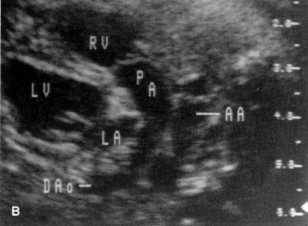

FIGURE 26–10. Magnified fetal long-axis view demonstrating the left atrioventricular and both ventriculoarterial connections. *A,* The left atrium (LA) drains into the left ventricle (LV) via the mitral valve. The ascending aorta (AAo) arises from the left ventricle. The innominate vein (IV) is seen coursing anterior to the aorta. The descending aorta (DAo) running posterior to the left atrium is imaged in cross-section. *B,* With slight angulation of the scan plane to the fetal left side the pulmonary artery (PA) is seen arising from the right ventricle (RV) and running below the aortic arch (AA).

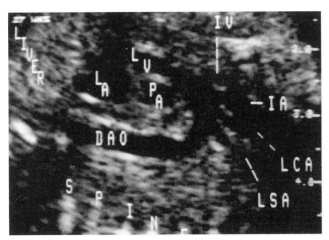

FIGURE 26-11. Fetal sagittal view of the entire fetal aortic arch. The arch with head and neck arteries (A) can be seen; the descending aorta (DAo) lies in front of the spine (S). The arteries arising from the aortic arch are the innominate (IA), the left carotid (LCA), and the left subclavian artery (LSA). In the concavity of this arch the left atrium (LA) and the right pulmonary artery (PA) are seen. Note that the "ductus-arch" cannot be seen in this plane. The mitral valve lies between the left atrium and the left ventricle (LV), and the aortic valve can be seen between the left ventricle and the ascending aorta. The innominate vein (IV) is seen coursing from the left to right in front of the aorta and innominate artery.

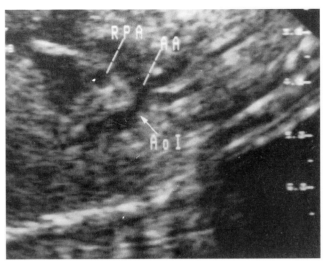

FIGURE 26-13. Magnified fetal sagittal view of the aortic arch (AA) demonstrating the normal aortic isthmus (AoI), which is relatively narrow. (RPA = right pulmonary artery.)

played, and the size and position of the great arteries assessed. Using high-resolution equipment, even the proximal coronary arteries may be displayed in this plane, thus helping to define the aortic vessel (Fig. 26–15). We have established a series of normal dimensions that can be read from the fetal scans rather than M-mode echocardiography, which can be used to assess whether the dimensions of a particular scan are within normal limits or fall outside the normal range (Fig. 26–16).

M-Mode Echocardiography

Real-time directed M-mode echocardiography in the fetus is a useful addition to cross-sectional imaging in the evaluation of ventricular cavity dimension and wall thickness, valve and wall motion, as well as cardiac

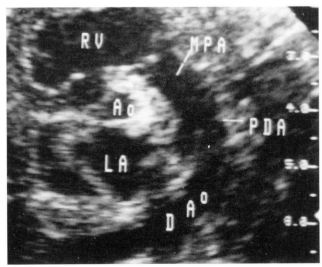

FIGURE 26-12. Magnified fetal sagittal view at 36 weeks' gestation demonstrating the continuation of main pulmonary artery (MPA), ductus arteriosus (PDA), and descending aorta (DAo), the so-called "ductus-arch." The ascending aorta (Ao) is seen in cross-section; the origin of the left pulmonary artery branch is seen, but the main continuation of the ductus continues as an arch into the descending aorta. Note that the ductus at this stage of gestation appears to be narrower than the caliber of pulmonary artery or the descending aorta. The other structures identified in this view are: the right atrium and right ventricle (RV), and a small portion of the left ventricle (LV).

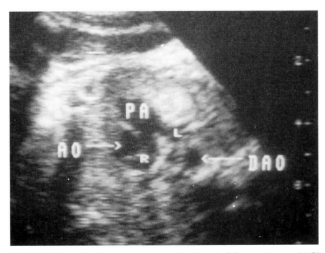

FIGURE 26-14. Short-axis view at the level of the aortic root (AO) in a fetus, depicting the pulmonary artery (PA) and its bifurcation into the right (R) and left pulmonary artery (L). The descending aorta (DAO) is seen in cross-section behind the bifurcating pulmonary branches.

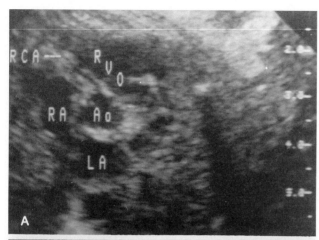

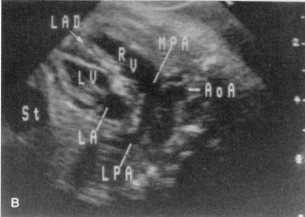

FIGURE 26–15. *A,* A magnified fetal short-axis view displays the right coronary artery (RCA), which arises from the aortic root (Ao). *B,* A long-axis view of the right ventricular (RV) outflow tract shows the left anterior descending coronary artery (LAD) running on the ventricular septum (AoA = aortic arch; LA = left atrium; LPA = left pulmonary artery; LV = left ventricle; MPA = main pulmonary artery; RA = right atrium; RVO = right ventricular outflow tract; St = stomach.)

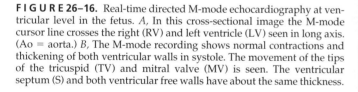

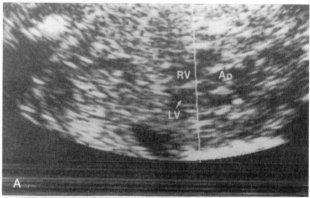

FIGURE 26–16. Real-time directed M-mode echocardiography at ventricular level in the fetus. *A,* In this cross-sectional image the M-mode cursor line crosses the right (RV) and left ventricle (LV) seen in long axis. (Ao = aorta.) *B,* The M-mode recording shows normal contractions and thickening of both ventricular walls in systole. The movement of the tips of the tricuspid (TV) and mitral valve (MV) is seen. The ventricular septum (S) and both ventricular free walls have about the same thickness.

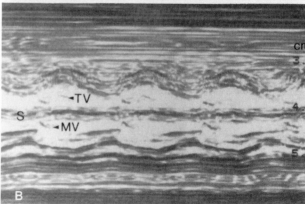

arrhythmias[12, 15, 18, 30–32, 36–38] (Figs. 26–17 and 26–18). Both long- and short-axis views at the level of the semilunar and atrioventricular valves allow the assessment of atrial and ventricular size (Figs. 26–19 and 26–20). Pericardial effusions, especially when small, are best substantiated by M-mode display where the separation of the parietal and visceral pericardium demonstrates how a pericardial effusion can be better distinguished from pleural effusions in the hydropic fetus (Figs. 26–19 and 26–20). For the exploration of fetal arrhythmias, M-mode recordings can be obtained from any plane, which allows simultaneous display of movements of an

(Text continued on page 394)

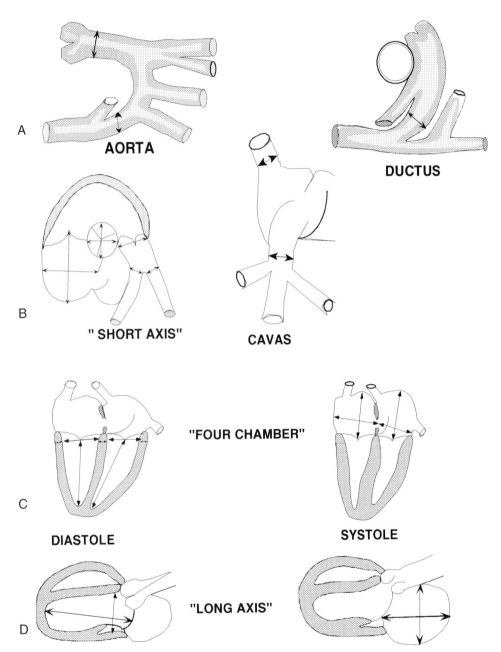

FIGURE 26–17. A graphic representation of the views that were used to obtain the dimensions (*arrows*) that were measured, which were graphed in the following figure. *A,* On the left, measurements made in the ascending and aortic isthmic region, and on the right, measurement of the ductus dimension. *B,* From the "short-axis" view (*left*), measurements of the right atrial, aortic root, pulmonary arterial, and branch left and right pulmonary arterial dimensions. The superior and inferior caval veins were measured (*right*) at the entrance of each cava into the right atrium. *C,* In the "four-chamber" view during diastole (*left*), the ventricular dimensions were measured just below the opposed tips of the atrioventricular valve leaflets; the ventricular lengths were also measured, as well as wall and septal thickness. In systole (*right*), the atrial dimensions were measured. *D,* On the left, measurements of the left heart in diastole obtained from "long-axis" equivalent and the left ventricular minor and major axis, and on the right, the left atrial dimensions from this view measured in systole. The arch of the aorta shown in the top left of the diagram was often seen from this plane.

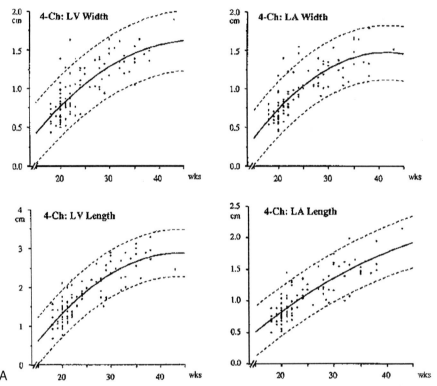

FIGURE 26–18. *A,* Left heart measurements from the four-chamber view (4-Ch). (LV = left ventricular; LA = left atrial.) *Note:* in each graph in this and the following figures, gestational age, in weeks, is displayed on the ordinate measurement, and ultrasound dimension, in centimeters, on the abscissa. Likewise, all graphs show the line of regression as a bold, continuous line, the 95% confidence intervals as dotted lines, and the data points for each fetus. (From Tan J, Silverman NH, Hoffman JIE, et al: Cardiac dimensions in the human fetus from 18 weeks to term: A cross-sectional echocardiographic study. Am J Cardiol 70: 1459–1467, 1992. Copyright 1992, Excerpta Medica Inc., with permission.)

Four-chamber view for:

Left ventricular width	n, 100 $y = -0.9478 + 0.1090 \times -0.001153 \times^2$ SEE, 0.200	r, 0.807
Left ventricular length	n, 100 $y = -2.318 \ + 0.2356 \times -0.002674 \times^2$ SEE, 0.308	r, 0.866
Left atrial width	n, 100 $y = -1.1246 + 0.1305 \times -0.001563 \times^2$ SEE, 0.181	r, 0.830
Left atrial length	n, 100 $y = -0.6508 + 0.0873 \times -0.000674 \times^2$ SEE, 0.196	r, 0.838

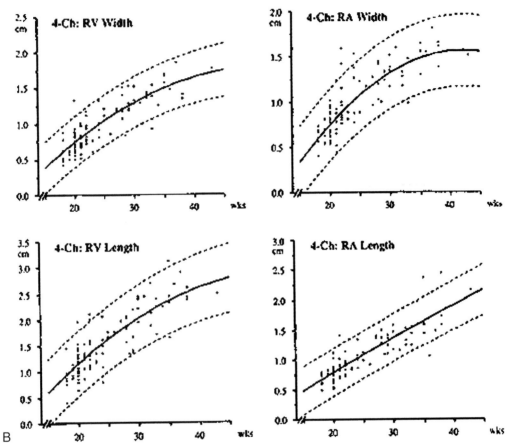

FIGURE 26–18 *Continued.* *B*, Right heart measurements from the four-chamber view (4-Ch). (RV = right ventricular dimensions; RA = right atrial dimensions.)

Four-chamber view for:

Right ventricular width	*n*, 100	y = −0.9869 + 0.1075 × −0.001036 ×² SEE, 0.179 *r*, 0.860
Right ventricular length	*n*, 100	y = −1.5082 + 0.1634 × −0.001514 ×² SEE, 0.316 *r*, 0.836
Right atrial width	*n*, 100	y = −1.4025 + 0.1410 × −0.001671 ×² SEE, 0.203 *r*, 0.826
Right atrial length	*n*, 100	y = −0.4873 + 0.06797 × −0.000202 ×² SEE, 0.199 *r*, 0.862

Illustration continued on following page

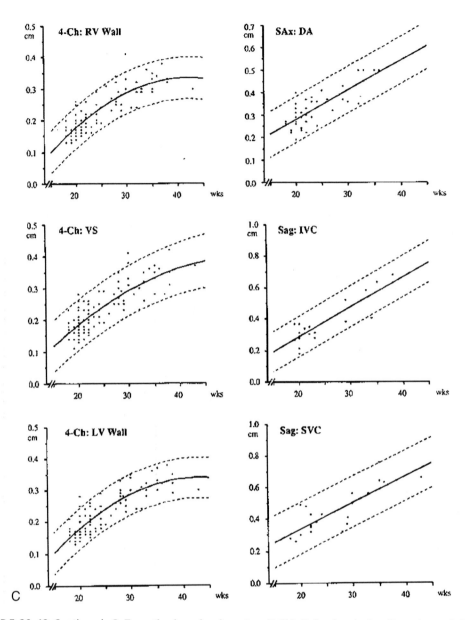

F I G U R E 26–18 *Continued. C,* From the four-chamber view (4-Ch) (*Left column*), the dimensions of the right ventricular (RV) wall, ventricular septum (VS), and left ventricular (LV) wall. *Right column,* From the short-axis view (SAx), the dimensions of the ductus arteriosus (DA), and from the sagittal view (Sag), the inferior vena cava (IVC) and superior vena cava (SVC).

Four-chamber view for:

Right ventricular wall	n, 100	$y = -0.2316 + 0.02677 \times -0.000316 \times^2$ SEE, 0.034 r, 0.857
Ventricular septum	n, 100	$y = -0.1415 + 0.0200 \times -0.000185 \times^2$ SEE, 0.040 r, 0.829
Left ventricular wall	n, 100	$y = -0.2136 + 0.02562 \times -0.000295 \times^2$ SEE, 0.033 r, 0.862

Short axis view for:

Ductus arteriosus	n, 38	$y = 0.01539 + 0.01325 \times$ SEE, 0.052 r, 0.787

Sagittal view for:

Inferior vena cava	n, 22	$y = -0.09012 + 0.01883 \times$ SEE, 0.065 r, 0.869
Superior vena cava	n, 22	$y = 0.004078 + 0.01673 \times$ SEE, 0.082 r, 0.815

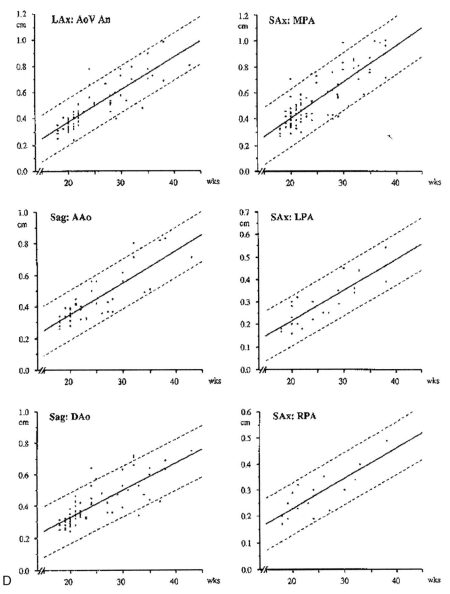

FIGURE 26-18 *Continued. D,* Measurements of the aortic and pulmonary arteries *Left column,* From the long-axis view (LAx), the diameter of the aortic valve annulus (AoV An), and from the sagittal view (Sag), the diameters of the ascending aortic root (AAo) and the descending aortic root (DAo). *Right column,* From the short-axis view (SAx), the diameter of the main pulmonary artery (MPA), left pulmonary artery (LPA), and right pulmonary artery (RPA).

Long-axis view:

Aortic valve annulus	$n = 71$ $y = -0.1278 + 0.02497 \times$ SEE, 0.089 r, 0.85	
Ascending aorta	$n = 45$ $y = -0.0523 + 0.0201 \times$ SEE, 0.081 r, 0.837	
Descending aorta	$n = 69$ $y = -0.0185 + 0.0173 \times$ SEE, 0.080 r, 0.801	

Short-axis view:

Main pulmonary artery	$n = 84$ $y = -0.1617 + 0.0279 \times$ SEE, 0.110 r, 0.825	
Left pulmonary artery	$n = 23$ $y = -0.0554 + 0.0136 \times$ SEE, 0.056 r, 0.839	
Right pulmonary artery	$n = 17$ $y = -0.0058 + 0.0117 \times$ SEE, 0.050 r, 0.817	

Illustration continued on following page

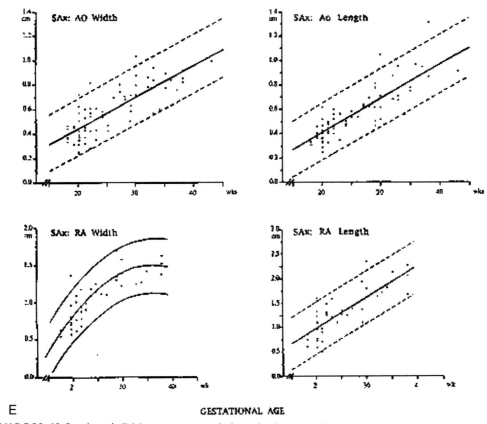

F I G U R E 26–18 *Continued. E,* Measurements made from the short axis (SAx). The top graphs show the dimension of the aorta (AO) from the horizontal plane (Width) on the left, and on the sagittal plane (Length) on the right. The bottom graphs show corresponding right atrial measurements (RA).

Short-axis view for:

Aortic width	$n = 75$ $y = -0.0545 + 0.257 \times$		SEE, 0.117 r, 0.807
Aortic length	$n = 75$ $y = -0.1502 + 0.02791 \times$		SEE, 0.114 r, 0.837
Right atrial width	$n = 43$ $y = -2.145 + 0.1976 \times -0.00273 \times^2$		SEE, 0.181 r, 0.853
Right atrial length	$n = 41$ $y = -0.293 + 0.06378 \times$		SEE, 0.279 r, 0.808

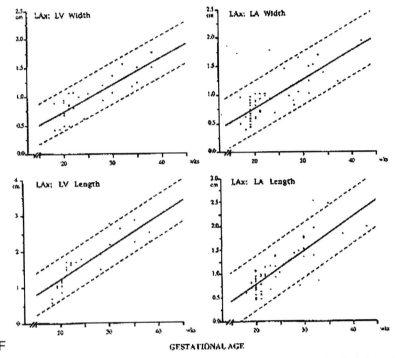

FIGURE 26-18 *Continued. F,* Left heart dimensions from the long-axis view (LAx). The left-hand graphs show the diastolic left ventricular (LV) minor axis (Width) and major axis (Length), while the graphs on the right show the left atrial (LA) anteroposterior dimension (Width) and superoinferior dimension (Length).

Long-axis view for:

Left ventricular width	$n = 31$	$y = -0.1739 + 0.0465 \times$	SEE, 0.180	r, 0.855
Left ventricular length	$n = 29$	$y = -0.4990 + 0.0868 \times$	SEE, 0.296	r, 0.887
Left atrial width	$n = 54$	$y = -0.3422 + 0.0498 \times$	SEE, 0.231	r, 0.778
Left atrial length	$n = 54$	$y = -0.6408 + 0.0707 \times$	SEE, 0.290	r, 0.810

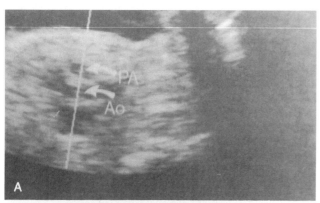

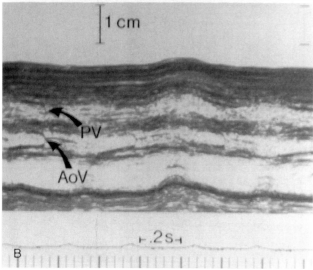

FIGURE 26–19. M-mode echocardiogram at the level of both great arteries. *A,* At the the base of the heart the M-mode reference line crosses the pulmonary artery (PA) and the aortic root (Ao). *B,* The typical systolic motion of both semilunar valves as open boxes is demonstrated. The *black arrows* indicate the closure of the pulmonary valve (PV) and of the aortic valve (AoV). The diameters of both great vessels can easily be measured from this M-mode recording. The depth and time markers in this figure relate to the bottom frame.

atrial and/or a ventricular wall, or of a semilunar valve and an atrioventricular valve. These features will be presented in the next chapter.

Doppler Echocardiography

Pulsed Doppler ultrasound demonstrates the direction and characteristics of blood flow within the fetal heart and the great vessels and allows qualitative and quantitative definition of flow disturbances such as those that occur with valvar stenotic or regurgitant lesions (Figs. 26–21 and 26–22). As is our practice after birth, pulsed Doppler ultrasound can also be used as a form of flow mapping, or "intracardiac stethoscope." Doppler ultrasound uses the principle of the change in frequency (the so-called Doppler shift) of sound waves reflected from the red blood cells within the cardiovascular system. If the red cells are traveling toward the transducer, the pitch increases, and if the cells are traveling away from the transducer, the pitch is lowered. These Doppler sig-

nals are displayed above or below the baseline, respectively. By timing the receiving period it is possible to "listen" at a specific distance from the transducer (range gating). This is displayed by a small line or box (so-called sample volume) on the cursor, which can be steered through any sector line or depth of the image. The size of the sample volume may vary from 1.5 mm to 9 mm in axial depth. Lateral resolution varies depending on the focal length of the transducer. The angle between blood flow and the path of the Doppler sound is called the angle θ. The more perpendicular the sound wave is to blood flow, the less the frequency (or velocity) changes. The ideal approach for sampling, then, is axial to blood flow. For practical purposes of measurement, it is desirable to keep the angle θ to less than 25 degrees. The Doppler carrier frequency we have used is 3 or 5 MHz, preferably the higher frequency to ensure lower ultrasound exposure of the fetus. Current state-of-the-art pulsed Doppler employing fast-Fourier analysis has become accepted standard. Currently, most ultrasound systems convert the frequency shift into a velocity display automatically from the formula:

$$v = \frac{f_d * c}{2.f_o * \cos \theta}$$

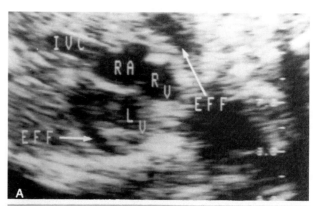

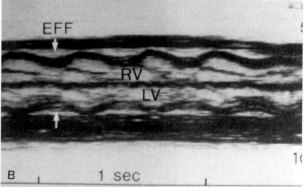

FIGURE 26–20. *A,* Magnified cross-sectional image of the heart at 22 weeks' gestation in a fetus with nonimmune hydrops. Although the pericardial effusion (EFF, *arrows*) may be seen, it can be better substantiated from the M-mode recording in the same fetus (*B*). The dense echoes of the pericardium and the rhythmically contracting ventricular myocardium are separated by the echo-free area of the effusion. (IVC = inferior vena cava; LV = left ventricle; RA = right atrium; RV = right ventricle.)

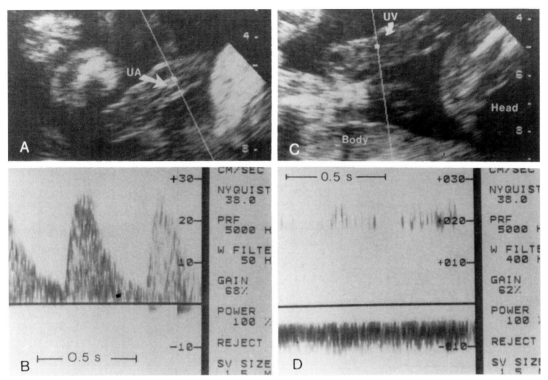

FIGURE 26–21. Pulsed Doppler interrogation at the site of the umbilical cord. *A,* The Doppler sample volume lies within the umbilical artery (UA, *arrow*). *B,* A characteristic umbilical arterial signal is displayed above the baseline demonstrating flow towards the transducer. *C,* The Doppler sample volume is now seen within the umbilical vein (UV, *arrow*); fetal body and head are also shown. *D,* A venous flow signal of fairly uniform low velocity throughout systole and diastole is demonstrated below the baseline; this flow is directed away from the transducer and towards the fetal body. Because the wall filter was set at 400 Hz compared to 50 Hz in the left panel, the origin of the spectral signals is blanked out.

where v is the velocity (m/s), f_d is the frequency shift (Hz), c is the conducting velocity of sound in water (1,500 m/sec), f_0 is the carrier frequency of the transducer (e.g., 3 or 5 MHz), and θ is the angle between the ultrasound beam and the direction of blood flow. One problem with pulsed Doppler ultrasound is that high-velocity flow cannot be determined accurately because of its finite-sampling rate. The frequency shift sampled from range-gating techniques can only be sampled at a rate that depends on the number of pulses of sound emitted by the transducer. If the frequency shift of the red blood cell targets exceeds the sampling frequency, aliasing of the signal occurs. This is analogous to observing a wagon wheel apparently spinning backwards as it is moving forward, which relates to optic sampling (27 cycles/sec for the human eye) being exceeded. To measure high velocities of flow, two alternatives are available: high-pulse-repetition frequency or continuous wave Doppler ultrasound. High-pulse-repetition frequency Doppler has an advantage in the fetus because the beam and the sample volume can be guided through the sector image to define the origin of the flow disturbance. Modern equipment allows continuous wave Doppler to be guided accurately through the sector image.

Doppler ultrasound, particularly the pulsed mode, exposes the fetus to higher levels of ultrasonic energy than M-mode or cross-sectional imaging. Although echocardiography, to date, has not been reported to have harmful effects on the developing fetus, Doppler ultrasonic energy should be kept at or below 100 mW/cm² (spatial peak-temporal average), and Doppler interrogation should be limited to as short a time as possible. On the other hand, Doppler ultrasound provides information unavailable with other techniques in the fetus and, despite the concern as to its bioeffects, remains a most valuable technique.

Color-coded Doppler flow mapping displays flow disturbance and flow direction and should be used where appropriate. In fact, rapid recognition of such disorders may limit the exposure time to Doppler ultrasound. Color-coded flow mapping is a most valuable technology for displaying flow information in real time, which provides some information about flow direction and the extent of flow disturbance. Flow mapping is a multigate Doppler technique where sampling along all the scan lines and depths in the field occurs simultaneously. No hard and fast standard of color Doppler display is in use; however, flow toward the transducer is commonly depicted as warm colors (orange, red), and flow away from the transducer is depicted as cool colors (blue). Disturbed flow signals are depicted as mixtures of these colors (e.g., yellow-green or turquoise). As these colors are displayed across the cross-sectional image in real time, not only can the direction of blood flow be mapped in time, but the direction and magnitude of flow disturbances such as leaks and stenoses also can be assessed.

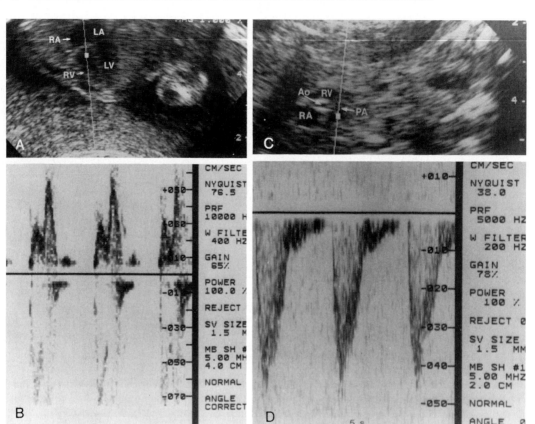

FIGURE 26–22. Normal fetal Doppler flow profiles across an atrioventricular and a semilunar valve are shown. *A*, In a four-chamber view the left atrium (LA), the right atrium (RA), the left ventricle (LV), and the right ventricle (RV) are seen. The sample volume lies below the tricuspid valve. The Doppler display (*B*) shows the diastolic inflow into the right ventricle above the baseline, indicating its direction towards the transducer. A biphasic signal is seen with a smaller v-component resulting from rapid venous filling, followed by a larger a-component (*black arrowheads*) resulting from atrial contraction. This pattern with predominant a-waves is typical for the fetus. The mirror-like display below the baseline is an artifact caused by too high a gain setting. *C*, In a fetal short-axis view, the right atrium (RA), right ventricle (RV), pulmonary artery (PA), and aorta (Ao) are seen. The sample volume lies distal to the pulmonary valve within the pulmonary artery. The Doppler flow signal below the baseline is directed away from the transducer (*D*).

This technique has been most valuable for the assessment of congenital heart disease in utero. Unfortunately, because the energy levels of this ultrasound method are higher than those of older, established modalities, certain manufacturers have recommended that this technique be curtailed in the fetus.

Doppler interrogation within vascular structures either at the level of the umbilical cord or within the fetal body identifies arterial or venous flow (Figs. 26–7 and 26–21), helping the ultrasonographer to distinguish arteries and veins and to evaluate the direction of blood flow in complex cardiovascular malformations. Normal flow velocity profiles across both the atrioventricular and the semilunar valves have been defined in the fetus[39–42] (Fig. 26–22); normal values for peak and mean temporal flow velocities as well as for volume flow across these valves have been established (Table 26–1). The flow velocity curve across a fetal atrioventricular valve normally is characterized by an early v-component (due to venous filling), which is followed by a higher and later a-component (due to atrial contraction) (Fig. 26–22, *left*). This pattern is different from that observed postnatally and in the adult, where the v-component is higher

than the a-component and may relate to the fetal ventricular size or to diminished fetal ventricular compliance. Because flow through the atrioventricular orifice relates to filling in that portion of diastole, the high fetal a-component suggests that a substantial amount of filling

TABLE 26–1. FLOW MEASUREMENT IN THE NORMAL FETAL HEART*

	PEAK VELOCITY (CM/S)	MEAN TEMPORAL VELOCITY (CM/S)
Tricuspid valve†	51 ± 9.1	11.8 ± 3.1
Mitral valve†	47 ± 8.3	11.2 ± 2.3
Pulmonary valve†	60 ± 12.9	16 ± 4.1
Aortic valve†	70 ± 12.2	18 ± 3.3
Right ventricular output‡	307 ± 127 mL/kg/min	
Left ventricular output‡	232 ± 106 mL/kg/min	

*Adapted from Reed KL, Meijboom EJ, Sahn DJ, et al: Cardiac Doppler flow velocities, in human fetuses. Circulation 73:41–46, 1986, with permission.
†Angle-corrected maximal and mean temporal flow velocities across the cardiac valves are expressed as mean ± SD.
‡Cardiac output derived from tricuspid and mitral valve area and mean velocities (mean ± SD).

occurs as a result of atrial contraction. This may explain why fetal tachycardia is so poorly tolerated in the fetus and may lead to the development of fetal hydrops.

The highest velocity in the fetal heart is recorded within the ductus arteriosus[43] (Fig. 26–22, *right*); color-coded Doppler flow mapping demonstrates aliased flow in the fetal ductus. By using Doppler interrogation in a direction where the blood flow velocity is axial to the sample volume, one may obtain high-velocity profiles across stenotic or regurgitant atrioventricular and semilunar valves, which permits estimation of the pressure difference across these valves (Fig. 26–23). The modified Bernoulli equation is used for this purpose, which states that the pressure drop (measured in mm Hg) across an orifice is proportional to four times the squared peak velocity (in m/sec) across that valve:

$$P = 4\,V_d^2,$$

where V_d is the high velocity in the jet distal to the stenotic orifice.[44, 45]

The characteristics of the pulse in the umbilical artery have been used to demonstrate altered flow dynamics in growth-retarded fetuses. The ratio of the peak systolic velocity divided by the minimal diastolic velocity is called the pulsatility index; it changes normally during gestation.[46, 47] Higher ratios reflecting increasing vascular resistance of the placental vascular bed suggest a decreased flow to the placenta, such as occurs in growth-retarded fetuses.[48] By using ratios, the measurements may be less dependent on the angle of insonification. In our experience, Doppler ultrasound was an essential feature in the examination of a fetus with congenital heart disease, enabling us to demonstrate stenotic and regurgitant lesions[49] and to diagnose arrhythmias. The use of this ultrasound modality allows detection of cardiac lesions not possible by other methods (e.g., mitral regurgitation in a cardiomyopathy).

Recently, the use of color flow mapping has added a dimension to cardiac evaluation, allowing rapid detection of stenotic or regurgitant jets, shunts, and normal and abnormal flow patterns, thereby diminishing the time required for Doppler interrogation (Fig. 26–24). Because energy levels of the Doppler output in the color flow mode are slightly higher than with B-mode ultrasound and other modes of Doppler ultrasound interrogation, its use should be curtailed. Doppler color flow mapping also provides information on a variety of flow disturbances, including valvar stenosis and regurgitation, abnormal flow patterns such as reversed atrial and ductus shunt flow, interventricular communications, ventricular shunting, and confirmation of vascular structures. It even can be used for calculating flow from umbilical venous velocity, as the product of the mean velocity and cross-sectional area.[50]

Although Doppler ultrasound readily defines stenotic and regurgitant lesions, one must be aware of certain pitfalls. Because of the physical principle of beam divergence, ambiguity in the position of the sample volume may occur in closely situated structures. For example, due to beam divergence, sampling within the right atrium close to the aorta may lead to the misinterpreta-

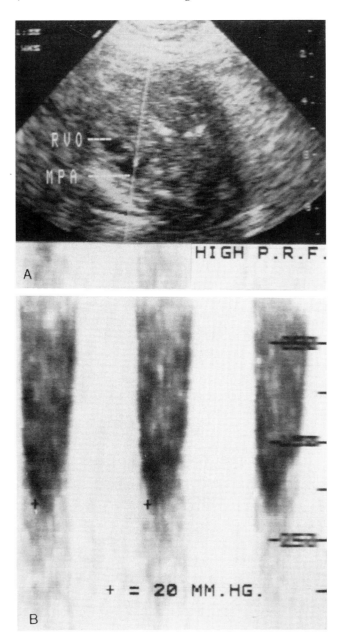

FIGURE 26–23. *A*, The Doppler sample volume is placed in the main pulmonary artery of this 23-week-old fetus whose mother was on high dosage of lithium. The Doppler sample volume lies just above the pulmonary valve in the ascending aorta (Ao). The right ventricular outflow tract (RVO) is labeled. *B*, Although the angle at the site of Doppler interrogation is more than 25 degrees, thus underestimating the flow velocity, high-pulse-repetition-frequency Doppler demonstrates a jet velocity of 2.2 m/sec, indicating a 20-mm Hg pressure gradient. The scale in the frame reads 50, 150, and 250 cm/sec.

tion of tricuspid regurgitation because, in fact, the signal of a normal flow in the ascending aorta was sampled. This becomes particularly important when short-focused high-frequency transducers are used because these frequencies have rapid far-field divergence of the sound beam. Unfavorable fetal position or a great distance from the transducer, as in cases of polyhydramnios, may limit the Doppler technique in certain cases. Attempts have been made to calculate fetal cardiac output from blood flow velocity profiles,[39, 42, 51] but this calcu-

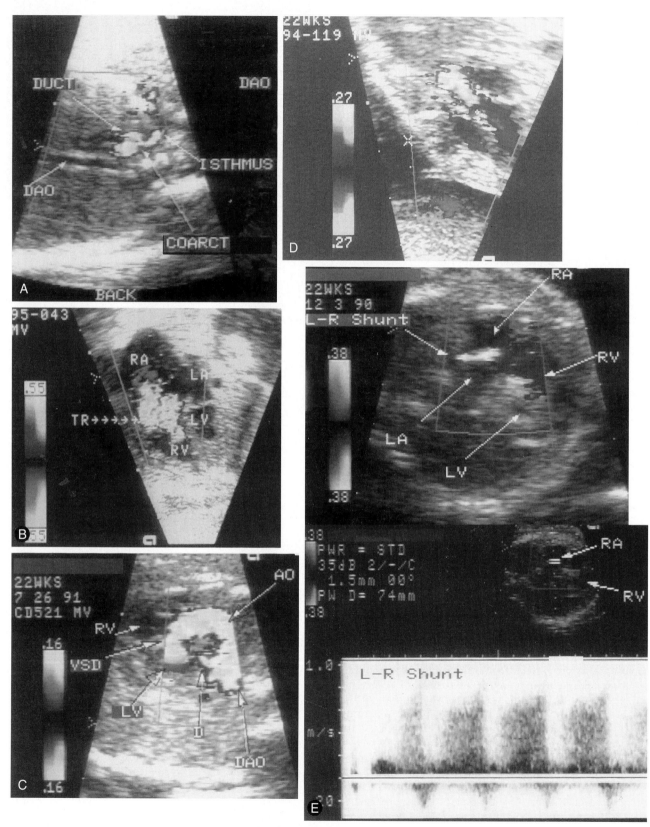

FIGURE 26–24. *See legend on opposite page*

lation unfortunately requires accurate measurement of valve or vessel diameters. Inaccuracy of even 1 mm may yield an unacceptably high error in the calculation of fetal cardiac output, particularly when the flow vessel diameter was small. The calculation of flow in experimental animal models, however, leads us to believe that valid measurements of aortic and pulmonic flow may be made, and combined cardiac output as well as left and right ventricular stroke volume may be obtained.

Detection of Structural Defects

Studies have shown a different spectrum of congenital heart disease in fetuses from the presentation at birth. Allan and colleagues have defined the incidence in 1,006 fetuses.[52] Table 26–2 demonstrates the reasons for referral, by diagnostic category. The outcome of these pregnancies is shown in Table 26–3. The spectrum of disease appears different from that seen after birth (Table 26–4). Previously, others[53] have shown that the outcome of lesions detected prenatally carried a poor prognosis for long-term survival, although recent studies suggest that some lesions detected by fetal ultrasound carry an improved prognosis.[54]

Among the 3,000 fetuses we have now studied, we have maintained an incidence of structural cardiac abnormalities in 9% of referrals and cardiac rhythm disturbances in 17%. The remaining studies were within normal limits. This description follows that of the frequency set out by Allan[52] (Table 26–3), with the exception that we have grouped common lesions together, such as left heart hypoplasia and conotruncal abnormalities.

Atrioventricular Septal Defect

The commonest serious structural abnormality found in Allan's series was atrioventricular septal defect (Fig. 26–25). The major reason for referral has been the associ-

ation of chromosomal abnormalities such as Down syndrome. This defect was less often part of a complex cardiac lesion including left atrial isomerism, complete heart block, and nonimmune hydrops.

Pathophysiology and Natural History

There is usually no left-to-right shunt in utero because of similar pressures in both atria and both ventricles. There is most frequently little atrioventricular valvar regurgitation in utero. As the ostium primum defect is close to the tricuspid valve, there may be some redirection of superior vena caval blood into the left atrium with a decrease of oxygen saturation between the ascending and descending aorta. Also, because of the potential mixing of blood from the atrial and ventricular defects, the Po_2 of the pulmonary arterial blood flow may increase and aortic blood flow may decrease. This would diminish the amount of blood flowing across the aortic isthmus and increase the likelihood of isthmic hypoplastic and aortic coarctation. As the fetus is sensitive to small increases in pulmonary arterial oxygen concentration, pulmonary blood flow may increase, and there may be a diminution of blood flow into the ascending aorta. All fetuses with this diagnosis should have chromosomal analysis, because of the high incidence in this condition.

Management Strategies

There is no reason to deliver these patients early, as surgical repair is easier in larger patients.

Hypoplasia of the Left Heart

The second most frequent lesion reported in Allan's series was hypoplastic left heart syndrome. When one considers mitral atresia and critical aortic stenosis and coarctation of the aorta together, this group of lesions

---

FIGURE 26–24. Five different examples of the use of Doppler color flow mapping. *A,* Aortic coarctation (Coarc.) demonstrated by Doppler color flow mapping in a 20-week-gestation fetus. The arch was imaged in its long axis showing the isthmus of the aorta, and the entrance of the arterial duct and the continuation as the descending aorta (DAO). *B,* Ebstein's malformation with severe pulmonary stenosis in a four-chamber view. The orientation shows the right atrium (RA), left atrium (LA), left ventricle (LV), and right ventricle (RV). The tricuspid regurgitation (TR) is shown in this systolic frame. Additionally, on the left, the Nyquist limit defines the range of velocities that may be defined by this Doppler method; here these are set at 55 cm/sec. *C,* A ductus arteriosus (D) as a sole supply of the minute pulmonary arteries in a patient with pulmonary atresia and a ventricular septal defect. There the signals are all aliased, that is, above the Nyquist limit of 16 cm/sec. Flow here is represented as a "color angiogram" showing the flow arising from the left ventricle (LV), through the ventricular septal defect (VSD), into the right ventricle (RV) and into the aorta (AO). The flow can be followed into the descending aorta (DAO) and through the small ductus (D) into the pulmonary circulation. The ductus flow is imaged and flowing in the opposite direction of normal fetal ductus flow, that is, left to right. *D,* Flow mapping in a fetus with aortic stenosis. Here the map shows acceleration in this systolic frame as blood is accelerated through the stenotic aortic valve. The blue blood exceeds the limit of the Nyquist range at 22 cm/sec. At this low velocity this does not indicate severe stenosis, which must always be assessed by Doppler techniques such as continuous wave Doppler ultrasound, which have the facility to define higher velocities. This map indicates the acceleration site was at the level of the valve. *E,* A flame-shaped jet from the left atrium projecting into the right atrium. This is the opposite direction of normal flow expected in the fetus. In this instance the fetus had hypoplastic left heart syndrome with associated mitral atresia. Pulmonary venous blood could only be directed across the atrial septum into the right atrium. The *middle* and *bottom* frames in *E* show the sample volume directed to the site of the flame, and the resulting left-to-right atrial shunt in the bottom frame shows the velocity of this left-to-right shunt rising to nearly 1 m/sec and indicating a substantial abnormality.

TABLE 26–2. REASONS FOR REFERRAL BY DIAGNOSTIC CATEGORY OF 1,006 FETUSES WHO HAD FETAL ECHOCARDIOGRAPHY*

DIAGNOSIS	REASON FOR REFERRAL†					FOLLOW-UP†		
	Positive Family History	Extracardiac Anomaly	Fetal Arrhythmia	Hydrops	Echo Suspected Heart Malformation	Follow-up Information Available	Additional Diagnosis after Birth	Incorrect Diagnosis or Central Diagnosis Unconfirmed
Atrioventricular septal defect	177	15	14	7	14	127	154	26
Hypoplastic left heart syndrome	161	11	6	1	6	137	127	3
Coarctation of the aorta	113	23	18	2	4	66	104	8
Tricuspid dysplasia/ Ebstein anomaly	75	6	0	2	1	66	66	6
Ventricular septal defect	60	10	17	3	5	25	52	3
Mitral atresia	60	5	5	0	0	48	50	0
Pulmonary atresia, IVS/critical PS	55	2	0	0	2	49	48	0
Tricuspid atresia	45	1	1	0	0	43	43	7
Critical aortic stenosis	41	0	1	0	1	39	40	0
Cardiomyopathies	41	0	13	1	7	20	37	0
Conotruncal abnormalities								
Double-outlet right ventricle	33	1	4	1	1	25	26	1
Tetralogy of Fallot	31	5	15	1	1	9	27	1
Complete transposition	20	6	1	0	0	12	20	0
Double-inlet ventricle	18	1	0	0	0	17	17	2
Tetralogy with pulmonary atresia	15	2	1	0	0	11	11	1
Common arterial trunk	14	7	1	0	0	6	14	0
Tumor	13	1	0	0	1	11	13	0
Conjoined twins and ectopia cordis	12	0	0	0	0	12	12	5
Absent pulmonary valve syndrome	10	0	0	0	0	10	7	0
Aortic–left ventricular tunnel	4	0	0	0	0	4	4	3
TAPVC	3	2	0	0	0	1	3	2
Congenitally corrected transposition	3	0	0	0	0	3	3	0
Miscellaneous	(5)							
Calcific arterial disease	2	1	0	0	1	0		
Interruption of the aorta	1	1	0	0	0	0		
Mitral stenosis	1	0	0	0	1	0		
Idiopathic right atrial enlargement	1	0	0	0	0	1		

* From Allan LD, Sharland GK, Milburn A, et al: Prospective diagnosis of 1,006 consecutive cases of congenital heart disease in the fetus. J Am Coll Cardiol 23:1452–1458, 1994. Copyright 1994, Excerpta Medica Inc., with permission.
†Data are the number of cases.
IVS, interventricular septum; PS, pulmonary stenosis; TAPVC, total anomalous pulmonary venous connection. See text for details of each diagnosis.

TABLE 26–3. OUTCOME OF 1,006 FETUSES WHO HAD FETAL ECHOCARDIOGRAPHY*

DIAGNOSIS	CHROMOSOMAL ANOMALY (%)	TERMINATION OF PREGNANCY (%)	INTRAUTERINE DEATH (%)	NEONATAL DEATH (%)	DEATH IN INFANCY OR CHILDHOOD (%)	SURVIVORS OF CONTINUING PREGNANCIES (%)
Atrioventricular septal defect	35	62	20	11	3	37
Hypoplastic left heart syndrome	4	72	5	20	0.6	4
Coarctation of the aorta	29	46	11	10	4	51
Tricuspid dysplasia/Ebstein anomaly	5	44	14	17	2	38
Ventricular septal defect	48	41	16	15	3	40
Mitral atresia	18	68	6	18	3	11
Pulmonary atresia, IVS/critical PS	5	50	9	7	1	63
Tricuspid atresia	2	53	4	4	6	61
Critical aortic stenosis		56	4	31	2	11
Cardiomyopathies	2	35	20	15	2	40
Double-outlet right ventricle	12	75	6	6	0	50
Tetralogy of Fallot	27	35	13	16	13	35
Complete transposition	0	40	0	5	0	92
Double-inlet ventricle	0	72	0	1	0	80
Tetralogy with pulmonary atresia	13	40	6	33	13	11
Common arterial trunk	14	50	0	40	30	0
Tumor	0	38	30	0	0	44
Conjoint twins and ecopia cordis	0	58	0	33	0	20
Absent pulmonary valve syndrome	20	30	30	30	10	0
Aortic–left ventricular tunnel	0	75	0	0	25	0
TAPVC	30	0	0	33	33	33
Congenitally corrected transposition	0	66	0	33	0	0
Miscellaneous	0	0	40	20	20	20

* From Allan LD, Sharland GK, Milburn A, et al: Prospective diagnosis of 1,006 consecutive cases of congenital heart disease in the fetus. J Am Coll Cardiol 23:1452–1458, 1994. Copyright 1994, Excerpta Medica Inc., with permission.
Abbreviations as in Table 26–2.

TABLE 26–4. COMPARISON OF DISEASES SEEN IN INFANT AND FETAL SERIES*

DIAGNOSIS	BROMPTON (%)	NERICP (%)	FETAL (%)
Ventricular septal defect	15.4	15.7	5
Complete transposition	10.4	9.9	2
Tetralogy of Fallot	9.9	8.9	3
Coarctation	10.5	7.5	11
Hypoplastic left heart syndrome	3.7	7.4	16
Mitral atresia	0	0	5
Critical aortic stenosis	1.1	1.9	4
Atrioventricular septal defect	3.9	5.0	17.5
Pulmonary stenosis/atresia	4.9	6.4	5
Atrial septal defect	0.5	2.9	0
Total anomalous pulmonary venous connection	3.6	2.6	<1
Cardiomyopathy	2.7	2.6	4
Tricuspid atresia	4.7	2.6	4
Double-inlet ventricle	4.3	2.4	2
Double-outlet right ventricle	3.0	1.5	3
Trunk	2.1	1.4	1.5
Ebstein malformation	0	0	7
Tumor	0	0	1
Corrected transposition	0.8	0.9	<1
Miscellaneous	11.3	10.4	<1

* From Allan LD, Sharland GK, Milburn A, et al: Prospective diagnosis of 1,006 consecutive cases of congenital heart disease in the fetus. J Am Coll Cardiol 23:1452–1458, 1994. Copyright 1994, Excerpta Medica Inc., with permission.
Brompton, Royal Brompton Hospital, London; NERICP, New England Regional Infant Cardiac Care Program.

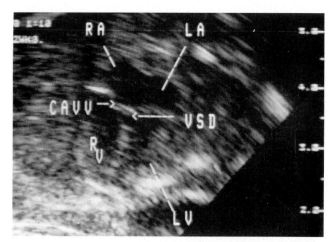

FIGURE 26–25. Fetal four-chamber view at 32 weeks' gestation. An atrioventricular (canal) septal defect is demonstrated. The common atrioventricular valve (CAVV, *white arrows*) straddles a common atrioventricular orifice dividing the large defect seen in this view into an atrial and a ventricular component. (LA = left atrium; LV = left ventricle; RA = right atrium; RV = right ventricle.)

may be the most frequently recognized group of fetal cardiac diseases. Classic cases of hypoplastic left heart syndrome can be recognized early in the second trimester (Fig. 26–26).

Pathophysiology and Natural History

Left heart hypoplasia may develop because of underdevelopment of the left ventricle or restriction of mitral inflow, or as a consequence of aortic stenosis. During development, the fetus with aortic stenosis may have some redistribution of cardiac output, thereby diminishing the left-sided stroke output and increasing the right-heart output. The obstruction takes extra force to overcome. As a consequence there is an increased workload. Because diastolic pressure in the fetus is low, myocardial blood supply is also low. The oxygen demand of the left ventricle is increased because of the workload necessary to overcome the aortic obstruction, and the ratio of myocardial oxygen demand to oxygen supply is compromised because of the high myocardial oxygen demand and the gradation of myocardial blood flow. If ischemia develops, it does so first in the inner layer because myocardial perfusion is lowest in the inner third of the myocardium and highest in the outer third. Perhaps that is why endocardial fibrosis develops in aortic stenosis. Once this has developed the inner layers of the myocardium may become restrictive to filling. As it is well known that form follows flow dynamics[55, 56] within the developing cardiovascular system, this inner layer may become restrictive, preventing filling of the ventricle and restricting further growth. There is now clear evidence for this phenomenon from measurements.

From our own experience, as well as the studies published by Sharland[57] and Hornberger et al.,[58, 59] aortic stenosis and hypoplastic left heart clearly may be progressive aspects of the same disease in certain cases. Intervention by means of catheter or direct surgical intervention has been contemplated.[54] Hypoplastic left

heart syndrome may develop for other reasons, such as mitral atresia. In such instances, the ventricle may fail to develop because it does not have any blood flow to change its size.

Management Strategies

In utero recognition has made several important potential contributions to future invasive management of the fetus with this lesion. We have directed our efforts at consideration of direct catheterization of umbilical vessels in an experimental model.[60] In aortic atresia or stenosis, the use of balloon valvuloplasty has been considered. In a recent study, Kohl polled the major centers regarding their use of balloon valvuloplasty in utero for this condition.[61] Only one of seven fetuses survived for any length of time.

In our own experience, prenatal recognition of hypoplastic left heart syndrome has led to postnatal survival of over 90% of referred patients.[54]

Pathophysiology and Natural History

With regard to mitral stenosis and mitral atresia, blood flow is redirected across the atrial septum from left to right. This has been observed by Doppler color flow mapping.[62] Unless the atrial septum becomes restrictive, there is no impact on development because the shifts of flow occur with a circulation in parallel. Restriction of atrial left-to-right shunt may occur, particularly when there is mitral regurgitation, which may lead to early and serious pulmonary edema as the pulmonary blood flow and venous return increase.

Ebstein Malformation and Associated Tricuspid Valve Dysplasia

Ebstein malformation was a commonly recognized abnormality (Fig. 26–27). It is clear that some may die with severe hydrops in utero, or early in postnatal life, which may account in part for the much lower frequency of this lesion in series gathered after birth, particularly after the period of early infancy. We have encountered fetuses that were products of mothers who had the same lesion; these mothers had taken high doses of lithium, a known cardiac teratogen,[23, 63] during early pregnancy.[49, 64]

Pathophysiology and Natural History

This lesion is one of the most significant causes of fetal hydrops, heart failure, and fetal loss.[49, 65] This lesion has at its core fetal atrioventricular valvar regurgitation, which leads to ineffective pulmonary flow. In fact, we have observed diminishing pulmonary forward flow from early studies using M-mode and subsequent studies with Doppler ultrasound. There is an increasing right-to-left atrial shunt. Because of diminished forward flow across the pulmonary valve, the increasing systemic flow, and the presence of systemic pressure within the pulmonary arterial ductus–pulmonary artery circulation, the pulmonary valve is held closed. This may

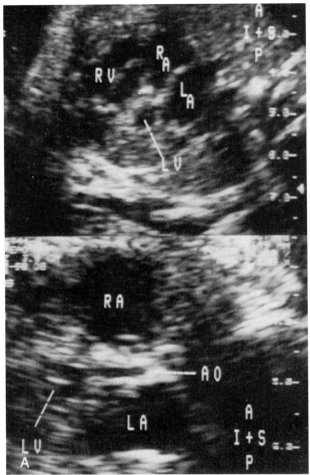

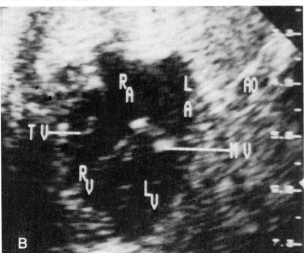

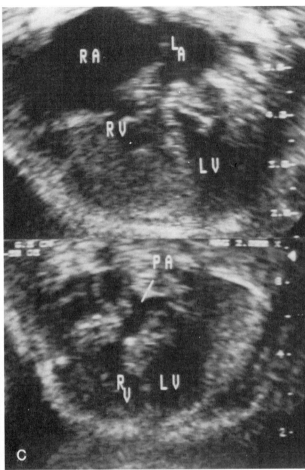

FIGURE 26–26. A composite figure showing various features of hypoplastic left and right ventricular lesions. *A,* The top frame shows a four-chamber view of the heart indicating a hypoplastic left ventricle (LV). The other chambers (RV = right ventricle; RA = right atrium; LA = left atrium) are seen. Note the diminutive but clear mitral valve between the left-sided atrium and ventricle. Orientation: A = anterior; I = inferior; P = posterior; S = superior. The bottom frame shows a magnified view in a similar plane but focusing on the minute left ventricle (LV); the extremely small left ventricular outflow and ascending aorta is less than 2 mm in diameter. *B,* This example in a 27-week-old fetus shows severe mitral stenosis due to a parachute mitral valve and an associated mid-muscular ventricular septal defect. Note that in this diastolic frame the tricuspid valve (TV) is opened widely, whereas the mitral valve (MV) appears as a dense white mass of echoes. The left atrium (LA) and left ventricle are of good size because of communications between both atria and ventricles. (Ao = aorta; RA = right atrium.) *C,* Composite four-chamber images of the heart in a fetus with a classic form of hypoplastic right ventricle (pulmonary atresia with intact ventricular septum). In the top frame, the right ventricular wall is hypertrophic and the right ventricular cavity is diminutive. The right atrium (RA) is enlarged, and a normal sized tricuspid valve lies between these chambers. The atrial septum bulges into the left atrium (LA); the left atrium and left ventricle (LV) are of normal size. In the bottom frame, the transducer has been angled superiorly to display the right ventricular outflow tract and the pulmonary artery (PA). Although the pulmonary artery is well developed (because it has been fed by the fetal ductus), there was evidence of pulmonary valve opening and only a dense white plate of echoes is seen in the region of the pulmonary annulus.

Illustration continued on following page

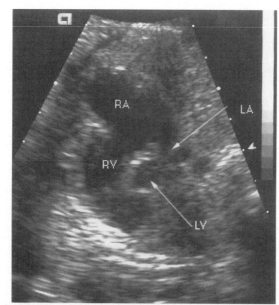

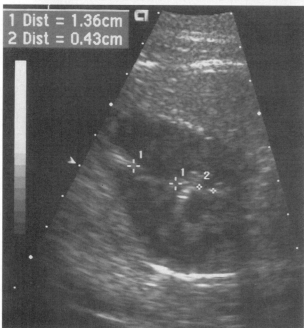

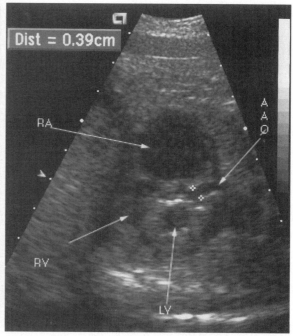

FIGURE 26–26 Continued. D, This 32-week-old fetus was sent for evaluation because the fetus was recognized to have a hypoplastic left ventricle and the physician and parents had requested surgical repair with the Norwood operation. The first two frames show the left ventricle shows bright endocardial outline, and a much smaller mitral valve than tricuspid valve (0.43 cm vs. 1.36 cm). The aorta shown in the subsequent frame shows a dimension of 0.39 cm, much below the expected aortic diameter for the aorta at this gestational age.

lead to the development of valvar synechia and acquired pulmonary valvar atresia.

Management Strategies

There is no treatment strategy for this lesion.

Ventricular Septal Defects

Ventricular septal defects were found with a fairly high frequency (Table 26–2, Fig. 26–28). We have observed two instances of spontaneous closure of ventricular septal defects on subsequent fetal examinations when there was no additional lesion.

Cardiomyopathy

We have encountered several cases of cardiomyopathy, more often the congestive form with dilated, poorly contracting ventricles and atrioventricular valve regurgitation associated with fetal hydrops (Figs. 26–29 and 26–30). In only one study did the abnormality begin as a predominantly right-sided lesion; in this family, a previous sibling had presented similarly. One fetus presented as a hypertrophic cardiomyopathy, clinically identified to have Noonan syndrome at birth. Two fetuses appeared to have normal cardiac function at 20 weeks' gestation but were recognized to have congestive cardiomyathy shortly after birth, suggesting that it may not always be possible to detect this abnormality prena-

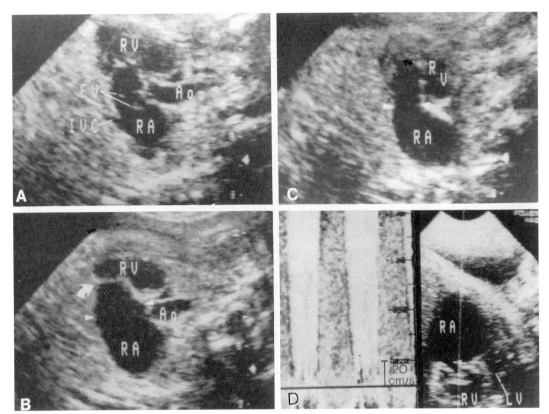

FIGURE 26–27. Magnified sagittal view in a fetus of 20 weeks' gestation with Ebstein anomaly. *A,* The inferior vena cava (IVC) drains into the dilated right atrium (RA); the eustachian valve (EV) can be seen marking the approximate position of the atrioventricular groove. The right ventricle (RV) and aorta (Ao) are also seen. *B,* The displacement of the valve leaflets, especially of the posteroinferior leaflet (*thick arrow*), is demonstrated during systole when the leaflets are apposed. The tricuspid valve ring, which is part of the atrioventricular groove is marked by *small arrowheads. C,* In a diastolic frame the displaced posteroinferior leaflet is shown tethered to the diaphragmatic surface of the right ventricular wall. *D,* On the right is a reference cross-sectional image with Doppler sample volume placed in the right atrium. (RA = right ventricle; LV = left ventricle.) The Doppler sample shows a high-velocity jet at over 150 cm/sec representing the tricuspid regurgitation.

tally, and that myocardial dysfunction may occur either after examination in utero or after birth.

Pulmonary Atresia with Intact Ventricular Septum or Critical Pulmonary Stenosis

Pulmonary atresia with intact ventricular septum or critical pulmonary stenosis was found in 5.5% of Allan's series.

Pathophysiology and Natural History

There is now evidence that this is a progressive lesion.[58, 66–68] Perhaps pulmonary stenosis develops first, which leads to progressive right ventricular hypertrophy. There is accompanying leak of the tricuspid valve, which has been observed in utero. The reason for the ventriculocoronary connections is less clearly established.

When this lesion is encountered early in the second trimester of gestation, the right ventricle may appear larger than the left. Later it appears to adopt the hypoplastic size associated with the postnatal appearance of the lesion (Fig. 26–26). The ventricle fills poorly, as for

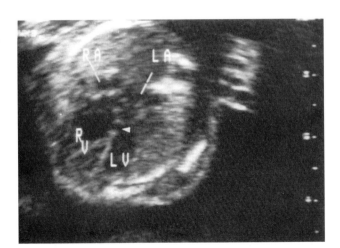

FIGURE 26–28. Fetal four-chamber view in a 32-week fetus. An isolated ventricular septal defect (VSD) is depicted in the apical muscular part of the ventricular septum (*arrow*). (LV = left ventricle; RA = right atrium; RV = right ventricle.)

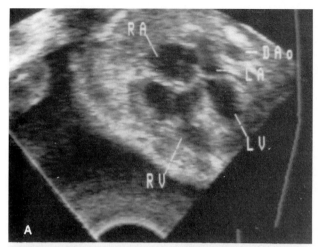

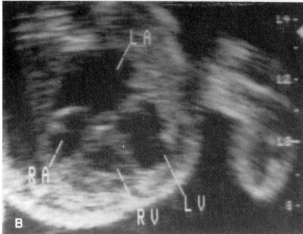

FIGURE 26–29. Four-chamber views in a 32-week fetus with familial right-sided cardiomyopathy (A) and in a 31-week fetus with cardiomyopathy, severe mitral regurgitation, and hydrops (B). In A, the right-sided chambers are enlarged. In the end-systolic frame (B), the left atrium (LA) and the left ventricle (LV) are considerably dilated, whereas the right atrium (RA) and the right ventricle (RV) appear to be of normal size. Ao indicates the descending aorta labeled in the top frame.

the left-sided obstructive lesions, and there is poorer perfusion of the endocardium with the development of right ventricular endocardial fibrosis, which contributes to a restrictive filling. This leads to inadequate right ventricular filling and, with the progressive ventricular hypertrophy, a hypoplastic ventricular cavity. The normal thebesian vessels, which communicate with the ventricular cavity, now act to decompress the ventricle, further limiting the right ventricular perfusion. Right-to-left atrial shunting increases and the perfusion across the ductus diminishes, until it is solely left-to-right. When the ductus fills in this direction, because the volume of blood required to perfuse the lungs is smaller than the usual ductus flow, the ductus is more vertically oriented and smaller than normal.[69] The type of right pulmonary atresia with a large right ventricle may have a pathogenesis similar to that in Ebstein malformation.

Management Strategies

As with the left-sided obstructive lesions, this lesion may well be one of those that when halted or palliated

by intervening in the gestation may prevent destruction of the ventricle and also prevent some of the right ventricular hypoplasia. Indeed, direct pulmonary perforation has already been attempted.[61] Experimental balloon valvotomy has successfully been performed in animals through videolaparoscopic techniques.[60, 70]

Conotruncal Abnormalities: Transposition, Double-Outlet Right Ventricle, Tetralogy, and Variants of these Lesions and Persistent Truncus Arteriosus

We have also encountered several fetuses with transposition of the great arteries with and without ventricular septal defect (Fig. 26–31) or with ventricular septal defect; one had pulmonary atresia in addition. We have also encountered corrected transposition in fetuses (Fig. 26–31B).

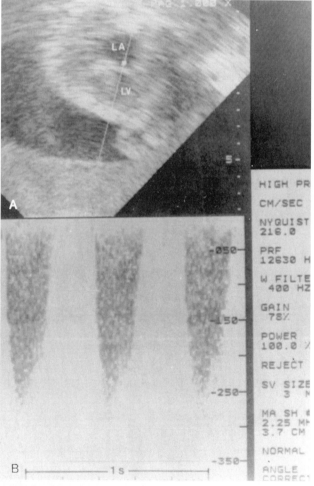

FIGURE 26–30. In a four-chamber view of a 28-week fetus with a cardiomyopathy, the Doppler sample volume is above the mitral valve within the left atrium, which is considerably dilated. A turbulent jet of high velocity directed away from the transducer is displayed on high-pulse-repetition-frequency Doppler in systole (B) indicating mitral insufficiency.

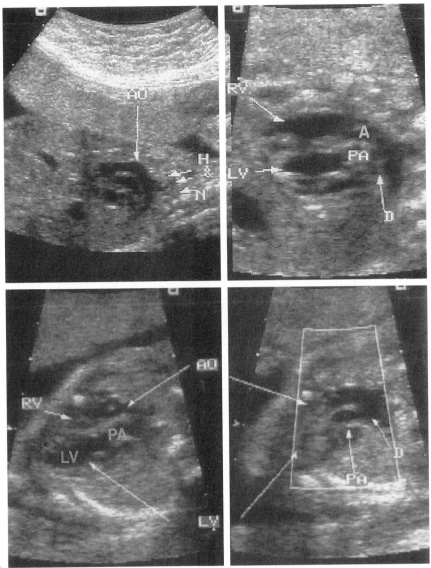

FIGURE 26–31. *A,* This fetus presented at 24 weeks with the features consistent with transposition. The aorta (AO) is anterior and arising from the right ventricle, (RV), and the pulmonary artery (PA) from the left ventricle (LV). *Top left,* The anterior vessel is the aorta because the head and neck vessels (H & N, *arrows*). The pulmonary artery (PA) can be seen arising from the left ventricle (LV) (*Top right and bottom left*). The ductus arteriosus (D) is seen below the arch connecting the aorta to the pulmonary trunk (*top right* and *bottom right*).

Illustration continued on following page

Pathophysiology and Natural History

This lesion is compatible with fetal survival and normal development, and changes in the circulation do not appear to affect fetal development adversely.

Tetralogy of Fallot has been found in 3% of Allan's large series. According to Rudolph,[69] this lesion has no adverse effect on the fetal or placental circulations.[71] In the situation of tetralogy with absent pulmonary valve, the enlarging pulmonary arteries encroach on the bronchi and destroy the cartilage. A dilemma in fetal management exists that relates to balancing the risk of prematurity from early delivery versus waiting too long for delivery, thus allowing continued bronchial destruction.

In addition to the patient we encountered with the absent pulmonary valve complex (Figs. 26–32 and 26–33),

several other forms of conoventricular abnormalities have been encountered in our population. These include several patients with diaphragmatic hernia, chromosomal abnormalities, and other associated lesions. These usually complex lesions need to be recognized in order to make an accurate prognosis. For example, in the patient shown in Figure 26–34, repair of the associated diaphragmatic hernia would leave severe pulmonary hypertension due to lung hypoplasia and serious congenital heart disease consisting of double-outlet right ventricle, Taussig-Bing malformation, and interrupted aortic arch.

Truncus arteriosus was found in several fetuses, of whom almost half had a chromosomal abnormality (Fig. 26–35). It is an advisable point of caution to question the differential diagnosis of aortic atresia with ventricular septal defect, without mitral atresia and adequate sized left ventricle.

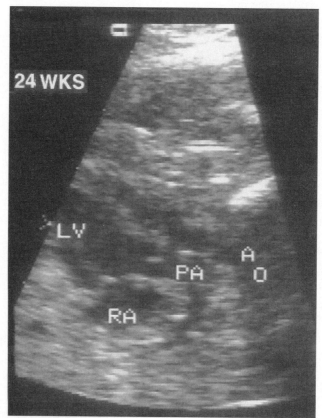

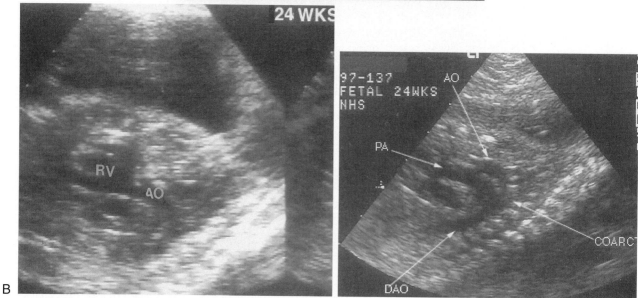

B

F I G U R E 26–31 *Continued.* *B,* Patient with situs solitus, atrioventricular, and ventriculoarterial discordance, known as corrected transposition. The top frame demonstrates the connection between the right atrium (RA), identified by four-chamber imaging previously, and the left ventricle (LV). The aorta (Ao) is seen arising anteriorly from the right ventricle (RV) in the middle frame. The bottom frame shows the aorta (AO) with head and neck vessels arising from it. In the bottom frame, the large pulmonary artery (PA) connects to the descending aorta, (DAO) and an area of aortic coarctation (COARCT) is shown.

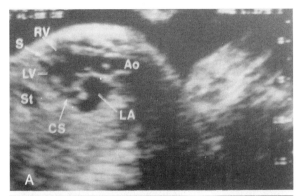

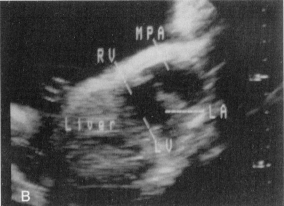

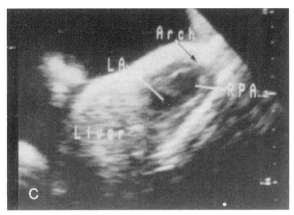

F I G U R E 26–32. Sagittal views in a fetus of 31 weeks' gestation with absent pulmonary valve complex and tetralogy of Fallot. *A,* The ascending aorta (Ao) is seen overriding a large ventricular septal defect. *B,* With the scan plane directed more to the left, the dysplastic pulmonary valve and the markedly dilated main pulmonary artery (MPA) are demonstrated. *C,* More to the right, the aortic arch is shown. Note the discrepancy between the size of the aortic arch and the right pulmonary artery (RPA), which lies underneath it. (CS = coronary sinus; LA = left atrium; LV = left ventricle; RV = right ventricle; S = ventricular septum; St = stomach.)

F I G U R E 26–33. Pulsed Doppler ultrasound examination in the same fetus shown in Figure 26–32. In the top left reference image, the Doppler sample volume lies in the pulmonary artery (PA) distal to the dysplastic pulmonary valve (*arrow*); the right ventricle (RV) is also seen. The spectral Doppler display is not corrected for angle. A diastolic signal of disturbed flow at a high velocity is demonstrated above the baseline (directed towards the transducer) and reflects pulmonary regurgitation, whereas the systolic signal below the baseline (directed away from the transducer) indicates pulmonary stenosis.

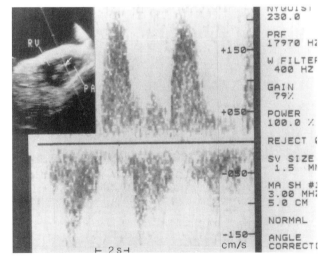

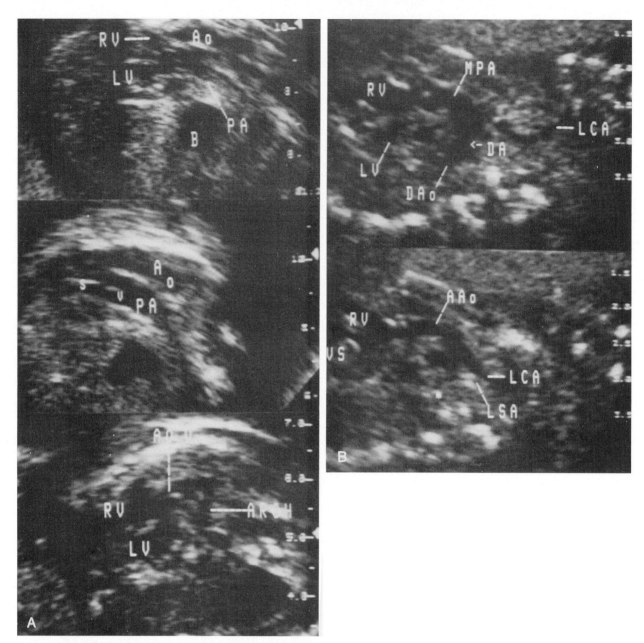

FIGURE 26–34. This series of long-axis scans was taken from a fetus recognized to have a diaphragmatic hernia and double-outlet right ventricle of the Taussig-Bing variety. *A,* The intracardiac anatomy. The top frame shows the small (ascending) aorta (Ao) arising from the right ventricle (RV) and the large pulmonary artery (PA) arising from both the left and right ventricles above a ventricular septal defect. The bowel (B) is seen lying posterior to the heart within the thorax. The left panel, middle frame of *A* shows a magnification of the aortopulmonary relationships. The apposed pulmonary valve leaflets lie almost directly above the rest of the ventricular septum, demonstrating the classic override of these associated with a conotruncal malformation. The ventricular septal defect is created by this malalignment. The left panel, bottom frame of *A* shows the diminutive aorta and arch arising from the right ventricle. The aortic valve (AoV) is seen arising from the right ventricle. *B,* The vessel morphology and aortic arch interruption is displayed. The top frame (in *B*) shows the main pulmonary artery (MPA) and the ductus arch (DA) as it arises from the right ventricle and then courses around to the descending aorta (DAo) as an uninterrupted arch. The left carotid artery (LCA) is seen but does not make contact with this arch. The bottom frame (in *B*) shows the ascending aorta (AAo) arising from the right ventricle as well (double-outlet right ventricle). It is considerably smaller than the pulmonary artery–ductus arch and ends at the left carotid artery (LCA). The left subclavian artery (LSA) arises from the descending aorta (*upper frame*), indicating that the aortic arch is interrupted between the left carotid and left subclavian arteries. (Vs = ventricular septum.)

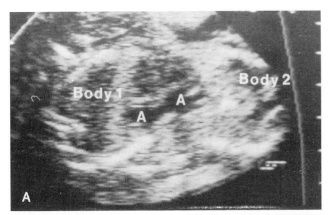

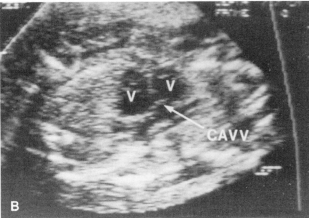

FIGURE 26–35. Long-axis orientation in a fetus of 32 weeks' gestation with truncus arteriosus. *A,* The single truncal vessel (Tr) is seen overriding a ventricular septal defect. The coronary sinus (CS) is dilated because of a left superior vena caval connection. *B,* After magnification and slight angulation of the transducer to the fetal left side, the common origin of a pulmonary artery from the truncus and its division into right and left pulmonary branches (R, L) can be seen. (DAo = descending aorta; LV = left ventricle; RV = right ventricle.)

Univentricular Atrioventricular Connections

Complex forms of cardiac defects were detected frequently. We have encountered several fetuses with a univentricular atrioventricular connection, presenting in one as an absent right-sided atrioventricular connection and ventriculoarterial discordance (Figs. 26–36 and 26–37), and hypoplastic or interrupted aortic arch. We have encountered several cases of hypoplastic left heart complex with aortic atresia (Fig. 26–36). Although some cases may be straightforward, presenting few diagnostic problems, others may present with features of a small left ventricle with marked endocardial fibroelastosis and a thick, immobile aortic valve. The ventricle, by comparison with the right ventricle, may not be as small, relatively, as in the classical hypoplastic left heart syndrome, but transitional variants of this disorder are well recognized postnatally. In addition, some of these infants have had premature closure of the foramen ovale without the presence of nonimmune hydrops. In this group, we have recognized one fetus who had Shone complex (parachute mitral valve, single left ventricular papillary muscle, bicuspid aortic valve, and ventricular and atrial septal defects).

Cardiac Tumors

Multiple rhabdomyomas as an expression of tuberous sclerosis were encountered on two occasions (Fig. 26–38). Multiple lesions were present in one fetus, and in another, an isolated lesion lying in the ventricular septum produced left ventricular outflow obstruction and left ventricular endocardial fibroelastosis. Several other lesions were encountered once, including pericardial teratomas, which presented with polyhydramnios, and have been treated with percutaneous pericardiocentesis.

Abnormalities of Situs; Left Isomerism (Polysplenia and Right Isomerism—Asplenia)

We have reviewed the reported cases of left and right isomerism in utero. These lesions have substantial mor-

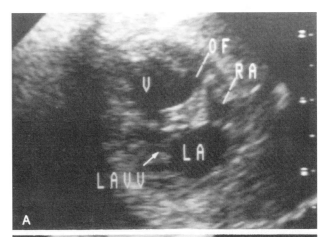

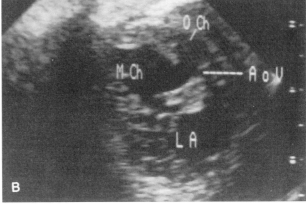

FIGURE 26–36. Long-axis orientation in a fetus of 38 weeks' gestation with tricuspid atresia (univentricular atrioventricular connection). *A,* Instead of a right atrioventricular valve there is echodense tissue between the right atrium (RA) and the dilated ventricle (V). The left atrium (LA) is enlarged and drains via a left atrioventricular valve (LAVV) into the ventricle. An outlet foramen (OF) is displayed anteriorly leading into an outlet chamber, which can be better appreciated in the bottom frame. *B,* This frame demonstrates a semilunar valve connected to the outlet chamber (OCh). Since the aorta arises anteriorly from that outlet chamber (see Figure 26–35), this is the aortic valve (AoV). The single atrioventricular valve is demonstrated lying between the left atrium and main chamber of left ventricular morphology.

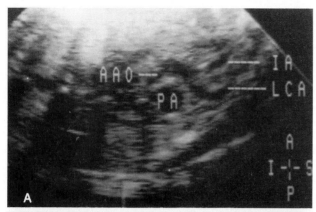

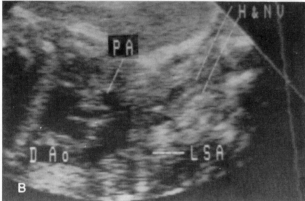

FIGURE 26–37. Sagittal view in a fetus of 34 weeks' gestation with absent left-sided atrioventricular connection, doublet-outlet right ventricle, and interrupted aortic arch. *A,* The ascending aorta (AAo) and the proximal arch, which runs on top of the right pulmonary artery (PA), is seen giving rise to the innominate artery (IA) and to the left carotid artery (LCA). *B,* After slight angulation of the transducer to the fetus' left side, the dilated pulmonary artery (PA) and its continuation via the ductus arteriosus into the descending aorta (DAo) are displayed. The left subclavian artery (LSA) can be seen arising from the descending aorta, which is separated from the arch and the head and neck vessels (HNV). (A = anterior; I = inferior; P = posterior; S = superior.)

bidity and mortality after birth, but before birth the risk appears to be with the development of complete heart block with left isomerism. The incidence of left isomerism appears somewhat greater than the postnatal appearance, suggesting a higher intrauterine mortality.[72]

Thoracopagus Twins

We have examined several sets of thoracopagus twins.[73] The outcome of these pregnancies has been uniformly fatal. Echocardiographic assessment is often difficult because of the superimposition of one twin's bony structures on the other; at autopsy the lesions are often more complicated than defined by ultrasound. In a thoracopagus twin detected as early as 16 weeks, we noted the hearts to be fused with shared atria and shared ventricles, one common atrioventricular valve, and only one dilated great artery in each body (pulmonary atresia in one, aortic hypoplasia with interrupted arch in the other) (Fig. 26–39).

Diagnostic Errors

Despite the increased resolution of ultrasound equipment, errors in interpretation or omission are possible, even inevitable. We made a false-negative diagnosis of a structurally normal heart in fetuses of our series that have had lesions as simple as a ventricular septal defect, aortic coarctation coupled with double-orifice mitral valve, or mild pulmonary stenosis. We have even falsely diagnosed pulmonary atresia in an infant subsequently born with pulmonary hypertension that resolved whose fetal study demonstrated tricuspid stenosis and tricuspid regurgitation with right ventricular contractions. We have falsely diagnosed normal situs when there was mirror-image dextrocardia. The latter error, which was made early in our experience, should not be if the correct

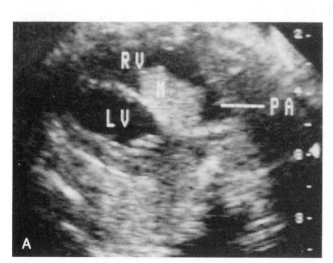

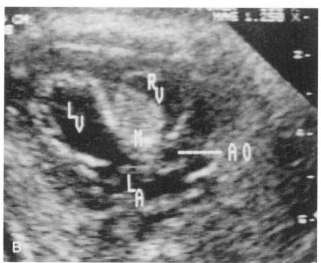

FIGURE 26–38. This example shows a rhabdomyoma. Large septal mass (M) is seen in this fetus in a long-axis cut. *A,* The relation of the mass to the underlying left and right ventricle (RV) and pulmonary artery is shown. There is no significant right ventricular outflow tract obstruction. *B,* The mass clearly encroaches on the underlying left ventricular outflow tract, almost separating the left ventricle from the aorta (Ao). (LA = left atrium.)

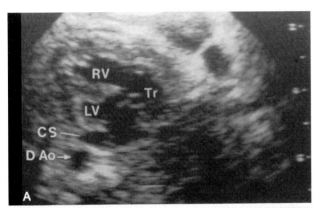

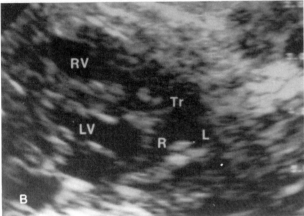

FIGURE 26–39. Thoracopagus twins at 24 weeks. Both bodies are visualized; the fused hearts share the atria (*A*) and the ventricles (*B*). Only one common atrioventricular valve (CAVV) shared between the two hearts can be seen.

position of the heart within the chest is determined first. We have encountered subsequent patients with situs inversus that has been correctly recognized prospectively. In complex cardiac defects the main lesion may be recognizable, but secondary lesions might be missed unless careful attention is paid to the entire examination. In general, experience suggests that prenatal findings in complex congenital abnormalities tend to underestimate the severity of the spectrum of abnormalities.

Both false-negative and false-positive findings have been reported previously.[7, 8, 11, 74] When evaluating the cause for errors we found that most of the serious ones had been made using older equipment that had poorer resolution, when magnification was not possible, and when the Doppler technique was not used. Other errors unrelated to equipment are beyond the ultrasonographer's control, including technical factors such as suboptimal imaging that occurs with gross maternal obesity, polyhydramnios, or fetal lie. Because the resolution of echocardiographic imaging is limited to distances of 1.0 to 1.5 mm, structural abnormalities such as relatively small ventricular septal defects may be technically impossible to image. The newer high-resolution ultrasound systems, which have greater penetration and resolution coupled with superior Doppler and color flow mapping, coupled with greater experience and skill, will minimize these errors.

Mild aortic or pulmonic stenosis may be difficult to detect, because valve morphology may not be resolved accurately enough to determine minor valve abnormalities, and blood flow velocity may be lower than after birth due to low ventricular pressures present in fetal life. Other defects such as mild aortic coarctation or a secundum atrial septal defect may be indistinguishable from normal anatomy in the fetus. Furthermore, cardiac lesions may develop or worsen later in pregnancy, as we have observed in cases of cardiomyopathy, and will be detected only if serial studies are performed. We have made it a practice to restudy fetuses later in gestation when there is doubt as to whether the study is normal. On the other hand, some lesions may disappear on subsequent studies, such as ventricular septal defects closing spontaneously.

Outcome of Fetuses with Structural Cardiac Defects

Reported experience that the overall outcome of a fetus with a structural cardiac abnormality is unfavorable[10, 49, 66, 74] was confirmed in our series (Table 26–3). Six pregnancies were terminated electively, two because of severe fetal cardiac defects, the others because of chromosomal abnormalities. There were 30 fetal or neonatal deaths, four fetuses are not yet born, and only 11 children (23%) were alive at the end of the neonatal period. Four of these underwent cardiac surgery within the first months of life, including one who had cardiac transplantation. The incidence of fetal death in those cases presenting with nonimmune hydrops and cardiac defects was high (16 out of 18 cases); ten of these fetuses had severe atrioventricular regurgitation, and all died either before birth or within the first week postnatally. Cardiac defects coupled with complete atrioventricular block were present in eight fetuses, seven of whom died prenatally or in the neonatal period. The prognosis for fetal survival appears to be poor in the presence of structural abnormalities coupled with atrioventricular valve regurgitation, complete heart block, or fetal hydrops. It is important to note that because the technique is in its early stages, those defects most likely to be symptomatic are more likely to have been recognized. It seems possible that the recognition of fetal heart disease may have a positive impact on survival of the newborn. Although this has not been noted previously, a recent study from our laboratory[54] showed an improved survival of prenatally diagnosed fetuses with hypoplastic left heart syndrome.

Comments

Incidence

The spectrum of abnormalities we found does not reflect the common incidence of the different types of congenital cardiac defects.[1, 2, 75, 76] On the contrary, rarer and more complex forms of congenital cardiac defects are detected, presumably because they are more likely to be symptomatic. Both the frequent diagnosis of complex lesions and the high incidence of structural cardiac defects may relate to the criteria we set for evaluation of the population for the development of congenital heart defects. The risk of developing congenital heart disease has been described to increase when there is a family history of either congenital heart defects or extracardiac malformations.[24–26,77,78] In particular, maternal congenital heart disease appears to be a risk factor as great as 10 to 15% for subsequent pregnancies, whereas the recurrence of congenital heart disease in the case of one affected sibling is about 2%.

Impact of Fetal Echocardiography on Obstetric Management

Fetal echocardiography may influence decisions on further obstetric management of the pregnancy. Because of its potential for prenatal distinction of simple and complex structural abnormalities of the heart, this information has been made available for genetic counseling, aiding in the decision for elective termination of pregnancy, as in 4% of our cases, where chromosomal defects were present. Elective termination of pregnancy based purely on morphologic information obtained by fetal echocardiography was performed in only 2% of fetuses in our series, although others have reported higher incidences[10]; however, the detection of serious cardiac defects may become a much more frequent reason for terminating pregnancy when the technique becomes more generally applied. The role of fetal echocardiography in detecting severe structural abnormalities as an adjunct to genetic counseling is therefore comparable to the role of amniocentesis or fetal blood sampling, which are used as diagnostic tools for the assessment of severe chromosomal or inborn metabolic disorders.[77] When terminating pregnancy is not an alternative, fetal echocardiography plays an important role in determining the course of appropriate management.[79, 80] If immediate neonatal support is contemplated, the delivery can also be planned at a center with facilities for medical and surgical cardiac treatment of these neonates. The detection of cardiac defects also may influence the route of delivery; for example, where prolonged labor may cause myocardial ischemia, cesarean section might be contemplated.[80]

In our series, most cases with major cardiac defects had had a prior examination by an obstetric ultrasonographer who recognized some cardiac disturbance. The impact of fetal echocardiography will be greater when it becomes an accepted and familiar technique for primary-care ultrasonographers. Since it appears that fetal echocardiography is considerably more complex than obtaining a fairly "normal looking" four-chamber view, further training of obstetric ultrasonographers in the recognition of structural abnormalities of the fetal heart seems warranted. When cardiac examination of the fetus becomes a routine part of the primary ultrasonographic examination, it is conceivable that an entirely new perspective may emerge on congenital heart disease including diagnosis and physiology, which may shift the emphasis for early treatment to the prenatal period.

Outlook

New therapeutic strategies may develop because of fetal echocardiography. Prenatal surgery, already an established treatment for hydrocephalus or hydronephrosis, may become an alternative approach for the treatment of congenital heart defects. Experimental data indicate the potential for performing certain forms of fetal cardiovascular surgery to palliate or remove severe right heart obstructive lesions,[21, 22] which may allow better development of these malformed hearts. For the same reason, interventional catheterization in the fetus has been proposed as a possible future therapeutic approach. Fetal echocardiography is the only technique currently available as a prenatal test for congenital heart defects. Although nuclear magnetic resonance has been used to demonstrate fetal cardiac anatomy,[81] its applicability and safety have obvious limitations.

Monitoring of the fetal cardiovascular function, arrhythmias, or congestive heart failure in the fetus where medication has been administered either by a maternal[12–15, 18–20, 82–85] or a direct fetal route[85, 86] may be expanded considerably in the future. Moreover, fetal echocardiography may allow the detection of undesired side effects of drugs taken for maternal indications such as the constriction of the ductus arteriosus after indomethacin therapy in the mother.[43]

Fetal echocardiography provides new information about the development of the heart in the presence of structural or functional disease,[49, 66, 87, 88] which will contribute to a better understanding of the natural history of congenital heart disease and open up the potential for fetal treatment.

Acknowledgments

We are indebted to Mrs. Heather Silverman and Mr. Paul Sagan for editorial assistance with this manuscript.

REFERENCES

1. Mitchell SC, Korones SB, Berendes HW: Congenital heart disease in 56,109 births. Incidence and natural history. Circulation 43:323–332, 1971.
2. Hoffman JIE, Christianson R: Congenital heart disease in a cohort of 19,502 births with long-term follow-up. Am J Cardiol 42:641–647, 1978.
3. Allan LD, Tynan MJ, Campbell S, et al: Echocardiographic and anatomical correlates in the fetus. Br Heart J 44:444–451, 1980.
4. Lange LW, Sahn DJ, Allen HD, et al: Qualitative real-time cross-sectional echocardiographic imaging of the human fetus during the second half of pregnancy. Circulation 62:799–806, 1980.
5. Sahn DJ, Lange LW, Allen HD, et al: Quantitative real-time cross-sectional echocardiography in the developing normal human fetus and newborn. Circulation 62:588–597, 1980.
6. Huhta JC, Hagler DJ, Hill LM: Two-dimensional echocardiographic assessment of normal fetal cardiac anatomy. J Reprod Med 29:162–167, 1984.
7. Allan LD, Crawford DC, Anderson RH, Tynan MJ: Echocardiographic and anatomical correlations in fetal congenital heart disease. Br Heart J 52:542–548, 1984.

8. Silverman NH, Golbus MS: Echocardiographic techniques for assessing normal and abnormal fetal cardiac anatomy. Bethesda Conference #14. J Am Coll Cardiol 5:20S–29S, 1985.

9. Fermont L, deGeeter B, Aubry MC, Sidi D: A close collaboration between obstetricians and pediatric cardiologists allows antenatal detection of severe cardiac malformations by two-dimensional echocardiography. In Doyle EF, Engle MA, Gersony WM, Rashkind WJ, Talner NS (eds): Pediatric Cardiology: Proceedings of the Second World Congress. New York: Springer, 1986, pp 34–37.

10. Allan LD, Crawford DC, Anderson RH, Tynan M: Spectrum of congenital heart disease detected echocardiographically in prenatal life. Br Heart J 54:523–526, 1985.

11. Sandor GGS, Farquarson D, Wittmann B, et al: Fetal echocardiography: Results in high-risk patients. Obstet Gynecol 67:358–364, 1986.

12. Kleinman CS, Donnerstein RL, Jaffe CC, et al: Fetal echocardiography. A tool for evaluation of in utero cardiac arrhythmias and monitoring of in utero therapy: Analysis of 71 patients. Am J Cardiol 51:237–243, 1983.

13. Allan LD, Anderson RH, Sullivan ID, et al: Evaluation of fetal arrhythmias by echocardiography. Br Heart J 50:240–245, 1983.

14. DeVore GR, Siassi B, Platt LD: Fetal echocardiography. III. The diagnosis of cardiac arrhythmias using real-time-directed M-mode ultrasound. Am J Obstet Gynecol 146:792–799, 1983.

15. Silverman NH, Enderlein MA, Stanger P, et al: Recognition of fetal arrhythmias by echocardiography. J Clin Ultrasound 13:255–263, 1985.

16. Strasburger JF, Huhta JC, Carpenter RJ Jr, et al: Doppler echocardiography in the diagnosis and management of persistent fetal arrhythmias. J Am Coll Cardiol 7:1386–1391, 1986.

17. Steinfeld L, Rappaport HL, Rossbach HC, Martinez E: Diagnosis of fetal arrhythmias using echocardiographic and Doppler techniques. J Am Coll Cardiol 8:1425–1433, 1986.

18. Kleinman CS, Donnerstein RL, DeVore GR, et al: Fetal echocardiography for evaluation of in utero congestive heart failure. N Engl J Med 306:568–575, 1982.

19. Wiggins JW, Bowes W, Clewell W, et al: Echocardiographic diagnosis and intravenous digoxin management of fetal tachyarrhythmias and congestive heart failure. Am J Dis Child 140:202–204, 1986.

20. Simpson PC, Trudinger BJ, Walker A, Baird PJ: The intrauterine treatment of fetal cardiac failure in a twin pregnancy with an acardiac, acephalic monster. Am J Obstet Gynecol 147:842–844, 1983.

21. Turley K, Vlahakes GJ, Harrison MR, et al: Intrauterine cardiothoracic surgery: The fetal lamb model. Ann Thorac Surg 34:422–426, 1982.

22. Slate RK, Stevens MB, Verrier ED, et al: Intrauterine repair of pulmonary stenosis in fetal sheep. Surg Forum 36:246–247, 1985.

23. Zierler S: Maternal drugs and congenital heart disease. Obstet Gynecol 65:155–165, 1985.

24. Allan LD, Crawford DC, Chita SK, et al: Familial recurrence of congenital heart disease in a prospective series of mothers referred for fetal echocardiography. Am J Cardiol 58:334–337, 1986.

25. Whittemore R, Hobbins JC, Engle MA: Pregnancy and its outcome in women with and without surgical treatment of congenital heart disease. Am J Cardiol 50:641–651, 1982.

26. Nora JJ, Nora AH: Maternal transmission of congenital heart diseases: New recurrence risk figures and the questions of cytoplasmic inheritance and vulnerability to teratogens. Am J Cardiol 59:459–463, 1987.

27. McCue CM, Mantakas ME, Tingelstad JB, Ruddy S: Congenital heart block in newborns of mothers with connective tissue disease. Circulation 56:82–90, 1977.

28. Scott JS, Maddison PJ, Taylor PV, et al: Connective-tissue disease, antibodies to ribonucleoprotein, and congenital heart block. N Engl J Med 309:209–212, 1983.

29. Yagel S, Weissman A, Rotstein Z, et al: Congenital heart defects: Natural course and in utero development. Circulation 96:550–555, 1997.

30. Allan LD, Joseph MC, Boyd EGC, et al: M-mode echocardiography in the developing human fetus. Br Heart J 47:573–583, 1982.

31. St. John Sutton MG, Gewitz MH, Shah B, et al: Quantitative assessment of growth and function of the cardiac chambers in the normal human fetus: A prospective longitudinal echocardiographic study. Circulation 69:645–654, 1984.

32. DeVore GR, Siassi B, Platt LD: Fetal echocardiography. IV. M-mode assessment of ventricular size and contractility during the second and third trimesters of pregnancy in the normal fetus. Am J Obstet Gynecol 150:981–988, 1984.

33. Anderson RH, Becker AE, Freedom RM, et al: Sequential segmental analysis of congenital heart disease. Pediatr Cardiol 5:281–287, 1984.

34. Silverman NH, de Araujo LML: An echocardiographic method for the diagnosis of cardiac situs and malpositions. Echocardiography 4:35–57, 1987.

35. de Araujo LML, Silverman NH, Filly RA, et al: Prenatal detection of left atrial isomerism by ultrasound. J Ultrasound Med 6:667–670, 1987.

36. Stewart PA, Tonge HM, Wladimiroff JW: Arrhythmia and structural abnormalities of the fetal heart. Br Heart J 50:550–554, 1983.

37. Kleinman CS, Donnerstein RL: Ultrasonic assessment of cardiac function in the intact human fetus. J Am Coll Cardiol 5(Suppl 1): 84S–94S, 1985.

38. Tan J, Silverman NH, Hoffman JIE, et al: Cardiac dimensions in the human fetus from 18 weeks to term: A cross-sectional echocardiographic study. Am J Cardiol 70:1459–1467, 1992.

39. Reed KL, Meijboom EJ, Sahn DJ, et al: Cardiac Doppler flow velocities in human fetuses. Circulation 73:41–46, 1986.

40. Huhta JC, Strasburger JF, Carpenter RJ, et al: Pulsed Doppler fetal echocardiography. J Clin Ultrasound 13:247–254, 1985.

41. Reed KL, Sahn DJ, Scagnelli S, et al: Doppler echocardiographic studies of diastolic function in the human fetal heart: Changes during gestation. J Am Coll Cardiol 8:391–395, 1986.

42. Maulik D, Nanda NC, Saini VD: Fetal Doppler echocardiography: Methods and characterization of normal and abnormal hemodynamics. Am J Cardiol 53:572–578, 1984.

43. Huhta JC, Moise KJ, Fisher DJ, et al: Detection and quantitation of constriction of the fetal ductus arteriosus by Doppler echocardiography. Circulation 75:406–412, 1987.

44. Hatle L, Brubakk A, Tromsdal A, Angelsen B: Noninvasive assessment of pressure drop in mitral stenosis by Doppler ultrasound. Br Heart J 40:131–140, 1978.

45. Hatle L, Angelsen BA, Tromsdal A: Non-invasive assesment of aortic stenosis by Doppler ultrasound. Br Heart J 43:284–292, 1980.

46. Stuart B, Drumm J, FitzGerald DE, Duignan NM: Fetal blood velocity waveforms in normal pregnancy. Br J Obstet Gynaecol 87:780–785, 1980.

47. Schulman H, Fleischer A, Stern W, et al: Umbilical velocity wave ratios in human pregnancy. Am J Obstet Gynecol 148:985–990, 1984.

48. Trudinger BJ, Giles WB, Cook CM, et al: Fetal umbilical artery flow velocity waveforms and placental resistance: Clinical significance. Br J Obstet Gynaecol 92:23–30, 1985.

49. Silverman NH, Kleinman CS, Rudolph AM, et al: Fetal atrioventricular valve insufficiency associated with nonimmune hydrops: A two-dimensional echocardiography and pulsed Doppler ultrasound study. Circulation 72:825–831, 1985.

50. Kohl T, Silverman NH: Evaluation of umbilical venous blood flow by Doppler color flow mapping and conventional ultrasonographic methods. J Ultrasound Med 15:465–473, 1996.

51. Huhta JC, Gutgesell HP, Nihill MR: Cross-sectional echocardiographic diagnosis of total anomalous pulmonary venous connection. Br Heart J 53:525–534, 1985.

52. Allan LD, Sharland GK, Milburn A, et al: Prospective diagnosis of 1,006 consecutive cases of congenital heart disease in the fetus. J Am Coll Cardiol 23:1452–1458, 1994.

53. Smythe JF, Copel JA, Kleinman CS: Outcome of prenatally detected cardiac malformations. Am J Cardiol 69:1471–1474, 1992.

54. Tworetzky W, McElhinney DB, Reddy VM, et al: Does prenatal diagnosis of hypoplastic left heart syndrome lead to improved surgical outcome? J Am Coll Cardiol 31(Suppl A): 71A, 1998.

55. Rudolph AM: Congenital Diseases of the Heart: Clinical-Physiologic Considerations in Diagnosis and Management. Chicago: Year Book Medical Publishers, 1974.

56. Somerville J: Congenital heart disease—changes in form and function. Br Heart J 41:1–22, 1979.

57. Sharland GK, Chita SK, Fagg NL, et al: Left ventricular dysfunction in the fetus: Relation to aortic valve anomalies and endocardial fibroelastosis. Br Heart J 66:419–424, 1991.

58. Hornberger LK, Bromley B, Lichter E, Benacerraf BR: Development of severe aortic stenosis and left ventricular dysfunction with endocardial fibroelastosis in a second trimester fetus. J Ultrasound Med 15:651–654, 1996.

59. Hornberger LK, Sanders SP, Rein AJ, et al: Left heart obstructive lesions and left ventricular growth in the midtrimester fetus. A longitudinal study. Circulation 92:1531–1538, 1995.

60. Kohl T, Szabo Z, Suda K, et al: Fetoscopic and open transumbilical fetal cardiac catheterization in sheep. Potential approaches for human fetal cardiac intervention. Circulation 95:1048–1053, 1997.

61. Kohl T, Sharland G, Chaoui R, et al: Percutaneous ultrasound-guided balloon valvuloplasty in human fetuses with severe semilunar valvar obstructions—early clinical experience and preliminary selection criteria for future procedures. J Am Coll Cardiol (in press).

62. Berning RA, Silverman NH, Villegas M, et al: Reverse shunting across the ductus arteriosus or atrial septum in utero heralds severe congenital heart disease. J Am Coll Cardiol 27:481–486, 1993.

63. Weinstein MR, Goldfield MD: Cardiovascular malformations with lithium use during pregnancy. Am J Psychiatry 132:529–531, 1975.

64. Oberhoffer R, Cook AC, Lang D, et al: Correlation between echocardiographic and morphological investigations of lesions of the tricuspid valve diagnosed during fetal life. Br Heart J 68:580–585, 1992.

65. Roberson DA, Silverman NH: Ebstein's anomaly: Echocardiographic and clinical features in the fetus and neonate. J Am Coll Cardiol 14:1300–1307, 1989.

66. Allan LD, Crawford DC, Tynan MJ: Pulmonary atresia in prenatal life. J Am Coll Cardiol 8:1131–1136, 1986.

67. Allan LD, Cook A: Pulmonary atresia with intact ventricular septum in the fetus. Cardiol Young 2:367–376, 1992.

68. Hornberger LK, Benacerraf BR, Bromley BS, et al: Prenatal detection of severe right ventricular outflow tract obstruction: Pulmonary stenosis and pulmonary atresia. J Ultrasound Med 13:743–750, 1994.

69. Rudolph AM (ed): Rudolph's Pediatrics. Stamford, CT: Appleton & Lange, 1996, p 2337.

70. Tometzki AJP, Suda K, Kohl T, et al: Accuracy of prenatal echocardiographic diagnosis and prognosis of fetuses with conotruncal anomalies. J Am Coll Cardiol 33:1696–1701, 1999.

71. Ettedgui JA, Sharland GK, Chita SK, et al: Absent pulmonary valve syndrome with ventricular septal defect: Role of the arterial duct. Am J Cardiol 66:233–234, 1990.

72. Phoon CK, Villegas MD, Ursell PC, Silverman NH: Left atrial isomerism detected in fetal life. Am J Cardiol 77:1083–1088, 1996.

73. Barth RA, Filly RA, Goldberg JD, et al: Conjoined twins: Prenatal diagnosis and assessment of associated malformations. Radiology 177:201–207, 1990.

74. Huhta JC, Strasburger JF, Carpenter RJ, Reiter A: Fetal echocardiography: Accuracy and limitations in the diagnosis of cardiac disease. J Am Coll Cardiol 5:387, 1985.

75. Scott DJ, Rigby ML, Miller GA, Shinebourne EA: The presentation of symptomatic heart disease in infancy based on 10 years' experience (1973–82). Implications for the provision of services. Br Heart J 52:248–257, 1984.

76. Fyler DC, Buckley LP, Hellenbrand WE, et al: Report of the New England Regional Infant Cardiac Program. Pediatrics 65:375–461, 1980.

77. Copel JA, Pilu G, Kleinman CS: Congenital heart disease and extracardiac anomalies: Associations and indications for fetal echocardiography. Am J Obstet Gynecol 154:1121–1132, 1986.

78. Nora JJ, Nora AH: The evolution of specific genetic and environmental counseling in congenital heart diseases. Circulation 57:205–213, 1978.

79. Sanders SP, Chin AJ, Parness IA, et al: Prenatal diagnosis of congenital heart defects in thoracoabdominally conjoined twins. N Engl J Med 313:370–374, 1985.

80. Huhta JC, Carpenter RJ, Moise KJ: Prenatal diagnosis and postnatal management of critical aortic stenosis. Circulation 75:573–576, 1987.

81. Lowe TW, Weinreb J, Santos-Ramos R, Cunningham FG: Magnetic resonance imaging in human pregnancy. Obstet Gynecol 66:629–633, 1985.

82. Kleinman CS, Copel JA, Weinstein EM, et al: Treatment of fetal supraventricular tachyarrhythmias. J Clin Ultrasound 13:265–273, 1985.

83. Dumesic DA, Silverman NH, Tobias S, Golbus MS: Transplacental cardioversion of fetal supraventricular tachycardia with procainamide. N Engl J Med 307:1128–1131, 1982.

84. Arnoux P, Seyral P, Llurens M, et al: Amiodarone and digoxin for refractory fetal tachycardia. Am J Cardiol 59:166–167, 1987.

85. Redel DA, Hansmann M: Prenatal diagnosis and treatment of heart disease. In Dellenbach P (ed): 1. Symposium International d'Echocardiologie Foetale, Vol. Strasbourg: Milupa Dietetique, 1982, pp 127–134.

86. Hansmann M, Redel DA: Prenatal symptoms and clinical management of heart disease. In Dellenbach P (ed): 1. Symposium International d'Echocardiologie Foetale, Vol. Strasbourg: Milupa Dietetique, 1982, pp 137–149.

87. Birnbaum SE, McGahan JP, Janos GG, Meyers M: Fetal tachycardia and intramyocardial tumors. J Am Coll Cardiol 6:1358–1361, 1985.

88. Allan LD, Crawford DC, Tynan M: Evolution of coarctation of the aorta in intrauterine life. Br Heart J 52:471–473, 1984.

CHAPTER *27*

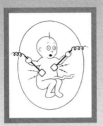

The Fetus with Cardiac Arrhythmia

CHARLES S. KLEINMAN, JOSHUA A. COPEL, and RODRIGO NEHGME

Irregularities of cardiac rhythm in the human fetus often lead to levels of anxiety among parents and treating physicians that are out of proportion to the clinical significance of the arrhythmias themselves. Most fetal cardiac arrhythmias result from isolated extrasystoles of the fetal heart, that are appreciated as skipped beats by the observer who is auscultating cardiac activity using a Doppler "listening device" that detects umbilical arterial blood flow. In most cases the skipping represents the pause following an extrasystole that has not reset the sinus node pacemaker of the fetal heart. Alternatively, an extrasystole occurring very soon after a normal beat may encounter the conduction system when it is still refractory, resulting in a "blocked" extrasystole, or may cause an early ventricular contraction, so soon after the last beat that diastolic filling is incomplete. The latter may result in a ventricular stroke volume that is too small to create an umbilical pulse of adequate volume for Doppler detection.

On occasion, sustained tachy- or bradyarrhythmias may be associated with important clinical consequences, including the development of nonimmune fetal hydrops.[1-21] In some situations the clinical status of the fetus and mother may suggest a role for in utero antiarrhythmic therapy. Such treatment should be administered in a well-monitored situation, using a treatment strategy that maximizes the likelihood of arrhythmia control, while minimizing risks to both the mother and her fetus. Such therapy should be logically planned, based on an understanding of the electrophysiologic mechanism of the arrhythmia, an understanding of fetal pharmacology, and the pharmacokinetics of the fetal-placental-maternal unit.[22-28]

This chapter provides a discussion of the pathophysiology of fetal cardiac arrhythmias, and discusses the natural history of these arrhythmias and the potential advantages and hazards of antiarrhythmic therapy, in order to provide a framework to allow the reader to formulate effective strategies for the management of these patients.

The Pathophysiology of Fetal Cardiac Arrhythmias

Atrial and Ventricular Extrasystoles

Abrupt alterations in cardiac rhythm in the fetus are most often the result of extrasystoles. In more than 90% of fetuses who have been referred for evaluation to the Yale Fetal Cardiovascular Center since 1977 for evaluation of fetal cardiac arrhythmias, the diagnosis has been isolated extrasystoles. These almost always have been perceived by the referring physician as intermittent pauses or "skipped beats" interposed into an otherwise regular fetal cardiac rhythm. In most such cases the pause represents the interval following a premature beat that has been interposed into the normal sinus rhythm of the fetus.

In most cases we have ascertained that these premature beats arise within one of the fetal atrial chambers. The premature beat stimulates an early ventricular contraction after it has passed through the atrioventricular node and the bundle of His. Atrial premature beats will usually depolarize the sinus node and cause it to "reset" itself. This results in an interval between the premature beat and the next sinus beat that is identical to the normal interval between sinus beats. The "pause" that is perceived by the clinician usually relates to the fact that when a premature atrial beat occurs soon after a normal sinus beat the premature contraction may occur at a time when diastolic filling has been incomplete, resulting in a ventricular ejection of inadequate stroke volume to create an umbilical arterial flow waveform that is audible to the usual Doppler "listening device." The clinician, therefore, hears no flow during the extrasystolic contraction and hears only the flow during the pre- and the postextrasystolic sinus beats. Alternatively, atrial premature contractions may occur with a coupling interval to the previous sinus beat that is so short that the impulse may encounter the atrioventricular (AV) node and bundle of His while they are still refractory following the previous sinus beat. Such extrasystoles will be nonconducted, and truly do represent intermittently skipped beats.

Most atrial extrasystoles are benign, and carry no ominous significance regarding fetal well-being or prognosis. These benign rhythm disturbances have been noted in 14% of all neonates, and in 13 to 21% of older children.[29-31] While premature atrial contractions occasionally occur in the presence of mechanical irritation of the atrial wall (e.g., in the presence of indwelling central venous catheters), electrolyte imbalances (hypokalemia or hypocalcemia), hypoxemia, hypoglycemia, or drug exposures (caffeine, amphetamines, sympathomimetics, digoxin), they most often are encountered in normal cardiovascular systems.

The only real potential consequence of such extrasystoles is that with the appropriate timing with relationship to the previous sinus beat, if there is an underlying anatomic substrate, there is the potential for one of these beats to initiate reentry tachycardia, either within the atrial muscle or at the atrioventricular junction (see "Supraventricular Tachycardia," below). For this reason we believe that such fetuses should be monitored twice weekly, in order to preclude the possible oversight of a sustained supraventricular tachyarrhythmia. The pre- and postnatal risk of sustained supraventricular tachycardia or atrial flutter in a fetus presenting with supraventricular extrasystoles is in the 0.5% range.[33-39]

Similarly, isolated ventricular extrasystoles in the absence of sustained episodes of ventricular tachycardia are considered benign, although if persistent should engender a search for evidence of myocardial ischemia, myocardial dysfunction, or segmental myocardial malformations such as tumor or scar. In most cases, however, isolated ventricular extrasystoles carry no more import than supraventricular extrasystoles, and we do not expend undue effort to distinguish the site of origin of isolated extrasystoles if the fetal heart is otherwise structurally and functionally normal, without evidence of sustained or nonsustained supraventricular or ventricular tachycardia.

Supraventricular Tachycardia

Supraventricular tachycardia (SVT) is the most commonly encountered fetal cardiac arrhythmia that is associated with important clinical consequences. While SVT may result due to a variety of electrophysiologic mechanisms, the most commonly encountered of these is "reciprocating" or "reentrant" tachycardia, arising from a circular circuit of electrical activity. This circular wavefront alternately stimulates the atrium and ventricle to contract at a rate that is faster than that of the intrinsic sinus pacemaker. There is, therefore, one atrial contraction for each ventricular contraction. The overall heart rate is dependent upon the size of the reentry pathway and the intrinsic electrical properties of the limbs of the circuit. In the human fetus with SVT the characteristic heart rate is 240 to 260 bpm. This electrophysiologic mechanism underlies SVT in over 90% of fetuses and neonates presenting with this arrhythmia. The other mechanisms that may cause SVT are considerably rarer

and more difficult to control. The latter include automatic tachycardia (arising within an irritable ectopic atrial focus, above the bundle of His), or atrial flutter or fibrillation.[40-54]

Atrioventricular reciprocating tachycardia requires an anatomic substrate in the electrical conduction system that results from the existence of at least two discrete pathways with differing conduction velocities and recovery times (Fig. 27–1). In this setting, an incidental extrasystole that occurs with a critical timing ("coupling interval") after the preceding sinus beat may encounter the atrioventricular junction at a time when one of the available conduction pathways has recovered its ability to conduct from atrium to ventricle. At the same time the second limb is still unable to conduct the impulse, due to its longer recovery or refractory period (Fig. 27–2). If the limb that conducts activity to the ventricle conducts the impulse slowly enough, the electrical impulse spreading through the ventricular muscle may reach the ventricular end of the slowly recovering limb after it has had an opportunity to recover its conductivity. The electrical impulse may then reenter the atrium (Fig. 27–3), by conducting upward, from ventricle to atrium, thus establishing a circular movement of electrical energy that enters and reenters atrium and ventricle (Fig. 27–4). Thus "reentry" or "reciprocating" tachycardia refers to the unidirectional block of conduction over one of the pathways, antegrade conduction over the second pathway, and then reentry over the initially refractory pathway. Such reciprocating tachycardias occur most often in fetuses and neonates using an accessory conduction ("Kent") bundle discretely separate from the atrioventricular node tissue, and which electrically connects the atrium and ventricle across the fibrous atrioventricular junction, bypassing the normal electrical delay in the AV node. This is the underlying mechanism for the Wolff-Parkinson-White (WPW) syndrome. Alternatively, some neonates and fetuses have atrioventricular reentry within the region of the AV node itself, where some of the electrically active tissue appears to have differing conduction velocities and refractory periods than neighboring tissue within the node itself. Such babies present with reciprocating supraventricular tachycardia, which has the same physiologic, albeit slightly different anatomic, substrate as those with discrete accessory conduction pathways (Fig. 27–5).

In both forms of reciprocating SVT (atrioventricular reentry [discrete conduction bundle-mediated] and AV *nodal* reentry), the arrhythmia depends upon a critical relationship between conduction velocity and refractory period in the two pathways conducting impulses. Therapeutic intervention is logically aimed at interrupting the delicate balance in timing between the two electrical pathways of reentry that are required to sustain the tachycardia[55-70] (Figs. 27–6 and 27–7).

Atrial Flutter

Atrial flutter is an arrhythmia that also arises due to reentry of electrical impulses around a circular circuit. In this case the reentry circuit involves pathways with

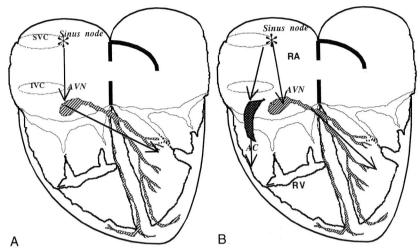

A   B

F I G U R E 27–1. *A,* Depiction of the conduction system in the normal fetal heart. The sinus node (*asterisk*) is the site of the fasted intrinsic pacemaker activity. The heart beats at the rate of the fastest intrinsic pacemaker that has intact electrical conduction to the ventricular muscle. In the normal situation, electrical impulses spread through the right and left atrial muscle and converge at the atrioventricular junction at the site of the atrioventricular node (AVN). The fibrous atrioventricular junction is electrically inert. Electrical conduction normally occurs from atrium to ventricle through the atrioventricular node, through the bundle of His, to enter the Purkinje fibers that make up the right and left bundle branches, that conduct the electrical impulse to the ventricular muscle, which contracts in response to electrical stimulation. The depolarization of the atrium appears on the electrocardiogram (ECG) as the P-wave. The depolarization of the ventricles is seen on the electrocardiogram as the QRS complex. The latter is usually narrow, representing relatively rapid conduction of electrical impulses through the ventricles via the conduction system. Conduction velocity through the atrioventricular node is relatively slow, and results in a delay between atrial and ventricular depolarization that is seen on the ECG as the PR interval. This results in coordinated mechanical responses of the atrium and ventricle. The active contraction of the atrium contributes to ventricular filling. A loss of the normal sequence of atrioventricular contraction results in a decrease of 15 to 20% in ventricular stroke volume and cardiac output. This decrease is of little significance postnatally in the normal cardiovascular system, but may be of great hemodynamic importance in the face of myocardial systolic or diastolic dysfunction, or in a cardiovascular system that has limited systolic or diastolic reserve, such as the cardiovascular system in the normal human fetus. The sinus node is located in the right atrium, at the junction of the superior vena cava (SVC). The atrioventricular node is normally located at the junction of the right atrium and the crest of the ventricular septum, medial to the inferior vena cava (IVC). *B,* In the presence of an accessory electrical connection (AC) at the atrioventricular junction there is an alternate pathway for electrical conduction, directly from atrial to ventricular muscle, outside of the AVN. In this situation the conduction velocity between atrium and ventricle is faster than that in the atrioventricular node. During normal sinus rhythm in the presence of such an accessory connection the heart rate and rhythm are governed by the pacemaker activity of the sinus node. The QRS complex on the electrocardiogram will reflect the early depolarization of the ventricular muscle at the distal end of the accessory connection as a slurred depolarization wave, or "delta" wave. The QRS complex will be wider than normal, due to the fact that the early depolarization into the ventricular muscle is occurring outside of the normal, rapid, conduction within the bundle branch system. The QRS complex is, therefore, wider than normal, with the early portion of the complex reflecting electrical depolarization through "preexcited" ventricular muscle. This depolarization then "fuses" with the normal, rapid, terminal depolarization of ventricular muscle through the bundle branch system that has occurred with the depolarization that was delayed in its passage through the normal atrioventricular nodal tissue. This accounts for the appearance of the electrocardiogram postnatally in the Wolff-Parkinson-White syndrome.

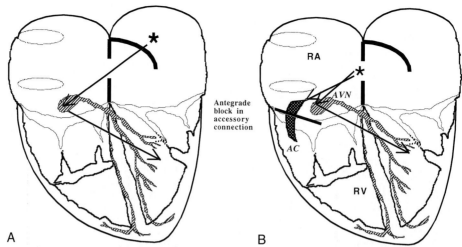

A   B

FIGURE 27–2. *A,* Depiction of the electrical conduction system in the fetal heart in the presence of a supraventricular premature contraction (*asterisk*). In this case an irritable ectopic pacemaker has depolarized prior to the anticipated depolarization of the sinus node. The electrical impulse from this early pacemaker spreads through the atrial tissue to arrive at the atrioventricular node, through which it courses to depolarize the ventricle. In this situation there will be an irregular rhythm, due to the early atrial and subsequent ventricular depolarization. If the premature contraction occurs early enough following the previous conducted impulse it may encounter the atrioventricular node during its recovery, or refractory, period, while it is unable to conduct electrical impulses. In this situation the "blocked extrasystole" will lead to a pause in fetal cardiac rhythm. *B,* Supraventricular extrasystole (*asterisk*) in a fetal heart with an accessory conduction pathway (AC). In this situation the refractory periods of the accessory pathway and the atrioventricular node usually differ from one another. Typically, the atrioventricular node conducts impulses slowly, but has a rapid recovery (short refractory period), whereas the accessory conduction pathways conduct impulses rapidly but have a longer recovery (long refractory period). In the case demonstrated in this figure the premature impulse encounters the atrioventricular node at a point when it has recovered its ability to conduct impulses, whereas the accessory connection is still refractory, and the premature impulse is not conducted through this pathway into the ventricular muscle.

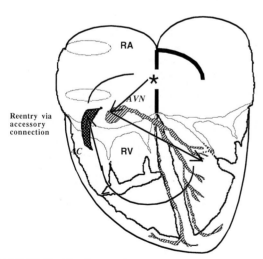

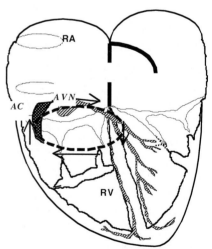

FIGURE 27–3. After having been conducted to the ventricle by way of the atrioventricular node, which conducts impulses slowly, the impulse spreads through the ventricular myocardium and encounters the distal (ventricular) end of the accessory connection. By this time the accessory connection has recovered its capacity to conduct impulses, and allows the electrical impulse to "reenter" the atrium in a retrograde direction.

FIGURE 27–4. Depiction of a fetal heart with reciprocating atrioventricular reentrant tachycardia. The electrical impulse that reentered the atrium spreads through the atrial muscle and reenters the atrioventricular node to stimulate the ventricle. This has established a circular ("circus") movement of electrical impulses that stimulates the atria and ventricles sequentially and repetitively at a rate that exceeds and usurps that of the intrinsic sinus node pacemaker. There is one atrial valve for each ventricular depolarization. The heart rate is dependent upon the size of the reentrant pathway and the conduction velocity within the involved circuits. In the human fetus the heart rate during reciprocating atrioventricular tachycardia is typically 240 to 260 bpm.

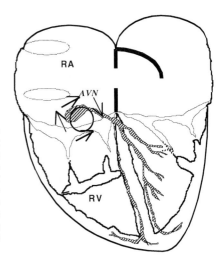

FIGURE 27–5. Depiction of a fetal heart with atrioventricular nodal reentry tachycardia. There is an obvious similarity to the electrophysiology of atrioventricular reentry tachycardia; using an accessory atrioventricular connection the tachycardia in this arrhythmia involves a circus movement of electrical stimulation at the atrioventricular junction. Atrioventricular conduction is via the slow pathway within the atrioventricular node. Unlike the situation with atrioventricular reciprocating tachycardia, however, the retrograde limb of the reentry circuit is not an anatomically discrete atrioventricular accessory connection, but rather rapidly conducting fibers within the atrioventricular junction itself, within or immediately adjacent to the atrioventricular node itself. Once again the rate of the tachycardia is dependent upon the size and intrinsic properties of the electrical conduction tissue comprising the reentry circuit, and there is a 1:1 relationship between atrial and ventricular stimulation.

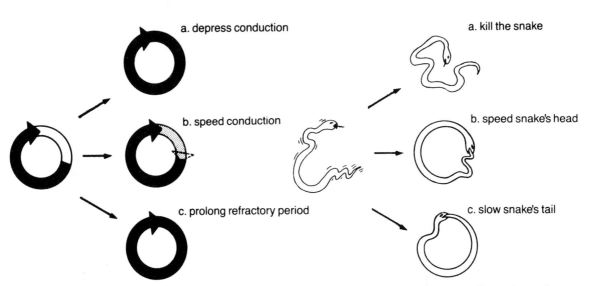

FIGURE 27–6. This diagram demonstrates the circular wavelet that sustains "circus movement" or reciprocating tachycardia. The circular movement of electrical energy occurs over intact electrical conduction tissue, around an electrically inert area. The latter may represent electrically isolated tissue at the atrioventricular junction, in the case of atrioventricular reciprocating tachycardia, or may represent fibrous or scar tissue within the atrial or ventricular myocardium. In order to sustain such a circuit the timing of electrical conduction and refractory periods must be maintained. Therapeutic strategies for antiarrhythmic therapy of such tachycardias are aimed at disturbing the delicate balance that must exist between electrical conduction and refractoriness. Dr. Katz, in this diagram, has likened this circular movement to a snake chasing its tail. In order to terminate electrical reentry one may depolarize the entire circuit simultaneously. This may be accomplished clinically with synchronized DC cardioversion. This would be the equivalent of killing the snake. Alternatively, by either speeding conduction in the slow limb, slowing it in the rapid limb, or by prolonging the refractory period in one or another limb of the conduction system the electrical wavefront will encounter refractory conduction tissue, and the electrical circuit will be interrupted. (From Katz AM: Physiology of the Heart, 2nd ed. New York: Raven Press, 1992, p 543, with permission.)

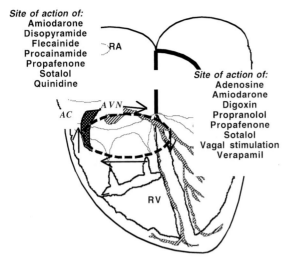

FIGURE 27–7. In this diagram the various antiarrhythmic agents that have been used for the therapy of atrioventricular reentry in the fetus are superimposed upon the diagram depicting atrioventricular reentry tachycardia via an accessory conduction pathway. The antiarrhythmic agents are listed according to the primary site of their action, that is, whether they slow conduction and/or recovery within the accessory connection or within the atrioventricular node.

distinct electrophysiologic properties separated by electrically inactive tissue (usually fibrous tissue or scar). The circuit is completely contained within the atrium, and does not involve ventricular muscle at all. The atrioventricular node is not part of the circuit, and serves only to transmit, with a variable degree of slowing or block, the atrial flutter waves to the ventricles (Fig. 27–8). Unlike reciprocating SVT, slowing or blocking conduction through the AV node does not terminate the arrhythmia, but decreases the ventricular response rate to the atrial flutter.[47]

The atrial rate in atrial flutter in the neonate is typically 300 to 400 bpm, whereas in the fetus atrial flutter rates up to 500 bpm may be seen. The varying degrees of AV block that may be associated with atrial flutter may result in varying ventricular response rates, which may be fixed at a given fraction of the atrial flutter rate (e.g., fixed 2:1, 3:1), or variable (with varying degrees of AV block) (Fig. 27–9). In either case the fetal heart rate does not respond in a regular 1:1 fashion to fetal atrial activity. Atrial flutter is an arrhythmia seen in later life in patients who have progressive dilation of the atria, for example, in cases of chronic mitral stenosis or insufficiency. In the fetus with atrial flutter the underlying substrate may also relate to atrial dilation, as seen in patients with right atrial enlargement secondary to tricuspid valve regurgitation in the Ebstein malformation of the tricuspid valve, or in fetuses with left atrial dilation, secondary to mitral insufficiency.

Atrial Fibrillation

Atrial fibrillation is an even rarer arrhythmia in the fetus than atrial flutter. This arrhythmia results from extremely rapid and disorganized electrical stimulation of the atrial chambers, which "writhe" at extremely rapid

rates. Atrioventricular conduction of atrial fibrillatory waves is blocked substantially in the AV node, resulting in variable ventricular response rates, with rhythms that are irregularly irregular (irregular without a fixed pattern to the irregularity).

Ventricular Tachycardia

These fetuses may present with intermittent or incessant tachycardia at rates varying from 180 to well over 300 bpm. While not invariably present, the finding of atrioventricular dissociation, with ventricular rates in excess of those in the atria, without a fixed relationship between atrial and ventricular mechanical (and presumably, electrical) activity, is highly suggestive of either ventricular or junctional origin of the arrhythmia. While ventricular tachycardia appears to be a more common (albeit, rare) fetal cardiac arrhythmia than junctional ectopic tachycardia, the distinction between these two arrhythmias is probably impossible using the echocardiographic techniques that are currently available for analysis of fetal arrhythmias. The underlying basis of this arrhythmia appears to be a reentrant electrical circuit that is contained within ventricular myocardium, with electrical circus movement around an electrically inert area of muscle (presumably fibrous tissue or scar). Such arrhythmias are significantly more common among adults, who have a propensity for the development of discrete areas of ventricular scar, relating to ischemic heart disease (Fig. 27–10). Fetuses and neonates, with a predilection for segmental abnormalities of myocardial oxygen supply/demand, such as those with severe ventricular hypertrophy secondary to semilunar valve stenosis, hypertrophic cardiomyopathy, coronary artery

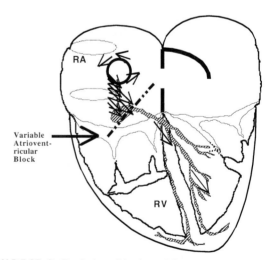

FIGURE 27–8. Depiction of fetal atrial flutter. In this situation the sinus pacemaker is usurped by a rapid circus movement of tachycardia in an electrical circuit that is completely contained within atrial tissue. The circuit occurs around an area of electrically inert atrial myocardium, presumably a site of fibrosis or scar within the atrium. Atrial stimulation typically occurs at rates between 360 and 500 bpm. There is almost always some degree of atrioventricular block, resulting in a regular or irregular ventricular response rate that is slower than the monotonous, very rapid, atrial rate.

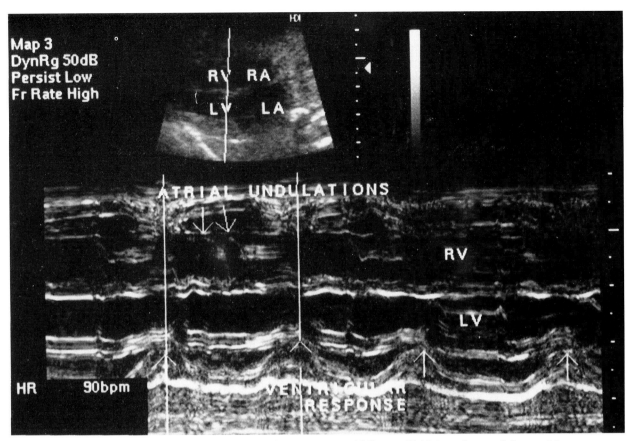

FIGURE 27–9. An M-mode echocardiogram demonstrating atrial flutter with high-grade second-degree atrioventricular block. The M-mode cursor is oriented through the ventricular body. The posterior wall of the left ventricle is seen at the lower aspect of the tracing, while the undulations of the tricuspid valve can be seen within the right ventricular cavity. The tricuspid valve is undulating rapidly and reflects an atrial flutter rate of 450 bpm. The 5:1 Mobitz type II atrioventricular block results in a regular fetal bradycardia at a rate of 90 bpm.

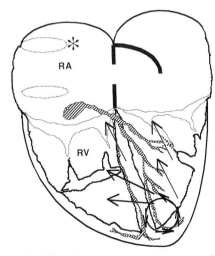

FIGURE 27–10. This diagram presents a representation of a fetal heart with ventricular tachycardia. Fetal ventricles are beating at a rate governed by a circus movement of electrical energy arising within the ventricular muscle. The circus movement occurs around an area of electrically inert ventricular myocardium, presumably an area of fibrosis or scar. In most cases the ventricular impulses are faster than the atrial impulses and are dissociated from the atrial rhythm, although there may, rarely, be retrograde ventriculoatrial conduction of ventricular beats into the atrium.

abnormalities, or cardiac tumors, may present with ventricular tachycardia. Alternatively, fetuses with genetic abnormalities of myocardial structure, such as those with "arrhythmogenic right ventricular dysplasia," or those with inborn abnormalities of ion channel function, resulting in prolongation and dispersion of ventricular repolarization (e.g., prolongation of the QTc interval [electrocardiographic QT interval corrected for pulse rate]) may present with ventricular tachycardia.[71–73]

Sinus Bradycardia

Bradycardia in the fetus may be found during labor, in the presence of placental insufficiency. On the other hand, fetal heart rates that vary rate normally around a baseline heart rate below 110 to 120 bpm may be encountered in otherwise normal fetuses. In such situations the potential for fetal hypothyroidism should be considered. In some fetuses, with structurally abnormal hearts, there may be anatomic absence of a dominant sinus node. In such cases the heart rate will be determined by a lower, slower, nonsinus pacemaker. Structural abnormalities such as bilateral superior venae cavae, atrioventricular septal defect, or inferior vena caval interruption, with azygous or hemiazygous continuation to the superior vena cava should be sought in such patients, to rule out the presence of left atrial isomerism. The latter is a syndrome in which atrial anatomy resembles that of bilateral left atria and, therefore, does not contain a normal sinus node (normally a right atrial structure).[74-80]

"Blocked Atrial Bigeminy"

Supraventricular extrasystolic beats may occur in a random or in a fixed relationship with the underlying sinus rhythm. In some cases the extrasystolic beat may result from "reentry" of electrical energy from the ventricular depolarization of the previous sinus beat into the atrium. If such a reentry occurs before the limb of the conduction system that conducts impulses in the antegrade direction (atrium to ventricle) has recovered its ability to conduct, the resulting rhythm will be irregular. The "echo" beat will have depolarized the atrium, but there will be no corresponding ventricular response. If such beats recur in a regular pattern (e.g., an echo beat follows alternately after each sinus beat [bigeminy]), the result will be to have a ventricular response that is regular, at a rate that is considerably lower than the intrinsic sinus rate. The result is fetal bradycardia.[81, 82] The pathology underlying this bradycardia does not involve an abnormality of AV nodal function, and each ventricular contraction is preceded by an atrial contraction. This rhythm can be distinguished from sinus bradycardia and from second-degree AV block by noting the pattern of atrial depolarization (electrocardiographically), or atrial contraction (echocardiographically). In sinus bradycardia the atrial rate is slow and equal to the ventricular rate. In second-degree AV block the atrial rate is normal or somewhat above normal, with a regular atrial rhythm. In this case the ventricle would not respond to every atrial contraction. In the case of blocked atrial bigeminy, or blocked atrial echo beats, the atrial contraction pattern is irregular, with a distinct pairing of atrial contractions, with a ventricular response occurring only after the first of the two paired atrial beats. The significance of this pattern of contraction relates to the potential for completion of a reentry circuit in response to one of the ectopic or echo beats, with the subsequent development of reciprocating supraventricular tachycardia. The presence of echo beats establishes the presence of an accessory conduction pathway, allowing electrical impulses to be conducted in the retrograde direction, from ventricle to atrium. It does not necessarily follow that the electrical properties of the two pathways can support a completed circus pathway for development of a sustained reciprocating supraventricular tachycardia.

Atrioventricular Block

Atrioventricular block represents an impairment in conduction between sinus node activation and ventricular activation. The various degrees of AV block vary in etiology and pathologic significance.[83]

First-Degree Atrioventricular Block

First-degree atrioventricular block refers to a greater than normal interval between the onset of sinus node activation and the first activation of the ventricular muscle (prolonged PR interval). Structural heart disease may contribute to first-degree heart block through dilation of the right atrium, through which the atrial activation must pass before reaching the AV node and the bundle of His. In most patients, however, first-degree atrioventricular block results from prolonged conduction within the AV node, itself. While first-degree block may be diagnosed by measurement of the PR interval on the neonatal electrocardiogram (ECG), in the mid-trimester fetus recordings of the fetal ECG signal, obtained from the maternal abdominal wall, do not provide high-quality recordings of atrial P waves. While gross abnormalities in the interval between atrial and ventricular wall activation may suggest the presence of first-degree atrioventricular block in the fetal echocardiogram, we have not been successful in diagnosing first-degree atrioventricular block in the human fetus.

Second-Degree Atrioventricular Block

Periodic pauses in ventricular activation in the presence of regular atrial stimulation result when there are occasional atrial electrical impulses that are nonconducted. Two patterns of such intermittent loss of conduction have been described. The first, described at the turn of the 20th century by Wenckebach, results when there is a progressive lengthening of the PR interval, with progressive shortening of the RR interval, until there is a skipped beat. While there are a number of potential explanations for the presence of Wenckebach-type, or "Mobitz type I," second-degree block, the frequent association of this conduction abnormality among patients with increased vagal tone suggests some involvement of the autonomic nervous system in its causation.

Mobitz type II atrioventricular block is the periodic loss of atrioventricular conduction without a progressive lengthening of PR interval. This may be manifest as occasional loss of atrioventricular conduction, or, in the presence of high-grade second-degree block, as several consecutive dropped beats. While the former may be associated with wide swings in vagal tone, high-grade second-degree block is usually associated with conduction system disease, and may presage the development of complete heart block. High-grade second-degree heart block may be associated with Stokes-Adams attacks and sudden death.

Second-Degree Heart Block and Congenital QT Prolongation

In infants with marked prolongation of the QT interval, the repolarization of the ventricle may be so prolonged that the ventricle remains refractory to the electrical stimulation of the subsequent sinus beat, resulting in a slowing of ventricular rate, due to the presence of 2:1 atrioventricular block. This represents a rare presentation of a rare genetic syndrome. Many of these cases present sporadically, and probably represent isolated genetic mutations. The potential for the development of polymorphic ventricular tachycardia and sudden death, secondary to dispersion of ventricular repolarization, is exceedingly high. Fetuses and neonates presenting with 2:1 atrioventricular block as a manifestation of prolonged QT-interval syndrome have mortality rates as high as 50% within the first months of life, and as high as 75%[84–89] within the first 18 months of life. This mortality rate is considerably higher than that reported in other pediatric studies of the prolonged QT interval.

Complete Heart Block

In complete atrioventricular block atrial electrical impulses are completely unable to propagate through the conduction system to activate the ventricles.[90–106] There is atrioventricular dissociation, with a regular atrial rate that is faster than the ventricular rate, without a fixed relationship between atrial and ventricular activation (Fig. 27–11). This conduction abnormality is invariably associated with an anatomic abnormality in the atrioventricular node, the penetrating bundle of His, or with extensive damage of the distal conduction system, involving the bundle branches.

In congenital complete atrioventricular block these structural abnormalities may accompany complex congenital heart disease, or may be associated with inflammatory damage to otherwise anatomically normal conduction systems.

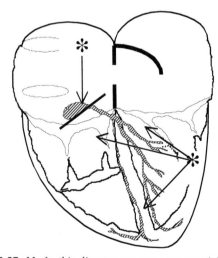

FIGURE 27–11. In this diagram we see a representation of fetal complete atrioventricular block. The ventricles are beating at the rate of the fastest intact intrinsic pacemaker. In this case that is depicted within the ventricular myocardium itself. The "lower" the escaping pacemaker within the cardiac conduction system, the slower the ventricular rate. There is atrioventricular dissociation, with a faster atrial than ventricular rate, due to a complete electrical disconnection between the atrium and ventricle, usually at the level of the atrioventricular node and/or the bundle of His. In the human fetus congenital complete atrioventricular block is usually either a manifestation of complex deformity of the anatomy of the atrioventricular node or a manifestation of autoimmune damage to the normally formed atrioventricular node.

Sustained Fetal Cardiac Arrhythmias and Congestive Circulatory Failure

The development of fetal and placental anasarca (nonimmune hydrops fetalis) represents an imbalance between serum oncotic pressure and transmural hydrostatic pressure, resulting in a net water flux into the interstitial tissue and third spaces. Hydrops fetalis may, therefore, result from cardiac systolic or diastolic pump failure; from hepatic dysfunction and secondary hypoalbuminemia and lowered oncotic pressure; from mechanical or hemodynamic obstruction to venous or lymphatic drainage; from endothelial dysfunction, allowing for abnormal fluid extravasation; or from altered physical properties of interstitial tissue.[107–110]

The intrinsic characteristics of the fetal heart and circulatory system render the fetus particularly susceptible to the development of hydrops fetalis as a manifestation of circulatory insufficiency. Studies performed over 20 years ago on the immature myocardium of the sheep demonstrated that the fetal heart has limited systolic reserve compared with that of mature myocardium. Furthermore, these studies demonstrated that at any given end-diastolic myocardial cell length the end-diastolic pressure was higher in the fetal heart than in the more mature heart (e.g., fetal myocardium is less compliant than mature myocardium).[111] Subsequent studies in the human fetus, using pulsed-Doppler echocardiography, have demonstrated evidence of diastolic filling characteristics of the fetal ventricles that strongly suggest that the fetal heart is dependent upon the active phase of ventricular filling, associated with atrial contraction.[112] These filling characteristics are quite similar to those noted postnatally in patients with restrictive cardiomyopathy,[113] in whom the onset of atrial fibrillation, with a loss of coordinated atrioventricular contractions, is accompanied by a precipitous drop (approximately 20%) in stroke output, and a remarkable increase in venous filling pressure.

The human fetal circulatory system has been demonstrated, using pulsed-Doppler techniques,[112, 114] to have the two ventricular circulations connected in parallel with one another, with communications at the level of the foramen ovale and the ductus arteriosus. As in the fetal lamb,[115] these parallel circuits support a circulation that is relatively right-ventricular dominant, with most left ventricular filling derived from shunting of inferior vena caval blood directly across the foramen ovale, into the left atrium. The systemic venous circulation of the fetus is, therefore, relatively volume overloaded compared with the pulmonary venous circulation, and any impairment in ventricular systolic or diastolic performance is apt to result in further volume loading of the systemic venous circulation. In light of the known restriction to diastolic filling of the fetal ventricles, this increase in systemic venous volume loading is accompanied by a dramatic increase in systemic venous pressure.

The association of sustained fetal supraventricular tachycardia with nonimmune hydrops fetalis has been well established,[116] as has the high fetal and neonatal mortality associated with hydrops fetalis of any cause.[107] It is reasonable to assume, therefore, that severely hydropic fetuses with fetal arrhythmias are at high mortality risk and that such fetuses might be considered candidates for in utero antiarrhythmic therapy, following a rational risk/benefit analysis.

Hydrops Fetalis with Supraventricular Tachycardia

The association between the development of hydrops fetalis and the presence of sustained fetal supraventricular tachycardia has been well described through the years. While some workers[39] have suggested that even intermittent fetal supraventricular tachycardia invariably eventuates in fetal congestive heart failure, we have not found this to be the case. While incessant supraventricular tachycardia in the fetus is often associated with hydrops fetalis, we have encountered many fetuses with frequent extrasystoles and short runs of nonsustained supraventricular tachycardia who neither present with fetal edema nor go on to develop congestive heart failure, under careful observation. We find it difficult, therefore, to advise all such parents that the finite risks involved in the ingestion of antiarrhythmic medications are outweighed by the benefit of doing so.

On the other hand, it does appear that there must be some threshold beyond which the duration of the episodes of tachycardia, or other factors regarding the tachycardia, overwhelm the "reserve" of the fetal cardiovascular system, with resulting congestive heart failure.[35] If it were possible to accurately predict which particular fetus is at highest risk for the development of hydrops fetalis, one would be able to optimize fetal therapy. This would avoid the unwarranted risk of exposing mother and fetus to potent antiarrhythmic agents in cases that are at low risk for the development of fetal congestive heart failure, while providing timely and effective therapy to the fetus at high risk. By providing antiarrhythmic therapy to the high-risk fetus without awaiting severe congestive heart failure one could conceivably avoid potential long-term complications that may accompany the altered fetal blood flow associated with incessant supraventricular tachycardia and congestive circulatory failure.[117] It has, for example, been suggested that fetal supraventricular tachycardia and hydrops fetalis may be associated with neurodevelopmental impairment of the neonate, secondary to impaired fetal cerebral perfusion associated with the fetal arrhythmia.[118–120]

We have recently reported[120] observations that suggest that the site of ectopic atrial stimulation or the location of the bypass tract mediating atrioventricular reentry, by preexciting the left atrium of the fetus (Fig. 27–12), may be predictive of a particularly high risk for the development of hydrops fetalis. This preexcitation of the fetal left atrium appears to transiently reverse the usual pressure gradient in utero that normally favors filling of the left atrium directly from the fetal inferior vena cava. By altering this pressure gradient, left atrial preexcitation results in partial closure of the fetal foramen ovale, thereby trapping venous return in the already volume-loaded fetal right atrium and right ventricle.[121] Since fetal cardiac ventricles are relatively restrictive, this additional volume loading results in a

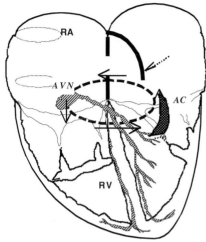

F I G U R E 27–12. In this fetal heart there is atrioventricular reciprocating tachycardia involving an accessory connection. Is this case, however, the accessory connection bridges the atrioventricular junction between the left atrium and left ventricle. In this situation the tachycardia is identical to that in the heart in Figure 27–6, but the retrograde ventriculoatrial conduction stimulates contraction of the left atrium a fraction of a second prior to the stimulation of the right atrium. This results in a transient reversal of the usual pressure relationship between the right atrium and systemic venous return and the left atrium. This reversal of pressure relationships results in partial closure of the foramen ovale, due to apposition of the atrial septum primum against the septum secundum rim of the foramen ovale. The premature narrowing of the foramen ovale results in "trapping" of systemic venous return in the right atrium and systemic venous circulation. The latter leads to increased hydrostatic pressure in the systemic venous circulation, and predisposes such fetuses to early accumulation of interstitial edema and fluid third-spacing.

dramatic increase in venous hydrostatic pressure, and leads to the early development of fetal hydrops.

We have adopted a policy of attempting to determine which of the two atria is being excited first. If we find evidence of left atrial preexcitation and, especially if we find evidence that the foramen ovale is smaller than normal (smaller than 30 to 35% of atrial septal area or less than aortic orifice size), we are more aggressive about initiating fetal antiarrhythmic therapy, even in the absence of overt fetal edema.

Observations in several laboratories[122, 123] have demonstrated that rapid atrial pacing of the fetal lamb quickly results in the accumulation of fetal edema and the development of hydrops fetalis. Such lambs immediately develop markedly elevated right atrial and central venous hypertension. This is associated with the immediate development of retrograde flow pulsations in the fetal inferior vena cava. These pulsations are detectable within the hepatic venous system. Such venous pulsations are associated with impaired hepatic synthesis of albumin. While not observed in all studies, Nimrod and associates noted the rapid development of fetal hypoalbuminemia. The rapidity with which hypoalbuminemia developed appears to rule out impaired synthesis of albumin as the sole cause of the decreased serum oncotic pressure, requiring that one invoke a poorly understood increase in transmural leakage of albumin into the interstitial tissue. With further tachycardia the development of tachycardia-induced myocardial dysfunction is found. We have been impressed that biatrial dilation and diminished atrial contraction may precede the development of biventricular dilation and diminished ventricular shortening. Atrial pump failure may accompany or even precede the development of ventricular systolic pump dysfunction, and lead to further circulatory impairment of the fetus with protracted, incessant supraventricular tachycardia or atrial flutter.

We have encountered two fetuses, and have recently been made aware of a third case[124] in which fetal hydrops resolved in fetuses with sustained supraventricular tachycardia following initiation of digoxin therapy, despite persistence of the tachycardia. Whether this relates to a slight (<10%) decrease in the heart rate, or to drug-induced enhancement of the ventricular inotropic state, is unclear.

In fetuses with atrial flutter and variable or fixed atrioventricular block the ventricular response rate may vary.[125, 126] Ventricular systolic pump failure may not be encountered when the degree of atrioventricular block prevents the development of incessantly rapid ventricular rates. Nonetheless, fetal atrial flutter may be associated with hydrops fetalis. In these fetuses the atrial flow characteristics and the retrograde flow in the inferior vena caval and hepatic circulations are manifest, just as they are observed in the ovine models. In such cases it is unclear whether the underlying etiology is solely related to the abnormal venous flow patterns and associated atrial pump failure or whether the hydrops fetalis developed at a time when the ventricular response rates were considerably higher, resulting in ventricular pump failure as well. In such cases, however, we have been impressed that simply ensuring that the atrioventricular block is maintained, preventing the development of rapid ventricular response rates, is an unsatisfactory treatment paradigm. Unlike the situation in adults with atrial flutter or fibrillation, in which symptoms of heart failure are usually resolved with ventricular rate control alone, when hydrops has developed in the fetus with atrial flutter it is necessary to restore a 1:1 relationship between atrial and ventricular contractions if the third-spaced fluid is to be resolved. We believe that this is related to the persistent presence of cannon waves, which occur when the atrium contracts against a closed or partially closed atrioventricular valve. This results in persistent elevation in the mean atrial and venous pressures. This persistent elevation of hydrostatic pressure, in the presence of decreased fetal osmotic pressure associated with fetal hypoalbuminemia, does not favor the resolution of fetal edema, and fluid third-spacing. In the fetal patient presenting with atrial flutter and atrioventricular block without fetal edema, we believe that control of atrioventricular conduction, to prevent overly rapid ventricular contraction rates, along with inotropic support of fetal systolic pump function associated with the administration of digoxin to the fetus, may prevent the deterioration in cardiovascular function that leads to hydrops fetalis.

Hydrops Fetalis in the Fetus with Complete Heart Block

The second group of fetuses who have demonstrated a proclivity for the development of hydrops fetalis in the presence of sustained fetal rhythm disturbances are those with congenital complete heart block.[127]

Many observers have confirmed that there are two relatively equal-sized groups of fetuses who present with congenital complete heart block. They are characterized as fetuses with major forms of congenital heart disease versus those with normal cardiac structure. In cases in which congenital complete heart block is associated with congenital heart disease the latter usually involves a complex abnormality of atrioventricular connection. The most commonly associated congenital cardiac malformation with complete heart block is left atrial isomerism. In these fetuses there is congenital absence of the sinoatrial node. The atria most often resemble bilateral left atria, lack a coronary sinus and triangle of Koch, and the atrioventricular connection is ambiguous. These patients often have complex intracardiac malformations, usually manifesting forms of atrioventricular septal defect, often with associated abnormalities of pulmonary venous return (partial anomalous) and systemic venous return (interrupted suprarenal segment of the inferior vena cava with azygous or hemiazygous continuation to right- or left-sided venae cavae). The second most common association between congenital complete heart block and congenital heart disease is found in fetuses with atrioventricular and ventriculoarterial discordant connections (physiologically corrected transposition) with or without associated ventricular septal defects and/or ventricular outflow tract obstruction. The atrioventricular discordant connection is associated with a congenitally malformed atrioventricular node and penetrating portion of the bundle of His. Other congenital malformations that are found in association with congenital complete heart block are complete atrioventricular septal ("canal") defects without atrial isomerism, and ventricular septal defects (the latter most frequently posterior inflow ["canal-type"]).

When congenital complete heart block is associated with complex congenital heart disease, it is not uncommon for the fetus to develop congestive heart failure and hydrops fetalis prior to delivery. In such cases there is almost always significant atrioventricular valve regurgitation detected, either through the common atrioventricular valve of the atrioventricular septal defect, or via a displaced and congenitally dysplastic left atrioventricular valve in the fetus with congenitally corrected transposition. The prognosis for survival of these fetuses is quite poor, regardless of the aggressiveness of prenatal or postnatal therapy. Most centers caring for infants with congenital heart disease and congenital heart block routinely place permanent pacemakers in infants with complete heart block and associated congenital heart disease, especially when the congenital heart disease is associated either with congestive heart failure or with significant cyanosis.

The second subgroup of fetuses with complete heart block have structurally normal hearts. In these fetuses there is almost always a significant titer of anti-RNA antibodies detectable in the mother.[128–146] These antibodies, SS-A (anti-Ro) and SS-B (anti-La), appear to cross the placenta and recognize certain fetal tissues as foreign material. The antibodies bind to fetal tissue, and the resulting inflammatory response and complement release result in tissue damage to fetal organs. These antibodies bind preferentially to fetal cardiac conduction tissue, contractile myocardium and, to a lesser extent, fetal adrenal cortex. While most fetuses presenting with congenital heart block from this etiology are not detected until there is a fixed fetal bradycardia secondary to complete heart block, some fetuses have been detected before complete heart block has been manifest. These fetuses may present with varying degrees of second-degree heart block, and presumably have immunoglobulin-mediated inflammatory damage to the conduction system that has not been completed. The potential for providing treatment aimed at ameliorating the immune-mediated inflammatory damage has been speculated upon by a number of workers. We have recently had a preliminary experience that suggests that in selected cases, detected early in the course of deterioration of the fetal conduction tissue, anti-inflammatory treatment may ameliorate the ongoing damage to the fetal conduction system and limit or reverse the heart block.[147]

It should be noted that while many of the mothers of these fetuses have some form of collagen vascular disease (e.g., Sjögren syndrome or systemic lupus erythematosis), many have been free of inflammatory disease and do not subsequently develop such symptoms. Not all offspring of affected mothers develop heart block, despite the detection of high antibody titers during subsequent pregnancies. It is unclear whether this is related to variable transplacental transfer of antibodies, and a dose-response effect at the level of the fetal heart, or whether other factors, such as HLA, are operative in determining which offspring will and which will not be affected.[148, 149]

In cases in which immune-complex–related congenital complete heart block is associated with hydrops fetalis, the outlook for fetal survival is bleak. In a multicenter study[127] it was found that fetal prognosis related to the ventricular escape rate, with 55 bpm appearing to be the critical ventricular rate, below which there was a high fetal mortality risk. In addition, we noted that slow fetal atrial rates, below 80 bpm were, for the overall group of patients with complete heart block, a negative prognostic finding. After further analysis of data, however, it was found that the slow atrial rates were found predominantly among fetuses with complete heart block and congenital heart disease and, within that group, in the fetuses with complete heart block and left atrial isomerism.[127] The slow atrial rate, therefore, was related to the prominence of nonsinus, ectopic atrial rhythm among the patients with left atrial isomerism and lacking a dominant sinus node pacemaker.

We reasoned that since ventricular rate appeared to be a prognostic indicator, therapy aimed at increasing ventricular escape rate might improve the fetus with complete heart block and hydrops fetalis. While some workers[96, 150–152] have found that the administration of β-mimetic agents increases fetal heart rate and improves hydrops fetalis, we have found that while there may be as much as a 50% increase in ventricular escape rate among fetuses exposed to maternally administered ter-

butaline, isoproterenol, or salbutamol, there has been no improvement in fetal fluid third-spacing. We have attributed the latter to the persistence of atrioventricular dissociation, with persistence of "cannon" a-waves, related to atrial contraction against closed atrioventricular valves. These waves result in an increase in mean right atrial and systemic venous pressure that does not result in a favorable relationship between hydrostatic and oncotic pressure for fetal edema to resolve. It is for this reason that we have not been surprised to find that fetal ventricular pacing for fetuses with complete heart block and hydrops fetalis has been unsuccessful.[153–156] We suspect that such efforts are doomed to failure unless two issues are addressed: (1) the need to reestablish a fixed relationship between atrial and ventricular contraction (i.e., with dual chamber pacing and sensing), and (2) inotropic support of failing fetal myocardium that is affected by immune-complex–mediated fetal cardiomyopathy. The latter may require the use of inotropic support, with medications such as digoxin or β-mimetics, anti-inflammatory therapy such as steroids, or an effort to either lower antibody titers (maternal plasmapheresis) or introduce "blocking antibodies" (fetal and/or maternal intravenous γ-globulin therapy).

Risk-Benefit Analysis in Considering Fetal Antiarrhythmic Therapy

The simple existence of techniques to diagnose and treat fetal cardiac arrhythmias is insufficient justification to expose a mother and fetus to potentially hazardous medications. The management schema for such patients should include an understanding of the natural history of the arrhythmia, a precise understanding of the electrophysiologic basis of the arrhythmia, and a detailed understanding of the pharmacokinetics and pharmacology of these antiarrhythmic agents in the fetus, mother, and placenta.[22–28, 157–216] These must be factored into a common-sense approach to a risk-benefit analysis. The risk to the neonate increases proportionately with the degree of prematurity and lung immaturity at the time of initial diagnosis.

If, for example, the diagnosis of supraventricular tachycardia without hydrops fetalis is made at a gestational age when pulmonary maturity of the fetus is likely (or at an earlier age, but with lung maturity documented by amniocentesis), delivery with postnatal treatment is advisable. At extreme levels of prematurity, immediate delivery may not be a viable option. In this setting, the decision with regard to administration of in utero therapy should consider (1) the potential risk for the development of hydrops fetalis, (2) the potential risks to mother and fetus inherent in antiarrhythmic therapy, and (3) individual issues including the ability to provide adequate monitoring of mother and fetus and maternal willingness to submit to therapy (maternal autonomy vs. fetal risk).

The frequent association of hydrops fetalis with sustained supraventricular tachyarrhythmias and the dismal prognosis for such fetuses and neonates, regardless of the underlying cause of fetal anasarca, probably justify vigorous efforts at in utero therapy, if such therapy can be offered with a reasonable expectation of success at a tolerably low risk to the mother. Even a moderate risk to the fetus would be justifiable in this setting, in light of the poor prognosis for the neonate if the arrhythmia and hydrops fetalis are unremitting.[48, 107, 147, 198, 217–221]

Proarrhythmia and Antiarrhythmic Therapy

While antiarrhythmic medications are administered with the hope of suppressing cardiac rhythm disturbances, virtually all of these agents have the potential to provoke new, or to exacerbate existing, arrhythmias. This proclivity for paradoxic arrhythmogenesis is referred to as "proarrhythmia."[97, 193, 222–233] These effects may occur "early" after initiation of therapy, and may vary from nonserious through potentially fatal rhythm disturbances. Late proarrhythmic complications may manifest as enhanced arrhythmic death. Among the agents that have been used for fetal antiarrhythmic therapy, only the class II (β-blocking) agents appear to lack the potential for late proarrhythmic mortality.

Digitalis glycosides and Vaughn-Williams class I, II, III, or IV antiarrhythmic agents can cause severe sinus or atrioventricular node dysfunction. Digoxin toxicity may be associated with atrial tachycardia with variable atrioventricular block and with junctional tachycardia. Type IA and III agents, by prolonging the QT interval, may be associated with torsades de pointes polymorphic ventricular tachycardia along with other medications that bind to ventricular muscle cell membrane sodium channels or are metabolized by the enzymes of the cytochrome P-450 pathway, including tricyclic antidepressants, histamine blockers, erythromycin, clarithromycin, ketoconazole, trimethoprim-sulfamethoxazole, and cisapride.[234]

Uniform ventricular tachycardia resistant to resuscitation is a characteristic proarrhythmic response to IC antiarrhythmic agents such as flecainide and propafenone.

Such hazards render fetal antiarrhythmic therapy, administered through maternal drug treatment, to have the potential for a 200% mortality.

These proarrhythmic complications are of greatest concern in the presence of congestive heart failure, or in the presence of drug- or dietary-induced hypokalemia, hypocalcemia, or hypomagnesemia. Therapy with potent antiarrhythmic agents should be initiated in an inpatient setting, with low doses of the antiarrhythmic agents. If drug dosages are escalated, such increases should be made incrementally, with careful monitoring of fetal and maternal drug responses. Special care should be taken to avoid potentially hazardous drug combinations, either purposely administered or inadvertently combined, if second or third agents are initiated prior to adequate clearance of agents included in the early phases of therapy. In such circumstances care should be taken to hold prior therapy for at least 3 drug half-lives (Table 27–1) before treatment with a new agent is initiated.

Specific Treatment Protocols

Arrhythmia Diagnosis and Monitoring Antiarrhythmic Therapy

While it would be ideal to use high-quality recordings of the fetal ECG signal to analyze fetal cardiac rhythm and to monitor the effects of in utero antiarrhythmic therapy, the technology required to provide high-fidelity recordings of fetal ECG, free of interference from the maternal ECG signal, is still lagging.[235, 236] Fetal magnetocardiography has recently been proposed as a means for evaluating fetal cardiac electrical activity. The utility of this technique for the analysis of complex fetal cardiac arrhythmias, and for monitoring fetal antiarrhythmic therapy, has yet to be proven.[237, 238]

In the absence of a reliable fetal electrocardiographic signal, echocardiographic strategies have been developed to provide information concerning cardiac mechanical activity against time, with the assumption that recordings of mechanical or flow activity against time reflect preceding electrical stimulation of atrial or ventricular contraction. Using M-mode recordings of ventricular wall, septal, or valve motion or Doppler flow within the cardiac chambers or great arteries and veins against time, an analysis of atrial and ventricular mechanical activity provides information concerning cardiac electrical activity in real time (Figs. 27–13 to 27–15). Detailed descriptions of the use of echocardiographic strategies for the analysis of fetal cardiac rhythm are available in a number of publications.[112, 114, 239–288]

Fetal Supraventricular Tachyarrhythmic Treatment Protocols

Antiarrhythmic therapy should be initiated on an inpatient basis. External fetal cardiac monitoring is carried out for 12 to 24 hours prior to initiating drug therapy, to determine the proportion of time that the fetus is tachycardic. This will determine the severity of the arrhythmia, and provides baseline information to gauge the effectiveness of antiarrhythmic treatments.

There are no universal algorithms for the treatment of fetal arrhythmias. Arrhythmias do not respond in a predictable fashion postnatally, with occasional patients requiring aggressive multidrug treatment protocols, or invasive catheter therapies and radiofrequency ablation. It is naive to assume that a single "magic bullet" will be found that will successfully treat all forms of fetal tachycardia, or even all cases of reentrant tachycardia.

With this caveat, the following protocols for treatment of fetuses who present with fetal tachycardia may be considered. The accompanying algorithms refer to the use of varying antiarrhythmic agents. Information concerning specific antiarrhythmic agents, dosages, routes of administration, maternal and fetal side effects, and desired maternal serum levels may be found in Table

TABLE 27–1. FETAL ANTIARRHYTHMIC AGENTS

DRUG	CLASS	ARRHYTHMIA	DOSE	METABOLISM	SIDE EFFECTS & PRECAUTIONS	PA (%)	CLINICAL EXPERIENCE
Quinidine	IA	Supraventricular tachyarrhythmias; ventricular tachyarrhythmias	See clinical experience	Hepatic	Hypotension; torsades de pointes; sudden death; monitor QRS and QTc intervals; increases digoxin levels	5–20	Increases mortality; should not be used
Procainamide	IA	Supraventricular tachyarrhythmias; ventricular tachyarrhythmias	IV: 100-mg bolus over 2 min; up to 25 mg/min to 1 g over first hour; Maintenance 2–6 mg/min PO: 1 g; then up to 500 mg q3h	Hepatic metabolism to N-acetyl-procainamide; rapid renal elimination; $t_{1/2}$ 3.5 hr; therapeutic level 4–10 ng/mL	Hypotension with IV; limit oral use to 3–6 mo (lupus), gastrointestinal symptoms; agranulocytosis; torsades de pointes rare; interacts with class III agents (torsades de pointes); fetal levels may exceed maternal	9–21	Rarely effective; frequency of oral dosing major limitation to compliance; gastrointestinal side effects often limit compliance
Disopyramide	IA	Supraventricular tachyarrhythmias; ventricular tachyarrhythmias	PO: loading dose, 300 mg; then 100–200 mg q6h	Hepatic 50%; renal excretion of unmetabolized drug 50%; $t_{1/2}$ 8 hr; therapeutic level 3–6 μg/mL; toxic > 7 μg/mL	Hypotension; torsades de pointes; negative inotropic agent; vagolytic side effects; interacts with class II agents (torsades de pointes)	1–6	Rarely used in children; limited experience in fetus; side effects limit compliance; may worsen signs of CHF; may stimulate uterine contraction
Flecainide	IC	Supraventricular tachyarrhythmias; ventricular tachyarrhythmias	IV:Not available in USA; PO: 100–400 mg bid	Hepatic 67%; 33% renally excreted as unmetabolized drug; $t_{1/2}$ 13–19 hr; therapeutic trough level <1 μg/mL	Narrow therapeutic range; visual disturbances; lightheadedness; nausea; important negative inotropic effect; proarrhythmia; increases mortality post-MI; interacts with many antiarrhythmic	4–33	Probably safe with structurally normal hearts; must monitor for proarrhythmia; contraindicated with cardiac pump failure
Propafenone	IC	Supraventricular tachyarrhythmias; ventricular tachyarrhythmias	IV: Not available in USA PO: 150–300 mg tid	Hepatic (cytochrome P-450) $t_{1/2}$ 2–10 hr, up to 32 hr in nonmetabolizers; therapeutic level 0.2–3.0 μg/mL	Increases digoxin level; Prolongs QRS duration; negative inotropic effect; proarrhythmia; gastrointestinal side effects	5–15	Gastrointestinal side effects common
Propranolol	II	Supraventricular tachyarrhythmias; ventricular tachyarrhythmias	IV: 1–6 mg, slowly; PO: 40–160 mg q6h	Hepatic $t_{1/2}$ 1–6 hr; serum levels not therapeutically useful	Bronchospasm; heart block; negative inotropic effect; drug interactions; CNS depression; may mask symptoms of hypoglycemia in diabetics; may impair glucose tolerance in non–insulin-dependent diabetics; contraindicated in Raynaud phenomenon; contraindicated in sick-sinus syndrome	?	May prefer longer acting β-blockers (inderal LA; atenolol); may prefer more cardioselective agents (labetolol; atenolol; metoprolol); has been useful to suppress ectopy in fetuses with recurrent SVT; may depress respirations or cause hypoglycemia or bradycardia in neonate; possible association with low birthweight
Amiodarone	III	Supraventricular tachyarrhythmias; ventricular tachyarrhythmias	IV: 5 mg/kg over 20 min; 500–1,000 mg over 24 hr, then oral; PO: (loading) 1,200–1,600 mg/d in 2 divided doses for 7–14	Hepatic lipid soluble, distributes extensively throughout body; $t_{1/2}$ 25–110 days; Therapeutic level 1.0–2.5 μg/mL	Increases digoxin level; interacts with type I agents to predispose to torsades de pointes; side effects fetal or maternal hypo- or	4–30	Drug of last resort for fetal treatment; should not be used unless adequate doses of other antiarrhythmics are

Drug	Class	Indications	Dose	Metabolism/excretion	Adverse effects	%*	Comments
			days, then 400–800 mg QD for 1–3 wk; maintenance, 200–400 mg/d		hyperthyroidism; corneal microdeposits; photosensitivity; life-threatening pulmonary alveolitis (not dose-related); hepatitis; myopathy; neuropathy; nausea; rash; alopecia; tremor; insomnia; nightmares		unsuccessful or poorly tolerated; adverse reactions require drug discontinuation in approximately 20% of patients; may be excreted in milk for several weeks
Sotalol	III	Supraventricular tachyarrhythmias; ventricular tachyarrhythmias	IV: Not available in USA PO: 80–320 mg bid	Not metabolized; renal excretion of intact drug; $t_{1/2}$ 15–17 hr; therapeutic levels not measured	Torsades de pointes with hypokalemia; negative inotropic effect; sinus bradycardia; atrioventricular block; proarrhythmia more common in renal failure; proarrhythmia more common in females	10–16	Limited fetal experience; should probably be considered for early inclusion in treatment protocol if β-blockade is not contraindicated
Verapamil	IV	Supraventricular tachyarrhythmias	IV: 5–10 mg over 30–60 sec PO: 80–160 mg tid	Renal 75%; gastrointestinal 25%; $t_{1/2}$ 3–7 hr; serum levels not clinically useful	Calcium-channel blocking agent; increases digoxin levels; depresses sinoatrial and atrioventricular node function; contraindicated in sinus node dysfunction; contraindicated with magnesium sulfate; interacts with β-blockers; may cause cardiovascular collapse if given to immature heart with CHF; may cause cardiovascular collapse if given to patient with ventricular tachycardia	18	Use of IV verapamil for supraventricular tachycardia with CHF in neonates considered contraindicated; use with caution, if at all, in fetuses
Adenosine	IV	Reentrant supraventricular tachycardia	IV: 100–200 μg/kg estimated fetal weight by rapid bolus into umbilical vein; fetal therapy by maternal IV administration not feasible; PO: Not available	Metabolized throughout body by conversion to ATP; $t_{1/2}$ 10–30 sec; therapeutic levels not measured	Bronchospasm, especially in asthmatics; transient arrhythmias after conversion; briefly increases atrioventricular block	?	May be useful as diagnostic test to identify reentrant SVT; may break incessant SVT; does not prevent recurrent SVT
Digoxin	Cardiac glycoside	Supraventricular tachyarrhythmias	IV: 1 mg divided over 24 hr to load only; PO: 0.25–1.0 mg daily in 2 divided doses	Most excreted unchanged in urine; approximately 30% nonrenal clearance, more in presence of renal failure; $t_{1/2}$ 36 hr; therapeutic levels 1–2 ng/mL	Toxicity results in arrhythmias, nausea, anorexia, vomiting, diarrhea, malaise, fatigue, confusion, facial pain, insomnia, depression, vertigo, colored vision; may be encountered at low drug serum levels with hypokalemia or hypomagnesemia; interacts with quinidine, verapamil, amiodarone, propafenone, erythromycin; dose should be adjusted downward in renal failure	?	Contraindicated with ventricular arrhythmias; Contraindicated in Wolff-Parkinson-White syndrome (impossible to detect in fetus prenatally; mother should have ECG prior to therapy); may be poorly absorbed by hydropic fetuses; should have frequent ECG monitoring for evidence of toxicity

* Percentage of patients reported to develop proarrhythmia when using this agent for postnatal antiarrhythmic therapy.
IV, intravenous; PO, oral; CNS, central nervous system; SVT, supraventricular tachycardia; CHF, congestive heart failure; ATP, adenosine triphosphate; ECG, electrocardiogram; MI, myocardial infarction.

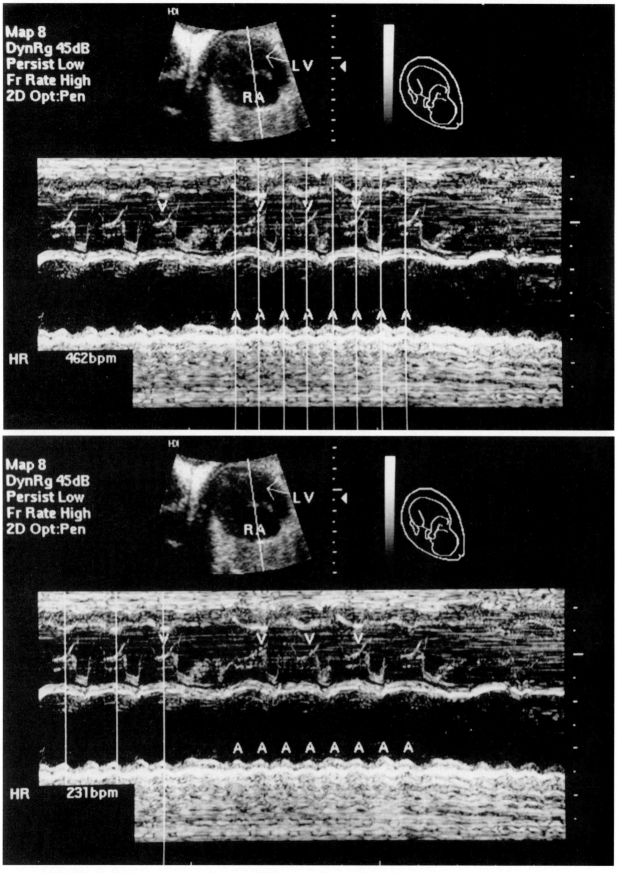

FIGURE 27–13. M-mode echocardiogram with M-mode cursor placed to intercept the left ventricle (at the upper aspect of the tracing) and the right atrial wall, at the lower aspect of the tracing. The atrial wall undulations demonstrate a rapid and monotonous atrial flutter rate of 462 bpm (*A*). Mobitz type II atrioventricular block (2:1) results in a monotonous tachycardic ventricular response rate of 231 bpm (*B*).

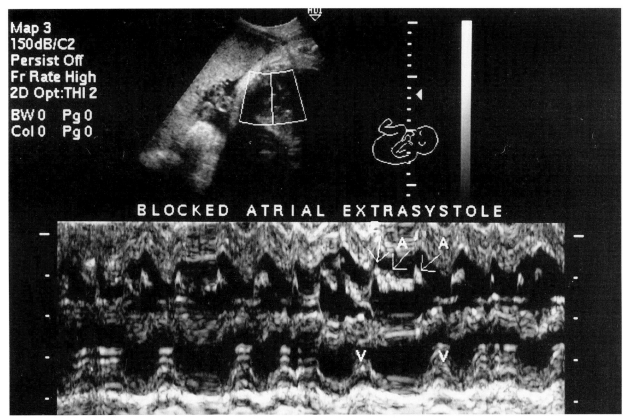

FIGURE 27–14. M-mode echocardiogram of a fetus who was referred for evaluation of an irregular fetal bradycardia. The referring physician planned premature cesarean delivery secondary to the assumption that the fetal bradycardia represented a manifestation of fetal distress. The fetal heart was structurally normal, with normal systolic pump function and no evidence of hydrops fetalis. The M-mode cursor transects the two ventricles. The posterior left ventricular wall demonstrates an irregular rhythm, with occasional premature beats. The bradycardia results from frequent blocked atrial extrasystoles. The tricuspid valve is seen within the superior right ventricle. The E-wave is followed by an early extrasystole (A') that is nonconducted, due to atrioventricular nodal refractoriness. The subsequent atrial depolarization (A) is conducted, resulting in the ventricular response (V). The resulting ventricular rate (distance between two ventricular contractions [V]) results in a perceived heart rate of 60 to 65 bpm.

27–1. It is important to recognize the potential for drug interactions. The half-lives of these drugs must be borne in mind when changing medications, and/or adding multiple drugs to the fetal treatment protocols.

Supraventricular Tachycardia

For the fetus with reentrant supraventricular tachycardia, there is a 1:1 relationship between atrial and ventricular activity, with a fetal heart rate of between 240 and 260 bpm. Episodic, reentrant supraventricular tachycardia is characterized as having sudden rather than gradual onset and termination (Fig. 27–16). With frequent episodes of tachycardia or incessant tachycardia in the extremely premature infant (<24 to 26 weeks' gestation), or in the presence of hydrops fetalis, in utero therapy may be considered but should never progress beyond the use of digoxin and/or propranolol to third- or fourth-line medications, unless there is evidence of hemodynamic decompensation.

Prior to initiating therapy, a maternal ECG should be obtained, to seek evidence of Wolff-Parkinson-White syndrome, or other contraindications to maternal digoxin loading. In addition, maternal serum electrolytes, blood urea nitrogen (BUN), creatinine, and serum calcium and magnesium levels should be evaluated. Intravenous "loading" of digoxin is administered to the mother, according to the standard recommended dosage. Continuous maternal ECG monitoring and daily 12-lead ECGs are obtained to search for electrocardiographic evidence of digoxin toxicity. The mother must be questioned daily concerning potential signs and symptoms of clinical digoxin toxicity, since this is a clinical, rather than a laboratory, diagnosis.

If tachycardia resolves on digoxin therapy, the drug is continued and no further therapy is initiated. Hydrops fetalis may take days or weeks to resolve.

If second-line agents are required, we introduce propranolol as the next agent. The mother and fetus are monitored for the development of bradycardia, and the mother is monitored for supine and orthostatic hypotension.

Under no circumstance should third-line agents be initiated, unless despite digoxin and propranolol therapy there is hydrops fetalis that is unremitting.

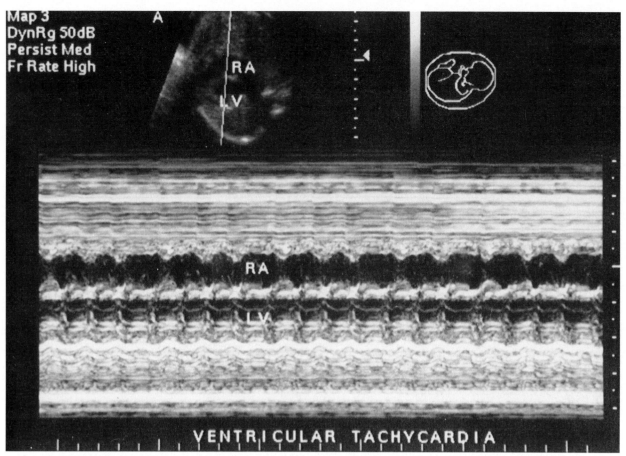

FIGURE 27–15. M-mode echocardiogram in a fetus with ventricular tachycardia. The M-mode cursor transects the right atrium at the upper aspect of the tracing, and the left ventricle, at the lower aspect. The ventricle is contracting at a regular tachycardia rate of approximately 190 bpm, whereas the atrium is contracting at a slower rate, with atrioventricular dissociation. The irregularity of the atrial rate is related to intermittent ventriculoatrial conduction of the ventricular beats.

In the event that digoxin and propranolol combined therapy is ineffective, the next agent in our treatment protocol is flecainide. Maternal ECG is carefully montored for QRS and total PT prolongation. There is a small but significant proarrhythmic danger to both mother and fetus.

Only if triple therapy is unsuccessful should one consider introduction of a fourth-line agent, such as sotalol or amiodarone (see Table 27–1).

Sotalol or amiodarone should not be introduced until flecainide and propranolol have been discontinued for at least 72 hours, to ensure that sufficient time has been allowed for clearance of these agents from the mother and fetus. Since digoxin bioavailability may be increased during concomitant amiodarone administration, the digoxin dosage should empirically be halved. Concerns about thyroid function of the mother, and especially of the fetus, should be considered in maternal, fetal, and neonatal monitoring.

Atrial Flutter

The treatment of fetuses with atrial flutter and associated hydrops fetalis is similar to the treatment of supraventricular tachycardia. An initial loading protocol of maternal digoxin is followed, as noted above.

Digoxin is administered to slow the ventricular response to the atrial flutter. Rarely, atrial flutter can be controlled with the simple administration of digoxin. Once digoxin loading is completed and maintenance is initiated, a second agent can be added. We have come to recognize that type III antiarrhythmic agents, such as sotalol and amiodarone, should be considered at this point.

Summary

Most fetal cardiac arrhythmias relate to relatively benign supraventricular or ventricular premature beats. Most of these resolve spontaneously, either later in gestation or during the neonatal period. Only rarely do these extrasystoles precipitate persistent supraventricular tachycardia, which may be of clinical import. Fetal arrhythmias are only rarely associated with structural congenital heart disease, but such an association does exist, especially with atrial flutter or with congenital complete heart block.

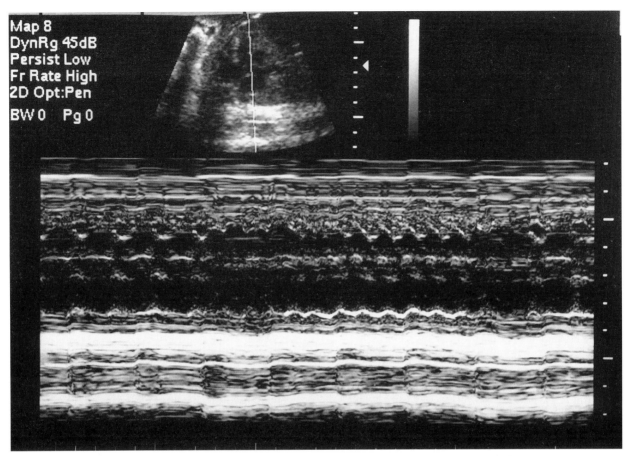

Map 8
DynRg 45dB
Persist Low
Fr Rate High
2D Opt:Pen
BW 0 Pg 0

FIGURE 27–16. An M-mode echocardiogram demonstrating ventricular wall motion in a fetus who has intermittent, self-limited episodes of atrioventricular reentry tachycardia. The episodes of tachycardia are of sudden onset and sudden termination. The onset of tachycardia begins with an extrasystole with a critical coupling interval following the previous sinus beat. This fetus has a heart rate of approximately 260 bpm during tachycardia.

Only in cases of sustained tachycardia in extremely early gestation, or in the presence of hydrops fetalis, should the use of antiarrhythmic therapy be considered. Fetal antiarrhythmic therapy must be undertaken with great respect for the potential for catastrophic proarrhythmic effects on the mother or fetus. Caution with regard to the use of these medications, alone and in combination, must be exercised, especially in light of the potential additive proarrhythmic or cardiac depressive effects of many of these agents.

A common sense risk-benefit analysis should be made before antiarrhythmic therapy is initiated; the presence or absence of hydrops fetalis and the fetal gestational age and pulmonary maturity must be weighed against the possible hazards of fetal antiarrhythmic therapy and the potential for premature delivery and postnatal treatment. In the absence of hydrops fetalis, and especially when the fetus is likely to be mature enough for independent survival, the administration of antiarrhythmic agents to mother and fetus is unwarranted.

All therapy should be grounded on a firm understanding of the electrophysiologic nature of the arrhythmia, and the pharmacology and pharmacokinetics of the antiarrhythmic agents in both mother and fetus, as well as in the placenta. Finally, therapy should be undertaken only in a close collaboration between obstetricians, pediatric cardiologists, and informed parents.

REFERENCES

1. James TN: Congenital disorders of cardiac rhythm and conduction. J Cardiovasc Electrophysiol 4:702–718, 1993.
2. Komaromy B, Gaal J, Mihaly G, et al: Data on the significance of fetal arrhythmia. Am J Obstet Gynecol 99:79–85, 1967.
3. Lingman G, Lundstrom NR, Marsal K: Clinical outcome and circulatory effects of fetal cardiac arrhythmias. Acta Paediatr Scand Suppl 329:120–126, 1986.
4. Maeno Y, Kiyomatsu Y, Rikitake N, et al: Fetal arrhythmias: Intrauterine diagnosis, treatment and prognosis. Acta Paediatr Jpn 37:431–436, 1995.
5. Maragnes P, Fournier A, Lessard M, Fouron JC: Evaluation and prognosis of fetal arrhythmias. J Peditrie (Bucur) 46:481–488, 1991.
6. Martin GR, Ruckman RN: Fetal echocardiography: A large clinical experience and follow-up. J Am Soc Echocardiogr 3:4–8, 1990.
7. Maxwell DJ, Crawford DC, Curry PVM, et al: Obstetric importance, diagnosis and management of fetal tachycardias. BMJ 297:107–110, 1988.
8. Naumburg E, Riesenfeld T, Axelsson O: Fetal tachycardia: Intrauterine and postnatal course. Fetal Diagn Ther 12:205–209, 1997.
9. Newburger JW, Keane JF: Intra-uterine supraventricular tachycardia. J Pediatr 95:780–786, 1979.
10. Owen J, Colvin EV, Davis RO: Fetal death after successful conversion of fetal supraventricular tachycardia with digoxin and verapamil. Am J Obstet Gynecol 158:1169–1170, 1988.

11. Perry JC: Fetal arrhythmias, pediatric arrhythmias, and pediatric electrophysiology. Curr Opin Cardiol 10:52–57, 1995.

12. Rane HS, Purandare HM, Chakravarty A: Type and significance of fetal arrhythmias. Indian Heart J 48:40–44, 1996.

13. Rasanen J, Juntunen K, Jouppila P: Clinical significance of fetal cardiac arrhythmias. Duodecim 110:575–583, 1994.

14. Respondek M, Wilczynski J: Clinical followup in a case of fetal arrhythmia—review of the literature. Ginekol Pol 65:714–718, 1994.

15. Schlotter CM, Uhlhorn G, Holzgreve W, et al: Difficulties in interpreting the cardiotocogram in atrioventricular arrhythmia of the fetal heart. Geburtshilfe Frauenheilkd 49:192–194, 1989.

16. Stewart PA, Wladimiroff JW: Cardiac tachyarrhythmia in the fetus: Diagnosis, treatment and prognosis. Fetal Ther 2:7–16, 1987.

17. Szabo I, Hajdu J, Csabay L, et al: Prenatal follow-up of fetal tachyarrhythmia. Orv Hetil 135:2603–2607, 1994.

18. Trigo C, Macedo AJ, Ferreira M, et al: Fetal arrhythmia. A case load of 4 years and an half. Acta Med Port 8:73–79, 1995.

19. VanEngelen AD, Weitjens O, Brenner JI, et al: Management outcome and follow-up of fetal tachycardia. J Am Coll Cardiol 24:1371–1375, 1994.

20. Wenicke K, Kubli F, Schmidt W, Boos R: Fetal arrhythmia. Z Geburtshilfe Perinatol 188:105–114, 1984.

21. Zielinsky P: Fetal heart rhythm disorders. Detection and prenatal management. Arq Bras Cardiol 66:83–86, 1996.

22. Juchau MR, Pedersen MG, Fantel A, Shepard TH: Drug metabolism by placenta. Clin Pharmacol Ther 14:673–679, 1973.

23. Krauer B, Krauer F: Drug kinetics in pregnancy. Clin Pharmacokinet 2:167–181, 1977.

24. Levy G: Pharmacokinetics of fetal and neonatal exposure to drugs. Obstet Gynecol 58:9S–16S, 1981.

25. McKercher HG, Radde IC: Placental transfer of drugs and fetal pharmacology. In McLeod SM, Radde IC (eds): Textbook of Pediatric Clinical Pharmacology. Littleton, MA: PSG Publishing, 1985, pp 293–307.

26. Mattison DR, Malek A, Cistola C: Physiological adaptations to pregnancy: Impact on pharmacokinetics. In Yaffe SJ, Aranda JV (eds): Pediatric Pharmacology: Therapeutic Principles in Practice. Philadelphia: WB Saunders Company, 1992, pp 81–96.

27. Pacifici GM, Nottoli R: Placental transfer of drugs administered to the mother. Clin Pharmacokinet 28:235–269, 1995.

28. Ward RM: Pharmacological treatment of the fetus: Clinical pharmacokinetic considerations. Clin Pharmacokinet 28:343–350, 1995.

29. Scott O, Williams GJ, Fiddler GI: Results of 24 hour ambulatory monitoring of electrocardiogram in 131 healthy boys aged 10–13 years. Br Heart J 44:304–308, 1980.

30. Southall DP, Richards J, Mitchell P, et al: Study of cardiac rhythm in healthy newborn infants. Br Heart J 43:14–20, 1980.

31. Southall DP, Johnston F, Shinebourne EA, et al: 24-hour electrocardiographic study of heart rate and rhythm patterns in population of healthy children. Br Heart J 45:281–291, 1981.

32. Tulzer G, Huhta JC, Gudmundsson S, et al: Fetal supraventricular extrasystole: Indication for fetal echocardiography? Klin Padiatr 206:430–432, 1994.

33. Gembruch U, Hansmann M, Bald R, Redel BA: Supraventricular tachycardia of the fetus in the 3d trimester of pregnancy following persistent supraventricular extrasystole. Geburtshilfe Frauenheilkd 47:656–659, 1987.

34. Itskovitz J, Timor-Tritsch I, Brandes JM: Intrauterine fetal arrhythmia: Atrial premature beats. Int J Gynaecol Obstet 16:419–421, 1979.

35. Kallfelz HC: Cardiac arrhythmias in the fetus: Diagnosis, significance and prognosis. In Goodman JM, Marquis RM (eds): Paediatric Cardiology, Vol 2. New York: Churchill Livingstone, 1979, pp 80–97.

36. Respondek M, Wloch A, Kaczmarek P, et al: Diagnostic and perinatal management of fetal extrasystole. Pediatr Cardiol 18:361–366, 1997.

37. Rice MJ, McDonald RW, Reller MD: Fetal atrial septal aneurysm: A cause of fetal atrial arrhythmias. J Am Coll Cardiol 12:1292–1297, 1988.

38. Simpson JM, Milburn A, Yates RW, et al: Outcome of intermittent tachyarrhythmia in the fetus. Pediatr Cardiol 18:78–82, 1997.

39. Strasburger JF: Cardiac arrhythmias in childhood. Diagnostic considerations and treatment. Drugs 42:974–983, 1991.

40. Dudorkinova D, Povysilova V, Skovranek J: Anomalies in the development of the sinus venosus as a probable cause of heart rhythm disorders and fetal hydrops. Cesk Pediatr 48:544–546, 1993.

41. Frassica JJ, Orav EJ, Walsh EP, Lipshultz SE: Arrhythmias in children prenatally exposed to cocaine. Arch Pediatr Adolesc Med 148:1163–1169, 1994.

42. Frohn-Mulder IM, Stewart PA, Witsenburg M, et al: The efficacy of flecainide versus digoxin in the management of fetal supraventricular tachycardia. Prenat Diagn 15:1297–1302, 1995.

43. Ludomirsky A, Garson A Jr: Supraventricular tachycardia. In Gillette PC, Garson A (eds): Pediatric Cardiac Dysrhythmias. Philadelphia: WB Saunders Company, 1990, pp 380–426.

44. Gillette PC: The mechanisms of supraventricular tachycardia in children. Circulation 54:133–139, 1980.

45. Gutierrez-Larraya Aguado F, Galindo Izquierdo A, Olaizola Llodio I, et al: Fetal supraventricular tachycardia. Rev Esp Cardiol 49:444–450, 1996.

46. Jacqz-Aigrain E, Azancot-Benisty A, Guirguis NM: Troubles du rythme supraventriculaire due foetus: diagnostic, prise en charge therapeutique, perspectives. Flammarian Medecine-Sciences. Journees Parisiennes de Pediatrie, Paris 1991:257–263.

47. Johnson WH Jr, Dunnigan A, Fehr P, Benson DW Jr: Association of atrial flutter with orthodromic reciprocating fetal tachycardia. Am J Cardiol 59:374–375, 1987.

48. Killeen AA, Bowers LD: Fetal supraventricular tachycardia treated with high-dose quinidine: Toxicity associated with marked elevation of the metabolite 3(S)-3-hydroxyquinidine. Obstet Gynecol 70:445–449, 1987.

49. Moak JP: Pharmacology and electrophysiology of antiarrhythmic drugs. In Gilette PC, Garson A Jr (eds): Pediatric Cardiac Dysrhythmias. New York: Grune & Stratton, 1990, pp 37–117.

50. Naheed ZJ, Strasburger JF, Deal BJ, et al: Fetal tachycardia: Mechanisms and predictors of hydrops fetalis. J Am Coll Cardiol 27:1736–1740, 1996.

51. Richards DS, Wagman AJ, Cabaniss ML: Ascites not due to congestive heart failure in a fetus with lupus-induced heart block. Obstet Gynecol 76:957–959, 1990.

52. Stewart PA, Wladimiroff JW: Fetal atrial arrhythmias associated with redundancy/aneurysm of the foramen ovale. J Clin Ultrasound 16:643–650, 1988.

53. Wu CT, Chen MR, Hon SH: Neonatal tuberous sclerosis with cardiac rhabdomyomas presenting as fetal supraventricular tachycardia. Jpn Heart J 38:133–137, 1997.

54. Zielinsky P, Firpo CM, de Lima RP, et al: Prenatal echocardiographic study of septum primum redundancy and its relationship to the genesis of atrial extrasystole in the fetus. Arq Bras Cardiol 65:153–157, 1995.

55. Blandon R, Leandro I: Fetal heart arrhythmia: Clinical experience with antiarrhythmic drugs. In Doyle EF, Engle MA, Gersony WM, et al (eds): Pediatric Cardiology: Proceedings of the Second World Congress. New York: Springer-Verlag, 1985, p 483.

56. Dumesic DA, Silverman NH, Tobias S, Golbus MS: Transplacental cardioversion of fetal supraventricular tachycardia with procainamide. N Engl J Med 307:1128–1131, 1982.

57. Fernandez C, DeRosa GE, Guevara E, et al: Reversion by vagal reflex of a fetal paroxysmal atrial tachycardia detected by echocardiography. Am J Obstetric Gynecol 159:860–861, 1988.

58. Given BD, Phillippe M, Sanders SP, Dzau VJ: Procainamide cardioversion of fetal supraventricular tachycardia. Am J Cardiol 53:1460–1461, 1984.

59. Guntheroth WG, Cyr DR, Mack LA, et al: Hydrops from reciprocating atrioventricular tachycardia in a 27-week fetus requiring quinidine for conversion. Obstet Gynecol 66:29S, 1985.

60. Hajdu J, Szabo I, Papp C, et al: Management of hemodynamically significant fetal arrhythmias. Orv Hetil 138:2335–2338, 1997.

61. Hamel P, Febbraro W, Barjot P, et al: Fetal supraventricular tachycardia with anasarca complicating benign extrasystole: Treatment with flecainide. Apropos of a case. Arch Mal Coeur Vaiss 90:407–410, 1997.

62. Hansmann M, Gembruch U, Bald R, et al: Fetal tachyarrhythmias: Transplacental and direct treatment of the fetus. A report of 60 cases. Ultrasound Obstet Gynecol 1:162–167, 1991.

63. Hourvitz A, Achiron R, Abraham A, et al: Induced cardioversion of fetal flutter by artificial rupture of membranes at term. J Perinat Med 23:403–407, 1995.
64. Katz AM: Physiology of the Heart, 2nd ed. New York: Raven Press, 1992, p 543.
65. Kofinas AD, Simon NV, Sagel H, et al: Treatment of fetal supraventricular tachycardia with flecainide acetate after digoxin failure. Am J Obstet Gynecol 165:630–632, 1991.
66. Martin CB Jr, Nijhuis JG, Weijer AA: Correction of fetal supraventricular tachycardia by compression of the umbilical cord: Report of a case. Am J Obstet Gynecol 150:324–326, 1984.
67. Prystowsky EN: Inpatient versus outpatient initiation of antiarrhythmic drug therapy for patients with supraventricular tachycardia. Clin Cardiol 17:II7–II10, 1994.
68. Rae AP, Webb CR: Management of supraventricular tachycardia. Cardiology in Practice, 197–204, November/December, 1974.
69. Wellens HJJ, Durrer D: Effect of digitalis on atrioventricular conduction and circus movement tachycardia in patients with the Wolff-Parkinson-White syndrome. Circulation 47:1229–1236, 1973.
70. Wunderlich M: Therapy of fetal cardiac arrhythmia antepartum and sub partu. Zentralbl Gynakol 110:1263–1271, 1988.
71. Brand JM, Friedberg DZ: Spontaneous regression of a primary cardiac tumor presenting as fetal tachyarrhythmias. J Perinat 12:48–50, 1992.
72. Hoadley SD, Wallace RL, Milelr JF, Murgo JP: Prenatal diagnosis of multiple cardiac tumors presenting as an arrhythmia. J Clin Ultrasound 14:639–643, 1986.
73. Lopes LM, Cha SC, Scanavacca MI, et al: Fetal idiopathic ventricular tachycardia with nonimmune hydrops: Benign course. Pediatr Cardiol 17:192–193, 1996.
74. Cha'ban FK, Cohen-Overbeek TE, Frohn-Mulder IM, Wladimiroff JW: Multiple intracardiac tumors: Spontaneous prenatal recovery of fetal bradyarrhythmias. Ultrasound Obstet Gynecol 8:120–122, 1996.
75. Engelhardt W, Lehnen H, Grabitz R, von Bernuth G: Diagnosis and therapy of fetal bradyarrhythmia. Z Geburtshilfe Perinatol 194:153–157, 1990.
76. Gardella C, Thoulon-Bosc JM, Charvet F: Fetal bradycardia during pregnancy. Apropos of 2 cases without fetal distress. Rev Fr Gynecol Obstet 82:111–114, 1987.
77. Hankins GD, Leicht T, Van Hook JW: Prolonged fetal bradycardia secondary to maternal hypothermia in response to urosepsis. Am J Perinatol 14:217–219, 1997.
78. Jan CJ, Wu FF, Sue WC, et al: Tuberous sclerosis with cardiac rhabdomyoma manifested by fetal bradycardia: Report of a case. Chung Hua Min Kuo Hsiao Erh Ko I Hseuh Hui Tsa Chih 32:183–190, 1991.
79. Minagawa Y, Akaiwa A, Hidaka T, et al: Severe fetal supraventricular bradyarrhythmia without fetal hypoxia. Obstet Gynecol 70:454–456, 1987.
80. Wladimiroff JW, Stewart PA, Tonge HM: Fetal bradyarrhythmia: Diagnosis and outcome. Prenat Diagn 8:53–57, 1988.
81. Col JY: Fetal bradycardia caused by arrhythmia. Apropos of a case of blocked staggered atrial extrasystole. J Gynecol Obstet Biol Reprod (Paris) 18:777–794, 1989.
82. Sohn C, Fendel H, Sohn G: Fetal functional atrioventricular blocks in pregnancies at risk. Z Geburtshilfe Perinatol 192:67–72, 1988.
83. Bridge JA, McManus BM, Remmenga J, Cuppage FP: Complete heart block in the 18p-syndrome. Congenital calcification of the atrioventricular block. Arch Pathol Lab Med 113:539–541, 1989.
84. Hofbeck M, Ulmer H, Beinder E, et al: Prenatal findings in patients with prolonged QT interval in the neonatal period. Heart 77:198–204, 1997.
85. Marks ML, Whisler SL, Clericuzio C, Keating M: A new form of long QT syndrome associated with syndactyly. J Am Coll Cardiol 25:59–64, 1995.
86. Presbitero P, Mangiardi L, Antolini R: Congenital long QT syndrome inducing 2:1 atrioventricular block: Early detection in fetal life. Int J Cardiol 24:109–112, 1989.
87. Trippel DL, Parsons MK, Gillette PC: Infants with long QT syndrome and 2:1 AV block. Am Heart J 130:1130–1134, 1995.
88. Van Hare GF, Franz MR, Roge C, Scheinman MM: Persistent functional atrioventricular block in two patients with prolonged QT intervals: Elucidation of the mechanism of block. PACE: Pacing Clin Electrophysiol 13:608–618, 1990.
89. Vigliani M: Romano-Ward syndrome diagnosed as moderate fetal bradycardia. A case report. J Reprod Med 40:725–728, 1995.
90. Agarwala B, Sheikh, Cibils LA: Congenital complete heart block. J Natl Med Assoc 88:725–729, 1996.
91. Assad RS, Jatene MB, Moreira LF, et al: Fetal heart block: A new experimental model to assess fetal pacing. Pacing Clin Electrophysiol 17:1256–1263, 1994.
92. Davison MB, Radford DJ: Fetal and neonatal congenital complete heart block. Med J Aust 150:192–198, 1989.
93. Donders GG, Delport SD, Potze F: Isolated complete congenital heart block diagnosed prenatally in Down's syndrome: A case report. Eur J Obstet Gynecol Reprod Biol 31:293–297, 1989.
94. Gembruch U, Hansmann M, Bald R: Fetal atrial flutter in complete atrioventricular canal and trisomy 18. Geburtshilfe Frauenheilkd 48:445–447, 1988.
95. Gembruch U, Manz M, Bald R, et al: Repeated intravascular treatment with amiodarone in a fetus with refractory supraventricular tachycardia and hydrops fetalis. Am Heart J 118:1335–1338, 1989.
96. Groves AM, Allan LD, Rosenthal E: Outcome of isolated congenital complete heart block diagnosed in utero. Heart 75:190–194, 1996.
97. Hohnloser SH: Proarrhythmia with class III antiarrhythmic drugs: Types, risks, and management. Am J Cardiol 80:82G–89G, 1997.
98. Ishikawa S, Yin J, Maeda H, et al: Successful intrauterine digoxin therapy for fetal complete atrioventricular block with endocardial cusion defect: A case report. Fukuoka Igaku Zasshi 83:315–318, 1992.
99. Machado MV, Tynan MJ, Curry PV, Allan LD: Fetal complete heart block. Br Heart J 60:512–515, 1988.
100. Michaelsson M, Engle MA: Congenital complete heart block: An international study of the natural history. Cardiovasc Clin 4:85–101, 1972.
101. Michaelsson M, Riesenfeld T, Jonzon A: Natural history of congenital complete atrioventricular block. Pacing Clin Electrophysiol 20:2098–2101, 1997.
102. Moodley TR, Baughan JE, Chuntarpursat I, et al: Congenital heart block detected in utero. A case report. S Afr Med J 70:433–434, 1986.
103. Prystowsky EN: Proarrhythmia during drug treatment of supraventricular tachycardia: Paradoxical risk of sinus rhythm for sudden death. Am J Cardiol 78:35–41, 1996.
104. Shaw CT: Polysplenia in a fetus with bradycardia from 26 to 36 weeks' gestation, complete cardiac malformations, and heart block. J Am Osteopath Assoc 90:1100–1102, 1990.
105. Sheley RC, Nyberg DA, Kapur R: Azygous continuation of the interrupted inferior vena cava: A clue to prenatal diagnosis of the cardiosplenic syndromes. J Ultrasound Med 14:381–387, 1995.
106. Takeyama Y, Murotsuki J, Kimura Y, et al: Three cases of congenital complete A-V block. Nippon Sanka Fujinka Gakkai Zasshi 45:267–270, 1993.
107. Andersen HM, Drew JH, Beischer NA, et al: Non-immune hydrops fetalis: Changing contribution to perinatal mortality. Br J Obstet Gynecol 90:636–639, 1983.
108. Knilans TK: Cardiac abnormalities associated with hydrops fetalis. Semin Perinatol 19:483–492, 1995.
109. Sperandeo V, Pipitone S: Physiopathology of cardiac decompensation in the fetus. G Ital Cardiol 21:1219–1227, 1991.
110. Stejskalova S, Dolezal Z, Nekvasil R: Non-immunologic fetal hydrops. Cesk Pediatr 48:410–414, 1993.
111. Freidman WF: The intrinsic physiologic properties of the developing heart. In Friedman WF, Lesch M, Sonnenblick EH (eds): Neonatal Heart Disease. New York: Grune & Stratton, 1973, pp 87–111.
112. Reed KL, Sahn DJ, Marx GR, et al: Cardiac Doppler flows during fetal arrhythmias: Physiologic consequences. Obstet Gynecol 70:1–6, 1987.
113. Snider AR, Serwer GA, Ritter SB: Assessment of ventricular function. In Echocardiography in Pediatric Heart Disease. St. Louis: Mosby, 1997, pp 195–223.
114. Reed KL, Appleton CP, Anderson CF, et al: Doppler studies of vena cava flows in human fetuses. Insights into normal and abnormal cardiac physiology. Circulation 81:498–505, 1990.

115. Rudolph AM: Congenital Diseases of the Heart. Chicago: Yearbook, 1974.
116. Kleinman CS, Donnerstein RL, DeVore GR, et al: Fetal echocardiography for evaluation of in utero congestive heart failure: A technique for study of nonimmune fetal hydrops. N Engl J Med 306:568–575, 1982.
117. Tweed WA, Davies JM, Alexander F, et al: Effects of isoproterenol-induced tachycardia on myocardial blood flow and glycogen in the fetal lamb. Biol Neonate 52:104–114, 1987.
118. Azarbayjani F, Danielsson BR: Pharmacologically induced embryonic dysrhythmia and episodes of hypoxia followed by reoxygenation: A common teratogenic mechanism for antiepileptic drugs? Teratology 57:117–126, 1998.
119. Riabykina TS, Zav'ialov AV, Osipova TP: Disorders of cardiac rhythm in children with pre- and perinatal damage of the brain. Pediatrica 4:14–18, 1989.
120. Kleinman CS, Dubin AM, Nehgme RA, et al: Left atrial tachycardia in the human fetus: Identifying the fetus at greatest risk for developing nonimmune hydrops fetalis. Proceedings of the Second World Congress of Pediatric Cardiology and Cardiac Surgery. Armonk: Futura, 1999 (in press).
121. Rudolph AM, Heymann MA: Cardiac output in the fetal lamb: The effect of spontaneous and induced changes of heart rate on the right and left ventricular output. Am J Obstet Gynecol 124:183–189, 1976.
122. Gest AL, Hansen TN, Moise AA, Hartley CJ: Atrial tachycardia causes hydrops in fetal lambs. Am J Physiol 258:H1159–H1163, 1990.
123. Nimrod C, Davies D, Harder J, et al: Ultrasound evaluation of tachycardia-induced hydrops in the fetal lamb. Am J Obstet Gynecol 157:655–661, 1987.
124. Platt L: Personal communication.
125. Gembruch U, Hansmann M, Redel DA, et al: Non-immunologically-induced hydrops fetalis in complete atrioventricular block of the fetus. A summary of 11 prenatally diagnosed cases. Geburtshilfe Frauenheilkd 48:494–499, 1988.
126. Payraudeau P, Ciaru-Vigneron N, Nguyen Tan Lung R, et al: Prenatal diagnosis and treatment of auricular flutter. Apropos of a case and review of the literature. J Gynecol Obstet Biol Reprod (Paris) 17:535–541, 1988.
127. Schmidt KG, Ulmer HE, Silverman NH, et al: Perinatal outcome of fetal congenital complete atrioventricular block: A multicenter experience. J Am Coll Cardiol 17:1360–1366, 1991.
128. Alexander EL, Buyon JP, Lane J, et al: Anti-SS-A/Ro SS-B/La antibodies bind to neonatal rabbit cardiac cells and preferentially inhibit in vitro cardiac repolarization. J Autoimmun 2:463–469, 1989.
129. Behan WM, Behan PO, Reid JM, et al: Family studies of congenital heart block associated with Ro antibody. Br Heart J 62:320–324, 1989.
130. Belhassen A, Vaksmann G, Francart C, et al: Value of amiodarone in the treatment of fetal supraventricular tachycardia. Apropos of a case. J Gynecol Obstet Biol Reprod (Paris) 16:795–800, 1987.
131. Boutjdir M, Chen L, Zhang ZH, et al: Arrhythmogenitcity of IgG and anti-52-KD SSA/Ro affinity-purified antibodies from mothers of children with congenital heart block. Circ Res 80:354–362, 1997.
132. Buyon JP, Swersky SH, Fox HE, et al: Intrauterine therapy for presumptive fetal myocarditis with acquired heart block due to a systemic lupus erythematosus. Experience in a mother with a predominance of SS-B (La) antibodies. Arthritis Rheum 30:44–49, 1986.
133. Buyon JP, Tseng CE, Di Donato F, et al: Cardiac expression of 52 beta, an alternative transcript of the congenital heart block-associated 52-id SS-A/Ro autoantigen, is maximal during fetal development. Arthritis Rheum 40:655–660, 1997.
134. Buyon JP, Winchester RJ, Slade SG, et al: Identification of mothers at risk for congenital heart block and other neonatal lupus syndromes in their children. Comparison of enzyme-linked immunosorbent assay and immunoblot for measurement of anti-SS-A/Ro and anti-SS-B/La antibodies. Arthritis Rheum 36:1263–1273, 1993.
135. Chitrit Y, Zorn B, Guillevin L, et al: Congenital auriculoventricular block and anti-Ro (SS-A)/anti-La (SS-B) antibody. J Gynecol Obstet Biol Reprod (Paris) 22:777–781, 1993.
136. Deng JS, Bair LW Jr, Shen-Schwarz S, et al: Localization of Ro (SS-A) antigen in the cardiac conduction system. Arthritis Rheum 30:1232–1238, 1987.
137. Finkelstein Y, Adler Y, Harel L, et al: Anti-Ro (SSA) and anti-La (SSB) antibodies and complete congenital heart block. Ann Med Interne (Paris) 148:205–208, 1997.
138. Garcia S, Nascimento JH, Bonfa E, et al: Cellular mechanism of the conduction abnormalities induced by serum from Anti Ro/SSA positive patients in rabbits hearts. J Clin Invest 93:718–724, 1994.
139. Horsfall AC, Li JM, Maini RN: Placental and fetal cardiac laminin are targets for cross-reacting autoantibodies from mothers of children with congenital heart block. J Autoimmun 9:561–568, 1996.
140. Horsfall AC, Rose LM: Cross-reactive maternal autoantibodies and congenital heart block. J Autoimmun 5:479–493, 1992.
141. Horsfall AC, Venables PJW, Taylor PV, et al: Ro and La antigens and maternal autoantibody idiotype in the surface of myocardial fibres in congenital heart block. J Autoimmun 4:165–176, 1991.
142. Li JM, Horsfall AC, Maini RN: Anti-La (SS-B) but not anti-Ro52 (SS-A) antibodies cross-react with laminin—a role in the pathogenesis of congenital heart block? Clin Exp Immunol 99:316–324, 1995.
143. Richards IS, Kulkarni AP, Bremner WF: Cocaine-induced arrhythmia in human foetal myocardium in vitro: Possible mechanism for foetal death in utero. Pharmacol Toxicol 66:150–154, 1990.
144. Steier JA, Akslen LA, Flesland O, Askvik K: Fetal heart block, anti-SSA and anti-SSB antibodies. Association with intra-uterine growth retardation, fetal death and lupus anticoagulant. Acta Obstet Gynecol Scand 66:737–739, 1987.
145. Taylor PV, Scott JS, Gerlis LM, et al: Maternal antibodies against fetal cardiac antigens in congenital complete heart block. N Engl J Med 315:667–672, 1986.
146. Wedeking-Schohl H, Maisch B, Schonian UH: Fetal arrhythmias—new immunologic studies and results. Z Geburtshilfe Perinatol 197:144–147, 1993.
147. Copel JA, Friedman AH, Kleinman CS: Management of fetal cardiac arrhythmias. Obstet Gynecol Clin North Am 24:201–211, 1997.
148. Lee LA, Bias WB, Arnett FC Jr, et al: Immunogenetics of the neonatal lupus syndrome. Ann Intern Med 99:502–596, 1983.
149. Scheib JS, Waxman J: Congenital heart block in successive pregnancies: A case report and evaluation of risk with therapeutic consideration. Obstet Gynecol 73:481–484, 1989.
150. Anandakumar C, Biswas A, Chew SS, et al: Direct fetal therapy for hydrops secondary to congenital atrioventricular heart block. Obstet Gynecol 87:835–837, 1996.
151. Harris JP, Alexson CG, Manning JA, Thompson HO: Medical therapy for the hydropic fetus with congenital complete atrioventricular block. Am J Perinatol 10:217–219, 1993.
152. Koike T, Minakami H, Shiraishi H, Sato I: Fetal ventricular rate in case of congenital complete heart block is increased by ritodrine. Case report. J Perinat Med 25:216–218, 1997.
153. Carpenter RJ, Strasburger JF, Garson A Jr, et al: Fetal ventricular pacing for hydrops secondary to complete atrioventricular block. J Am Coll Cardiol 8:1434–1436, 1986.
154. Kikuchi Y, Shiraishi H, Igarashi H, et al: Cardiac pacing in fetal lambs: Intrauterine transvenous cardiac pacing for fetal complete heart block. Pacing Clin Electrophysiol 18:417–423, 1995.
155. Mrotsuki J, Okamura K, Watanabe T, et al: Production of complete heart block and in utero cardiac pacing in fetal lambs. J Obstet Gynaecol 21:233–239, 1995.
156. Walkinshaw SA, Welch CR, McCormack J, et al: In utero pacing for fetal congenital heart block. Fetal Diagn Ther 9:183–185, 1994.
157. Antman EM, Stone PH, Muller JE, Braunwald E: Calcium channel blocking agents in the treatment of cardiovascular disorders. Part I: Basic and clinical electrophysiologic effects. Ann Intern Med 93:875, 1980.
158. Bauman J: Class III antiarrhythmic agents: The next wave. Pharmacotherapy 17:76S–83S, 1997.
159. Bourget P, Pons JC, Delouis C, et al: Flecainide distribution, transplacental passage, and accumulation in the amniotic fluid during the third trimester of pregnancy. Ann Pharmacother 28:1031–1034, 1994.

160. Camm AJ, Garratt CJ: Adenosine and supraventricular tachycardia. N Engl J Med 325:1621–1626, 1991.

161. Chiba Y: Therapy of fetal diseases. Nippon Sanka Fujinka Gakkai Zasshi 47:845–851, 1995.

162. Cockrell JL, Scheinmann MM, Titus C, et al: Safety and efficacy of oral flecainide therapy in patients with atrioventricular reentrant tachycardia. Ann Intern Med 114:189–194, 1991.

163. Colin A, Chabaud JJ, Poinsot J, et al: Les tachycardies supraventriculaires foetales et leur traitement. A propos de 23 cas. Arch Fr Pediatr 46:335–340, 1989.

164. Cottril CM, McAllister A, Gettes CG, Noonan JA: Propranolol therapy during pregnancy: Evidence for transplacental transfer. Pediatrics 91:812–814, 1977.

165. Cox JL, Gardner MJ: Treatment of cardiac arrhythmias during pregnancy. Prog Cardiovasc Dis 36:137–178, 1993.

166. Deloof E, Devlieger H, Van Hoestenberghe R, et al: Management with a staged approach of the premature hydropic fetus due to complete congenital heart block. Eur J Pediatr 156:521–523, 1997.

167. de Wolf D, de Schepper J, Verhaaren H, et al: Congenital hypothyroid goiter and amiodarone. Acta Paediatr Scand 77:616–618, 1988.

168. Dildy GA, Louckys CA, Clark SL: Intrapartum fetal pulse oximetry in the presence of fetal cardiac arrhythmia. Am J Obstet Gynecol 169:1609–1611, 1993.

169. Epstein AE: Flecainide for pediatric arrhythmias: Do children behave like little adults? Am J Cardiol 14:192–193, 1989.

170. Erkkola R, Lammintausta R, Liukko P, Antiila M: Transfer of propranolol and sotalol across the human placenta: Their effect on maternal and fetal plasma renin activity. Acta Obstet Gynaecol Scand 61:31–34, 1982.

171. Evans MI, Pryde PG, Reichler A, et al: Fetal drug therapy. West J Med 159:325–332, 1993.

172. Gembruch U, Hansmann M, Redel DA, et al: Fetal complete heart block: Antenatal diagnosis, significance and management. Eur J Obstet Gynecol Reprod Biol 31:9–22, 1989.

173. Gladstone GR, Hordof A, Gersony WM: Propranolol administration during pregnancy: Effects on the fetus. J Pediatr 86:962–964, 1975.

174. Golichowski AM, Caldwell R, Hartsough A, Peleg D: Pharmacologic cardioversion of intrauterine supraventricular tachycardia. A case report. J Reprod Med 30:139–144, 1985.

175. Habib A, McCarthy JS: Effects on the neonate of propranolol administered during pregnancy. J Pediatr 91:808–811, 1977.

176. Hijazi Z, Rosenfeld LE, Copel JA, Kleinman CS: Amiodarone therapy of intractable atrial flutter in a premature, hydropic neonate. Pediatr Cardiol 13:227–229, 1992.

177. Janousek J, Paul T: Safety of oral propafenone in the treatment of arrhythmias in infants and children (European retrospective multicenter study). Working Group on Pediatric Arrhythmias and Electrophysiology of the Association of European Pediatric Cardiologists. Am J Cardiol 81:1121–1124, 1998.

178. Janousek J, Paul T, Reimer A, Kallfelz HC: Usefulness of propafenone for supraventricular arrhythmias in infants and children. Am J Cardiol 72:294–300, 1993.

179. Kauffman KS, Seidler FJ, Slotkin TA: Prenatal dexamethasone exposure causes loss of neonatal hypoxia tolerance: Cellular mechanisms. Pediatr Res 35:515–522, 1994.

180. Kerenyi TD, Gleicher N, Meller J, et al: Transplacental cardioversion of intrauterine supraventricular tachycardia with digitalis. Lancet 2:393–394, 1980.

181. Laurent M, Betremieux P, Biron Y, Lehelloco A: Neonatal hypothyroidism after treatment by amiodarone during pregnancy [letter]. Am J Cardiol 60:942, 1987.

182. Lazzara R: From first class to third class: Recent upheaval in antiarrhythmic therapy—lessons from clinical trials. Am J Cardiol 78:28–33, 1996.

183. Lie KI, Kuren DR, Manger CV, et al: Long-term efficacy of verapamil in the treatment of paroxysmal supraventricular tachycardias. Am Heart J 105:688–671, 1983.

184. Lima JJ, Kuritzky PM, Schentag JJ, et al: Fetal uptake and neonatal disposition of procainamide and its acetylated metabolite: A case report. Pediatrics 61:491, 1978.

185. Lingman G, Ohrlander S, Ohlin P: Intrauterine digoxin treatment of fetal paroxysmal tachycardia. Br J Obstet Gynaecol 87:340–342, 1980.

186. Luderitz B, Jung W, Manz M: Combination anti-arrhythmic drug therapy. Z Kardiol 81:157–161, 1992.

187. Lusson JR, Beytout M, Jacquetin B, et al: Traitment d'une tachycardie supraventriculaire foetale: association digoxin-amiodarone. Coeur 15:315–317, 1985.

188. MacNeil DJ: The side effect profile of class III antiarrhythmic drugs: Focus on d, l-sotalol. Am J Cardiol 80:90G–98G, 1997.

189. Magee LA, Dowar E, Sermer M, et al: Pregnancy outcome after gestational exposure to amiodarone in Canada. Am J Obstet Gynecol 172:1307–1311, 1995.

190. O'Hare MF, Leahey W, Murnaghan GA, McDevitt DG: Pharmacokinetics of sotalol during pregnancy. Eur J Clin Pharmacol 24:521–524, 1983.

191. Perry JC, Ayres NA, Carpenter RJ: Fetal supraventricular tachycardia treated with flecainide acetate. J Pediatr 118:303–305, 1991.

192. Perry JC, Garson A Jr: Flecainide acetate for treatment of tachyarrhythmias in children: Review of world literature on efficacy, safety, and dosing. Am Heart J 124:1614–1621, 1992.

193. Pfammatter JP, Paul T, Lehmann C, Kallfelz HC: Efficacy and proarrhythmia of oral sotalol in pediatric patients. J Am Coll Cardiol 26:1002–1007, 1995.

194. Pinsky WW, Rayburn WF, Evans MI: Pharmacologic therapy for fetal arrhythmias. Clin Obstet Gynecol 34:304–309, 1991.

195. Reiffel JA: Impact of structural heart disease on the selection of class III antiarrhythmics for the prevention of atrial fibrillation and flutter. Am Heart J 135:551–556, 1998.

196. Rogers MC, Willerson JT, Goldblatt A, Smith TW: Serum digoxin concentrations in the human fetus, neonate and infant. N Engl J Med 287:1010–1014, 1972.

197. Saarikoski S: Placental transfer and fetal uptake of ^{3}H-digoxin in humans. Br J Obstet Gynaecol 83:879–884, 1976.

198. Rotmensch HH, Belhassen B, Ferguson RK: Amiodarone: Benefits and risks in perspective. Am Heart J 104:1117–1119, 1982.

199. Rotmensch HH, Elkayem U, Frishman W: Antiarrhythmic drug therapy during pregnancy. Ann Intern Med 98:487–497, 1983.

200. Rotmensch HH, Rotmensch S, Elkayam U: Management of cardiac arrhythmias during pregnancy. Current concepts. Drugs 33:623–633, 1987.

201. Rubin PC: Beta-blockers in pregnancy. N Engl J Med 305:1323–1326, 1981.

202. Spinnato JA, Shaver DC, Flinn GS, et al: Fetal supraventricular tachycardia: In utero therapy with digoxin and quinidine. Obstet Gynecol 64:730, 1984.

203. Strigl R, Pfeiffer U, Erhardt W, et al: Does the administration of the calcium antagonist verapamil in tocolysis with beta sympathomimetics still make sense? J Perinat Med 9:235, 1981.

204. Teuscher A, Bossi E, Imhof P, et al: Effect of propranolol on fetal tachycardia in diabetic pregnancy. Am J Cardiol 42:304–307, 1978.

205. Valensise H, Civitella C, Garzetti GG, Romanini C: Amiodarone treatment in pregnancy for dilatative cardiomyopathy with ventricular malignant extrasystole and normal maternal and neonatal outcome. Prenat Diagn 12:705–708, 1992.

206. Vlahot N, Morvan J, Bernard AM, et al: Tachycardie supraventriculaire foetale: Traitement antenatal par l'association digoxine-amiodarone. J Gynecol Obstet Biol Reprod (Paris) 16:393–400, 1987.

207. Wagner X, Jouglard J, Moulin M, et al: Coadministration of flecainide acetate and sotalol during pregnancy: Lack of teratogenic effects, passage across the placenta, and excretion in human breast milk. Am Heart J 119:700–702, 1990.

208. Weindling SN, Saul JP, Walsh EP: Efficacy and risks of medical therapy for supraventricular tachycardia in neonates and infants. Am Heart J 131:66–72, 1996.

209. Weiner CP, Thompson MIB: Direct treatment of fetal supraventricular tachycardia after failed transplacental therapy. Am J Obstet Gynecol 158:570–573, 1988.

210. Witter FR, King TM, Blake DA: Adverse effects of cardiovascular drug therapy on the fetus and neonate. Obstet Gynecol 58:100S–105S, 1981.

211. Wladimiroff JW, Stewart PA: Treatment of fetal cardiac arrhythmias. Br J Hosp Med 34:134–140, 1985.

212. Wolff F, Breuker KH, Schlensker KH, Bolte A: Prenatal diagnosis and therapy of fetal heart rate anomalies with a contribution on the placental transfer of verapamil. J Perinatol Med 8:203–208, 1980.

213. Wren C, Hunter S: Maternal administration of flecainide to terminate and suppress fetal tachycardia. BMJ 296:249–253, 1988.

214. Wu D, Denes P, Dhingra R, et al: The effects of propranolol on induction of AV nodal reentrant paroxysmal tachycardia. Circulation 50:665–667, 1974.

215. Yankowitz J, Weiner C: Medical fetal therapy. Baillieres Clin Obstet Gynecol 9:553–570, 1995.

216. Younis JS, Granat M: Insufficient transplacental digoxin transfer in severe hydrops fetalis. Am J Obstet Gynecol 157:1268–1269, 1987.

217. Arnoux P, Seyral P, Llurens M, et al: Amiodarone and digoxin for refractory fetal tachycardia. Am J Cardiol 59:166–167, 1987.

218. Auzelle MP, Menstre A, Lachassine E: Traitement in utero des tachycardies foetales par l'association digitalique-beta bloquants. A propos de deux cas. J Gynecol Obstet Biol Reprod (Paris) 16:383–391, 1987.

219. Garson A Jr: Medicolegal problems in the management of cardiac arrhythmias in children. Pediatrics 79:84–88, 1987.

220. Roden DM: Risks and benefits of antiarrhythmic therapy. N Engl J Med 305:785–791, 1994.

221. Rovet J, Ehrlich R, Sorbac D: Intellectual outcome in children with fetal hypothyroidism. J Pediatr 110:700–704, 1987.

222. Bassett AL, Chakko S, Epstein M: Are calcium antagonists proarrhythmic? J Hypertens 15:915–923, 1997.

223. Bigger JT Jr, Sahar DI: Clinical types of proarrhythmic response to antiarrhythmic drugs. Am J Cardiol 59:2E–9E, 1987.

224. The Cardiac Arrhythmia Suppression Trial (CAST) Investigators: Preliminary report: Effect of encainide and flecainide on mortality in a randomized trial of arrhythmia suppression after myocardial infarction. N Engl J Med 3:406–412, 1989.

225. Exner DV, Muzyka T, Gillis AM: Proarrhythmia in patients with the Wolff-Parkinson-White syndrome after standard doses of intravenous adenosine. Ann Intern Med 122:351–352, 1995.

226. Faber TS, Zehender M, Just H: Drug-induced torsade de pointes. Incidence, management and prevention. Drug Saf 11:463–476, 1994.

227. Falk RH: Proarrhythmia in patients treated for atrial fibrillation or flutter. Ann Intern Med 117:141–150, 1992.

228. Haverkamp W, Wichter T, Chen X, et al: The pro-arrhythmic effects of anti-arrhythmia agents. Z Kardiol 83 (Suppl 5):75–85, 1994.

229. Horowitz LN: Proarrhythmia—taking the bad with the good. N Engl J Med 319:304–305, 1988.

230. Makkar RR, Fromm BS, Steinman RT, et al: Female gender as a risk factor for torsades de pointes associated with cardiovascular drugs. JAMA 270:2590–2597, 1993.

231. Morganroth J: Risk factors for the development of proarrhythmic events. Am J Cardiol 59:32E–37E, 1987.

232. Morganroth J: Early and late proarrhythmia from antiarrhythmic drug therapy. Cardiovasc Drugs Ther 6:11–14, 1992.

233. Morganroth J: Proarrhythmic effects of antiarrhythmic drugs: Evolving concepts. Am Heart J 123:1137–1139, 1992.

234. Martyn R, Somberg JC, Kerin NZ: Proarrhythmia of nonantiarrhythmic drugs. Am Heart J 126:201–205, 1993.

235. Arulkumaran S, Nicolini U, Fisk NM, et al: Direct antenatal fetal electrocardiographic waveform analysis. Br J Obstet Gynaecol 98:829–831, 1991.

236. Frank TH, Blaumanis OR, Gibbs RK, Wells RK: Adaptive filtering in ECG monitoring of the fetal heart rate. J Electrocardiol 20 (Suppl):108–113, 1987.

237. Quinn A, Weir A, Shahani U, et al: Antenatal fetal magnetocardiography: A new method for fetal surveillance? Br J Obstet Gynaecol 101:866–870, 1994.

238. Van Leeuwen P, Schussler M, Bettermann H, et al: Magnetocardiography for assessment of fetal heart actions. Geburtshilfe Frauenheilkd 55:642–646, 1995.

239. Allan LD, Anderson RH, Sullivan ID, et al: Evaluation of fetal arrhythmias by echocardiography. Br Heart J 50:240–245, 1983.

240. Allan L, Chita S, Sharland GK, et al: Flecainide in the treatment of fetal tachycardias. Br Heart J 65:46–48, 1991.

241. Amano K, Harada Y, Shoda T, et al: Successful treatment of supraventricular tachycardia with flecainide acetate. Fetal Diagn Ther 12:328–331, 1997.

242. Bollmann R, Chaoui R, Schilling H, et al: Prenatal diagnosis and management of fetal arrhythmias. Z Geburtshilfe Perinatol 192:266–272, 1988.

243. Brown DL: Sonographic assessment of fetal arrhythmias. Am J Roentgenol 169:1029–1033, 1997.

244. Calvin SE, Gaziano EP, Bendel RP, et al: Evaluation of fetal cardiac arrhythmias. Ultrasound findings and neonatal outcome. Minn Med 75:29–31, 1992.

245. Cameron A, Nicholson S, Nimrod C, et al: Evaluation of fetal cardiac dysrhythmias with two-dimensional, M-mode, and pulsed-Doppler ultrasonography. Am J Obstet Gynecol 158:286–290, 1988.

246. Chan FY, Woo SK, Ghosh A, et al: Prenatal diagnosis of congenital fetal arrhythmias by simultaneous pulsed Doppler velocimetry of the fetal abdominal aorta and inferior vena cava. Obstet Gynecol 76:200–205, 1990.

247. Chaoui R, Bollmann R, Hoffmann H, Goldner B: Fetal echocardiography: Part III. Fetal arrhythmia. Zentralbl Gynakol 113:1335–1350, 1991.

248. Chorro FJ, Santonja J, Merino J, et al: Fetal cardiac arrhythmia characterized by Doppler echocardiography. Rev Esp Cardiol 45:215–218, 1992.

249. Crowley DC, Dick M, Rayburn WF, Rosenthal A: Two-dimensional and m-mode echocardiographic evaluation of fetal arrhythmia. Clin Cardiol 8:1–8, 1985.

250. Cullen T: Evaluation of fetal arrhythmias. Am Fam Physician 46:1745–1749, 1992.

251. Deng J: Echocardiographic detection of fetal arrhythmias. Chung Hua Fu Chan Ko Tsa Chih 26:75–77, 1991.

252. DeVore GR, Horenstein J: Simultaneous Doppler recording of the pulmonary artery and vein: A new technique for the evaluation of a fetal arrhythmia. J Ultrasound Med 12:669–671, 1993.

253. DeVore GR, Siassi B, Platt LD: Fetal echocardiography III. The diagnosis of cardiac arrhythmias using real-time-directed M-mode ultrasound. Am J Obstet Gynecol 146:792–798, 1983.

254. Dunnigan A: Signs and symptoms associated with cardiac rhythm disorders in the fetus, infant, and child. Compr Ther 15:27–37, 1989.

255. Eik-Nes SH, Marsal K, Kristoffersen K: Methodology and basic problems related to blood flow studies in the human fetus. Ultrasound Med Biol 10:329, 1984.

256. Fermont L: Recherche, identification, pronostic et traitement des troubles due rythme et de la conduction chez le foetus. In Doin (ed): Troubles due rythme cardiaque chez l'enfant. 1987, pp 37–54.

257. Fyfe DA, Meyer KB, Case CL: Sonographic assessment of fetal cardiac arrhythmia. Semin Ultrasound CT MR 14:286–297, 1993.

258. Gai MY: Fetal arrhythmia. Chung Hua Fu Can Ko Tsa Chih 26:355–357, 1991.

259. Gembruch U, Bald R, Hansmann M: Color-coded M-mode Doppler echocardiography in the diagnosis of fetal arrhythmia. Geburtshilfe Frauenheilkd 50:286–290, 1990.

260. Gembruch U, Somville T: Intrauterine diagnosis and therapy of fetal arrhythmias. Gynakologe 28:329–345, 1995.

261. Gonser M, Dietl J, Pfeiffer K, Clees JP: Evaluation of fetal heart rate artifacts, hemodynamics and digoxin treatment in fetal tachyarrhythmia by Doppler measurement of fetal blood flow—case report of a pre-excitation syndrome. J Perinat Med 17:411–416, 1989.

262. Hawrylyshyn PA, Miskin M, Gilbert BW, et al: The role of echocardiography in fetal cardiac arrhythmias. Am J Obstet Gynecol 141:223–225, 1981.

263. Hirose O: Fetal arrhytmmia. Ryoikibetsu Shokogun Shirizu 12:370–372, 1966.

264. Kachaner J, Fermont L, Villain E, Pedroni E: Clinical evaluation and treatment of rhythm and conduction disorders in the fetus. Pediatr Med Chir 9:527–534, 1987.

265. Kadar K, Papp Z: Diagnosis and treatment of fetal and neonatal tachycardia. Orv Hetil 134:811–814, 1993.

266. Kleinman CS, Copel JA, Hobbins JC: Combined echocardiographic and Doppler assessment of fetal congenital atrioventricular block. Br J Obstet Gynaecol 94:967–974, 1987.

267. Kleinman CS, Copel JA: Electrophysiologic principles and fetal antiarrhythmic therapy. Ultrasound Obstet Gynecol 1:286–297, 1991.

268. Kleinman CS, Donnerstein RL, Jaffe CC, et al: Fetal echocardiography. A tool for evaluation of in utero cardiac arrhythmias and

monitoring of in utero therapy: Analysis of 71 patients. Am J Cardiol 51:237–243, 1983.

269. Kleinman CS, Hobbins JC, Jaffe CC, et al: Echocardiographic studies of the human fetus: Prenatal diagnosis of congenital heart disease and cardiac dysrhythmias. Pediatrics 65:1059–1067, 1980.

270. Kleinman CS, Valdes-Cruz LM, Weinstein EM, Sahn DJ: Two-dimensional Doppler echocardiographic analysis of fetal cardiac arrhythmias. Pediatr Res 18:124A, 1984.

271. Knudson JM, Kleinman CS, Copel JA, et al: Ectopic atrial tachycardia in utero. Obstet Gynecol 84:686–689, 1994.

272. Lingman G, Marsal K: Fetal cardiac arrhythmias: Doppler assessment. Semin Perinatol 11:357–361, 1987.

273. Lopes LM, Kahhale S, Barbato A, et al: Prenatal diagnosis of congenital heart diseases and cardiac arrhythmias by Doppler echocardiography. Arq Bras Cardiol 54:121–125, 1990.

274. Munoz H, Loureiro O, Brugere S, et al: Fetal echocardiography. III. The antenatal diagnosis of structural and rhythm changes. Rev Chil Obstet Ginecol 57:16–21, 1992.

275. Oberhansli I, Extermann P, Extermann D: Prenatal diagnosis of arrhythmias and associated congenital cardiac abnormalities using ultrasonography. Schweiz Med Wochenschr 123:537–541, 1993.

276. Piela A, Kuzniar J, Skret A, et al: Fetal echocardiography. 6. Ultrasonic evaluation of fetal arrhythmia. Ginekol Pol 56:459–765, 1985.

277. Pizzuto F, Lancia O, Miceli S, et al: Prenatal diagnosis of cardiac arrhythmia using fetal echocardiography. Cardiologia 33:175–181, 1988.

278. Respondek A, Huhta JC, Wood D, Respondek M: Echocardiographic evaluation of fetal arrhythmias. Kardiologia Polska 33:136–149, 1990.

279. Silverman NH, Enderlein MA, Stanger P, et al: Recognition of fetal arrhythmias by echocardiography. J Clin Ultrasound 13:255–263, 1985.

280. Simpson LL, Marx GR: Diagnosis and treatment of structural fetal cardiac abnormality and dysrhythmia. Semin Perinatol 18:215–227, 1994.

281. Smith GC, Fleming JE, Whitfield CR: Post-extrasystolic potentiation in a human fetus detected during measurement of systolic time intervals in labour. Eur J Obstet Gynecol Reprod Biol 37:205–210, 1990.

282. Stewart PA, Tonge HM, Wladimiroff JW: Arrhythmia and structural abnormalities of the fetal heart. Br Heart J 50:550–554, 1983.

283. Strasburger JF, Huhta JC, Carpenter RJ Jr, et al: Doppler echocardiography in the diagnosis and management of persistent fetal arrhythmias. J Am Coll Cardiol 7:1386–1391, 1986.

284. Tonge HM, Wladimiroff JW, Noordam MJ, Stewart PA: Fetal cardiac arrhythmias and their effect on volume blood flow in descending aorta of human fetus. J Clin Ultrasound 14:607–612, 1986.

285. van den Berg P, Gembruch U, Schmidt S, et al: Continuous fetal intrapartum monitoring in supraventricular tachycardia by atraumatic measurement of transcutaneous carbon dioxide tension. J Perinat Med 17:371–374, 1989.

286. Wladimiroff JW, Struyk P, Stewart PA, et al: Fetal cardiovascular dynamics during cardiac dysrhythmia. Case report. Br J Obstet Gynaecol 90:573–574, 1983.

287. Zhou AC, Lu SK, Fan P: The spectral characters of pulsed Doppler in fetal arrhythmia. Chung Hua Fu Chan Ko Tsa Chih 29:468–470, 1994.

288. Zhu WL: Identification of congenital cardiac malformation and in utero arrhythmia by fetal echocardiography. Chung Hus I Hseuh Tsa Chih 69:684–686, 1989.

ADDITIONAL READINGS

Andersen JL: Reassessment of benefit-risk ratio and treatment algorithms for antiarrhythmic drug therapy after the cardiac arrhythmia suppression trial. J Clin Pharmacol 30:981–989, 1990.

Assad RS, Aiello VD, Jatene MB, et al: Cryosurgical ablation of fetal atrioventricular node: New model to treat fetal malignant tachyarrhythmias. Ann Thorac Surg 60:S629–S632, 1995.

Azancot A: The determinants of cardiac failure in utero: The case of fetal tachycardias. Arch Pediatr (Paris) 3:354S–355S, 1996.

Azancot-Benisty A, Jacqz-Aigrain E, Guirguis NM, et al: Clinical and pharmacological study of fetal supraventricular tachyarrhythmias. J Pediatr 121:608–613, 1992.

Bergmans MGM, Jonker GJ, Kock HCLV: Fetal supraventricular tachycardia. Review of the literature. Obstet Gynecol Surv 40:61–68, 1985.

Buis-Liem TN, Ottenkamp J, Meerman RH, et al: The concurrence of fetal supraventricular tachycardia and obstruction of the foramen ovale. Prenat Diagn 7:425–431, 1987.

Copel JA, Buyon JP, Kleinman CS: Successful in utero therapy of fetal heart block. Am J Obstet Gynecol 173:1384–1390, 1995.

Erskine L: Placental compliance—inferences from Doppler studies of umbilical blood flow during cardiac arrhythmia. Acta Obstet Gynecol Scand 66:301–304, 1987.

Groves AM, Allan LD, Rosenthal E: Therapeutic trial of sympathomimetics in three cases of complete heart block in the fetus. Circulation 92:3394–3396, 1995.

Kanzaki T, Murakami M, Kobayashi H, et al: Hemodynamic changes during cardioversion in utero: A case report of supraventricular tachycardia and atrial flutter. Fetal Diagn Ther 8:37–44, 1993.

Karrer G, Baumann H, Vetter K, et al: Hydrops fetalis in tachycardia: Diagnostic and therapeutic procedures. Gynakol Rundsch 30:28–29, 1990.

Kim CJ, Cho JH, Chi JG, Kim YJ: Multiple rhabdomyoma of the heart presenting with a congenital supraventricular tachycardia—report of case with ultrastructural study. J Korean Med Sci 4:143–147, 1989.

Koyanagi T, Hara K, Satoh S, et al: Relationship between heart rate and rhythm, and cardiac performance in the human fetus in utero. Int J Cardiol 28:163–171, 1990.

Krapp M, Gembruch U, Baumann P: Venous blood flow pattern suggesting tachycardia-induced 'cardiomyopathy' in the fetus. Ultrasound Obstet Gynecol 10:32–40, 1997.

MacNeil DJ, Davies RO, Deitchman D: Clinical safety profile of sotalol in the treatment of arrhythmias. Am J Cardiol 72:44A–50A, 1993.

Morganroth J: Drug-induced early and late proarrhythmia. Cardiol Clin 10:397–401, 1992.

Petrikovsky B, Schneider E, Ovadia M: Natural history of hydrops resolution in fetuses with tachyarrhythmias diagnosed and treated in utero. Fetal Diagn Ther 11:292–295, 1996.

Pfammatter JP, Paul T: New antiarrhythmic drug in pediatric use: Sotalol. Pediatr Cardiol 18:28–34, 1997.

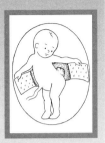

CHAPTER *28*

The Fetus with a Myelomeningocele

MARTIN MEULI

T his chapter summarizes the current knowledge of whether fetal surgery could reduce the devastating neurologic deficit associated with myelomeningocele (MMC).

The hypothesis is that the neural damage is predominantly due to a secondary, in utero acquired injury to the openly exposed neural elements. Fetal animal models demonstrated that spinal cord tissue, if exposed to the amniotic cavity, undergoes significant morphologic changes and suffers progressive loss of function as gestation continues. At birth, a human-like MMC with a characteristic neurologic impairment is present. If such a developing experimental MMC is covered in a timely manner in utero, then the spinal cord destruction is stopped, and the newborn animal is neurologically normal.

Some morphologic and scant functional data from human fetuses with MMC support the concept of progressive intrauterine damage to the unprotected spinal cord tissue potentially preventable by early prenatal intervention.

Although there is considerable experimental and some clinical evidence that fetal surgery might be the only way to reduce the neurologic deficit of MMC, several medical problems and ethical issues must be solved prior to routinely treating selected human fetuses with MMC.

Being born with a myelomeningocele (MMC) is a disastrous start of life. If given urgent state-of-the-art care, most children with this common malformation (1 in 2,000 live births worldwide) will survive, but crippling physical handicaps including paralysis, hydrocephalus, parenchymal brain anomalies, bladder and bowel incontinence, sexual dysfunction, and skeletal deformities will all be part of their future lives. Additionally, about 15% of these unfortunate children will exhibit severely impaired intelligence and cognitive development mandating some form of custodial care.[1-5]

Although many of these physical and psychosocial problems can be ameliorated surgically[1] and through extensive rehabilitation,[6] providing the patients with the potential to enjoy an acceptably productive and fulfilling life, the neurologic deficit is irremediable and remains a core problem throughout life.

While it appears clear that all neural damage is irreversibly established when the baby is born, the question is unanswered what exactly causes the loss of spinal cord function and when during embryogenesis or fetal life these processes take place. It is generally accepted that most cases of MMC are the result of failed neurulation (i.e., folding of the neural plate into the neural tube does not occur during the fourth week of gestation).[7-10] In a few cases the pathogenic mechanism is a failure of mesoderm migration over a closed neural tube resulting in an open spine and missing soft tissue coverage. In any case, however, the affected neural elements are openly exposed to the amniotic cavity for the remainder of gestation.[10, 11]

The fact that extremely friable fetal spinal cord tissue remains completely unprotected for approximately 8 months of intrauterine life in a potentially inhospitable environment has generated the working hypothesis detailed below.

The Hypothesis

The hypothesis is that the neurologic deficit is not (entirely) an intrinsic feature of the primary malformation itself, but rather a consequence of functional, nonneurulated or neurulated, spinal cord tissue being pathologically exposed to the intrauterine environment. Consequently, the fragile neural tissue is progressively damaged by mechanical and/or chemical factors during gestation, labor, and passage of the fetus through the narrow birth canal. If the hypothesis of a significant *secondary* and thus potentially *preventable* neural damage with loss of function proves correct, then protective in utero coverage of the lesion might be a way to reduce or even obviate the neurologic deficit at birth.

Animal Models for In Utero Creation and Repair of MMC

Early experimental work investigated surgical creation of a spina bifida–like lesion followed by *instant* repair

443

of the bony defect in monkey fetuses.[12] Fetal lumbar laminectomy (L3–L5) and displacement of the spinal cord from the spinal canal was followed by immediate reconstruction of the dorsal vertebral column using an allogeneic bone paste. Control fetuses were left unrepaired (i.e., with the spinal cord exposed to the intrauterine environment). At birth, the repaired animals were neurologically normal while the unrepaired animals exhibited an MMC-like back lesion and a neurologic deficit like the one found in natural MMC.

Similarly, *late* gestational surgical creation of a spina bifida–type lesion with open exposure of the undamaged spinal cord in rat fetuses led to pups born with severe deformity and weakness of hindlimbs and tail, indicating substantial in utero acquired spinal cord damage. Histologically, the exposed part of the cord revealed extensive erosion and necrosis consistent with *secondary* intrauterine spinal cord injury.[13] Immediate or slightly delayed (24 hours) skin coverage of these lesions led to pups without detectable neurologic deficit.[14] The same investigators reported on analogous experiments using pig fetuses. Spinal cord exposure relatively late in gestation resulted in impaired motor and sensory hindlimb function postnatally. In one pig fetus, immediate coverage of spina bifida was successfully performed using cadaver allodura.

These experiments show that fetal spinal cord exposure results in significant *in utero acquired* neural tissue damage and, correspondingly, in significant loss of neurologic function by the time of birth. Also, they demonstrate that *immediate* in utero repair of spina bifida–like lesions is feasible and not associated with impaired neurology of the newborn animals. However, these studies have not dealt with the crucial biologic dynamics of creation and in utero repair of experimental MMC. In order to appropriately test the potential benefit of prenatal MMC repair, a large animal model with long-term gestation must be used. Such a model should be able to mimic human MMC in terms of both morphologic and functional features. Most importantly, this fetal animal model should permit *early* gestational MMC creation and a significantly *delayed* repair of an evolving MMC thereafter so as to simulate an assumed human fetal MMC repair as closely as possible.

In the recent past, we developed such a model using fetal sheep.[15, 16] The fetal ovine model perfectly meets the criteria for technically demanding and delicate experiments because it offers the unique possibilities of repeated fetal surgical interventions with long fetal exposure times in fetuses of suitable size. Moreover, fetal morbidity and mortality is low and retention of pregnancy is usually warranted.

In midgestational fetuses (term = 150 days), a human-like spina bifida defect was surgically created (Fig. 28–1). Over the lumbar spine, a circular skin excision was made, the median portions of the paraspinal musculature were excised, and a complete laminectomy of L1–L4 was performed. Finally, the dorsal portion of the dura mater between the dorsal roots from L1–L4 was removed so as to expose the normal and undamaged lumbar spinal cord directly to the amniotic cavity. Pregnancy was continued until near term and the animals were born via cesarean section. At birth, the lambs exhibited a human-like MMC with the severely altered cord tissue resting on the dorsal aspect of a fluid-filled cystic sac (Figs. 28–2 and 28–3). Clinically, they all had sensorimotor flaccid paraplegia and were incontinent of urine and stool. Electrophysiologic examination revealed absent somatosensory evoked potentials (SEPs) from hindlimbs, confirming lack of sensation. Histologically, there was significant or even total loss of neural tissue in the center of the experimental MMC. In other parts, the neural remnants demonstrated most severe alterations including abrasion, avulsion, disruption, and necrosis, leading to a complete loss of the characteristic cytoarchitecture (Fig. 28–4). Interestingly, there were striking histomorphologic similarities between our experimental MMC and

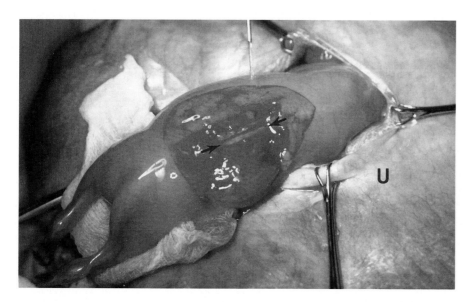

FIGURE 28–1. Human-like spina bifida–type defect created at 75 days' gestation. The normal and undamaged spinal cord is openly exposed between lumbar levels 1 and 4 (*arrows*). (U = uterus.)

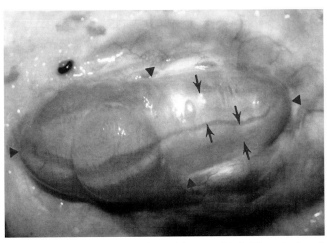

FIGURE 28–2. Experimental MMC lesion at birth. The spinal cord remnants rest on the dorsal aspect of a fluid-filled cystic sac (*markers*) and appear as two separated and extremely flattened parts ("hemicords") (*paired arrows*). See Color Plate 3

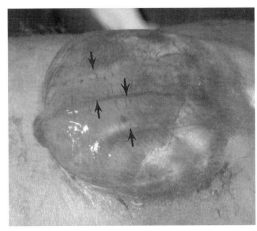

FIGURE 28–3. Human MMC lesion at birth. Note the striking similarities between the experimental and the naturally occurring phenotypes. The severely altered spinal cord tissue also appears split into two separate parts (*paired arrows*). See Color Plate 3

a comparable human MMC (see below and Fig. 28–5). Some fetuses were examined morphologically 4 weeks after creation of spina bifida (i.e., at 100 days of gestation). Here, the back lesions were smaller and the destructive changes within the neural tissue were much less severe, indicating that spinal cord destruction in this context is a relatively slowly progressing phenomenon. This model of early gestational creation of spina bifida demonstrates that exposure of the normal lumbar spinal cord to the intrauterine environment for the second half of pregnancy leads to an experimental MMC at birth that shares most of the functional and morphologic characteristics with the naturally occurring human MMC.

The same model was used to answer the question whether in utero coverage of developing MMC can salvage neurologic function.[17, 18] In 75-day-old sheep fe-

tuses, the above-described spina bifida–type defect was made and the fetuses were replaced into the uterus and underwent repair when they were 100 days old. At this timepoint, the exposed part of the spinal cord was macroscopically intact but flattened and herniated slightly out of the spinal canal (Fig. 28–5). The lesion itself was left unmanipulated. It was covered with two layers consisting of a distally pedicled latissimus dorsi flap (Figs. 28–6 and 28–7),[19] and the skin. After delivery by cesarean section near term, the back wounds were perfectly healed and the animals were neurologically normal. They were able to stand and walk (Fig. 28–8); hindlimb sensibility was normal and so were SEPs (Fig. 28–9). Micturition and defecation were normal. Histology revealed a mildly deformed but grossly intact spinal cord, a viable muscle flap covering the entire lesion, and healed skin (Figs. 28–10 and 28–11). This study very

FIGURE 28–4. Transverse histologic section through the center of the experimental lesion shown in Figure 28–2. The spinal cord remnants are exposed on the surface and show massive alterations and complete loss of the characteristic cytoarchitecture. Each arrow points at one "hemicord." (V = vertebral body.) For comparison with an analogous human lesion, see Figure 28–12. *See Color Plate 3*

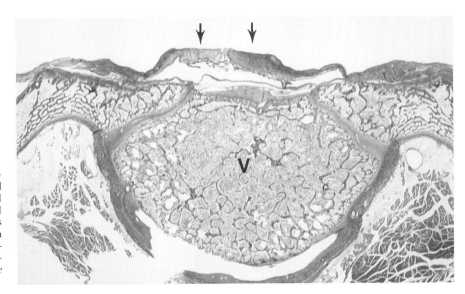

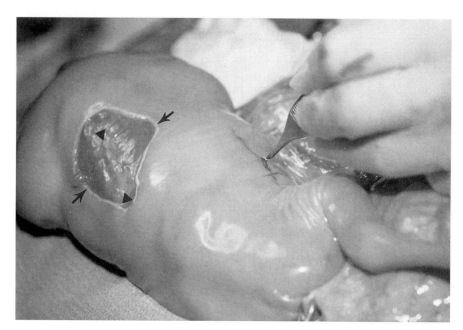

FIGURE 28–5. Developing MMC lesion at 100 days' gestation prior to repair (defect creation at 75 days). *Arrows* delineate the large skin defect. Note the slight herniation of the spinal cord (*markers*) out of the spinal canal. Otherwise, the cord appears grossly intact. Skin incision where flap will be raised.

clearly demonstrates that timely and reliable in utero coverage of *experimental* MMC stops the otherwise ongoing spinal cord destruction and saves neurologic function by the time of birth.

Although these experiments have produced strong evidence in support of the initially formulated hypothesis, they do not provide enough evidence that *human* fetuses with MMC should now be repaired routinely. The main concern with our animal model is that it does not exactly replicate human MMC. For instance, MMC is surgically created and not the result of a developmental disorder. Also, the experimental MMC starts to develop around midgestation, while the natural MMC starts to evolve after the first month of gestation. Finally,

our model did not produce any of the spinal cord or brain anomalies like hydromyelia, diplomyelia, Arnold-Chiari malformation, or hydrocephalus, frequently associated with human MMC. It is mandatory, therefore, to study further the prenatal natural history of human MMC so as to corroborate or invalidate our hypothesis.

Human Studies with Implications for Fetal Surgery

Before fetal surgery was a reality, investigations of human embryos, fetuses, and children with MMC were rare and did not explicitly focus on what is the main

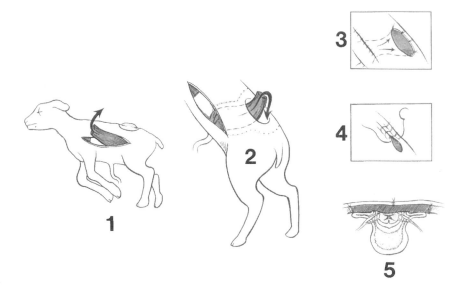

FIGURE 28–6. Schematic representation of the repair procedure. A distally based latissimus dorsi flap is raised (1), flipped over and pulled through a subcutaneous tunnel (2) over the lesion where it is sutured in place (3). Skin closure (4). Cross-sectional view of completed repair (5).

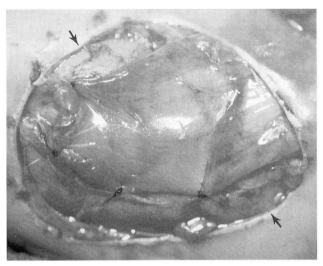

FIGURE 28-7. View of the latissimus dorsi muscle flap covering the entire lesion. Skin defect is delineated by *arrows.*

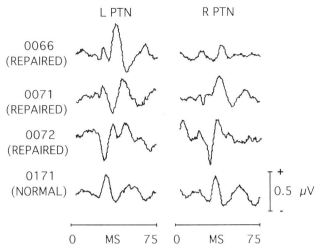

FIGURE 28-9. Electrophysiologic investigation of sensory function in three repaired animals and one control. Shown are the responses to left (L PTN) and right (R PTN) posterior tibial nerve stimulation. All potentials from experimental animals were in the normal range, indicating intact sensory function. (MS = milliseconds; μV = microvolts; + = positivity; − = negativity.)

field of interest here. However, some studies report relevant data.

In 1953, Patten described two human embryos and one human fetus with lumbar MMC.[20] In all three specimens, the exposed part of the cord was not neurulated but was otherwise well developed anatomically, especially in the fetus, and grossly undamaged. The lack of apparent tissue alterations led to the conclusion that the neural tissue degeneration present postnatally must be a *secondary* and relatively *late* occurring phenomenon.

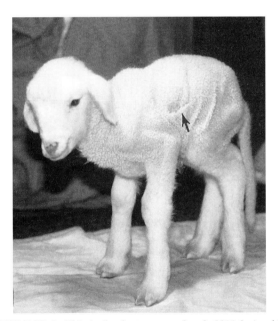

FIGURE 28-8. This is the first success. Lamb 0066 (spina bifida creation at 75 days and in utero repair at 100 days of gestation) a few hours after birth. The (hardly visible) back wound is healed; note the slight scarring on the left flank where the flap was raised (*arrow*).

Cameron (1956) reported on six newborn babies with MMC where the nonneurulated spinal cord remnants formed a thin tissue ribbon exposed on the *external* surface of the cystic sac in much the same way as an unclosed embryologic neural plate. Occasionally, ependyma remained on the external surface.[21]

Emery and Lendon (1973) studied postnatal MMC morphology in 100 patients, 90 of whom had undergone postnatal repair.[10] In most cases, the cord had failed to neurulate, whereas in a few, neurulation had occurred, but the spine was open and the meninges were missing. It could not be discerned clearly whether the varying degrees of spinal cord injuries to the dorsal neural elements were "intrinsic," handling related, or postoperative in nature.

Osaka (1978) published the largest series of human embryos and fetuses with neural tube defects (96 specimens).[22] In the 18 embryos with the classic caudal MMC, he found an everted neural plate with the basic cellular orientation and most of the membrane coverings preserved. Interestingly, there was *no* Arnold-Chiari malformation in these embryos, whereas it was present in the two fetuses with caudal myeloschisis. Similarly, hydrocephalus was not present in the embryos, but was found in one fetus.

Marin-Padilla (1978) studied an array of human dysraphic disorders and concluded that the primary anomaly was a disturbance of the axial chordomesodermal tissues (i.e., the embryologic forerunner of the spine and the meninges) to provide adequate lodging and protection to the developing nervous system, and that the degeneration and destruction of the neural tissue were *secondary* events.[23]

Copp (1990) wrote the most recent as well as the most comprehensive review article about the development of mammalian neural tube defects.[9] He stated that during

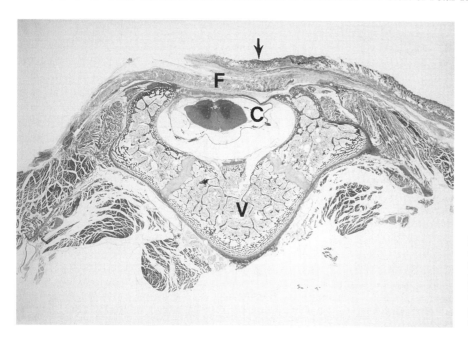

FIGURE 28–10. Histologic overview of cross section through repair site. The spinal cord (C) is somewhat deformed when compared to the normal situation (see Fig. 28–11), but the anatomic hallmarks are preserved. The muscle flap (F) and the healed skin (*arrow*) cover the defect completely. (V = vertebral body.)

in utero development, these malformations usually involve defective folding and fusion of a *normal* neural plate and that the nervous tissue *degenerates* as a result of its abnormal exposure.

Taken together, the above-mentioned studies indicate that early stages of MMC development are characterized by nonneurulated but otherwise (near) normal spinal cord tissue. There is consensus that pathologic exposure

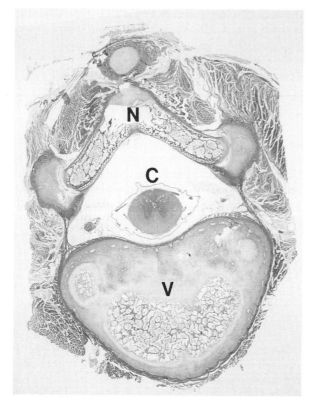

FIGURE 28–11. Cross section through normal lumbar spine. (N = neural arch; C = spinal cord; V = vertebral body.)

of cord tissue leads to *secondary* and rather *late*-occurring degeneration. Finally, the typically associated central nervous system (CNS) malformations emerge rather late in gestation.

With fetal surgery as a potential therapy in mind, our group investigated a total of 18 human fetuses (gestational ages ranging from 19 to 25 weeks, thoracolumbosacral lesions) with MMC.[24, 25] This appears to be the largest fetal series published, and it provides the first detailed description of the relationship between meninges and spinal cord in MMC. The lesions (a representative example is shown in Fig. 28–12) were characterized by skin and soft tissue defects, deficiency of the dorsal bony arch of the vertebrae, and open defects of all meninges. More precisely, the open periosteum of the vertebral canal fused to the fascia of the paraspinal musculature, the open dura mater fused to the deep dermis, and the open pia mater fused to the superficial dermis and epidermis of the surrounding skin. The spinal cord was lying unprotected and devoid of any covering on the dorsal aspect of the pathologically configured arachnoid space, which was enclosed by the open pia (dorsally) and the open dura (ventrally), both fused laterally to the skin. The spinal cords exhibited varying degrees of recent traumatic injuries ranging from perfect preservation to total destruction or loss of neural elements. In most cases, the spinal cord had a winged appearance and an open central canal lined with ependyma. This configuration is consistent with failed neurulation. In those cases with preserved neural tissues, ventral and dorsal roots, spinal ganglia, gray and white matter, as well as normal looking motor neurons were discernible, reflecting a high degree of normal cord development. The cord proximal and distal to the lesion was normal in some cases, while in a majority, focal hemorrhages or anomalies such as hydromyelia, syringomyelia, duplication, or diastematomyelia were found. Interestingly, there was no detectable difference in skeletal mus-

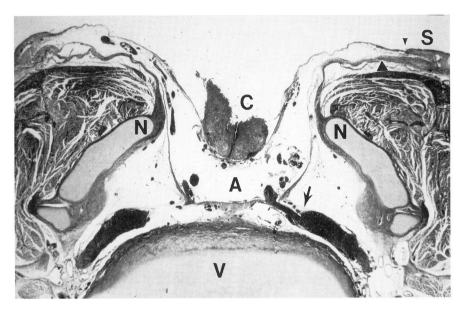

FIGURE 28–12. Classic morphology of human fetal MMC (23 gestational weeks) (histologic cross section). The exposed spinal cord tissue (C) appears grossly normal ventrally, while the dorsal part is lost (avulsion injury). The open pia fuses laterally to the epidermis (*small marker*), the open dura to the dermis (*large marker*) of the skin (S), thereby enclosing the enlarged and abnormally configured arachnoid space (A). Spinal nerve and dorsal root ganglia look normal (*arrow*). (N = open neural arch; V = vertebral body.) *See Color Plate 4*

culature and peripheral nerves between upper and lower extremities. This study demonstrates that except from disordered neurulation, there is near normal cord development within the MMC lesion in most cases. It also supports the hypothesis that *secondary* spinal cord injury, incurred relatively *late* in gestation or during birth, may significantly contribute to the loss of neurologic function. Thus, the assumption is tenable that early intrauterine coverage might efficiently protect the cord and prevent further damage.

Most recently, we looked at potential differences between the lower genitourinary tract and rectum of male fetuses (mean age, 20 gestational weeks) with MMC and age-matched controls.[26] In MMC fetuses, innervation of bladder, prostate, and rectum was markedly decreased. MMC bladders contained less smooth muscle fibers and more collagen than controls; however, the external sphincters were similar in both groups. Finally, bladders and prostates of affected and control fetuses showed a disparate expression pattern of transforming growth factor (TGF)-α, TGF-β_1, TGF-β_2, and TGF-β_3. These purely morphologic findings indicate that by midgestation visceral organ alterations are already present. Certainly, this field needs further elucidation, especially regarding the question of whether there is significant and irreversible bladder and rectum dysfunction around midgestation.

Information regarding *neurologic function* in MMC fetuses is scarce. Korenromp reported leg movements in four fetuses aged between 16 and 17 weeks' gestation who had neural tube defects ranging from small to very large.[27] In three of the four fetuses, movements appeared no different from those observed in normal fetuses of less than 20 weeks' gestational age; in one, the frequency of movements seemed slightly lower than in the others. There is no follow-up, since all pregnancies were interrupted (M. J. Korenromp, personal communication, 1994). These observations do not prove, but are consistent with the view, that the neurologic deficit may be acquired predominantly during the late second and

third trimester of pregnancy. Of note, even sonographers extremely experienced in fetal ultrasound find it difficult to differentiate between spontaneous and reflex-associated fetal movements.[28]

Luthy, Shurtleff, and Scheller found that elective cesarean section before rupture of amniotic membranes and before onset of labor decreased the degree of paralysis in infants with MMC.[29–31] They concluded that this delivery mode averted trauma to the exposed neural tissue resulting from labor and passage through the birth canal. Other investigators are skeptical as to whether this strategy affects neurologic outcome.[32, 33]

Preliminary Data from Human Fetal Surgery

Allegedly, successful in utero repair of two human fetuses has been performed using endoscopic techniques to place a maternal skin allograft over the MMC lesion (J. P. Bruner, personal communication, 1996). While one fetus died shortly after the procedure, the other was born by cesarean section at 35 weeks' gestation. However, the authors failed to produce evidence that the graft stayed in place and, more importantly, that the procedure affected neurologic outcome. Also, we remain unconvinced that gluing skin allografts over the lesion is appropriate for protective coverage. Ideally, prenatal repair should provide definitive, robust, multilayered autologous coverage of the lesion and be performable safely, quickly, and easily. We have shown experimentally[19] and in a postmortem study of human fetuses[34] that latissimus dorsi flap procedures meet these criteria.

The latest news is that the first *open* fetal surgery for human MMC was performed on March 21, 1998, by Adzick and Sutton at the Children's Hospital of Philadelphia (N. S. Adzick, personal communication, 1998). A 23-week-old male fetus with a thoracolumbosacral MMC underwent in utero coverage of the MMC lesion with local skin flaps. Preoperatively, this fetus demonstrated normal hip, knee, ankle, and toe movements and no club feet on serial ultrasound investigations. Although there was an Arnold-Chiari malformation, ventriculomegaly was not found. At 4 months of age, the level of neurologic impairment was L5–S1 for the left leg and L3 for the right leg. The right foot was clubbed. There was no ventriculomegaly and the previously described Arnold-Chiari malformation had resolved. Micturition and defecation were in portions. At present, the neurologic level appears to be markedly better (low lumbosacral) than one would expect from the lesion (low thoracic). This case is an encouraging start of a new experimental therapy.

Conclusions and Future Directions

Despite intense research and remarkable progress in understanding, fetal surgery for MMC is still lacking solid justification. Most importantly, the prenatal natural history of human MMC is not known in detail. While it is generally accepted that the pathogenesis is a defective neurulation in most cases and a failed mesoderm migration over a normally neurulated cord in a few, it is not understood *what* exactly causes the neurologic deficit and *when* during gestation it is established. Clearly, both pathogenic mechanisms lead to spinal cord tissue being openly exposed to the amniotic cavity for the entire duration of gestation. Very likely, this arrangement is the reason for in utero acquired, progressive chemical, degenerative, and traumatic neural damage. However, there is not yet conclusive evidence that the loss of spinal cord function is exclusively the consequence of *late* occurring, *secondary* and thus potentially preventable events. It is also conceivable that an important proportion of the secondary damage happens so *early* in pregnancy that fetal surgery, currently feasible around midgestation,[35] is no option. Finally, the functional deficit may be mainly caused by the primary malformation itself. Then, fetal surgery would not likely impact on neurologic outcome either. These considerations imply that we must gain more insight, especially into the time course of the neurologic deficit.

Other critical issues must be addressed. For example, how can prenatal diagnosis accurately determine that there *is* spinal cord function worth salvaging? What are the criteria for patient selection? Is fetal surgery ethically justifiable for non–life-threatening conditions, especially when unsolved problems like preterm labor are associated with considerable fetal morbidity and mortality?[35]

If fetal surgery is to be performed, how should repair be accomplished? Is skin coverage alone sufficient? If not, is a multilayer soft tissue coverage sufficient, or is it even necessary to reconstruct the missing bony parts? Is resection of the cystic sac, reconstruction of the neural plate into a tube, and closure of the dura mater mandated as in postnatal repair?[1] And if so, is it technically feasible around midgestation? What is the impact of prenatal repair on hydrocephalus, hydromyelia, and other associated cerebral or spinal anomalies?

If these gaps of knowledge can be filled with *sound and favorable* data generated from laboratory and experimental clinical work, then parents of an MMC fetus might be offered a revolutionary alternative to the currently dismal choice between termination of pregnancy and multiple handicaps of their yet-to-be-born child.

Acknowledgments

My thanks go to my wife, Claudia Meuli, MD, who plays a pivotal role in our myelomeningocele research, and to Louis Burger for technical assistance and art work.

REFERENCES

1. McLone DG: Care of the neonate with a myelomeningocele. Neurosurg Clin North Am 9:111, 1998.
2. Lemire RJ: Neural tube defects. JAMA 259:558, 1988.
3. McLaughlin JF, Shurtleff DB, Lamers JY, et al: Influence of prognosis on decisions regarding the care of newborns with myelodysplasia. N Engl J Med 312:1589, 1985.
4. Rekate HL: To shunt or not to shunt: Hydrocephalus and dysrhaphism. Clin Neurosurg 32:593, 1985.
5. Karol LA: Orthopedic management in myelomeningocele. Neurosurg Clin North Am 6:259, 1995.
6. McDonnell CM: Rehabilitation of children with spinal dysrhaphism. Neurosurg Clin North Am 6:393, 1995.
7. Copp AJ: Neural tube defects. Trends Neurosci 16:381, 1993.
8. Campbell LR, Dayton DH, Sohal GS: Neural tube defects: A review of human and animal studies on the etiology of neural tube defects. Teratology 34:171, 1986.
9. Copp AJ, Brook FA, Estibeiro JP, et al: The embryonic development of mammalian neural tube defects. Prog Neurobiol 35:363, 1990.
10. Emery JL, Lendon RG: The local cord lesion in neurospinal dysrhaphism (meningomyelocele). J Pathol 110:83, 1973.
11. Hutchins GM, McGowan KD, Blakemore KJ: Spinal dysrhaphia: Not a neural tube defect? Am J Hum Genet 51(Suppl 1):A319, 1992.
12. Micheida M: Intrauterine treatment of spina bifida: Primate model. Z Kinderchir 39:259, 1984.
13. Heffez DS, Aryanpur J, Hutchins GM, Freeman JM: The paralysis associated with myelomeningocele: Clinical and experimental data implicating a preventable spinal cord injury. Neurosurgery 26:987–992, 1990.
14. Heffez DS, Aryanpur J, Rotellini NA, et al: Intrauterine repair of experimental surgically created dysrhaphism. Neurosurgery 32:1005, 1993.
15. Meuli M, Meuli-Simmen C, Yingling CD, et al: A new model of myelomeningocele: Studies in the fetal lamb. Surg Forum 45:587, 1994.
16. Meuli M, Meuli-Simmen C, Yingling CD, et al: Creation of myelomeningocele in utero: A model of functional damage from spinal cord exposure in fetal sheep. J Pediatr Surg 30:1028, 1995.
17. Meuli M, Meuli-Simmen C, Hutchins GM, et al: In utero surgery rescues neurological function at birth in sheep with spina bifida. Nat Med 1:342, 1995.
18. Meuli M, Meuli-Simmen C, Yingling CD, et al: In utero repair of experimental myelomeningocele saves neurologic function at birth. J Pediatr Surg 31:397, 1996.
19. Meuli-Simmen C, Meuli M, Hutchins GM, et al: Fetal reconstructive surgery: Experimental use of the latissimus dorsi flap to correct myelomeningocele in utero. Plast Reconstr Surg 96:1007, 1995.
20. Patten BM: Embryological stages in the establishing of myeloschisis with spina bifida. Am J Anat 93:365, 1953.
21. Cameron AH: The spinal cord lesion in spina bifida cystica. Lancet 2:171, 1956.
22. Osaka K, Tanimura T, Hirayama A, Matsumoto S: Myelomeningocele before birth. J Neurosurg 49:711, 1978.

23. Marin-Padilla M: Spina bifida. *In* Vinkin EL, Bruyn G W (eds): Handbook of Clinical Neurology. New York: Elsevier Publishers, 1978, pp 159–191.
24. Hutchins GM, Meuli M, Meuli-Simmen C, et al: Acquired spinal cord injury in human fetuses with myelomeningocele. Pediatr Pathol Lab Med 16:701, 1996.
25. Meuli M, Meuli-Simmen C, Hutchins GM, et al: The spinal cord lesion in human fetuses with myelomeningocele: Implications for fetal surgery. J Pediatr Surg 32:448, 1997.
26. Shapiro E, Seller MJ, Steiner MS, et al: Altered smooth muscle development and growth factor expression in the lower genitourinary tract of the male fetus with myelomeningocele. J Urol 160:1047, 1998.
27. Korenromp MJ, Van Gool JD, Bruinese HW, Kriek R: Early fetal leg movements in myelomeningocele. Lancet 1:917, 1986.
28. Filly RA: Ultrasound evaluation of the fetal neural axis. *In* Callen PW (ed): Ultrasonography in Obstetrics and Gynecology. Philadelphia: WB Saunders Company, 1994, pp 189–234.
29. Luthy DA, Wardinsky T, Shurtleff DB, et al: Cesarean section before the onset of labor and subsequent motor function in infants with meningomyelocele diagnosed antenatally. N Engl J Med 324:662, 1991.
30. Shurtleff DB, Luthy DA, Nyberg DA, et al: Meningomyelocele: Management in utero and post natum. Ciba Foundation Symp 181:270, 1994.
31. Scheller JM, Nelson KB: Does cesarean delivery prevent cerebral palsy or other neurologic problems of childhood? Obstet Gynecol 83:624, 1994.
32. Hill AE, Beattie F: Does cesarean section delivery improve neurologic outcome in open spina bifida? Eur J Pediatr Surg 4 (Suppl 1):32, 1994.
33. Cochrane D, Aronyk K, Sawatzky B, et al: The effects of labor and delivery on spinal cord function and ambulation in patients with myelomeningocele. Childs Nerv Syst 7:312, 1991.
34. Meuli-Simmen C, Meuli M, Adzick NS, Harrison MR: Latissimus dorsi flap procedures to cover myelomeningocele in utero: A feasibility study in human fetuses. J Pediatr Surg 32:1154, 1997.
35. Adzick NS, Harrison MR: Fetal surgical therapy. Lancet 343:897, 1994.

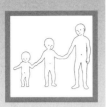

Intrauterine Myelomeningocele Repair

NOEL B. TULIPAN and JOSEPH P. BRUNER

Background

Myelomeningocele is the most common congenital malformation of the central nervous system. With an incidence of 4.4 to 4.6 cases per 10,000 live births, 1,500 to 2,000 babies with myelomeningocele are delivered in the United States annually.[1] Affected infants exhibit varying degrees of somatosensory loss, neurogenic sphincter dysfunction, paresis, and skeletal deformities.[2] Virtually all such infants also have the Chiari II malformation. In addition, up to 95% of infants with myelomeningocele require ventriculoperitoneal shunt placement for management of hydrocephalus.[3] The Centers for Disease Control (CDC) estimates that myelomeningocele and its associated abnormalities consume more than $200 billion in health care costs per year.[4] Thus myelomeningocele remains, at present, a major public health problem.

Myelomeningocele results from the failure of caudal neural tube closure during the fourth week of gestation. The lesion is characterized by protrusion of the meninges through a midline bony defect of the spine forming a sac containing cerebrospinal fluid (CSF) and dysplastic neural tissue. This malformation is inherited in a multifactorial fashion. Known environmental factors include viruses, vitamin and mineral deficiencies, chemicals, drugs, and maternal disease such as diabetes.[5] The most widely recognized environmental trigger for myelomeningocele is a deficiency of folic acid, a common water-soluble vitamin that acts as a cofactor for enzymes involved in DNA and RNA biosynthesis and as a methyl donor in the methylation cycle.[6] The etiologic role of folic acid was demonstrated in a randomized, double-blind clinical trial conducted by the Medical Research Council that demonstrated a 70% reduction in the recurrence of myelomeningocele after periconceptual administration of 4 mg of folic acid daily.[7] A preventive effect of folate-containing multivitamins on the first occurrence of myelomeningocele has also been confirmed.[8] It is not likely that myelomeningocele is caused by maternal deficiency of folic acid, since mothers of affected fetuses have been shown to have normal or near-normal red blood cell and serum folate levels.[6] Instead, attention has focused on genetically controlled defects of folate metabolism in the developing embryo.[9] Another possible interaction between an environmental factor and a genetic predisposition to myelomeningocele was recently discovered. Administration of myoinositol to pregnant curly tail mice at the time of neural tube closure resulted in a significant reduction in the incidence and severity of myelomeningocele.[10]

Numerous gene mutations leading to myelomeningocele in mice have been identified. The gene loci are widely distributed throughout the genome.[11] Early progress has been hampered by the complexity of the process, which is apparently both heterogeneous and genetically multifactorial.[12] However, many specific gene loci whose defective function may lead to myelomeningocele have been identified both in mice and in humans, and more will undoubtedly be found. In summary, a number of gene loci and environmental factors have been identified that appear to contribute to the formation of myelomeningocele in humans and mice, but the mechanisms by which they exert their actions remain unclear.

With widespread maternal serum screening and the use of high-resolution ultrasonography, most cases of myelomeningocele are now detectable in the second trimester of pregnancy. The only management options currently available, however, are either abortion or continuation of the pregnancy with neonatal therapy. These management strategies are based, in part, on the historical belief that the neurologic deficits seen in patients with myelomeningocele result solely from an embryologic error that is already complete by the fourth week of gestation. But a growing body of experimental evidence suggests that in addition to the embryologic defects, many of the neurologic deficits associated with myelomeningocele may be caused by prolonged exposure of the dysplastic spinal cord to the intrauterine environment. For instance, Michejda induced a spina bifida–like condition in eight *Macaca mulatta* fetuses by performing intrauterine lumbar laminectomy and displacing the spinal cord from the central canal.[13] This condition was repaired in utero in five animals. All of the monkey fetuses were delivered by cesarean section near term. After delivery, the five animals whose lesion was covered developed normally, while those with open lesions were paraplegic with incontinence and lower extremity somatosensory loss.

In a similar study performed in pregnant rats by Heffez et al., spinal dysraphism was created surgically in 14 rat pups, while identical lesions in nine control pups were covered in utero.[14] Those pups whose spinal cords were intentionally exposed to the amniotic fluid were born with severe deformity and weakness of the hindlimbs and tail. By contrast, control rats were normal at birth. Histologic studies of the exposed spinal cords revealed pathology similar to that described in children with myelomeningocele. Analogous studies have been performed in fetal pigs[15] and lambs[16] with similar findings. The results of these animal studies led to development of the "two-hit" hypothesis.[14] The first "hit" is the embryologic spinal cord malformation. The second "hit" is the spinal cord injury resulting from prolonged exposure of the neural elements to the intrauterine environment. The implication of the two-hit hypothesis is that intrauterine protection of the exposed spinal cord might prevent some or all of the hypothetical secondary neurologic injury.

Although data from the above-mentioned studies support the occurrence of intrauterine damage to exposed spinal elements, the timing and pathophysiology of such injury are unknown. One suspected mechanism of injury is direct toxicity of the amniotic fluid.[14] Early in gestation, the composition of the amniotic fluid reflects its origins from both maternal and fetal plasma.[17] By the end of the first trimester, however, the fetal kidneys become functional[18] followed by keratinization of the fetal skin after 22 weeks' gestation.[19] In the second half of pregnancy, therefore, amniotic fluid becomes progressively more hypotonic as the contribution of fetal urine increases. These biochemical changes in the composition of amniotic fluid with advancing gestation may result in injury to exposed spinal tissue. An alternative, or additional, mechanism of injury may be direct trauma to unprotected neural tissue or unsupported vascular structures by the uterine wall as the fetus moves about during pregnancy.[16]

Until the present time, fetal surgery has most often been performed to treat malformations that would otherwise result in the death of the fetus or newborn infant. This was due, in large part, to the fact that the inherent risks of fetal surgery were unknown, thus a risk/reward ratio could not be postulated. Lethal anomalies were therefore selected for intervention because the theoretical benefits of operation clearly outweighed the certainty of death without intervention. But as the cumulative experience of centers worldwide has clarified many of the anticipated risks and benefits of fetal surgical procedures,[20] attention has turned to nonlethal anomalies as potential targets for fetal therapeutics.[21] While spina bifida is usually not lethal, it can nonetheless be severely disabling, resulting in a large burden for affected individuals, their families, and society in general. In addition, the diagnosis of myelomeningocele antenatally is rarely ambiguous. The combined use of high-resolution ultrasonography and amniotic fluid analysis for α-fetoprotein and acetylcholinesterase results in the certain diagnosis of myelomeningocele in almost every case. Furthermore, myelomeningocele is relatively easy to repair, requiring a minimum of exposure and dissection. If, as suggested above, the spinal cord sustains progressive damage as gestation progresses, then myelomeningocele might be the ideal candidate for fetal surgical repair. It was therefore the consensus of the Fetal Diagnosis and Therapy group at Vanderbilt that the potential for decreasing the burden of disability resulting from myelomeningocele might well outweigh the risks of antepartum intervention to the extent that they are currently known. Thus in 1992 we launched a program of laboratory and clinical studies to explore the feasibility of intrauterine myelomeningocele repair.

Laboratory Studies

Developing the Endoscopic Model

The goal of our research group is to understand the mechanisms of secondary damage to the dysplastic neural components of a myelomeningocele, and to utilize this knowledge to perfect techniques for fetal surgical therapy with the goal of preventing such injury. Our initial efforts focused on developing an appropriate animal model for intrauterine protection of the exposed spinal elements.[22] Although a substantial body of evidence supported the theory that the neural elements of a myelomeningocele are secondarily damaged as the result of exposure to the intrauterine environment, the critical time at which this secondary insult might occur was not clearly defined.[13–16] Based on the limited data available, it seemed reasonable to assume a progressive injury and attempt intervention as soon as possible after detection. Since maternal serum screening for fetal spina bifida (maternal serum α-fetoprotein) is recommended between 15 and 18 gestational weeks, and obstetric ultrasound screening is commonly performed at 20 weeks' gestation, most cases of myelomeningocele are diagnosed in the mid trimester. The earliest opportunity for intrauterine coverage of the open spinal lesion is therefore about 21 to 22 weeks.

The sheep was initially chosen as an experimental model for two reasons. First, facilities for ovine surgery and postsurgical care were readily available at Vanderbilt, and second, the midgestational fetal lamb is similar in size to the 22-week human fetus. Given the extensive literature suggesting that fetal exposure via a hysterotomy led to a high incidence of preterm labor and delivery, it was decided at the outset to attempt an endoscopic surgical approach. It was anticipated that by avoiding hysterotomy the risk of preterm labor might be reduced. During our initial experiments with the endoscopic approach we immediately encountered two technical difficulties. First, we quickly concluded that a standard suture repair would be impossible given the technology currently available. In particular, the intrauterine space was too restricted and the current endoscopic suture technology too crude to allow for adequate dissection and suture closure of the fetal dural sac and skin in the routine fashion. Furthermore, at 22 weeks' gestation fetal skin is just beginning to keratinize, and we were concerned that the tissue might lack the integrity required for dissection and suture placement. Therefore, the most practical approach to early intervention with endoscopic surgery seemed to be coverage of the lesion with some type of graft.[22] Eventually it was decided to use a maternal skin graft. This would achieve the goal of protecting the exposed spinal cord from amniotic fluid and/or trauma while avoiding the need for meticulous endoscopic dissection and suturing. The second technical problem that we encountered was that the turbidity of the amniotic fluid hampered the already limited visibility afforded by a small-diameter endoscope. Replacement of the amniotic fluid with either saline or Hartmann's solution was attempted but visualization was not greatly enhanced. Furthermore, the use of any liquid environment would impede attachment of the autologous skin graft with a biologic adhesive. For these reasons, a CO_2 environment was eventually chosen.

Several successful endoscopic procedures were then performed. Briefly, the uterus was insufflated with CO_2. Three endoscopic ports were then inserted into the uterus, one for a 4-mm rigid endoscope and two for instruments. Amniotic fluid was then withdrawn until the fetus was fully exposed. A 1-cm^2 patch of full-thickness skin was removed from the fetus' back and a full-thickness skin graft, obtained from the mother, was applied to the resulting skin defect. Several different methods of achieving graft adherence were tried. It was concluded that optimal graft adherence could be obtained by covering the graft with woven oxidized cellulose (Surgicel, Johnson & Johnson, Arlington, TX), a common hemostatic agent, and then covering the entire construct with fibrin glue consisting of human cryoprecipitate activated with bovine thrombin. Using this method excellent graft survival was achieved as confirmed by histologic studies performed subsequent to the birth of the lamb. Furthermore, both the ewe and fetus tolerated the procedures well. In each case the pregnancy proceeded normally to a term delivery.

Demonstration of Amniotic Fluid Toxicity In Vitro

As mentioned above, it has been postulated that the myelodysplastic components of a myelomeningocele are secondarily damaged as the result of exposure to amniotic fluid, the so-called two-hit hypothesis.[14] However, amniotic fluid toxicity to spinal cord tissue has not been demonstrated experimentally in vitro. Furthermore, the critical time at which this secondary insult might occur has not been previously defined. Research from our laboratory has addressed these issues by quantitatively assessing the toxic effects of human amniotic fluid of various gestational ages upon organotypic cultures of rat spinal cord.[23] Organotypic cultures of spinal cord were derived from 18-day-old rat fetuses. Each spinal cord was dissected out of the spinal canal, and

sections were cultured in feeding medium for a total of 6 days. At that time, cultures were examined by light microscopy to assess viability and adequacy of tissue volume for experiments. Those cultures showing even distribution of early neuritic outgrowth and well-formed translucent cell mass were exposed to either nutritive medium or human amniotic fluid from 15, 19, 28, 34, 37, or 38 weeks' gestation. After 48 hours of incubation, medium from each culture was assayed for lactate dehydrogenase (LDH) efflux. LDH activity was used as a marker for neuronal and glial injury according to methods described by Koh and Choi,[24] who showed that neurons contain relatively high levels of LDH, and that spontaneous efflux of LDH from uninjured cells is relatively low. Their method has since been cited in well over 300 scientific publications and has become one of the proven standards for evaluating neurotoxicity in a variety of experimental models.

The LDH assay results are illustrated in Figure 29–1. In the experimental group, the cultures exposed to amniotic fluid from the second trimester (15 to 28 weeks) demonstrated levels of LDH activity similar to controls. However, the LDH activity increased significantly ($p < 0.002$) at the 34-week time point in 18 individual cultures using amniotic fluid from two different patients. This trend persisted with 37-week amniotic fluid exposure ($p < 0.025$) and then returned to control levels with the 37 5/7-week and 38-week groups.

These findings indicate that organotypic spinal cord cultures may provide a reliable in vitro tissue substrate for assessing the toxic effect of amniotic fluid on spinal cord tissue. Use of the LDH assay allows simple quantitative analysis of toxicity, and represents an improvement over other assays of neurotoxicity. These preliminary results suggest that amniotic fluid becomes toxic to spinal cord tissue at a relatively specific time during gestation, here shown to be 34 weeks. In order to confirm these results, a larger series of amniotic fluid samples from a wide variety of gestational ages will be tested. If our findings are confirmed by such a study, they would suggest that progressive damage to human myelodysplastic tissue might be prevented by early delivery of the child. However, the potential benefits of early delivery would have to be weighed against the attendant risks of prematurity. Alternatively, intrauterine repair of the defect sometime prior to 34 weeks might be therapeutic.

Clinical Studies

The Endoscopic Approach Applied to Human Myelomeningocele

Technique

Utilizing the techniques developed in the sheep model, intrauterine coverage of a myelomeningocele was performed by our Fetal Diagnosis and Therapy group in four human fetuses (Table 29–1).[25, 26] The procedure consisted of maternal laparotomy under both general and epidural anesthesia, with exposure of the gravid uterus. Endoscopic ports were placed in the uterine wall for a

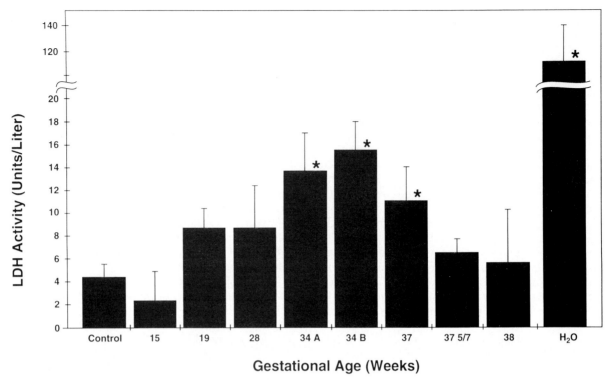

FIGURE 29–1. The average LDH activity of culture supernatants following a 48-hour incubation with amniotic fluid and serum-free medium, or serum-free medium alone (control).

camera and operating instruments (Fig. 29–2). Amniotic fluid was removed and replaced with CO_2 while maintaining ambient intrauterine pressure. The fetus was then positioned and a maternal split-thickness skin graft placed over the exposed neural elements (Fig. 29–3). The skin graft and a covering of Surgicel were attached with fibrin glue prepared from autologous cryoprecipi-

tate (Fig. 29–4). The fetal age at the time of surgery was between 22 and 24 weeks.

Results

The first infant was born via uncomplicated cesarean delivery at 35 weeks after documentation of fetal lung

TABLE 29–1. PERIOPERATIVE DATA FOR THE FOUR PATIENTS WHO UNDERWENT ENDOSCOPIC MYELOMENINGOCELE REPAIR

CASE	DESCRIPTION OF LESION	EGA AT GRAFT PLACEMENT (WK)	EGA AT DELIVERY (WK)	OUTCOME
1	L4–S3 Mild hydrocephalus Chiari II No talipes	22 3/7	35 1/7	Neonatal myelomeningocele closure/shunt placement L4 neurologic level Now 18 months old
2	L3–S2 Mild hydrocephalus Chiari II Bilateral talipes	23 6/7	24 5/7	Amnionitis Unable to resuscitate newborn in delivery room
3	T12–S5 Mild hydrocephalus Chiari II No talipes	22 4/7	28 1/7	Disruption of membranes Neonatal myelomeningocele closure/shunt placement
4	T12–S3 Hemivertebra L3 Mild hydrocephalus Chiari II Bilateral talipes	24 3/7	24 3/7	Placental abruption Intrauterine fetal demise

EGA, estimated gestational age.

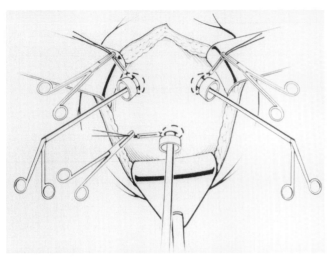

FIGURE 29–2. Schematic view of the camera and instrument ports for an endoscopic myelomeningocele repair.

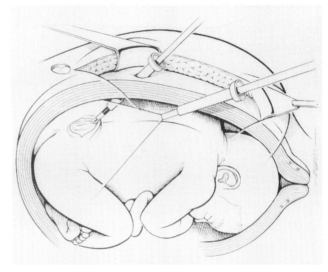

FIGURE 29–3. Cutaway schematic view of the myelomeningocele sac being prepared for placement of a maternal skin graft.

maturity by transabdominal amniocentesis (Table 29–1). On physical examination the myelomeningocele appeared unrepaired. There was no evidence of residual skin graft and histologic evaluation of samples of the tissue surrounding the lesion failed to reveal any evidence of mature maternal skin.

The myelomeningocele was repaired in routine fashion soon after birth, and a ventriculoperitoneal shunt was placed at 6 days of life. The second patient returned approximately 1 week after surgery with fever and uterine cramping. Gram stain of amniotic fluid obtained by amniocentesis revealed gram-positive cocci, and the previable fetus was delivered that day. Subsequent cultures grew *Staphylococcus*. The third patient underwent uncomplicated repair, but shortly after surgery ultrasonographic examination revealed that the amnion had partially separated from the uterine wall. Fluid began

leaking through the cervical os during the 26th week of gestation, presumably from the high leak, and the patient was admitted for inpatient care. Preterm labor occurred at 28 weeks' gestation, and a 1,040-g male infant was delivered by cesarean section. The myelomeningocele defect once again appeared undisturbed. There was no evidence of a skin graft. Multilayered closure was performed at 3 days of age, and a ventriculoperitoneal shunt was placed on day 5. In the fourth patient, epidural blockade was not maintained after induction of general endotracheal anesthesia. As the skin graft was being attached, strong, coordinated uterine contractions began. The epidural was redosed and intravenous tocolytics were administered, but by the time uterine relaxation was achieved, the placental edge was bleeding. A fetal heartbeat could not be detected in the recovery

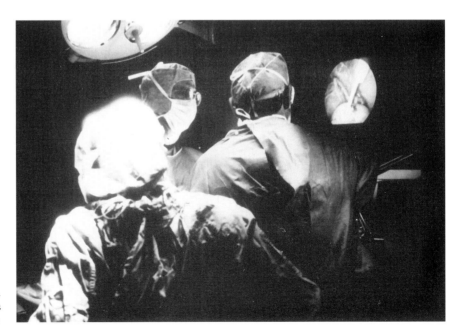

FIGURE 29–4. Surgeons observe endoscopic image projected on a video monitor as fibrin glue is being applied to the skin graft.

T A B L E 29–2. PRENATAL ULTRASONOGRAPHIC FINDINGS PRIOR TO INTRAUTERINE MYELOMENINGOCELE REPAIR

CASE	EXTENT OF LESION*	VENTRICULAR DIAMETER†	CHIARI II‡	TALIPES	OTHER
1	L5–S1	21.9	Present	None	None
2	S1–S5	13.6	Present	None	SUA
3	L5–S5	10.7	Present	None	None
4	L5–S5	10.5	Present	None	None
5	L2–S3	14.8	Present	Bilateral	None
6	L3–S5	10.7	Present	None	None
7	L4–S5	12.6	Present	Bilateral	None
8	L4–S4	20.2	Present	None	Large third ventricle
9	L3–S4	15.1	Present	Left	Polyhydramnios
10	L4–S5	13.2	Present	Bilateral	None
11	L4–S3	21.1	Present	None	None
12	L4–S4	6.6	Present	None	IUGR
13	L3–S5	12.3	Present	Bilateral	None
14	T12–S2	21.6	Present	None	None
15	S1–S5	13.7	Present	None	None
16	L2–S4	14.8	Present	Right	Rachischisis
17	S1–S3	10.1	Present	None	Rachischisis
18	L3–S4	30.3	Present	None	None
19	L3–S4	23.4	Present	Left	None
20	L3–S5	16.4	Present	Bilateral	None
21	L3–S5	11.5	Present	None	Rachischisis
22	L3–S5	13.3	Present	None	Rachischisis
23	L3–S4	13.6	Present	None	Rachischisis
24	L3–S4	14.8	Present	None	None
25	S1–S4	10.1	Present	None	Rachischisis

* Determined by careful inspection of the lesion in multiple viewing planes using standard anatomic landmarks.
† Transverse diameter of the atria of the lateral cerebral ventricles.
‡ Presence of small posterior fossa in association with absence of the cisterna magna in the axial view.
EGA, estimated gestational age. SUA, single umbilical artery; IUGR, intrauterine growth retardation.

room, and intrauterine fetal demise secondary to placental abruption was diagnosed. A stillborn female infant was delivered the same day. The skin graft was still attached, and a blood clot covered approximately 50% of the placental surface.

Discussion

Unfortunately, fetal morbidity and mortality related to the endoscopic procedure were disappointingly high. Two fetal losses occurred, and a third infant was delivered prematurely after an extended period of membrane disruption. With further experience, it is likely that these complications could be reduced or avoided entirely, but other issues also argued against further development of this technique. First, the endoscopic approach to intrauterine coverage of myelomeningocele is cumbersome and time consuming, making it unlikely to achieve popular acceptance. Second, the skin grafting technique is not definitive, only palliative. The skin grafts did not appear to survive, but even if they had a standard neurosurgical closure would probably still have been required after delivery. Definitive closure of fetal myelomeningocele under endoscopic guidance would eliminate the need for postpartum repair, but our experience with the four procedures convinced us that such an approach was not possible at any gestational age given the current state of endoscopic technology. In spite of the limitations of the endoscopic approach to myelomeningocele repair, it did have certain advantages. Placement of multiple

endoscopic ports seemed to be well tolerated by the gravid uterus, and except for the single case of intraoperative abruption, subjects experienced minimal postoperative contractions despite placement of up to four ports. However, after careful consideration of the advantages and disadvantages, we concluded that the endoscopic technique should be abandoned.[27] In the future, further refinements in endoscopic technology might one day make the procedure an attractive alternative to other techniques.

Open Intrauterine Repair of Myelomeningocele

Technique

Because of the difficulties encountered in performance of the endoscopic surgery, and based on our laboratory evidence that most secondary spinal cord damage may occur in the third trimester, we chose to revise our protocol and attempt myelomeningocele repair under direct vision through a hysterotomy in the 22- to 30-week fetus.[21] Pregnant patients with ultrasonographically confirmed fetal myelomeningocele are evaluated according to an institutional review board (IRB)-approved protocol that includes extensive counseling by members of the multidisciplinary Fetal Diagnosis and Therapy team. After initial patient interest is established, genetic amniocentesis is performed.[28] Patients whose fetus has either ultrasonographic or chromosomal evidence of abnormalities other than those usually associated with myelomeningocele are excluded from the study. Patients who elect to enter the study are scheduled for surgery at a time selected by the parents after careful consideration of the potential risks and benefits, so far as they are known. Initially, because of the limited information available, procedures were performed at 28 to 30 weeks in order to minimize the risk to the fetus if premature delivery became necessary. With a growing experience, the average gestational age at the time of repair has steadily decreased (Table 29–3).

On the day of operation, the mother is taken to a standard obstetric operating room. An epidural catheter is placed and, after induction of general endotracheal anesthesia, she is prepared as for a cesarean section. The combination of general and epidural anesthesia is used because of evidence suggesting that this combination is superior to either individually in preventing unwanted uterine contractions.[29] The epidural catheter also enables the administration of continuous postoperative analgesics. The gravid uterus is exposed via a Pfannenstiel incision and exteriorized. The fetus and placenta are then localized using a sterile ultrasound transducer. Initial uterine entry is obtained through the use of a specialized trocar developed by the authors with the technical assistance of Cook Incorporated (Bloomington, IN). The Tulipan-Bruner trocar reduces operative time and blood loss while providing relatively atraumatic entry into the uterus in comparison to routine electrocautery. The device consists of a tapered central introducer covered

by a Peel-Away sheath (Fig. 29–5). Two through-and-through chromic sutures are passed through the uterine wall and membranes on either side of the selected entry point. The introducer is then passed into the uterine cavity under ultrasonographic guidance using the Seldinger technique. As this maneuver is performed, the sutures are elevated by an assistant to provide countertraction. The central introducer is then withdrawn leaving only the Peel-Away sheath. Most of the amniotic fluid is withdrawn and retained in warm, sterile syringes. The foot plate of a U.S. Surgical CS-57 autostapling device (United States Surgical Corporation, Norwalk, CT) (Fig. 29–6) is then passed into the uterine cavity through the Peel-Away sheath, and the sheath is removed leaving the stapler in proper position. The stapler is then activated to create a 6-cm uterine incision. The fetus is directly visualized and manually positioned within the uterus such that the myelomeningocele sac is in the center of the hysterotomy incision (Fig. 29–7). The fetus is exposed to the same volatile anesthetic gases inhaled by the mother, and therefore does not move during surgery. Proper positioning is maintained by grasping the fetal head and trunk through the flaccid uterine wall.

The myelomeningocele is closed in routine neurosurgical fashion. The neural placode is sharply dissected from surrounding arachnoidal tissue and allowed to drop into the spinal canal. The dura is then identified and freed from the skin and lumbodorsal fascia. It is reflected over the placode and closed using a running 7-0 Vicryl suture. A 1.5-mm-diameter Spetzler catheter

T A B L E 29–3. PERIOPERATIVE DATA FOR THE 25 PATIENTS WHO HAVE UNDERGONE INTRAUTERINE MYELOMENINGOCELE REPAIR TO DATE

CASE	EGA AT SURGERY	EGA AT DELIVERY	COMPLICATIONS	VP SHUNT PLACEMENT (AGE)
1	29 4/7	35 4/7	None	Yes (3 wk)
2	28 5/7	34	None	No
3	28 2/7	33	Hysterotomy dehiscence	Yes (3 mo)
4	28 2/7	35 4/7	None	No
5	26 2/7	33	Vaginal breech delivery	No
6	27 5/7	36 3/7	None	No
7	26 4/7	35	None	No
8	29 3/7	35	None	Yes (9 d)
9	28 3/7	28 3/7	Placental abruption	No
10	26 2/7	34 3/7	None	No
11	26	31	Small bowel obstruction	Yes (6 d)
12	27 5/7	35 2/7	None	No
13	26 1/7	29 2/7	Severe preeclampsia	No
14	28 6/7	34 5/7	None	Yes (2 d)
15	26 1/7	32	None	No
16	26 3/7	34 6/7	None	Yes (2 d)
17	26 2/7	32 4/7	None	No
18	26 3/7	32 5/7	None	No
19	26 3/7	Expecting		
20	25 4/7	Expecting		
21	26 3/7	Expecting		
22	27 4/7	Expecting		
23	26 1/7	Expecting		
24	25 6/7	Expecting		
25	24 4/7	Expecting		

EGA, estimated gestational age; VP, ventriculoperitoneal.

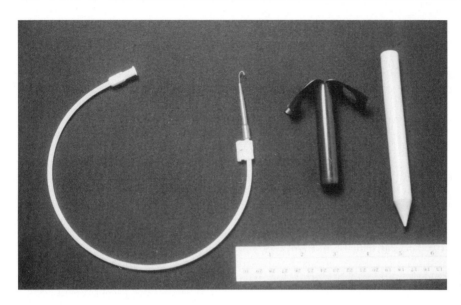

FIGURE 29–5. Tulipan-Bruner trocar used to introduce the stapling device into the uterus.

(Heyer-Schulte NeuroCare., Pleasant Prairie, WI) is then trimmed and placed next to the dural sac and brought out through a stab incision lateral to the myelomeningocele defect (Fig. 29–8). This catheter is placed to provide egress for any cerebrospinal fluid that might potentially accumulate at the site. The skin is mobilized and closed using a single 5.0 PDS suture and the drain secured using a 5.0 nylon suture (Fig. 29–9). During the procedure the fetal heartbeat is intermittently monitored by direct ultrasonographic visualization. The uterus is closed in layers using No. 1 PDS suture. The first layer incorporates the absorbable polyglycolic acid staples left by the autostapling device. As the last stitches of this layer are placed, the reserved amniotic fluid mixed with 500 mg of nafcillin is returned to the uterus. Next, commercially available fibrin glue (Tisseel Fibrin Sealant, Baxter Healthcare Corp., Glendale, CA) is applied to the suture line in an attempt to provide a watertight seal.

Finally, an imbricating layer of No. 1 PDS suture is added. This layer is also treated with fibrin glue, and a sheet of Interceed absorbable adhesion barrier (Johnson & Johnson Medical, Inc., Arlington, TX) is attached over the incision to prevent adhesion formation. The uterus is returned to the abdomen. The fascial layer is closed in routine fashion, and the dermis closed with a running subcuticular suture or staples. The fetus is monitored postoperatively using continuous electronic fetal monitoring (EFM) and intermittent transabdominal ultrasonography.

Postoperative uterine contractions are monitored using continuous EFM. Uterine contractions are initially controlled with intravenous magnesium sulfate and oral or rectal indomethacin, and subsequently with subcutaneous terbutaline. Each patient is discharged from the hospital with a subcutaneous terbutaline pump (Matria Healthcare, Inc., Atlanta, GA) supplemented by oral

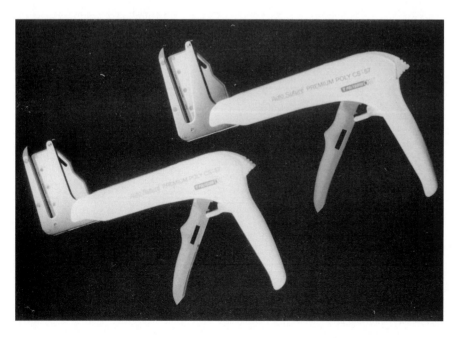

FIGURE 29–6. U.S. Surgical CS-57 autostapling device used to incise the uterus.

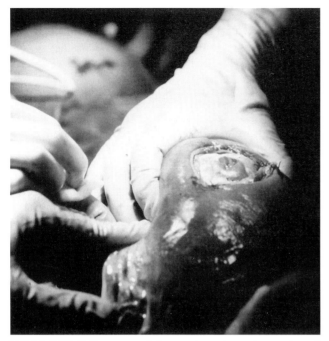

FIGURE 29–7. Exposure of the myelomeningocele sac through the hysterotomy.

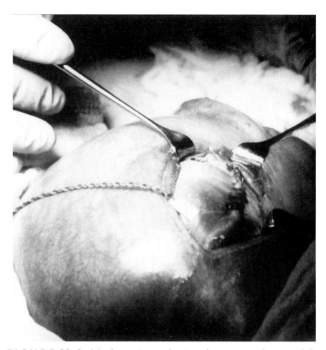

FIGURE 29–9. Myelomeningocele site after suture closure of the dura and skin.

magnesium oxide and indomethacin as needed. The terbutaline pump is used because the lower dose administered in this fashion may delay the onset of β-adrenergic receptor desensitization, also known as tachyphylaxis.[30] Patients are monitored with weekly transabdominal ultrasonographic examinations. Delivery of each child is accomplished via standard cesarean section. This is because of evidence suggesting that children with myelomeningocele have fewer neurologic deficits if delivered in this fashion,[31,32] but is also necessitated by the presence

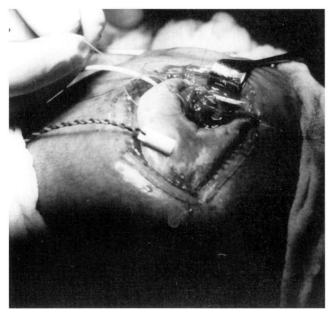

FIGURE 29–8. Placement of the Spetzler catheter in the epidural space.

of the fundal hysterotomy incision. Although the same abdominal incision is used for the cesarean section as for the fetal surgery, the fetus is preferably delivered via a lower uterine segment incision. The uterine and abdominal incisions are closed in routine fashion.

Results

Open intrauterine repair of myelomeningocele has been performed by our Fetal Diagnosis and Therapy team in 25 patients (Table 29–3). Preoperative ultrasonographic studies revealed no major abnormalities other than those usually associated with myelomeningocele, namely, the Chiari II malformation, hydrocephalus, and talipes (Table 29–2). In each case except one the mother underwent uncomplicated uterine exposure, hysterotomy, and closure once the fetus had reached 24 to 30 weeks of gestation (Table 29–3). Maternal vital signs remained stable and no uterine contractions were appreciated intraoperatively. In a patient (case 9) with polyhydramnios the uterus felt unusually firm upon exteriorization. Removal of the large amount of amniotic fluid initiated spontaneous uterine contractions that in turn led to precipitous extrusion of the fetus through the hysterotomy at the time of surgery. This subsequently led to placental abruption, which necessitated definitive delivery. The infant was easily resuscitated and underwent uncomplicated myelomeningocele repair on the fifth day of life. He was subsequently discharged healthy after an uneventful hospital stay. There was no evidence of either lung disease or intraventricular hemorrhage. The baseline moderate hydrocephalus remained stable and no shunting procedure was performed. The mother suffered no ill effects.

Estimated blood loss ranged from 50 to 100 mL in each of the other cases. Each fetus' myelomeningocele was successfully repaired as described above. Intraoperative monitoring of the fetal heartbeat revealed no prolonged bradycardic episodes or other untoward events throughout any of the procedures. Postoperative maternal monitoring demonstrated mild, irregular uterine contractions for up to 6 hours in approximately half of the patients. These contractions gradually subsided, and had ceased by the first postoperative day. Continuous monitoring of the fetal heartbeat revealed no periodic decelerations in any of the fetuses. The only obvious ultrasonographic abnormality was a marked paucity of amniotic fluid in the earlier cases. In the first three patients oligohydramnios became evident within 24 hours and persisted for several weeks. Serial speculum examinations of the cervical os could discern no evidence of fluid leakage, and ultrasonography revealed no signs of membrane disruption, fetal edema, or extrauterine fluid collection. Hourly fetal urine production was unchanged before and after repair. Finally, measurements of amniotic fluid pressure performed before hysterotomy and after uterine closure demonstrated a marked reduction in intrauterine pressure. In subsequent patients a deliberate attempt was made to capture and replace as much of the amniotic fluid as possible, and additional warmed saline was added to reproduce the preoperative uterine volume and turgor. Oligohydramnios has not been as serious a problem since that time. The patients and their apparently healthy fetuses were discharged between the third and fifth postoperative days.

Posthospitalization monitoring with transabdominal ultrasonography confirmed ongoing fetal well-being in each case. Persistent oligohydramnios remained the only appreciable abnormality as mentioned above. At approximately 5 weeks postoperatively (33 weeks' gestation), the third woman in the series experienced a brief episode of sharp abdominal pain. Ultrasonography at an outside hospital showed that one of the fetal legs had protruded through the hysterotomy into the peritoneal cavity. Neither the mother nor the fetus showed any signs of distress, but the decision was made to deliver the fetus. At surgery, the fetal leg was found protruding through the partially healed uterine incision. A healthy infant was delivered through the dehiscence without incident. The uterus was repaired, and the mother recovered uneventfully.[33] It was felt that the problem in this case might have resulted from the use of inadequately long lasting suture, namely chromic gut. In all subsequent procedures PDS has been used instead of chromic.

The 11th patient developed signs and symptoms of a small bowel obstruction approximately 5 weeks after surgery. She eventually required exploration. At surgery a small hysterotomy dehiscence with adherent bowel was found. The fetus was delivered without incident and is doing well. Subsequent culture of the resected hysterotomy edge revealed mucormycosis. The mother recovered uneventfully. The other infants were delivered at an average of 34 ± 2 weeks of gestation after the onset of spontaneous labor or fluid leakage. Prior to delivery, a few of the patients experienced preterm uterine contractions leading to hospital admission, although none had any demonstrable cervical change. In

no case did the preterm labor necessitate delivery until after tocolysis had been discontinued at 34 to 35 weeks.

On physical examination, most newborns had a well-healed myelomeningocele scar (Fig. 29–10). One infant had a small area of skin dehiscence at the lower end of the myelomeningocele repair. This was closed primarily in the operating room without complication. Another infant had an even smaller open area that healed without intervention. Each of the fetal epidural catheters was also still in place save four which were never located and which were presumably discarded with the uterine contents. Each of the other catheters was removed without complication within 24 hours of delivery. Since delivery most of the infants have done well from a medical perspective. However, one infant born at 35 weeks developed pulmonary problems soon after delivery. These problems required temporary mechanical ventilation and have since necessitated several hospitalizations. The child was subsequently diagnosed as having cellular interstitial pneumonitis, a rare, idiopathic pulmonary disease probably unrelated to prematurity or the fetal surgery.

Little can be said at this time about the effect of intrauterine myelomeningocele repair on leg or bladder function. As this chapter is written the eldest child is only 16 months old and seven remain unborn. No clear trend toward improvement can yet be discerned, but neither is any child worse than might be predicted from the anatomic level of his or her lesion. By contrast, we have noted a marked reduction in the incidence of the hindbrain herniation normally associated with the Chiari II malformation. None of the first five patients successfully treated in utero has any evidence of hindbrain herniation on postnatal ultrasound or magnetic resonance imaging (MRI) scan (Figs. 29–11 and 29–12).[34] This is markedly unusual considering the fact that in large series greater than 95% of patients with myelomeningocele

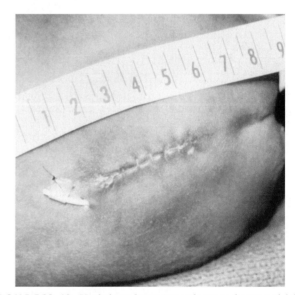

F I G U R E 29–10. Healed myelomeningocele sac at the time of delivery. Note the epidural catheter still in place.

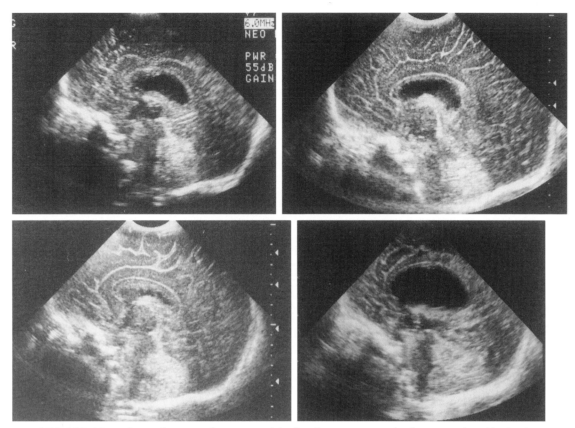

FIGURE 29–11. Midsagittal sonographic images of the first four experimental subjects in order of birth. There is no evidence of cerebellar herniation through the foramen magnum.

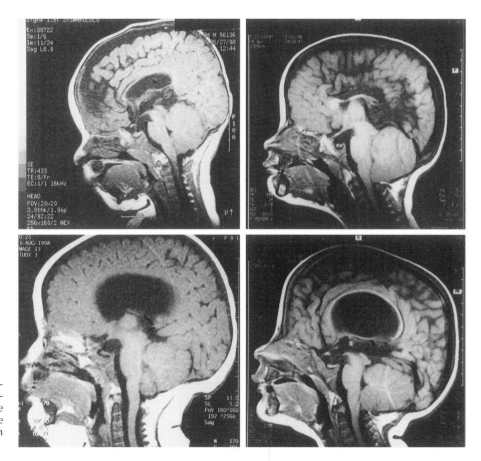

FIGURE 29–12. Midsagittal T1-weighted images of the first four experimental subjects in order of birth. Note the normal position of the fourth ventricle and the absence of cerebellar herniation in each.

have some evidence of such herniation.[35-37] The remainder of the infants have yet to be studied; but if this finding is consistent, then it suggests that intrauterine repair of a myelomeningocele may reduce the degree of cerebellar and brainstem herniation normally seen in association with the Chiari II malformation. Of additional interest is the fact that only 6 of the 18 (33%) born so far have required a ventriculoperitoneal shunt, four at 1 week, one at 3 weeks, and one at 3 months. Any bias toward avoiding a shunt has been reduced by the fact that only five of the infants have been managed postnatally by the authors. The remainder have been born elsewhere and managed by local neurosurgeons. These data would therefore suggest that the need for shunting is also reduced by intrauterine repair.

Discussion

It has been postulated that many of the anatomic defects associated with the Chiari II malformation result from persistent leakage of spinal fluid through the neural placode. This leakage sets into motion a complex series of embryologic events that result not only in hindbrain herniation, but the other stigmata of the malformation as well.[38] That this process seems to progress during gestation is suggested by published series of prenatal ultrasounds that indicate that the degree of cerebellar compression and herniation becomes more severe at later gestational ages.[39] In fact, it would appear that cerebellar herniation can progress or recede even after birth. Ruge et al. reported progression of the Chiari II malformation in 18 of 22 patients studied.[40] Reports of acquired Chiari defects of the type I variety after lumbar peritoneal (LP) shunting also support the notion that constant drainage of lumbar CSF may promote cerebellar herniation through the foramen magnum.[41] There are even reports of resolution of acquired Chiari malformations after removal of LP shunts.[42] It is therefore possible that by closing the myelomeningocele defect earlier in development the hindbrain herniation may be either prevented or reversed. This process may be aided by the pliability of the fetal skull and perhaps by the consistency of the fetal brain, which is poorly myelinated and therefore more deformable than mature brain. These results will necessarily need to be confirmed in a larger group of patients, but if true may have important implications with regard to prognosis. In particular, a reduction in the degree of hindbrain herniation may reduce the incidence of symptoms related to brain stem compression, and might also reduce the incidence of associated syringomyelia.

A less obvious but perhaps more important implication of these results is the possibility of reducing the incidence of hydrocephalus. It has been suggested by some that the hydrocephalus seen in association with myelomeningocele is at least in part due to the Chiari malformation.[43] It is postulated that the malformation may result in obstruction of the normal flow of fluid at the skull base. Once again, prenatal ultrasound lends credence to this theory. In a series of 51 fetuses with myelomeningocele the incidence and severity of ventriculomegaly increased later in gestation concomitant with a general worsening of the cerebellar abnormalities.[44] If, in fact, hindbrain herniation can be reduced by intrauterine myelomeningocele repair there might be a proportionate reduction in the incidence of hydrocephalus. The unusually long interval between birth and shunting in two of the six patients requiring shunting suggests that even in those there might have been a milder degree of CSF malabsorption than is commonly seen.

These results suggest that intrauterine myelomeningocele repair can be performed with a minimum of morbidity to both the mother and her unborn child. The most serious complication remains the single premature intraoperative delivery. This might potentially have resulted in significant complications related to prematurity but did not. Greater attention is now being paid to the turgor of the uterus intraoperatively. It is our plan in the future to terminate the procedure if adequate uterine relaxation cannot be obtained by administration of additional anesthetics or tocolytics. The other significant complications to date relate to dehiscence of the hysterotomy. This potentially serious complication represents a diagnostic challenge because the small hysterotomy is not easily visualized with real-time ultrasonography. The first instance was diagnosed antenatally because a fetal small part was protruding through the defect. The second case was diagnosed intraoperatively during exploratory laparotomy for small bowel obstruction. This has implications for obstetric management near delivery. At present, patients are delivered with the onset of labor or amniorrhexis after 34 weeks' gestation. Expectant management is followed because of our interest in determining the natural interval between intrauterine surgery and delivery. Since patients thus far have tended to begin labor or leak amniotic fluid around 34 weeks, we anticipate elective delivery around that gestational age in the future. One reasonable approach would be to continue tocolysis until 34 or 35 weeks, then schedule elective cesarean delivery prior to the onset of labor. An alternative would be to perform amniocentesis at 34 or 35 weeks and deliver after documentation of fetal lung maturity. Either approach would balance the risk of hysterotomy dehiscence against that of iatrogenic fetal immaturity.

Ethical Considerations

Open fetal surgery for the treatment of nonlethal malformations such as myelomeningocele opens a new chapter in the ethical debate over prenatal therapy.[45] Until recently, such surgery was only performed for lethal anomalies. The ethical considerations were therefore relatively simple. In the absence of intervention, fetal or neonatal mortality is inevitable. Presumably, when faced with the decision of life with surgery or death without, the fetus would choose life in almost every case. Thus when a correctable lethal malformation is identified in a fetus, the role of the objective fetal advocate is straightforward. This focuses the bulk of ethical decision making around the mother and the potential risks to her health. When nonlethal fetal abnormalities are treated, the focus shifts. By definition, all affected fetuses will survive, although severe disability may result. Participants in the decision-making process are then faced with the challenge of balancing the likelihood of improved lifestyle for the unborn child against the risks of fetal and maternal morbidity and mortality if surgery is performed.

The largest obstacle to meaningful dialogue within this new paradigm is failure of the involved parties to recognize that the ethical context has changed. When asked to reveal their greatest fear about their unborn child's welfare, potential candidates for intrauterine surgery invariably answer "the death of my baby," yet even brief reflection will reveal that this cannot be the case. If this were truly their greatest fear, then parents of a fetus with a nonlethal malformation should decline fetal therapy, since in the absence of any intrauterine treatment their child would almost certainly be born alive. The most serious risk of fetal death in fact results directly from the attempted intrauterine surgery. What these frightened parents are unable to articulate is that their real fear is of severe disability with all of the attendant ramifications that such a handicap entails. This fear is so great, in fact, that they are willing to risk the death of their fetus in an effort to reduce the potential disability. The challenge to medical ethicists and fetal surgeons alike is to recognize the changing landscape in which ethical discourse is now taking place, so that the opportunity for informed decision making can be fully enhanced.

Summary

It remains to be seen whether any substantial neurologic benefit can be ascribed to this surgery. So far, no firm conclusions can be drawn with respect to the effect of intrauterine myelomeningocele repair on leg and bladder function. However, it can now be stated with some assurance that the severity of the Chiari II malformation and the incidence of shunt-dependent hydrocephalus are reduced by intrauterine repair. Whether these patients will suffer fewer of the symptoms of these abnormalities remains unknown. One of the many interesting questions raised by these data is whether additional benefits might result from even earlier surgery. The answer is probably yes. Myelomeningocele can now be reliably diagnosed as early as the first trimester of pregnancy. But as the surgery is performed earlier the risks associated with extreme prematurity also increase exponentially. How then will we weigh the potential benefits of ever-earlier surgery with the increasing risk of prematurity or death? Questions such as these await further study but if, as the preceding data suggest, intrauterine treatment of myelomeningocele can significantly reduce the burden of this problem, it will give prospective parents an attractive third alternative to abortion or conventional treatment. Intrauterine myelomeningocele repair may offer the fetal surgery team the exciting ability to alter the natural history of this otherwise devastating disease.

REFERENCES

1. Lary JM, Edmonds LD: Prevalence of spina bifida at birth—United States, 1983–1990: A comparison of two surveillance systems. MMWR Morb Mortal Wkly Rep 45:15–26, 1996.
2. Steinbok P, Irvine B, Cochrane DD, Irwin BJ: Long-term outcome and complications of children born with meningomyelocele. Childs Nerv Syst 8:92–96, 1992.
3. McLone DG: Continuing concepts in the management of spina bifida. Pediatr Neurosurg 18:254–256, 1992.
4. Economic burden of spina bifida—United States, 1980–1990. MMWR Morb Mortal Wkly Rep 38:264–267, 1989.
5. Mitchell LE: Genetic epidemiology of birth defects: Nonsyndromic cleft lip and neural tube defects. Epidemiol Rev 19:61–68, 1997.
6. Scott JM, Weir DG, Molloy A, et al: Folic acid metabolism and mechanisms of neural tube defects. In Bock G, Marsh J (eds): Neural Tube Defects (Ciba Foundation Symposium 181) Chichester: John Wiley & Sons, 1994.
7. Wald N, Sneddon J, Densem J, et al: MRC Vitamin Study Research Group. Prevention of neural tube defects: Results of the Medical Research Council Vitamin Study. Lancet 338:131–137, 1991.
8. Czeizel AE, Dudas I: Prevention of the first occurrence of neural tube defects by periconceptual vitamin supplementation. N Engl J Med 327:1832–1835, 1992.
9. Copp AJ: Prevention of neural tube defects: Vitamins, enzymes and genes. Curr Opin Neurol 11:97–102, 1998.
10. Greene NDE, Copp AJ: Inositol prevents folate-resistant neural tube defects in the mouse. Nat Med 3:60–66, 1997.
11. Harris MJ, Juriloff DM: Genetic landmarks for defects in mouse neural tube closure. Teratology 56:177–187, 1997.
12. Campbell LR, Dayton DH, Sohal ES: Neural tube defects: A review of human and animal studies on the etiology of neural tube defects. Teratology 34:171–187, 1986.
13. Michejda M: Intrauterine treatment of spina bifida: Primate model. Z Kinderchir 39:259–261, 1984.
14. Heffez DS, Aryanpur J, Hutchins GM, Freeman JM: The paralysis associated with myelomeningocele: Clinical and experimental data implicating a preventable spinal cord injury. Neurosurgery 26:987–992, 1990.
15. Heffez DS, Aryanpur J, Cuello-Rotellini NA, et al: Intrauterine repair of experimental surgically created dysraphism. Neurosurgery 32:1005–1010, 1993.
16. Meuli M, Meuli-Simmen C, Yingling CD, et al: Creation of myelomeningocele in utero: A model of functional damage from spinal cord exposure in fetal sheep. J Pediatr Surg 30:1028–1033, 1995.
17. Lind T, Parkin FM, Cheyne GA: Biochemical and cytological changes in liquor amnii with advancing gestation. Br J Obstet Gynaecol 76:673–680, 1969.
18. Lind T, Kendall A, Hytten FE: The role of the fetus in the formation of amniotic fluid. Br J Obstet Gynaecol 79:289–298, 1972.
19. Wallenburg HCS: The amniotic fluid. I. Water and electrolyte homeostasis. J Perinatol Med 5:191–205, 1977.
20. Harrison MR: Fetal surgery. Am J Obstet Gynecol 174:1255–1264, 1996.
21. Tulipan N, Bruner JP: Myelomeningocele repair in utero: A report of three cases. Pediatr Neurosurg 28:177–180, 1998.
22. Copeland ML, Bruner JP, Richards WO, et al: A model for in utero endoscopic treatment of myelomeningocele. Neurosurgery 33:542–544, 1993.
23. Drewek MJ, Bruner JP, Whetsell WO, Tulipan N: Quantitative analysis of the toxicity of human amniotic fluid to cultured rat spinal cord. Pediatr Neurosurg 27:190–193, 1997.
24. Koh JY, Choi DW: Quantitative determination of glutamate-mediated cortical neuronal injury in cell culture by lactate dehydrogenase efflux assay. J Neurosci Meth 20:83–90, 1987.
25. Bruner JP, Richards WO, Tulipan NB, Arney T: Endoscopic coverage of fetal myelomeningocele in utero. Am J Obstet Gynecol 180:153–158, 1999.
26. Bruner JP: Fetal surgery. In Sutton C, Diamond MP (eds): Endoscopic Surgery for Gynecologists. Philadelphia: WB Saunders Company, 1998, pp 651–667.
27. Bruner JP, Tulipan N, Richards WO, et al: In utero repair of myelomeningocele: A comparison of endoscopy and hysterotomy. Fetal Diagn Ther (in press).

28. Babcook CJ, Goldstein RB, Filly RA: Prenatally detected fetal myelomeningocele: Is karyotype analysis warranted? Radiology 194:491–494, 1995.
29. Thorp JA, Meyer BA, Cohen GR, et al: Epidural analgesia in labor and cesarean delivery for dystocia. Obstet Gynecol Surv 49:362–369, 1994.
30. Iams JD, Johnson FF, O'Shaughnessy RW, West LC: A prospective random trial of home uterine activity monitoring in pregnancies at increased risk of preterm labor, II. Am J Obstet Gynecol 159:595–603, 1988.
31. Luthy DA, Wardinsky T, Shutleff DB, et al: Cesarean section before the onset of labor and subsequent motor function in infants with meningomyelocele diagnosed antenatally. N Engl J Med 324:662–666, 1991.
32. Kuller JA, Katz VL, Wells SR, et al: Cesarean delivery for fetal malformations. Obstet Gynecol Surv 51:371–375, 1996.
33. Ranzini AC, White M, Guzman ER, Scorza WE: Prenatal sonographic diagnosis of uterine rupture following open fetal surgery. Obstet Gynecol 29:274–278, 1999.
34. Tulipan N, Hernanz-Schulman M, Bruner JP: Reduced hindbrain herniation after intrauterine myelomeningocele repair: A report of four cases. Pediatr Neurosurg 29(5):274–278, 1998.
35. El Gamma T, Mark EK, Brooks BS: MR imaging of Chiari II malformation. AJR Am J Roentgenol 150:163–170, 1988.
36. Wolpert SM, Scott RM, Platenberg C, Runge VM: The clinical significance of hindbrain herniation and deformity as shown on MR images of patients with Chiari II malformation. AJNR Am J Neuroradiol 9:1075–1078, 1988.
37. Curnes JT, Oakes WJ, Boyko OB: MR imaging of hindbrain deformity in Chiari II patients with and without symptoms of brainstem compression. AJNR Am J Neuroradiol 10:293–302, 1989.
38. McLone DG, Knepper PA: The cause of the Chiari II Malformation: A unified theory. Pediatr Neurosci 15:1–12, 1989.
39. Van den Hof MC, Nicolaides KH, Campbell J, Campbell S: Evaluation of the lemon and banana signs in one hundred thirty fetuses with open spina bifida. Am J Obstet Gynecol 162:322–327, 1990.
40. Ruge JR, Masciopinto J, Storrs BB, McLone DG: Anatomical progression of the Chiari II malformation. Childs Nerv Syst 8:86–91, 1992.
41. Chumas PD, Armstrong DC, Drake JM, et al: Tonsillar herniation: The rule rather than the exception after lumboperitoneal shunting in the pediatric population. J Neurosurg 78:568–573, 1993.
42. Pyner TD, Prenger E, Berger TS, Crone KR: Acquired Chiari malformations: Incidence, diagnosis, and management. Neurosurgery 34:429–434, 1994.
43. Russell DS, Donald C: The mechanism of hydrocephalus in spina bifida. Brain 58:203–215, 1935.
44. Babcook CJ, Goldstein RB, Barth RA, et al: Prevalence of ventriculomegaly in association with myelomeningocele: Correlation with gestational age and severity of posterior fossa deformity. Radiology 190:703–707, 1994.
45. Bliton MJ, Zaner RM: Ready or not, everything is different now: Revisiting ethical considerations and the "new" fetal surgery. (Submitted).

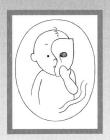

CHAPTER 30

The Fetus with Cleft Lip/Palate and Craniofacial Anomalies

MICHAEL T. LONGAKER

Fetal Wound Repair

The unique ability of early gestation fetal skin wounds to heal without scarring has for a long time captured the attention of pediatric and plastic surgeons. While experimental studies of fetal wound healing have made substantial progress over the past decade, the biomolecular regulation of scarless repair remains largely unknown. This chapter will briefly review fetal repair and discuss experimental work describing the in utero creation and reconstruction of craniofacial anomalies in animal models.

In broad terms, the unique fetal ability to heal early gestation skin wounds without scarring may be due to differences between fetal and adult cells, the fetal environment, or a combination of both.[1-3] Several studies have helped clarify the role of the intrauterine environment in fetal repair. Simply placing adult skin into the intrauterine environment, where it was bathed by amniotic fluid and perfused by fetal serum, did not modulate adult repair to become scarless in nature.[4] More importantly, it has been shown that human fetal skin can heal without scarring outside of the intrauterine environment using a nude mouse model.[5] Therefore, it appears that the fetal environment alone is not responsible for the ability to heal early gestational skin wounds without a scar. This finding is encouraging to investigators who desire to manipulate wound repair in children and adults to become more fetal-like. In contrast to studies investigating the role of the wound environment in fetal repair, differences between fetal and adult cells remain unknown, but remain an intense area of research.

While much descriptive work has been reported, the biomolecular regulation of fetal repair remains elusive. The more we learn about fetal repair, the more specific one must be when describing "scarless fetal wound healing." Specificity regarding species, gestational age, organ and wound type, and size have now been described for fetal repair (Table 30–1). The following broad characteristics have emerged regarding fetal wound healing.

Species Specificity

Awareness of species-specific differences is important when reviewing fetal repair literature. Differences between species include the length of gestation, manner of placentation, and intrinsic wound healing characteristics.[2, 6] The most dramatic demonstration of these differences relates to wound contraction. For example, fetal rabbit wounds do not contract in the presence of amniotic fluid, but do contract when excluded from amniotic fluid.[7, 8] These differences are believed to be due to a characteristic of amniotic fluid that inhibits fetal fibroblast contraction. In contrast, excisional fetal lamb wounds do contract in utero.[9] In addition, sheep amniotic fluid stimulates in vitro fibroblast populated collagen lattice contraction in a dose-responsive manner.[10] Furthermore, wounds in an embryonic chicken model contract by undergoing a unique purse-string closure by contraction of actin cables, demonstrating yet another method of fetal wound closure.[11] Therefore, it is important to remember that the characteristics of fetal repair can be unique to the animal model used to study fetal wound healing. Caution must be exercised when comparing fetal wound repair data between species. However, the unifying aspect in all animal models of fetal wound healing is that incisional wounds made early in gestation heal without the scar formation seen in adult incisional wounds.

Organ Specificity

Different fetal tissues appear to possess different healing patterns. Human fetal surgery has demonstrated that intra-abdominal adhesions can occur following fetal diaphragmatic hernia repair.[12-15] In support of clinical observations, studies in fetal lambs show that the diaphragm heals with scar formation.[16] Furthermore, even if the diaphragm is marsupialized and exposed to amniotic fluid, healing is not modulated and maintains a scar pattern. Of interest, several studies have demonstrated that the fetal gastrointestinal tract heals with scar formation and adhesions.[17, 18] In addition, fetal long bone heal-

T A B L E 30–1. BROAD CHARACTERISTICS OF FETAL REPAIR

Species specificity
Organ specificity
Gestational age specificity
Wound type and size specificity

ing proceeds rapidly and without a cartilaginous intermediate. Finally, fetal long bone healing can successfully overcome what would be a critical size gap in postnatal bone.[19] These findings suggest that there may be differences in the timing or mechanism of repair in wounds from tissues of different embryonic origins. A thorough understanding of the types of repair in various organ systems will be crucial in the potential planning of any human fetal operation that is performed to harness the unique qualities of fetal skin repair.[20] Fortunately, early gestation incisional skin wounds heal without scarring in the fetal animal models reported to date. This observation is important when considering fetal surgery for craniofacial anomalies such as cleft lip/palate.[21]

Gestational Age Specificity

Fetal skin undergoes a dramatic change in architecture, progressing from a simple epithelial covering with absorptive qualities early in development to a complex organ containing epidermis, dermis, hair follicles, and sebaceous and sweat glands that by birth acts as a barrier.[22] It is not surprising that these dramatic changes in differentiation, physiology, and architecture may be associated with a change in the quality and organization of repair. This hypothesis is supported by studies in fetal sheep, monkey, rat, and opossum demonstrating a transition from scarless healing to scar formation as a function of gestational or early postnatal age.[2, 23–26] In the lamb model, the transition for incisional wound healing occurs early in the third trimester.[23] Similarly, in primates histologic changes with the gradual loss of scar-free healing have also been described.[24] Initially, fetal primate incisional wounds lose the ability to regenerate dermal elements such as hair follicles, but retain the ability to heal the dermis without a scar. This has been defined by Lorenz et al. as the "transition wound."[24] Subsequently, wounds made later in gestation are characterized by disorganized dermis resulting in a scar with densely packed collagen deposition.

The observation of a transition from scar-free repair to healing with scar occurring prior to birth has important implications for the timing of when any potential fetal procedure that attempts to "harness" scarless repair should be performed. Specifically, with the transition for human fetal wound healing as yet undefined, at what fetal age should surgery be considered for cleft lip/palate? This issue must be addressed prior to clinical attempts to correct cleft lip/palate in utero.[20, 21]

Wound Size Specificity

A recent report by Cass et al. addressed the effects of both gestational age and excisional wound size on fetal repair.[27] At 60, 70, 80, and 90 days' gestation, incisional wounds and excisional wounds that were 2, 4, 6, and 10 mm in diameter were created on fetal lambs. Scar formation was seen in 3% of incisional, as well as 2- and 4-mm^2 excisional wounds. In contrast, scar was present in 28% of 6-mm^2 and 59% of 10-mm^2 excisional wounds. In general, as fetal lambs progressed in gestation, there was a decrease in the ability to heal without a scar and an increase in transitional repair and scarring. Thus, there appeared to be a change from scar-free healing to repair with scar formation between wounds of 4-mm and 10-mm diameter. These data suggest that there is a developmentally regulated threshold for scarless healing based on *both* gestational age and the size of injury. The study by Cass et al. may help shed some light on the findings of Horne et al., who demonstrated scar formation with 2-cm incisional and 2.5-cm^2 excisional wounds in fetal lambs.[28]

In summary, the fetal wound healing "story" has become more complex. The scarless nature of fetal repair depends on how, when, and where the fetus is wounded. Most importantly, it is essential that surgeons and scientists continue to investigate the mechanisms underlying scarless repair because of the ultimate clinical aim of manipulating wound healing in children and adults to become more fetal-like. A thorough understanding of the scarless fetal "blueprint" will provide the ideal target as we attempt to modulate wound healing clinically. Finally, the alluring quality of scarless repair remains a driving force behind experimental studies into fetal surgery to correct craniofacial anomalies (Fig. 30–1).

Fetal Models and Surgery for Craniofacial Anomalies

Fetal surgery for craniofacial disorders has captured the attention of pediatric and plastic surgeons for several reasons: (1) early gestation fetal skin heals without scarring; (2) fetal surgery may interrupt the cascade of detrimental scarring and secondary effects of various craniofacial disorders; and (3) fetal surgery may eliminate secondary operations ultimately required to correct craniofacial deformities.

Fetal Surgery for Cleft Lip and Palate

Many different animal models have been used for the study of fetal surgery of cleft lip and palate. In general, these animals can be divided into two groups: (1) small, short gestation; and (2) large, long gestation.[6] Small, short-gestation animals like mice and rats offer the advantages of large experimental numbers, low costs, and widely available molecular reagents such as gene sequences, specific antibodies, knockouts, and transgenic animals. These models are ideal for sophisticated anal-

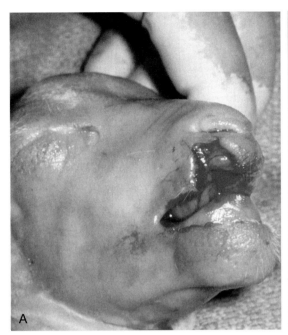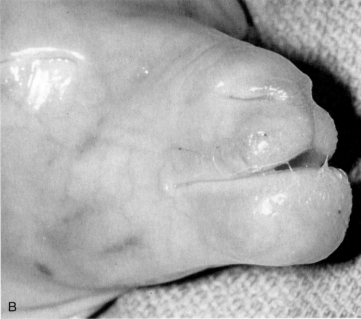

F I G U R E 30–1. Photographs of scarless fetal lamb wound healing. *A*, Excisional cleft lip wound created on fetal lamb at 70 days' gestation. This wound was closed in layers, and the fetus was returned to the uterus. *B*, Appearance of wound 14 days after repair. Note suture in skin of upper lip.

ysis of the biomolecular mechanisms of fetal wound healing and may provide insight to targeted therapeutic manipulations designed to improve the quality of repair for neonatal and adult wounds. In addition, numerous spontaneously clefting lip and palate models have been described in small animals, thus potentially making the repair of these defects more clinically relevant. Small animal models, however, are complicated by the fact that fetal manipulation is only possible late in gestation, thus limiting the postoperative, intrauterine period. This shortcoming is particularly important, since scarless fetal wounds can undergo a transition to healing by scar during the late stages of gestation. In addition, because of their small size, surgical manipulation in these models can be technically challenging. Thus, while small animal models are useful for sophisticated biomolecular analyses of wound healing in the context of spontaneously formed cleft lip and palate, the clinical relevance of these models to human fetal surgery may be somewhat decreased when compared to larger animal models due to the technical challenges inherent to fetal surgery in small animals.

Large, long-gestation animal models such as primates and lamb, are useful models to evaluate fetal healing, since these animals have a significantly longer postoperative intrauterine period. This period of time is crucial in fetal cleft lip repair since, as previously described, scarless healing in fetal wounds is gestational age dependent. Thus, wounds created during late gestation are more likely to take on an adult phenotype with scarring, whereas wounds created earlier during gestation heal without the detrimental effects of scar formation. In ad-

dition, because of their relatively long gestation, these large animal models permit multiple intrauterine procedures, allowing for formation and subsequent repair of surgically created defects. Finally, the larger size of these animals facilitates surgical manipulation, making complex surgical procedures such as multilayered repairs and endoscopic fetal surgery technically feasible.

The most commonly described small animal model of cleft palate repair is the A/J mouse. These animals are useful, since they display a high rate of spontaneous cleft palate formation (7 to 12%) that can be increased to nearly 100% when pregnant mice are treated with Dilantin. Hallock was the first to describe the use of these animals in fetal cleft lip repair by demonstrating that cleft lip repair can be performed on gestational day 17 (term gestation = 19 days) animals.[29] Repairs were performed by freshening the cleft edges followed by a simple, straight-line closure using interrupted 10-0 sutures. Hallock reported complete epithelialization with minimal scar formation 24 to 48 hours after surgery. Subsequently, Sullivan, in an interesting and important experiment, demonstrated that simply approximating the cleft edges without de-epithelialization resulted in wound healing without evidence of grossly visible scar.[30] More recently, Oberg et al. reported the use of microclips for the repair of surgically created cleft lips in Swiss-Webster mice.[31] These authors noted excellent healing of surgically created cleft lip defects without evidence of excess collagen accumulation or inflammatory reaction in defects closed by clips. However, slight asymmetry of repaired lips with some evidence of epidermal deformation at the site of clip application was noted. Examination of a small number of animals born after in utero repair demonstrated excellent lip continuity with minimal lip asymmetry as compared with unrepaired animals. In addition, Oberg et al. reported a significant decrease in operating time with an average of 7 ± 2 seconds for animals treated with clips as compared with 90 ± 15 seconds in sutured animals. The reduction in surgical time is important because decreased fetal exposure time may lead to a decreased incidence of fetal demise. Finally, these findings were significant, since they demonstrated that microclips can be used successfully in fetal repair and set the stage for minimally invasive treatment of fetal cleft lip using an endoscopic approach.

Rabbit cleft lip and palate models have also been extensively described. These models provided an important alternative to mouse models because their larger size decreased the technical challenges of intrauterine surgery. Unlike the A/J mouse, however, spontaneous cleft formation has not been reported in rabbits, thus necessitating the creation of a surgical cleft and limiting their clinical relevance. Longaker et al. reported a rabbit model for fetal cleft lip repair by creating a 1-mm full-thickness excisional defect of the fetal lip and anterior maxillary alveolus midway between the midline and the labial commissure on the 24th day of gestation (term gestation = 32 days).[32] Repaired animals demonstrated an excellent survival rate (75%) and epithelial continuity without scar formation across the cleft lip in wounds analyzed at 4 and 7 days following repair. In contrast, unrepaired animals demonstrated minimal healing with open epithelialized clefts. In addition, repaired animals demonstrated decreased facial asymmetry as compared with unrepaired controls. When the animals were allowed to survive for 19 days postoperatively, the authors noted symmetric lips that healed without scarring and with only a small linear depression in the area of the cleft.

Stern et al. used the same surgically created cleft model to examine the histologic characteristics of fetal rabbit cleft lip repair.[33] These authors demonstrated that healing of both repaired and unrepaired cleft wounds occurred without scar formation and inflammatory cell infiltration. Interestingly, complete regeneration of muscle fibers across the wound was noted in repaired animals. These findings led the authors to hypothesize that the lack of scarring secondary to in utero repair may support normal maxillary growth postnatally.

Dodson et al. and Kaban et al. tested the hypothesis that scarless healing following the repair of surgically created cleft lip defects may support subsequent normal midface growth. They evaluated postnatal maxillary growth of repaired and unrepaired surgically created rabbit cleft lips.[34, 35] Interestingly, these authors demonstrated that although in utero repair of a cleft lip defect significantly decreased facial asymmetry, surgically created in utero fetal cleft lip with or without repair did not cause long-term postnatal maxillary growth disturbances. These findings led the authors to conclude that the lack of scarring and fibrosis in repaired and unrepaired surgical fetal cleft lip animals was not followed by the midface growth impairment noted in surgically

created defects in postnatal animal models of cleft lip repair.[36–40]

Ovine models of surgically created fetal cleft lip and palate repair have also been extensively described. Beck et al. described the surgical creation of a 4-mm × 2-cm intraoral defect extending from the second deciduous molar to an area approximately 2 cm posterior to the anterior pad of the palate between the midline and posterior alveolar crest on gestation day-120 lambs (term gestation = 145 days).[41] Defects were left unrepaired and animals were examined after 8, 16, and 24 weeks. In this study, histologic examination failed to demonstrate scarless repair of the defect. In addition, the authors noted a significant decrease in anterior and total posterior palatal width in animals that had a surgically created cleft when these measurements were compared with unoperated controls. Thus, this study did not support the findings of scarless fetal repair and normal postnatal palatal growth noted in smaller animal models. It is believed that these data were largely due to the late gestational age of the experimental animals used.

Longaker et al. evaluated fetal cleft lip repair in lambs, however, unlike Beck et al., fetal surgery was performed on gestational day 75.[42] In this study, a 3-mm-wide left paramedian section of the fetal lip and premaxilla was excised, thus creating a full-thickness oronasal fistula (Fig. 30–2). Control animals were left unrepaired, whereas experimental animals underwent a multilayer closure of the defect. Wounds were harvested 1, 2, and 3 weeks postoperatively, and at term for histologic analysis. After 1 week, the defect in the unrepaired fetuses was patent with incomplete reepithelialization. In contrast, wounds in animals that underwent intrauterine repair were grossly invisible except for a small indentation of the alveolus. In animals examined at 2 or 3 weeks postoperatively or at term, the defect in unrepaired animals was completely reepithelialized, but remained

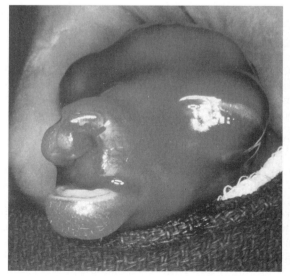

FIGURE 30–2. Photograph of excisional cleft lip wound created on a fetal lamb at 75 days' gestation.

widely patent. In addition, these animals demonstrated asymmetry of the maxilla. In contrast, repaired fetuses demonstrated nearly scarless healing of the lip and pre-maxilla defects (Fig. 30–3). Thus, this study in the lamb model demonstrated that scarless repair of a fetal lip is not limited to small animal models. These findings were supported by a more thorough experiment by Canady and colleagues examining the healing of surgically cre-ated cleft palates in fetal lambs ranging in age from gestational age 70 to 133 days.[43] Interestingly, scar for-mation in late-gestation fetal lamb cleft palate repair did *not* cause disturbances in midface growth in animals studied only 1 month after birth.[44]

Estes et al. expanded on the findings of the above studies by demonstrating the utility of endoscopic fetal surgery in a lamb model of surgically created cleft lip. This study for the first time provided a minimally invasive experimental approach for the treatment of nonlethal congenital malformations. The authors hy-pothesized that such minimally invasive operations may decrease the incidence of preterm labor and fetal and maternal complications.[45] The results indicated that en-doscopic techniques are possible in the repair of fetal cleft lip. However, it remains unknown whether such minimally invasive techniques are indeed safer for the mother and the unborn fetus when applied to fetal cleft lip repair.

In an effort to facilitate minimally invasive fetal surgi-cal procedures, the use of a microclip repair of surgically created cleft lip-like defects in lambs was explored by Evans et al.[46] The authors utilized fetal lambs at 124 days' gestation with an open or endoscopic approach and reported minimal scar formation at birth. In addi-tion, similar to the findings of Oberg et al. in mice, the authors reported a striking decrease in operative time with the use of microclips. Furthermore, microclip repair was not associated with the "modest" inflammatory response noted in lips repaired with Prolene sutures. The authors concluded that decreased operating time, in combination with ease of use and lack of inflammatory reaction associated with the use of microclips, makes the use of these devices ideal for endoscopic fetal sur-gery. They subsequently tested this hypothesis in a sur-gically created incisional model of endoscopic fetal lamb cleft lip repair.[47] Endoscopic operative procedures were performed on fetal lambs at 95 days' gestation using a harmonic scalpel and compared endoscopic clip place-ment with endoscopic suture repair. As expected, clip repairs were significantly faster (2.7 minutes) than su-ture repair (24 minutes). However, clip placement through the endoscope was reportedly more difficult than the open approach. Although the use of the har-monic scalpel in the creation of a lip defect was thought to minimize intraoperative hemorrhage, this device was also associated with increased scar formation and in one case reportedly resulted in a failed repair. Thus, this study provided further evidence that endoscopic proce-dures with microclip placement are feasible in large animal models.

A major criticism of the fetal lamb model of cleft lip and palate repair has been the surgical creation and immediate repair used in most experiments. Thus, it has been proposed that this model is not clinically relevant, since wound edges are not epithelialized at the time of the repair and the "cleft" is really a surgical lip wound. To address this shortcoming, Hedrick et al. described a lamb model in which delayed in utero repair of a surgi-cally created fetal cleft lip was performed.[48] In this study, a surgically created cleft lip was created on gestational days 58 through 62 using either a 2-mm excisional defect or an incisional defect using an amniotic bubble or "space helmet" technique (Fig. 30–4). Surgically created clefts were subsequently repaired on gestational days 73 through 75 (2 weeks after cleft creation). At the time of cleft lip repair, lambs with incisional defects demon-strated a significant degree of autorepair, and at harvest (6 weeks after cleft lip creation) both repaired and unre-paired incisional defect animals demonstrated scarless repair. In contrast, in the excisional group, no evidence of autorepair was noted at the time of the repair when epithelialized wound edges were freshened and closed primarily. At harvest, unrepaired excisional defect ani-mals demonstrated a widely patent cleft lip reminiscent of defects observed clinically. In contrast, repaired exci-sional defect animals demonstrated healing of the defect with minimal scar formation. Healing in these lambs was less than ideal, however, since the area of repair was thinned, lacked hair follicles and glandular ele-ments, and failed to demonstrate lip muscle regenera-tion. These deficiencies resulted in ipsilateral nostril widening and flaring. In addition, this study was further complicated by a relatively high fetal loss rate of approx-imately 40%, possibly due to the early gestational age of the first operative procedure. Thus, although this study represented an advance in the study of fetal cleft lip

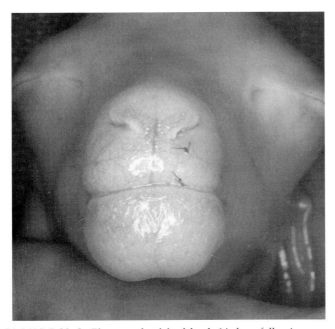

FIGURE 30–3. Photograph of fetal lamb 14 days following crea-tion and repair of left-sided cleft lip at 75 days' gestation. Note scarless repair and sutures in skin.

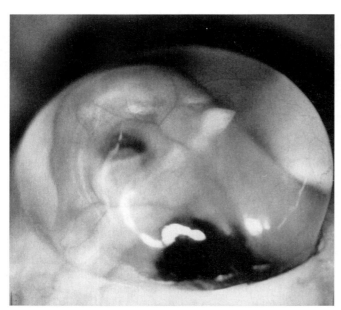

F I G U R E 30–4. Photograph of fetal lamb head and neck at 60 days' gestation inside an amniotic bubble or "space helmet."

repair, it highlighted the potential difficulties of these procedures in human fetal operations.

A large animal model in which spontaneous cleft lip and palate formation occurs would be ideal for the study of fetal repair. However, fetal repair of spontaneous clefts or clefts secondary to teratogen exposure (i.e., cyclophosphamide, phenytoin) has not been reported in fetal lambs. Recently, Weinzweig et al. described the effect of anabasine treatment on fetal goats.[49] Anabasine, a neuromuscular blocking agent with potent teratogenic effects, has been noted to cause cleft palate formation in goats, sheep, and swine.[50–52] This effect is thought to be due to an impairment of tongue motion resulting in the inhibition of palatal shelf closure. Weinzweig et al. reported a 100% incidence of cleft palate formation in anabasine-treated goat fetuses resulting in a phenotype that closely resembles human clinical cases. Preliminary results of fetal repair in this important model of nonsurgically created clefts suggests that in utero repair is feasible and results in healing without scar formation.[53] Furthermore, preliminary data also support that in utero repair results in palate mobility and velopharyngeal closure postnatally. Further work in this model will yield important data on the efficacy of in utero cleft palate repair.

Fetal Surgery for Lateral Facial Clefts

The potential advantages of fetal surgery (i.e., scarless repair and avoidance of secondary deformities) have also led to experimental work in the development of fetal models for other craniofacial disorders, including lateral facial clefts and craniosynostoses.

Lateral oblique facial clefts are a disfiguring group of rare malformations that occur with relatively low frequency.[54] Several hypotheses have been advanced to explain the etiopathogenesis of these rare clefts including abnormal mesodermal migration, disruption of neural crest cell development along normal fusion planes, and external restrictive forces such as amniotic bands.[55–57] Support for the latter hypothesis can be derived from fetal lamb studies in which Tessier No. 5 and 7 clefts were created in fetal lambs at 70 days' gestation when a nylon suture served as a constriction band.[58] In this study, 2-0 nylon sutures were placed circumferentially around the zygomatic arch and the infraorbital rim to the oral commissure in utero at 70 days' gestation (Fig. 30–5). At term, the authors noted macrostomia and partial bony cleft formation in the malar or zygomatic regions (Fig. 30–6). These studies demonstrated that lateral facial clefting can occur after the period of primary facial morphogenesis, and that external compression of developing facial structures (i.e., an amniotic band) may serve as an initiating event. The authors hypothesized that lateral facial clefting secondary to external compression in this model resulted from abnormal tissue migration due to direct tethering as well as cellular ischemia and necrosis secondary to external pressure from the suture band.

As a follow-up to these studies, Stelnicki et al. attempted an in utero repair of suture-induced Tessier No. 7 lateral clefts using the above model.[59] In this experiment, external compression was initiated as described above using a nylon suture on gestational day 70, followed by repair 2 weeks postoperatively by excising

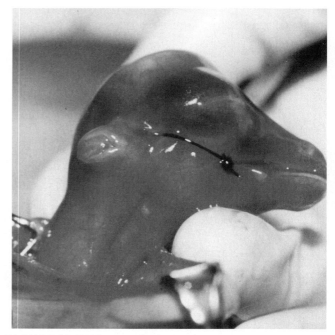

F I G U R E 30–5. Photograph of 2-0 nylon suture placed around the right zygomatic arch and oral commissure on a fetal lamb at 70 days' gestation.

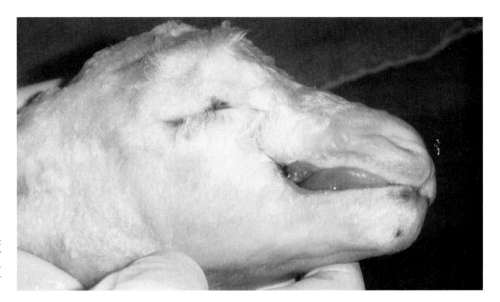

F I G U R E 30–6. Photograph of lamb at term with lateral facial cleft created by suture band placed at 70 days' gestation. Note macrostomia and decreased oculo-oral distance.

the constricting band and primarily approximating the epithelialized cleft edges. Control animals were left with the constricting band in place. All animals were sacrificed postnatally at 3 months of age and examined grossly, histologically, and anthropometrically. Interestingly, animals repaired in utero demonstrated symmetric faces without bony or soft tissue clefts (Fig. 30–7). Furthermore, no evidence of scar formation was noted histologically. In contrast, control (unrepaired) animals demonstrated a phenotype similar to what is seen clinically in Tessier No. 7 lateral facial clefts including macrostomia and soft and bony tissue clefting (Fig. 30–6). The authors concluded that lateral facial clefts may be treated successfully in utero and that early intervention

may prevent the potentially devastating facial asymmetry seen in these abnormalities. This conclusion is particularly important because current childhood reconstructions of these disorders often fail to restore facial symmetry.

Fetal Surgery for Craniosynostosis

Fetal surgery for the treatment of craniosynostosis has also been studied experimentally. Perhaps the most well-described animal model of congenital craniosynostosis is a strain of New Zealand white rabbits with an autosomal dominant mutation associated with coronal

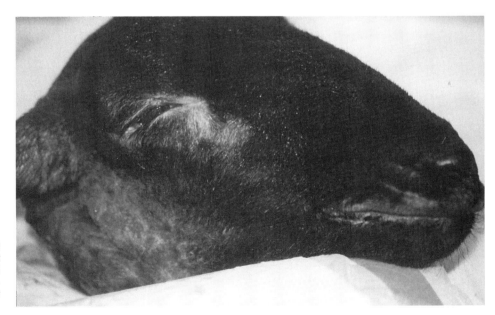

F I G U R E 30–7. Photograph of lamb at 3 months of age. This animal underwent in utero creation (70 days' gestation) and repair (14 days later) of lateral facial cleft. Note normal appearing oral commissure without macrostomia.

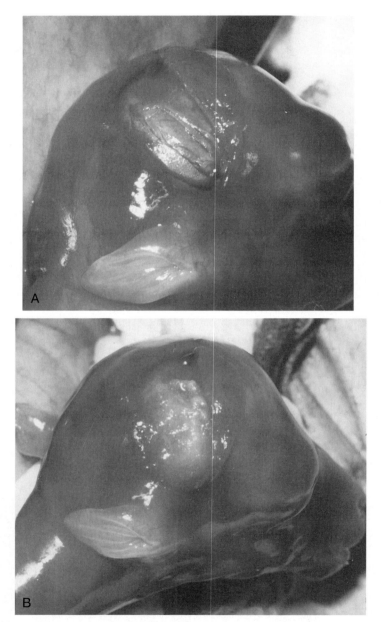

F I G U R E 30–8. Photograph of right side of fetal lamb head at 70 days' gestation during creation of right coronal synostosis. *A*, Right coronal suture excised. *B*, Cranial defect packed with demineralized bone matrix, bone morphogenetic protein-2, and transforming growth factor-β_1.

suture synostosis.[60–64] Approximately 30 to 40% of animals exhibit some degree of coronal suture craniosynostosis, and analysis of the pattern of inheritance suggests an autosomal dominant transmission with high penetrance and variable expressivity.[60–64] Due to the variable expression of this mutation, a range of phenotypes are observed experimentally, including partial, unilateral, and complete bilateral coronal suture synostoses. Recently, it has been reported that in its severe form (i.e., bilateral complete coronal suture synostosis), the mutation can be diagnosed ultrasonographically prior to birth (gestational day 25; term gestation = 31 to 32 days).[65] Thus, these studies have paved the way for potential in utero experimental manipulation of affected animals.[66] Such experiments have been hampered, however, by an unusually high fetal loss rate following in utero reconstruction.

Several surgically induced models of fetal craniosynostosis have also been reported.[67, 68] Duncan et al. reported a surgically induced fetal model of craniosynostosis by excising the coronal suture of New Zealand white rabbits at 25 days' gestation and filling the resultant bony gap with demineralized bone matrix (DBM).[67] Animals were studied 6, 10, 21, and 28 days postoperatively. The authors reported an in utero fetal demise rate of approximately 53%. Of the animals that survived vaginal delivery, both control and experimental animals demonstrated a high mortality rate, with evidence of central nervous system dysfunction and only 28% surviving long-term postoperatively. Histologic and gross examination of experimental animals revealed ablation of the coronal sutures 28 days postoperatively (i.e., 3 weeks after delivery). In contrast, operated controls (strip craniectomy without DBM implantation) had persistent defects in the area of the coronal suture. Although this model was successful in simulating a synostosed coronal suture, its utility was greatly diminished by the high mortality rate and the relatively late fetal stage of the primary operation. Thus, the relatively late gestational age of the primary operation essentially precluded subsequent in utero repair.

In order to address the shortcomings associated with the rabbit model cited above, Stelnicki et al. reported a fetal lamb model of coronal suture fusion.[68] In this model, the right coronal suture of 70-day-gestation fetal lambs was excised and packed with demineralized bone matrix (25 mg), bone morphogenetic protein-2 (50 μg) and transforming growth factor-β_1 (1 μg) (Fig. 30–8). Lambs were studied on gestational day 90 (20 days postoperatively) and at birth. On gestational day 90, experimental animals were noted to have completely obliterated coronal sutures. This obliteration led to significant flattening of the ipsilateral forehead, posterior and superior placement of the ipsilateral orbit, and deviation of the snout away from the side of the defect (Fig. 30–9). Interestingly, significant alterations in the cranial base of experimental animals, including rotation toward the side of the defect and flattening of the anterior and middle cranial fossas, were also noted. Furthermore, unlike the surgically induced fetal rabbit model, the fetal lamb model had acceptable operative morbidity and mortality.

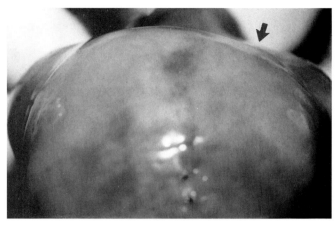

FIGURE 30–9. Superior-posterior photograph of fetal lamb with synostosed right coronal suture at 90 days. Note flattening of right side of forehead (*arrow*).

In utero repair of coronal synostosis in the fetal lamb model has been recently reported.[69] In this study, the right coronal suture was induced to undergo fusion using the same methods described previously on gestational day 70. Twenty-one days postoperatively (gestational day 91) the fetal lambs were reoperated, the synostosed right coronal suture was resected, and the edges of the excision were wrapped with Gore-Tex sheets to prevent reossification (Fig. 30–10). Control animals were left untreated and all animals were sacrificed at term. All in utero treated animals demonstrated widely patent strip craniectomy sites without evidence of bone formation. In addition, animals reconstructed in utero demonstrated a marked improvement in craniofacial morphology with correction of dysmorphic orbital position, skull height, and frontal bone shape (Fig. 30–11). In contrast, untreated controls (i.e., unrepaired coronal synostosis) demonstrated ipsilateral marked orbital elevation, vertical expansion of the cranial vault, and ipsilateral frontal bone flattening (Fig. 30–12). Thus, in utero correction of craniosynostosis, in this model, resulted in a marked improvement in craniofacial morphology, leading the authors to conclude that fetal surgery may in the future hold promise in the treatment of selected cases of severe cranial suture fusion. This conclusion requires evaluation in a nonsurgical or endogenous model of craniosynostosis, however, since it is unclear if similar results would be obtained in genetically abnormal animals.

Conclusions

The unique ability of early gestation fetal animals to heal without scar formation makes fetal surgery for craniofacial anomalies appealing. As progress is made in the treatment of preterm labor, the indications for fetal surgery may expand to include craniofacial anomalies such as cleft lip/palate, lateral facial clefts, and severe craniosynostoses.

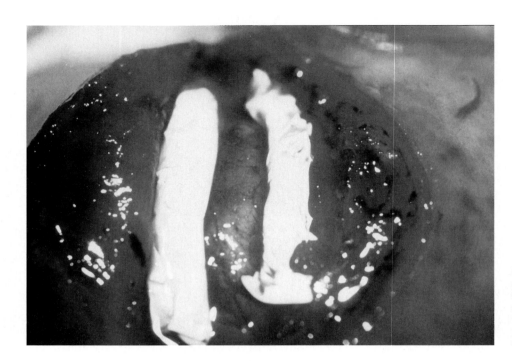

F I G U R E 30–10. Up-close photograph of fetal lamb cranium at 90 days' gestation. The right coronal suture has been resected and the bony edges have been wrapped with Gore-Tex. This animal had previously undergone creation of right coronal suture fusion at 70 days of age.

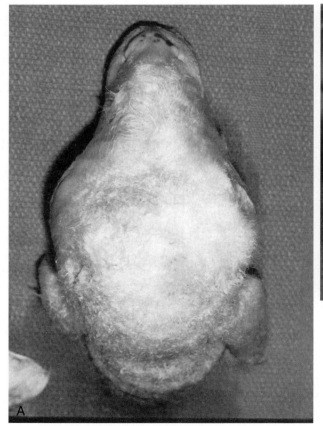

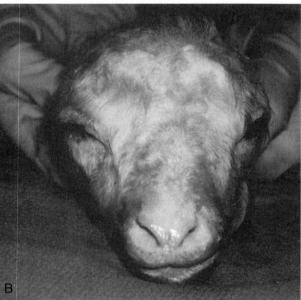

F I G U R E 30–11. Photographs of term lamb that underwent creation (70 days' gestation) and reconstruction (91 days' gestation) of right coronal suture fusion. *A,* Superior view. Note improved symmetry in forehead, orbits, and cranium. *B,* Frontal view. Note symmetry in forehead and orbits.

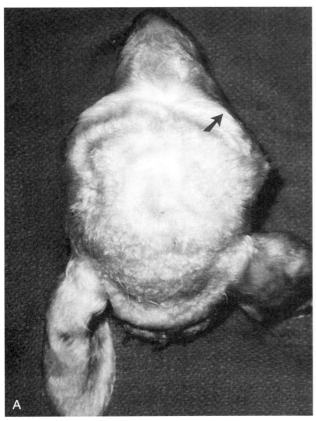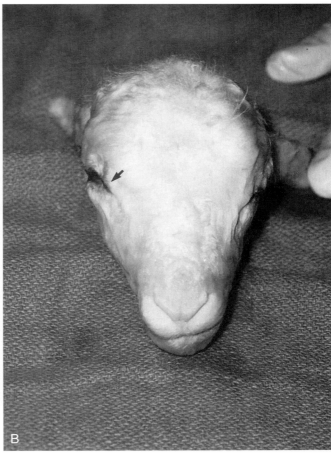

FIGURE 30–12. Photographs of term lamb with right coronal suture fusion created at 70 days' gestation. *A,* Superior-posterior view. Note flattening right side of forehead (*arrow*). *B,* Superior-frontal view. Note cranial asymmetry and posterior and superior displacement of right eye (*arrow*).

REFERENCES

1. Longaker MT, Adzick NS: The biology of fetal wound healing: A review. Plast Reconstr Surg 87:788–798, 1991.
2. Ferguson MWJ, Whitby DJ, Shah M, et al: Scar formation: The spectral nature of fetal wound repair. Plast Reconstr Surg 97:854–860, 1996.
3. Olutoye OO, Cohen IK: Fetal wound healing: An overview. Wound Rep Reg 4:66–74, 1996.
4. Longaker MT, Whitby DJ, Ferguson MWJ, et al: Adult skin wounds in the fetal environment heal with scar formation. Ann Surg 219:65–72, 1994.
5. Lorenz HP, Longaker MT, Perkocha LA, et al: Scarless wound repair; a human fetal skin model. Development 114:253–259, 1992.
6. Adzick NS, Longaker MT: Animal models for the study of fetal tissue repair. J Surg Res 51:216–222, 1991.
7. Somasundarm K, Prathap K: Intra-uterine healing of skin wounds in rabbit foetuses. J Pathol 100:81–86, 1970.
8. Somasundaram K, Prathap K: The effect of exclusion of amniotic fluid on intrauterine healing of skin wounds in rabbit foetuses. J Pathol 107:127–130, 1992.
9. Longaker MT, Burd DAR, Gown AM, et al: Midgestation fetal lamb excisional wounds contract in utero. J Pediatr Surg 26:942–948, 1991.
10. Rittenberg T, Longaker MT, Adzick NS, et al: Sheep amniotic fluid has a protein factor which stimulates human fibroblast populated collagen lattice contraction. J Cell Physiol 149:444–450, 1991.
11. Martin P, Lewis J: Actin cables and epidermal movement in embryonic wound healing. Nature 360:179–182, 1992.
12. Harrison MR, Adzick NS: The fetus as a patient: Surgical considerations. Ann Surg 213:279, 1991.
13. Harrison MR, Adzick NS, Flake AW: Congenital diaphragmatic hernia: An unsolved problem. Semin Pediatr Surg 2:109–112, 1993.
14. Harrison MR, Adzick NS, Flake AW, et al: Correction of congenital diaphragmatic hernia in utero VIII: Response of the hypoplastic lung to tracheal occlusion. J Pediatr Surg 31:1339, 1996.
15. Harrison MR: Personal communication, 1998.
16. Longaker MT, Whitby DJ, Jennings RW, et al: Fetal diaphragmatic wounds heal with scar formation. J Surg Res 50:375–385, 1991.
17. Meuli M, Lorenz HP, Hedrick MH, et al: Scar formation in the fetal alimentary tract. J Pediatr Surg 30:392–395, 1995.
18. Mast BA, Albanese CT, Kapadia S: Tissue repair in the fetal intestinal tract occurs with adhesions, fibrosis and neovascularization. Ann Plast Surg 41:140–144, 1998.
19. Longaker MT, Moelleken BRW, Cheng JC, et al: Fetal fracture healing in a lamb model. Plast Reconstr Surg 90:161–171, 1992.
20. Longaker MT, Whitby DJ, Adzick NS, et al: Fetal surgery for cleft lip: A plea for caution. Plast Reconstr Surg 88:1087–1093, 1991.
21. Lopoo J, Hedrick MH, Chasen S, et al: Natural history of fetuses with cleft lip. Plast Reconstr Surg 103:34–38, 1999.
22. Lane AT: Human fetal skin development. Pediatr Dermatol 3:487, 1986.
23. Longaker MT, Whitby DJ, Adzick NS, et al: Studies in fetal wound healing: VI. Second and early third trimester fetal wounds demonstrate rapid collagen disposition without scar formation. J Pediatr Surg 25:63–69, 1990.
24. Lorenz HP, Whitby DJ, Longaker MT, et al: Fetal wound healing. The ontogeny of scar formation in the non-human primate. Ann Surg 217:391–396, 1993.
25. Ihara S, Motobayashi Y, Nagao E, Kistler A: Ontogenetic transition of wound healing pattern in rat skin occurring at the fetal stage. Development 110:671–680, 1990.

26. Armstrong JR, Ferguson MWJ: Ontogeny of the skin and transition from scar-free to scarring phenotype during wound healing in the pouch young of a marsupial, *Mondoelphis domestica*. Dev Biol 169:242–260, 1995.

27. Cass DL, Bullard KM, Sylvester KG, et al: Wound size and gestational age modulate scar formation in fetal wound repair. J Pediatr Surg 32:411–415, 1997.

28. Horne RS, Hurley JV, Crowe DM, et al: Wound healing in the fetal sheep: A histological and electron microscope study. Br J Plast Surg 45:333–344, 1992.

29. Hallock GG: In utero cleft lip repair in A/J mice. Plast Reconstr Surg 75:785–790, 1985.

30. Sullivan WG: In utero cleft lip repair in the mouse without an incision. Plast Reconstr Surg 84:723–730, 1989.

31. Oberg KC, Evans ML, Nguyen T, et al: Intrauterine repair of surgically created defects in mice (lip incision model) with a microclip; preamble to endoscopic intrauterine surgery. Cleft Palate Craniofac J 32:129–137, 1995.

32. Longaker MT, Dodson TB, Kaban LB: A rabbit model for fetal cleft lip repair. J Oral Maxillofac Surg 48:714–719, 1990.

33. Stern M, Dodson TB, Longaker MT, et al: Fetal cleft lip repair in lambs: Histologic characteristics of the healing wound. Int J Oral Maxillofac Surg 22:371–374, 1993.

34. Dodson TB, Schmidt B, Longaker MT, Kaban LB: Fetal cleft lip repair in rabbits: Postnatal facial growth after repair. J Oral Maxillofac Surg 49:603–611, 1991.

35. Kaban LB, Dodson TB, Longaker MT, et al: Fetal cleft lip repair in rabbits: Long-term clinical and cephalometric results. Cleft Palate Craniofac J 30:13–21, 1993.

36. Bardach J, Eisbach K: The influence of primary unilateral cleft lip repair on facial growth. Part 1. Lip pressure. Cleft Palate J 14:88–97, 1977.

37. Bardach J, Klausner E, Eisbach K: The relationship between lip pressure and facial growth after cleft lip repair: An experimental model. Cleft Palate J 16:137–146, 1997.

38. Bardach J, Mooney M, Bardach E: The influence of two-flap palatoplasty on facial growth in beagles. Plast Reconstr Surg 69:927–936, 1982.

39. Bardach J, Mooney M, Giedrojc-Juraha Z: A comparative study of facial growth following cleft lip repair with or without soft-tissue undermining: An experimental model study in rabbits. Plast Reconstr Surg 69:745–753, 1982.

40. Bardach J, Mooney M: The relationship between lip pressure following lip repair and craniofacial growth: An experimental study in beagles. Plast Reconstr Surg 73:544–555, 1984.

41. Beck G, Bruce R, Fonseca R: The effect of antenatal surgery on postnatal palatal growth in sheep. J Oral Maxillofac Surg 46:217–223, 1988.

42. Longaker MT, Stern M, Lorenz HP, et al: A model for fetal cleft lip repair in lambs. Plast Reconstr Surg 90:750–756, 1993.

43. Canady JW, Landas SK, Morris H, Thompson SA: In utero cleft palate repair in the ovine model. Cleft Palate Craniofac J 31:37–44, 1994.

44. Canady JW, Thompson SA, Colburn A: Craniofacial growth after iatrogenic cleft palate repair in a fetal ovine model. Cleft Palate Craniofac J 34:69–72, 1997.

45. Estes JM, Whitby DJ, Lorenz HP, et al: Endoscopic creation and repair of fetal cleft lip. Plast Reconstr Surg 90:743–749, 1992.

46. Evans ML, Oberg KC, Kirsch W, et al: Intrauterine repair of cleft lip-like defects in lambs with a novel microclip. J Craniofac Surg 6:126–131, 1995.

47. Oberg K, Robles A, Ducsay C, et al: Endoscopic excision and repair of simulated bilateral cleft lips in fetal lambs. Plast Reconstr Surg 102:1–9, 1998.

48. Hedrick MH, Rice HE, Vander Wall KJ, et al: Delayed in utero repair of surgically created fetal cleft lip and palate. Plast Reconstr Surg 97:900–905, 1996.

49. Weinzweig J, Sullivan P, Panter K, et al: The fetal cleft palate: *In utero* repair of a true congenital model. Plast Surg Forum 20:25–27, 1997.

50. Keeler RF, Crowe MW: Teratogenicity and toxicity of wild tree tobacco, Nicotiana glauca in sheep. Cornell Vet 74:50–59, 1994.

51. Keeler RF, Crowe MW, Lambert EA: Teratogenicity in swine of the tobacco alkaloid anabasine isolated from Nicotiana glauca. Teratology 30:61–69.51, 1984.

52. Panter KE, Keeler RF, Bunch TD, Callan RJ: Congenital skeletal malformations and cleft palate induced in goats by ingestion of Lupinus, Conium and Nicotiana species. Toxicon 28:1377–1385, 1990.

53. Weinzweig J, Panter K, Pantaloni M, et al: The fetal cleft palate: A histomorphologic study of palatal development and function following in utero repair of a congenital model. Plast Surg Forum 21:27–29, 1998.

54. Longaker MT, Lipshutz GS, Kawamoto HK: Reconstruction of Tessier No. 4 clefts revisited. Plast Reconstr Surg 99:1501–1507, 1997.

55. Pitanguy I: Facial Clefts As Seen in a Large Series of Untreated Adults and their Later Management. London: Pitman, 1968.

56. Popescu V: Congenital transverse facial clefts. Stomatologia 15:75, 1968.

57. Johnson M: Morphogenesis and malformation of the face and brain. Birth Defects 11:1, 1975.

58. Stelnicki EJ, Hoffman WY, Vanderwall K, et al: A new in utero model for lateral facial clefts. J Craniofac Surg 8:460–465, 1997.

59. Stelnicki E, Hoffman W, Foster R, Longaker MT: The in utero repair of Tessier 7 lateral facial clefts created by amniotic band-like compression. J Craniofac Surg 9:557–562, 1998.

60. Mooney MP, Aston CE, Siegel MI, et al: Craniosynostosis with autosomal dominant transmission in New Zealand white rabbits. J Craniofac Genet Dev Biol 16:52–63, 1996.

61. Mooney MP, Losken HW, Siegel MI, et al: Development of a strain of rabbits with congenital simple nonsyndromic coronal suture synostosis. Part II: Somatic and craniofacial growth patterns. Cleft Palate Craniofac J 31:8–16, 1994.

62. Mooney MP, Losken HW, Siegel MI, et al: Development of a strain of rabbits with congenital simple nonsyndromic coronal suture synostosis. Part I: Breeding demographics, inheritance pattern, and craniofacial anomalies. Cleft Palate Craniofac J 31:1–7, 1994.

63. Mooney MP, Losken HW, Tschakaloff A, et al: Congenital bilateral coronal suture synostosis in a rabbit and craniofacial growth comparisons with experimental models. Cleft Palate Craniofac J 30:121–128, 1993.

64. Mooney MP, Smith TD, Burrows AM, et al: Coronal suture pathology and synostotic progression in rabbits with congenital craniosynostosis. Cleft Palate Craniofac J 33:369–378, 1996.

65. Stelnicki EJ, Mooney MP, Losken HW, et al: Ultrasonic prenatal diagnosis of coronal suture synostosis. J Craniofac Surg 8:252–258, 1997.

66. Longaker MT: Commentary on ultrasonic prenatal diagnosis of coronal suture synostosis. J Craniofac Surg 8:259–260, 1997.

67. Duncan BW, Adzick NS, Moelleken BR, et al: An in utero model of craniosynostosis. J Craniofac Surg 3:70–78, 1992.

68. Stelnicki EJ, Vanderwall K, Hoffman WY, et al: A new in utero sheep model for unilateral coronal craniosynostosis. Plast Reconstr Surg 101:278–286, 1998.

69. Stelnicki EJ, Vanderwall K, Harrison MR, et al: The in utero correction of unilateral coronal craniosynostosis. Plast Reconstr Surg 101:287–296, 1998.

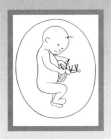

CHAPTER 31

The Fetus with an Abdominal Wall Defect

JACOB C. LANGER

Abdominal wall defects encompass a number of related but distinct anomalies. These include omphalocele, gastroschisis, and exstrophy. These conditions are common enough to be seen in most prenatal diagnosis units at least occasionally. They are usually detectable during a detailed sonographic examination, and therefore the sensitivity of ultrasound is extremely high. In addition, ultrasound is usually accurate in differentiating one abdominal wall defect from another (Table 31–1). There is a wide range of prognosis in fetuses with abdominal wall defects, depending on the type of defect, severity of organ injury, and the presence and severity of associated chromosomal and structural anomalies.[1, 2] A detailed understanding of the natural history of these conditions is imperative in order to appropriately counsel affected families.[3]

As with many other types of congenital anomaly, prenatal diagnosis of an abdominal wall defect creates a potential opportunity to influence neonatal outcome through changes in the management of the pregnancy or delivery, and by prenatal education and counseling of the family. Decisions should be made by a team consisting of obstetric, surgical, and pediatric specialists, in consultation with the family.[4] The optimal management of an individual fetus depends on careful prenatal assessment of the defect and knowledge of the natural history and expected outcome for that particular lesion.

The Fetus with Omphalocele

During normal development, the intestine and liver grow rapidly around the eighth menstrual week (sixth week after conception). Since the abdominal cavity cannot accommodate this growth, the viscera migrate into the umbilical cord, and then move back around the 12th menstrual week.[5] Omphalocele (also called exomphalos) is caused by failure of the viscera to return to the abdominal cavity. Infants with omphalocele have a membranous sac covering the herniated viscera, which consists of Wharton's jelly. The abdominal wall defect may range from very large to very small (Fig. 31–1). The intestines and liver remain morphologically and functionally normal.[6, 7] Because bowel within the umbilical cord is a normal phenomenon between 8 and 12 menstrual weeks, omphalocele cannot be reliably identified earlier than approximately 10 weeks.

Associated structural malformations are common in infants with omphalocele, with an incidence ranging from 37 to 81%.[8–12] Examples include cardiac, renal, limb, and facial anomalies,[11, 13, 14] as well as syndromes such as Beckwith-Wiedemann, pentalogy of Cantrell (omphalocele, ectopia cordis, Morgagni diaphragmatic hernia, cardiac anomalies, and sternal/pericardial defects), and OEIS (*o*mphalocele, *e*xstrophy, *i*mperforate anus, and *s*pinal anomalies). Chromosomal anomalies are also commonly associated with omphalocele; this is particularly true of small omphaloceles that do not contain liver.[15, 16]

Prognosis for the child with omphalocele is related to the presence of associated chromosomal and structural anomalies[9, 17–20] and the size of the defect.[6, 21] It is therefore important to obtain as much information as possible using karyotype analysis and high-level sonography.[22] If life-threatening abnormalities are detected, and the fetus is still previable, pregnancy termination can be offered. In all cases, prenatal diagnosis permits education and counseling for the family, and their involvement in this difficult decision-making process.

If the pregnancy is carried to term, a decision must be made regarding route of delivery. Fetuses with a small omphalocele can be delivered vaginally without undue risk. Many obstetricians perform cesarean delivery for infants with a large omphalocele, to minimize the risk of damage to the sac and liver.[23, 24] This approach has never been subjected to a prospective or randomized study, but routine cesarean delivery is not supported by most of the published retrospective literature.[17, 20, 25–31]

All infants with omphalocele should be delivered at a perinatal center, so that neonatal and surgical expertise are immediately available. This permits early diagnosis and management of previously unrecognized anomalies, as well as evaluation and appropriate surgical treatment of the abdominal wall defect. In addition, some infants with large omphaloceles have significant respira-

TABLE 31–1. DIFFERENTIATING FEATURES BETWEEN TYPES OF ABDOMINAL WALL DEFECT

	OMPHALOCELE	GASTROSCHISIS	EXSTROPHY
Sac	Present	Absent	Sometimes early
Associated anomalies	Common	Uncommon	Common
Location of defect	Umbilicus	Right of umbilicus	Below umbilicus
Maternal age	Average	Younger	Average
Pubic symphysis	Normal	Normal	Diastasis
Bladder	Normal	Normal	Not seen

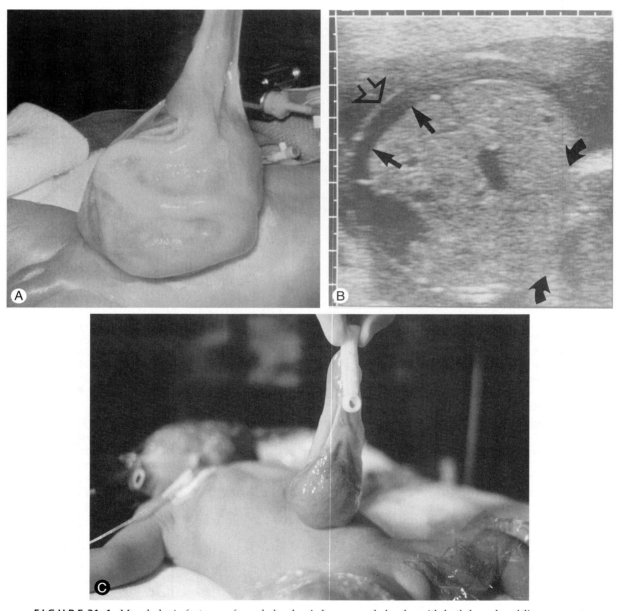

FIGURE 31–1. Morphologic features of omphalocele. *A,* Large omphalocele, with both bowel and liver present within the sac. The umbilical vessels travel over the surface of the sac. *B,* Sonogram of a large omphalocele, demonstrating liver and bowel within the sac. The abdominal wall defect is shown by the *curved arrows,* and ascites is also present. *C,* Small omphalocele, containing only bowel.

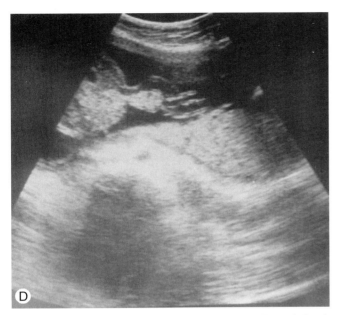

FIGURE 31–1 *Continued. D,* Sonogram of a small omphalocele. Absence of liver in the sac implies a higher risk of chromosomal anomalies.

tory insufficiency, which may require urgent intubation and ventilation at the time of birth.[32]

The Fetus with Gastroschisis

Gastroschisis is characterized by an abdominal wall defect that is lateral to the umbilicus, almost always on the right side. The embryology of gastroschisis is unknown, but the prevaling theory suggests that it is caused by abdominal wall ischemia due to involution of the vitelline artery[33] or the right umbilical vein.[34] Other possibilities include interruption of mesenchymal somatic migration during abdominal wall development,[35] and rupture of a previous omphalocele.[36] Epidemiologic studies have shown that mothers of infants with gastroschisis tend to be young,[37] and may have been more likely to use vasoactive drugs such as decongestants.[38] The etiologic implications of these observations are unclear. Occasionally gastroschisis may occur as a result of amniotic band syndrome,[39] where the defect is presumably due to mechanical disruption of the abdominal wall by the amniotic band.

The diagnosis of gastroschisis has been made sonographically as early as 12 menstrual weeks using a transvaginal probe.[40] In contrast to omphalocele, the bowel in infants with gastroschisis is exposed to amniotic fluid during fetal life. At delivery, the bowel may exhibit shortening, thickening, and the development of a thick fibrous peel (Fig. 31–2). Because the intestine is exposed, the maternal level of α-fetoprotein (AFP) is usually elevated.[41] In areas where screening for maternal AFP is routine, the vast majority of cases are identified prenatally.

Intestinal atresia is seen in approximately 10% of infants with gastroschisis, but it is unclear whether this represents a common vascular etiology of the two lesions[33] or is the result of intestinal ischemia secondary to constriction at the abdominal wall.[42] Atresia is often suspected in cases where there is dilatation of the small bowel or polyhydramnios early in gestation, particularly if the dilatation is intra-abdominal.

Prognosis for the infant with gastroschisis is primarily determined by the condition of the exteriorized bowel at the time of delivery.[19, 21, 43, 44] These infants almost universally experience problems with absorptive function and prolonged hypomotility.[45–47] Prenatal diagnosis theoretically could provide an opportunity for intervention designed to minimize the damage that leads to these problems. However, the etiology of intestinal damage in gastroschisis remains unclear.

Etiology of Intestinal Damage: Analysis of Human Tissue

Histologic evaluation of tissue from human fetuses and newborns with gastroschisis has been difficult, since the only indication for neonatal resection is severe ischemic bowel damage. Tibboel and co-workers found no histologic evidence of enteric nervous system abnormalities in either prenatal or postnatal specimens,[48] and they noted that the fibrous peel appeared at approximately 30 weeks' gestation.[49] Ischemic changes were not seen in any of the fetuses studied, but were seen in postnatal cases suffering from hypoperistalsis, suggesting that bowel constriction at the abdominal wall defect caused damage through an ischemic mechanism late in gestation.[48] In a similar study, Amoury and associates characterized the peel as consisting of type I collagen and fibrin, and noted that it dissolves after repair postnatally.[50] In addition, the lack of ischemic changes (except in specimens with atresia), or abnormalities in ganglion cell appearance led these authors to conclude that the motility disorder is entirely attributable to the peel.

In order to further define the etiology of intestinal damage in gastroschisis, a number of investigators have developed experimental models in the chick embryo, the fetal rabbit, and the fetal lamb. Using these models, two etiologic hypotheses have been tested: (1) damage is due to contact between the bowel and the amniotic fluid, and (2) damage is due to constriction of the bowel at the abdominal wall defect.

Etiology of Intestinal Damage: Amniotic Fluid Exposure

In the chick embryo, bowel exposed to allantoic contents becomes thickened, edematous, and covered with a fibrous peel, whereas bowel bathed in amniotic fluid alone is normal, suggesting that bowel damage is most likely caused by urine in the amniotic fluid.[51] This is supported by a more recent study using a similar model, in which amnioallantoic fluid exchange prevented bowel damage.[52]

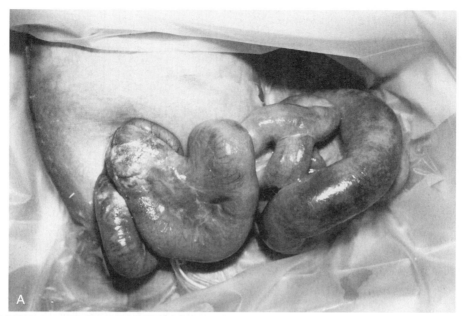

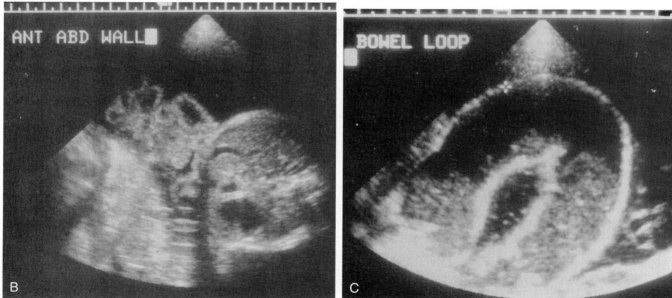

F I G U R E 31–2. Morphologic features of gastroschisis. *A,* The bowel is matted, thickened, and covered by a fibrous peel. *B,* Ultrasound early in gestation shows exteriorized bowel loops that are decompressed and thin walled. *C,* Ultrasound late in gestation demonstrates a dilated, thickened bowel loop containing echogenic material.

Further evidence for the role of amniotic fluid in the etiology of intestinal damage comes from the rabbit and sheep models, in which defects in mucosal absorption of proline and glucose[53] and decreases in mucosal enzyme function[54] and gene expression[55] have been documented. Other studies have demonstrated increased collagen production[56] and decreased smooth muscle function[57] in response to amniotic fluid exposure. Finally, bowel damage does not occur in a rabbit model of gastroschisis in which the lower half of the fetus is placed in an extrauterine position, thus avoiding contact with amniotic fluid.[58]

Etiology of Intestinal Damage: Constriction at the Abdominal Wall Defect

Evidence that amniotic fluid exposure is not the only factor affecting bowel damage comes from several sources. In an early study in fetal rabbits,[59] injection of amniotic fluid into the peritoneal cavity, without creation of an abdominal wall defect, did not result in any bowel abnormalities. A recent case reported bowel typical of gastroschisis inside an intact omphalocele sac.[60] Using the fetal lamb model, we sought to define the roles of amniotic fluid exposure and constriction at the abdominal wall defect.[57] In a series of experiments, we found that the peel was primarily caused by amniotic fluid exposure, and the bowel wall thickening and dilatation were due to constriction at the abdominal wall defect. Decreased smooth muscle contractility was due to both factors, acting in an additive fashion. In further studies we determined that the mechanism of constriction-induced bowel damage was through mechanical obstruction,[61] rather than ischemia.[62] The latter finding is supported by a recent clinical study in which there was no evidence of intestinal ischemia in fetuses with gastroschisis using Doppler velocimetry.[63]

Timing of Intestinal Damage

Early work in the lamb model suggested that the bowel damage increased in severity with time of exposure to amniotic fluid.[64] Subsequent studies specifically examining this issue found that both histologic and contractility changes were most severe toward the end of gestation.[54] Simulated "repair" of the abdominal wall defect was able to partially reverse these changes (Fig. 31–3). These data suggested that there was no role for fetal repair of gastroschisis, but that there may be some rationale for preterm delivery in fetuses at high risk for ongoing intestinal damage. Recently, some investigators have suggested that prenatal amniotic fluid exchange late during gestation, to minimize exposure of the bowel to amniotic fluid, may prevent intestinal damage in these fetuses.[65]

Identification of the High-Risk Fetus

Since most of the bowel damage in fetuses with gastroschisis occurs late in pregnancy, and is associated with bowel dilatation and thickening in animal models, there is a theoretical rationale for preterm delivery for fetuses with ongoing bowel dilatation and thickening. An early clinical study found an increased incidence of intestinal necrosis and atresia and a longer period of hypoperistalsis in fetuses who were found subjectively to have dilatation and thickening of the bowel wall.[66] However, other authors found these characteristics to be unreliable.[67–69] Several subsequent studies have attempted to develop objective sonographic parameters that could be used to predict outcome, and have suggested that bowel diameter may be predictive of outcome.[63, 70, 71] Various thresholds have been suggested, ranging in diameter from 10 to 18 mm. We found that bowel diameter was particularly useful when plotted against gestational age (Fig. 31–4), and Abuhamad and associates found that a diameter of 10 mm between 28 and 32 weeks' gestation was highly predictive of outcome.[63] In addition, the presence of dilated intra-abdominal bowel loops associated with polyhydramnios has been reported to be associated with short bowel syndrome in several fetuses with gastroschisis.[72]

Options for Management In Utero

Accurate prenatal diagnosis may provide an opportunity to prevent intestinal damage by altering either the mode or timing of delivery. Thus far, no studies have clearly demonstrated an advantage to routine cesarean delivery for gastroschisis.[17, 20, 25–31, 71, 73–76] Some authors have suggested that elective delivery by cesarean section may prevent ongoing damage and result in improved outcome, but it is likely the timing rather than the mode of delivery[77–81] or the need for postnatal transport of the infant[82] that has affected outcome in these series. There is inadequate evidence, however, that preterm delivery actually improves outcome, and it remains clear that

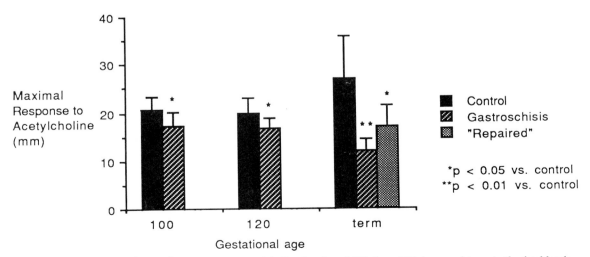

FIGURE 31–3. Smooth muscle response to acetylcholine in vitro at 100 days, 120 days, and term in the fetal lamb model. In an additional group, the defect was "repaired" at 120 days by removing the constrictor and placing a Silastic pouch over the bowel to protect it from amniotic fluid. These studies demonstrated that most of the intestinal damage occurred late in gestation, and that "repair" at 120 days ameliorated, but did not completely prevent, the damage.

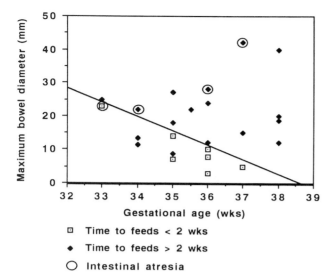

☐ Time to feeds < 2 wks

◆ Time to feeds > 2 wks

◯ Intestinal atresia

FIGURE 31-4. Effect of gestational age and maximal bowel diameter on intestinal motility in 24 fetuses with gastroschisis. A "threshold" line has been drawn, above which all infants had prolonged hypoperistalsis, and below which only 30% of infants had prolonged hypoperistalsis. The four fetuses with intestinal atresia are also shown.

the risks of prematurity must always be weighed against the potential advantages of preterm delivery for these infants.[70]

The use of amnioinfusion or amniotic fluid exchange to prevent bowel damage is supported by the experimental work of Aktug in fetal rabbits.[52] In a preliminary case report, the same authors have documented a decrease in intestinal damage using this technique at 29 weeks' gestation.[65] Further studies are necessary to con-

firm these results and to ensure the safety of this technique.

Finally, there is some evidence that at least part of the intestinal damage in infants with gastroschisis may occur early postnatally, since immediate repair of the defect in the delivery room has been associated with improved outcome in a retrospective noncontrolled study.[83] Our preliminary experience with immediate placement of a spring-loaded silo soon after birth has also resulted in excellent outcomes.[84] Prospective controlled studies are needed to further define the role of fetal ultrasound in the decision-making process during the management of these fetuses.

The Fetus with Bladder or Cloacal Exstrophy

Bladder and cloacal exstrophy are rare anomalies that occur as a result of failed closure of the anterior abdominal wall at the ventral end of the cloacal membrane. The precise embryology of these anomalies is unclear, but experimental studies suggest failure of the primitive streak mesoderm to invade the allantoic extension of the cloacal membrane around 4 weeks after conception.[85] Bladder exstrophy involves the bladder, urethra, penis, and pubic ramus (Fig. 31–5), but is often associated with other genitourinary anomalies.[86] Cloacal exstrophy is a more complex anomaly (Fig. 31–6), which is accompanied by omphalocele, imperforate anus, diastasis of the pubis, and absent or diminutive genitalia. A neural tube defect is present in 50% of infants and congenital short bowel syndrome in 20%.[87] Although surgical recon-

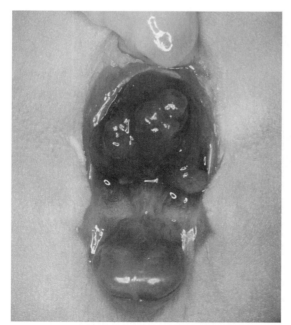

FIGURE 31-5. Bladder exstrophy. The bladder is open, the pubic rami are widely separated, there is no urethra, and the penis is diminutive. (Courtesy of Dr. D. Coplen.)

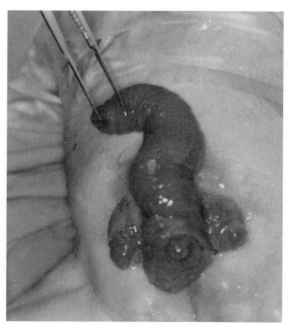

FIGURE 31-6. Cloacal exstrophy. There is a central bowel plate consisting of the exstrophied cecum, with one or two appendiceal orifices. There is a prolapsed ileum at the top and a diminutive hindgut at the bottom that ends blindly in the pelvis. There is a bladder plate on either side, each with a ureteral orifice. Also note the wide separation of the pubis, ambiguous genitalia, and a small omphalocele.

struction can be accomplished in most cases of bladder and cloacal exstrophy, many children have long-term problems with urinary continence. Most authors advocate sex reassignment in male infants with cloacal exstrophy.[88]

Bladder exstrophy may be recognized sonographically due to absence of the bladder, as well as recognition of associated genitourinary anomalies.[90–91] Cloacal exstrophy has been identified because of associated neural tube defects, omphalocele, or splaying of the pubis rami.[91–94] Several cases of fetal cloacal exstrophy have been described in which the cloacal membrane persisted until the second trimester, and there was sonographic evidence of a large cystic mass in the lower abdomen.[95, 96] The membrane subsequently ruptured, resulting in the typical findings of cloacal exstrophy at birth (Fig. 31–7).

Prenatal diagnosis of bladder or cloacal exstrophy should lead to a careful search for associated chromosomal and structural anomalies. Parental counseling by a multidisciplinary team is mandatory, particularly addressing the issues of continence and possible sex reassignment. There is no evidence to support routine cesarean section in these cases, but it is preferable for delivery to occur at a perinatal center where appropriate neonatal and surgical expertise are available.

Summary

Our approach to the perinatal management of the fetus with an abdominal wall defect is summarized in Figure 31–8. The first issue is to determine the type of abdominal wall defect. The presence of a sac, the location of

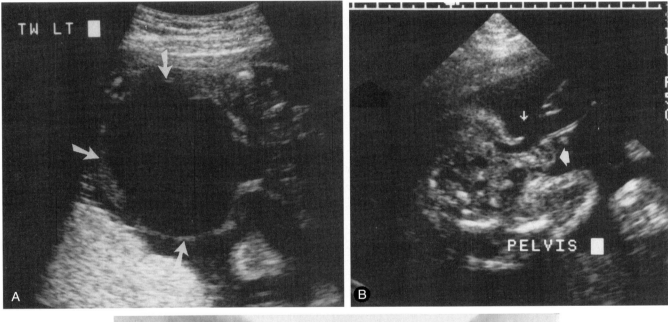

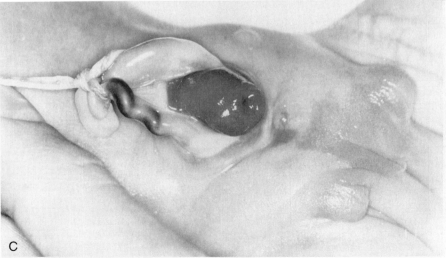

FIGURE 31–7. Prenatal diagnosis of cloacal exstrophy. *A,* At 22 weeks there is a large cystic mass in the pelvis. *B,* At 26 weeks the cystic mass has disappeared, there is no bladder visualized, and a small omphalocele is seen (*arrowhead*). *C,* At birth the infant had typical cloacal exstrophy with wide separation of the pubic rami, a small bladder plate and lateral bowel plates, small omphalocele, imperforate anus, and ambiguous genitalia.

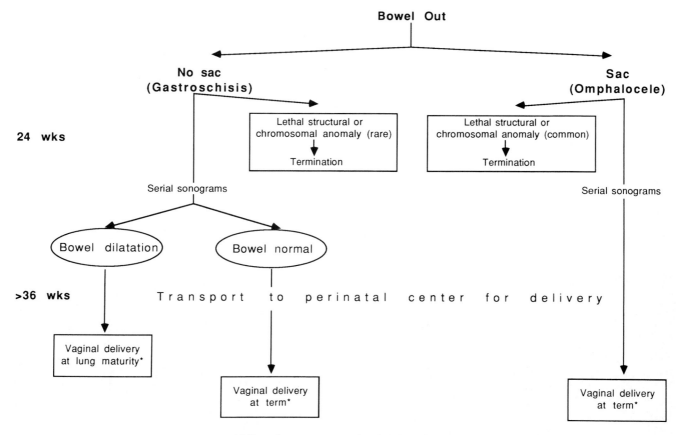

FIGURE 31–8. Algorithm for the management of a prenatally diagnosed abdominal wall defect.

the defect with respect to the umbilical cord, and identification of extruded liver are important features. In omphalocele, the size of the defect should be estimated.

The second task is careful sonographic assessment for associated structural anomalies, and in high-risk cases amniocentesis or chorionic villus sampling should be done for karyotype analysis. For fetuses in whom lethal anomalies are detected, elective termination may be offered.

For those fetuses without lethal associated anomalies, serial sonograms should be done, as previously unrecognized anomalies may become apparent. Transport to a perinatal center should be encouraged prior to delivery,[97] although a good outcome can be achieved with postnatal transfer if excellent neonatal care is available and the transport distance is not too great.[98, 99]

Appropriate timing and mode of delivery remain controversial. There is no convincing evidence to support routine cesarean section for most abdominal wall defects. In fetuses with gastroschisis, preterm delivery or amniotic fluid exchange may be advisable for cases with evidence of worsening bowel damage, and objective criteria are still being developed for selecting appropriate patients. The risks of the intervention must be weighed against the potential advantages on an individual basis. In all cases of abdominal wall defects, prenatal diagnosis should be followed by parental counseling by a multi-disciplinary team consisting of obstetricians, neonatologists, and pediatric surgeons.

REFERENCES

1. Langer JC: Fetal abdominal wall defects. Semin Pediatr Surg 2:121–128, 1993.
2. Dykes EH: Prenatal diagnosis and management of abdominal wall defects. Semin Pediatr Surg 5:90–94, 1996.
3. Boyd PA, Bhattacharjee A, Gould S, et al: Outcome of prenatally diagnosed anterior abdominal wall defects. Arch Dis Child Fetal Neonatal Ed 78:F209–F213, 1998.
4. Crombleholme TM, D'Alton M, Cendron M, et al: Prenatal diagnosis and the pediatric surgeon: The impact of prenatal consultation on perinatal management. J Pediatr Surg 31:156–162, 1996.
5. Langer JC: Normal fetal development. In Oldham KT, Colombani PM, Foglia RP (eds): Surgery of Infants and Children. Philadelphia: Lippincott-Raven Publishers, 1997, pp 41–48.
6. Seashore JH: Congenital abdominal wall defects. Clin Perinatol 5:61–77, 1978.
7. Mayer T, Black R, Matlak ME, et al: Gastroschisis and omphalocele, An eight-year review. Ann Surg 192:783–787, 1980.
8. Moore TC: Gastroschisis and omphalocele: Clinical differences. Surgery 82:561–568, 1977.
9. Venugopal S, Zachary RB, Spitz L: Exomphalos and gastroschisis: A 10-year review. Br J Surg 63:523–525, 1976.
10. Lindham S: Omphalocele and gastroschisis in Sweden 1965–1976. Acta Paediatr Scand 70:55–60, 1981.
11. Moore TC, Nur K: An international survey of gastroschisis and omphalocele (490 cases) I. Nature and distribution of additional malformations. Pediatr Surg Int 1:461–50, 1986.

12. Cooney DR: Defects of the abdominal wall. *In* O'Neill JA, Rowe MI, Grosfeld JL, et al (eds): Pediatric Surgery, 5th ed. St. Louis: Mosby, 1998, pp 1045–1070.
13. Greenwood RD, Rosenthal A, Nadas AS: Cardiovascular malformations associated with omphalocele. J Pediatr 85:818–821, 1974.
14. Nicolaides KH, Snijders RJM, Cheng HH, et al: Fetal gastrointestinal and abdominal wall defects: Associated malformations and chromosomal abnormalities. Fetal Diagn Ther 7:102–115, 1992.
15. Nyberg DA, Fitzsimmons J, Mack LA, et al: Chromosomal abnormalities in fetuses with omphalocele: The significance of omphalocele contents. J Ultrasound Med 8:299–308, 1989.
16. Benacerraf BR, Saltzman DH, Estroff JA, et al: Abnormal karyotype of fetuses with omphalocele: Prediction based on omphalocele contents. Obstet Gynecol 75:317–319, 1990.
17. Carpenter MW, Curci MR, Dibbins AW, et al: Perinatal management of ventral wall defects. Obstet Gynecol 64:646–651, 1984.
18. Bair JH, Russ PD, Pretorius DH, et al: Fetal omphalocele and gastroschisis: a review of 24 cases. AJR Am J Roentgenol 147:1047–1051, 1986.
19. Moore TC, Nur K: An international survey of gastroschisis and omphalocele (490 cases) III. Factors influencing outcome of surgical management. Pediatr Surg Int 2:27–32, 1987.
20. Sermer M, Benzie RJ, Pitson L, et al: Prenatal diagnosis and management of congenital defects of the anterior abdominal wall. Am J Obstet Gynecol 156:308–312, 1987.
21. Stringel G, Filler RM: Prognostic factors in omphalocele and gastroschisis. J Pediatr Surg 14:515–519, 1979.
22. Hughes MD, Nyberg DA, Mack LA, et al: Fetal omphalocele: Prenatal US detection of concurrent anomalies and other predictors of outcome. Radiology 173:371–376, 1989.
23. Cameron GM, McQuown DS, Modanlau HD, et al: Intrauterine diagnosis of an omphalocele by diagnostic ultrasonography. Am J Obstet Gynecol 131:821–822, 1978.
24. Hasan S, Hermansen MC: The prenatal diagnosis of ventral abdominal wall defects. Am J Obstet Gynecol 155:842–845, 1986.
25. Kirk EP, Wah RM: Obstetric management of the fetus with omphalocele or gastroschisis: A review and report of one hundred twelve cases. Am J Obstet Gynecol 146:512–518, 1983.
26. Davidson JM, Johnson TRB, Rigdon DT, et al: Gastroschisis and omphalocele: Prenatal diagnosis and perinatal management. Prenat Diagn 4:355–363, 1984.
27. Calisti A, Manzoni C, Perrelli L: The fetus with an abdominal wall defect: Management and outcome. J Perinat Med 15:105–111, 1987.
28. Lewis DF, Towers CV, Garite TJ, et al: Fetal gastroschisis and omphalocele: Is cesarean section the best mode of delivery? Am J Obstet Gynecol 163:773–775, 1990.
29. Moretti M, Khoury A, Rodriguez J, et al: The effect of mode of delivery on the perinatal outcome in fetuses with abdominal wall defects. Am J Obstet Gynecol 163:833–838, 1990.
30. Sipes SL, Weiner CP, Sipes DR, et al: Gastroschisis and omphalocele: Does either antenatal diagnosis or route of delivery make a difference in perinatal outcome? Obstet Gynecol 76:195–199, 1990.
31. van de Geijn EJ, van Vugt JMG, Sollie JE, et al: Ultrasonographic diagnosis and perinatal management of fetal abdominal wall defects. Fetal Diagn Ther 6:2–10, 1991.
32. Hershenson MB, Brouillette RT, Klemka L, et al: Respiratory insufficiency in newborns with abdominal wall defects. J Pediatr Surg 20:348–353, 1985.
33. Hoyme HE, Higginbottom MC, Jones KL: The vascular pathogenesis of gastroschisis: Intrauterine interruption of the omphalomesenteric artery. J Pediatr 98:228–231, 1981.
34. deVries PA: The pathogenesis of gastroschisis and omphalocele. J Pediatr Surg 15:245–251, 1980.
35. Duhamel B: Embryology of exomphalos and allied malformations. Arch Dis Child 38:142–147, 1963.
36. Glick PL, Harrison MR, Adzick NS, et al: The missing link in the pathogenesis of gastroschisis. J Pediatr Surg 20:406–409, 1985.
37. Nichols CR, Dickinson JE, Pemberton PJ: Rising incidence of gastroschisis in teenage pregnancies. J Matern Fetal Med 6:225–229, 1997.
38. Werler MM, Mitchell AA, Shapiro S: First trimester maternal medication use in relation to gastroschisis. Teratology 45:361–367, 1992.
39. Higginbottom MC, Jones KL, Hall BD, et al: The amniotic band disruption complex: Timing of amniotic rupture and variable spectra of consequent defects. J Pediatr 95:544–549, 1979.
40. Guzman ER: Early prenatal diagnosis of gastroschisis with transvaginal ultrasonography. Am J Obstet Gynecol 162:1253–1254, 1990.
41. Palomaki GE, Hill LE, Knight GJ, et al: Second-trimester maternal serum alpha-fetoprotein levels in pregnancies associated with gastroschisis and omphalocele. Obstet Gynecol 71:906–909, 1988.
42. van Hoom WA, Hazebroek FWJ, Molenaar JC: Gastroschisis associated with atresia—a plea for delay in resection. Z Kinderchir 40:368–370, 1985.
43. van der Zee DC, Zwierstra RP, Kootstra G, et al: Gastroschisis and intestinal obstruction. Z Kinderchir 31:111–116, 1980.
44. Luck SR, Sherman JO, Raffensperger JG, et al: Gastroschisis in 106 consecutive newborn infants. Surgery 98:677–683, 1985.
45. O'Neill JA, Grosfeld JL: Intestinal malfunction after antenatal exposure of viscera. Am J Surg 127:129–132, 1974.
46. Oh KS, Dorst JP, Dominguez R, et al: Abnormal intestinal motility in gastroschisis. Radiology 127:457–460, 1978.
47. Rubin SZ, Martin DJ, Ein SH: A critical look at delayed intestinal motility in gastroschisis. Can J Surg 21:414–416, 1978.
48. Tibboel D, Kluck P, van der Kamp AWM, et al: The development of the characteristic anomalies found in gastroschisis—experimental and clinical data. Z Kinderchir 40:355–360, 1985.
49. Tibboel D, Vermey-Keers C, Kluck P, et al: The natural history of gastroschisis during fetal life: Development of the fibrous coating on the bowel loops. Teratology 33:267–272, 1986.
50. Amoury RA, Beatty EC, Wood WG, et al: Histology of the intestine in human gastroschisis—relationship to intestinal malfunction: Dissolution of the ''peel'' and its ultrastructural characteristics. J Pediatr Surg 23:950–956, 1988.
51. Kluck P, Tibboel D, van der Kamp AWM, et al: The effect of fetal urine on the development of the bowel in gastroschisis. J Pediatr Surg 18:47–50, 1983.
52. Aktug T, Erdag G, Kargi A, et al: Amnio-allantoic fluid exchange for the prevention of intestinal damage in gastroschisis: An experimental study on chick embryos. J Pediatr Surg 30:384–387, 1995.
53. Shaw K, Buchmiller TL, Curr M, et al: Impairment of nutrient uptake in a rabbit model of gastroschisis. J Pediatr Surg 29:376–378, 1994.
54. Langer JC, Bell JG, Castillo RO, et al: Etiology of intestinal damage in gastroschisis. II: Timing and reversibility of histologic changes, mucosal function, and contractility. J Pediatr Surg 25:1122–1126, 1990.
55. Srinathan SK, Langer JC, Wang J, et al: Enterocytic gene expression is altered in experimental gastroschisis. J Surg Res 68:1–6, 1997.
56. Srinathan SK, Langer JC, Botney M, et al: Submucosal collagen in experimental gastroschisis. J Surg Res 65:25–30, 1996.
57. Langer JC, Longaker MT, Crombleholme TM, et al: Etiology of bowel damage in gastroschisis. I: Effects of amniotic fluid exposure and bowel constriction in a fetal lamb model. J Pediatr Surg 24:992–997, 1989.
58. Albert A, Julia MV, Morales L, et al: Gastroschisis in the partially extraamniotic fetus: Experimental study. J Pediatr Surg 28:656–659, 1993.
59. Sherman NJ, Asch MJ, Isaacs H, et al: Experimental gastroschisis in the fetal rabbit. J Pediatr Surg 8:165–169, 1973.
60. Steinbrecher HA, Hanna M, Burge DM: Gastroschisis bowel in an intact exomphalos: Implications for etiology and possible prevention. J Pediatr Surg 31:342–343, 1996.
61. Srinathan SK, Langer JC, Blennerhassett MG, et al: Etiology of intestinal damage in gastroschisis. III: Morphometric analysis of the smooth muscle and submucosa. J Pediatr Surg 30:379–383, 1995.
62. Langer JC: Fetal abdominal wall defects. Semin Pediatr Surg 2:121–128, 1993.
63. Abuhamad AZ, Mari G, Cortina RM, et al: Superior mesenteric artery Doppler velocimetry and ultrasonographic assessment of fetal bowel in gastroschisis: A prospective longitudinal study. Am J Obstet Gynecol 176:985–990, 1997.
64. Haller JA, Kehrer BH, Shaker IJ, et al: Studies of the pathophysiology of gastroschisis in fetal sheep. J Pediatr Surg 9:627–632, 1974.
65. Aktug T, Demir N, Akgur FM, et al: Pretreatment of gastroschisis with transabdominal amniotic fluid exchange. Obstet Gynecol 91:821–823, 1998.
66. Bond SJ, Harrison MR, Filly RA, et al: Severity of intestinal damage in gastroschisis: Correlation with prenatal sonographic findings. J Pediatr Surg 23:520–525, 1988.

67. Sipes SL, Weiner CP, Williamson RA, et al: Fetal gastroschisis complicated by bowel dilation: An indication for imminent delivery? Fetal Diagn Ther 5:100–103, 1990.
68. Lenke RR, Persutte WH, Nemes J: Ultrasonographic assessment of intestinal damage in fetuses with gastroschisis: Is it of clinical value? Am J Obstet Gynecol 163:995–998, 1990.
69. Babcook CJ, Hedrick MH, Goldstein RB, et al: Gastroschisis: Can sonography of the fetal bowel accurately predict postnatal outcome? J Ultrasound Med 13:701–706, 1994.
70. Langer JC, Khanna J, Caco C, et al: Prenatal diagnosis of gastroschisis: Development of objective sonographic criteria for predicting outcome. Obstet Gynecol 81:53–56, 1993.
71. Adra AM, Landy HJ, Nahmias J, et al: The fetus with gastroschisis: Impact of route of delivery and prenatal ultrasonography. Am J Obstet Gynecol 174:540–546, 1996.
72. McMahon MJ, Kuller JA, Chescheir NC: Prenatal ultrasonographic findings associated with short bowel syndrome in two fetuses with gastroschisis. Obstet Gynecol 88:676–678, 1996.
73. Mercer S, Mercer B, D'Alton MEG, et al: Gastroschisis: Ultrasonographic diagnosis, perinatal embryology, surgical and obstetric treatment and outcomes. Can J Surg 31:25–26, 1988.
74. Bethel CAI, Seashore JH, Touloukian RJ: Caesarean section does not improve outcome in gastroschisis. J Pediatr Surg 24:1–4, 1989.
75. Chescheir NC, Azizkhan RG, Seeds JW, et al: Counseling and care for the pregnancy complicated by gastroschisis. Am J Perinatol 8:323–329, 1991.
76. Stringer MD, Brereton RJ, Wright VM: Controversies in the management of gastroschisis: A study of 40 patients. Arch Dis Child 66:34–36, 1991.
77. Moore TC: Elective preterm section for improved primary repair of gastroschisis. Pediatr Surg Int 4:25–26, 1988.
78. Lenke RR, Hatch EJ: Fetal gastroschisis: A preliminary report advocating the use of caesarean section. Obstet Gynecol 67:395–398, 1986.
79. Fitzsimmons J, Nyberg DR, Cyr DR, et al: Perinatal management of gastroschisis. Obstet Gynecol 71:910–913, 1988.
80. Moore TC: The role of labor in gastroschisis bowel thickening and prevention by elective preterm and pre-labor cesarean section. Pediatr Surg Int 7:256–259, 1992.
81. Swift RI, Singh MP, Ziderman DA, et al: A new regime in the management of gastroschisis. J Pediatr Surg 27:61–63, 1992.
82. Sakala EP, Erhard LN, White JJ: Elective caesarean section improves outcomes of neonates with gastroschisis. Am J Obstet Gynecol 169:1050–1053, 1993.
83. Coughlin JP, Drucker DEM, Jewell MR, et al: Delivery room repair of gastroschisis. Surgery 114:822–827, 1993.
84. Minkes RK, Langer JC, Mazziotti MV, et al: Routine insertion of a silastic spring-loaded silo for infants with gastroschisis. J Pediatr Surg (in press).
85. Ambrose SS, O'Brien DP: Surgical embryology of the exstrophy-epispadias complex. Surg Clin North Am 54:1379–1390, 1974.
86. Duffy PG: Bladder exstrophy. Semin Pediatr Surg 5:129–132, 1996.
87. Molenaar JC: Cloacal exstrophy. Semin Pediatr Surg 5:133–135, 1996.
88. Diamond DA, Jeffs RD: Cloacal exstrophy: A 22-year experience. J Urol 133:779–782, 1985.
89. Mirk P, Calisti A, Fileni A: Prenatal sonographic diagnosis of bladder exstrophy. J Ultrasound Med 5:291–293, 1986.
90. Gearhart JP, Ben-Chaim J, Jeffs RD, et al: Criteria for the prenatal diagnosis of classic bladder exstrophy. Obstet Gynecol 85:961–964, 1995.
91. Pinette MG, Pan YQ, Pinette SG, et al: Prenatal diagnosis of fetal bladder and cloacal exstrophy by ultrasound. A report of three cases. J Reprod Med 41:132–134, 1996.
92. Gosden C, Brock DJH: Prenatal diagnosis of exstrophy of the cloaca. Am J Med Genet 8:95–109, 1981.
93. McLaughlin JF, Marks WM, Jones G: Prospective management of exstrophy of the cloaca and myelocystocele following prenatal ultrasound recognition of neural tube defects in identical twins. Am J Med Genet 19:721–727, 1984.
94. Kutzner DK, Wilson WG, Hogge WA: OEIS complex (cloacal exstrophy): Prenatal diagnosis in the second trimester. Prenat Diagn 8:247–253, 1988.
95. Langer JC, Brennan B, Lappalainen RE, et al: Cloacal exstrophy: Prenatal diagnosis before rupture of the cloacal membrane. J Pediatr Surg 27:1352–1355, 1992.
96. Bruch SW, Adzick NS, Goldstein RB, et al: Challenging the embryogenesis of cloacal exstrophy. J Pediatr Surg 31:768–770, 1996.
97. Harris BA, Wirtschafter DD, Huddleston JF, et al: In utero versus neonatal transportation of high-risk perinates: A comparison. Obstet Gynecol 57:496–499, 1981.
98. Stoodley N, Sharma A, Noblett H, et al: Influence of place of delivery on outcome in babies with gastroschisis. Arch Dis Child 68:321–323, 1993.
99. Nicholls G, Upadhyaya V, Gomall P, et al: Is specialist centre delivery of gastroschisis beneficial? Arch Dis Child 69:71–73, 1993.

CHAPTER 32

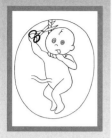

The Fetus with Amniotic Band Syndrome

TIMOTHY M. CROMBLEHOLME

The amniotic band syndrome (ABS) is a group of sporadic congenital anomalies involving the limbs, craniofacial regions, and trunk. These anomalies include constrictive bands of the extremities with effects ranging from pseudosyndactyly to amputation, as well as multiple craniofacial, visceral, and body wall defects.[1-9] ABS has become a grab bag of congenital anomalies that have been referred to with numerous names, including amniotic band disruption complex[1]; amniochorionic mesoblastic fibrous strings[7]; aberrant tissue bands[8]; amniotic deformity, adhesions, and mutilations (ADAM) complex[9]; amniotic adhesion malformation syndrome[10]; and the limb and/or body wall defect.[11]

The fetal malformations that can occur as a result of ABS can be categorized into neural tube–like defects, craniofacial anomalies, limb anomalies, and constrictive.[2, 5, 13, 14] The neural tube–like defects include cases of anencephaly and encephalocele, which may be asymmetric or multiple. The craniofacial anomalies include facial clefts, nasal deformity, asymmetric microphthalmia, and abnormal cranial calcification. Limb anomalies may be multiple and asymmetric including limb or digital amputation, pseudosyndactyly, abnormal dermatoglyphics, and some cases of clubbed feet (Fig. 32–1). Constrictive bands involving the extremities are the most common defects associated with the ABS.[15] Abdominal wall and thoracic wall defects can occur and some cases are mistaken for gastroschisis or ruptured omphalocele. The most puzzling component of the ABS is the associated visceral anomalies including bladder exstrophy; vertebral hypoplasia; and other renal, gonadal, cardiac, and pulmonary defects.[12]

Variations in manifestations of the ABS are thought to be due to differences in timing of amniotic rupture and the degree to which the fetus becomes entangled by strands of amnion.[1, 2] The effect the amniotic bands have on the developing fetus have been classified into malformation, disruption, and deformation.[1] Amniotic bands that interrupt the normal sequence of embryologic development lead to malformations such as cleft lip and palate, and abdominal wall defects. In contrast, bands may tear normally developed structures, leading to disruption such as central nervous system or calvarial defects, acrosyndactyly, amputations, and nonanatomic facial clefts.[4] The effects of fetal compression and tethering may lead to deformations such as clubbing of the feet and angulation of the spine.

Etiology of Amniotic Bands

Several theories have been advanced to explain the occurrence of these anomalies, but two are most commonly held. In 1930, Streeter proposed that a disruption in embryogenesis at the time of formation of the germ disc and the amniotic cavity initiated a chain of events leading to the multiple defects.[16] He suggested that amniotic bands were the result, not the cause, of the pathologic process. Bamforth, reviewed this theory in 1992 in a series of 54 cases of ABS and concluded it may be caused by a localized disturbance in establishment of basic embryonic organization.[12] The most widely accepted theory was proposed by Torpin in 1965.[7] He examined the placenta and fetal membranes in a number of affected individuals and concluded that the disorder was caused by primary rupture of the amnion early in gestation.[1, 2, 10, 11]

The timing of amnion rupture has been suggested to occur between 28 days following conception to 18 weeks' gestation. If amnion rupture occurs prior to 45 days' gestation the results are likely to be devastating, including severe skull defects and major visceral defects.[15] Rupture occurring after 45 days' gestation is likely to result in more limited defects.

The etiologies of amnion rupture and band formation are not well understood but have been observed following amniocentesis.[17] Late-gestation bands, even without amniocentesis, can also occur. Lage et al. reported ABS presenting at birth with multiple abnormalities of the extremities despite a normal appearance sonographically at 21 weeks' gestation.[17] There have also been cases of ABS associated with underlying disease. Young et al. reported two cases in fetuses with a vascular form of Ehlers-Danlos syndrome and one with osteogenesis imperfecta.[18] They speculated that the premature amnion

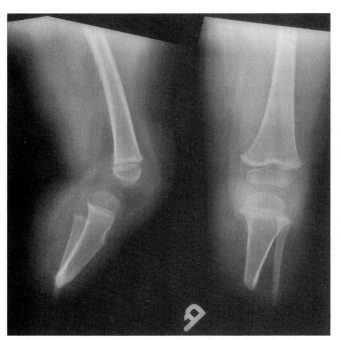

FIGURE 32–1. Plain radiograph of the right leg of a newborn who sustained amputation in utero of the right leg and foot from amniotic bands. (Courtesy of Benjamin Alman, MD.)

rupture may have been due to reduced or abnormal collagen in the amnion. There have been rare familial cases of ABS, and some teratogens have been reported in association with the syndrome.[14] Lysergic acid diethylamide and methadone as well as other teratogens have been reported, but these do not account for many cases of ABS.[19, 20]

More recently, Moerman et al. proposed that the ABS is a collection of three distinct entities which can reconcile Streeter's and Torpin's hypotheses.[21] They suggested that ABS consists of three distinct lesions: (1) constrictive tissue bands; (2) amniotic adhesions; and (3) the more complex pattern of anomalies designated the limb–body wall complex (LBWC). In this report of the fetopathologic evaluation of 18 cases of ABS, four cases had clearly constrictive bands that formed as a result of the amnion rupture sequence. The bands that result from amnion rupture encircle limbs, resulting in annular constrictions, secondary syndactyly, and intrauterine amputations (Fig. 32–1). In addition to their effect on extremities, constrictive amniotic bands of the umbilical cord can cause fetal death.[7, 8, 22]

Moerman et al. distinguish cases caused by constrictive bands from those caused by broad amniotic adhesions, and the group suggested that adhesive amniotic bands were morphologically and pathogenetically different from constrictive bands. These adhesive amniotic bands are usually associated with severe defects such as encephalocele and facial clefts. This group demonstrated pathologically the cranioplacental adhesions to be broad adhesions with the fetal skin fused to the amnion at the margins of the cranial defect. They speculated that the amnion covering the placenta or membranes seals the cranial defect separating the protruding brain from the chorion. Van Allen et al. proposed that the amnion becomes adherent to the embryo in areas of ischemic necrosis following vascular disruption.[23] In short, the amniotic adhesions are secondary to fetal defects.

In their classification Moerman et al. consider the LBWC to be due to both band-related and non–band-related defects. The band-related defects include limb defects such as club foot, while non–band-related defects occur as a result of vascular disruptions or from compression.[24] The thoracoabdominoschisis of LBWC is characterized by an anterolateral body wall defect with evisceration of abdominal and/or thoracic organs. The eviscerated organs are in an extra-amniotic sac bounded by the chorionic plate, a persistent extraembryonic coelom. The amnion is continuous with the skin. The umbilical cord is extremely short with umbilical vessels running in the amniotic sac, often with an absent umbilical artery. The severe scoliosis is a postural deformity caused by abnormal fixation of the fetus to the placenta. They also cite the high incidence of internal structural defects such as cardiac anomalies, unilateral absence of a kidney, or intestinal atresia, which do not fit with simple amnion rupture.

ABS is often misdiagnosed, especially in cases of early amniotic band rupture. Infants affected by early amniotic rupture present with anencephaly, encephaloceles, abdominal or thoracic wall defects, and severe limb abnormalities. The severity of the anomalies obscure the etiology, especially if the amniotic bands are not evident at birth. It has been estimated that a correct neonatal diagnosis of ABS is made in only 24 to 50% of patients without specialized genetic consultation.[2]

Because of difficulties in accurately diagnosing ABS, the estimates of its incidence vary widely. The incidence reported ranges from 1 in 1,200 to 1 in 15,000 live births.[2, 3, 13, 19] More recent estimates place the incidence of ABS at 1 in 1,200, due to a more frequent recognition of amniogenic etiology of congenital anomalies.[2, 25]

Sonographic Features

ABS has numerous sonographic features, as there are numerous forms of the syndrome, and these features may occur as isolated problems or in combination. The earliest that amniotic bands have been seen is 12 weeks by endovaginal sonographic probe. The bands can be extremely difficult to detect sonographically, and ABS is more often diagnosed by the effect that they have on fetal anatomy. The effect of amniotic bands on the extremities may be manifested by absent digits or portions of limbs, or swollen distal arm or leg secondary to constrictive amniotic bands (Fig. 32–2). The face may be affected in ABS with cleft lip or palate, asymmetric microphthalmia, and severe nasal deformity. Encephalocele may be a manifestation of ABS, especially when eccentrically positioned off the midline (Fig. 32–3). Abdominal wall defects can be the result of ABS, typically with large defects with free-floating intestine but large

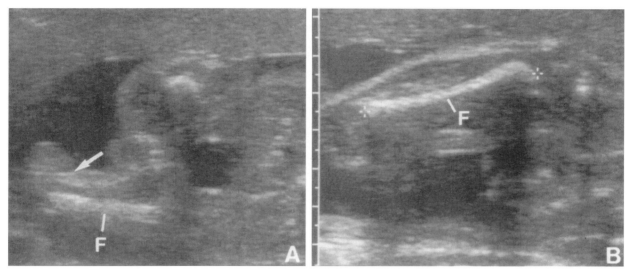

F I G U R E 32–2. Ultrasound of a fetus with a constricting amniotic band of an extremity. *A*, Amniotic bands resulting in amputation of the lower extremity immediately above the knee (*arrow*). *B*, The normal contralateral femur (F) is shown for comparison. (Courtesy of Roy Filly, MD, used with permission of WB Saunders Company.)

enough for the lines to herniate outside the abdomen (Fig. 32–4).

The characteristic appearance of an aberrant sheet or band of amnion attached to the fetus with resultant deformity and restriction of motion allows a diagnosis of ABS to be made. This is the exception rather than the rule, however. The findings in ABS may be limited to isolated defects including isolated facial cleft, digital amputation, or mild elephantiasis of an extremity beyond a constrictive band. These isolated features may be difficult to diagnose sonographically because the detailed fetal visualization required is beyond the scope of routine obstetric ultrasound examinations. At the worst end of the spectrum, the fetus may be so severely deformed by the amniotic bands that the spine is contorted and organs are formed in bizarre proportions. The head may be completely misshapen or absent. The bands responsible for these deformities are rarely seen, and a presumptive diagnosis of ABS is made based on deformities commonly associated with ABS.

The spinal deformities in ABS can be severe, manifesting as kyphotic lordosis or scoliosis, as well as severe rotational abnormalities or even spinal amputation. While spinal deformity can be seen in other syndromes,

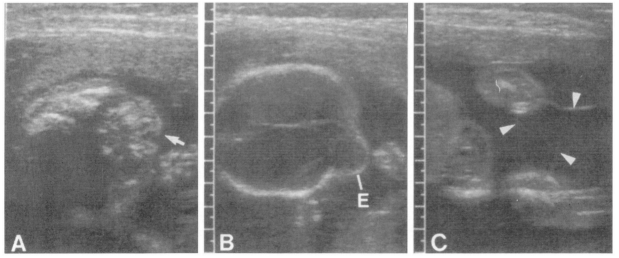

F I G U R E 32–3. Ultrasound of a fetus with amniotic band syndrome manifesting as (*A*) a "slash" defect in the maxillary region and (*B*) as an asymmetric encephalocele (E). *C*, Amniotic bands were also noted to be attached to the extremities (*arrowheads*). (Courtesy of Roy Filly, MD, used with permission of WB Saunders Company.)

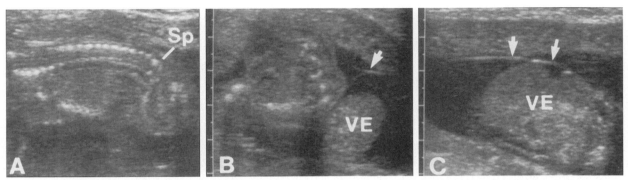

FIGURE 32–4. Ultrasound of a fetus with limb–body wall complex showing severe twisting deformity of the spine associated with gastropleuroschisis and amniotic bands attached to the extremities. *A,* The fetal spine (SP) has a severe twisting deformity. *B,* The twisting deformity is so severe that the viscera (VE) herniated through the gastropleuroschisis are found posterior to the fetus. *C,* The amnion (*arrows*) encircles the exteriorized viscera. (Courtesy of Roy Filly, MD, used with permission of WB Saunders Company.)

severe spinal deformity should suggest the possibility of ABS. Spinal deformity associated with an abdominal wall defect is particularly suggestive of ABS. While typical appearing omphalocele is possible, the more common body wall defect in ABS is a large slash-like defect of both the thoracic and abdominal cavities with evisceration. These defects have exteriorized bowel, liver, and sometimes heart without an enveloping membrane. When associated with limb abnormalities, this is characteristic of the limb–body wall complex form of ABS.

The deformation of the calvarium is another group of anomalies characteristic of ABS. If complete, the fetus may appear anencephalic; if partial, the fetus may appear to have an encephalocele. The distinguishing features that characterize these defects as ABS are the asymmetric nature of these defects and associated spinal deformity or abdominal wall defects. In classic anencephaly the calvarial bones are symmetrically absent. In anencephaly caused by ABS there is some portion of calvarium present, usually near the base of the skull or an orbit. Similarly, classic encephaloceles occur near the midline, while ABS causes encephaloceles off the midline.

The presence of bands is unnecessary for the diagnosis of ABS in the presence of characteristic fetal anomalies. The sonographic detection of bands is helpful in confirming the diagnosis of ABS as the cause of fetal deformity. However, observation of these bands without fetal abnormality is not ABS. It is important for the sonographer to distinguish amniotic bands from other membranes and separations within the amnion. Separation of amnion and chorion is normal in early pregnancy until fusion occurs at approximately 16 weeks' gestation.[26–28]

Chorioamniotic separation may occur as a result of amniocentesis, and extrachorionic hemorrhage may separate the chorioamniotic membrane from the uterine wall.[26, 29] In both of these instances a membrane may be sonographically observed. Other causes of membranes within the developing gestation include septate uterus, blighted twin, and circumvallate placenta.[30]

Adhesions that form in the uterus as a result of curettage, cesarean section, myomectomy, or fetal surgery may cause sheets of amnion that protrude into the lumen of the amniotic cavity.[30–34] Randel et al. found that 76% of patients with amniotic sheets had undergone instrumentation.[34] This results in an adhesion that becomes covered by chorion and amnion and has a thickness similar to the intertwin membrane of dichorionic diamniotic twins. These amniotic sheets do not adhere to the fetus because the amnion is intact. The uterine adhesion may rupture with growth of the pregnancy. Filly et al. have described the sonographic appearance of these synechiae as having a thickened base and has a fine edge that undulates.[30] There may be a bulbous edge, presumably due to the synechiae. There are no associated fetal abnormalities and there is free fetal movement around the sheet. The synechiae may not be seen in the third trimester, due to either rupture or compression by the growing fetus.

In the limb–body wall complex form of ABS there is a constellation of abnormalities including meningomyeloceles or caudal regression, thoracoabdominoschisis or abdominoschisis, and limb defects. A diagnosis of LBWC requires two of three of the following abnormalities: (1) meningomyelocele or caudal regression, (2) abdominal wall or thoracoabdominal wall defect, and (3) limb defects. The main differential are cases of isolated neural tube defects or ruptured omphalocele that do not meet the criteria for LBWC. The umbilical cord is usually short or absent with the placenta attached to the fetus. If present, there may only be a two-vessel cord. The limbs may be missing or the feet clubbed. The spine is often short and curved, and sacral regression is common. There may be Arnold-Chiari malformation and hydrocephalus associated with the meningomyelocele. There may be ectopia cordis as part of the thoracoabdominoschisis. Facial clefts may also be seen in association with LBWC.

The differential diagnosis in ABS depends on the sonographic findings. In isolated constrictive amniotic bands associated with distal limb edema, possible vascular malformations should be considered. However, color Doppler should clearly show the flow characteristics of a vascular malformation. Constrictive bands involving the upper extremity should suggest the possibility of the VACTERL (*v*ertebral, *a*nal, *c*ardiac, *t*racheal, *e*sophageal, *r*enal, and *l*imb) association if the radius is affected or Fanconi syndrome if radial hypoplasia or absent thumbs are observed.

Antenatal Natural History

There is great controversy about the pathogenesis of the various forms of ABS. Part of this controversy involves the timing in gestation of the development of amniotic bands. However, in constrictive amniotic bands of the extremities the progression of constriction combined with fetal growth has resulted in extremity amputation.[35] However, the poorly characterized pathogenesis of this syndrome and limited sonographic surveillance limit our understanding of its prenatal natural history.

Although constrictive amniotic bands of the extremities were presumed to progress to amputation, sonographic demonstration of this natural history had been lacking. Reports of the sonographic prenatal diagnosis of the amniotic band syndrome usually involved pregnancies in the second or third trimester in which the anomalies were already present when they were diagnosed.[35–39] Similarly, reports of amniotic band syndrome associated with amniocentesis have assumed the sequence of events but lacked serial sonographic examinations demonstrating the progression of the amniotic band sequence.[36–38] Tadmor et al. followed a fetus from 21 weeks' gestation with marked edema of both feet secondary to an amniotic band surrounding both limbs.[39] While color Doppler demonstrated arterial blood flow distal to the amniotic band at 21 weeks' gestation, this was lost by 24 weeks' gestation. By 30 weeks' gestation amputation of the right leg was evident and by delivery at 38 weeks' gestation there was partial amputation of the left leg with an extremely edematous and partly necrotic foot. Takenori made similar observations in a late first-trimester fetus.[40] Similarly, Laberge et al. described a case which, on ultrasound at 18 weeks' gestation, was noted to have his left hand attached to an amniotic band. At birth the infant had deformity of that hand typical of the amniotic band sequence.[41] As there are few serial sonographic data available for extremity amniotic band syndrome, there are even fewer documenting the progression of limb–body wall complex and amniotic bands associated with facial clefts and encephaloceles.

Chorioamniotic separation, occurring spontaneously or as a consequence of invasive procedures, is a potential cause of the amniotic band syndrome. The incidence of chorioamniotic separation diagnosed by ultrasound is reported to range from 1 in 187 to 1 in 4,333.[42–44] The natural history of chorioamniotic separation occurring in normal pregnancies was thought to be benign, as no case resulted in amniotic band formation. However, Graf et al. reported a case of chorioamniotic separation that resulted in the formation of amniotic bands involv-

ing the umbilical cord resulting in fetal demise.[45] The incidence of chorioamniotic separation may be even higher in cases of fetal surgery. In the same report, Graf described five cases of chorioamniotic separation occurring in a series of 40 patients undergoing open fetal surgery.[45] Three of the five fetuses had amniotic bands involving the umbilical cord leading to fetal death in one. This report speculated that because the amnion is adherent and fixed to the umbilical cord, once formed, amniotic bands may retract to the cord, causing strangulation. Heifetz, in a review of amniotic band syndrome, reported that as many as 10% of cases had umbilical cord strangulation.[46]

In managing a pregnancy with suspected ABS, it is essential to have a detailed sonographic fetal survey to accurately assess any anomalies present and include commonly associated ones. Fetal echocardiography is indicated in cases of abdominal wall or abdominothoracic wall defects because of increased incidence of associated cardiac defects. Amniocentesis is not necessary in clear-cut cases of ABS, as these are sporadic deformations with no association with chromosome abnormalities. However, in instances where the diagnosis is uncertain, genetic amniocentesis should be considered. For example, in cases of abdominal wall defects in which a ruptured covered omphalocele cannot be excluded, a genetic amniocentesis is indicated.

A fetus with ABS should pose no increased risk for the mother in the management of the pregnancy. ABS can be associated with oligohydramnios. Despite the severity of some forms of ABS, there is no adverse maternal consequences for this diagnosis and no apparent increase in the incidence of intrauterine fetal demise. There is no indication for cesarean section, except for routine obstetric indications. In severe cases of ABS, such as LBWC in which survival is not anticipated, unmonitored vaginal delivery without intervention for fetal distress should be considered.

Pathophysiology of Amniotic Band Syndrome

Constrictive bands are primarily responsible for manifestations of the ABS involving the extremity. The morbidity of constrictive amniotic bands involving the extremity can range from relatively minor, as in syndactyly, to significant when they result in elephantiasis or amputation.[2, 4, 7, 27, 31] Most information about ABS reflects only clinical, sonographic, and pathologic observations.[2, 4, 7, 20, 22, 26, 31, 47–49] Little experimental work has been done, and what is available has focused primarily on the pathogenesis of the amniotic bands themselves and not their pathologic sequelae in the fetal limb.[50–57] No appropriate animal model has been available to specifically study the pathophysiology of fetal extremity constriction by bands. Our group developed a model of ABS in the fetal lamb in order to study the effects of extremity constriction in utero and assess the morphologic, histologic, and functional response of the fetal limb to fetoscopic release of constrictive bands.[52]

T A B L E 32–1. FETOSCOPIC RELEASE OF CONSTRICTIVE BANDS

ANIMAL GROUP	LIMBS BANDED	LIMBS RELEASED	LIMBS LOST TO SAB	LIMBS EVALUATED AT TERM DELIVERY
Group 1	21	6	6*	15
Group 2	4	0	0	4
Sham-operated controls	7	0	2*	5
Nonoperated controls	8	0	0	8
Total Limbs	40	6	8	32

* Two lambs aborted each with three banded limbs and one sham-operated control limb.
SAB, spontaneous abortion.

Four time-dated, twin-gestation pregnant ewes obtained at 100 days' gestation (term = 145 days) were studied (Table 32–1). In addition, two unoperated neonatal lambs served as controls (n = 10; eight fetal and two neonatal lambs). A Dacron pledgeted purse-string suture of 2-0 silk was placed in the uterus through which a 4-cm hysterotomy was made to allow the exteriorization of the fetal limbs (Fig. 32–5). Baseline blood flow was measured in the extremities of each of eight fetal lambs by laser Doppler flowmeter once a steady state had been reached.[59] Laser Doppler was used to ensure that the umbilical tape bands were applied with uniform constriction in each limb. In 21 fetal limbs (group 1), the umbilical tape was applied as tightly as possible without affecting the extremity blood flow (0% reduction in blood flow). The mean blood flow prior to band application was 32.09 ± 8.9 mL/min/100 g tissue (± SD) and 32.12 ± 8.1 mL/min/100 g tissue following band application. In four lambs (group 2), umbilical tapes were applied sufficiently tightly to fore- and hindlimbs with the goal of effecting a 10 to 25% reduction in extremity blood flow from baseline. Band application actually resulted in a 18.7% reduction in blood flow from a mean of 33.7 ± 10.8 mL/min/100 g tissue (± SD) to 27.4 ± 8.9 mL/min/100 g of tissue (p < 0.003). Seven fetal

limbs were not banded and served as sham-operated controls. The progression of limb deformity was monitored by interval ultrasound scanning (Fig. 32–6.).

At 125 days' gestation the midline laparotomy incision was reopened, and the fetal orientation was determined by palpation. A Dacron pledgeted purse-string of 2-0 silk was placed in a position on the uterus to avoid placental cotyledons and allow fetoscopic access to all four extremities. A Veress needle was introduced into the amniotic cavity and position confirmed by aspirating amniotic fluid and the purse-string was then cinched tight in a Rummel clamp. Insufflation with CO_2 or helium (in order to avoid fetal acidosis[60]) was begun at a slow rate with a pressure limit of 4 cm H_2O. After adequate pneumoamnion had been achieved, a 2-mm 0-degree telescope was introduced through the Veress needle or a 4-mm 0-degree telescopic lens was placed through a separate purse-string and connected to a xenon light source (Fig. 32–7). Inspection of the fetus con-

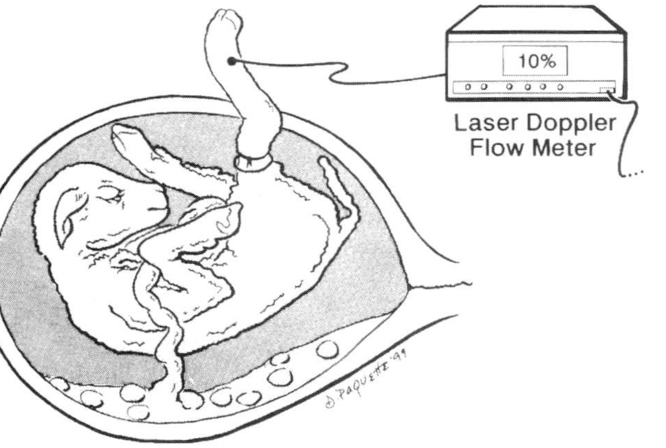

FIGURE 32–5. Schematic representation of the initial procedure, performed at 100 days' gestation. The fetal limb is exteriorized through a small hysterotomy and the umbilical tape is applied as a constrictive band. The laser Doppler is used to quantify the reduction of extremity blood flow induced by the constrictive band.

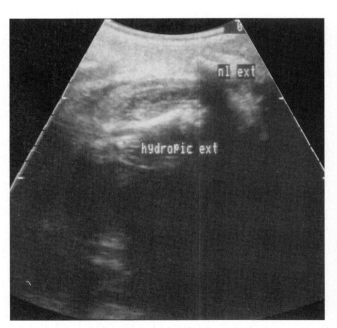

FIGURE 32–6. Ultrasound of a fetal lamb at 114 days' gestation 14 days following banding of the extremities. The leg is grossly hydropic distal to the level of the band mimicking the appearance of constrictive amniotic bands in human fetuses.

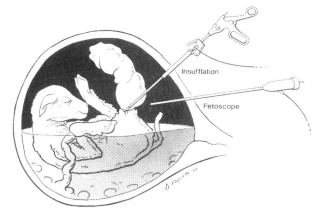

FIGURE 32–7. Schematic representation of the fetoscopic procedure. A Veress needle has been introduced into the amniotic cavity and pneumoamnion induced by insufflation with CO_2 or helium (pneumoamnion is dark and the lightly shaded area represents amniotic fluid). A 2-mm videofetoscope has been introduced through the Veress needle and a 5-mm operating trocar has been placed for continued insufflation and the passage of the endoshears. The constrictive band, often embedded in the fetal tissue is identified, cut, and removed.

firmed the presence of the umbilical tape bands with distal edema and deformity that had been noted sonographically. The videofetoscope was then used to place the 5-mm operating cannula through a second Dacron pledgeted purse-string in the uterus avoiding placental cotyledons and optimally positioned to cut the extremity bands. Endoshears were introduced and the umbilical tape bands were released (Fig. 32–8). The umbilical tapes were removed from six fetal limbs. Each newborn

lamb underwent morphometric measurements including segmental limb lengths; segmental limb circumference; and joint range of motion at the knee, ankle, and phalangeal joints. Soft tissue biopsies were performed on each extremity.

Banding the limbs of fetal lambs at 100 days' gestation replicated all of the clinical features of the extremity amniotic band syndrome (Fig. 32–9). Sonographic evaluation of fetal lambs following application of the constrictive bands demonstrated hydropic extremities distal to the bands similar to prenatal ultrasounds of human fetuses with ABS (Fig. 32–6). The newborn lambs were found to have severely deformed limbs, with pitting edema, venous congestion, and the absence of normal wool. Histologically, hematoxylin and eosin–stained biopsy sections of the banded extremities demonstrated increased subcutaneous tissue due to edema, venous and lymphatic congestion, and fibrosis (Fig. 32–10). The results of banding in group 2 (with reduction in blood flow) were worse than group 1 lambs (banded without reduction in blood flow) in both appearance and histologic changes.

Banding of the fetal limb resulted in a significant reduction in the segmental limb length of the distal forelimb compared to controls in both groups ($p < 0.05$; Table 32–2). Banding of the fetal limb resulted in significant increases in the segmental limb circumference in group 2 lambs in the distal-1 ($p < 0.03$) and distal-2 ($p < 0.003$) circumferences (Table 32–3).

The deformity caused by the banding resulted in significant reduction in joint range of motion in the group 2 limbs at both the ankle ($p < 0.003$) and phalangeal joints ($p < 0.003$; Table 32–4). There was a direct correlation between increasing severity of band constriction

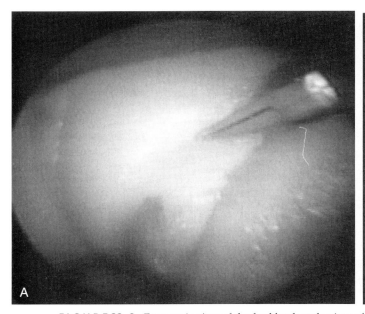
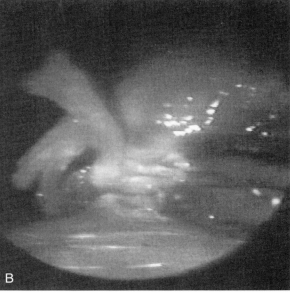

FIGURE 32–8. Fetoscopic view of the fetal lamb at the time of release of the bands. *A,* The panel on the left shows the crease at the level of the band with a severely edematous limb distal to it and a notable absence of wool. *B,* The panel on the right shows the endoscissors poised to cut the umbilical tape used to mimic the amniotic band.

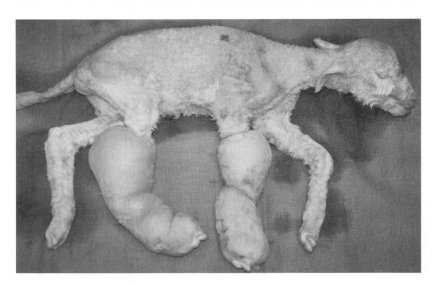

FIGURE 32–9. Photograph of newborn lamb that underwent banding of all four limbs at 100 days' gestation and fetoscopic release of the bands around the left fore- and hindlimbs at 125 days' gestation. The limbs are markedly edematous and deformed, with absence of wool affecting the hindlimb more than the forelimb.

and increasing limb circumference and an inverse relationship with joint range of motion (Tables 32–3 and 32–4). Radiographs demonstrated marked bowing and demineralization (Fig. 32–11). Banded limbs at term showed progression in these findings, especially the demineralization of bones and bowing with fractures at, or distal to, the site of banding. Banded limbs had increased hoof circumference and reduced joint range of motion compared to controls. In marked contrast, there were

no differences between limbs that were fetoscopically released and control limbs.

Fetoscopic release of bands at 125 days' gestation reversed the limb deformity, forelimb shortening, loss of joint range of motion, and absence of wool. The fetoscopically released limbs were grossly indistinguishable from normal control limbs (Fig. 32–9). However, histologic changes including mild venous and lymphatic congestion and increased fibrosis were noted on trichrome

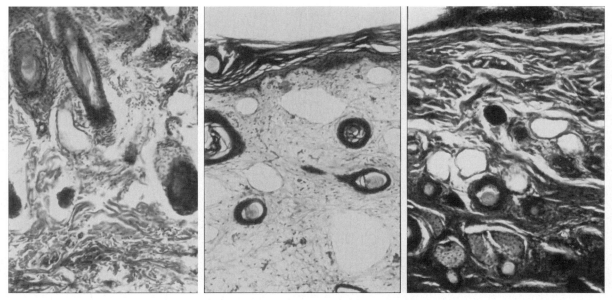

FIGURE 32–10. Trichrome stain of histologic sections of biopsies taken from the newborn limbs of normal control lambs (*left*), lambs that were banded and fetoscopically released (*middle*), and lambs that were banded and allowed to go to term (*right*). Banding of the extremity has resulted in marked increase in fibrosis, dilated venous and lymphatic channels, and dropout of hair follicles compared to normal control. The fetoscopically released limbs show less fibrosis but have persistence of lymphatic and venous ectasia compared to normal controls.

TABLE 32–2. SEGMENTAL LIMB LENGTHS

	CONTROL (cm)	GROUP 1 (cm)	GROUP 2* (cm)	FETOSCOPICALLY RELEASED (cm)
Forelimb				
Proximal	11.97 ± 0.97	12.13 ± 0.5	10.5 ± 1	11.0 ± 0.6
Distal	12.98 ± 0.69	10.97 ± 0.59†	10.8 ± 0.07†	11.9 ± 1.85
Hoof	5.43 ± 0.28	5.59 ± 0.18	5.5 ± 0.3	5.95 ± 0.05
Hindlimb				
Proximal	13.95 ± 0.05	13.18 ± 0.8	NA	13.9 ± 0.52
Distal	14.4 ± 1.1	13.9 ± 0.5	NA	13.9 ± 0.66
Hoof	5.75 ± 0.2	5.6 ± 0.34	NA	5.8 + 0.28

* The limbs in these groups had umbilical tape bands applied sufficiently tight to reduce blood flow by 18% as indicated by laser Doppler flowmetry.
†$p < 0.05$.

staining in the fetoscopically released limbs (Fig. 32–10). The distal forelimbs, which were significantly shortened in group 1 and 2 limbs, were normal length in limbs that were fetoscopically released (Table 32–2). There was no difference between controls and the fetoscopically released group in distal limb circumferences and joint range of motion at the ankle and phalangeal joints.

This model of amniotic band syndrome in fetal lambs replicates all the clinical features of ABS in human fetuses affected by constrictive extremity bands. Previous experimental models reported focused on the teratogenic induction of amniotic bands in an attempt to elucidate their origin and explain the myriad presentations of this syndrome.[50–57] Rowsell did report using constrictive bands in fetal mice, but the bands were placed on day 19 of a 21-day gestation, severely limiting the utility of the model.[57] This model of ABS in fetal lambs is the first reported in an animal of sufficiently long gestation to permit the study of the pathophysiologic sequelae of constrictive extremity bands and the potential for morphologic, histologic, and functional recovery of the fetal limbs after release in utero.

The sonographic appearance of banded limbs was identical to the prenatal sonographic appearance of extremity ABS and the clinical groups described by Hall for mild, moderate, and severe ABS.[31, 34, 48, 62] We observed no amputations, but the banded limbs demonstrated elephantiasis, most with an intact blood supply, consistent with Hall's moderate ABS.[4]

Fetoscopic release of the constrictive bands in this model reversed the hydropic changes in the limbs and prevented the other sequelae of banding including distal forelimb shortening, loss of joint mobility, and absence of wool. Postnatally, the fetoscopically released limbs were grossly indistinguishable from normal control limbs. A potential benefit of fetoscopic release of extremity amniotic bands is the unique healing property of fetal tissue, which provides an opportunity for dramatic restoration of form and function that may be lost by the time the infant is delivered.[57]

In our model of extremity ABS umbilical tape is not amnion, but it does replicate the inelastic constrictive properties of amniotic bands.[22] The application of bands without affecting the blood flow to the extremity in group 1 mimicked the passive encirclement of the fetal limb by amniotic bands, resulting in significant constriction with fetal growth from the unyielding nature of the band. The sequelae of the constrictive band must relate to the gestational age at which they occur. In this study, the bands were placed at 100 days' gestation, the equivalent of 27 weeks of gestation in humans. The earlier in gestation an inelastic band is applied, the more fetal growth will occur, and consequently the more severe the sequelae from the band in the developing limb. In addition, as demonstrated in our group 2 limbs, the more tightly applied the band is initially, the more severe the consequences. It is likely that in human fetuses, the earlier that amniotic band constriction occurs and

TABLE 32–3. SEGMENTAL LIMB CIRCUMFERENCE*

	CONTROL (cm)	GROUP 1 (cm)	GROUP 2 (cm)	FETOSCOPICALLY RELEASED (cm)
Proximal	17.9 ± 1.2	14.3 ± 0.3	11.75 ± 1.0	14.7 ± 0.9
Distal-1	10.5 ± 0.4	9.1 ± 1.7	13.9 ± 2.5†	6.8 ± 0.1‡
Distal-2	7 ± 0.4	8.45 ± 1.0	10.25 ± 1.89†	6.7 + 0.46‡
Hoof	9.5 ± 0.6	7.72 ± 0.2	11.18 ± 1.7	7.3 ± 0.1

* The controls included two neonatal lambs that averaged 1.5 kg larger than the experimental lambs. The larger values in the control group reflect this and may account for the lack of significance in the differences between the banded limbs and control animals. Despite this the limb circumference values for distal-1 and distal-2 in the 10 to 25% reduction group did achieve statistical significance. In the group of fetoscopically released limbs the values for distal-1 and distal-2 approached statistical significance.
† $p < 0.03$.
‡ $p = 0.06$.

T A B L E 32–4. JOINT RANGE OF MOTION (IN DEGREES)

JOINT	CONTROL	GROUP 1	GROUP 2	FETOSCOPICALLY RELEASED
Knee	128.8 ± 5.4	110 ± 14.7	126.2 ± 5.5	140 ± 10.6
Ankle	150 ± 8.2	127 ± 17	78.7 ± 26*	151 ± 13.5†
Phalangeal	99.6 ± 2.1	94 ± 8	60 ± 17*	99 ± 4†

* $p < 0.003$ versus control.
† $p < 0.03$ versus group 2.

the more tightly the band is applied, the greater the likelihood of infarction and autoamputation later in gestation.

Clinical Experience with Fetoscopic Release of Amniotic Bands

Indications for fetal surgery are, with few exceptions, only for life-threatening conditions such as cystic adenomatoid malformation of the lung with hydrops, diaphragmatic hernia with a low lung/head circumference ratio, bladder outlet obstruction with oligohydramnios, or sacrococcygeal teratoma with placentomegaly (see Chapters 18, 19, 20, and 21). However, as experience with the techniques of fetal surgery has grown and the natural histories of certain non–life-threatening conditions have been better defined, the indications for fetal surgery have been extended. Two examples of this are in utero repair of meningomyelocele to prevent the devastating neurologic injury to the spinal cord[63] and fetoscopic cord ligation in monochorionic twins with imminent co-twin demise to prevent neurologic injury in the surviving twin.[64] The indications for fetal surgery in the amniotic band syndrome may be either for a life-threatening condition if it involves constriction of the umbilical cord or, more commonly, threatened limb amputation in constrictive extremity ABS.[7, 39, 40, 45, 65]

Torpin reported 36 cases of fetal demise due to cord constriction from amniotic bands.[7] In each case the diagnosis was made retrospectively, however. Recognition of amniotic bands constricting the umbilical cord was recently reported by Kanayama et al., who were able to document fetal compromise by reversal of diastolic flow in the umbilical artery by color Doppler.[65] Graf similarly reported a case of amniotic bands involving the umbilical cord following the development of chorioamniotic separation.[45] Despite initially normal umbilical artery Doppler waveforms, this fetus died within 2 weeks from a constrictive amniotic band of the umbilical cord. It is in cases like those reported by Graf and Kanayama that fetoscopic lysis of amniotic bands could be lifesaving.

Based on their experience with fetoscopy for cord ligation in TRAP sequence[66] and the experimental work by Crombleholme et al.[58] demonstrating the potential for functional recovery of banded extremities once released,

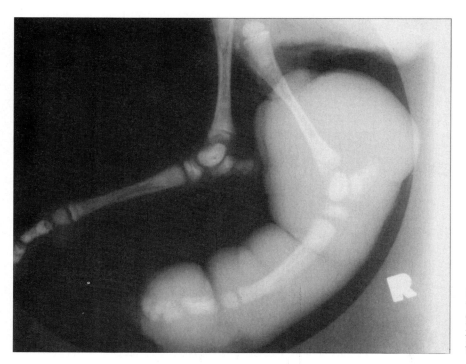

F I G U R E 32–11. Plain radiograph of the extremity of a newborn lamb that underwent banding at 100 days' gestation and that was followed to term demonstrating marked abnormal bowing and demineralization of the bones of the banded extremity.

Quintero et al., performed the first fetoscopic lysis of amniotic bands in human fetuses.[67] Their first case was a fetus at 21 weeks' gestation with bilateral cleft lip and bands attached to the face and left upper extremity with distal limb edema. In order to avert limb amputation, fetoscopic lysis of bands was attempted at 22 weeks' gestation using a two-port technique. However, due to bleeding encountered upon insertion of the second operating port it was removed. The endoscissors were passed through the port used for the fetoscope and the lysis performed with ultrasound guidance. There was resolution of the distal edema within 6 days of the procedure. At 32 weeks' gestation microphthalmia and anophthalmia of the right orbit were first noted at the site of the previously attached amniotic band. The patient delivered at 39 weeks' gestation and was found to have a Tessier type 4 craniofacial cleft and right microphthalmia. The extremity showed minimal residual scarring where the band had been attached and lysed. The hand had radial paresis and mild hypoplasia.

The second case was a fetus at 23 weeks' gestation with a thick amniotic band constricting the left ankle of the fetus. There was marked edema distal to the band, and minimal blood flow to the foot was observed by color and pulsed Doppler. Fetoscopy was performed using a 2.7-mm 5-degree endoscope confirming the sonographic findings. Again bleeding was encountered upon insertion of the operating port, necessitating its removal. Attempts at ultrasound-guided lysis using endoscissors were unsuccessful. A 2.4-mm 0-degree operating scope with a 400-μm contact yttrium-aluminium-garnet (YAG) laser fiber was used to lyse approximately 85% of the band. Complete lysis of the band was not achieved for fear of injury to "important elements in the ankle." Postoperatively the edema markedly improved, as did distal arterial blood flow, and there was return of flexion and extension on follow-up ultrasounds. The mother was hospitalized 8 weeks postoperatively at 31 weeks' gestation with premature rupture of membranes and delivered at 34.5 weeks of gestation. The infant underwent Z-plasties for residual effects of the amniotic band and full functional recovery is anticipated.

The rationale for performing fetoscopic lysis of constricting extremity amniotic bands is based on the natural history that progressive compromise with fetal growth leads to amputation. However, this assumes that the procedure can be accomplished with no maternal morbidity and minimal fetal morbidity. This procedure would be hard to justify in the face of a serious maternal complication or a fetal death due to severely premature delivery at 21 or 23 weeks' gestation even in the face of certain fetal limb amputation. While these two cases demonstrate the feasibility of fetoscopic lysis of amniotic bands, limiting application of these techniques to cases of umbilical cord constriction would be on more solid ground given the potential risks to mother and fetus.

Conclusions

While extremity ABS may have devastating morphologic and functional effects on a limb, possibly resulting in amputation, it is not lethal. Extremity ABS would not be an indication for fetoscopic surgery unless maternal risks and incidence of preterm labor could be markedly reduced from those seen now with open fetal surgery. However, there are forms of ABS that are lethal or have devastating neurologic sequelae, which may justify the current risks of intervention. Torpin has reported 36 cases of constrictive amniotic bands of the umbilical cord, which is uniformly fatal.[8] Although more rare than other forms of ABS, umbilical cord constriction once diagnosed sonographically may be amenable to fetoscopic release to avert fetal demise.

ABS is a relatively common, if underappreciated, cause of fetal and neonatal morbidity and mortality. The fetal lamb model of ABS will be useful to better define the pathophysiology of ABS, and to provide a tool to understand the unique fetal response to tissue injury, repair, and regeneration. Sonographic identification of ABS affecting the umbilical cord may be an indication for fetoscopic surgical intervention. In the future, intervention for nonlethal limb deformation may also be considered if maternal risk is sufficiently lowered. ABS is another in a growing list of conditions for which fetal surgery may be considered.

REFERENCES

1. Higginbottom MC, Jones KL: The amniotic band disruption complex. Timing of amniotic rupture and variable spectra of consequent defects. J Pediatr 96:544–549, 1979.
2. Seeds JW, Cefalo RC, Herbert WNP: ABS. Am J Obstet Gynecol 144:243–248, 1982.
3. Ray M, Hendrick SJ, Raimer SS, et al: ABS. Int J Dermatol 27:312–314, 1988.
4. Lockwood C, Ghidini A, Romero R, et al: Amniotic band syndrome: Reevaluation of its pathogenesis. Am J Obstet Gynecol 160:1030–1033, 1989.
5. Seidman JD, Abbonddanzo SL, Watkin WG, et al: Amniotic band syndrome: A report of two cases and a review of the literature. Arch Pathol Lab Med 113:891–897, 1989.
6. Kulkarni ML, Gopal PV: Amniotic band syndrome. Indian Pediatr 27:471–476, 1990.
7. Torpin R: Amniochorionic mesoblastic fibrous strings and amniotic bands. Am J Obstet Gynecol 91:65–75, 1965.
8. Torpin R: Fetal Malformations Caused by Amnion Rupture During Gestation. Springfield, IL: Charles C Thomas, 1968, pp 1–42.
9. Jones KL, Smith DW, Hall BD, et al: A pattern of craniofacial and limb defects secondary to aberrant tissue bands. J Pediatr 84:90–95, 1974.
10. Keller H, Neuhauser G, Durkin-Stamm MV, et al: "ADAM complex" (amniotic deformity, adhesions, mutilations): A pattern of craniofacial and limb defects. Am J Med Genet 2:81–98, 1978.
11. Herva R, Karkinen-Jaaskelainen M: Amniotic adhesion malformation syndrome: Fetal and placental pathology. Teratology 29:11–19, 1984.
12. Bamforth JS: Amniotic band sequence: Streeter's hypothesis reexamined. Am J Med Genet 44:280–287, 1992.
13. Ho DM, Liu HC: The ABS: Report of two autopsy cases and review of the literature. Clin Med J 39:429–436, 1987.
14. Lubinsky M, Sujansky E, Sanders W, et al: Familial amniotic bands. Am J Med Genet 14:81–87, 1983.
15. Huang CC, Eng HL, Chen WJ: Amniotic band syndrome: Report of two autopsy cases. Chang Gung Med J 18(4):371–377, 1995.
16. Streeter GL: Focal deficiencies in fetal tissues and their relation to intrauterine amputations. Contrib Embryol Carnegie Inst 22:1–44, 1930.
17. Lage JM, VanMarter LJ, Bieber FR: Questionable role of amniocentesis in the etiology of amniotic band formation: A case report. J Reprod Med 33:71–73, 1988.

18. Young ID, Lindenbaum RH, Thompson EM, et al: Amniotic bands in connective tissue disorders. Arch Dis Child 60:1061–1063, 1985.

19. Chemke J, Gaff G, Hurwitz N, et al: The amniotic band syndrome. Obstet Gynecol 41:332–336, 1973.

20. Daly CA, Freeman J, Weston W, et al: Prenatal diagnosis of ABS in a methadone user: Review of the literature and a case report. Ultrasound Obstet Gynecol 8:123–125, 1996.

21. Moerman P, Fryns JP, Vandenberghe K, et al: Constrictive amniotic bands, amniotic adhesions, and limb-body wall complex: Discrete disruption sequence with pathogenetic overlap. Am J Med Genet 42:470–479, 1992.

22. Hong CY, Simon MA: Amniotic bands knotted about umbilical cord: A rare cause of fetal death. Obstet Gynecol 22:667–670, 1963.

23. Van Allen MI, Curry C, Gallagher L: Limb body wall complex: I. Pathogenesis. Am J Med Genet 28:529–548, 1987.

24. Miller ME, Graham JM Jr, Higginbottom MC, et al: Compression-related defects from early amnion rupture: Evidence for mechanical teratogenesis. J Pediatr 98:292–297, 1981.

25. Ossipoff V, Hall BD: Etiologic factors in the ABS: A study of twenty-four patients. Birth Defects 13:117–121, 1977.

26. Burrows PE, Lyons EA, Phillips HJ, et al: Intrauterine membranes: Sonographic findings and clinical significance. J Ultrasound 10:1–8, 1982.

27. Patten RM, Van Allen M, Mack LA, et al: Limb body wall complex: In utero sonographic diagnosis of a complicated fetal malformation. AJR Am J Roentgenol 146:1019–1022, 1986.

28. Sauerbrei E, Cooperberg PL, Poland BJ: Ultrasound demonstration of the normal fetal yolk sac. J Clin Ultrasound 8:217–220, 1980.

29. Spirit BA, Kagan EH, Rozanski RM: Abruptio placenta: Sonographic and pathologic correlation. AJR Am J Roentgenol 133:877–881, 1979.

30. Filly RA, Golbus MS: The fetus with amniotic band syndrome. In Harrison MR, Golbus MS, Filly RA (eds): The Unborn Patient, 2nd ed. Philadelphia: WB Saunders Company, 1991, pp 440–447.

31. Comninos AC, Zourlas PA: Treatment of intrauterine adhesions (Asherman's syndrome). Am J Obstet Gynecol 105:862–867, 1969.

32. Asherman JG: Amenorrhoea traumatic. Br J Obstet Gynaecol 55:23–27, 1948.

33. Mahoney BS, Filly RA, Callen PW, et al: The amniotic band syndrome: Antenatal diagnosis and potential pitfalls. Am J Obstet Gynecol 152:63–68, 1985.

34. Randel SB, Filly RA, Callen PW, et al: Amniotic sheets. Radiology 166:633–636, 1988.

35. Hill L, Kislak S, Jones N: Prenatal ultrasound diagnosis of a forearm constrictive band. J Ultrasound Med 7:293–295, 1988.

36. Moessinger AC, Blanc WA, Byrne J: Amniotic band syndrome associated with amniocentesis. Am J Obstet Gynecol 141:588–592, 1981.

37. Rehder H, Weitzel H: Intrauterine amputations after amniocentesis. Lancet 1: 382–383, 1987.

38. Ashkenazy M, Borenstein R, Katz Z: Constriction of the umbilical cord by an amniotic band after midtrimester amniocentesis. Acta Obstet Gynecol Scand 61:89–91, 1982.

39. Tadmor OP, Kreisberg GA, Achiron R, et al: Limb amputation in amniotic band syndrome: Serial ultrasonographic and Doppler observations. Ultrasound Obstet Gynecol 10:312–315, 1997.

40. Takenori N, Ryosuke N: Amniotic band syndrome: Serial ultrasonographic observations in the first trimester. J Clin Ultrasound 22:275–278, 1994.

41. Laberge LC, Ruszkowski A, Morin F: Amniotic band attachment to a fetal limb: Demonstration with real-time sonography. Ann Plast Surg 35:316–319, 1995.

42. Burrows PE, Lyons EA, Phillips HJ, et al: Intrauterine membranes: Sonographic findings and clinical significance. J Clin Ultrasound 10:1–8, 1982.

43. Kaufman AJ, Fleischer AC, Thieme GA, et al: Separated chorioamnion and elevated chorion: Sonographic features and clinical significance. J Ultrasound Med 4:119–125, 1985.

44. Borlum KG: Second trimester chorioamniotic separation and amniocentesis. Eur J Obstet Gynecol Reprod Biol 30:35–38, 1989.

45. Graf JL, Bealer JF, Gibbs DL, et al: Chorioamniotic membrane separation: A potentially lethal finding. Fetal Diagn Ther 12:81–84, 1987.

46. Heifetz SA: Strangulation of the umbilical cord by amniotic bands. Pediatr Pathol 2:285–304, 1984.

47. Hall EJ, Johnson-Giebink R, Vasconez LO: Management of ring-constriction syndrome. Plast Reconstr Surg 69:532–538, 1982.

48. Patterson TJS: Congenital ring-constriction. Br J Plast Surg 14:1–5, 1961.

49. Kalousek P: Amniotic band syndrome in pre-viable fetuses. Pediatr Pathol 7:488–492, 1987.

50. DeMyer W, Baird O: Mortality and skeletal malformations from amniocentesis and oligohydramnios in rats: Cleft palate, club foot, microstomia, and adactyly. Teratology 2:33–37, 1969.

51. Love AM, Vickers TH: Amniocentesis dysmelia in rats. J Exp Pathol 53:435–444, 1972.

52. Poswillo D, Sopher D: Malformation and deformation of the animal embryo. Teratology 4:498–502, 1971.

53. Trasler DG, Walker BE, Fraser FC: Congenital malformations produced by amniotic-sac puncture. Science 124:439–440, 1956.

54. Kino Y: Clinical and experimental studies of the congenital constriction band syndrome with emphasis on its etiology. J Bone Joint Surg 57A:636–643, 1975.

55. Clavert JM, Clavert A, Issa WN, et al: Experimental approach to the pathogenesis of the anomalies of amniotic disease. J Pediatr Surg 15:63–67, 1980.

56. Rowsell AR: The amniotic band disruption complex: The pathogenesis of oblique facial clefts; an experimental study in the fetal rat. Br J Plast Surg 42:291–295, 1989.

57. Rowsell AR: The amniotic band disruption complex: The pathogenesis of congenital ring-constrictions; an experimental study in the fetal rat. Br J Plast Surg 41:45–51, 1988.

58. Crombleholme TM, Dirkes K, Whitney TM, et al: Amniotic band syndrome in fetal lambs I: Fetoscopic release and morphometric outcome. J Pediatr Surg 30(7):974–978, 1995.

59. Heden PG, Hamilton R, Arnander C, et al: Laser Doppler surveillance of the circulation of free flaps and replanted digits. Microsurgery 6:11–19, 1985.

60. Luks FI, DePrest J, Marcus M, et al: Carbon dioxide pneumoamnios causes fetal acidosis. Fetal Diagn Ther 9:105–109, 1994.

61. Burton DJ, Filly RA: Sonographic diagnosis of the amniotic band syndrome. AJR Am J Roentgenol 156:555–558, 1991.

62. Adzick NS, Lorenz HP: Cells, matrix, growth factors, and the surgeon. The biology of fetal wound repair. Ann Surg 220:10–18, 1994.

63. Adzick NS, Sutton LN, Crombleholme TM, et al: Successful fetal surgery for spina bifida. Lancet 350:1675–1676, 1998.

64. Crombleholme TM, Robertson FM, Marx G, et al: Fetoscopic cord ligation to prevent neurologic injury in monozygous twins. Lancet 348:191, 1996.

65. Kanayama MD, Gaffey TA, Ogburn PL Jr: Constriction of the umbilical cord by an amniotic band, with fetal compromise illustrated by reverse diastolic flow in the umbilical artery. A case report. J Med 40:71–73, 1995.

66. Quintero RA, Reich H, Puder K, et al: Umbilical cord ligation of an acardiac twin by fetoscopy at 19 weeks of gestation. N Engl J Med 330:469–471, 1994.

67. Quintero RA, Morales WJ, Phillips J, et al: In utero lysis of amniotic bands. Ultrasound Obstet Gynecol 10:316–320, 1997.

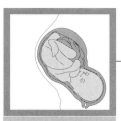

P A R T   IV

Fetal Metabolic and Cellular Defects Amenable to Treatment: The Art of Fetal Treatment

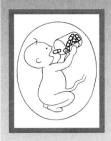

CHAPTER 33

The Fetus with a Biochemical Disorder

MARK I. EVANS

Over the past 15 years there have been tremendous strides in the prenatal treatment of a number of fetal abnormalities. In general, structural problems such as diaphragmatic hernia, urethral obstructions, and pleural effusion have lent themselves to surgical approaches, whereas metabolic disorders such as congenital adrenal hyperplasia and cardiac arrhythmias have responded to pharmacologic interventions.[1, 2] This chapter will focus on the fetus with a metabolic defect for which pharmacologic therapy is possible. Some of these follow mendelian inheritance, and others are polygenic/multifactorial. Some of these disorders may ultimately be best treated by genetic approaches, which are described in another chapter. Others are often purely physiologic, such as the cardiac arrhythmias, and are likewise described elsewhere.

For decades, drugs and other agents have also been administered to pregnant women for treatment of fetal disorders not usually classified as metabolic in the hope of improving the capacity for postnatal adaptation. Well-known examples include exchange transfusions in Rh disease, the administration of corticosteroids for the prevention of respiratory distress syndrome in premature infants, and the administration of phenobarbital prior to birth in the hope of inducing liver enzymes for postnatal reduction of serum bilirubin concentration. However, there are only a very few examples of attempted prenatal treatment for genetically determined metabolic defects (Table 33–1).

Endocrine Disorders

Congenital Adrenal Hyperplasia

Congenital adrenal hyperplasia (CAH) is the best described and most clearly successful example of pharmacologic prevention of fetal pathophysiology to prevent a birth defect. CAH comprises a group of autosomal recessive disorders characterized by a deficiency in one or more of the enzymes required for adrenal cortisol biosynthesis. There are several different levels of CAH phenotype, which have different degrees of pathophysiology and clinical implications (Table 33–2). The most common abnormality, responsible for more than 90% of patients with CAH, is caused by a deficiency of the enzyme 21-hydroxylase (21-OH), also known as p450c21, which results in defective transportation of cholesterol across mitochondrial membranes.[3–5] Other, less common, causes for CAH include enzyme deficiencies in 11α-hydroxylase, 17β-hydroxylase, p450scc deficiency, and 3β-OH-dehydrogenase. Diminished 21-OH activity results in accumulation of 17-hydroxyprogesterone (17-OHP) due to a decrease in its conversion to 11-deoxycorticosterone. The excess 17-OHP is then converted via androstenedione to androgens, the levels of which increase by as much as several-hundredfold (Fig. 33–1). The excess androgens cause masculinization of the undifferentiated female external genitalia. The degree of masculinization may vary from clitoral hypertrophy to complete formation of a phallus and scrotum. By contrast, genital formation in male fetuses is normal, but signs of androgen excess develop in childhood, and may manifest in precocious masculinization and accelerated growth and development. The "classic" form of CAH involves an almost complete block of enzyme activity and is clinically present at birth. The "nonclassic" form involves only partial blockade of the enzymatic activity and is usually clinically apparent only later in life. 21-OH deficiency is inherited as an autosomal recessive trait in close linkage to the HLA major histocompatibility complex on the short arm of chromosome 6.[6] The gene for 21-OH (CYP21B) has been mapped, allowing direct mutation analysis in informative families.[7]

Historically, in the late 1970s and early 1980s, diagnosis of CAH was made on amniocentesis by the finding of elevated levels of 17-OHP in the supernatant. With the development of chorionic villus sampling (CVS) in the 1980s, linkage-based diagnosis in the first trimester became available. Since discovery and mapping of the allelic variants in the 1980s, direct DNA analysis has become the routine approach. In addition, the sonographic detection of an abnormally enlarged phallus should alert the physician to investigate for CAH.[8]

The fetal adrenal gland can be pharmacologically suppressed by maternal replacement doses of dexametha-

TABLE 33–1. PHARMACOLOGIC FETAL THERAPIES

Congenital adrenal hyperplasia
Cardiac arrhythmias
Multiple carboxylase deficiency
Methylmalonic aciduria
Hypothyroidism
Hyperthyroidism
Smith-Lemli-Opitz syndrome
Neural tube defects

TABLE 33–2. CAH SPECTRUM OF SEVERITY

	NONCLASSIC	CLASSIC	
	Excess Androgen	Clitoral Hypertrophy	Virilized
Phenotype Classification		Non–salt wasting	Salt wasting
Mutation	Mild	Moderate → severe	Null

CAH, congenital adrenal hyperplasia.

sone.[9] In the first attempt to prevent female genital birth defects, Evans et al. in 1982 administered dexamethasone at a dose of 0.25 mg qid to a mother known to be at-risk for CAH, beginning at 10 weeks of gestation.[9] Serial maternal estriol and cortisol levels indicated that adrenal gland suppression had been achieved. The fetus, ultimately found to be a compound heterozygote, was born at 39 weeks' gestation with normal external genitalia. Forrest and David then employed a similar protocol beginning at 9 weeks' gestation to treat several fetuses known to be at risk for CAH.[10] Subsequently, those female fetuses confirmed to be clinically affected with the severe form of CAH were spared masculinization of the external genitalia. Several hundred pregnant women and their fetuses have been treated, with masculinization prevented in the vast majority.

Since the differentiation of the external genitalia begins at about 7 weeks' gestation, diagnosis by amniocentesis or even CVS comes far too late to prevent masculinization. Thus for patients at risk of having an affected fetus, pharmacologic therapy has to be initiated prior to diagnosis. This implies that therapy needs to be administered to all patients at risk despite the fact that the chance of an affected female fetus for carrier parents is only 1 in 8 (i.e., ¼ affected × ½ female). Direct DNA diagnosis or linkage studies may then be performed by CVS in the first trimester. Thus, for seven out of eight patients, therapy can be discontinued as soon as the diagnosis of male sex or CAH is ruled out. If the fetus is indeed found to be an affected female, then therapy

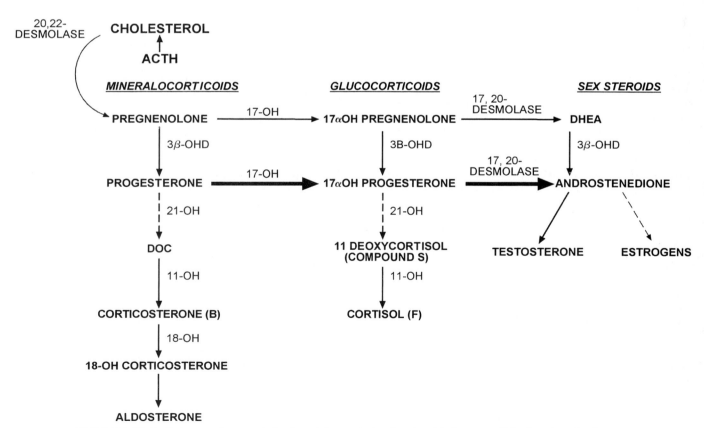

FIGURE 33–1. Pathway of congenital adrenal hyperplasia showing blockage at 21-hydroxylase leading to excess androgens.

is continued throughout gestation. Stress-dose corticosteroids should be given to the mother during labor and tapered gradually postpartum. If, however, the fetus is a male or is unaffected, then therapy can be discontinued at the time of diagnosis.

To date, dozens of infants who have inherited the classic CAH mutation, and who clearly would have been masculinized, have been born with normal genitalia. In a few cases, some masculinization has still been observed following this regimen beginning at 9 weeks. Our current protocol, therefore, is to begin at 7 weeks, although there have been too few cases to assess this modification.[11, 12] These events represent the first prevention of a birth defect and serve as the prototype for other attempts at pharmacologic fetal therapy.

Although this therapy is widely accepted, it is still considered experimental by some, especially insurance companies. A recently published commentary written in the *Journal of the American Medical Association* advocates IRB approval be obtained on all patients offered this treatment. As long-term follow-up has not been documented on individuals who received in utero steroid treatment for CAH, a registry has been proposed by the Lawson Wilkins Pediatric Endocrine Society for studies in North America.[13] This should help to assess the long-term outcome of fetuses exposed to high-dose steroids.

Hyperthyroidism

Neonatal hyperthyroidism is rare, with an incidence of 1 in 4,000 to 40,000 live births.[14] Fetal thyrotoxic goiter is usually secondary to maternal autoimmune disease, principally Graves disease or Hashimoto thyroiditis. As many as 12% of infants of mothers with a known history of Graves disease are affected with neonatal thyrotoxicosis, which may even occur despite the fact that the mother may be euthyroid.[15] As with hypothyroidism, inherent to the underlying mechanism is the transplacental passage of maternal immunoglobulin G (IgG) antibodies. In this case, the antibodies, known as TSAb (or TSI), are predominantly directed against the TSH receptor.

Usually, the investigation of fetal hyperthyroidism begins only after the discovery of fetal goiter. Often, the goiter is diagnosed on ultrasound in patients referred due to elevated thyroid-stimulating antibodies. In some cases, fetal goiters are realized serendipitously on routine ultrasonography. Others may be discovered in patients referred for scan because fundal height measures greater than expected by gestational age. In these cases there is often polyhydramnios as a result of the goiter. Once a fetal goiter is identified, biochemical evaluation is indicated. Historically, amniotic fluid levels of TSH and free thyroxine (FT_4) were used as potential indicators of fetal thyroid function. These, however, proved inconsistent in that amniotic fluid levels of these hormones do not always correlate with their serum levels. Some controversy still exists regarding their use; however, they may be of some benefit in centers that do not have cordocentesis available.[16] With the advent of cordocentesis, fetal thyroid status can be reliably documented[17, 18]; treatment can be planned according to the fetal blood results.

Once the diagnosis of fetal hyperthyroidism is confirmed, fetal treatment should be initiated. Authors have attempted treating fetal hyperthyroidism with maternally administered antithyroid drugs. Porreco has reported maternal treatment of fetal thyrotoxicosis with propylthiouracil (PTU), which led to a good outcome.[19] The initial dose used was 100 mg PO three times a day, which was later decreased to 50 mg PO three times a day. Wenstrom et al. described a favorable outcome using maternal methimazole to treat fetal hyperthyroidism in a patient who could not tolerate PTU.[20] Hatjis also treated fetal goitrous hyperthyroidism with a maternal dose of 300 mg PTU. This patient, however, required supplemental synthroid to remain euthyroid. There was good fetal outcome in this case as well.[21]

Hypothyroidism

Fetal hypothyroidism may have severe fetal and neonatal consequences. Fetal esophageal obstruction secondary to a goiter can lead to polyhydramnios, and may result in preterm delivery. Furthermore, a fetal goiter can cause extension of the fetal neck, leading to dystocia. The effects of hypothyroidism can be devastating. Without treatment, postnatal growth delay and severe mental retardation can ensue. Even with immediate diagnosis and treatment at birth, long-term follow-up of children with congenital hypothyroidism has shown them to have lower scores on perceptual-motor, visuospatial, and language tests.[22]

Maternal hyperthyroidism is often associated with fetal hypothyroidism. This may be secondary to the suppression of the fetal thyroid by maternally administered PTU. Conversely, fetal hypothyroidism may also result from transplacental passage of maternal blocking antibodies. These antibodies, known as TB1Ab or TBII, block thyroid-stimulating hormone (TSH) binding. Occasionally, fetal hypothyroidism is the result of inadvertent use of iodine-131 (^{131}I) in pregnant women, maternal ingestion of amiodarone or lithium, or excessive maternal iodine intake, sometimes in the form of vaginal douching. Fetal hypothyroidism caused by an intrinsic fetal abnormality is uncommon, occurring in 1 in 4,000 to 5,000 births.[23] The most common form of such permanent hypothyroidism in infants is thyroid dysgenesis. This may include hypoplastic and ectopic thyroid, or the total absence of thyroid tissue (athyreosis), which is associated with undetectable levels of thyroglobulin. Congenital hypothyroidism is only rarely associated with errors of thyroid hormone synthesis, TSH insensitivity, or absence of the pituitary gland.

Inquiry regarding a history of maternal hypothyroidism is considered as routine. In patients with this history, routine maternal thyroid hormone levels as well as blocking immunoglobulin levels should be measured. In addition, all women with a history of any thyroid disease (both hypothyroidism and hyperthyroidism) are advised to have monthly fetal ultrasound to screen for goiter, polyhydramnios, or fetal tachycardia.[17]

Fetal goitrous hypothyroidism is initially identified by ultrasound. Most commonly, the indication for the ultrasonographic scan is a fundal height greater than expected by gestational age. In such cases the increased uterine size is caused by polyhydramnios, resulting from esophageal obstruction and impaired swallowing. Sometimes, a fetal goiter is incidentally discovered on a routine scan. Finally, some cases are diagnosed on serial scans in fetuses with either known elevated maternal thyroid immunoglobulins or maternal treatment with antithyroid medications. Before the advent of cordocentesis, amniotic fluid levels of TSH and FT$_4$ were used as potential indicators of fetal thyroid function; however, these proved inconsistent.[16] With cordocentesis, fetal thyroid status can be directly and accurately evaluated; fetal response to therapy can therefore be reliably measured using available nomograms.[17, 18] Fetal hypothyroidism is diagnosed by measuring fetal serum levels of free T$_4$, total T$_4$, free T$_3$, total T$_3$, and TSH.

In utero treatment was initially suggested by Van Herle et al. using intramuscular (IM) injection of levothyroxine sodium.[24] Subsequent studies, however, have indicated that intra-amniotic (IA) administration of thyroxine is superior. The doses commonly used for treatment range from 200 to 500 mg IA every week.[25] More recently, it has been recommended that the dosage be adjusted for the fetal weight using 10 mg/kg, similar to the recommended dose for neonates.[26] With this regimen, fetal goiters have been shown to regress, and fetal and newborn TSH levels have normalized.

Inborn Errors of Metabolism

Methylmalonic Acidemia

Methylmalonic acidemia is related to a functional vitamin B$_{12}$ deficiency. Coenzymatically active B$_{12}$ is required for the conversion of methylmalonyl-coenzyme A to succinyl-coenzyme A. Several genetically determined etiologies for methylmalonic acidemia include defects in methylmalonyl-coenzyme A mutase or in the metabolism of vitamin B$_{12}$, to the coenzymatically active form, adenosylcobalamin by the converting enzyme. Some patients may respond to administration of large doses of B$_{12}$, which can enhance the amount of active holoenzyme (mutase apoenzyme plus adenosylcobalamin) (Fig. 33–2).

More than 20 years ago, Ampola et al. first attempted prenatal diagnosis and treatment of a B$_{12}$-responsive variant of methylmalonic acidemia.[27] They followed the pregnancy of a patient who had previously suffered the loss of a child to severe acidosis and dehydration at the age of 3 months. The diagnosis of methylmalonic acidemia was only made posthumously by chemical analysis of blood and urine. In the pregnancy they followed, an amniocentesis was performed at 19 weeks' gestation. An elevated methylmalonic acid content was documented in the cell-free amniotic fluid. Cultured amniotic fluid cells had defective propionate oxidation and undetectable levels of adenosylcobalamin, but there was normal succinate oxidation and methylmalonyl-coenzyme A mutase activity in the presence of added adenosylcobalamin. These studies established by ap-

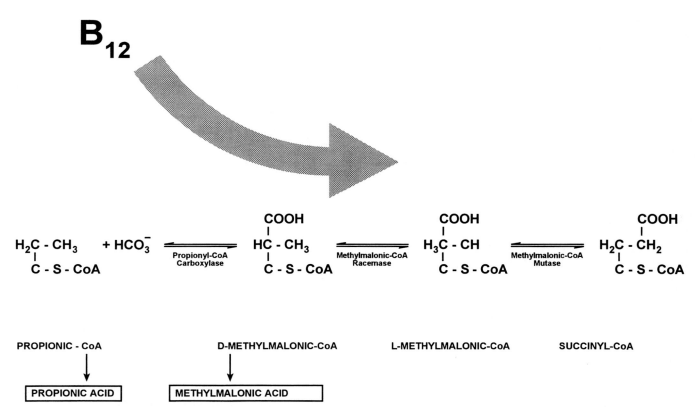

FIGURE 33–2. Pathway of methylmalonic aciduria showing reaction driven by excess B$_{12}$.

proximately 23 weeks' gestation that the fetus suffered from methylmalonic acidemia seemingly due to deficient synthesis of adenosylcobalamin.

It was already known that fetal methylmalonic acidemia is associated with increased methylmalonic acid excretion in maternal urine. Ampola and colleagues documented increased methylmalonic acidemia in a maternal urine sample first collected at 23 weeks' gestation[27]; the methylmalonic acid excretion per milligram of creatinine was approximately twice the upper normal limit and demonstrated a further rise by 25 weeks. Urinary methylmalonate excretion is not abnormal in heterozygous females carrying a normal fetus, as shown subsequently by these same investigators.

Very late in pregnancy, cyanocobalamin (10 mg/day) was orally administered to the mother in divided doses. The treatment only marginally altered the maternal serum B_{12} level; however, there was a slight reduction of urinary methylmalonic acid excretion that remained severalfold above normal. At approximately 34 weeks' gestation, 5 mg of cyanocobalamin per day intramuscularly was begun. The maternal serum B_{12} level then rose gradually to more than sixfold above normal and was accompanied by a progressive decrease in urinary methylmalonic acid excretion. Maternal urinary methylmalonate was only slightly above the normal range when delivery occurred at 41 menstrual weeks. Amniotic fluid methylmalonic acid concentrations were three times the normal mean at 19 menstrual weeks and four times the normal mean at term, despite prenatal treatment.

Postnatally, the diagnosis of methylmalonic acidemia was confirmed. The infant suffered no acute neonatal complications and had an extremely high serum B_{12} level. Long-term postnatal management involved protein restriction; however, no continuous B_{12} treatment was required.

In this instance, prenatal treatment certainly improved the fetal and, secondarily, the maternal biochemistry. Whether there was any significant clinical benefit to the fetus by in utero treatment cannot be assessed adequately. It seems likely that reducing the fetal burden of methylmalonic acid should have some beneficial effect on fetal development and could reduce the risks in the neonatal period; however, this is only speculation.

Evans et al. have documented the changing dose requirements necessary over the course of pregnancy to maintain adequate levels of B_{12}. They sequentially followed maternal plasma and urine levels in a prenatally treated pregnancy.[28] Data such as these suggest that modulation of maternal-fetal pharmacologic interchange of therapeutic drugs will be difficult to precisely control.

Multiple Carboxylase Deficiency

Biotin-responsive multiple carboxylase deficiency is an inborn error of metabolism in which the mitochondrial biotin-dependent enzymes, pyruvate carboxylase, propionyl-coenzyme A carboxylase, and α-methylcrotonyl-coenzyme A carboxylase have diminished activity (Fig. 33–2). Affected patients present as newborns or in the early childhood period with dermatitis, severe

metabolic acidosis, and a characteristic pattern of organic acid excretion. Metabolism in patients or in their cultured cells can be restored toward normal levels by biotin supplementation. There have been two reports of prenatal administration of biotin to fetuses affected with this disorder.

Roth and colleagues treated a fetus without the benefit of prenatal diagnosis in a case in which two siblings of the fetus had died of multiple carboxylase deficiency.[29] The first sibling had died within 3 days of birth, and in the second the diagnosis of biotin-responsive carboxylase deficiency was made posthumously.

The patient was first seen at 34 weeks' gestation. Prenatal diagnosis was not attempted because of the late stage of pregnancy. The maternal urinary organic acid profile was normal throughout the final 4 weeks of pregnancy. Because of severe neonatal manifestations in the previous siblings and the probable harmlessness of biotin, oral administration of this compound to the mother was begun at a dose of 10 mg/day. There were no apparent untoward effects; maternal urinary biotin excretion increased by a factor of approximately 100 during biotin administration.

Nonidentical twins were subsequently delivered at term. Cord blood and urinary organic acid profiles were normal, and cord blood biotin concentrations were four to seven times greater than normal. The neonatal course for both twins was unremarkable. Subsequent study of the cultured fibroblasts of both twins compared under biotin-rich and biotin-depleted growth conditions indicated that in biotin-depleted medium, the cells of twin B (but not of twin A) had virtually complete deficiency of all three carboxylase activities. Genetic complementation studies confirmed that despite the normal clinical presentation during the newborn period, twin B was homozygous for the disease mutation.

Packman and colleagues have also reported prenatal diagnosis and treatment of biotin-responsive multiple carboxylase deficiency for a mother who had previously given birth to a male with the neonatal-onset form of this disease.[30] In the next pregnancy, maternal urine organic acid profiles were normal. The three carboxylase activities were assayed in cultured amniotic fluid cells obtained by amniocentesis at 17 menstrual weeks. In biotin-restricted medium, the amniotic cells demonstrated the characteristic severe reduction in carboxylase activities.

The preceding two cases provide compelling evidence that biotin administration effectively prevents neonatal complications in certain patients with biotin-responsive multiple carboxylase deficiency. No toxicity from treatment was observed. At this time, it is not possible to assess definitively the relative advantages or disadvantages of prenatal treatment, although such therapy appears both effective and logical.

Smith-Lemli-Opitz Syndrome

Smith-Lemli-Opitz syndrome (SLOS) was first reported in 1964.[31] The reported incidence is approximately 1 in 20,000, established from patients that have been clinically diagnosed. The true incidence may be different now that a biochemical test is available to confirm the diagnosis. In 1993, an inborn error of cholesterol biosynthesis in a patient with SLOS was confirmed to be a deficiency of the enzyme 7-dehydrocholesterol (7-DHC) reductase in a liver specimen.[32-34]

Characteristic features include facial phenotype; growth and mental retardation; and anomalies of the heart, kidneys, central nervous system, and limbs. Cleft palate, postaxial polydactyly, syndactyly of the second and third toes, and cataracts are often seen in affected patients. The syndactyly of the second and third toes is very specific for this disorder and is seen in more than 90% of affected patients. The facial phenotype is absolutely characteristic of the syndrome. Affected patients typically present with a narrow forehead, ptosis, anteverted nares, low-set ears, and micrognathia.

The ambiguous genitalia seen in SLOS are the opposite of CAH. Patients with SLOS are deficient in cholesterol, and therefore also most likely have low levels of steroid hormones, which are necessary for masculinization of male genitalia. Therefore, the ambiguous genitalia that one sees in SLOS is the result of undermasculinization of male genitalia.

The biochemical defect in SLOS comes from X deficiency of 7-DHC reductase. This enzyme is responsible for the conversion of 7-DHC to cholesterol in the last step of cholesterol biosynthesis. This enzyme deficiency results in the characteristic biochemical pattern of low cholesterol and elevated 7-DHC and 8-dehydrocholesterol (8-DHC), its isomer, seen in affected patients. This pattern of decreased cholesterol and elevated 7-DHC and 8-DHC can be seen in multiple compartments from affected patients. These specimens include plasma, red cells, tissues (including brain and cataracts), fibroblasts, amniotic fluid, and chorionic villus. The diagnosis can even be made retrospectively in fixed tissue in paraffin blocks.

The exact values seen in affected patients are extremely variable. The diagnosis is made primarily by the presence of the cholesterol precursor, 7-DHC, and not by the deficiency of cholesterol. The level of 7-DHC in affected patients is 100 to 1,000 times normal. Unaffected individuals have levels of 7-DHC and 8-DHC of less than 1 mg/dL. Patients with SLOS have levels of 7 to 20 or greater. Clinical manifestations correlate with cholesterol levels. Those with severe manifestations are quite low (usually <10 to 15 mg/dL), while those with more mild manifestations may present with levels of 40 to 70 mg/dL.

Prenatal diagnosis of SLOS has now been available since 1994.[35-45] Prenatal diagnosis is possible by either amniocentesis (13+ weeks on) or chorionic villus sampling (10 to 12 weeks). Since identification of the cholesterol metabolic defect in a child with SLOS whose cholesterol level was 8 mg/dL (normal, >100 mg/dL), a treatment protocol has been tried providing exogenous cholesterol to affected patients. This form of therapy has now been provided to many patients with SLOS for the past several years in many centers in the United States and internationally,[46-48] with the goal of raising cholesterol levels and decreasing the precursors, 7-DHC and 8-DHC.

Fetal therapy strategies include providing cholesterol to the mother or to the fetus. The former is not possible because cholesterol does not cross the placenta well in the third trimester. Also, cholesterol is available only in a crystalline form, which cannot be given intravenously or intramuscularly. It also cannot be injected into amniotic fluid because it would precipitate, so this option is not feasible. However, cholesterol can be given to the fetus by giving fresh frozen plasma in the form of low-density lipoprotein (LDL) cholesterol. The group at Tufts has attempted treatment in two patients. Both cases have started late in pregnancy, and the results are inconclusive. Therefore, a major relevant principle is that in order for fetal therapy to be successful, the earlier the diagnosis, the better.

Galactosemia

Galactosemia is an inborn error of metabolism caused by diminished activity of the enzyme galactose-1-phosphate uridyltransferase. It is inherited in an autosomal recessive manner and results in cataracts, growth deficiency, and ovarian failure. Galactosemia can be diagnosed prenatally by study of cultured amniocytes and chorionic villi. Clinical symptoms appear in the neonatal period and can be largely ameliorated by elimination of galactose from the diet. However, oocytes have already been damaged irreversibly long before birth. Cellular damage in galactosemia is thought to be mediated by accumulation of galactose-1-phosphate intracellularly and of galactitol in the lens.

There are suggestions that even the early postnatal treatment of galactosemic individuals with a low-galactose diet may not be sufficient to ensure normal development. Some have speculated that prenatal damage to galactosemic fetuses could contribute to subsequent abnormal neurologic development and to lens cataract formation. Furthermore, it has been recognized recently that female galactosemics, even when treated from birth with galactose deprivation, have a high frequency of primary or secondary amenorrhea because of ovarian failure. There also may be some subtle abnormalities of male gonadal function.

Exposure to a high-galactose diet has been considered to represent an animal model for human galactosemia. Chen and colleagues have observed a reduction in the oocyte content of rat ovaries after prenatal exposure to a 50% galactose diet.[49] No analogous alterations in the testes were observed in prenatally treated males. Experiments in rats suggest that toxicity to the female gonads from galactose or its metabolites is most obvious during the premeiotic stages of ovarian development.

These observations in animals and human beings have led to speculation that galactose restriction during pregnancy may be desirable if the fetus is affected with galactosemia. In the human female, ovarian meiosis begins at 12 weeks and is complete by 28 menstrual weeks. Thus, ovarian damage, and perhaps neurologic or lens abnormalities, might occur prior to the usual time when prenatal diagnosis by amniocentesis can be accomplished. Thus, anticipatory treatment in pregnancies at risk for having a galactosemic fetus might best be initiated very early in gestation or even preconceptionally.

Despite these experiments and speculations, we are unaware of studies that adequately assess the impact of prenatal administration of a low-galactose diet to galactosemic infants. For obvious reasons such data, especially controlled, will be difficult to obtain. Nevertheless, prenatal galactose restriction is probably desirable in galactosemia and should be harmless. There is little reason to suppose that galactose restriction would have adverse consequences, since galactosemic and normal fetuses are both capable of some endogenous galactose synthesis.

Abnormalities of Mineral Metabolism

Specific prenatal mineral supplementation has yet to be reported for prevention of human fetal disease. However, such additives have been used in animals with genetic deficiencies. Animal studies are of considerable interest and suggest the possibility of analogous human treatment.

Copper

Hurley and colleagues, more than 20 years ago, investigated possible deleterious effects of prenatal copper administration on mice with the recessive mutant "crinkled" gene.[50] They have suggested that the "crinkled" gene produces many phenotypic characteristics common to patients with Menkes kinky-hair syndrome. Dietary supplementation of pregnant mice with copper sulfate partially ameliorated the effects of the crinkled gene in the offspring. Different prenatal copper regimens have resulted in varying degrees of success. Copper nitrilotriacetate appeared to be superior to copper sulfate in increasing postnatal survival and body copper content of the mutant offspring of heterozygous dams. Postnatal supplementation with copper did not increase survival of the mutants.

These studies may lead to insights possibly relevant to prenatal treatment of Menkes syndrome, a sex-linked disorder characterized by progressive degeneration of neurologic function in infants. Alterations suggestive of functional copper deficiency are present in affected infants. Fibroblasts from patients with Menkes disease accumulate excess copper probably present in an abnormally bound form. Menkes disease has been refractory to postnatal therapy with copper; and it is conceivable that by analogy to the crinkled mutation, prenatal treatment might be of benefit.[1]

Despite apparent responses to prenatal mineral administration of pallid and crinkled mutations, the relationships of these mutants, if any, to ocular albinism and Menkes disease, respectively, remain speculative. Although animal studies have proved encouraging, they have not yet led to trials of prenatal mineral supplementation in genetically defective human beings.

Manganese

The effects of prenatal manganese supplementation on the prevention of otolith defects in mice affected with the pallid mutation have been investigated. Pallid mice have defective pigmentation, including an absence of pigment from the membranous labyrinth. This pigmentary characteristic is fully penetrant in the pallid homozygous recessive, whereas another manifestation, impaired otolith formation, is variably expressed. A significant correlation between litter size and the expression of the otolith abnormalities in the offspring has been known for decades; the otolith defect may be influenced by competition in utero for an unidentified substance.

Hurley and colleagues showed that development of the inner ear in normal rats and mice to be affected by decreased manganese.[50] In mice, experimental in utero manganese deprivation induced a defect of the inner ear that was morphologically and behaviorally indistinguishable from pallid, although manganese deficiency did not mimic the effect of the mutant gene on pigmentation. Subsequently, these investigators observed that manganese supplementation of pallid mice throughout gestation with a diet containing from 45 to 2,000 parts per million of manganese yielded a dose-dependent decrease in the percentage of abnormal otoliths.

These data have been extended to a genetic basis for susceptibility. In several studies on prenatal manganese restriction, the percentage of otolith abnormalities was influenced by the strain of mice studied. Thus, interactions of manganese intake and genetic predisposition influence otolith development in several strains. These observations suggest that at low or borderline levels of dietary intake of many nutrients, the genotype of the fetus can substantially alter fetal responses.

There are a number of genetic defects in animals with associated pigmentary and inner ear abnormalities. Some data suggest that manganese may play a role in modifying the expression of such defects. Hurley and colleagues have suggested that a sex-linked form of ocular albinism in humans, associated with labyrinthine dysfunction, may be analogous to some of these animal models.[50] We are unaware of any studies of manganese metabolism in human ocular albinism, or of attempts to administer manganese prenatally in the hope of ameliorating expression of any associated labyrinthine defects.

Pharmacologic and Nutritional Approaches

It might be appropriate to consider suppressing excessive cholesterol production prenatally in severe hypercholesterolemia when a safe and effective agent for accomplishing this becomes available (although there is no clear evidence for hypercholesterolemic prenatal damage). If cysteamine or related agents were to prove an effective treatment for lethal variants of cystinosis, prenatal therapy might be considered, because excessive and possibly harmful cystine accumulation is evident even in cystinotic fetuses. Cysteamine levels have been detected in chorionic villi, and significant elevations even at 10 weeks' gestation have been hypothesized. Inhibitors of γ-glutamyl transpeptidase, if safe, would elevate intracellular glutathione levels and inhibit oxoproline production in glutathione synthase deficiency, thereby averting the characteristic neonatal acidosis. In theory, it would be desirable to minimize copper accumulation in Wilson disease as early as possible. If and when reliable prenatal diagnosis of Wilson disease is possible, cautious administration of penicillamine prenatally might be considered. This would be a double-edged sword, however, as the teratogenic and lathyritic potential of penicillamine would demand careful evaluation. Batshaw and colleagues have treated certain urea cycle defects by administering arginine and benzoate. Since hyperammonemia in some of these entities develops very acutely after birth, it might be desirable to consider pretreating the fetus with these compounds just prior to or during labor to minimize postnatal hyperammonemia.[51] Conversely, it may be desirable to consider drug avoidance as an approach to fetal treatment. For example, fetuses with glucose-6-phosphate dehydrogenase deficiency are sensitive to a variety of drugs that induce hemolysis. It would probably be appropriate to avoid administering such agents to women carrying or known to be at risk for carrying fetuses deficient in glucose-6-phosphate dehydrogenase.

Umbilical cord catheterization under ultrasound guidance may lead to the development of other types of fetal treatment.[52] Systems such as gene replacement are being developed for certain lysosomal storage disorders. Progress is being made in postnatal experimental models on administration of thymic cells for certain immune deficiency states, bone marrow transplantation for a variety of genetic disorders, and gene transfer. The development of better and earlier techniques for prenatal treatment will be complex, especially with regard to gene transfer; but progress will be made, and access to the fetal vasculature may be required for these methods to have a chance for success.

Bone marrow transplantation or thymic cell infusion is actually only a specialized example of organ transplantation. In the future, fetal organ transplantation may become possible and may open many prospects for surgical treatment of certain biochemical genetic disorders.

One can also speculate about the therapeutic possibilities involving compounds administered directly into the amniotic fluid or into the fetal intestinal tract. It might be possible, for example, to administer thyroid hormone in this fashion or to prevent meconium ileus in cystic fibrosis by instilling not yet determined enzymes into the fetal intestinal tract.

Multifactorial Disorders

Cardiac Fetal Therapy

Although great strides have been made in the diagnosis of fetal cardiac anatomic and functional abnormalities, in utero cardiac therapy currently is limited to the treatment of significant arrhythmias. In the future, treatment of some congenital anomalies, particularly valvular anomalies, may be attempted prenatally. Treatment of fetal arrhythmias is discussed extensively in Chapter 27.

Neural Tube Defects

Animal studies suggest that neural tube defects (NTDs) can arise from a variety of vitamin or mineral deficiencies. There are historical data in humans suggesting increased NTD frequencies in subjects with poor dietary histories or with intestinal bypasses. Biochemical evidence of suboptimal nutrition is present in some women bearing infants with NTDs. In 1980, Smithells et al. suggested that vitamin supplementation containing 0.36 mg folate could reduce the frequency of NTD recurrence by sevenfold in women with one or more prior affected children.[53, 54] For almost a decade, there has been a great deal of controversy regarding the benefit of folate supplementation for the prevention of NTDs.[55-58] Finally, in 1991, a randomized double-blinded trial designed by the MRC Vitamin Study Research Group demonstrated that preconceptional folate reduces the risk of recurrence in high risk patients.[59] Subsequently, it was shown that preparations containing folate and other vitamins also reduce the occurrence of first-time NTDs.[60] In response to these findings, guidelines were issued calling for consumption of 4.0 mg/day folic acid by women with a prior child affected with an NTD, for at least 1 month prior to conception through the first 3 months of pregnancy. In addition, 0.4 mg/day folic acid is recommended to all women planning a pregnancy to be taken preconceptionally. The data on NTD recurrence prevention is now very well established, and became routine for high-risk cases. The question of primary prevention is more difficult to prove because of the enormity of the size of the study that would be needed to have sufficient power. However, the majority of experts in the field believe that the primary incidence could be cut by perhaps half. As of January 1998, the United States Food and Drug Administration has mandated that breads and grains be supplemented with folic acid. It is one of the largest public health experiments ever performed. It is hoped that a 30 to 50% reduction of NTDs will be seen.

Conclusion

Metabolic disorders do not have the "sexiness" of those requiring surgical or genetic therapies, but they do contribute an important group of treatable conditions. Many of these occur in pregnancies not suspected a priori to be at risk, so in most cases, therapy is targeted to prevent recurrences in given families. As carrier detection strategies unfold, there will be a greater proportion of these cases that may yet be treated without the tragedy of first having an affected, phenotypically abnormal child.

REFERENCES

1. Evans MI, Pinsky WW, Johnson MP, Schulman JD: Medical fetal therapy. *In* Evans MI (ed): Reproductive Risks and Prenatal Diagnosis. Norwalk, CT: Appleton & Lange, 1992, p 236.
2. Johnson MP, Evans MI, Quintero RA, Flake AW: In utero therapy of the fetus. *In* Gleisher N, Buttino L Jr, Elkayam U, et al (eds). Principles and Practice of Medical Therapy in Pregnancy, 3rd ed. Norwalk, CT: Appleton & Lange, 1998, pp 223–235.
3. New MI, White PC, Pang S, et al: The adrenal hyperplasis. *In* Scriver CR, Beaudet AL, Sly WS, Valle D (eds): The Metabolic Basis of Inherited Disease, 7th ed. New York: McGraw-Hill, 1995, pp 2950–2951.
4. Miller WL, Morel Y: The molecular genetics of 21 hydroxylase deficiency. Ann Rev Genet 23:371–379, 1989.
5. Hughes IA: Congenital adrenal hyperplasia—a continuum of disorders. Lancet 352:752–754, 1998.
6. Dupont B, Oberfield SE, Smithwick EM, et al: Close genetic linkage between HLA and congenital adrenal hyperplasia (21-hydroxylase deficiency). Lancet 2:1309–1311, 1977.
7. White PC, Grossberger D, Onufer BJ, et al: Two genes encoding steroid 21-hydroxylase are located near the genes encoding the fourth component of complement in man. Proc Natl Acad Sci U S A 82:1089–1093, 1985.
8. Mandell J, Bromley B, Peters CA, Benacerraf BR: Prenatal sonographic detection of genital malformations. J Urol 153:1994–1996, 1995.
9. Evans MI, Chrousos GP, Mann DL, et al: Pharmacologic suppression of the fetal adrenal gland in utero: Attempted prevention of abnormal external genital masculinization in suspected congenital adrenal hyperplasia. JAMA 253:1015, 1985.
10. Forrest M, David M: Prenatal treatment of congenital adrenal hyperplasia due to 21-hydroxylase deficiency. 7th International Congress of Endocrinology, Abstract y11, Quebec, Canada, 1984.
11. Shulman DI, Mueller OT, Gallardo LA, et al: Treatment of congenital adrenal hyperplasia in utero. Pediatr Res 25:2, 1989.
12. Pang S, Pollack MS, Marshall RN, Immken L: Prenatal treatment of congenital adrenal hyperplasia due to 21-hydroxylase deficiency. N Engl J Med 22:111, 1990.
13. Seckl JR, Miller WL: How safe is long-term prenatal glucocorticoid treatment? JAMA 13:1077–1079, 1997.
14. Fisher DA: Neonatal thyroid disease of women with autoimmune thyroid disease. Thyroid Today 9:1–7, 1986.
15. Bruinse HW, Vermeulen-Meiners C, Wit JM: Fetal treatment for thyrotoxicosis in nonthyrotoxic pregnant women. Fetal Ther 3:152–157, 1988.
16. Sack J, Fisher DA, Hobel CJ, Lam R: Thyroxine in human amniotic fluid. J Pediatr 87:364–368, 1975.
17. Thorpe-Beeston JG, Nicolaides KH, McGregor AM: Fetal thyroid function. Thyroid 2:207–217, 1992.
18. Ballabio M, Nicolini U, Jowett T, et al: Maturation of thyroid function in normal human fetuses. Clin Endocrinol 31:565–571, 1989.
19. Poreco RP, Bloch CA: Fetal blood sampling in the management of intrauterine thyrotoxicosis. Obstet Gynecol 76:509–512, 1990.
20. Wenstrom KD, Weiner CP, Williamson RA, Grant SS: Prenatal diagnosis of fetal hyperthyroidism using funipuncture. Obstet Gynecol 76(3 Pt 2):513–517, 1990.
21. Hatjis CG: Diagnosis and successful treatment of fetal goitrous hyperthyroidism caused by maternal Graves' disease. Obstet Gynecol 81(Pt2):837–839, 1993.
22. Rovet J, Ehrlich R, Sorbara D: Intellectual outcome in children with fetal hypothyroidism. J Pediatr 110:700–704, 1987.
23. Trainer TD, Howard PL: Thyroid function tests in thyroid and nonthyroid disease. CRC Crit Rev Clin Lab Sci 19:135–171, 1983.
24. Van Herle AJ, Young RT, Fisher DA, et al: Intra-uterine treatment of a hypothyroid fetus. J Clin Endocrinol Metab 40:474–477, 1973.
25. Abuhamad AZ, Fisher DA, Warsof SL, et al: Antenatal diagnosis and treatment of fetal goitrous hypothyroidism: Case report and review of the literature. Ultrasound Obstet Gynecol 6:368–371, 1995.
26. Hadi HA, Strickland RT: In utero treatment of fetal goitrous hypothyroidism caused by maternal Graves' disease. Am J Perinatol 12:455–458, 1995.

27. Ampola MG, Mahoney MI, Nakamura E, et al: Prenatal therapy of a patient with vitamin B responsive methylmalonic acidemia. N Engl J Med 293:313, 1975.
28. Evans MI, Duquette DA, Rinaldo P, et al: Modulation of B12 dosage and response in fetal treatment of methylmalonic aciduria (MMA): Titration of treatment dose to serum and urine MMA. Fetal Diagn Ther 12:21–23, 1997.
29. Roth KS, Yang W, Allen L, et al: Prenatal administration of biotin: Biotin responsive multiple carboxylase deficiency. Pediatr Res 16:126, 1982.
30. Packman S, Cowan MJ, Golbus MS, et al: Prenatal treatment of biotin responsive multiple carboxylase deficiency. Lancet 1:1435, 1982.
31. Smith DW, Lemli L, Opitz JM: A newly recognized syndrome of multiple congenital anomalies. J Pediatr 64:210–217, 1964.
32. Irons M, Elias ER, Salen G, et al: Defective cholesterol biosynthesis in Smith-Lemli-Opitz syndrome. Lancet 341:1414, 1993.
33. Tint GS, Irons M, Elias E, et al: Defective cholesterol biosynthesis associated with the Smith-Lemli-Opitz syndrome. N Engl J Med 330:107–113, 1994.
34. Shefer S, Salen G, Batta AK, et al: Markedly inhibited 7-dehydrocholesterol-reductase activity in liver microsomes from Smith-Lemli-Opitz homozygotes. J Clin Invest 96:1779–1785, 1995.
35. Gelman-Kohan Z, Nisani R, Chemke J, et al: Prenatal detection of recurrent SLOS type 2. Am J Hum Genet 47:A57, 1990.
36. Hobbins JC, Jones OW, Gottesfeld MD, Persutte W: Transvaginal ultrasonography and transabdominal embryoscopy in the first-trimester diagnosis of Smith-Lemli-Opitz syndrome, type II. Am J Obstet Gynecol 171:546–549, 1994.
37. Johnson JA, Aughton DJ, Comstock CH, et al: Prenatal diagnosis of Smith-Lemli-Opitz syndrome, type II. Am J Med Genet 49:240–243, 1994.
38. Abuelo DN, Tint GS, Kelley R, et al: Prenatal detection of the cholesterol biosynthetic defect in the Smith-Lemli-Opitz syndrome by the analysis of amniotic fluid sterols. Am J Med Genet 56:281–285, 1995.
39. Dallaire L, Mitchell G, Giguere R, et al: Prenatal diagnosis of Smith-Lemli-Opitz syndrome is possible by measurement of 7-dehydrocholesterol in amniotic fluid. Prenat Diagn 15:855–858, 1995.
40. Hyett JA, Clayton PT, Moscoso G, Nicolaides KH: Increased first trimester nuchal translucency as a prenatal manifestation of Smith-Lemli-Opitz syndrome. Am J Med Genet 58:374–376, 1995.
41. Kelley RI: Diagnosis of Smith-Lemli-Opitz syndrome by gas chromatography/mass spectrometry of 7-dehydrocholesterol in plasma, amniotic fluid and cultured skin fibroblasts. Clin Chim Acta 236:45–58, 1995.
42. McGaughran JM, Clayton PT, Mills KA, et al: Prenatal diagnosis of Smith-Lemli-Opitz syndrome. Am J Med Genet 56:269–271, 1995.
43. Rossiter JP, Hofman KJ, Kelley RI: Smith-Lemli-Opitz syndrome: Prenatal diagnosis by quantification of cholesterol precursors in amniotic fluid. Am J Med Genet 56:272–275, 1995.
44. Mills K, Mandel H, Montemagno R, et al: First trimester prenatal diagnosis of Smith-Lemli-Opitz syndrome (7-dehydrocholesterol reductase deficiency). Pediatr Res 39:816–819, 1996.
45. Sharp P, Haan E, Fletcher JM, et al: First trimester diagnosis of Smith-Lemli-Opitz syndrome. Prenat Diagn 17:355–361, 1997.
46. Irons M, Elias E, Tint GS, et al: Abnormal cholesterol metabolism in the Smith-Lemli-Opitz syndrome: Report of clinical and biochemical findings in 4 patients and treatment in 1 patient. Am J Med Genet 50:347–352, 1994.
47. Irons M, Elias ER, Abuelo D, et al: Treatment of Smith-Lemli-Opitz syndrome: Results of a multicenter trial. Am J Med Genet 68:311–314, 1997.
48. Elias ER, Irons MB, Hurley AD, et al: Clinical effects of cholesterol supplementation in six patients with the Smith-Lemli-Opitz syndrome (SLOS). Am J Med Genet 68:305–310, 1997.
49. Chen YT, Mattison DR, Feigenbaum L, et al: Reduction in oocyte number following prenatal exposure to a high galactose diet. Science 314:1145, 1981.
50. Hurley LS, Bell LT: Genetic influence on response to dietary manganese deficiency in mice. J Nutr 104:133, 1974.
51. Batshaw M, Brusilow S, Waber L, et al: Treatment of inborn errors of urea synthesis: Activation of alternative pathways of waste nitrogen synthesis and excretion. N Engl J Med 306:1387, 1982.

52. Nicolaides KH, Thorpe-Beeston JG, Noble P: Cordocentesis. *In* Eden RD, Boehm FH (eds): Assessment and Care of the Fetus: Physiological, Clinical and Medicolegal Principles. Norwalk, CT: Appleton & Lange, 1990, p 291.

53. Smithells RW, Sheppard S, Schorah CJ, et al: Possible prevention of neural tube defects by preconceptual vitamin supplementation. Lancet 1:399–340, 1980.

54. Smithells RW, Nevin NC, Seller MJ, et al: Further experience of vitamin supplementation for prevention of neural tube defect recurrences. Lancet 1:1027, 1983.

55. Younis JS, Granat M: Insufficient transplacental digoxin transfer in severe hydrops fetalis. Am J Obstet Gynecol 157:1268, 1987.

56. Mills JL, Rhoads GG, Simpson JL, et al: The absence of a relation between the periconceptional use of vitamins and neural-tube defects. N Engl J Med 321:430, 1989.

57. Mulinare J, Cordero JF, Erickson JD, Berry RJ: Periconceptional use of multivitamins and the occurrence of neural tube defects. JAMA 260:3141, 1988.

58. Schulman JD: Treatment of the embryo and the fetus in the first trimester: Current status and future prospects. Am J Med Genet 35:197, 1990.

59. MRC Vitamin Study Research Group: Prevention of neural tube defects: Results of the MRC Vitamin Study. Lancet 338:132–137, 1991.

60. Czeizel AE, Dudas I: Prevention of the first occurrence of neural-tube defects by preconceptional vitamin supplementation. N Engl J Med 327:1832–1835, 1992.

CHAPTER 34

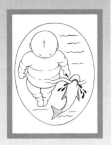

The Fetus with Immune Hydrops

KENNETH J. MOISE, JR.

The fetus with hydrops fetalis secondary to maternal red cell alloimmunization represents a true challenge in perinatal management. Often this situation is the result of late entry into prenatal care; less commonly it is secondary to late referral to perinatal centers experienced with the early detection of fetal anemia. The hydropic fetus represents an end-stage anemic state with a worse prognosis than its nonhydropic counterpart. In a recent review, the overall survival after intrauterine transfusion for hydrops fetalis was 74% as compared to 94% when no hydrops was present.[1] Clearly, the management of hemolytic disease of the fetus/newborn (HDN) entails the early detection of fetal anemia with intervention prior to the advent of hydrops.

Evaluation of the Sensitized Pregnancy

Maternal Antibody Measurement

The typical fetus becomes at risk for anemia once an antibody screen (indirect Coombs) is determined to be positive for 1 of more than 43 antibodies associated with HDN (Table 34–1). In England, anti-D levels are measured and compared to a standard and reported as international units per milliliter (IU/mL). In North America, maternal antibody titers are used to assess the degree of risk for fetal disease. Maternal antibody determinations are repeated at 2- to 4-week intervals until a threshold value is reached. Most centers will use a titer value between 8 and 32 (dilution: 1 : 8 and 1 : 32) as their definition of a critical value. Once a patient is found to have this titer, invasive fetal testing is indicated. An anti-D antibody level of greater than 4 IU/mL has been recommended as the threshold to initiate amniocentesis.[2]

Fetal Antigen Testing

Once a clinically significant antibody is detected, paternal evaluation is the next step in management. If the partner is negative for the particular red cell antigen involved and paternity is ensured, then further evaluation of the fetus is unnecessary. In other cases, paternal phenotype testing will reveal a heterozygous state (Table 34–2). With the advent of the cloning of many of the genes responsible for the blood group antigens associated with HDN, amniocentesis can now be performed to obtain fetal DNA. Polymerase chain reaction (PCR) primers can then be used to determine the blood type of the fetus. This approach is now available for the D,[3] C/c,[4] E/e,[4] and Kell (K1)/Cellano (K2),[5] Jk^a/Jk^b,[6] Fy^a/Fy^b,[7] M/N,[8] S/s[8] antigens. Typically, a reference laboratory will require a sample of maternal blood as a negative control and a sample of paternal blood as a positive control. The results of the PCR testing on amniotic fluid that indicates an antigen-negative fetus should be viewed with some degree of suspicion when paternity is not ensured or the patient's partner is unavailable for testing. In rare cases a paternal gene rearrangement could lead to an incorrect correlation between fetal serology (phenotype) and PCR results (genotype). In one review of 500 cases, this rate of error was reported to be 1.3%.[9] Two fetuses died, one neonate required exchange transfusions, another neonate needed phototherapy in conjunction with a simple transfusion, and the remaining infant was lost to follow-up. Many laboratories have resorted to the use of multiple sets of PCR primers in an effort to reduce this possibility. Another strategy that has been suggested when the fetus is determined to be antigen-negative by PCR and paternity is in question is to repeat the maternal titer in 6 weeks. A rising titer (more than a two-dilution increase) should lead one to suspect the PCR diagnosis. Cordocentesis for direct acquisition of fetal blood for serologic testing should be considered in these cases.

Clearly, a noninvasive technique for determining the fetal blood type would negate the risks of fetal loss and enhanced maternal sensitization associated with cordocentesis or amniocentesis. Lo and co-workers[10] were the first to study maternal blood for the presence of RhD-positive DNA of fetal origin. The technique proved accurate in detecting an RhD-positive fetus in eight of ten cases; however, in 3 of 11 cases in which the fetus was

TABLE 34–1. ANTIBODIES ASSOCIATED WITH HEMOLYTIC DISEASE OF THE NEWBORN*

BLOOD GROUP SYSTEM	ANTIGEN	BLOOD GROUP SYSTEM	ANTIGEN
Rhesus	D	Public antigens	Yt^a
	C		Lan
	c		En^a
	E		Ge
	e		Jr^a
			Co^a
Kell	K		Co^3
	k		Wright^b
Duffy	Fy^a	Private antigens	Batty
			Becker
Kidd	Jk^a		Berrens
	Jk^b		Biles
			Evans
MNSs	M		Gonzales
	N		Good
	S		Heibel
	s		Hunt
			Jobbins
Lutheran	Lu^a		Radin
	Lu^b		Rm
			Ven
Diego	Di^a		Wright^a
	Di^b		Zd
Xg	Xg^a		
P	PP$_1$P^k		

* Modified from Weinstein L: Irregular antibodies causing hemolytic disease of the newborn: A continuing problem. Clin Obstet Gynecol 25:321–332, 1982, with permission.

RhD-negative, a false-positive result was obtained. A follow-up study from these same investigators yielded a sensitivity of only 32% for detecting the RhD-positive fetus.[11] Geifman-Holtzman et al.[12] utilized fluorescent-activated cell sorting of maternal blood for fetal erythroblasts and correctly determined the fetal blood RhD type in 16 of 19 cases. More recently, Al-Mufti et al.[13] sorted maternal blood using triple-density gradient centrifugation. Reverse transcriptase-PCR for fetal RNA was more sensitive for the prediction of the fetal RhD status (28 of 35 cases) when compared to standard genomic-PCR for fetal DNA (22 of 35 cases correctly predicted).

The prenatal diagnosis of the fetal Rhc antigen status has also been undertaken using fetal erythroblasts sorted from the maternal circulation.[14] A positive fetal Rhc genotype was found in seven of eight samples.

Diagnosis of Fetal Anemia

Once the fetus is determined to be antigen positive, there are at least three approaches that are used to predict fetal anemia. Based on the rate of fetal loss associated with the various invasive procedures, the most conservative approach advocates the use of serial ultrasounds. A "middle-of-the-road" approach involves the use of serial amniocenteses to detect elevations in amniotic fluid bilirubin levels measured as the ΔOD_{450}. The most aggressive approach (highest background rate of fetal loss) involves the use of serial cordocenteses.

Ultrasound

Several investigators have advocated the use of serial ultrasound examinations to detect signs of impending hydrops. Once hydrops is noted, the fetal hemoglobin deficit is typically more than 7 g/dL below the mean value for gestational age.[15] However, in one series, ultrasound evidence of hydrops was noted in only two thirds of fetuses with this severe a degree of anemia.[15] Earlier studies that evaluated umbilical venous diameter, abdominal circumference, and placental thickness proved to be very disappointing.[16] More recent attention has turned to assessment of the fetal liver and spleen, sources of extramedullary hematopoiesis in response to fetal anemia. Two studies[17, 18] have proposed that an increase in the length of the right hepatic lobe is a good predictor of fetal anemia. Oepkes and co-workers[19] mea-

TABLE 34–2. PATERNAL ANTIGEN AND ZYGOSITY STATUS FOR COMMON ANTIGENS ASSOCIATED WITH HDN*

	CAUCASIAN		AFRICAN AMERICAN	
	Antigen Positive	Heterozygous	Antigen Positive	Heterozygous
D	85%	50%	93%	41%
C	70%	50%	30%	32%
c	80%	50%	96%	32%
E	30%	25%	20%	20%
e	98%	25%	99%	20%
K	9%	97.8%	2%	100%
k	99.8%	8.8%	100%	2%
Fy^a	66%	26%	10%	90%
Fy^b	83%	41%	23%	96%
Jk^a	77%	36%	91%	63%
Jk^b	72%	32%	43%	21%
M	78%	64%	70%	63%
N	77%	65%	74%	60%
S	55%	80%	31%	90%
s	89%	50%	97%	29%

* Modified from Vengelen-Tyler V: Technical Manual, 12th ed. Bethesda, MD: American Association of Blood Banks, 1996, with permission.

sured the fetal splenic perimeter with ultrasound and noted that splenomegaly was present in all nonhydropic, anemic fetuses. Splenomegaly predicted a hemoglobin deficit in excess of 5 standard deviations (SD) from the norm for gestational age with a sensitivity of 93%. Another line of investigation for the noninvasive prediction of fetal anemia has centered on the use of Doppler ultrasound to assess an increased fetal blood velocity in various vessels. This concept is based on animal data indicating that fetal blood velocities become elevated in response to an increase in cardiac output and a decline in blood viscosity when the fetus becomes anemic.[20] Initial reports utilizing such fetal vessels as the umbilical vein,[21] descending thoracic aorta,[22] and common carotid artery[23] were disappointing in the prediction of fetal hematocrit. These results are not surprising, as the majority of these vessels are found in the fetus perpendicular to the insonating Doppler beam. Peak velocities are therefore underestimated even utilizing such techniques as electronic angle correction. Mari et al.[24] were the first to suggest that the fetal middle cerebral artery (MCA) could represent the optimal vessel for obtaining a peak Doppler velocity for the detection of fetal anemia. These investigators determined a nomogram from 135 normal fetuses and then measured the peak systolic velocity in 16 fetuses at risk for anemia that underwent cordocentesis. All nonanemic fetuses were noted to exhibit a peak MCA velocity below the mean value for the corresponding gestational age; all anemic fetuses were found to have values above the mean.

More recently, Mari and co-workers[24a] evaluated the definition of fetal anemia in 265 normal fetuses. Mild anemia was defined as 0.84 to 0.65 MoM for gestational age, moderate anemia was 0.65 to 0.55 MoM, and severe anemia less than 0.55 MoM. One hundred eleven at-risk fetuses were then evaluated prospectively. An MCA velocity of greater than 1.50 MoM detected all cases of moderate to severe anemia with a 10% false-positive rate. Our current protocol is to begin fetal MCA velocity

determinations at 16 to 18 weeks' gestation. Doppler studies are repeated every 4 to 14 days based on the anemia prediction zone (Fig. 34–1). Color flow or power Doppler is used to locate the MCA over the anterior wing of the fetal sphenoid bone. All attempts are made to place the Dopper gate in the proximal portion of the MCA just distal to its origin from the carotid siphon. The MCA closest to the ultrasound transducer is used except in cases where the posterior MCA presents a less acute angle of insonation (Fig. 34–2). Color enhancement of the Doppler tracing should be used, as the true peak velocity is better recognized than with gray scale alone. In cases of a rapid rise of the MCA peak velocity into the "transfuse" zone, cordocentesis is undertaken with blood readily available for intrauterine transfusion should a fetal hematocrit of less than 30% be detected (Fig. 34–3).

Amniocentesis

Serial amniocentesis is still probably the most widely used diagnostic modality after a critical maternal titer is detected. First reported by Liley[25] in 1961, some confidence was lost in this method when Nicolaides et al.[26] reported that "modified" Liley curves extrapolated back from 27 weeks' gestation missed 70% of anemic fetuses between 18 and 25 weeks' gestation. Queenan et al.[27] published normal ΔOD_{450} values between 14 and 40 weeks' gestation based on 520 unaffected pregnancies (Fig. 34–4). A further analysis of 163 amniotic fluid samples in 75 alloimmunized pregnancies resulted in the development of four new zones of management: an "Rh-negative, unaffected" zone; an "indeterminate" zone, an "Rh-positive, affected" zone; and an "intrauterine death risk" zone. The authors recommended serial amniocenteses in the lower three zones and intrauterine transfusion or early delivery in the uppermost zone. Although these data have not been confirmed prospectively, a retrospective analysis of one center's data has

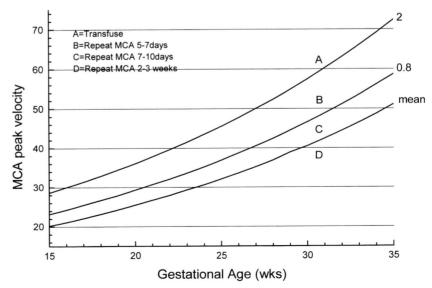

FIGURE 34–1. Management zones based on the peak MCA Doppler velocity.

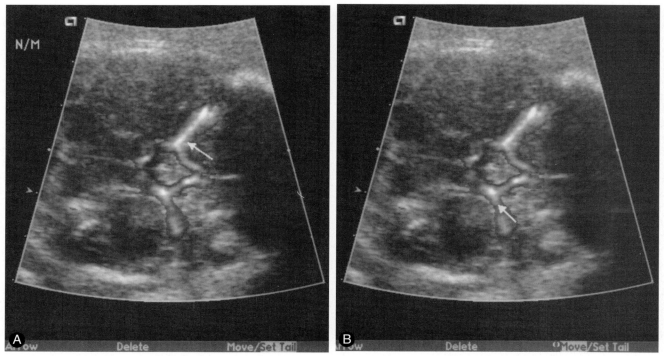

FIGURE 34–2. *A,* Doppler flow in fetal middle cerebral artery. *Arrow* notes location for Doppler gate when using the anterior vessel. *B,* Doppler flow in fetal middle cerebral artery. *Arrow* notes location for Doppler gate when using the posterior vessel.

been undertaken using the Queenan graph. Fernandez et al.[28] analyzed alloimmunized pregnancies and found that 14 antigen-positive fetuses had initial ΔOD_{450} values in the unaffected zone. Four of these fetuses required intrauterine transfusions and one required neonatal exchange transfusion. Unfortunately, the authors did not report how many of these 14 pregnancies involved alloimmunization to red cell antigens other than the RhD. If one elects to use serial amniocenteses, the Queenan graph should be used between 18 and 27 weeks' gesta-

tion; the use of the standard Liley curve thereafter would appear appropriate. Amniocenteses are repeated at 1- to 3-week intervals based on the initial value of the ΔOD_{450} and subsequent trends. All attempts should be undertaken to avoid transplacental puncture so as to avert an amnestic response and resultant worsening fetal hemolytic disease. Amniocenteses should be continued until fetal lung maturity is documented, at which time induction of labor would appear to be a more reasonable approach than continued amniocenteses. The

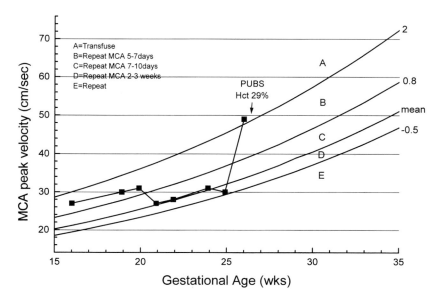

FIGURE 34–3. Case representation of using serial peak Doppler assessments in a case of Kell alloimmunization to detect fetal anemia. *Arrow* indicates percutaneous blood sampling with finding of fetal hematocrit of 29%.

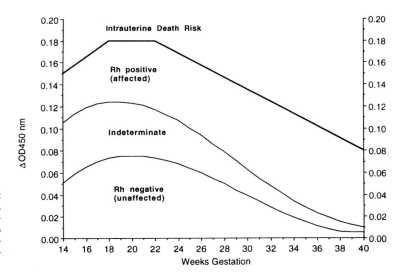

FIGURE 34–4. Amniotic fluid ΔOD_{450} value management zones based on gestational age. (From Queenan JT, Tomai TP, Ural SH, King JC: Deviation in the amniotic fluid optical density at a wavelength of 450 nm in Rh-immunized pregnancies from 14 to 40 weeks' gestation: A proposal for clinical management. Am J Obstet Gynecol 168:1370–1376, 1993, with permission.)

lecithin/sphingomyelin ratio should be used to determine fetal lung maturity, as diagnostic tests that utilize polarized light (Tdx-FLM) will yield falsely elevated results secondary to the presence of fetal bilirubin. Cordocentesis should be undertaken when the ΔOD_{450} value reaches the 80th percentile of the "Rh-positive, affected" zone (Queenan graph) or the 80th percentile of zone 2 of the Liley graph. Blood should be readied for intrauterine transfusion if the fetal hematocrit is found to be less than 30%.

Cordocentesis

Weiner and co-workers[29] have advocated the routine use of serial cordocenteses to detect fetal anemia. Fetal hematocrit, reticulocyte count, and direct Coombs results were analyzed and four distinct patterns were generated (Table 34–3). This algorithm was tested prospectively in 44 pregnancies at their center.[30] Two cases of

unexpected neonatal anemia occurred in the series. Further review revealed that one case was incorrectly managed according to their protocol secondary to an erroneous assessment of the fetal reticulocyte count. A fetal serum total bilirubin value of greater than 3 mg/dL has also been associated with the subsequent need for intrauterine transfusion.[31]

Kell Alloimmunization

The management of Kell (K1) alloimmunization deserves special mention. Bowman et al.[32] found that only 5% of live offspring born to sensitized Kell-negative women were affected by HDN. This is not unexpected in view of the fact that 91% of paternal blood typing will reveal a Kell-negative status. Early paternal testing for the Kell antigen will therefore eliminate the need for further diagnostic evaluation in the great majority of cases. Maternal antibody titers as low as 8 have been

TABLE 34–3. DIAGNOSTIC MANAGEMENT SCHEME USING SERIAL CORDOCENTESES*

HEMATOCRIT	RETICULOCYTE COUNT	DIRECT COOMBS	INTERVAL FOR CORDOCENTESIS (WK)	INTERVAL FOR ULTRASOUND (WK)	COMMENTS
Normal	Normal	Neg–Trace	—	4	If initial titer <128; repeat titer in 4 weeks. If titer doubles, repeat cordocentesis.
Normal	Normal or decreased	1+ to 2+	5–6	2	Do not repeat cordocentesis after 32 weeks; deliver at term.
Normal	Elevated	3+ to 4+	2	1	Repeat cordocentesis through 34 weeks if hematocrit stable; deliver after pulmonary maturity.
<2 SD	Any	Any	1–2	1	Repeat cordocentesis if hematocrit remains >30%; deliver after pulmonary maturity.
<30%	Any	Any	—	—	Intrauterine transfusion

* Modified from Weiner CP, Williamson RA, Wenstrom KD, et al: Management of fetal hemolytic disase by cordocentesis I. Prediction of fetal anemia. Am J Obstet Gynecol 165:546–553, 1991, with permission.

associated with hydrops fetalis.[30] Several clinical investigations have pointed to a unique pathophysiology of the fetal anemia in Kell alloimmunization. Two investigations compared Kell-affected fetuses to matched Rh-affected fetuses and noted a reduced hematopoietic response in association with the Kell-positive fetus.[33, 34] In addition, Vaughan et al.[33] noted lower ΔOD_{450} values associated with Kell disease. Other authors have also reported cases of low ΔOD_{450} values in association with severe fetal anemia in Kell alloimmunization.[33, 34] More recently, in vitro studies by Vaughan et al.[37] have further delineated the differences in fetal effects from Kell antibody as compared to anti-D antibody. Erythroid cell cultures were developed from cord blood samples from Kell-positive and Kell-negative infants. Serum samples from Kell-alloimmunized women markedly suppressed the development of Kell-positive but not Kell-negative erythroid cells. Monoclonal anti-Kell antibody suppressed erythropoieis in a dose-related fashion; monoclonal anti-D antibody had little effect on culture growth. These data led Vaughan et al.[37] to conclude that modalities other than amniocentesis for ΔOD_{450} should be used to assess the severity of fetal anemia in cases of Kell alloimmunization. Our center has elected to use serial Doppler assessments of the MCA to decide when to perform the first cordocentesis in the Kell-sensitized gestation. After an elevated MCA velocity is noted, blood is available in the room when the procedure is scheduled in the event that fetal anemia is detected.

Other Antibodies Associated with HDN

Due to the infrequency of other Rh antibodies (C, c, E, e) and other non-Rh red cell antibodies, diagnostic protocols are notably lacking from the literature. In these cases most centers follow a diagnostic algorithm similar to rhesus disease.

Intrauterine Transfusion

Historical Perspectives

The earliest attempts at fetal therapy involved the treatment of fetal anemia secondary to rhesus disease. As early as 1964, Freda and Adamsons[38] performed hysterotomy with placement of a catheter into the fetal femoral artery. Other centers attempted access to the fetal saphenous vein[39] and internal jugular vein[40] with little success. A less radical approach was proposed by Liley[41] in 1963 when he introduced the concept of infusing red cells into the fetal peritoneal cavity using a radiographically guided needle. The intraperitoneal transfusion (IPT) remained the mainstay of treatment for the anemic fetus until the early 1980s. In 1981, Rodeck et al.[42] described the first intravascular transfusion (IVT) of the fetus by directing a needle into chorionic plate vessels under visualization through a fetoscope. The following year, a Danish group reported the first successful intravascular transfusion of a fetus by umbilical venous puncture under ultrasound guidance.[43] By 1986, two schools of

thought had emerged regarding the optimal method for IVT. Grannum et al.[44] proposed an exchange intravascular technique similar to that used to treat HDN in the neonate, while Berkowitz and co-workers[44] advocated a direct intravascular transfusion technique. As more experience was gained with the two techniques, the direct IVT has been accepted worldwide as the procedure of choice for the treatment of fetal anemia.

Intrauterine Transfusion Method

Serial hematocrits from fetuses transfused with IVTs alone exhibit a decline between procedures of approximately 1% per day.[45] In an effort to allow for a reasonable interval between procedures, many centers will transfuse to a final hematocrit value of 50 to 65%. However, caution should be exercised in transfusing the fetus to nonphysiologic values of hematocrit. Welch et al.[46] demonstrated that a marked rise in whole blood viscosity is associated with fetal hematocrits above 50%. In order to avoid this problem, we began to evaluate whether a combined IPT/IVT technique would result in a more stable fetal hematocrit between intrauterine transfusions.[47] Our technique involved administering enough packed red cells (hematocrits, 75 to 85%) by IVT to achieve a final fetal hematocrit of 35 to 40%. A standard IPT was then undertaken. Our hypothesis was that the intraperitoneal infusion of blood would serve as a reservoir allowing the slow absorption of red cells between procedures. Four transfusion techniques in 19 fetuses were compared. A combined direct IVT/IPT achieved a more stable fetal hematocrit as compared to direct IVT alone. The combined method resulted in a decline in hematocrit of 0.01% per day between transfusions as compared to a decline of 1.14% per day with direct IVT alone. Nicolini et al.[48] also studied this technique. A final fetal hematocrit of 40% was achieved by IVT. Assuming complete absorption of the blood infused into the peritoneal cavity, a theoretical final hematocrit of 50 to 60% was used by these investigators to determine the volume for the IPT. Although the decline in hematocrit per day was identical for IVT and IVT/IPT, the combined procedure achieved a significantly longer interval between transfusions and also maintained a higher initial fetal hematocrit at subsequent transfusion. At our center, we perform an IVT with a final target hematocrit of 35 to 40%. The volume of red blood cells to be transfused is calculated by first determining the estimated fetal weight by ultrasound in grams. The hematocrit of the donor blood is measured and should approximate 75%. A transfusion coefficient is then used to calculate the volume of donor blood needed to achieve the desired final fetal hematocrit (Table 34–4).[49] A standard IPT is then undertaken using the following formula: volume of blood to be transfused (mL) = (gestational age in weeks -20) $\times$ 10.[50] Because the blood in the peritoneal reservoir will be absorbed over a 7- to 10-day period, fetal hyperviscosity can be prevented while maintaining a stable hematocrit between procedures. Subsequent intrauterine transfusions are scheduled at 14-day intervals until suppression of fetal erythropoiesis is noted on

TABLE 34–4. CALCULATION OF DONOR VOLUME AT INTRAVASCULAR TRANSFUSION*

TARGET INCREASE IN FETAL HEMATOCRIT	TRANSFUSION COEFFICIENT
10%	0.02
15%	0.03
20%	0.04
25%	0.05
30%	0.06

* From Giannina G, Moise KJ, Dorman K: A simple method to estimate volume for fetal intravascular transfusions. Fetal Diagn Ther 13:94–97, 1998, with permission.

Kleihauer-Betke (K-B) stains. This usually occurs by the third intrauterine transfusion. Thereafter, the interval for repeat procedures can be determined based on the decline in hematocrit for the individual fetus, usually a 3- to 4-week interval.

Transfusion of the Hydropic Fetus

The transfusion of the hydropic fetus requires several special considerations. It has been generally accepted that hydrops fetalis is associated with poor absorption of red cells from the peritoneal cavity.[51] Harman et al.[52] compared the experience at one referral center with IVT and IPT techniques for the treatment of the hydropic fetus using historical controls. Survival of the hydropic fetus was improved from 48% with IPT to 86% with IVT. It would therefore appear that IVT should be the primary modality for the management of the hydropic, anemic fetus. The severely anemic fetus at 18 to 24 weeks' gestation is less able to adapt to the acute complete correction of its anemia by IVT. Monitoring of the umbilical venous pressure during IVT has been found useful in such cases.[53] An increase of greater than 10 mm Hg predicted fetal death within 24 hours after transfusion with a sensitivity of 80%. Radunovic et al.[54] noted a 37% mortality within 72 hours of IVT in fetuses presenting with severe anemia and hydrops. Based on their data, these authors recommended that in the severely anemic fetus, the final posttransfusion hematocrit after IVT should not exceed a value of 25% or a fourfold increase from the pretransfusion value. At our center, we have chosen to use the umbilical venous pressure to determine when to conclude an IVT in the very anemic fetus in the early second trimester. Periodic evaluation of the pressure is undertaken and the procedure concluded when the change in pressure approaches 10 mm Hg. A second IVT is performed within 48 hours to correct the fetal hematocrit into the normal range; the third procedure is scheduled 7 to 10 days later. Thereafter, repeat transfusions are undertaken based on fetal hematocrits and K-B stains. Fetal thrombocytopenia can complicate the transfusion of a hydropic fetus through bleeding problems at the umbilical cord puncture site. In one series of 37 hydropic fetuses, Saade and co-workers[55] noted that 19% of these fetuses had a platelet count of less than 100,000/mm[3], while 8% of the population had a platelet count of less than 50,000/mm[3]. It would therefore appear prudent to obtain an initial platelet count at the same time the fetal hematocrit is measured during the introduction of the needle into the fetal vascular space at IVT. We have found the use of a portable automated cell hemocytometer to be invaluable during these procedures. Quality control is maintained by the hospital laboratory personnel, who also provide assistance during the intrauterine transfusion procedure. Random donor platelets are available in the procedure room. If the initial fetal platelet count returns at less than 50,000/mm[3], a platelet transfusion is administered before removal of the needle from the fetal umbilical cord. The volume of platelet concentrate to be transfused is calculated by first estimating the fetoplacental volume (FPV).[56] This volume in milliliters is equal to 1.0 + ultrasound estimated fetal weight (in grams) × 0.14. The following formula is then used:

$$\text{Volume of platelets to transfuse (mL)} = \frac{\text{FPV} \times 2 \times \text{desired platelet increment}}{\text{platelet count of the concentrate}}[57]$$

Fetal Paralysis and Antibiotics

Other adjuncts are helpful during intrauterine transfusion procedures. Maternal sedation, once routinely used, is no longer necessary, since temporary fetal paralysis can be effected with such short-acting agents as atracurium or vecuronium.[58, 59] These agents do not appear to cause the fetal tachycardia and loss of short-term heart rate variability associated with once commonly used pancuronium.[60] A vecuronium dose of 0.1 mg/kg of fetal weight estimated using ultrasound produces almost immediate cessation of fetal movement after intravascular injection at the start of the intrauterine transfusion. Fetal paralysis can be expected for 1 to 2 hours. Paralysis should be undertaken even when there is decreased fetal movement associated with fetal hydrops. We have anecdotally noted a marked increase in fetal movement as the fetal anemia is acutely corrected during the IVT. Such excessive movement can result in fetal or umbilical cord injury. The use of prophylactic antibiotics to prevent cases of chorioamnionitis is advocated by some centers, although this has not been systematically studied. An agent effective against typical skin flora should be selected. We currently do not routinely employ prophylactic antibiotics. Our routine practice is to always use a new procedure needle for each new skin puncture.

Gestational Age for Delivery

When IPTs were used as the sole means of in utero therapy, fetuses were routinely delivered at 32 weeks' gestation. Hyaline membrane disease and the need for neonatal exchange transfusions for the treatment of hyperbilirubinemia were common. As experience with IVT became widespread, pregnancies were delivered at later gestational ages. It now appears reasonable to perform the final intrauterine transfusion as late as 35 weeks' gestation, with delivery anticipated at 37 to 38 weeks. After a viable gestational age is attained, performing the transfusion in immediate proximity to the labor and delivery suite appears prudent so that operative delivery can be undertaken if fetal distress should occur. We routinely begin maternal oral phenobarital (30 mg tid) approximately 10 days prior to delivery. This enhances the ability of the neonatal liver to conjugate bilirubin and has negated the need for exchange transfusion after birth.

Maternal Blood as the Red Cell Source for Intrauterine Transfusion

In the past, O-negative, CMV-negative, allogeneic red blood cells were used as the primary source of blood for intrauterine transfusion. Patient concern regarding the transmission of human immunodeficiency virus (HIV) has led some to use maternal blood for intrauterine transfusion. Advantages include the availability of fresh blood and the decreased chance for sensitization to new red cell antigens if some of the transfused blood escapes back into the maternal circulation. In a series of 21 patients, up to 6 units of blood per patient were harvested for intrauterine transfusion.[61] Supplementation with prenatal vitamins, folate, and ferrous sulfate prevented maternal anemia in all cases. No serious maternal or fetal effects were noted. The mother should undergo routine donor screening for syphilis, HIV, HTLV-1, and hepatitis B and C. The red cells are washed to remove the offending antibody, tightly packed to achieve a final hematocrit of 75 to 85%, and then filtered through a leukocyte poor filter. Because the mother and fetus will share HLA antigens at many loci, the possibility of a graft-versus-host reaction must be considered. In order to avoid this complication, the maternal red cells are irradiated wth 2,500 Gy of external beam radiation. If the mother has antibody to the CMV virus, the blood may still be used, as the dormant CMV virus resides in the white blood cells that have been removed by the filtering process. On some occasions an ABO incompatibility may be detected between the mother and her fetus after the initial cordocentesis. We have used maternal blood in two such cases with no deleterious effects observed in the fetus. Follow-up at 3 years of age in these infants revealed anti-A and anti-B titers that were appropriate for age.

Neonatal Follow-up (Short and Long Term)

Immediate follow-up studies of infants treated with IVTs in utero have revealed a need for "top-up" transfusions in the early months of life. Typically, these infants are born with a virtual absence of reticulocytes with a red cell population consisting mainly of transfused red cells containing adult hemoglobin. Exchange transfusions for hyperbilirubinemia are rarely necessary. However, at 1 month of age these infants often require a simple transfusion due to symptoms associated with anemia. In our own series of 36 infants that had undergone intrauterine transfusions, 50% required top-up transfusions at a mean age of 38 days (range, 20 to 68 days).[62] Eleven of the 15 fetuses required only one transfusion, while two fetuses required two transfusions and an additional two needed three transfusions. Studies of these infants indicate erythroid hypoplasia of the bone marrow accompanied by low levels of circulating erythropoietin and reticulocytes.[63] This led Ovali et al.[64] to study the use of exogenous erythropoietin in neonates after intrauterine transfusions. Twenty infants were randomized to receive 200 U/kg of recombinant human erythropoietin or saline placebo subcutaneously three times a week between the second and eighth weeks of life. Infants in the treatment group required a mean of 1.8 red cell transfusions as compared to a mean of 4.2 transfusions in the placebo group. Two patients in the treatment group did not require transfusions while four others needed only two. In the control group, only one patient required one transfusion, one required two, and the remaining infants required three or more. Because of this phenomenon, weekly hematocrit and reticulocyte determinations are recommended for the first 1 to 2 months of life in infants who have undergone intrauterine transfusions.[65] One proposed criterion for transfusion includes a hemoglobin less than 5 to 6 g/dL in the symptom-free infant. In addition, any infant with symptoms related to anemia such as poor weight gain, lethargy, or feeding difficulties should be transfused. If erythropoietin is to be used, we suggest that it be used in the first week of life in the infant with a persistently low circulating reticulocyte count. Supplemental iron therapy is unnecessary due to the high levels of circulating iron in these infants secondary to ongoing hemolysis in utero.[66] Supplemental folate therapy (0.5 mg/day) should be considered.

Investigations regarding the long-term neurologic evaluation of infants that have been treated with IVTs are limited. These data are especially important in view of the likelihood that more moribund fetuses now survive due to advancements in treatment techniques. Doyle et al.[67] described an overall survival rate of 73% after IVT. In the 38 surviving infants, the authors noted one case of cerebral palsy, one case of severe developmental delay, one case of spastic hemiplegia, and one case of severe developmental delay associated with seizures. Janssens and co-workers[68] reported an overall perinatal survival of 79% after IVT. Sixty-nine infants were followed up to 6 months to 6 years of age. Seven percent of the children exhibited some evidence of neurologic handicap; three infants (4%) were diagnosed with cerebral palsy. Sixteen percent of the children were noted to have developmental delay; six cases showed mild delay, while five additional cases exhibited severe delay. Hydrops fetalis was not associated with a poorer prognosis for normal neurodevelopmental outcome. We recently reported an overall survival of 80% after intrauterine transfusion.[69] Forty surviving infants were followed up to 62 months of age. One case of severe bilateral hearing loss and one case of spastic hemiplegia were detected. Gesell and McCarthy developmental scores were similar to norms for the general population.

More importantly, neonates that were noted to present with hydrops fetalis in utero had developmental scores similar to neonates that did not develop hydrops. These data are reassuring in counseling the couple that presents with the severely anemic fetus. They can be reassured that a normal neurologic outcome can be expected in over 90% of surviving infants even if hydrops fetalis is noted at the time of the first IUT.

The Patient with Recurrent Hydrops Fetalis

The patient that presents with recurrent immune hydrops fetalis at less than 20 weeks' gestation is a true perinatal challenge. Technical limitations make umbilical cord puncture difficult. On occasion, an intraperitoneal transfusion can be attempted before the overt development of hydrops; however, formulas for calculating the correct volume for transfusion do not exist. Since the late 1960s, plasmapheresis has been suggested as a modality that may have a role in the treatment of severe rhesus disease.[70] Most literature reports involve single cases or small case series; the modality has never been studied in a systematic fashion. Odendaal et al.[71] reported the largest series of nine patients. Five of the nine patients had experienced a previous intrauterine death, while two others lost infants soon after birth secondary to hydrops fetalis. Intensive plasmapheresis led to a perinatal survival of 89% without the use of IUT. Bowman[68] has suggested that plasmapheresis may have a role in the management of select cases of red cell alloimmunization in that it may allow time for gestation to advance to a point when intravascular transfusion is technically possible. Intravenous γ-globulin is another treatment modality that has generated extreme interest for the treatment of severe fetal hemolytic disease. Several mechanisms of action have been postulated including decrease of maternal antibody levels through anti-idiotype suppression, blockade of the placenta Fc receptor sites, and fetal reticuloendothelial blockade. Recent evidence would suggest that the latter is the most probable explanation. Gottvall and Selbing[72] noted that the fetal/maternal ratio of anti-D antibodies increased with advancing gestational age in cases of RhD-negative fetuses. In contrast, the fetal/maternal ratio in cases of RhD-positive fetuses remained constant at 10%, indicating that the maternal antibody was actively bound to fetal red cells. In cases of alloimmunized pregnancies treated with intravenous immunoglobulin (IVIG), the fetal/maternal antibody ratio in cases of RhD-positive fetuses more closely approximated that seen in the case of RhD-negative fetuses. This led the authors to conclude that IVIG's major mechanism of action is to block the fetal reticuloendothelial system. Voto and co-workers[73] compared the outcome of 30 patients receiving IVIG before 20 weeks' gestation followed by IUTs after 20 weeks to a group of 39 patients treated with only IUTs between 20 and 25 weeks' gestation. Hydrops fetalis was less frequent in the IVIG/IUT group as compared to the IUT-only group (27% vs. 74%; RR = 0.36). In addition, the incidence of fetal death was markedly decreased

with the addition of IVIG (20% vs. 51%; RR = 0.39). These data would suggest that both plasmapheresis and IVIG could play a role in the prolongation of pregnancy in case of severe red cell alloimmunization with a history of second-trimester hydrops fetalis. Studies in other immunologic diseases such as Guillain-Barré syndrome have suggested an additive effect.[74] Besalduch et al.[75] have reported such combination therapy in a case of severe anti-E alloimmunization with good outcome. We have therefore elected to offer a combined treatment program of plasmapheresis and IVIG to patients with a history of recurrent early second-trimester hydrops fetalis. At 10 weeks' gestation, the patient undergoes a single-volume plasmapheresis every other day for three procedures. After the third procedure, the first half of a 2-g/kg loading dose of IVIG is administered. The following day, the second half of the loading dose (1 g/kg) of IVIG is given. The patient is maintained on weekly infusions of 1 g/kg of IVIG until 20 weeks' gestation (Fig. 34–5). All doses of IVIG are administered in the blood bank outpatient donor center or the outpatient oncology chemotherapy suite. Although the majority of the literature proposes a dose of 200 mg/kg each day for 5 successive days, we have elected to infuse the total amount in a single dose by slow infusion over 4 to 6 hours.[73] This appears to be well tolerated with the exception of severe headache. Premedication with two extra-strength capsules of acetaminophen seems to be effective in preventing this complication. An additional problem with the use of IVIG has been the conversion of serologic testing for viral infections such as hepatitis B. Although this does not indicate the acquisition of active infection, the presence of these viral markers precludes the patient from donating red cells according to Food and Drug Administration standards should IUTs later become necessary. We therefore usually have the patient donate 1 unit of red cells prior to receiving IVIG. The unit is fractionated into two subunits and frozen for later use. After 20 weeks' gestation, the patient's pregnancy is then managed with serial amniocenteses,

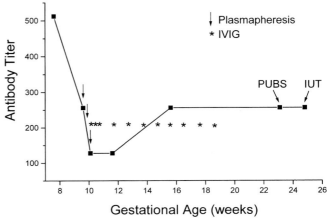

FIGURE 34–5. Graphic representation of maternal titer in a patient treated with combined plasmapheresis and intravenous immunoglobulin. *Vertical arrows* indicate plasmaphereses. *Asterisks* indicate doses of intravenous immune globulin. (PUBS = percutaneous umbilical blood sampling; IUT = intrauterine transfusion.)

cordocenteses, or Doppler assessments of the middle cerebral artery.

Conclusion

Intrauterine transfusion for severe fetal anemia can be touted as the first attempt at in utero therapy. Today it still holds the claim at being the most successful. Future efforts in the treatment of fetal HDN secondary to maternal red cell alloimmunization must focus on the down-regulation of the maternal antibody response once prophylactic immune globulin has failed the patient.

REFERENCES

1. Schamacher B, Moise KJ: Fetal transfusion for red cell alloimmunization in pregnancy. Obstet Gynecol 88:137–50, 1996.
2. Bowell P, Wainscoat JS, Peto TE, et al: Maternal anti-D concentrations and outcome in rhesus haemolytic disease of the newborn. Br Med J 285:327–379, 1987.
3. Bennett PR, Kim CL, Colin Y, et al: Prenatal determination of fetal RhD type by DNA amplification following chorion villus biopsy or amniocentesis. N Engl J Med 329:607–610, 1993.
4. Yankowitz J, Li S, Weiner CP: Polymerase chain reaction determination of RhC, Rhc, and RhE blood types: An evaluation of accuracy and clinical utility. Am J Obstet Gynecol 176:1107–1111, 1997.
5. Hessner MJ, McFarland JG, Endean DJ: Genotyping of KEL1 and KEL2 of the human Kell blood group system by the polymerase chain reaction with sequence-specific primers. Transfusion 36:495–499, 1996.
6. Hessner MJ, Pircon RA, Johnson ST, Luhm RA: Prenatal genotyping of Jka and Jkb of the human Kidd blood group system by alelle-specific polymerase chain reaction. Prenat Diagn 18:1225–1231, 1998.
7. Hessner MJ, Pircon RA, Johnson ST, Luhm RA: Prenatal genotyping of the Duffy blood group system by alelle-specific polymerase chain reaction. Prenat Diagn 19:41–45, 1999.
8. Eshleman JR, Shakin-Eshleman SH, Church A, et al: DNA typing of the human MN and Ss blood group antigens in amniotic fluid following massive transfusion. Am J Clin Pathol 103:353–357, 1995.
9. Van den Veyver IB, Moise KJ: Fetal RhD typing by polymerase chain reaction in pregnancies complicated by rhesus alloimmunization. Obstet Gynecol 88:1061–1067, 1996.
10. Lo Y-M D, Bowell PJ, Selinger M, et al: Prenatal determination of the fetal RhD status by analysis of peripheral blood of rhesus negative mothers. Lancet 341:1147–1148, 1993.
11. Lo YM, Noakes L, Bowell PJ, et al: Detection of fetal RhD sequence from peripheral blood of sensitized RhD-negative pregnant women. Br J Haematol 87:658–660, 1994.
12. Geifman-Holtzman O, Bernstein IM, Berry SM, et al: Fetal RhD genotyping in fetal cells flow sorted from maternal circulation. Am J Obstet Gynecol 174:818–822, 1996.
13. Al-Mufti R, Howard C, Overton T, et al: Detection of fetal messenger ribonucleic acid in maternal blood to determine the fetal RhD status as a strategy for noninvasive prenatal diagnosis. Am J Obstet Gynecol 179:210–214, 1998.
14. Geifman-Holtzman O, Kaufman L, Gonchoroff N, et al: Prenatal diagnosis of the fetal Rhc genotype from peripheral maternal blood. Obstet Gynecol 91:505–510, 1998.
15. Nicolaides KH, Thilaganathan B, Rodeck CH, Mibashan RS: Erythroblastosis and reticulocytosis in anemic fetuses. Am J Obstet Gynecol 159:1063–1065, 1988.
16. Nicolaides KH, Fontanarosa M, Gabbe SG, Rodeck CH: Failure of ultrasonographic parameters to predict the severity of fetal anemia in rhesus isoimmunization. Am J Obstet Gynecol 158:920–926, 1988.
17. Vintzileos AM, Campbell WA, Storlazzi E, et al: Fetal liver ultrasound measurements in isoimmunized pregnancies. Obstet Gynecol 68:162–167, 1986.
18. Roberts AB, Mitchell JM, Pattison NS: Fetal liver length in normal and isoimmunized pregnancies. Am J Obstet Gynecol 161:42–46, 1989.
19. Oepkes D, Meerman RH, Vandenbussche FP, et al: Ultrasonographic fetal spleen measurements in red blood cell alloimmunized pregnancies. Am J Obstet Gynecol 69:121–128, 1993.
20. Fan F-C, Chen RY, Schuessler GB, Chien S: Effects of hematocrit variations on regional hemodynamics and oxygen transport in the dog. Am J Physiol 238:H545–H552, 1980.
21. Warren PS, Gill RW, Fisher CC: Doppler flow studies in rhesus isoimmunization. Semin Perinatol 11:375–38, 1987.
22. Rightmire DA, Nicolaides KH, Rodeck CH, Campbell S: Fetal blood velocities in Rh isoimmunization: Relationship to gestational age and to fetal hematocrit. Obstet Gynecol 68:233–236, 1986.
23. Bilardo CM, Nicolaides KH, Campbell S: Doppler studies in red cell isoimmunization. Clin Obstet Gynecol 32:719–727, 1989.
24. Mari G, Adrignolo A, Abuhamad Z, et al: Diagnosis of fetal anemia with Doppler ultrasound in the pregnancy complicated by maternal blood group immunization. Ultrasound Obstet Gynecol 5:400–405, 1995.
24a. Mari G and the Collaborative Group for Doppler Assessment of the Blood Velocity in Anemic Fetuses: Noninvasive diagnosis by Doppler ultrasonography of fetal anemia due to maternal red-cell alloimmunization. N Eng J Med 342:9–14, 2000.
25. Liley AW: Liquor amnii analysis in the management of the pregnancy complicated by rhesus sensitization. Am J Obstet Gynecol 82:1359–1370, 1961.
26. Nicolaides KH, Rodeck CH, Mibashan RS, Kemp JR: Have Liley charts outlived their usefulness? Am J Obstet Gynecol 155:90–94, 1986.
27. Queenan JT, Tomai TP, Ural SH, King JC: Deviation in the amniotic fluid optical density at a wavelength of 450 nm in Rh-immunized pregnancies from 14 to 40 weeks' gestation: A proposal for clinical management. Am J Obstet Gynecol 168:1370–1376, 1993.
28. Fernandez CO, Wendel PJ, Brown CL: Rh-immunization: An evaluation of a proposed new clinical management protocol. 41st Annual Meeting of the Society for Gynecologic Investigation. Chicago, Illinois, 1993.
29. Weiner CP, Williamson RA, Wenstrom KD, et al: Management of fetal hemolytic disease by cordocentesis I. Prediction of fetal anemia. Am J Obstet Gynecol 165:546–553, 1991.
30. Weiner CP, Wenstrom KD: Outcome of alloimmunized fetuses managed solely by cordocentesis but not requiring antenatal transfusion. Fetal Diagn Ther 9:233–238, 1994.
31. Weiner CP: Human fetal bilirubin levels and fetal hemolytic disease. Am J Obstet Gynecol 166:1449–1454, 1992.
32. Bowman JM, Pollock JM, Manning FA, et al: Maternal Kell blood group alloimmunization. Obstet Gynecol 79:239–244, 1992.
33. Vaughan JI, Warwick R, Letsky E, et al: Erythropoietic suppression in fetal anemia because of Kell alloimmunization. Am J Obstet Gynecol 171:247–252, 1994.
34. Weiner C, Wildness J: Decreased erythropoiesis and hemolysis in Kell hemolytic disease. Am J Obstet Gynecol 172:277, 1995.
35. Berkowitz RL, Beyth Y, Sadovsky E: Death in utero due to Kell sensitization without excessive elevation of the ΔOD_{450} value in amniotic fluid. Obstet Gynecol 60:746–749, 1982.
36. Barss VA, Benacerraf BR, Greene MF, et al: Sonographic detection of fetal hydrops. J Reprod Med 30:893–894, 1985.
37. Vaughan JI, Manning M, Warwick RM, et al: Inhibition of erythroid progenitor cells by anti-Kell antibodies in fetal alloimmune anemia. N Engl J Med 338:798–803, 1998.
38. Freda VJ, Adamsons K: Exchange transfusion in utero. Report of a case. Am J Obstet Gynecol 89:817–821, 1964.
39. Asensio SH, Figueroa-Longo JG, Pelegrina IA: Intrauterine exchange transfusion. Am J Obstet Gynecol 95:1129–1133, 1966.
40. Asensio SH, Figueroa-Longo JG, Pelegrina IA: Intrauterine exchange transfusion. A new technic. Obstet Gynecol 32:350–355, 1968.
41. Liley AW: Intrauterine transfusion of foetus in haemolytic disease. Br Med J 2:1107–1109, 1963.
42. Rodeck CH, Kemp JR, Holman CA, et al: Direct intravascular fetal blood transfusion by fetoscopy in severe rhesus isoimmunization. Lancet 1:625–627, 1981.
43. Bang J, Bock JE, Trolle D: Ultrasound-guided fetal intravenous transfusion for severe rhesus haemolytic disease. Br Med J 284:373–374, 1982.
44. Grannum PA, Copel JA, Plaxe SC, et al: In utero exchange transfusion by direct intravascular injection in severe erythroblastosis fetalis. N Engl J Med 314:1431–1434, 1986.

45. Berkowitz RL, Chitkara U, Goldberg JD, et al: Intrauterine intravascular transfusions for severe red blood cell isoimmunization: Ultrasound-guided percutaneous approach. Am J Obstet Gynecol 155:574–581, 1986.

46. Welch R, Rampling MW, Anwar A, et al: Changes in hemorheology with fetal intravascular transfusion. Am J Obstet Gynecol 170:726–732, 1994.

47. Moise KJ, Carpenter RJ, Kirshon B, et al: Comparison of four types of intrauterine transfusion: Effect on fetal hematocrit. Fetal Ther 4:126–137, 1989.

48. Nicolini U, Kochenour NK, Greco P, et al: When to perform the next intrauterine transfusion in patients with Rh allo-immunization: Combined intravascular and intraperitoneal transfusion allows longer intervals. Fetal Ther 4:14–20, 1989.

49. Giannina G, Moise KJ, Dorman K: A simple method to estimate volume for fetal intravascular transfusions. Fetal Diagn Ther 13:94–97, 1998.

50. Bowman JM: The management of Rh-isoimmunization. Obstet Gynecol 52:1–16, 1978.

51. Lewis M, Bowman JM, Pollock J, Lowen B: Absorption of red cells from the peritoneal cavity of an hydropic twin. Transfusion 13:37–40, 1973.

52. Harman CR, Bowman JM, Manning FA, Menticoglou SM: Intrauterine transfusion-intraperitoneal versus intravascular approach: A case-control comparison. Am J Obstet Gynecol 162:1053–1059, 1990.

53. Hallak M, Moise KJ, Hesketh DE, et al: Intravascular transfusion of fetuses with rhesus incompatibility: Prediction of fetal outcome by changes in umbilical venous pressure. Obstet Gynecol 80:286–290, 1992.

54 Radunovic N, Lockwood CJ, Alvarez M, et al: The severely anemic and hydropic isoimmune fetus: Changes in fetal hematocrit associated with intrauterine death. Obstet Gynecol 79:390–393, 1992.

55. Saade GR, Moise KJ, Copel JA, et al: Fetal platelet counts correlate with the severity of the anemia in red-cell alloimmunization. Obstet Gynecol 82:987–991, 1993.

56. Mandelbrot L, Daffos F, Forestier F, et al: Assessment of fetal blood volume for computer-assisted management of in utero transfusion. Fetal Ther 3:60–66, 1988.

57. Waters AH: Prenatal management of fetal alloimmune thrombocytopenia. Vox Sang 65:180–189, 1993.

58. Bernstein HH, Chitkara U, Plosker H, et al: Use of atracurium besylate to arrest fetal activity during intrauterine intravascular transfusions. Obstet Gynecol 72:813–816, 1988.

59. Daffos F, Forestier F, Mac Alesse J, et al: Fetal curarization for prenatal magnetic resonance imaging. Prenat Diagn 8:311–114, 1988.

60. Pielet BW, Socol ML, MacGregor SN, et al: Fetal heart rate changes after fetal intravascular treatment with pancuronium bromide. Am J Obstet Gynecol 159:640–643, 1988.

61. Gonsoulin WJ, Moise KJ, Milam JD, et al: Serial maternal blood donations for intrauterine transfusion. Obstet Gynecol 75:158–162, 1990.

62. Saade GR, Moise KJ, Belfort MA, et al: Fetal and neonatal hematologic parameters in red cell alloimmunization: Predicting the need for late neonatal transfusions. Fetal Diagn Ther 8:161–164, 1993.

63. Koenig JM, Ashton RD, DeVore GR, Christensen RD: Late hypogenerative anemia in Rh hemolytic disease. J Pediatr 115:315–318, 1989.

64. Ovali F, Samanci N, Dağoğlu T: Management of late anemia in rhesus hemolytic disease: Use of recombinant human erythropoietin (a pilot study). Pediatr Res 39:831–834, 1996.

65. Millard DD, Gidding SS, Socol ML, et al: Effects of intravascular, intrauterine transfusion on prenatal and postnatal hemolysis and erythropoiesis in severe fetal isoimmunization. J Pediatr 117:447–454, 1990.

66. Nasrat HA, Nicolini U, Nicolaidis P, et al: The effect of intrauterine intravascular blood transfusion on iron metablosim in fetuses with Rh alloimmunization. Obstet Gynecol 77:558–562, 1991.

67. Doyle LW, Kelley EA, Rickards AL, et al: Sensorineural outcome at 2 years for survivors of erythroblastosis treated with fetal intravascular transfusions. Obstet Gynecol 81:931–935, 1993.

68. Janssens HM, de Haan MJ, van Kamp IL, et al: Outcome for children treated with fetal intravascular transfusions because of severe blood group antagonism. J Pediatr 131:373–380, 1997.

69. Hudon L, Moise KJ, Hegemier SE, et al: Long-term neurodevelopmental outcome after intrauterine transfusion for the treatment of fetal hemolytic disease. Am J Obstet Gynecol 179:859–863, 1998.

70. Bowman JM, Peddle LJ, Anderson C: Plasmapheresis in severe Rh isoimmunization. Vox Sang 15:272–277, 1968.

71. Odendaal HJ, Tribe R, Kriel CJ, et al: Successful treatment of severe Rh iso-immunization with immunosuppression and plasmapheresis. Vox Sang 60:169–773, 1991.

72. Gottvall T, Selbing A: Consumption of anti-D in the erythroblastotic fetus. Acta Obstet Gynecol Scand 77:500–503, 1998.

73. Voto LS, Mathet ER, Zapaterio JL, et al: High-dose gammaglobulin (IVIG) followed by intrauterine transfusions (IUT's): A new alternative for the treatment of severe fetal hemolytic disease. J Perinat Med 25:85–88, 1997.

74. Plasma Exchange/Sandoglobulin Guillain-Barré Syndrome Trial Group: Randomised trial of plasma exchange, intravenous immunoglobulin, and combined treatments in Guillain-Barré syndrome. Lancet 349:225–230, 1997.

75. Besalduch J, Forteza A, Durán MA: Rh hemolytic disease of the newborn treated with high-dose intravenous imunoglobulin and plasmapheresis. Transfusion 31:380–381, 1991.

76. Weinstein L: Irregular antibodies causing hemolytic disease of the newborn: A continuing problem. Clin Obstet Gynecol 25:321–332, 1982.

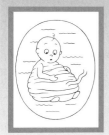

CHAPTER 35

The Fetus with Nonimmune Hydrops Fetalis

ULRICH GEMBRUCH and WOLFGANG HOLZGREVE

The Greek-Latin term "hydrops fetalis" refers to pathologically increased accumulations of interstitial fluid in fetal soft tissues and serous cavities (Fig. 35–1).[1] Hydrops is characterized as being "nonimmune" if there is no evidence of blood group incompatibility (isoimmunization), and it occurs in association with an extremely wide variety of conditions. The term "immune hydrops fetalis," which is covered in Chapter 34, is used in cases of hydrops caused by alloimmune hemolytic anemia in the presence of circulating maternal antibodies against fetal erythrocytes. The incidence of nonimmune hydrops (NIHF) varies between 1 in 1,500 and 1 in 4,000 deliveries.[2–4] Because of the high intrauterine loss rate among hydropic fetuses, the true occurrence rate most likely is higher; in some instances, however, fetal hydrops can also regress during gestation. Especially in chromosomally abnormal fetuses there is a high spontaneous abortion rate between the first and second or third trimesters of pregnancy[5] following an early appearance of hydrops in late first and early second trimesters, whereas in chromosomally normal fetuses the hydrops often develops much later.[6–9] When comparing the large variability of the reported NIHF series it is important to realize that the incidence and etiology are strongly influenced by ethnic background (e.g., homozygous α-thalassemia is the most common cause of nonimmune hydrops in Southeast Asia, whereas cardiac diseases are the most common cause in Caucasians). Furthermore, the incidence and the distribution of causative and associated diseases in the reported series are strongly influenced by factors such as the presence of a general ultrasound screening program, the gestational age windows of the screening examinations, and the specific referral patterns in any region. The same influences are relevant for the reported survival rates, which vary between 10 and 60% in the literature.[1, 4, 6, 7, 10–16]

The intrauterine diagnosis of hydrops fetalis is achieved by ultrasound, which demonstrates the skin edema and fluid accumulations in serous cavities, such as abdominal ascites, pleural and/or pericardial effusion in the fetus, and/or hydrops placentae. There is some confusion in the literature about the precise definition of the term "hydrops." Classically, hydrops was defined by the demonstration of fluid accumulations in at least two fetal sites; but some series also included cases of isolated pleural effusion, abdominal ascites, or generalized skin edema, because a fluid accumulation in one site may represent an early stage of a disease, which may lead to fluid accumulation in several sites at a more advanced stage. Although polyhydramnios is associated in 30 to 75% of cases with nonimmune hydrops,[4, 6] the amniotic sac should not be considered one of the serous cavities for the diagnosis of hydrops, because the pathophysiologic mechanisms of the occurrence of polyhydramnios can differ from the increased rate of interstitial fluid accumulation causing hydrops fetalis and placentae. Sometimes hydrops may even be associated with oligohydramnios (e.g., in some preterminal fetuses with Turner syndrome, where the cystic hygroma seems to fill the whole amniotic cavity or in cases with intrauterine cytomegaloviral infection).

The list of disorders associated with fetal hydrops comprises far more than 150 fetal conditions, but for many of these the association is only based on one or few case reports.[1, 11–15, 18] In previous reviews about nonimmune hydrops,[1, 11, 13, 15, 17–19] a classification was chosen based mainly on the most affected organ system (Table 35–1). In this chapter the different diseases and associations are additionally grouped and analyzed according to their prevalence, and the pathophysiologic mechanisms that lead to NIHF, and the possibility of their intrauterine management. Specific diseases associated with hydrops fetalis and their management are discussed in the following chapters of this book: Cardiac arrhythmia (Chapter 27), pulmonary diseases (Chapter 19), hydro-/chylothorax (Chapter 13), sacrococcygeal teratoma (Chapter 21), and the twin-twin transfusion syndrome (Chapter 23). The beginning or the increased risk of a generalized hydrops can sometimes be the indication for open fetal surgery, which is covered elsewhere in this book (see Chapter 5).

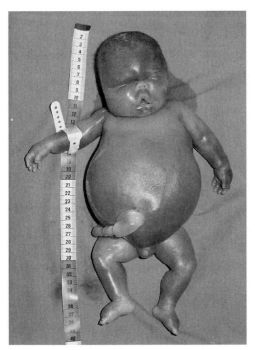

FIGURE 35–1. Third-trimester fetus with generalized NIHF who died in utero.

Pathophysiology

The extracellular fluid compartment is divided into an intravascular and interstitial compartment of which the latter consists of the transcellular and lymphatic fluid components. There is a constant exchange of fluids between both these compartments. Fetal fluid accumulation and hydrops generally originate from an imbalance between the rate of interstitial fluid formation by capillary ultrafiltration exceeding the rate of interstitial fluid return through the venule side of the capillary bed and the lymphatic system back to the circulation. The regulation of fluid movements between vascular and interstitial spaces and its alterations have been elegantly reviewed in detail.[20] The six classically postulated mechanisms for development of fetal hydrops can be explained by the concept of disturbed interstitial fluid balance: (1) primary myocardial failure; (2) high output cardiac failure; (3) decreased colloid oncotic plasma pressure; (4) increased capillary permeability especially secondary to tissue hypoxia or sepsis; (5) obstruction of venous flow; and (6) obstruction of lymphatic flow.[15, 20, 21]

The Starling hypothesis (Fig. 35–2) describes the regulation of fluid movement across the capillary membrane expressed by the following equation[20, 22]:

$$J_v = CFC \left[(P_c - P_i) - \sigma(\pi_c - \pi_i) \right]$$

The total flow of fluid (J_v) across the capillary membrane is influenced by the two driving forces for capillary ultrafiltration into the interstitial fluid: the intracapillary hydrostatic pressure (P_c) and the colloid oncotic pressure of the interstitial fluid (π_i). The interstitial hydrostatic pressure (tissue turgor tension) (P_i) and the plasma colloid osmotic pressure (π_c) are the opposite Starling forces. The fluid filtration coefficient (CFC) represents the net amount of fluid crossing the capillary membrane for a given imbalance of the Starling forces, and is affected by both the conductance of the capillary wall and the ease of fluid movement in the interstitial space. Furthermore, changes of the permeability of a particular capillary bed change the reflection coefficient for oncotically active solute (σ) and, therefore, the influence of a given colloid osmotic pressure differs between both compartments. Thus, an increased capillary permeability allows water and protein to leak easier into the interstitial space of the fetus and/or placenta. Under normal conditions, the differences of the hydrostatic and colloid oncotic pressure in the intracapillary and interstitial fluid cause a fluid shift into the interstitial compartment on the arteriolar side of the capillary bed and a flux back into the intravascular compartment on the venule end. Abundant fluid in the interstitial compartment is returned to the vascular space via the lymphatic system. The outflow pressure for the lymphatic flow is the central venous pressure, which determines the capacity of drainage of the interstitial space by the lymphatic system.[20, 22, 23]

In addition, regulation of fluid distribution in the fetus may be modified by the placental circulation receiving about 40% of the fetal combined cardiac output. Increased hydrostatic pressure or decreased plasma colloid oncotic pressure in the fetus enhance the transcapillary fluid filtration into the interstitial compartment of the fetus and the placenta; in the placenta this would also drive fluid into the maternal vascular space, at least partially counteracting the fluid retention by the fetus. On the other hand, studies in fetal sheep show that the fetal placental postcapillary resistance is quite large,[24] while the somatic postcapillary resistance is very low.[25] In other words, placental capillary pressure may be protected from an elevation of the venous pressure by a small decrease in placental flow, whereas somatic capillary pressure tightly reflects the systemic venous pressure.[26] Therefore, an elevation of venous pressure cannot result in a compensatory increased fetal fluid flux into the mother. In addition, tissue hypoxia may result in a slight increase of fetal serum lactate as a powerful osmotic agent.[27] Other osmotically active fetal waste products such as CO_2 and K^+ may be increased in the hydropic fetus too.[28] The presence of hydrops and polyhydramnios suggests that the net rate of fluid flux from the mother to the fetus must be increased in conditions with hydrops fetalis.[28] Furthermore, alterations of the frequently hydropic placenta may occur (e.g., an increased capillary permeability with loss of protein into the interstitial mesenchymal space of the villi). Data from fetal sheep also suggest a decrease in cardiac output in many fetuses with hydrops of different etiology resulting in an increased fluid rate from the mother to the fetus caused by the reduced hydrostatic pressure on the fetal side of the placenta.[28] In a primary lymphatic obstruction of the fetus, protective placental mechanisms against elevation of venous pressure cannot be effective.

TABLE 35–1. NONIMMUNE HYDROPS: CAUSES AND ASSOCIATIONS*†

FOCAL ABNORMALITIES IN THE FETUS

1. Cranial

Fetal intracranial hemorrhage   *low*
Vein of Galen aneurysm   *low*
Cerebral tumor   *low*

2. Thorax

2.1. Cardiac

Structural defects:
  Atrioventricular septal defect, isolated or in association with M.
    Down   *low*
  Atrioventricular septal defect in combination with heterotaxia
    syndrome (situs ambiguus, left atrial isomerism, right atrial
    isomerism) and bradyarrhythmia   *high*
  Tricuspid dysplasia and Ebstein anomaly   *low*
  Severe obstruction of right ventricular outflow tract by pulmonary
    stenosis, pulmonary atresia, and premature obstruction of
    ductus arteriosus (spontaneously or by indomethacin)   *low*
  Absent pulmonary valve syndrome (mostly combined with
    tetralogy of Fallot and/or agenesis of ductus arteriosus)   *low*
  Aortico-left ventricular channel   *low*
  Truncus arteriosus communis with insufficiency of the truncal
    valve   *low*
  Premature closure of foramen ovale   *unknown*
  Severe obstruction of left ventricular outflow tract by aortic
    stenosis and atresia leading to interatrial left-to-right shunt or
    premature closure of foramen ovale   *low*
Cardiac tumors:
  Rhabdomyoma, often as part of tuberous sclerosis   *low*
  Hemangioma
  Hamartoma
  Intrapericardial teratoma
Cardiomyopathy
  Dilated
  Restrictive
Myocarditis
Myocardial infarction
Idiopathic arterial calcification   *high*
Arrhythmias:
  Tachyarrhythmias   *high*
    Supraventricular tachycardia
    Atrial flutter
    Ventricular tachycardia
  Bradyarrhythmias:
    Sinus bradycardia   *low*
    Complete heart block
      Combined with atrial isomerism and structural defect (see
        above)   *high*
      In the presence of maternal autoimmune antibodies (anti-
        SSA, anti-SSB)   *low*

2.2. Pulmonary and Mediastinal

Primary uni- or bilateral hydro-/chylothorax   *high*
Congenital cystic adenomatoid malformation
  Macrocystic CCAML   *high*
  Microcystic CCAML   *low*
Extralobar pulmonary sequestration   *high*
Laryngeal atresia (CHAOS)
Mediastinal teratoma
Fibrosarcoma
Intrathoracic alimentary tract duplication cyst
Diaphragmatic hernia   *low*
Pulmonary lymphangiectasia

3. Gastrointestinal

Diaphragmatic hernia   *low*
Meconium peritonitis caused by bowel perforation: spontaneously,
  bowel obstruction (various types of atresia of the intestinal tract,
  volvulus), or infection   *low*
Intestinal hemorrhage caused by bowel perforation   *low*
Hepatitis
Hepatic fibrosis
Hemochromatosis
Cholestasis

Cirrhosis with portal hypertension
Congenital portal dysplasia
Polycystic disease of the liver
Giant cell hepatitis
Torsion of an ovarian cyst

4. Renal

Congenital nephrosis (Finnish type)   *low*
Urethral obstruction with rupture of bladder   *low*
Polycystic kidney diseases (ARCKD, ADCKD)   *low*
Renal vein thrombosis

5. Tumors and Vascular Disorders

Teratoma (sacrococcygeal, mediastinal, intracerebral,
  intrapericardial)   *low*
Mediastinal fibrosarcoma
Disseminated congenital neuroblastoma
Hepatoblastoma
Hamartoma
Mesoblastic nephroma
Arteriovenous malformation
  Fetal hemangioma (liver, neck, chest)   *low*
  Diffuse neonatal hemangiomatosis   *high*
  Klippel-Trenaunay-Weber syndrome   *low*
  Umbilical cord hemangioma   *low*
  Chorioangioma   *low*
Vena cava inferior thrombosis
Renal vein thrombosis
Idiopathic arterial calcification   *high*

GENERALIZED ABNORMALITIES IN THE FETUS

1. Hematologic Disorders Causing Fetal Anemia

Excessive erythrocyte loss
  Intrinsic hemolysis or abnormal hemoglobins
    α-Thalassemia   *high*
    Erythrocyte enzyme disorders: Glucose-6-phosphate
      dehydrogenase deficiency, pyruvate kinase deficiency, glucose
      phosphate isomerase deficiency, congenital erythropoietic
      porphyria   *low*
    Erythrocyte membrane disorders: abnormalities of
      spectrin   *low*
  Extrinsic hemolysis:
    Kasabach-Merritt sequence (arteriovenous malformations and
      tumors)
  Hemorrhage
    Fetomaternal hemorrhage   *high*
    Fetal closed-space hemorrhage (bowel, intracranial,
      tumor)   *low*
    Twin-to-twin transfusion (including acardiac parasitic
      twin)   *low*
Erythrocyte underproduction
  Liver and bone marrow replacement syndromes
    Transient myeloproliferative disorder
    Congenital leukemia
  Red cell aplasia and dyserythropoiesis
    Parvovirus B19 infection   *high*
    Blackfan-Diamond syndrome   *low*
    Dyserythropoietic anemias   *low*

2. Infectious Causes

Parvovirus B19   *high*
Cytomegalovirus   *low*
Syphilis   *low*
Toxoplasmosis   *low*
Herpes simplex virus   *low*
Adenovirus   *low*
Coxsackievirus   *low*
Varicella   *low*
Hepatitis A   *low*
Rubella   *low*
Respiratory syncytial virus   *low*
Listeriosis   *low*
Chagas diasease   *low*
Leptospirosis   *low*

Table continued on following page

TABLE 35–1. NONIMMUNE HYDROPS: CAUSES AND ASSOCIATIONS*† Continued

3. Skeletal Dysplasias   *low*

Achondrogenesis type I (Parenti-Fraccaro)
Achondrogenesis type II (Langer-Saldino)
Short-rib polydactyly syndromes
  Saldino-Noonan
  Majewski
  Verma-Naumoff
  Beemer
Osteogenesis imperfecta type II
Lethal osteopetrosis
Asphyxiating thoracic dysplasia (Jeune syndrome)
Thanatophoric dysplasia
Achondroplasia
Koide osteochondrodystrophy
McGuire osteochondrodysplasia
Intrauterine dwarfism with thin bones and fractures (Kozlowski-Kan
  syndrome)
Greenberg-Rimoin chondrodystrophy
Lethal chondrodysplasia with spondylocostal dysostosis and major
  non-skeletal anomalies (Moerman-Vandenberghe-Fryns syndrome)
Lethal Kniest-like dysplasia
Chondrodysplasia punctata, Conradi-Hünermann variant
Pyknoachondrogenesis
Wegmann-Jones-Smith syndrome
Boomerang skeletal dysplasia
Lethal chondrodysplasia with advanced bone age (Blomstrand
  syndrome)
Herva-Leisti-Kirkinen syndrome (contractures, congenital lethal
  Finnish type)
Congenital infantile cortical hyperostosis (Caffey syndrome)

4. Metabolic Disorders   *low*

Lysosomal storage diseases: *low*
  Sphingolipidoses:
    GM₁ gangliosidosis
    Galactosialidosis
    Farber disease (disseminated lipogranulomatosis)
    Gaucher disease (glucocerebrosidase deficiency)
    Niemann-Pick disease type A
  Mucopolysaccharidoses:
    Mucopolysaccharidosis type I (Hurler syndrome)
    Mucopolysaccharidosis type IVa (Morquio A syndrome)
    Mucopolysaccharidosis type VII (β-glucuronidase deficiency)
  Mucolipidoses:
    Mucolipidosis type I (sialidosis)
    Mucolipidosis type II (I-cell disease)
  Transport defects:
    Sialic acid storage disease
    Salla disease
    Niemann-Pick disease type C
  Other lysosomal storage diseases:
    Wolman disease
Carbohydrate-deficient gycoprotein syndrome   *low*
Glycogen storage disease type II (Pompe)   *low*
Cardiac glycogen storage disease with normal maltase
  activity   *low*
Carnitine deficiency   *low*
Erythrocyte enzyme disorders:
  Glucose-6-phosphate dehydrogenase deficiency   *low*
  Pyruvate kinase deficiency   *low*
  Glucose phosphate isomerase deficiency   *low*

Fetal hyperthyroidism (maternal Graves disease)   *low*
Fetal hypothyroidism   *low*

5. Syndromes   *low*

Autosomal dominant inheritance
  G.-syndrome (Optiz-Frias syndrome)
  Congenital myotonic dystrophy
  Cornelia de Lange syndrome
  Noonan syndrome
  Yellow nail syndrome
  Tuberous sclerosis (already in utero with rhabdomyomata)
Autosomal recessive inheritance
  Arthrogryposis multiplex congenita
  Pena-Shokeir syndrome
  Lethal multiple pterygium syndrome
  Neu-Laxova syndrome
  Recurrent isolated hydrops
  Cryptophthalmos-syndactyly syndrome (Fraser syndrome)
  Cumming syndrome
  Polysplenia syndrome (left atrial isomerism)
  Orofaciodigital syndrome type II (Mohr syndrome)
  Isolated recurrent cystic hygroma
  Elejalde syndrome
  McKusick-Kaufman syndrome
  Hypophosphatasia
Angioosteohypertrophy syndrome (Klippel-Feil-Trenaunay)   *low*
Wiedemann-Beckwith syndrome   *low*

6. Chromosomal Aberrations   *low*

Trisomy 21
Trisomy 18
Trisomy 13
Turner syndrome
Trisomy 15
Trisomy 16
Triploidy
Tetraploidy
Trisomy 10 mosaicism
46,XX/XY mosaic
49,XXXXY
Partial duplication of chromosome 5
Partial duplication of chromosome 11
Partial duplication of chromosomes 15 and 17
Partial duplication of chromosome 18
Partial deletion of the short arm of chromosome 13
Partial deletion of the short arm of chromosome 18
Rearrangement of the long arm of chromosome 22

7. Placental and Umbilical Cord Anomalies   *low*

Chorioangioma
Chorioangioma as part of Wiedemann-Beckwith syndrome
Subchorial placental hematoma
Hemorrhagic endovasculitis of the placenta
Chorionic vein thrombosis
Placental and umbilical vein thrombosis
True knots of the cord
Angiomyxoma of the umbilical cord
Aneurysm of the umbilical artery
Umbilical cord torsion

---

* This table is modified from corresponding tables in the following publications: Holzgreve et al. 1984[11], 1985[12]; Machin, 1989[15]; Holzgreve, 1990[1]; Hansmann et al., 1990[13]; Jones, 1995[18]; and Arcasoy & Gallagher, 1995.[200]
† The statement *low* and *high* behind the particular disease indicates the rate of the occurrence of hydrops if the fetus has the respective disease. In the vast majority of causes and associations the incidences of these diseases are too low for giving reliable information.

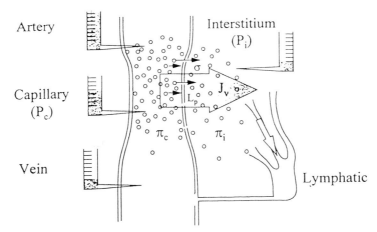

FIGURE 35–2. The Starling hypothesis of fluid distribution between blood plasma and interstitial compartments. Capillary ultrafiltration is driven between capillary (P_c) and interstitial (P_i) hydrostatic pressures. Fluid reabsorption by the capillary is driven by the difference between the capillary (π_c) and interstitial (π_i) colloid oncotic pressures, measures of the concentrations of oncotically active molecules. The reflection coefficient for oncotically active solute (σ) and the hydraulic permeability (L_p) are intrinsic properties of the capillary wall that characterize the efficacy of such driving forces to produce water flux (J_v). The capillary fluid filtration coefficient, CFC, is the product of capillary surface area and hydraulic conductivity (L_p) and represents the net amount of fluid crossing the capillary bed for a given imbalance in the Starling forces. Interstitial fluid is returned to the circulation via the lymphatic system. The outflow pressure for the lymphatic flow is the venous pressure. The "manometers" indicate the relative pressures in each compartment. Thus, the overall flux across the capillary (J_v), can be expressed by the equation: $J_v = \text{CFC}\,[(P_c - P_i) - \sigma(\pi_c - \pi_i)]$. (From Apkon M: Pathophysiology of hydrops fetalis. Semin Perinatol 19:437–446, 1995, with permission.)

Data on fluid distribution and regulation of the intercompartmental flow under normal and pathologic circumstances, however, are almost exclusively based on studies in the sheep and only allow a cautious extrapolation to other species, especially the human fetus. Furthermore, the relevance of the different endocrine, paracrine, and neuronal factors that may generally and locally govern the regulation of body fluid distribution by changes of the Starling forces and the lymphatic drainage are very difficult to study and at present poorly understood. Physiologically, the interstitial space of the fetus seems to be substantially large in comparison to the postpartum situation. The ratio of interstitial fluid volume to plasma volume in fetal sheep is about 3:1, which is similar to that of adult sheep. But considering that roughly 30% of the fetal plasma volume is outside of the fetal body, it becomes evident that the fetal interstitial volume is increased relative to the adult sheep with an elevated ratio of about 4.4:1.[23]

According to fetal lamb studies, several factors facilitate transcapillary fluid filtration into the interstitial space during fetal compared to adult life.[20, 22]

1. Especially, the permeability of the capillary membrane for plasma proteins is 15 times higher than in adult sheep[29]; this decreases the reflection coefficient for the colloids (σ), impairing the effect of the colloid oncotic pressure difference between fetal vascular and interstitial space and, therefore, the driving force of fluid flux back into the vascular space. On the other hand, this lower effect of the colloid oncotic pressure difference on the transcapillary fluid flux in the fetus seems to relatively protect the fetus against the negative effect of a hypoproteinemia.

2. Furthermore, the fluid filtration coefficient (CFC) of the capillary bed is roughly fivefold higher in fetal than in adult sheep, facilitating and increasing the fluid flow for any given imbalance in the Starling forces.[30]

3. In addition, the compliance of the interstitial space of the fetus is higher than in the adult sheep. Therefore, a greater accumulation of interstitial fluid is necessary in the fetus to increase the interstitial hydrostatic pressure or, expressed in another way, smaller changes in the hydrostatic pressure difference between capillary and interstitial space ($\Delta P = \Delta P_c - \Delta P_i$) lead to a larger fluid flow across the capillary membrane.[30] The increase of both the fluid filtration coefficient and the compliance of the interstitial space facilitate the transcapillary fluid flow and allow the fetus a more rapid restoration of blood volume after acute blood volume loss and expansion caused by acute hemorrhage and infusion, respectively.[20, 23] Changes of the transplacental fluid transfer seem to be without relevance in this context.

The lymphatic system allows the return of fluid and the oncotic active proteins to the vascular space. Studies in sheep have elucidated the importance of this system for the fluid balance between the intravascular and interstitial compartment.[23] Basal lymph flow rates in the fetus are substantially higher than postpartum, reflecting the enhanced transcapillary flow into the interstitial space.[23, 31] In fetal sheep, vascular volume load increases the lymph flow rate, and draining via the thoracic duct to the outside decreases the blood volume.[23] There is a uniform relationship between thoracic duct lymph and plasma protein concentration of around 50 to 75% in the sheep fetus, newborn, and adult.[23] Very important for the pathogenesis of hydrops is the observation that the lymphatic drainage of the interstitial space is not impeded at a normal outflow pressure for the lymphatic system, which represents the central venous pressure.[23, 31, 32] The lymphatic flow rate in the thoracic duct of fetal sheep is four- to fivefold higher than in adult sheep.[23, 31] If the venous pressure increases over the physiologic value of 3 to 4 mm Hg, the lymphatic flow rate in the fetus is substantially reduced and ceases at only 16 mm Hg[23, 31, 32] (Fig. 35–3). In adult sheep the flow is relatively constant up to 8 mm Hg and only stops at 26 mm Hg. This delicate relationship between venous pressure and lymphatic flow represents one important pathophysiologic mechanism for the occurrence of fetal hydrops.[23, 31, 32]

Elevation of the systemic venous pressure due to circulatory dysfunction seems to be the most important pathogenetic mechanism for the development of hydrops even if increased capillary permeability, decreased plasma oncotic pressure, and obstruction of lymphatic return may also contribute to the fluid accumulation in fetal soft tissue and serous cavities.[20] An increase of venous pressure may be considered as a consequence of homeostatic mechanisms serving to preserve adequate systemic delivery of metabolic substrate when cardiocirculatory function is impaired. Decreased intravascular volume may occur due to blood loss as a result of fetofetal or fetomaternal transfusion or fetal hemorrhage or due to a relative deficiency of intravascular volume as a result of an increased fluid loss into the interstitial space by increased capillary permeability or

decreased plasma oncotic pressure. Tissue hypoxia may cause capillary damage; hepatocellular injury can lead to hypoproteinemia. Furthermore, local hypoxia may lead to tissue lactate accumulation, a powerful osmotic agent. Diminished venous return may be caused by local obstruction of venous flow, but more often by a decreased ventricular compliance and by significant shortening of the diastolic period in tachyarrhythmia. Inadequate oxygen supply during the advanced stage of various alterations may decrease the ventricular compliance, possibly also in tachyarrhythmia, which may lead to inadequate myocardial blood flow because of the substantially shortened duration of the diastole. In consequence, diastolic cardiac dysfunction and decreased venous return may result in low cardiac output due to inadequate ventricular filling. Primary myocardial dysfunction may also impair stroke volume and cardiac output (e.g., in cases of myocarditis, myocardial infarction, or myocardial hypoxia). Furthermore, systolic cardiac dysfunction can occur when right and left ventricular afterload are increased, which is very poorly tolerated by the fetus. In this group, obstructive lesions of the semilunar valves, premature constriction of the ductus arteriosus, and arterial hypertension in the recipient fetus of a fetofetal transfusion syndrome and in cases with hypoxemia-induced arterial blood flow redistribution with peripheral vasoconstriction increasing significantly the right ventricular afterload can be included. Because of the low heart rate, the cardiac output may be diminished in fetuses with complete heart block, even if the stroke volume is compensatorily increased. Furthermore, diminished supply of organs with oxygen and nutrients may be compensated for by an increase of cardiac output, the product of stroke volume and heart rate leading to high output cardiac failure (e.g., in cases of decreased hemoglobin saturation and/or hemoglobin concentration, in cases of maldistribution of flow, such as tumors and arteriovenous malformations, or in cases of metabolic disorders such as thyrotoxicosis).[20, 21]

In all of these pathologic conditions local and systemic compensatory mechanisms become effective and may help the fetus to survive. On the other hand, some of these mechanisms at the same time increase the imbalance of Starling forces, resulting in enhanced interstitial fluid accumulation. In advanced disease an increase of hydrops and fetal deterioration may occur when the compensatory mechanisms become exhausted, resulting in further elevation of venous pressure by secondary volume overload or myocardial dysfunction with occurrence of atrioventricular valve regurgitation.[20, 21] Compensatory mechanisms are:

1. The opening of additional capillaries may increase the exchange area between vascular and interstitial space, improving the extraction of oxygen and nutrients.
2. The distribution of arterial and venous blood flow by selective vasoconstriction maintains the supply of heart, brain, and adrenal glands with oxygen and nutrients at the expense of other organs. This selective reaction of the vascular bed is triggered

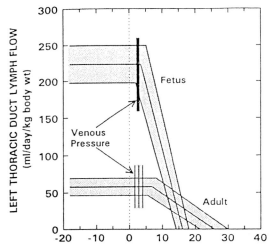

FIGURE 35–3. Comparison of lymphatic flow function curves for the left thoracic duct in unanesthetized fetal and adult sheep. The outflow pressure for the lymphatic system is central venous pressure which is the same in near-term ovine fetus and adult and averages 3 to 4 mm Hg (*Stippled area covers* ± 2 SE). In the ovine fetus, any increase in venous pressure reduces lymphatic flow, which ceases when venous pressure nears 16 mm Hg. In adult sheep the flow is relatively constant up to 8 mm Hg and only stops at 26 mm Hg. (From Brace RA: Fluid distribution in the fetus and neonate. *In* Polin RA, Fox WW [eds]: Fetal and Neonatal Physiology. Philadelphia: WB Saunders Company, 1998, pp 1703–1713, with permission.)

by chemoreceptors followed by neuronal and endocrine-mediated stimulation of vasoconstriction and by local autoregulation.

3. The increase of blood flow and better supply of oxygen and nutrients to organs may result from elevation of the cardiac output, which can be achieved by increase of the heart rate and/or systolic ventricular function as well as by an increase of intravascular blood volume and/or venous pressure.

An increase of intravascular volume may be achieved by fluid retention by the kidneys and/or by transcapillary reabsorption, especially in cases of lowered intravascular volume and venous pressure. Elevation of venous pressure by volume increase or increase of venous tone leads to an improved ventricular filling. However, because of the diminished preload reserve and Frank-Starling mechanism of the fetal heart, which seems to operate near to the top of its ventricular function curve, it seems to be difficult for the fetus to convert any increase of myocardial filling into an appropriate augmentation of cardiac output, which limits this compensatory mechanism. Above this limit, atrial distention may lead to release of atrial natriuretic factor, which may increase not only the production of urine but also the capillary permeability. In the fetal lamb, transient right atrial pacing inducing hydrops causes a three- to fourfold increase in atrial natriuretic peptide concentration, which normalizes parallel to the clearance of hydrops.[33] In human fetuses, increased concentrations of atrial natriuretic factor were demonstrated by cordocentesis in conditions associated with atrial distention (e.g., in anemic and acidemic fetuses, in fetuses with congestive heart failure, in the recipient fetus with twin-twin transfusion syndrome, and in fetuses after volume expansion by intrauterine blood transfusion).[34, 35] Furthermore, aldosterone levels are increased in hydropic fetuses when compared with normal grown and growth-restricted fetuses.[36] In the fetus, the renin-angiotensin system controls the intravascular volume by modulating placental capillary blood pressure, but in adults by affecting urine excretion.[37] By blocking the renin-angiotensin system in the hydropic ovine fetus, a substantial increase of placental blood flow at the expense of somatic flow was followed by a considerable reduction of the degree of hydrops.[37] Disturbances of other factors such as vasopressin, endothelin, and prostaglandins may also occur in some hydropic fetuses and be relevant as pathogenetic mechanisms.[37] Thyroid hormones may regulate the activity of the adrenergic receptors in the lymphatic system. In thyroid hormone deficiency, reduced adrenergic stimulation of the lymphatic system may delay the return of lymphatic fluid to the vascular compartment and may be a possible pathophysiologic explanation for the association between congential hypothyroidism and hydro-/chylothorax with hydrops.[38]

Cardiovascular Anomalies

Because fetal cardiac arrhythmias are covered in detail in Chapter 27 and congenital heart diseases in Chapter 26, we concentrate here on the association of cardiac diseases with nonimmune hydrops fetalis.

With documented incidences between 20 and 40%, cardiac anomalies are the defects most commonly associated with nonimmune hydrops.[11, 13, 14, 39] Sustained arrhythmia and/or structural cardiac defects can cause congestive heart failure and resultant nonimmune hydrops.[39] Because of the parallel arrangement of the fetal circulation, anomalies of the right and left ventricular flow may elevate the right atrial and systemic venous pressure. Soft tissue edema and effusion into the serous cavities, but not pulmonary edema, are the consequence. On the other hand, the parallel flow circuitry protects the fetus against cardiac decompensation; isolated structural cardiac defects very seldom lead to interstitial fluid accumulation and hydrops. Therefore, it is incorrect from a pathophysiologic point of view that in many published reports a causative relationship between the cardiac lesion and the hydrops is postulated (e.g., in cases with ventricular or atrial septal defects, tetralogy of Fallot, or transposition of the great arteries). In these cases, different reasons may have led to hydrops, especially in fetuses with autosomal trisomies and Turner syndrome. Therefore, in many cases with hydrops and heart defect there is only a coincidental, not causal, relationship between the cardiac abnormality and the nonimmune hydrops.[39, 40]

Cardiomegaly and severe atrioventricular valve regurgitation (tricuspid and/or mitral regurgitation) are often demonstrated if a primary or secondary congestive heart failure is present. Common examples would be cases of malformations of the atrioventricular valve, arteriovenous malformations, tumors, anemia, or hypervolemia due to twin-twin transfusion sequence. Structural cardiac defects more frequently causing hydrops are malformations of the atrioventricular (AV) valve apparatus, such as tricuspid dysplasia, Ebstein anomaly, and atrioventricular septal defects (AV canal defect). In the presence of severe atrioventricular regurgitation there is an elevation of atrial pressure during the regurgitation and during the diastolic period due to increased filling volume. The severity of the atrioventricular valve incompetence (Fig. 35–4), or even diminished function of the left ventricle and/or a relatively small opening of the foramen ovale in the cases of tricuspid dysplasia/Ebstein anomaly and the coexistence of atrioventricular conduction block in cases of atrioventricular septal defect, determine whether a congestive heart failure occurs in the individual case.[41–45] Rare structural abnormalities with severe insufficiency of the semilunar valve, such as truncus arteriosus communis with severe incompetence of truncal valve and the absent pulmonary valve syndrome, may cause severe atrioventricular regurgitation with consecutive elevation of the right atrial and venous pressure. Absent pulmonary valve syndrome, however, is most commonly associated with tetralogy of Fallot and mostly with agenesis of ductus arteriosus.[46] In these fetuses, pressure and volume overload due to pulmonary stenosis and insufficiency may cause tricuspid incompetence and sometimes hydrops.[47, 48] Constriction of ductus arteriosus leads to acute afterload mismatch, elevation of right ventricular pressure, and

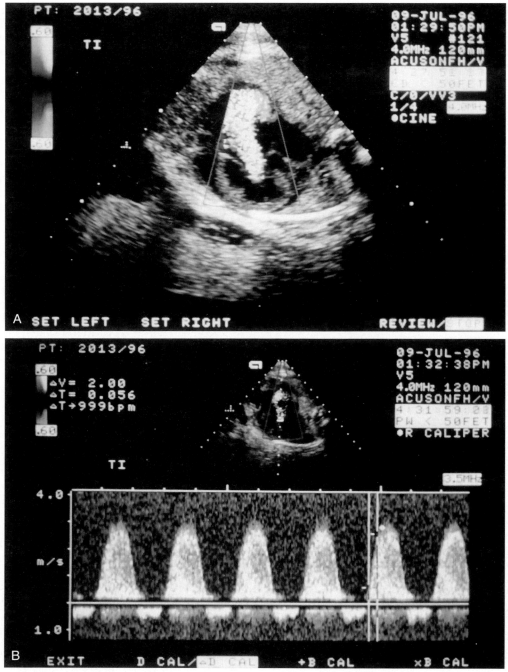

FIGURE 35–4. *A,* In a 28-week fetus with pericardial perfusion, polyhydramnios, and placentomegaly, fetal echocardiography showed cardiomegaly, tricuspid dysplasia, and pulmonary atresia. Holosystolic tricuspid regurgitation was demonstrated by color flow Doppler mapping. The mosaic pattern of the jet filled the major part of the dilated right atrium. *B,* The investigation by a continuous wave Doppler confirmed the diagnosis of severe tricuspid insufficiency demonstrating the high velocity (maximal velocity, 3.15 m/sec; pgrad = 40 mm Hg; $\Delta p/\Delta t$ = 286 mm Hg/sec) and turbulent character (high variance of the Doppler shift frequencies within the jet) of the tricuspid regurgitant jet.

severe tricuspid regurgitation, probably caused by papillary muscle dysfunction and/or dilatation of the tricuspid annular ring.[49] Rarely, there is a spontaneous constriction and closure of the ductus arteriosus.[50, 51] In the vast majority of cases ductal constriction or closure is caused by transplacental transfer of indomethacin or other prostaglandin synthesis inhibitors applied to the mother for treatment of premature contractions and/or polyhydramnios.[49, 52, 53] In the same way, afterload mismatch by structural right ventricular outflow tract obstruction (pulmonary atresia with intact interventricular septum and severe pulmonary stenosis) and, rather rarely, left ventricular outflow tract (aortic atresia and severe aortic stenosis) obstruction may cause severe insufficiency of tricuspid or mitral valves, respectively. In severe mitral regurgitation, elevation of the right atrial pressure may be caused by substantial alteration of flow via the foramen ovale with appearance of left to right shunt or complete closure of the foramen ovale.[54–56] The existence of a primary premature closure of the foramen ovale as an occasional cause of a secondary hypoplastic left heart syndrome has been abandoned in the meantime. A few case reports, however, describe an isolated restriction and premature closure of the foramen ovale in association with a nonimmune hydrops,[57, 58] also in association with tachyarrhythmia.[59] In those cases initial left atrial depolarization may result in a premature pressure increase in the left atrium, which lowers the interatrial shunt during the short diastole or may lead to premature closure of the foramen ovale. On the other hand, premature closure of the foramen ovale has also been reported in nonhydropic fetuses[60] and, in an autopsy series, was not significantly increased among hydropic infants compared to nonhydropic controls, indicating that factors other than premature closure of the foramen ovale are operative in the pathogenesis of nonimmune hydrops.[40] Primary myocardial dysfunction may be caused by myocarditis[61] and dilated or restrictive cardiomyopathies and may lead to hydrops by reduced cardiac output because of an impairment of the diastolic and/or systolic ventricular function and, consequently, generalized circulatory failure.[62–64] As a secondary consequence, cardiomegaly and atrioventricular valve regurgitation may occur under these circumstances. Myocardial infarction is very rare during fetal life, and seems to be mostly induced by coronary thromboembolism.[65] Due to the parallel circuitry, fetuses with the left coronary artery originating from the pulmonary trunk stay compensated until birth. Postpartum, the resulting hyp-

oxia can cause myocardial infarction. Dependent on their localization, size, and number, cardiac tumors may cause hydrops by impeding diastolic filling, by altering the function of atrioventricular valves, or by obstructing the outflow tract,[66] sometimes indirectly by induction of sustained tachyarrhythmia. The majority of fetal intracardiac tumors are rhabdomyomata (Fig. 35–5) without and with tuberous sclerosis, which is present in around 50% of fetuses with rhabdomyomata.[67–69] In case of rhabdomyoma, a definitive exclusion of tuberous sclerosis is impossible by prenatal ultrasound, because the pathognomonic giant cell astrocytomata are almost always undetectable by sonography of fetal brain. However, successful in utero diagnosis of associated intracerebral lesions indicating tuberous sclerosis has been reported by magnetic resonance imaging.[70] Furthermore, development of fetal hydrops has been seen in one fetus with a right atrial hemangioma[71] and in another with a hamartoma of the conduction system in association with tachyarrhythmia and structural heart defect.[72] More often, a pericardial teratoma may induce hydrops by cardiac compression.[73–76] In some cases of cardiac defects with AV valve regurgitation, atrial dilatation may induce tachyarrhythmia, which may contribute to fetal hydrops.[77–79] Eventually, various extracardiac diseases may secondarily cause cardiomegaly and significant atrioventricular valve regurgitation (e.g., high-cardiac-output failure, increased afterload, and hypoxemia). The idiopathic arterial calcification has an unknown etiology and is characterized by generalized calcification, especially of the wall in the arterial trunk of the pulmonary artery and aorta.[80] Most commonly, the coronary arteries are affected, but peripheral arteries of the gastrointestinal tract, kidneys, extremities, brain, and placenta may also be involved (Fig. 35–6). In these fetuses myocardial dysfunction may cause severe hydrops, tissue ischemia, and fetal death in the late second or third trimester.[80, 81]

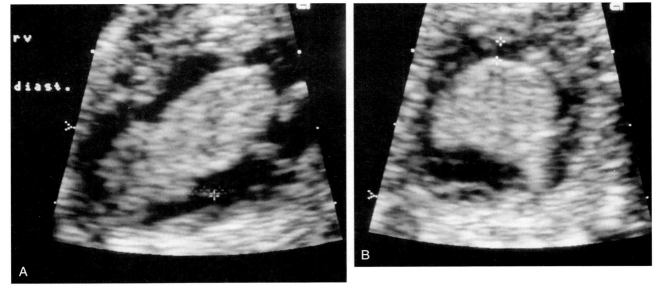

FIGURE 35–5. *A*, In a fetus of 23 weeks' gestation, the four-chamber view shows a large rhabdomyoma involving the interventricular septum and the major part of the right ventricle and extending to the valve ring. *B*, Short-axis view of the same fetus at 23 + 0 weeks' gestation showing that the rhabdomyoma almost fills the whole right ventricle.

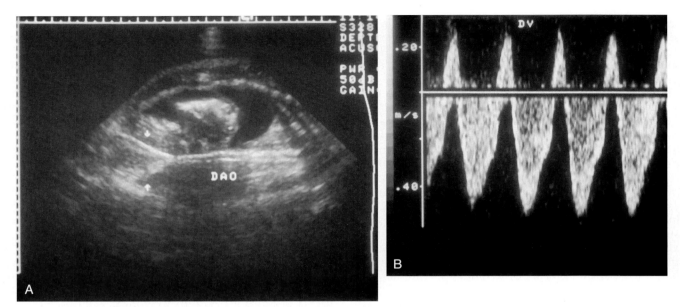

FIGURE 35–6. *A,* In this severe hydropic fetus of 29 weeks' gestation, idiopathic arterial calcification was correctly diagnosed by demonstration of the characteristic calcifications in the walls of the arteries in this fetus not only in the central arteries but also in the coronary, renal, hepatic, mesenteric, and extremity arteries. The ultrasound figure showed the calcified walls of the descending aorta and its bifurcation, the iliac arteries, and in the hepatic arteries. Ascites and skin edema are also visible on this picture. *B,* The blood flow velocity waveform in the ductus venosus shows a distinct reverse blood flow during atrial contraction indicating the severe cardiac dysfunction.

In less severe cases, especially if no hydrops is present, palliative treatment postpartum with steroids and diphosphonates may stop the progression of the disease.[80] However, most infants with idiopathic arterial calcification die within the first year of life complicated by cardiac and pulmonary failure, renal infarction, peripheral gangrene, and bowel infarction.[80]

As there are no curative in utero treatment options for fetal hydrops caused by cardiac defects, only palliative treatment is indicated in selected cases. Complete or partial remission or prevention of congestive heart failure by improvement and maintenance of normal cardiac function is a very important part of intrauterine therapy in these diseases. Currently, transplacental and sometimes direct application of digoxin seems to be the only approach for a nonspecific palliative treatment.

Sustained fetal tachyarrhythmia (supraventricular tachycardia with 1:1 AV conduction and atrial flutter) may cause congestive heart failure leading to elevated right atrial and systemic venous pressure and may be followed by nonimmune hydrops, placental edema, and polyhydramnios (Fig. 35–7). In fetuses supraventricular tachycardia is more frequent than atrial flutter independent of the presence or absence of hydrops, whereas ventricular tachycardia is very rare.[82] Between 80 and 90% of cases with this supraventricular tachycardia are AV reentrant tachycardias based on an accessory atrioventricular conduction pathway beside the AV node, whereas an ectopic tachycardia and an AV nodal reentrant tachycardia are not often the electrophysiologic mechanism of perinatal supraventricular tachycardia.[79, 83–85] An accessory atrioventricular connection seems also to be present in the majority of fetuses with atrial flutter.[79] Pathophysiologically, there is a substantial shorten-ing of the diastolic period of the cardiac cycle that prevents adequate early diastolic filling of the ventricles. Furthermore, it is suggested that initial left atrial depolarization can be tolerated to a lesser degree by the fetus, because the left ventricular output is diminished and the interatrial right-to-left shunt is disturbed. Due to the relative stiffness of the fetal myocardium, ventricular filling is predominantly dependent on the atrial systole and a regular 1:1 AV conduction sequence. Intermittent atrial contraction against a closed AV valve may predispose some fetuses with atrial flutter to the development of hydrops. Although there are important differences between atrial pacing in animal models, on the one hand, and supraventricular reentrant tachycardia, atrial flutter, and rapid sinus tachycardia in human fetus, on the other hand, atrial pacing studies in fetal lamb models still give important insights into the pathogenetic mechanisms of the development of fetal hydrops.[28, 86–89] In atrial pacing at rates up to 300 bpm there is an increase of ventricular output and a decrease of ventricular end-diastolic pressure. Prolonged left atrial pacing at rates of 300 to 320 bpm results in a decrease of cardiac output and in the development of hydrops within 4 to 48 hours; this confirms the suggestion that above a critical heart rate diastolic filling is impeded, especially for the ipsilateral ventricle. In these situations, cardiomegaly and hepatomegaly develop, arterial oxygen tension remains unchanged, and protein as well as albumin concentration stay stable or decrease slightly later on in the disease process.[28, 86–89] Because no or only a slight, nonsignificant hypoproteinemia may be observed, there is no evidence for an increase of capillary permeability for albumin. In advanced stages of congestive heart failure, however, there may be a more distinct hypoproteinemia due to

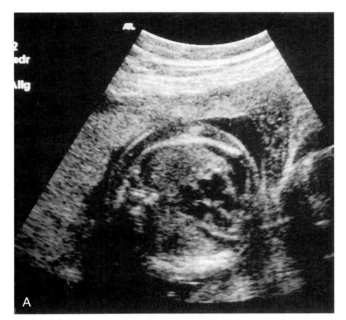

FIGURE 35–7. *A,* A hydropic fetus with supraventricular 1:1 re-entrant tachycardia of 250 bpm showed bilateral marked pleural effusions and cardiomegaly, visualized in the transverse scan of the thorax. Marked ascites, polyhydramnios, and placental hydrops were also visible at 21 + 5 weeks' gestation. *B,* Pulsed wave Doppler sonography of the ductus venosus showing the abrupt change from the normal biphasic forward flow pattern to the monophasic forward flow pattern with antegrade flow during systole and a reverse flow during diastole. This abrupt change from a biphasic to monophasic flow pattern is associated with an increase of inferior vena cava blood pressure of about 75% in fetal sheep.

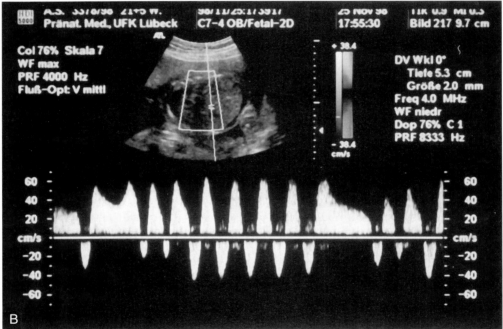

disturbed hepatic synthesis. The aortic pressure remains unchanged, while the mean venous pressure in the inferior vena cava increases by 75%.[89] This elevation may reflect a compensatory increase of venomotoric tone for maintenance of adequate cardiac output by an elevation of the preload. However, the abrupt elevation of venous pressure is associated with an immediate appearance of pulsatile reversal of blood flow occurring during diastole.[89] This is observed above a "critical" heart rate of 310 bpm. Below this heart rate, the venous flow is biphasic, with a systolic and diastolic forward surge that also occurs immediately after the pacing is stopped.[89] Besides the direct impeding of diastolic filling when the diastolic interval is critically shortened, the abrupt occurrence of

changes—reduction of ventricular output, the immediate elevation of venous pressure, and the appearance of pulsatile venous blood flow above a "critical" pacing rate—suggests ventricular dysfunction consistent with alteration of the pressure-volume relationship in association with impaired ventricular relaxation at high pacing rates. The most likely explanation is that oxygen supply to the myocardium by coronary blood flow is inadequate for the increased requirement of the myocardium during tachycardia.[90] Myocardial blood flow is maintained primarily by the pressure gradient across the vascular bed, extravascular pressure, and local autoregulation. Since the extravascular pressure is considerably lower in diastole than in systole, the major portion of coronary blood flow occurs in diastole. In tachycardia, however, the diastolic period is significantly shortened. Furthermore, with increased atrial pressure, the myocardial pressure gradients decrease. Severe ventricular dysfunction and even injury of the myocardium may occur in prolonged tachycardia and may cause reversible tachycardia-induced "cardiomyopathy" in humans and animals.[90–92] In conjunction with the enormous cardiac dilatation in fetuses with sustained supraventricular tachycardia, functional incompetence, as indicated by annular enlargement of both AV valves, may be observed, suggesting structural remodeling of the ventricles in the presence of tachycardia-induced "cardiomyopathy." In pigs, recovery from tachycardia-induced "cardiomyopathy" was accompanied by persisting chamber dilatation, significant myocardial hypertrophy, and persisting diastolic dysfunction.[93] During early recovery, left ventricular function and myocardial blood flow normalize at no exertion, but stress results in marked systolic and diastolic left ventricular dysfunction and reduced myocardial blood flow.[90, 92] In human fetuses, after termination of supraventricular tachycardia, cardiac dilatation, myocardial hypertrophy, AV valve incompetence, and hydrops disappear with immense interindividual differences, which could be explained by different stages of progression of tachycardia-induced "cardiomyopathy" at the time of drug-induced cardioversion.[78] Venous blood flow studies in the human fetus with supraventricular tachycardia demonstrate the occurrence of monophasic forward and pulsatile reversal blood flow during diastole in the inferior vena cava and ductus venosus (Fig. 35–7B) above a critical heart rate of approximately 210 to 220 bpm,[94] which is in accordance with the fetal lamb studies, where this change of venous blood flow pattern was associated with a considerable elevation of venous pressure.[89] Furthermore, in addition to persistence of cardiomegaly and atrioventricular valve regurgitation, abnormal indices of venous blood flow during sinus rhythm indicate the existence of altered myocardial function, suggesting the presence of a reversible tachycardia-induced "cardiomyopathy" in the human fetus too.[95] Time for remission of hydrops, disappearance of AV valve regurgitation, and normalization of the venous blood flow indices show a good correlation with immense interindividual differences, in which first the hydrops disappears, then the AV valve incompetence recovers, and, finally, the venous Doppler indices become normal.[78, 95, 96] In conclusion, the pathophysiologically most important mechanism in supraventricular tachycardia of the human fetus is an impeded ventricular filling due to an inadequately short diastolic interval that may directly alter the ventricular filling and/or by changes of diastolic ventricular function due to inadequate oxygen supply by reduced myocardial blood flow. Both mechanisms result in an elevation of venous pressure with a subsequently increased transcapillary fluid filtration rate into the interstitial space and significant reduction of lymphatic flow inadequate for drainage of the increasingly produced interstitial fluid back into the vascular space. Data of studies in animals and humans suggest that in not-so-advanced stages of disease the elevation of the venous

pressure results in a substantially increased transcapillary fluid filtration rate. Furthermore, the impaired lymphatic drainage is the most important pathophysiologic mechanism in sustained tachyarrhythmia, while hypoxia-induced increase of capillary permeability to water and proteins and alterations of the hepatic protein synthesis are not relevant for the development of hydrops.[86] Therefore, it seems advisable to treat fetuses with tachyarrhythmia in utero, because the congestive heart failure and elevation of venous pressure are reversible after drug-induced cardioversion, while tissue hypoxia damaging capillary membranes and/or liver cells seems not to be present in these fetuses.

Complete heart block may also cause fetal hydrops (Fig. 35–8). The combination of fetal complete heart block and AV septal defect in fetuses with left atrial isomerism especially seems to have a very poor prognosis, with appearance of hydrops and intrauterine death in the majority of fetuses.[41, 97, 98] The combination of malformed and most severely incompetent AV valve with ventricular bradycardia causing high stroke volume and increase of ventricular pressure is the pathophysiologic mechanism explaining the most common appearance of hydrops in these fetuses. In contrast, occurrence of hydrops in fetuses with AV block and "corrected" transposition of the great arteries is very rare because the AV valve apparatus is generally intact in these fetuses.[41,63] This is also the reason why in fetuses with complete heart block without congenital heart disease appearance of hydrops is much less frequently observed, occurring in only approximately 10 to 20% of the fetuses.[99] In these fetuses, complete heart block is not caused by a malformation of the conduction system, but follows an inflammatory destruction of conduction pathways especially in the AV-nodal region induced by a transplacental transfer of maternal autoimmune antibodies. Hydrops may occur when the ventricular escape rhythm is very low; furthermore, a widespread myocarditis and/or a generalized extracardiac inflammation may contribute to the occurrence of hydrops in some of these fetuses. Sometimes, hydrops only develops after 30 weeks' gestation, because at this time the required increase of the combined cardiac output cannot be produced by these fetuses. Another cause may be a progression of a more generalized myocarditis and/or inflammation of other fetal tissues due to autoimmune antibodies.[100, 101]

If hydrops develops as a result of a structural cardiac defect, the prognosis is very poor and intrauterine death often occurs. Especially postpartum, if switching of circulation and a substantial increase of cardiac work take place, these hydropic neonates with cardiac malformation will die. Therefore, in most cases of congenital heart defects causing hydrops, intrauterine treatment and preterm cesarean section seem not to be indicated. The same is true for cases with cardiac tumors and significant nonimmune hydrops. In some cases heart transplantation may be a therapeutic option, but the difficulties in the primary resuscitation of hydropic fetuses have to be considered. Furthermore, in cases of rhabdomyomata a tuberous sclerosis can never be completely excluded prenatally. In very special situations, particular considerations may lead to attempting palliative treatment of congestive

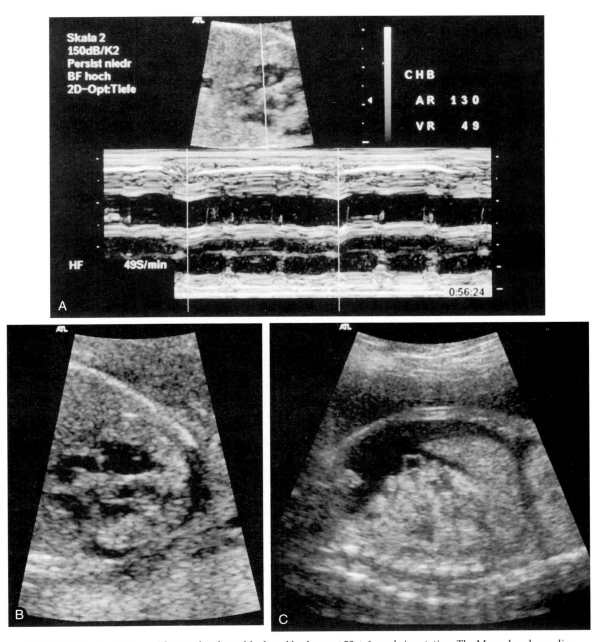

F I G U R E 35–8. *A,* Fetus with complete heart block and hydrops at 23 + 1 weeks' gestation. The M-mode echocardiogram shows a ventricular rate of 49 bpm and an atrial rate of 130 bpm; the ventricular systoles are independent of the atrial systoles. *B,* In the four-chamber view, cardiomegaly, distinct biventricular myocardial hypertrophy, and a mild pericardial effusion are visible. *C,* Marked ascites was present in this fetus with complete heart block already at 23 + 1 weeks' gestation.

heart failure by digoxin, if parents favor a more aggressive management. For example, both in tricuspid dysplasia and/or Ebstein anomaly with open pulmonary valve and in absent pulmonary valve syndrome, a distinct decrease of the right ventricular afterload may occur postnatally if the physiologic pulmonary hypertension present during fetal life disappears, inducing a significant reduction in the severity of tricuspid insufficiency. However, in many fetuses with these diseases, there is not only a severe pulmonary valve obstruction, but also lung hypoplasia and a maldevelopment of the pulmo-

nary arteries that cause persistent pulmonary hypertension and neonatal death. In a fetus with aortic stenosis and hydrops treated with digoxin, delivery by cesarean section, and balloon dilatation of the stenotic aortic valve in the neonatal period resulted in a successful outcome.[56] In the rare situation of isolated premature closure of the foramen ovale, delivery may be the best treatment[57] except for fetuses with tachyarrhythmia; in these latter fetuses prenatal normalization of cardiac rhythm may lead to a "reopening" of the foramen ovale. In rare individual cases of cardiac defects with consecutive hydrops, if the fetus is too immature for delivery, a palliative treatment with digoxin, which sometimes results in a transient stop of progression or a remission of hydrops by the positive-inotropic effect on the myocardium, may be applied in some selected cases, considering the generally very poor prognosis. However, because in the majority of cases the prognosis is very poor, termination of pregnancy or avoidance of aggressive in utero treatment and of an unnecessary cesarean section may be considered.

For fetal tachyarrhythmia, however, pathophysiologic data indicate that hydrops results from elevated venous pressure and consecutive obstruction of lymphatic drainage, but not from hypoxic damage of capillaries or other tissues. Due to the various problems postpartum in managing premature hydropic fetuses (postpartum increase of cardiac work, regulation of body temperature, mechanical ventilation; repetitive pleural drainage; simultaneous occurrence of lung edema and hyaline membrane disease, which reduce the effectiveness of surfactant therapy; tachyarrhythmia), iatrogenic preterm delivery of hydropic fetuses for better control of arrhythmia often results in a poor outcome. Treatment in utero for adequate control of the arrhythmia and remission of hydrops is prudent in sustained tachyarrhythmia of fetuses with and also without hydrops. In hydropic fetuses with tachyarrhythmia, intrauterine treatment with digoxin alone and in combination with different antiarrhythmic drugs (flecainide, propranolol, sotalol, amiodarone) is the best approach for almost all fetuses, as elaborated in Chapter 27. Transplacental treatment is successful in the majority of the cases.[83, 84, 102–104] Atrial flutter may be successfully suppressed by digoxin alone in only 50% of fetuses, but this therapy may be useful for its positive inotropic and negative chronotropic properties.[105] Also, in the absence of cardioversion and 1:1 AV conduction, hydrops does not often occur, presumably because atrial flutter seems to mostly start after 30 weeks of gestation.[105] Therefore, a second-line therapy is not commonly indicated in fetuses with atrial flutter.[105] In fetuses with supraventricular tachycardia refractory to transplacental therapy, the direct intravascular application of antiarrhythmic drugs to the fetus as an ultimate method may be successful.[102, 106, 107] In fetuses with complete heart block without structural cardiac malformation, intrauterine treatment of hydropic fetuses may be successful by transplacental infusion with salbutamol and isoprenaline (positive chronotropic and positive inotropic effects),[108] by treatment with digoxin (positive inotropic effect),[41, 109, 110] and by dexamethasone[100, 101] and/or plasmapheresis impairing the severity of inflammation, which may be not only in the conductive tissue but also in the myocardium and other fetal organs (see Chapter 27). In a few reported cases direct intrauterine pacing was technically successful, but only for hours.[111, 112]

Pulmonary Causes

The most frequent causes for pleural effusions are primary hydro-/chylothorax, congenital cystic adenoma-

toid malformation of the lung (CCAML), and extralobar pulmonary sequestration. Generalized hydrops may occur in all of these diseases. In contrast, pulmonary lymphangiectasia, laryngeal atresia, pulmonary hamartoma, mediastinal teratoma, intrathoracic alimentary tract duplication cyst, and diaphragmatic hernia are relatively rare causes of pleural effusion and hydrops. In all these cases the nonimmune hydrops most likely results from obstruction of the venous and/or lymphatic return. Some aspects of these diseases are discussed in this chapter. More information can also be found in the chapters about hydro-/chylothorax (Chapter 25), lung masses (Chapter 19), shunting (Chapter 23), and sonography for fetal thoracic surgery (Chapter 7).

Isolated uni- and often bilateral hydro-/chylothoraces are thought to result from a failure of the lymphatic drainage of the pleural space, most likely by maldevelopment of local lymph vessels, especially of the thoracic duct. The high frequency of pleural effusions in other fetal diseases associated with a maldevelopment of the lymphatic system such as Turner syndrome, Noonan syndrome, fetal lymphatic dysplasia, multiple pterygium colli syndrome, and pulmonary lymphangiectasia support the validity of this pathogenic mechanism. In addition, familiar occurrence of hydro-/chylothorax due to maldeveloped lymphatic organs was reported with isolated pleural effusion and generalized hydrops. In these disorders manifestation of pleural effusion and consecutive hydrops most commonly occurred during the late first and early second trimesters of pregnancy. Hydro-/chylothorax may result in generalized hydrops, especially with ascites and skin edema (Fig. 35–9), most likely by obstruction of abdominal lymph drainage—the thoracic duct transports the intra-abdominal interstitial fluid back into the superior vena cava—and increased venous pressure by excessive mediastinal shifting. In primary fetal hydrothorax, occurrence of hydrops is associated with a poor prognosis.[113] On the other hand, small primary uni- or bilateral hydrothoraces may be well tolerated, often followed by spontaneous regression later in gestation.[113]

In cases with pulmonary sequestration, however, increased production of pleural fluid may take place beyond 16 to 18 weeks' gestation (most likely due to the increasing production of pulmonary fluid). Increase of fluid retention with consecutive shifting and compression of other intrathoracic structures usually appears after 16 to 18 weeks in cases of CCAML and complete laryngeal atresia because of the increasing production of lung fluid. All these occupying processes in the intrathoracic space impede the thoracic and abdominal lymphatic drainage and, if further increase of intrathoracic pressure occurs, the venous return by compression and mediastinal shifting.[114] A compression of the fetal heart with consecutive restrictive cardiac failure in cases of massive bilateral pleural effusions and laryngeal atresia may be a further but rather rare pathogenic mechanism leading to generalized fluid accumulation only in an extremely advanced stage. Polyhydramnios, which is usually associated in these cases, seems to be the consequence of esophageal compression rather than of cardiac failure, especially in cases of microcystic CCAML and

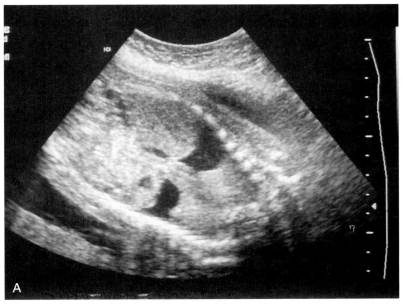

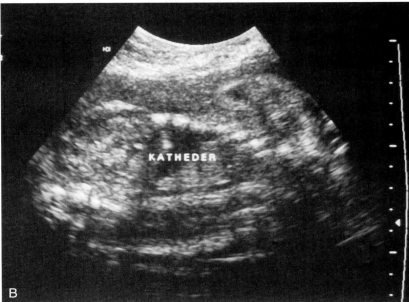

FIGURE 35–9. *A*, Fetus with bilateral hydrothoraces at 27 weeks' gestation. *B*, In the same fetus, after placement of bilateral pleural amniotic shunts in the following pregnancy, remission of hydrops was achieved. After birth the baby was treated because of development of chylothorax.

laryngeal atresia. In addition to the development of hydrops, all of these diseases except for laryngeal atresia may result in hypoplasia of the lung with consecutive respiratory distress after birth. For these lung masses, the survival rate is over 90% when hydrops is absent, but very low in hydropic fetuses.[115]

Pulmonary sequestration is characterized by masses of nonfunctional lung tissue supplied by an anomalous systemic artery. Extralobar sequestration mostly occurs intrathoracically, but also sometimes subdiaphragmatically. Sonographically, it is characterized as a well-defined, echodense, homogeneous mass similar to the microcystic type of CCAML (Fig. 35–10). Color flow Doppler mapping demonstrates the arterial supply coming from the descending aorta or intercostal arteries and venous return in the opposite direction into the azygos or hemiazygos veins. Intralobar sequestration also receives arterial supply from the systemic circulation, but venous drainage leads into the pulmonary vein. Retention of secretion and increased ipsilateral production of pleural fluid may reflect an inadequate lymphatic drainage of the sequestrum. In many cases, however, spontaneous involution of the pulmonary sequestration and accompanying pleural effusion may occur.[116] On the other hand, few cases with extralobar pulmonary sequestration may result in massive ipsilateral pleural effusion with subsequent mediastinal shifting, hypoplasia of ipsilateral and also contralateral lung, as well as generalized hydrops.[116, 117]

Congenital cystic adenomatoid malformations of the lung (CCAML) are classified by Stocker and co-workers into three types based primarily on cyst size.[118] Sono-

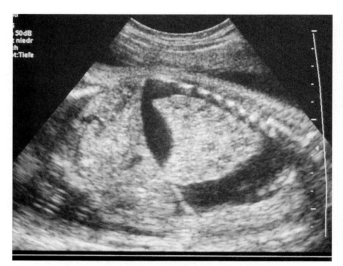

F I G U R E 35–10. In this fetus of 29 weeks' gestation, a hyperecho-genic sequestration of the right lung was demonstrated leading to massive hydrothorax with mediastinal shifting and downward bulging of the diaphragm.

graphically, types I and II are difficult to distinguish; therefore, in prenatal diagnosis, most authors differentiate only between the macrocystic type (single or multiple cysts with diameter of ≥5 mm) (Fig. 35–11) and the microcystic type (echodense homogeneous lung) (Fig. 35–12). Independent from the presence or absence of hydrops, the prognosis is much better for fetuses with macrocystic CCAML than for fetuses with microcystic CCAML, with survival rates of approximately 90% and 20%, respectively.[119] The most important prognostic factor of both diseases is the occurrence of hydrops; less important are mediastinal shifting and polyhydram-

nios.[115, 116, 119–121] Once the fetus develops hydrops prior to 28 weeks' gestation, the condition will usually be fatal unless treated in time.[116, 120] Because of the increase in lung fluid production, distention and hyperechogenicity are usually detectable from 16 to 18 weeks onwards. In contrast to the macrocystic type, microcystic CCAML is often associated with severe complications like pulmonary hypoplasia, hydrops fetalis, polyhydramnios, and placentomegaly. Especially for the macrocystic type of CCAML, however, partial involution and even disappearance, probably resulting from decompression into the bronchial tree or by outgrowth, have often been reported over the course of the pregnancy. Therefore, termination of pregnancy, but also intrauterine treatment, seems not to be necessary in fetuses with CCAML of the macrocystic type except for the rare cases with hydrops.[116, 121]

On the other hand, large pleural effusions in uni- or bilateral hydro-/chylothoraces present before 30 weeks may result in pulmonary compression and pulmonary hypoplasia of both lungs or of the remaining healthy lung tissue; furthermore, development of hydrops and polyhydramnios may decrease the survival rate and may lead to preterm labor or iatrogenic preterm delivery because of fetal distress. Therefore, an intrauterine treatment by decompression for prevention of lung hypoplasia seems to be indicated in such fetuses, especially if hydrops occurs. Although spontaneous resolution of primary hydrothorax is not rare, it seems to be unlikely if hydrops fetalis is already present.[113]

Intrauterine treatment of primary and also secondary hydrothorax resulting from a lung mass by repeated thoracocentesis has been reported and may lead to an improvement of the fetal condition documented by fetal heart rate monitoring and an increase in fetal move-

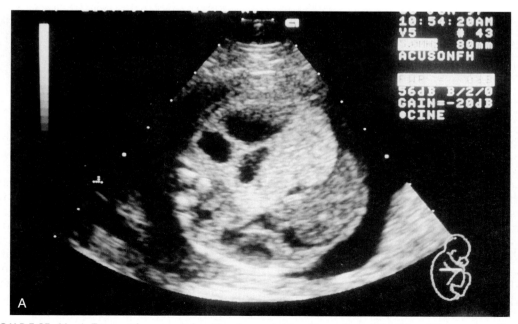

F I G U R E 35–11. *A,* Fetus with congenital cystic adenomatoid malformation of the lung of the macrocystic type at 20 + 3 weeks' gestation leading to massive shifting of mediastinum and to moderate ascites.

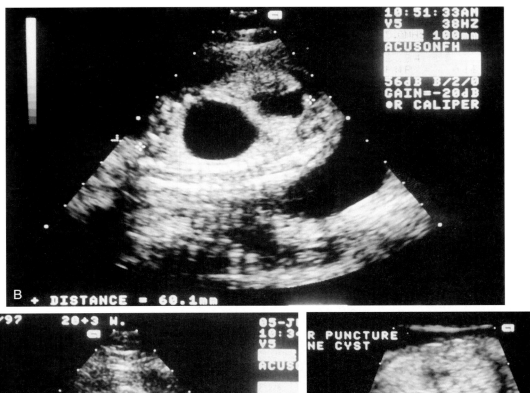

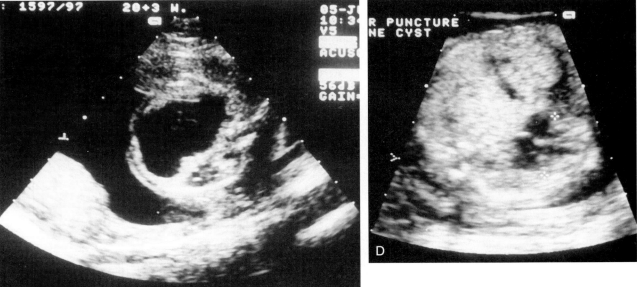

FIGURE 35–11 *Continued. B,* Sagittal scan of the same fetus showing the macrocystic malformed lung bulging the diaphragm downward. *C,* Large cyst extending to both sides of the thorax. *D,* After voiding of the cyst by needle thoracocentesis, the mediastinal shifting decreased. In the following gestation, spontaneous regression of the size of malformed lung occurred, hydrops disappeared, and a healthy baby was born. Postpartum lobectomy was successfully performed.

ments. In some cases of hydrothorax, fluid accumulation stops after only one thoracocentesis. In the vast majority of cases, however, single aspiration of pleural effusion is usually followed by rapid reaccumulation of pleural fluid within 24 hours. Therefore, single aspiration does not lead to an adequate continuous drainage of the pleural space. It may have (1) a diagnostic value, because it has been recognized that in hydro-/chylothorax almost all cells are lymphocytes, and (2) a prognostic value showing the potential of lung dilatation after decompression. Most centers recommend the placement of

pleuroamniotic shunts, unilateral or, if necessary, bilateral, for continuous decompression of the thoracic space[113, 122] (Fig. 35–13). In hydro-/chylothorax the reexpansion of the lung after aspiration and/or shunting seems to be an important prognostic sign. In cases of failed reexpansion, severe pulmonary hypoplasia must be expected. Successful drainage of fluid leading to remission of hydrops has been reported in a case of congenital diaphragmatic hernia too.[123] Also, in a fetus with an intrathoracic duplication cyst of the stomach, needle aspirations resulted in a rapid resolution of mediastinal

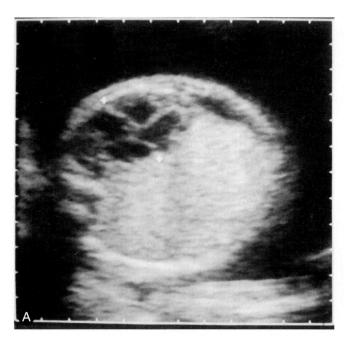

FIGURE 35–12. *A,* In a 24-week severely hydropic fetus, transverse scan of thorax showing a CCAML of the microcystic type (CCAML type III of the classification of Stocker[118]) of the right lung. Heart and mediastinum are shifted to the left side, and the hypoplastic left lung is not detectable. *B,* Doppler waveform profile of an intrapulmonary artery in a fetus with CCAML type III (microcystic type).

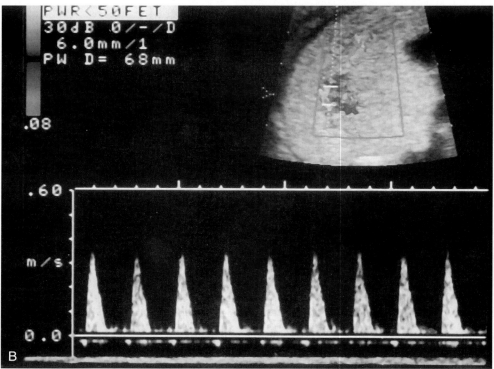

shift and hydrops, but in another fetus a reaccumulation of fluid in the alimentary tract duplication cyst was observed.[124] In macrocystic CCAML, puncturing and subsequent shunt placement in a large cyst may be successful; on the other hand, in the macrocystic type of CCAML spontaneous regression is relatively common and development of hydrops is rare; and therefore the prognosis is relatively good.[116] Puncturing and/or shunting of a large cyst in cases of CCAML are only justified in the presence of hydrops[116, 121] and in cases of extensive compression of other intrathoracic structures.

To the contrary, in fetuses with the microcystic CCAML development of hydrops is more frequent, mediastinal shifting and compression of the contralateral lung are more pronounced, and the prognosis is worse than in the microcystic type. In comparison with normal fetuses and fetuses with CCAML without progression to hydrops, increased mesenchymal production of platelet-derived growth factor-B was demonstrated in cases with CCAML with rapid growth and development of hydrops, requiring in utero resection, and may be responsible for the autonomous growth and proliferation in these

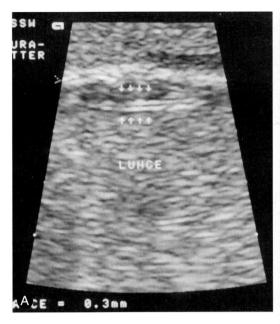
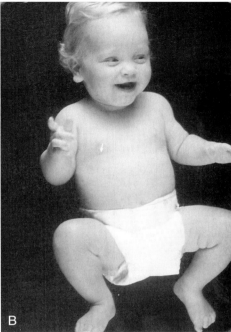

FIGURE 35–13. *A,* Successful in utero drainage of hydrothorax by a pleuroamniotic shunt in a fetus at 32 weeks' gestation; the pigtail catheter is marked by the *arrows. B,* After in utero placement of a pleuroamniotic shunt, the healthy infant showed only a small scar below his right nipple where the catheter was located, marked by the *arrow. See Color Plate 4*

cases.[125] In the absence of large cysts, puncturing and/or pleuroamniotic shunting is not possible. Therefore, in microcystic CCAML and development of hydrops prior to 30 weeks' gestation surgical resection by fetal lobectomy in utero was attempted and successfully performed, allowing expansion of the normal lung tissue in the following weeks still in utero.[116] After 30 weeks' gestation, early delivery following lung resection may be indicated in hydropic fetuses.

The sonographic findings of laryngeal atresia are very similar to microcystic CCAML, but always bilateral. Because of the retention of lung fluid under pressure, the expanded lungs are homogeneously echodense and may be diagnosable from 16 weeks' gestation onwards[126] (Fig. 35–14). There is a massive hyperplasia of lungs and an accelerated air space development. In contrast to the rare bilateral microcystic CCAML, the large bronchi are dilated in isolated laryngeal atresia. In fetuses with incomplete laryngeal atresia, pulmonary distention may fail and prenatal diagnosis may be impossible. In cases of complete atresia, compression of the lymphatics, the heart, and the venous return often results in hydrops. In the presence of an additional fistula, such as a tracheoesophageal fistula or persistent pharyngotracheal duct, regression of hydrops has been described.[126] Prognosis in fetuses with hydrops in general is poor. Neonatal management demands urgent tracheostomy to prevent asphyxia.[126] In these fetuses the EXIT (ex utero intrapartum treatment) procedure, which is applied to deliver fetuses with congenital diaphragmatic hernia after fetal surgical tracheal occlusion and fetuses with congenital high airway obstruction syndrome (CHAOS) by laryngeal atresia and large neck tumors, seems to be the optimal way to maintain an adequate uteroplacental perfusion and maternal oxygen support to the fetus until the fetal airway is secured and ventilation is established before dividing the cord.[127] Exact and comprehensive prenatal diagnosis is mandatory, because approximately 50% of fetuses have associated anomalies.[126] The autosomal recessive inherited cryptophthalmos-syndactyly syndrome (Fraser syndrome) is characterized by cryptophthalmos, abnormal genitalia, syndactyly of fingers and toes, uni- and bilateral renal agenesis, and/or multicystic renal dysplasia, often associated with laryngeal obstruction. In spite of severe oligohydramnios and other symptoms of the oligohydramnios sequence, the lungs are overdistended and hydrops may subsequently appear in these fetuses.[128]

Gastrointestinal Disorders

Omphalocele, different types of gastrointestinal obstruction, and bowel volvulus may be associated with isolated ascites as well as diaphragmatic hernia. Local obstruction of lymphatic drainage and venous obstruction may be possible pathogenic mechanisms for the occasional development of ascites in these disorders. Various, mostly secondary hepatic disorders are reported in association with hydrops, especially hepatitis, cirrhosis, necrosis, increased extramedullary hematopoiesis, and hemochromatosis.[15, 17, 18, 129–132]

More common is an isolated ascites caused by meconium peritonitis that may be caused by obstructive

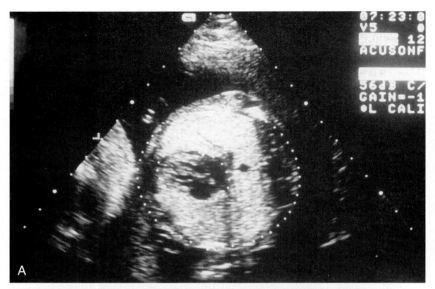

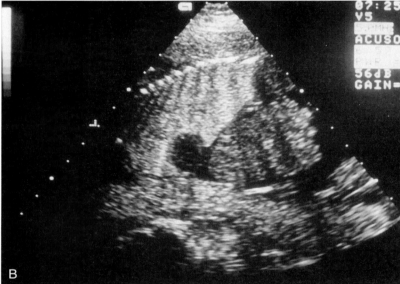

FIGURE 35–14. *A,* Transverse scan of the thorax in a fetus of 24 weeks' gestation shows bilateral hyperechogenic lungs compressing the fetal heart. Laryngeal atresia was correctly diagnosed. *B,* The sagittal scan revealed, in addition, a moderate ascites.

bowel disorders, cystic fibrosis, or viral diseases such as cytomegaly, hepatitis A, and parvovirus B19 infection.[133–136] The meconium produces a chemical peritonitis characterized by numerous intra-abdominal calcifications on the surface of the liver, the bowel wall, and the mediastinum (Fig. 35–15). If the accompanying ascites is still present, fibrin fibers (in particular, between the liver and parietal peritoneum of the anterior abdominal wall) are typical. In some fetuses intestinal perforation by volvulus or other alterations causing meconium peritonitis may be associated with a severe fetal hemorrhage and subsequent generalized hydrops.[137–140] In these cases, in utero treatment by transfusion of packed erythrocytes may be successful (U. Gembruch, unpublished observation). Furthermore, protein loss and subsequent hypoproteinemia is another mechanism suspected to rarely cause generalized hydrops in fetuses with meconium peritonitis.

Renal Diseases

Renal diseases rarely cause hydrops except in cases of congenital nephrosis of the Finnish type leading to the congenital nephrotic syndrome, which can result in hydrops most likely due to hypoproteinemia. Massive proteinuria and progressive renal failure characterize this autosomal recessive disorder, which occurs not only in the Finnish population.[141] Placentomegaly is also sonographically detectable in nonhydropic fetuses. Excessively elevated α-fetoprotein concentrations are present in the maternal blood and amniotic fluid.[142] Furthermore, hydrops has been very rarely reported in association with the autosomal recessive[143] and autosomal dominant cystic kidney diseases.[144] The exact pathogenic mechanism is unclear in these cases.

Isolated ascites, however, may be caused by rupture of the fetal urinary bladder caused by subvesical urinary

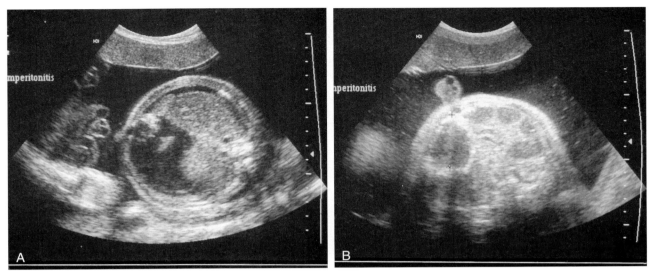

FIGURE 35–15. *A,* Ultrasound at 29 + 4 weeks' gestation demonstrates marked ascites, perihepatic and mesenteric calcifications, and dilated bowel loops as well as polyhydramnios. *B,* Six weeks later, ascites had disappeared, but dilatation of the intestine and calcifications resulting from meconium peritonitis were observed. Postnatal laparotomy in the newborn showed an ileal atresia as the cause of an in utero spontaneous bowel perforation and meconium peritonitis.

obstruction.[141] This form of urinary ascites must be distinguished from nonimmune hydrops. Furthermore, urinary ascites may appear in fetuses with complex urogenital malformations (e.g., hydrometrocolpos and fistula between the genital and urinary tracts), especially in fetuses with the autosomal recessive McKusick-Kaufman syndrome[145] (Fig. 35–16). Through the tubes, both urine and the watery-mucoid fluid of the genital tract may lead to a protein-rich intra-abdominal free fluid accumulation.

Skeletal Dysplasia

In skeletal dysplasias, development of hydrops fetalis is a rare complication. The occurrence of hydrops presumably results from an extramedullary hematopoiesis with obstructive effects. On the other hand, the frequent association of skeletal dysplasias with a more local edema of fetal neck and cranium causing thickened "nuchal translucency" in early pregnancy suggests interstitial fluid accumulation resulting from altered properties of the connective tissue, especially of the extracellular matrix. The vast majority of skeletal dysplasias that are reportedly associated with hydrops are lethal due to thoracic and lung hypoplasia (e.g., achondrogenesis type I and II), various short rib-polydactyly syndromes (Saldino-Noonan, Majewski, Naumoff, and Beemer), Jeune syndrome, thanatophoric dysplasia, osteogenesis imperfecta, osteopetrosis, nonrhizomelic chondrodysplasia punctata, congenital infantile cortical hyperostosis (Caffey disease), and Cumming syndrome.[1, 13–15, 18, 146–148] Polyhydramnios is present in the absence of hydrops too, especially in the second and third trimesters, probably resulting from an impaired fetal swallowing.

Because of the lethal prognosis in most cases with skeletal dysplasia, in utero treatment in these cases of NIFH is not appropriate.

Tumors

The most common tumors in the fetus are teratomata, which are composed of tissues from the three primitive germ layers. Approximately 80% of teratomata are localized at the sacrococcygeal site; other locations include the neck area. Intracranial, mediastinal, intrapericardial, and ovarian teratomas occur less often (Figs. 35–17 and 35–18). The associated complications depend on the location, the size of tumor, and the percentage of the solid and cystic components. Malignancy of teratoma, however, is very rare in utero and at birth. Enormously large tumors with a high proportion of solid tissue demand high amounts of blood supplying the tumor with nutrients and oxygen. Therefore, a high percentage of combined cardiac output is sacrificed only for the perfusion of the teratoma (in fetuses with sacrococcygeal teratoma primarily derived from the middle sacral artery), causing high cardiac output; furthermore, increased cardiac output may occur due to intratumoral arteriovenous shunting. Development of high output cardiac failure as demonstrated by Doppler techniques may occur in about one third of the cases with sacrococcygeal teratoma. Not so common is the subsequent development of generalized hydrops fetalis et placentae, which is correlated with a very high spontaneous death rate.[149] Hydrops has also been reported in fetuses with teratoma of other locations.[73–76, 150–154] Furthermore, in some fetuses a mostly mild or moderate anemia may be detected that is caused by spontaneous hemorrhages into the tumor or

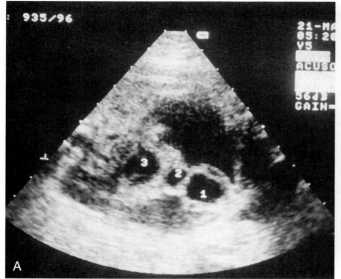

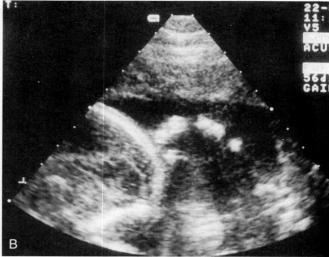

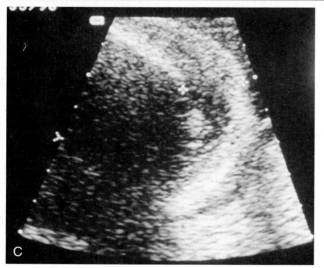

FIGURE 35–16. *A,* Fetus at 28 weeks' gestation showing the ascites and three cystic structures in the lower abdomen interpreted as urine bladder (1), uterus (2), and vagina (3), characteristic for a hydrometrocolpos. *B,* The demonstration of a bilateral postaxial hexadactyly of the upper extremities in association with the hydrometrocolpos leads to the correct diagnosis of McKusick-Kaufman syndrome. *C,* Later in the pregnancy the fetus also developed a skin edema.

Kasabach-Merritt sequence with signs of consumption coagulopathy. In utero treatment of a fetus with teratoma developing hydrops depends on several factors. In particular, cases with a large intracorporeal portion compressing and displacing other organs have a poorer prognosis than cases with predominantly extracorporeal components. In fetuses with sacrococcygeal teratoma of the extracorporeal type, the presence of a completely solid tumor with its risk for malignancy and hypervascularization seems to be an important negative prognostic factor.[155] Intrauterine transfusion of packed erythrocytes for correction of anemia and transplacental digitalization may be considered. Ligation, embolization, perivascular sclerosis, and coagulation of the supplying arteries interrupting the blood supply or resection of the tumor by open fetal surgery or fetoscopy seem to be a more curative treatment approach, correcting the high output cardiac failure in immature fetuses; these approaches are discussed elsewhere in this book. Prenatal debulking of the tumor and devascularization in premature fetuses with sacrococcygeal teratoma develop-

ing hydrops may significantly reduce the cardiac output and thus be the best treatment option. Disappearance of malignant elements, tumor maturation, and complete disappearance of tumor despite incomplete resection in utero have been observed in cases with sacrococcygeal teratoma.[156] A poor prognostic sign is the development of hydrops in a teratoma localized elsewhere especially in a mediastinal[150, 153] or intrapericardial teratoma,[73–76] where local compression of the heart, cardiac tamponade, lymphatic drainage, and venous return may occur in addition, similar to other thoracal masses with origin from the lungs or mediastinum such as fibrosarcoma.[157]

Disseminated congenital neuroblastoma of the fetus may lead to hydrops and placentomegaly by the added effect of several pathomechanisms. These are liver destruction by metastases or excessive extramedullary hematopoiesis resulting in hypoproteinemia, obstruction of venous and/or lymphatic return by large tumors and/or tumor cell emboli, and in anemia by bone marrow invasion.[158–160] Furthermore, other liver tumors that have been rarely reported to cause hydrops fetalis in-

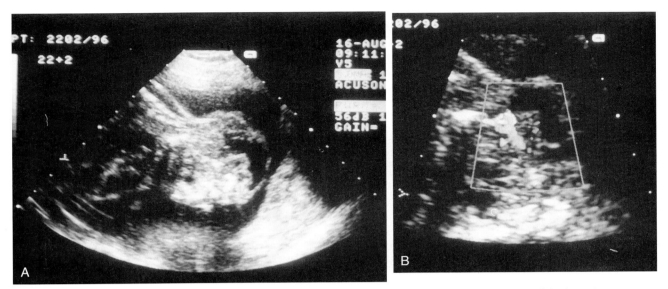

FIGURE 35–17. *A,* Large cystic-solid sacrococcygeal teratoma in a fetus with cranial skin edema, polyhydramnios, and placentomegaly. *B,* The blood flow in the solid area of the teratoma is demonstrated by color Doppler flow mapping.

clude mesenchymal hamartoma[161, 162] and hepatoblastoma.[163] In all these tumors, development of hydrops fetalis is a poor prognostic sign for perinatal survival as well as in other rare fetal tumors if complicated by hydrops fetalis such as mesoblastic nephroma.[164]

Vascular tumors and arteriovenous malformations that may also cause hydrops include liver hemangiomas, cavernous hemangiomata of the chest, nuchal hemangiomata, diffuse neonatal hemangiomatosis[165] (Fig. 35–19), intracerebral hemangioma,[166] umbilical cord hemangioma,[167, 168] and placental chorioangioma[169–171]; the most important pathomechanism is a high output cardiac failure due to massive arteriovenous shunts inside the tumor. In addition, anemia due to a Kasabach-Merritt sequence and/or a hemorrhage may occur in these tumors and further enhance the hyperdynamic state. Fetuses with a giant hemangioma of the liver[172–176] or neck,[177] with a diffuse hemangiomatosis,[165] and with Klippel-Trenaunay syndrome[178] (Fig. 35–20) especially may develop hydrops and Kasabach-Merritt sequence, with microangiopathic hemolytic anemia, thrombocytopenia, and consumptive coagulopathy. In these situations, treatment options for immature fetuses developing hydrops may be transfusion of packed erythrocytes if anemia is present, and of thrombocytes if severe thrombocytopenia is present, digitalization, and high doses of placenta-crossing corticosteroids.[179, 180]

Intracerebral arteriovenous malformations may involve and dilate the vein of Galen ("aneurysm" of the vein of Galen), resulting in a significant shunting of blood volume and high output cardiac failure characterized by cardiomegaly, AV valve insufficiency, and development of hydrops fetalis et placentae as well as polyhydramnios.[181, 182] In addition, brain damage may occur if there is a relevant arteriovenous blood shunting that bypasses the brain parenchyma ("steal" phenomenon). Sinus venosus atrial septal defect with partially anomalous pulmonary venous return and discrete aortic coarctation are associated, most likely due to the increased blood flow through the low-resistance circuit of the vein of Galen early in gestation.[183] Palliative treatment with digoxin seems to be the only sensible approach in immature nonviable fetuses with high output cardiac failure.

Agenesis of the ductus venosus with anomalous return of umbilical venous blood bypassing the liver may increase preload and can result in congestive heart failure. In this context, entering of the umbilical vein into iliac vein, inferior vena cava, and the right atrium are described.[184] Absence of the ductus venosus with a normal course of the umbilical vein without bypassing the hepatic circulation was reported in association with hydrops, which may occur by portal hypertension, liver cell injury with consecutive hypoproteinemia, or hypoxia-induced capillary damage.[185, 186] The causal relationship, however, is not evident in the reported cases, and agenesis of the ductus venosus without bypassing the liver was also prenatally diagnosed in fetuses without hydrops and hypoxia.[187]

Cardiac tumors, most commonly rhabdomyomata, and intrapericardial tumors may directly or indirectly impair the cardiac function and result in the development of hydrops fetalis as mentioned above. Whereas it is a rare complication in fetuses with rhabdomyomata caused either by obstruction or by tachyarrhythmia,[66–68, 102] development of hydrops is more common in fetuses with intrapericardial teratoma.[73–76] Pericardiocentesis for cardiac decompression may be appropriate for these fetuses in which a significant pericardial effusion accompanies the intrapericardial teratoma. In such fetuses with cardiac tamponade by a massive pericardial effusion, stabilization of cardiac function may be achieved by single or repeated pericardiocenteses.[188, 189] In utero open fetal surgery may be indicated in very

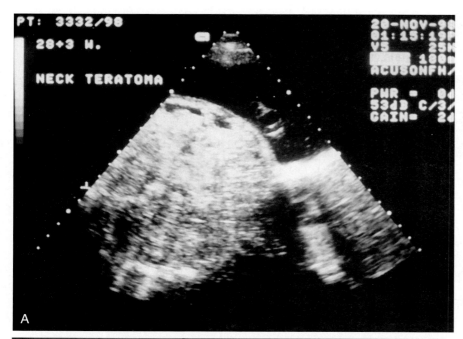

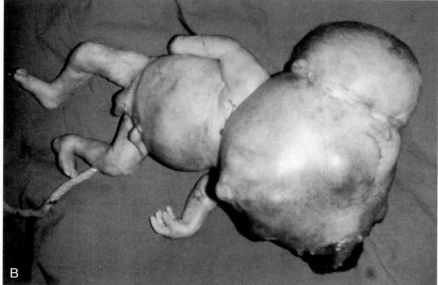

FIGURE 35–18. *A,* Sagittal scan of a fetus at 28 + 3 weeks' gestation with skin edema, severe polyhydramnios, and hydrops placentae demonstrating a large neck teratoma with a diameter of 12 cm. *B,* After a premature rupture of membranes and birth at 29 weeks' gestation, the intubation and ventilation of this newborn with neck teratoma were impossible. *See Color Plate 4*

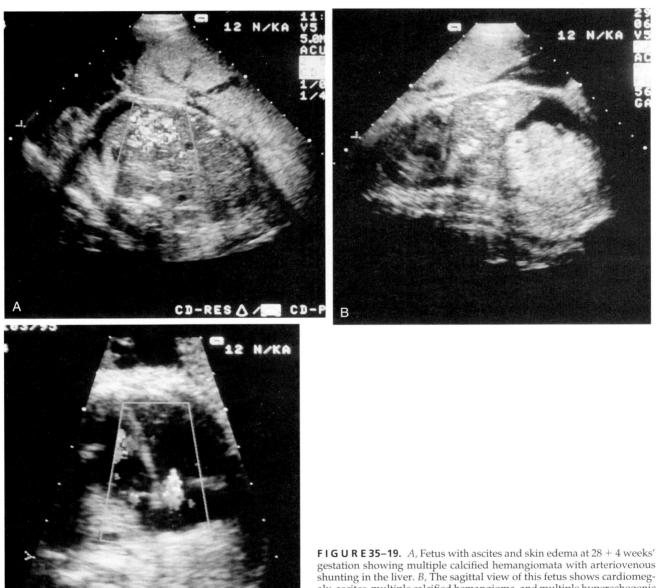

FIGURE 35–19. *A,* Fetus with ascites and skin edema at 28 + 4 weeks' gestation showing multiple calcified hemangiomata with arteriovenous shunting in the liver. *B,* The sagittal view of this fetus shows cardiomegaly, ascites, multiple calcified hemangioma, and multiple hyperechogenic hemangiomata in the liver. *C,* Fetal echocardiography shows cardiomegaly, high output cardiac failure, and tricuspid regurgitation.

Illustration continued on following page

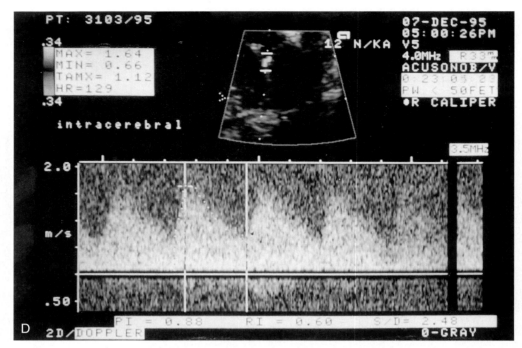

FIGURE 35–19 *Continued. D,* The diagnosis of a diffuse hemangiomatosis was supported by the demonstration of two intracerebral arteriovenous shunts with high-velocity turbulent blood flow during systole and diastole and with low pulsatility (systolic peak velocity, 164 cm/sec; diastolic velocity, 66 cm/sec; PI, 0.88). After spontaneous delivery at 29 weeks' gestation the baby died after 4 minutes. Kasabach-Merritt syndrome with hemolytic anemia, severe thrombocytopenia, and disseminated intravascular coagulation was already demonstrated before by fetal blood sampling. Autopsy revealed multiple hemangiomata in the liver, pancreas, lungs, brain, kidneys, and testes.

immature fetuses with hydrops caused by an intraperi-cardial teratoma.[75, 76]

Cystic lymphangioma, most commonly occurring in the head and neck regions, may also be associated with hydrops.[190] Because of the special location in the cervical region, planned delivery and prompt resuscitation, if necessary by emergency tracheostomy, may improve the perinatal outcome.[190] On the other hand, cases of cystic nuchal hygromata colli especially are most frequently associated with chromosomal abnormalities, most commonly Turner syndrome (Fig. 35–21), and with the development of hydrothoraces and generalized hydrops as a consequence of a more generalized malformation of the lymphatic system. These fetuses usually die during the second trimester as well as the majority of chromosomally normal fetuses with cystic nuchal hygromata colli followed by development of hydrops.[191]

Hematologic Disorders

In general, among the hematologic etiologies of nonimmune hydrops genetic causes such as specific hemoglobinopathies, Diamond-Blackfan syndrome, and glucose-6-phosphate dehydrogenase (G6PD) deficiency have to be differentiated from acquired ones, such as some forms of hemolysis or fetal hemorrhage. Regarding the pathophysiology in fetal anemia, several alterations of circulation and of oxygen transport and metabolism occur. High cardiac output develops because the arterial oxygen content decreases. Furthermore, in animal studies

anemia leads to some degree of arterial blood flow redistribution with increase of blood flow to the brain, heart, and adrenals and decrease of blood flow to the nonvital organs.[192] There are, however, distinct differences between fetuses with a more rapid and those fetuses with a delayed development of anemia. In fetal lamb studies where nonimmune anemia was induced by partial exchange transfusions there was a lack of correlation between the degree of anemia and hydrops.[193] Hydrops only occurred in fetuses that became anemic rapidly. Umbilical venous pressure was elevated in both the hydropic and the nonhydropic lambs, but the central venous pressure became elevated only in the hydropic fetuses after rapid onset of anemia.[193] This difference between umbilical venous pressure and central venous pressure is in accordance with data of cordocenteses in human fetuses with alloimmune hemolytic anemia where a fixed relationship between umbilical venous pressure and hydrops is missing.[194] An elevation of umbilical venous pressure may be induced by increased cardiac output, but only elevation of central venous pressure leads to an increased transcapillary fluid filtration rate and to an impaired lymphatic drainage of the interstitial space. This is also in accordance with Doppler examinations in anemic fetuses showing a hyperdynamic circulation with increased venous, intracardiac, and arterial blood flow velocities.[195] Even in hydropic fetuses pulsatility of venous blood flow velocity waveforms may be normal, indicating a relatively unchanged central venous and atrial pressure and showing that heart failure is not the primary mechanism for develop-

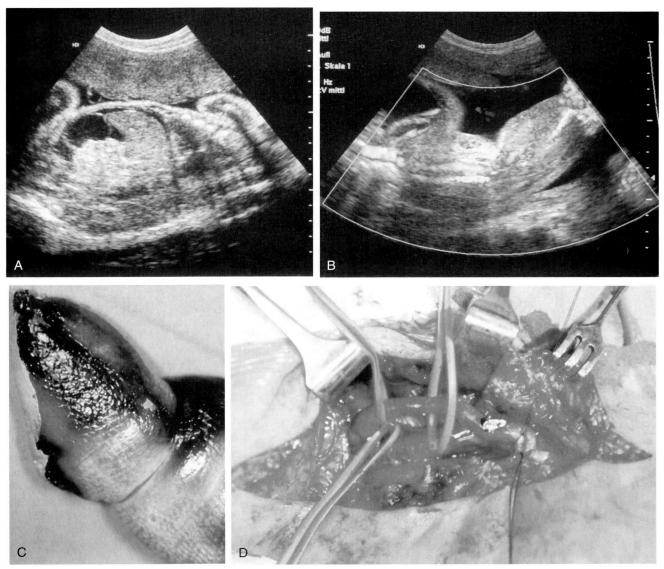

FIGURE 35–20. *A*, This fetus with Klippel-Trenaunay syndrome shows ascites, skin edema, and polyhydramnios at 29 weeks' gestation. *B*, B-mode ultrasound and power Doppler showed edematous left leg that seems to show an increased blood flow to the proximal part of the leg. *C* and *D*, Postpartum examination confirmed the prenatal diagnosis of Klippel-Trenaunay syndrome showing unilateral hypertrophy of the whole left leg, cutaneous "port-wine" hemangiomas; furthermore, arteriovenous fistula was diagnosed and successfully operated. *See Color Plate 5*

ment of hydrops in chronic anemia.[195] Hypoxia-induced capillary damage and reduced colloid oncotic pressure may be more relevant. In the advanced stage of chronic anemia, however, congestive heart failure may occur in addition, detectable by an increase of pulsatility of venous blood flow waveforms,[195–197] cardiomegaly, and AV valve regurgitation. A compensatory elevation of venomotoric tone may be present in anemia that may also contribute to the increased preload, leading to congestive heart failure. Conditions of rapid blood loss in human fetuses that correspond to the animal model of more acute onset of anemia may be a fetomaternal or a fetal hemorrhage into the brain or abdomen. The fetus can well tolerate considerable amounts of blood loss by rapidly restoring the intravascular volume through

mobilization of interstitial fluid and protein, too, but not by a net movement of fluid across the placenta.[23, 198, 199]

The hematologic findings in fetuses with anemia and hydrops due to severe alloimmune hemolytic anemia confirm the relevance of reduced oxygen delivery to tissues, demonstrating extramedullary erythropoiesis; high concentration of erythroblasts, reticulocytes, and erythropoietin; and further neutropenia, thrombocytopenia and significant hypoalbuminemia. However, anemia due to alloimmune antibodies, chronic hemolysis, infection, Kasabach-Merritt sequence, repeated fetomaternal bleeding, or erythrocyte underproduction considerably differ from the animal model of repeated hemodilution, because the significantly slower decrease of hemoglobin concentration allows for various adaptive

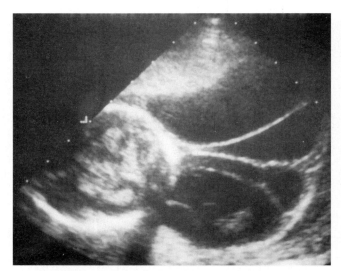

FIGURE 35–21. Fetus with Turner syndrome (45,X) at 18 weeks' gestation showing the nuchal hygromata colli with large fluid-filled lymphatic cysts in the dorsal neck and occiput area of the fetus. In addition, bilateral pleural effusions and severe oligohydramnios were present.

reactions of the fetus. Doppler studies in anemic fetuses by alloimmunization failed to show an increased pulsatility of venous blood flow as a sign for elevated central venous pressure.[195] In cases of a slower development of anemia, alteration of hepatic protein synthesis by tissue hypoxia or by stimulation of the extramedullary erythropoietic system and/or a capillary damage with an increase of permeability for water and protein seem to be important pathogenic mechanisms. When anemia is associated with other disorders, hydrops may appear even in cases of mild anemia at hemoglobin concentrations of 7 to 8 g/dL. Examples are a severe tissue hypoxia due to abnormal oxygen carrier function (e.g., homozygous α-thalassemia), high output cardiac failure (such as in arteriovenous malformations with Kasabach-Merritt sequence), or myeloblast proliferation in the medullary and extramedullary tissue (such as in transient myeloproliferative disorders associated with Down syndrome).

The most common hematologic disorders causing anemia and subsequent nonimmune hydrops are excessive erythrocyte loss by hemolysis or by chronic hemorrhage and rarely an insufficient production of erythrocytes,[200] except for epidemics of parvovirus infection which are covered later in this chapter.

Excessive Erythrocyte Loss by Intrinsic Erythrocyte Abnormalities

Hemoglobinopathies

Hemoglobin in its different ontogenic stages consists of a tetramer of two α-like (α and ζ) and two β-like (ε, δ, γ, or β) globin chains.[200] Synthesis of individual globin in regulated during normal development according to a precise time sequence. Early embryonic hemoglobin is made up of two ζ- and two ε-globin chains; during

the sixth and seventh weeks following conception, as erythropoiesis shifts from yolk sac to the fetal liver, transcription of the ζ-globin gene decreases and the transcription of both α-globin genes begins and persists during lifetime. Therefore, the α-globin is essential for the fetus, neonate, and adult. Whereas fetal hemoglobin consists of two α- and two γ-chains (HbF), adult hemoglobin is comprised of two α- and two β-chains (HbA).[200]

The inherited hemoglobinopathies are a heterogeneous group of recessive disorders including sickle cell anemia and thalassemias. Among all hemoglobinopathies, only the α-thalassemia, which is characterized by a deficiency of α-globin chain synthesis, leads to hydrops fetalis. This α^0-thalassemia which leads to fetal hydrops and intrauterine demise due to this etiology remains an important health problem in Southeast Asia. Inherited defects in the α-globin gene located on chromosome 16 result in decreased or absent synthesis of the α-chain of hemoglobin.[200] The α-globin gene cluster is made up of one embryonic globin gene, two α-globin genes (α_1- and α_2-gene), and four pseudogenes.[200] Therefore, α-globin genes are duplicated, and thus a normal person has four functional α-globin genes in the diploid cell (gene status: $\alpha\alpha/\alpha\alpha$). The vast majority of cases of α-thalassemia are based on different types of gene deletions; only in rare instances, may nondeletion mutations cause α-thalassemia.[200, 201] Therefore, we can distinguish clinical phenotypes of α-thalassemia according to the number of functional α-globin genes (i.e., 3, 2, 1, and 0, respectively)[200, 201]:

1. The homozygous α- or α^0-thalassemia has no functional α-gene (gene status: --/--) with a complete absence of α-globin synthesis. There is a synthesis of homotetrameric hemoglobin molecules consisting of four γ-chains (Hb Barts) with an extreme high affinity to and an impaired delivery of oxygen. This results in severe tissue hypoxia, shortened life span of erythrocytes, and possibly ineffective erythropoiesis.[200]

2. The hemoglobin H (Hb H) disease (gene status: --/-α) with one functional α-gene results from the heterozygous state for α^0- and α^+-thalassemia, or a combination of two globin gene deletions and a point mutation of the third globin gene. Hb H disease is associated with a mild or moderate hypochromic microcytic anemia and is characterized by precipitated β-globin chains (Hb H) in red cells.[200] In rare instances, Hb H disease may cause hydrops fetalis and severe anemia, probably due to a nondeletional $\alpha\alpha^+$-thalassemia.[202]

3. α-Thalassemia traits with two functional genes—α^0-thalassemia trait (heterozygous α^0-thalassemia trait) with both α-genes deleted from the same chromosome 16 (gene status: --/$\alpha\alpha$) and α^+-thalassemia trait (-α/-α)—are clinically insignificant. Only mild hypochromic microcytic anemia with normal iron levels may be present; differentiation between these two genotypes of α-thalassemia trait can only be achieved by DNA-analysis. The majority of cases with α^+-thalassemia result from deletions of one of the two globin genes; five different deletions have been characterized al-

ready.[200, 201] α^+-Thalassemia due to nondeletion mutations—17 different nondeletion mutations have been characterized to date—are much less frequent, but show a more severe reduction in the α-globin chain synthesis than in a deletional α^+-thalassemia, because all of the mutations except one are located on the dominant α_2-globin gene.[200, 201]

4. The so-called silent carrier state with three functional genes (gene status: -α/$\alpha\alpha$) is not associated with anemia.

In Southeast Asia, the heterozygous α^0-thalassemia carrier status (--/) occurs in 5 to 15% of the population, in the Mediterranean population in less than 1%.[201, 203] Therefore, homozygous α^0-thalassemia or Hb Bart disease is the most common cause of hydrops in Southeast Asia, accounting for 60 to 90% of cases with nonimmune hydrops and for up to one in four perinatal deaths in this region.[200, 203] After the shift away from the embryonic hemoglobin (Hb Portland 1), which is normally com-

pleted by the sixth to seventh week following conception, Hb Bart becomes predominant with approximately 80% and only 10 to 20% embryonic hemoglobin (Hb Portland 1), while Hb A, Hb A2, and Hb F are absent.[200, 203] The small proportion of Hb Portland 1 keeps the fetus alive until the third trimester. The peripheral smear of fetal blood reveals hypochromic and anisopoikilocytic erythrocytes as well as a large number of reticulocytes and nucleated red blood cells. Markers indicating hemolysis are increased, especially lactate dehydrogenase and bilirubin. Already in the first and early in the second trimester of pregnancy, the homozygous α^0-thalassemia results in a severe tissue hypoxia, which can adversely affect organogenesis and in utero development.[203] Symptoms are anemia ranging from 3 to 10 g/dL, cardiomegaly, hepatosplenomegaly, hydrops fetalis and placentae, and poly- and later oligohydramnios (Fig. 35–22). Intrauterine death generally occurs between 30 and 40 weeks' gestation or shortly after birth even if not all affected newborns are grossly hydropic.[203]

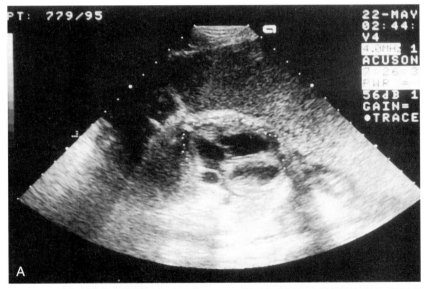

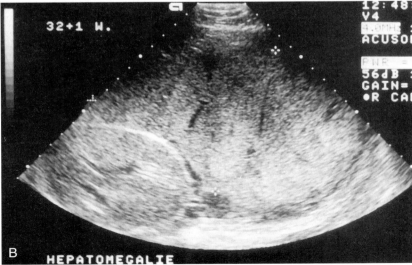

FIGURE 35–22. *A,* Fetus of 32 + 1 weeks' gestation showing the severe cardiomegaly, generalized skin edema, hydrops placentae, and oligohydramnios caused by α-thalassemia in a couple coming from Vietnam. *B,* In the fetus with α-thalassemia (32 + 1 weeks' gestation), the severe hydrops placentae (placental thickness of 98 mm) and hepatosplenomegaly are demonstrated.

In the majority of cases additional maternal obstetric complications appear, especially pregnancy-induced hypertension and preeclampsia and associated complications such as abruptio placentae and postpartum hemorrhage.[203] As in other diseases, placentomegaly is likely an important factor for the maternal hyperdynamic and hypertensive state, the so-called mirror syndrome. Therefore, prenatal diagnosis is always indicated to avoid these maternal complications. A thickened placenta seems to be the first sonographic marker detectable from 10 to 18 weeks' gestation, followed by cardiomegaly, hepatosplenomegaly, and fetal hydrops, which may present as early as the 12th week of gestation and most commonly beyond the 20th week of gestation.[204–207] Polyhydramnios, but also oligohydramnios, may be present.[203, 205] Demonstration of placentomegaly, cardiomegaly resulting in an increased cardiothoracic ratio, and hydrops are used not only alternatively in Southeast Asia if DNA-based prenatal diagnosis is not readily available, but also as alternative diagnostic means avoiding the risks related to invasive procedures.[203, 205–208] Measurement of cardiothoracic ratio by transvaginal sonography can distinctively identify the affected fetuses at 12 to 13 weeks' gestation.[208] After sonographic detection, diagnosis is confirmed by fetal blood sampling showing hemolytic anemia, abnormal hemoglobin, and hypoxemia.[207, 208] Although some anemic fetuses show increased peak velocities at the pulmonary valve and a larger pulmonary valve diameter at 12 to 13 weeks' gestation, there is an extensive overlap between anemic and nonanemic.[209] Also, nuchal translucency thickness, nuchal edema, and hydrops, respectively, seem to be not useful for prediction of anemic fetuses in early gestation.[210]

DNA-based diagnostic techniques from fetal tissue (i.e., blood, amniotic fluid, and chorionic villi, respectively) allow the prenatal diagnosis of all the α-thalassemia deletions and of mutations of genes by Southern blotting and some by polymerase chain reaction (PCR)-based strategies.[201, 203] In α^0-thalassemia, at least 14 different deletions of both α-globin genes have been characterized by restriction enzyme mapping.[201] A quicker diagnosis is possible by selective PCR amplification of DNA fragments. But the gap PCR can diagnose only the most common alleles, the Southeast Asian deletion, $--^{SEA}$, and the two Mediterranean deletions, $--^{MED}$ and $-(\alpha)^{20.5}$.[201, 203]

If there are typical anomalies demonstrated by ultrasound, which is in part performed as a screening method for homozygous α^0-thalassemia in Southeast Asia, definitive diagnosis is then achieved by demonstration of Hb Bart through hemoglobin electrophoresis in fetal blood or by DNA analysis on any prenatally obtainable cells.[203, 207] Especially, chorionic villus sampling at around 10 weeks' gestation allows DNA-based early prenatal diagnosis in high-risk families. Screening for heterozygous α^0-thalassemia carriers is effectively performed among the high-risk population in Southeast Asia and in other parts of the world using hematologic (microcytosis and hypochromia, hemoglobin electrophoresis, Hb H inclusion bodies, and embryonic ζ-globin chains) and subsequent DNA-based techniques

for definitive diagnosis resulting in the prepregnancy identification of high-risk couples.[203, 211] Chorionic villus sampling can then be offered already in the first pregnancy of an at-risk couple.[203] Meanwhile, successful single-cell DNA-based diagnosis of homozygous α^0-thalassemia by the technique of preimplantation diagnosis using single cells from the blastocyst and by isolation of single nucleated red blood cells from maternal circulation[212] have been reported.

Although the outcome of homozygous α^0-thalassemia is generally the intrauterine demise, survival is possible after aggressive treatment by intrauterine and neonatal packed red cell transfusions, followed by bone marrow transplantation.[203, 213, 214] Such intensive active prenatal and postnatal treatment, however, cannot be recommended as routine clinical practice and should remain experimental until the questions of long-term mortality, morbidity, associated anomalies, and especially neurodevelopmental outcome are answered.[203, 214, 215] In the future, in utero hematopoietic stem cell transplantation or gene therapy may become an alternative approach for in utero treatment of fetuses with this otherwise lethal condition.[216]

Red Blood Cell Enzymopathies

Although red blood cell enzymopathies frequently lead to hemolytic anemia in newborns and adults, fetal hydrops caused by inherited deficiency of red blood cell enzymes seems to be very rare.[200] In only a few case reports severe fetal anemia and hydrops are associated with autosomal recessively inherited deficiencies of pyruvate kinase[217, 218] and glucose phosphate isomerase,[219] resulting in a disturbance of anaerobic glycolysis with consecutive deficiency of erythrocyte adenosine triphosphate (ATP). The autosomal-recessively inherited G6PD deficiency also leads to an alteration of erythrocyte glucose metabolism via the hexose monophosphate shunt generating NADPH and thus maintaining adequate levels of reduced glutathione, which protects the erythrocyte against oxidants. In cases of G6PD deficiency, contact with oxidants by ingestion of foods (fava beans), drugs, surgery, or infection leads to acute hemolytic anemia in adults, rarely in neonates. Fetal hydrops, however, is very rarely caused by G6PD deficiency. Only three cases of G6PD deficiency associated with fetal hydrops are reported, the first after maternal ingestion of sulfisoxazole,[220] and the second after maternal ingestion of fava beans and ascorbic acid.[221] In a third case, spontaneous resolution of second-trimester hydrops and recurrence at 34 weeks' gestation was observed.[222] Ingestion of oxidant drugs and foods should be avoided by pregnant women in populations at risk of G6PD deficiency. Treatment of fetal anemia and hydrops caused by red blood cell enzymopathies consists of repeated intrauterine blood transfusions and, if necessary exchange blood transfusions after birth.[222] In utero hemolysis resulting in fetal hydrops may rarely occur in cases of congenital erythropoietic porphyria, an autosomal-recessive disorder, caused by a profound deficiency of uroporphyrinogen III synthase, the fourth enzyme in the heme synthesis pathway.[223]

In one case, fetal hydrops was suggested to be the result from a methemoglobinemia after combustion gas intoxication; it seems possible that a physiologically low level of cytochrome-b_5 reductase causes fetal susceptibility to oxidants and acquired methemoglobinemia.[224]

Defects of the Red Cell Membrane Skeleton

Fetal hemolytic anemia and hydrops seem to be very rarely caused by defects of the red cell membrane skeleton.[200] Two cases with defects of the membrane skeleton protein spectrin have been reported[225, 226]; one of these was successfully treated by ante- and postnatal red cell transfusions.[226]

Excessive Erythrocyte Loss by Extrinsic Hemolysis

Kasabach-Merritt Sequence

In cases of arteriovenous malformations, hemolytic anemia, thrombocytopenia, and consumptive coagulopathy may occur. Classic cases are large cavernous hemangiomas. This so-called Kasabach-Merritt sequence may be complicated by the additional appearance of a high output cardiac failure by arteriovenous fistula and severe anemia secondary to bleeding within the hemangioma. Fetal nonimmune hydrops and Kasabach-Merritt sequence have been described in cases of large nuchal hemangiomata,[177] large liver hemangiomata,[172, 174] in diffuse neonatal hemangiomatosis,[165] and in severe cases of Klippel-Trenaunay-Weber syndrome.[178] Chorioangiomata may also lead to fetal Kasabach-Merritt sequence with and without hydrops.[169, 170] In other fetuses with arteriovenous malformations, massive arteriovenous blood shunting can cause high output cardiac failure and hydrops without or in the presence of only a mild degree of Kasabach-Merritt sequence.

Excessive Erythrocyte Loss by Hemorrhage

Acute massive fetomaternal hemorrhage may lead to fetal death without the appearance of hydrops. If there is a more chronic or repetitive fetomaternal transfusion, severe fetal anemia can be associated with hydrops fetalis and placentae; an increase of medullary and extramedullary erythropoiesis with hepatosplenomegaly and cardiomegaly due to high output cardiac failure may be present (Fig. 35–23). Maternal serum α-fetoprotein levels are elevated in cases of fetomaternal bleeding. The demonstration of fetal erythrocytes containing fetal hemoglobin (Hb F) by the Kleihauer-Betke acid-elution staining or channelyzer analysis confirms the diagnosis. This test is based on a maternal blood sample and should be performed in all fetuses with hydrops and in cases of intrauterine fetal death. Due to a very short life span of fetal mature erythrocytes in the maternal circulation, the Kleihauer-Betke test becomes uninformative a few days after fetomaternal transfusion, dependent on its volume and on the presence of an additional ABO-

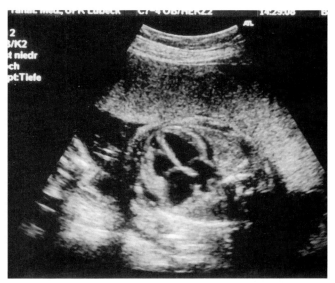

FIGURE 35–23. Fetus with severe anemia (hemoglobin 2.0 g/dL) and thrombocytopenia (8,000 thrombocytes/μL) resulting from fetomaternal transfusion. Severe cardiomegaly, bilateral pleural effusions, ascites, polyhydramnios, and hydrops placenta were present. The percentage of HbF in the maternal blood was 3%.

incompatibility. Furthermore, other factors influence the accuracy of the Kleihauer-Betke test for estimation of the volume of fetomaternal transfusion, especially variations in the individual maternal blood volume.[227] Measurements of α-fetoprotein concentration in the maternal blood show great inter- and intraindividual variations during pregnancy, and are therefore not useful for estimation of the severity of fetal bleeding. Sinusoidal heart rate pattern and decreased or absent fetal movements may indicate severe anemia[227] in combination with the sonographic demonstration of hydrops, cardiomegaly, hydrops placentae, and polyhydramnios. Fetal blood sampling shows severe anemia without signs of hemolysis and a large number of reticulocytes and nucleated red blood cells. Sometimes, relevant thrombocytopenia may also occur. Treatment of fetomaternal transfusion included intrauterine blood transfusion for prolongation of the pregnancy,[226–228] and infusion of platelets, if relevant thrombocytopenia is present. Close fetal surveillance by daily fetal heart rate monitoring, by biophysical profile, and by Doppler blood flow velocimetry for detection of high-cardiac-output state are mandatory, as fetomaternal hemorrhage may often be chronic and/or intermittent.[227, 228] Therefore, repeated fetal blood sampling or transfusion has been recommended. Dependent on the fetal maturation, preterm delivery may be safer for these fetuses.

Fetal hemorrhage in association with hydrops is described in only a few case reports[200] of intracranial bleeding, especially subdural hematoma[229, 230] (Fig. 35–24), liver hematoma,[231] diffuse neonatal hemangiomatosis,[165] and small bowel volvulus.[137, 138, 140] Severe trauma, thrombocytopenia, coagulopathy, arteriovenous malformations, and also perforation of bowel may be possible causes for those bleedings. Fetal blood sampling reveals different degrees of anemia with a compensatory eleva-

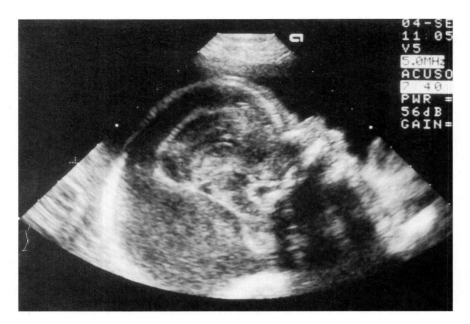

FIGURE 35–24. Fetus at 21 + 5 weeks' gestation showing a massive bilateral subdural hematoma compressing the fetal brain causing anemia, cardiomegaly, skin edema, polyhydramnios, and hydrops placentae. There were no maternal antibodies against fetal thrombocytes, coagulation disorders, trauma, cerebral malformations, and infection.

tion of the number of reticulocytes and nucleated red blood cells, as well as signs of consumption coagulopathy (thrombocytopenia, prolonged prothrombin time/partial thromboplastin time [PT/PTT], and hypofibrinogenemia). By ultrasound, hematoma and/or hyperechogenic ascites may be detectable; furthermore, polyhydramnios, cardiomegaly, and AV valve insufficiencies can be found. Elevated blood flow velocities and interstitial fluid accumulation in the fetus and the placenta may be indirect signs for high output cardiac failure.

Erythrocyte Underproduction

One of the most common causes for an erythrocyte underproduction is a parvovirus B19 infection characterized by a diminished number of erythrocyte precursors in the bone marrow and severe reticulocytopenia; sometimes, underproduction of leukocytes and thrombocytes is also present. Hydrops caused by aplastic or hypoplastic anemia is extremely unusual and is described in only few case reports (e.g., Diamond-Blackfan syndrome, pure red cell aplasia, and congenital dyserythropoietic anemia). A pure red cell aplasia acquired by the mother may repetitively cause severe anemia and hydrops[232] and was treated successfully with intrauterine intravascular transfusion in another case.[233] Dyserythropoietic anemias seem to be a rare cause of nonimmune hydrops fetalis.[234–238] The Diamond-Blackfan syndrome usually leads to anemia in the first year of life.[200, 239] Under rare conditions, however, it seemed to be the cause of severe anemia and reticulocytopenia, sometimes with subsequent hydrops already in utero.[239–241] Another case of hydrops has been reported in association with an aplastic anemia of unknown etiology.[242]

Transient myeloproliferative disorders (TMD) are a much more common cause of erythrocyte underproduction,[200, 243] whereas the true malignant congenital leuke-

mia is very rare.[244, 245] Both hardly distinguishable disorders are characterized by the presence of myeloblasts in the peripheral blood and by the proliferation of myeloblasts within the bone marrow and extramedullary sites of erythropoiesis, leading to fetal liver and bone marrow replacement by myeloblasts. TMD, however, leads to spontaneous remission in utero or postpartum without an infiltration of nonhematopoietic tissues, whereas the true malignant leukemia shows widespread visceral and placental infiltration.[200, 243] Furthermore, TMD and leukemia must be distinguished from the leukemoid reactions as a result of infections, hypoxia, or hemolysis. TDM is rare in genetically normal neonates and is almost universally associated with Down syndrome, where blast cells carry a third chromosome 21, and with cases of additional transient clonal cytogenetic abnormalities.[243] It appears that the additional chromosome 21 is the key for the leukemic reaction. TMD in fetuses and neonates is characterized by high levels of circulating blast cells, but sometimes may also be associated with pancytopenia,[246] hepatomegaly, splenomegaly, hydrops fetalis, hydrops placentae, cardiomegaly, AV valve insufficiencies, polyhydramnios, and oligohydramnios[246–250] (Fig. 35–25). Morphologic and immunologic examinations predominately reveal blast cells similar to a subtype of acute megakaryoblastic leukemia of the French-American-British (FAB) classification M7.[243] The risk of acute myeloid leukemia in fetuses with TMD, especially of the subtype M7, is greatly increased during infancy. The pathogenesis of this transient leukemic reaction is unknown. Clinically, TMD is indistinguishable from an acute myelogenous leukemia and shows spontaneous remission without any chemotherapy,[243] which may also occur in utero[248] and may be accompanied by a remission of hydrops. On the other hand, TMD may run a fulminate course with marked organ involvement, cardiac failure, and even intrauterine fetal death.[246, 250]

In fetuses with TDM and congenital leukemia, several pathogenetic mechanisms predispose to the develop-

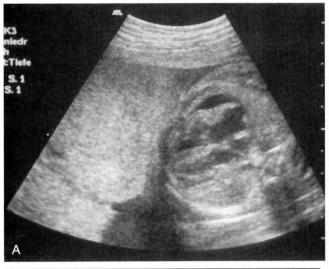

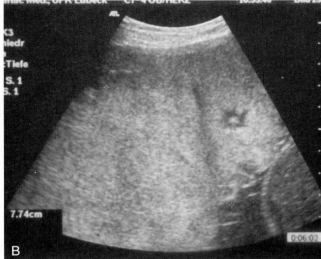

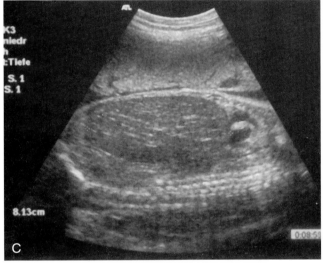

FIGURE 35–25. *A,* Fetus with trisomy 21 mosaicism and transient myeloproliferative disorder at 28 + 0 weeks' gestation showing a severe cardiomegaly, pericardial effusion, and hydrops placentae. *B,* Placentomegaly due to hydrops placentae was demonstrated at 28 + 0 weeks' gestation. The placental thickness was 77.4 mm. *C,* The sagittal scan of this fetus showing massive hepatomegaly. Splenomegaly was also present.

ment of hydrops: mild to moderate anemia with hemoglobin concentrations between 6 and 10 g/dL causing high cardiac output, capillary damage by hypoxia resulting from anemia and hyperviscosity, increased vascular resistance, extramedullary megakaryoblastic proliferation, liver fibrosis as a consequence of growth, and increased collagen synthesis by fibroblasts stimulated through cytokines produced by the abnormal blasts in TMD.[243, 246] Myelofibrosis, however, is related to megakaryoblastic leukemia in patients with and without Down syndrome and is generally absent in TMD.[243]

Infection

Infectious causes of nonimmune hydrops due to maternal-fetal transmission are reported for many viral (parvovirus B19, cytomegalovirus, adenovirus, herpes simplex, varicella-zoster [Fig. 35–26], coxsackie, hepatitis A, rubella, polio, influenza B, respiratory syncytial virus), bacterial (*Treponema pallidum, Listeria monocytogenes, Leptospira interrogans*), parasitic (*Toxoplasma gondii,*

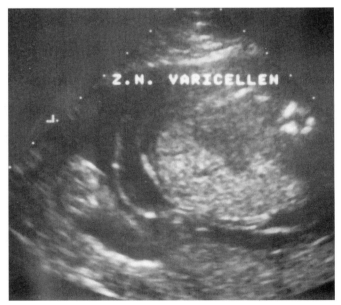

FIGURE 35–26. NIHF in a fetus with varicella infection.

Trypanosoma cruzii), and other (*Chlamydia, Ureaplasma urealyticum*) maternal infections.[1, 13–15, 17, 18, 134, 136, 251–253] For some of these infections, however, only associations between maternal and/or fetal infection with hydrops have been reported. Although in some cases of hydrops the causative infectious disease remains undetected, especially in older series of hydrops, it is estimated that fetal infections account for approximately 5 to 10% of cases with nonimmune hydrops. It may be speculated that the increase in application of highly sensitive PCR techniques in cases of hydrops will result in an increased detection of nonimmune hydrops cases with infectious etiology, which has already been demonstrated for parvoviral[254, 255] and other viral infections.[256]

The vast majority of these NIHF cases are caused by parvovirus B19, cytomegalovirus, syphilis, and toxoplasmosis, much more rarely by herpes simplex type 1 or adenovirus. These specific infectious diseases should be discussed in more detail later in the chapter. There are only a few reports on other infectious diseases such as various types of hepatitis infection associated with hydrops. In these cases the suggested causative relationship seems not evident.

In general, in these infectious disease cases, there are different pathogenic mechanisms responsible for the development of nonimmune hydrops that occur alone or in combination[253]:

1. High output cardiac failure by anemia due to hemolytic destruction of erythrocytes or erythroid progenitor cells.
2. Hepatitis leading to decreased hepatic red cell production and to hypoproteinemia.
3. Myocarditis.
4. Fetal sepsis with hypoxia-induced endothelial damage and increased transcapillary filtration of interstitial fluid and proteins. To date, intrauterine treatment seems to be feasible only in cases of nonimmune hydrops due to parvovirus B19 and syphilis.

Parvovirus B19

Fetal infection by parvovirus B19 shows a tropism for fetal erythroid progenitor cells with subsequent lytic destruction or stimulation of apoptosis.[253, 257, 258] The virus binds to a specific glycoside cellular receptor (erythrocyte P antigen), which is usually present on the erythropoietic cells but also on other cells, such as endothelial and myocardial cells.[259] The lack of this virus receptor seems to cause a resistance to parvovirus B19 infection in some people.[260] Occasionally, viral infections may cause pancytopenia and myocarditis.[261, 262] The highest susceptibility of the fetuses seems to be between 14 and 24 weeks' gestation because of the distinct increase of erythropoiesis during the second trimester.[253, 257] Meanwhile, few cases of hydrops caused by parvovirus B19 in the late first trimester have been reported.[263, 264] The transplacental virus transmission rate is approximately 30% and the risk for fetal death seems to be between 5 and 10%.[253, 257] It was estimated that more than one half of cases with intrauterine infection are unrecognized.[253, 257]

Fetal infection by parvovirus B19 causing aplastic anemia leads to compensatory high cardiac output and extramedullary hematopoiesis with hepatosplenomegaly. Furthermore, polyhydramnios, placental hydrops, cardiomegaly, and high-cardiac-output congestive heart failure with fetal fluid accumulation may occur; in most advanced stages bilateral AV valve insufficiencies and abnormal venous Doppler studies indicate cardiac failure (Fig. 35–27). In some fetuses viral myocarditis may be a very important additional pathogenetic mechanism for congestive heart failure.[261, 262, 265–268] Spontaneous re-

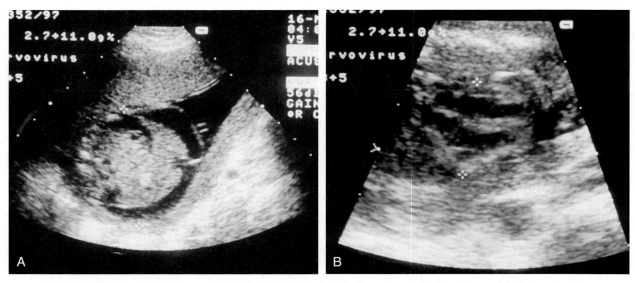

FIGURE 35–27. *A,* Fetus presenting with ascites and pleural effusions, polyhydramnios, and hydrops placentae at 17 + 6 weeks' gestation resulting from a parvovirus B19 infection. By two transfusions of O Rh negative packed erythrocytes the hemoglobin could be elevated from 2.7 g/dL to 11.0 g/dL. In the following weeks the hemoglobin concentrations remained constant and hydrops showed a complete remission within 6 weeks. A healthy newborn was spontaneously born at term. *B,* In the same fetus, a cardiomegaly was also present.

mission of anemia and hydrops is possible because the aplastic state lasts around 7 to 10 days and bone marrow recovery takes 2 to 3 weeks.[253, 257, 269, 270] These cases are characterized by a high number of reticulocytes and nucleated red cells in the fetal blood and an erythroid hyperplasia in the bone marrow.[253, 257]

In accordance with the shortened life span of normal fetal erythrocytes ranging from 45 to 70 days, the maximal anemia and the appearance of hydrops usually occurs 4 to 8 weeks after maternal infection—and potentially longer. Maternal infection is asymptomatic or symptomatic with the typical rash on the face, the trunk, or extremities (erythema infectiosum) and/or symptoms of arthritis in different joints.[253, 257, 271]

Diagnosis by serology of maternal blood is obtained by positive immunoglobulin M (IgM) antibodies in combination with high or increasing IgG titers.[253, 257, 272] Elevated maternal serum α-fetoprotein (MSAFP) has been reported to indicate the fetuses developing hydrops, but this correlation is as poor for clinical use as the determination of maternal serum human chorionic gonadotropin[273, 274]; furthermore, elevated MSAFP showed only a weak association to parvovirus B19 infection not useful for a routine screening program.[275] In cases of NIHF due to parvovirus B19 infection, fetal blood sampling revealed aplastic anemia without reticulocytosis. There may be a few nucleated red blood cells with characteristic intranuclear inclusions (lantern cells) visualized by microscopy[276] (Fig. 35–28). Lantern cells are usually present in the stroma of various fetal tissues, especially in the fetal bone marrow, liver, and spleen.[276] The detection of specific IgM antibodies is quite specific but not sensitive and reliable enough in fetal blood, because IgM antibody response may be especially poor or absent before 18 to 22 weeks' gestation.[257, 277] More accurate is the demonstration of viral DNA by in situ hybridization and PCR in the amniotic fluid or in the fetal compartments, such as blood and ascites.[277–280] Parvoviral infection could be demonstrated in 10 to 15%

of cases with "idiopathic" nonimmune hydrops using PCR-based methods.[254, 255] Furthermore, in investigating abortion and stillbirth specimens from unexplained nonimmune hydrops cases, PCR analysis for parvoviral DNA of paraffin-embedded liver tissue[281] may be more successful than the microscopic identification of inclusions in routine histologic sections and the immunohistochemistry using monoclonal antibodies against parvoviral protein.[281, 282] On the other hand, not only specific IgM but also parvoviral B19 DNA may be no more detectable in the maternal blood if the interval between infection and manifestation of fetal anemia and hydrops is longer than 4 to 6 weeks.[283] Later again IgM and parvoviral B19 DNA may also be undetectable in the fetal blood.[283] In such cases diagnosis can only be established by demonstration of persistent specific IgG antibodies in the infant blood beyond the sixth to eighth months of life because the catabolism of passively acquired antibodies would be expected by age 3 to 4 months.

In the case of primary maternal infection in pregnancy, weekly fetal surveillance by serial ultrasound scanning up to 8 (rarely to 12) weeks—and potentially longer—after maternal infection has been recommended[284, 285] for the early detection of development of polyhydramnios, placental hydrops, and fetal hydrops; additional measurement of blood flow velocities in the ascending aorta, pulmonary trunk and/or middle cerebral artery may offer an earlier diagnosis of anemia. Because the prevalence of hydrops after maternal infection with parvovirus B19 is as low as 1 or 2%, invasive procedures such as amniocentesis or cordocentesis are not feasible in the initial management and should be reserved for cases of hydrops or other signs of anemia.[285]

In fetuses with severe hydrops and anemia, therapy consists of intrauterine transfusion of packed red cells into the umbilical vein.[253, 257, 280, 286] An additional transfusion of packed thrombocytes may be considered in fetuses with severe thrombocytopenia,[280] which may also cause exsanguination after funipuncture. A high reticu-

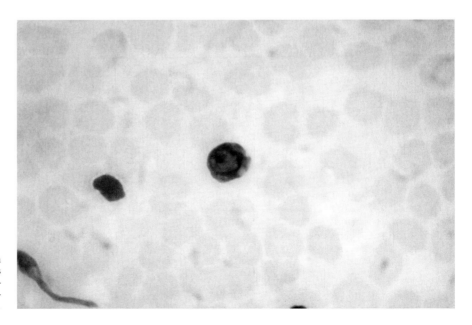

F I G U R E 35–28. Blood smear of a fetus with parvovirus B19–induced anemia and hydrops showing typical "lantern cells," which are nucleated red blood cells with amphophilic intranuclear inclusions visualized by microscopy.

locyte count indicates that spontaneous remission has already begun and transfusions might be avoidable depending on the extent of the anemia. According to the results of a retrospective study performed in several centers in North America,[287] in the presence of hydrops due to parvovirus B19 infection hydrops spontaneously resolves in approximately 34% and in a further 29% after intrauterine transfusion. Without intrauterine transfusion, about 30% of the hydropic fetuses die; in the group of transfused fetuses 83.5% survived.[287] Long-term neurologic outcome of children exposed to parvovirus B19 infection in utero seems to be normal,[287, 288] whereas data about outcome of hydropic fetuses have not been systematically obtained. This was also observed in fetuses with red cell alloimmunization, where no significantly worse long-term neurologic outcome in the group of hydropic and severely anemic fetuses compared to the nonhydropic fetuses was observed.[289]

Cytomegalovirus

Cytomegalovirus (CMV) is the most common congenital viral infection. In the United States and Europe, where 50% of pregnant women are CMV seronegative, it has a prevalence of approximately 1% per pregnancy.[290, 291] In primary infection during pregnancy, the risk of a vertical maternal-fetal transmission through the placenta is approximately 40 to 50% at any gestational age,[290, 291] whereas the rate of fetal infection after recurrent infection by reactivation or by reinfection with a different strain of the virus is less than 1%.[290, 291] The severity of disease seems to be independent of the gestational age at infection.[291] Between 10 and 20% of infected neonates are symptomatic at birth, 50% of these with severe disease.[290, 291] Around 70% of those with moderate symptoms and around 10% of the asymptomatic neonates exhibit psychomotoric retardation, visual and/or hearing impairment later on.[290, 291] Therefore, 1 of 20 to 30 pregnancies with primary CMV infection results in an infant with significant sequelae.[290, 291]

Sonographic signs of a fetal CMV infection are not specific, but suggest the presence of a severe fetal infection. In cases of documented seroconversion or in other cases they may be the primary finding resulting in the diagnosis of fetal CMV infection. The sensitivity of ultrasound findings, however, seems to be relatively low for detection of infected fetuses.[292] Among the signs are intrauterine growth retardation, oligohydramnios, ventriculomegaly, microcephaly, hydrocephalus, cerebral calcifications, echogenic vessels in the fetal thalami and basal ganglia due to vasculitis, hyperreflectoric and sometimes dilated bowel due to viral enterocolitis, hepatosplenomegaly with echogenic foci, and nonimmune hydrops.[290-294] Fetal meconium peritonitis caused by CMV infection[133] and the association of CMV infection and fetal supraventricular tachycardia[295] have been observed. Intrauterine resolution of hydrops has also been reported in association with fetal CMV infection.[296, 297, 298] Thrombocytopenia causing petechial skin bleedings, anemia, and hepatitis with elevated liver enzymes may be present in utero too.[290, 292] Hepatic destruction, vasculitis, with capillary damage and also anemia are

the pathogenic mechanisms for the development of hydrops in cases of fetal CMV infection.

Diagnosis of maternal infection is obtained by demonstration of CMV-IgM and seroconversion of CMV-IgG and by virus isolation from urine and other body secretions.[290, 291] For the diagnosis of fetal infection, invasive techniques are necessary because of the low sensitivity of the ultrasound findings. Due to delayed fetal immune response fetal blood sampling with specific IgM assessment has low sensitivity and should only be performed after 22 weeks' gestation.[299] Therefore, isolation of the virus and amplification of viral DNA by PCR from amniotic fluid and fetal blood is the best method to diagnose a fetal infection.[290, 291] Diagnosis by PCR from amniotic fluid should be performed after 20 weeks' gestation[300, 301] and at least 6 weeks after maternal infection when fetal viral excretion is starting. In some cases a second amniocentesis may be needed some weeks later.[291] In addition to the sonographically detectable abnormalities, hemolytic anemia, thrombocytopenia, and elevated liver enzymes in the fetal blood may suggest severe disease.

Antiviral treatment of CMV-infected newborns by gancyclovir has been reported and seems to decrease viral excretion and to have positive effects on the hearing capabilities.[290] However, the effectiveness of a transplacental and/or direct intrauterine treatment of fetal CMV infection with or without NIHF is not proven. Manifestation of hydrops seems to occur late, indicating a severe fetal CMV infection, and irreversible damages of organs with significant sequelae must be expected. Therefore, intrauterine antiviral therapy seems to be unjustified in those severely affected fetuses diagnosed by ultrasound. To date, there is no evidence at all for the effectiveness of treatment with gancyclovir during pregnancy for prevention of fetal infection or for avoidance of irreversible damages due to progressive fetal infection after proven maternal CMV infection. Recently, a cytomegalovirus infection of a twin fetus seems to be successfully treated by administration of cytomegalovirus hyperimmunoglobulin, both intravenously to the mother and intra-amniotically, resulting in a decrease of placental edema and an improvement of fetal growth.[302]

Syphilis

Maternal infection by *Treponema pallidum* can result in fetal transmission at any gestational age especially in mothers with primary and secondary syphilis. The reported transmission rates vary between 50 and 80%.[303] The perinatal mortality of early congenital syphilis is around 50%; some of its classical signs are sonographically detectable, such as nonimmune hydrops most often as ascites and skin edema, hepatosplenomegaly, hyperechogenic and/or dilated bowel, placentomegaly, and polyhydramnios. Other symptoms are profound anemia and thrombocytopenia, skin lesions, rash, ostitis and periostitis, pneumonia and hepatitis, disseminated intravascular coagulation, and sepsis.[253, 303] Important pathogenetic mechanisms for hydrops in fetal syphilis are hepatic destruction, sepsis with capillary damage, and anemia.

Serologic diagnosis from maternal and fetal blood is achieved through the positive result of a screening test, either a Venereal Disease Research Laboratories (VDRL) or a rapid plasma reagin (RPR) test with a subsequent confirmation by a specific treponema test such as fluorescent treponemal antibody absorption test (FTA-ABS) or microhemagglutination for *Treponema pallidum* (MHATP).[303] Occasionally, false-negative maternal serology screening for syphilis may occur despite overwhelming infection seen during primary and secondary syphilis, a condition that has been termed the "prozone effect" occurring because a higher than optimal amount of antibodies in the tested sera prevents the characteristic flocculation reaction. The prozone phenomenon has also been reported in a case of fetal hydrops.[304, 305] Detection of *Treponema pallidum* in the amniotic fluid may be achieved by PCR[306] and by rabbit infectivity test (RIT),[307] which was found to correlate well with the sonographically measured hepatomegaly.[307] Specific IgM and positive PCR in the fetal blood obtained by cordocentesis proves fetal involvement.[308]

As in the nonpregnant state, penicillin G is the therapy of choice in pregnancy.[303] But the common treatment with a single dose of benzathine penicillin, 2.4 million units, intramusculary or weekly for 3 weeks in cases with syphilis of undetermined length or with latent syphilis for longer than 1 year must be modified for fetuses with hydrops.[253] In those fetuses maternal penicillin therapy and delivery is recommended, and for very premature fetuses a prolonged high-dose maternal penicillin therapy (e.g., 2.4 million units benzathine penicillin G weekly) should be applied until a more advanced gestational age is achieved.[253, 303] With this treatment regimen remission of hydrops and good outcome can be achieved in some fetuses,[309] although the outcome in this group of hydropic fetuses is rather poor, complicated by stillbirth and premature labor.[303] For patients with penicillin allergy, desensitization and use of penicillin is recommended and was successfully performed in a hydropic fetus, because of the unacceptably high failure rate (11%) of erythromycin treatment.[303] In more mature fetuses, delivery followed by postnatal antibiotic treatment of newborn and mother seems to be safer.

Toxoplasmosis

Toxoplasmosis is a systemic disease caused by the protozoan *Toxoplasma gondii*. In the case of primary infection with seroconversion of the mother in pregnancy the risk of transmission to the fetus, which can occur with a 1- to 4-month delay, is below 15% in the first, 25% in the second, and 65% in the third trimester, but the severity of fetal disease is the highest with first-trimester infection.[310–312] Hydrocephalus, cerebral calcifications, and chorioretinitis are the classical triad in the newborn.[311] Generalized hydrops may uncommonly occur in some of the affected fetuses.[253, 313] Hepatitis, elevated liver enzymes, hypoproteinemia, hemolytic anemia, thrombocytopenia, hepatosplenomegaly with diffuse extramedullary hematopoiesis, and sometimes myocarditis are common findings.[311] Sonographically, hepatosplenomegaly, cardiomegaly, hydro- and/or microcephaly

and cerebral calcifications, ascites, hydrops placentae, and oligohydramnios have been observed.[311, 314–316] The sensitivity of the ultrasound findings for the diagnosis of fetal toxoplasmosis infection is very low; the sonographic signs are more prevalent in fetuses with infection in early gestation.[314–316] Toxoplasma cysts and tachyzoites are found in placenta, organs, endothelial, and phagocytic cells.[311]

Diagnosis of toxoplasmosis infection is obtained by serologic testing of maternal and fetal blood for IgM and IgG. Long-time persistence of maternal IgM and variability of host antibody response and in laboratory analysis often cause confusion in interpretation of the test. Repeated sampling of maternal blood for evaluation of IgG titers, additional study of IgA and IgE antibodies, and the IgG avidity test are useful for a more accurate determination of the time of the infection.[311] In the fetus, however, there is a delayed antibody response, especially before 20 weeks. After that, in fetal blood sensitivity for IgM and IgA was 50% and 80%, respectively.[315] The "gold standard" of the diagnostic tests is the mouse inoculation by fetal blood sample and amniotic fluid specimens, but this test requires at least 3 weeks. More rapid diagnosis with a sensitivity over 95% may be achieved by amplification of toxoplasma DNA by PCR from amniotic fluid.[311, 312, 317] Current practice is to advise all women with seroconversion to have amniocentesis, and to suggest termination only if there is a diagnosis of fetal infection and detection of abnormalities by ultrasound, because even children with chorioretinitis and intracerebral calcifications may have a normal neurologic development.[312] PCR can also be performed in fetal blood. In addition, nonspecific signs of fetal infection are the presence of thrombocytopenia, eosinophilia, increased lactate dehydrogenase, and increased γ-glutamyl transferase in the fetal blood.[315, 316]

Toxoplasmosis during pregnancy is prenatally treated by spiramycin and/or by a combination of pyrimethamine and sulfadiazine. To decrease toxicity from pyrimethamine to the developing fetus folic acid is added. Most centers prefer an alternating treatment with both regimens.[311, 318–321] Pyrimethamine and sulfonamide, however, cross the placenta and seem to be more effective than spiramycin in reducing the severity of fetal infections.[319, 321] Prenatal antibiotic treatment, which should start as soon as possible after diagnosis of maternal infection, reduces the frequency and the severity of sequelae among infected. Antibiotic treatment of congenitally infected infants should be started soon after birth and should be continued for 1 year for avoidance of further deterioration in the symptomatology.[322] Normal ultrasound findings in the late second trimester followed by prenatal antibiotic therapy is most commonly associated with normal neurodevelopmental outcome.[312, 314] In addition, prenatal antibiotic treatment has been shown to prevent vertical maternofetal transmission of the protozoa,[318] but this could not be confirmed in a recent multicenter study.[320] There is not enough experience concerning the antibiotic treatment of fetuses with hydrops. In one case, resolution of hydrops and normal short-term outcome were observed after prenatal antibiotic treatment.[323] Anyway, the decision for or against treatment in these few cases must be achieved individually in order to avoid a very severe degree of illness and irreversible sequelae.

Herpes Simplex Virus

Primary maternal infection with herpes simplex virus is associated with an increased risk of spontaneous abortion, intrauterine growth retardation, and preterm labor.[324–326] Approximately 90% of neonatal HSV infection is acquired sub partu, 5% postpartally, and 5% during pregnancy by transplacental transmission causing congenital HSV infection, which is characterized by skin vesicles and scarring, chorioretinitis, microphthalmia, microcephaly, and brain defects.[324–326] Nonimmune hydrops is reported only in a few case reports in which hydrops was the only manifestation of fetal infection.[10, 328] Diagnosis of fetal infection is based on viral culture and more recently on amplification of viral DNA by PCR.[329] Antiviral treatment with acyclovir is successful in neonatal HSV infections and is recommended in generalized HSV infection in pregnancy.[327] There are no data about antiviral treatment in HSV-infected fetuses with nonimmune hydrops.

Adenovirus

There are a few case reports on adenoviral infection associated with hydrops. In one case myocarditis seemed to cause hydrops[330]; in another case, presumably, tachyarrhythmia caused by myocarditis led to hydrops and was successfully treated in utero by transplacental digitalization.[331] In a twin pregnancy, adenovirus was exclusively demonstrated in the amniotic fluid of the twin afflicted with hydrops using PCR, whereas the other severely growth-restricted twin was not hydropic and his amniotic fluid was negative for adenoviral DNA. This proves the differential transmission of adenovirus in a twin pregnancy.[332] The etiologic relationship between hydrops and adenoviral infection, however, seems to be unproved in the reported case, because a twin-twin transfusion syndrome could not definitively be excluded. As for other infections, it may be speculated that the application of highly sensitive PCR techniques in cases of hydrops will result in an increased proportion of infectious etiologies among all cases with nonimmune hydrops as demonstrated in a recent report.[256] On the other hand, various viruses, especially adenovirus, sometimes seem to be present in amniotic fluid without negative effects on the pregnancy outcome as demonstrated in amniotic fluid samples for genetic second-trimester amniocenteses by PCR-based methods.[333]

Genetic Disorders

Chromosomal Abnormalities

The vast majority of genetic disorders that occur in association with hydrops are chromosomal abnormalities, especially monosomy X (Turner syndrome), trisomy 21, trisomy 18, trisomy 13, and triploidy, but also rare trisomies, mosaicisms, and chromosomal rearrangements such as translocations, deletions, inversions, rings, and markers.[1, 14, 15, 17, 18, 334–338] In total, chromosomal abnormalities are reportedly present in 10 to 35% of the fetuses with NIHF.[1, 14, 15, 17, 18, 336] The rates of numerical chromosomal abnormalities most commonly depend on the gestational age at diagnosis, because there is a very high spontaneous abortion rate between first trimester, second trimester, third trimester, and term,[339] and the occurrence of hydrops seems to markedly increase the risk of in utero deaths in fetuses with chromosomal abnormalities. Therefore, a high percentage of chromosomal abnormalities is found in series of nonimmune hydrops in early pregnancy.[8]

Hydrops in fetuses with Turner syndrome results from a maldevelopment of the lymphatic vessels and is mostly combined with a cystic nuchal hygroma colli that extends to the posterior as well as lateral aspects of the head and the back (Fig. 35–21). In contrast to the transient nuchal edema ("nuchal translucency"), which

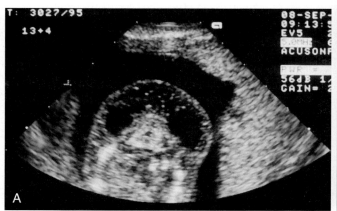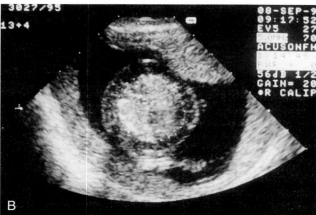

FIGURE 35–29. *A,* Fetus at 13 + 4 weeks' gestation with bilateral hygromata colli and generalized skin edema. Chorionic villus sampling revealed Turner syndrome (45,X). Two days later the fetus spontaneously died. *B,* The same fetus showed generalized skin edema on the transverse scan of the fetal abdomen.

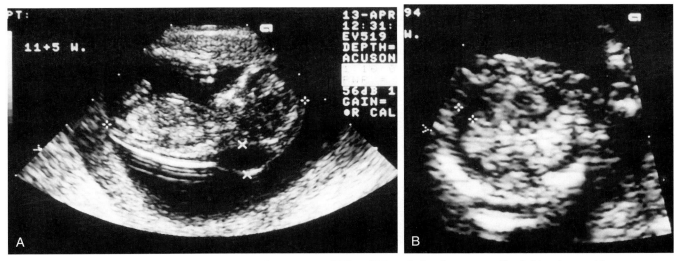

FIGURE 35–30. *A,* Fetus at 11 + 4 weeks' gestation (CRL = 53.8 mm) showing a generalized skin edema with a sick nuclei translucency of 8.0 mm. Chorionic villus sampling revealed Turner syndrome (45,X). *B,* The same fetus had bilateral hydrothoraces. In this picture, the distance between the left lung and the lateral thoracic wall are 0.8 mm.

is an excellent sonographic marker for autosomal trisomies between 10 and 14 weeks' gestation,[339] the lymph accumulations in Turner syndrome are often progressive, followed by the appearance of bilateral pleural effusions, ascites, and generalized skin edema (Figs. 35–29 through 35–32). In only a few fetuses does the hygromata colli remain isolated or spontaneously disappear later in gestation.[191, 340, 341] Redundant nuchal skin and lymphedema of the hands and feet are common findings in newborns with Turner syndrome, as are, sometimes, chylothorax and lymphangiectasia. Coarctation of the aorta and other obstructions of the left ventricular outflow tract are the commonest cardiac malformations associated with Turner syndrome in utero as well

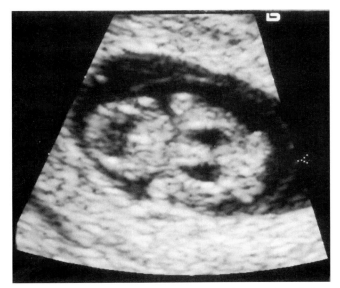

FIGURE 35–31. Bilateral hydrothoraces in a fetus at 10 weeks' gestation.

as postpartum.[342, 343] These defects are associated with diminished blood flow through the left ventricle and are more common in cases of Turner syndrome with hygromata colli than in those without hygromata colli. Clark[344] speculated that increased lymphatic pressure associated with jugular sac obstruction also distends thoracic lymph vessels at the base of the ascending aorta. This compression may result in decreased left-sided and subsequent diminished blood flow through the ascending aorta. Maintenance of adequate head growth causes a redistribution of aortic blood flow and flow across the aortic arch; thus, coarctation of the aorta may occur and persist.[342] On the other hand, the presence of hygromata colli indicates poor prognostic outcome in Turner syndrome and most commonly progresses to generalized hydrops. Intrauterine fetal death usually ensues at the latest in midtrimester in these cases, explaining the higher incidence of cardiac anomalies in Turner syndrome in early gestation than in live births. Presumably, there is a correlation between the degree of lymphatic obstruction causing hydrops with consecutive fetal death and the severity of left heart obstruction. Therefore, the left ventricular outflow tract obstruction seems not to be the cause of hydrops or a lethal factor, but rather an indicator of the degree of lymphatic obstruction.

Hydrops may occur in fetuses with trisomy 21 in the presence as well as in the absence of cardiovascular malformations. In early pregnancy fetuses with trisomy 21 very often have a transient nuchal edema,[339] but in some cases a generalized skin edema and hydrops fetalis may occur (Fig. 35–33). Both groups contain fetuses without cardiac defects, although the incidence of atrioventricular septal defects and ventricular septal defects is much higher in fetuses with increased "nuchal translucency," and the degree of hydrops can be correlated with "nuchal translucency" thickness.[342, 345] In the majority of both the chromosomally abnormal and normal

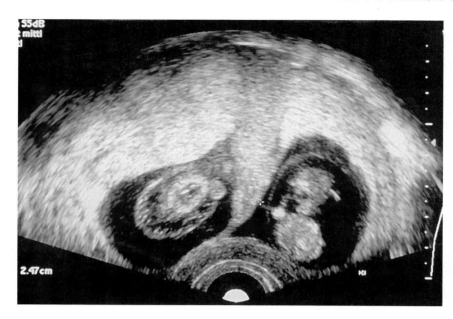

FIGURE 35–32. Dichorionic twin pregnancy at 11 weeks' gestation showing a normal developed twin and a severely hydropic fetus that spontaneously died a short time later. The cause of the hydrops remains unknown.

fetuses with isolated increased nuchal translucency the fluid accumulation disappears after 14 weeks, most likely because of a more sufficient drainage of the interstitial fluid by the lymphatic system and/or by the drop in peripheral arterial resistance. In some of the hydropic fetuses, but also in fetuses with isolated nuchal edema, AV valve regurgitation and abnormal venous Doppler flow velocity waveforms suggest cardiac congestive heart failure as a pathomechanism for the development of hydrops.[346–348] Furthermore, in fetuses with atrioventricular septal defect with and without trisomy 21, severity of AV valve incompetence correlates with the occurrence of hydrops in the second and third trimesters.[43] On the other hand, in some hydropic fetuses with trisomy 21

cardiac defects seem to be only associated. In these fetuses and the hydropic trisomy 21 fetuses without cardiac anomalies other pathomechanisms have to be discussed, including a maldevelopment of lymphatic vessels especially in cases of isolated hydro-/chylothorax that may be found in fetuses with trisomy 21 (Figs. 35–34 and 35–35), a hypoxia-induced capillary damage, a transient myeloproliferative disorder, and/or an altered collagen formation due to a dose effect from responsible genes on chromosome 21.

Nuchal edema and hydrops may be associated with other autosomal trisomies (e.g., trisomies 18 and 13) and triploidy.[339] Although the isolated nuchal edema may be transient, hydrops already occurring in the first and

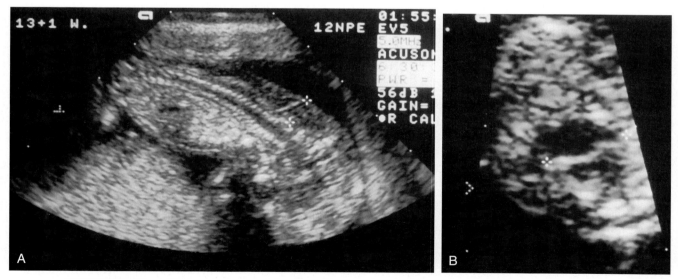

FIGURE 35–33. *A,* Transvaginal sonography showed increased nuchal edema in a fetus at 13 + 1 weeks' gestation. *B,* A complete atrioventricular septal defect was diagnosed by transvaginal echocardiography. The four-chamber view during diastolic period demonstrated a common atrium, a closed common AV valve, and a large ventricular septal defect. Trisomy 21 was diagnosed by chorionic villus sampling.

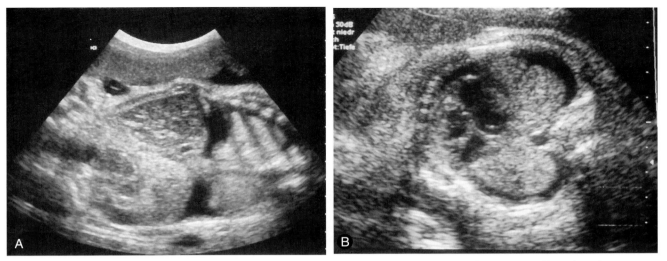

FIGURE 35–34. *A,* Trisomy 21 fetus with bilateral moderate hydrothoraces at 29 weeks' gestation. Skin edema is also present. *B,* Four-chamber view additionally revealed a complete atrioventricular septal defect (AV canal), suggesting a trisomy 21, which was confirmed by fetal blood sampling.

early second trimesters is associated with spontaneous abortion in the vast majority of these fetuses.

Hereditary Syndromes

Diseases with Altered Lymphatic Drainage

Noonan syndrome, multiple pterygium syndrome, Fryns syndrome, congenital pulmonary lymphangiectasia, and hydro-/chylothorax are hereditary diseases with familial recurrence.[349–352] In these disorders hydrops seems to result from a local or a more generalized lymphatic dysplasia. In Noonan, multiple pterygium, and Fryns syndrome cystic nuchal hygromata colli are fre-

quently present (Fig. 35–36). In the Noonan syndrome, congenital heart diseases, especially valvular pulmonary stenosis, and cryptorchidism are present. In the Fryns syndrome, a lethal autosomal-recessive inherited disorder with diaphragmatic hernia, cerebral anomalies, abnormal facies and corneas, and digit anomalies, the cystic hygromata colli seems to be a valuable diagnostic feature already in the late first trimester.[353, 354] For isolated hydro-/chylothorax, intrauterine treatment may also be successful in cases of familial occurrence. A detailed familial history with a search for discrete signs of lymphatic dysfunction among the relatives is very important for adequate genetic counseling.[17]

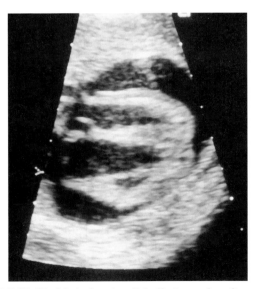

FIGURE 35–35. Marked pericardial effusion and cardiomegaly in a fetus with trisomy 21 mosaicism and mild hemolytic anemia of unknown cause at 31 + 2 weeks' gestation.

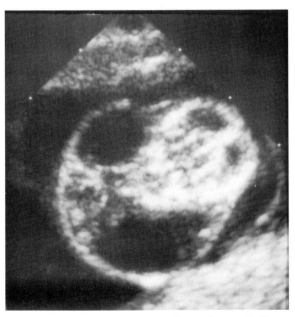

FIGURE 35–36. Cystic hygromata colli in a fetus with Fryns syndrome at 12 weeks' gestation.

Diseases with Fetal Hypo- and Akinesia

Congenital myotonic dystrophy is characterized by hypotonia and respiratory insufficiency at birth; moderate mental retardation is common for children with congenital myotonic dystrophy. This autosomal dominant disease is almost exclusively inherited from the mother and caused by amplification of an unstable cytosine-thymidine-guanine (CTG) nucleotide repeat upstream to the myotonin protein kinase gene.[355] Due to the phenomenon of "anticipation," each successive generation inheriting the affected allele on the long arm of chromosome 19 has an increased number of triplet repeats and correspondingly a more severe phenotype.[355, 356] Excessive polyhydramnios due to poor fetal swallowing, skin edema of the fetal head, and less often generalized hydrops as well as reduced fetal breathing movements and activity due to weakness of muscles and malpresentation are the sonographically detectable symptoms of this disease[356-359]; additionally, in some cases severe cardiomyopathy has been reported.[360, 361] The rate of intrauterine death is increased in the congenital cases. Careful examination of the pregnant woman and family history provide clues for diagnosis. Meanwhile, DNA-based diagnosis using mutation analysis on maternal and fetal DNA and detection of the CTG repeat expansion is possible for congenital myotonic dystrophy using fetal tissue.[336] Cases symptomatic already prenatally most commonly show a severe disease postpartum that demands mechanical ventilatory support even in newborns at term. Recently, successful weaning from prolonged respiratory support over several months was reported.[362]

Similar to the congenital myotonic dystrophy, other rare disorders with decreased fetal movements are often associated with skin edema and severe polyhydramnios, in a few cases also with nonimmune hydrops and placentomegaly, such as lethal multiple pterygium syndrome,[363] Pena-Shokeir syndrome,[364] nemaline myopathy,[365, 366] amyoplasia,[367] other fetal akinesia deformation sequences with and without arthrogryposis caused by various neuronal and/or muscular diseases,[334, 365, 368] and Neu-Laxova syndrome.[369] It has been suggested that fetal hypo- and akinesia with poor body and breathing movements may preferentially lead to a skin edema and in early pregnancy to nuchal edema with increased nuchal translucency thickness.[370]

Metabolic Disorders

Lysosomal Storage Diseases

Inborn errors of metabolism and other single-gene defects cause only about 1% of cases of nonimmune hydrops, but their exact diagnosis is very important, because there is a substantial risk of recurrence due to their mostly autosomal recessive inheritance. In particular, a large number of lysosomal storage diseases may present as fetal ascites or generalized hydrops with placentomegaly and polyhydramnios, although the prenatal manifestation of these storage diseases is rather uncommon. Hydrops is suggested as a consequence of hepato-

cellular damage due to lysosomal storage disease resulting in a local obstruction with ascites and, thus, generalized hydrops similar to cases with increased extramedullary hematopoiesis. Lysosomal storage diseases reportedly associated with hydrops are some sphingolipidoses (gangliosidoses such as GM_1-gangliosidosis, galactosialidosis, and Farber disease; visceral storage diseases such as Gaucher disease [glucocerebrosidase deficiency], and Niemann-Pick disease type A), mucopolysaccharidoses (MPS type I [Hurler syndrome], MPS IVa [Morquio A syndrome], MPS VII [β-glucuronidase deficiency, or Sly syndrome]), mucolipidoses (mucolipidosis type I [sialidosis], mucolipidosis type II [I-cell disease]), transport defects (sialic acid storage disease, Salla disease, Niemann-Pick disease type C), and other storage diseases (Wolman disease, glycogen storage disease type II [Pompe])[371-377] (Fig. 35-37). Furthermore, fetal hydrops has been reported in one case of carbohydrate-deficient glycoprotein syndrome[378] and in one case of a cardiac glycogenosis without acid maltase deficiency.[62] Diagnosis is very difficult and often fails, especially if there is not an index case, and the clinical spectrum may vary.[371, 376] Abnormalities of white blood cell morphology in fetal blood sample obtained by cordocentesis[377] and detection of sialic acid, glycosaminoglycans, or oligosaccharides in amniotic fluid samples may suggest the presence of a fetal metabolic disorder as the cause of hydrops.[371] Positive family history or consanguinity, however, may lead more directly to adequate diagnostic steps. However, their definitive diagnosis demands a lot of special pathohistologic examinations using light and also electron microscopy, and histochemical and biochemical examinations with attention to the liver, spleen, heart, bone marrow, and especially placenta, which have been recently reviewed in detail by Lake and co-workers.[371]

In subsequent pregnancies, once the diagnosis is confirmed in the affected index case, evidence of the gene defect on a biochemical or DNA level permits prenatal diagnosis by biochemical (enzyme activity or storage product), histochemical, molecular genetic, and morphologic studies in fetal tissue and/or amniotic fluid obtained by chorionic villus sampling or amniocentesis, respectively. Combination of these independent methods (enzyme assay, morphology, and DNA analysis) is recommended for correct diagnosis and should only be performed in a laboratory with high competence in this diagnostic field.[371] Analysis of fetal blood demonstrating white blood cell anomalies in some of the lysosomal storage diseases may be useful for primary diagnosis in hydropic fetuses of unclear etiology where fetal blood sampling is an essential diagnostic step, but is unnecessary in subsequent pregnancies at risk, if the definitive diagnosis is known from the index case. Although DNA-based diagnosis can be performed in families with specific mutations, to date, biochemical enzyme assay is sometimes still the quickest and most accurate method for prenatal diagnosis, particularly since mutations can be quite specific to a particular family. In the future, however, DNA-based diagnosis of lysosomal storage diseases may surely become possible in more cases, including the possibility of preimplantation diagnosis

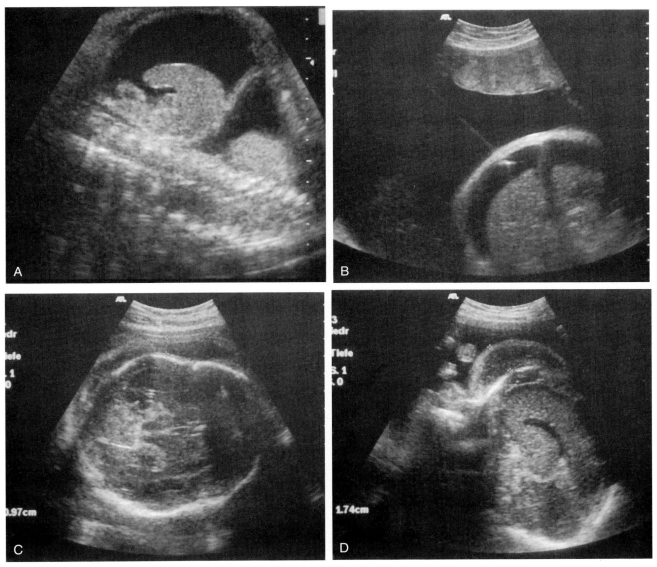

F I G U R E 35–37. *A,* Left-sided pleural effusion, ascites, and splenomegaly were demonstrated in the severe hydropic fetus of 32 + 1 weeks' gestation showing massive skin edema, bilateral pleural effusion, ascites, cardiomegaly, polyhydramnios, and hydrops placentae. The extent of fluid accumulation remained constant from 24 to 32 weeks' gestation and normal biophysical profile was always demonstrated in this period of gestation. Fetal blood sampling revealed a normal hemoglobin content. Postpartum, a mucopolysaccharidosis type VII (Sly syndrome) was diagnosed. *B,* Transverse scan through the abdomen shows massive ascites and hepatomegaly. A diagnostic puncture of the ascites was performed. *C,* The transverse scan of the fetal head demonstrates a massive skin edema. *D & E,* Sagittal scan of the fetal head shows the massive skin edema in the frontal and face area.

from a single blastomere[379] or from a single fetal cell isolated from the maternal circulation.[380]

Disorders of Fetal Thyroid Function

Fetal hyperthyroidism and thyrotoxicosis are generalized metabolic disorders with increased fuel metabolism and high cardiac output caused by thyroid stimulatory and thyroid-binding inhibitory immunoglobulin G antibodies in maternal Graves disease, and also in euthyroid gravidae. Fetal tachycardia between 170 and 190 bpm, fetal thyroid goiter, growth retardation, and sometimes hydrops were reported. Maternal propylthiouracil treat-

ment may normalize fetal thyroid size and function, as indicated by a decrease of heart rate and resolving fetal hydrops.[381-383]

Twin Pregnancies

In twin pregnancies the most common cause of nonimmune hydrops is the chronic twin-twin syndrome (TTTS), which complicates between 10 and 15% of the monochorionic twin pregnancies.[384] TTTS occurs on the basis of a monochorionic placenta where superficial arterioarterial and venovenous vascular connections and sometimes deep unidirectional arteriovenous anastomoses between the two twins are present. Placental studies in monochorionic twins with and without chronic TTTS suggest an imbalance between these anastomoses, especially a paucity of compensatory superficial anastomoses in the presence of a deep arteriovenous anastomosis causing an unbalanced unidirectional shunt leading to chronic donor and recipient twins.[385–388] Furthermore, other factors may contribute to the development of chronic TTTS (e.g., an absolutely and relatively small placental portion of the donor twin,[385] marginal and velamentous cord insertion,[389] discordance in cord diameter, and reduced umbilical coiling index in the donor twin[390]). The donor fetus becomes hypovolemic and oligouric, growth-restricted, and sometimes anemic (Fig. 35–38). The chronic recipient fetus develops hypervolemia and polyuria with subsequent polyhydramnios, normal growth, and sometimes plethora. Doppler studies often demonstrate increased placental resistance in the donor fetus, whereas the main problems for the recipient are diminished cardiac function due to high preload and afterload conditions with volume overload and systemic arterial hypertension, respectively.[391–393] In the recipient, increased pulsatility of the systemic veins implicate elevated venous blood pressure. Biventricular myocardial hypertrophy, cardiomegaly, and AV valve incompetence signify cardiac compromise and usually appear before the development of hydrops.[391, 392] In contrast, generalized hydrops, AV valve incompetence, and increased pulsatility of venous blood flow are extremely rare in the donor fetus, which may show only isolated mild to moderate pericardial effusion occasionally.

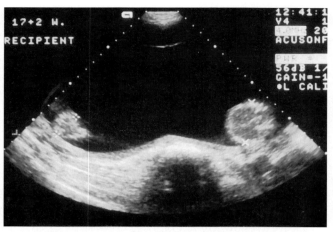

F I G U R E 35–39. Chronic twin-twin transfusion syndrome at 17 + 2 weeks' gestation. Severe polyhydramnios of the recipient twin is present, whereas the donor twin has anhydramnios ("stuck twin" phenomenon). A growth discrepancy is also demonstrated; the abdominal transverse diameter was 40 mm for the recipient fetus and 25 mm for the donor fetus, respectively.

Therefore, diagnosis of chronic TTTS is based on the demonstration of monochorionicity, which can most accurately and quickly be assessed in the first trimester,[386] and on the detection of gross polyhydramnios and severe oligohydramnios causing the "stuck twin" phenomenon in the absence of other causes for abnormal amniotic fluid volume[387] (Fig. 35–39). Further sonographic criteria are intertwin growth discordance, different echogenicity of both portions of the placenta, dilated bladder, and signs of cardiac overload in the recipient fetus (e.g., biventricular myocardial hypertrophy; cardiac dilatation; uni- or bilateral AV incompetence; congestive heart failure; and, in a much advanced stage, reverse perfusion of ductus arteriosus, main pulmonary trunk, pulmonary valve, and the right ventricle[387,391–393]). Increased nuchal translucency in monochorionic twins between 10 and 14 weeks' gestation seems to predict severe TTTS in later gestation.[387] Fetal blood sampling may show a high intertwin hemoglobin difference, but mostly only mild differences less than 5 g/dL occur.[394–396] Atrial natriuretic hormone is elevated, especially in the recipient fetus.[34, 35]

The mortality and morbidity is very high in chronic TTTS.[384, 387] The sequelae of very early prematurity, intrauterine death of one or both fetuses, in utero ischemic or thromboembolic brain damage, cardiac dysfunction, and pulmonary hypertension are the most common complications.[386, 387] Postnatally, hypertrophic cardiomyopathy may complicate the neonatal course; in some of these neonates, subpulmonic[393] and subaortic obstruction[391] have been observed. Increased nuchal translucency thickness may be an early indicator for development of chronic TTTS in monochorionic twins.[397] A reduction of mortality and morbidity can be achieved by intrauterine treatment reducing the mortality rate from 80 to 100% to around 35 to 50%. The most effective methods of treatment, confirmed in large series, are serial amnioreduction[398–400] and laser coagulation of placental vascular anastomoses.[401–405] The selective fetocide of one twin[406] involves the risk of exsanguination of the surviving co-twin and should always be combined with an occlusion of the

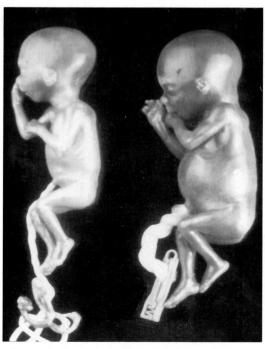

F I G U R E 35–38. Spontaneous abortion of monochorionic, diamniotic twins with twin-twin tranfusion syndrome. At 23 weeks' gestation the normally grown recipient fetus shows the signs of polyglobuly. The growth-retarded donor twin was severely anemic.

umbilical vessels. These techniques are discussed in more detail in Chapter 23. In addition, transplacental treatment with digoxin may help to improve myocardial function of the recipient fetus.

The twin reversed arterial perfusion (TRAP) sequence is a rare complication of a monochorionic placenta. The pump twin perfuses a mostly acardiac parasitic twin and in consequence develops a high-cardiac-output failure. A mortality of 50% due to prematurity and cardiac dysfunction of the pump twin has been reported. The mortality is substantially increased if the acardiac/ pump twin weight ratio is more then 50%. Intrauterine therapeutic options therefore include digitalization, tocolysis, indomethacin, and amnioreduction as palliative treatment on the one hand, and on the other cord embolization (Fig. 35-40), cord ligation, fetoscopic laser coagulation of the cord, and thermocoagulation of the aorta of the parasitic twin by monopolar wire electrode as curative treatment.[13, 402, 407–412] These therapeutic options have to be carefully evaluated. Treatment should preferentially be considered in cases of cardiac decompensation of the pump twin indicated by elevated pulsatility of the venous blood flow velocity waveforms in the ductus venosus and the vena cava inferior, AV valve insufficiency, and/or hydrops.

Placenta and Umbilical Cord Abnormalities

Chorioangioma as a benign AV malformation of the placenta is the most common placental tumor, with an incidence of 1% on microscopic examination of randomly selected placentas.[413, 414] Only large chorioangiomata, however, which are detectable by ultrasound, seem to have clinical significance. Bypassing the normal placenta, tumors act as an arteriovenous shunt in the fetal circulation causing compensatory high cardiac output, cardiomegaly, AV valve insufficiency, and sometimes congestive heart failure and placental hydrops.[170, 171] Polyhydramnios is most commonly present. Furthermore, the development of hydrops is favored, because varying degrees of a Kasabach-Merritt sequence with microangiopathic hemolytic anemia are often present in those cases.[169, 170, 416] The resulting hemolytic anemia not only increases the fetal cardiac output, but also may lead to hypoxia and capillary damage together with placental shunting of unoxygenated blood. Chorioangioma in Wiedemann-Beckwith syndrome was reported and interpreted as a part of this syndrome, which may be associated with nonimmune hydrops fetalis.[417]

Several disorders of the umbilical cord in association with fetal hydrops have been described in individual case reports including angiomyxoma and hemangioma of the umbilical cord,[167] aneurysm of the umbilical artery, umbilical vein thrombosis,[418] and true knot of the cord,[419] but the exact pathogenic mechanism in some of these cases is speculative.[420, 421]

Independent of the different causes of nonimmune hydrops, microscopic examination of the placenta in cases of fetal hydrops often reveals a similar pattern with edematous villi, many Hofbauer cells, persisting cytotrophoblasts, sparse and small fetal vessels, immature red blood cells, and foci of erythropoiesis. Villous stem vessels may be obliterated. Additional thrombosis and extravasation of erythrocytes characterize the "hemorrhagic endovasculitis" of the placenta,[422] a misnomer, because there is no inflammatory component.[423] It was speculated that in some cases this conditon may first cause fetal hydrops either by fetal hypoxia or by fetoplacental hemorrhage, but it may more likely be interpreted as a general result of chronic low-blood-flow states in the placenta.[423] Furthermore, a case with large subchorial hematoma of the placenta has been reported in association with reversible NIHF.[424]

Idiopathic Hydrops

The term "idiopathic" hydrops is often applied in those cases in which no causes for fetal hydrops can be found despite extensive investigations. The development of better diagnostic techniques, detailed pre- and postnatal investigations, and also pathoanatomic examinations of fetus and placenta markedly decrease and will further decrease the proportion of idiopathic causes in series of nonimmune hydrops. The improvement of microbiologic techniques, in particular DNA-based techniques, and their consistent application not only in maternal blood samples but also in fetal tissue samples or as part of an autopsy, for example, lead to the recognition that a large portion of the cases primarily classified as idiopathic result from a fetal parvovirus B19 infection[254] or from other viral infections.[256] In addition, diagnosis of some other viral infections and inborn errors of metabolism is difficult to establish, but very important because of the recurrence risk of metabolic storage diseases.[371]

Similar to the theories about an immunologic origin of abortion, of fetal growth restriction, and preeclamp-

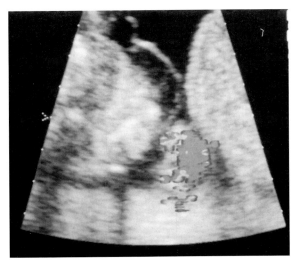

FIGURE 35–40. In utero aspect of an acardius acranius (left side) where the cord was successfully blocked by cordocentesis and application of alcoholized suture material. Doppler color flow mapping demonstrated blood flow only in the umbilical cord of the previously pumping twin (right side). The twin reversed arterial perfusion of the parasitic twin was successfully interrupted.

sia, an immunologic origin may also be present in some cases of idiopathic nonimmune hydrops. This could be shown in an investigation comparing fetuses with idiopathic hydrops to fetuses with nonimmune hydrops of known etiology.[425] In the group of idiopathic hydrops, the proportion of parents sharing four or five HLA antigens was significantly increased. Furthermore, the incidence and percentage of lymphocytotoxic antibodies were decreased in the pregnant women of the idiopathic hydrops group. Further investigations have to be performed to evaluate possible immunologic causes of nonimmune hydrops fetalis and to perform immunotherapy in appropriate cases.[425]

Maternal Complication in Nonimmune Hydrops

Preeclampsia and all related complications such as placental abruption and HELLP (hemolysis, elevated liver enzymes, and low platelet count) syndrome are more common in hydropic than in nonhydropic fetuses. Presumably, placentomegaly may have a causative relationship to these maternal diseases and the terms "mirror syndrome," Ballantyne syndrome, and maternal hydrops syndrome have been applied for this association. The maternal hyperdynamic and hypertensive state seem to be most common in cases of α-thalassemia,[203] but also in other hydropic fetal diseases with placentomegaly such as sacrococcygeal teratoma, tachyarrhythmia, aneurysm of the vein of Galen, chorioangioma, and rhesus incompatibility.[181, 426–429] Polyhydramnios, preterm labor, and postpartum hemorrhage are other common complications in fetal hydrops. Despite a recently reported case,[430] it still remains unclear whether disappearance of hydrops—after intrauterine therapy or spontaneously—regularly leads to an improvement or complete remission of the preeclamptic symptoms of the mother.

Diagnostic Approach to NIHF

The prognosis in cases of nonimmune hydrops mainly depends on the underlying disease. Further prognostic indicators are: distribution as well as extent of fluid accumulation and edema, degree of cardiac decompensation, and the gestational age at the time of manifestation. Therefore, correct assignment of the precise diagnosis in each case of nonimmune hydrops is mandatory for an adequate management of the pregnancy and counseling of the parents. Diagnostic methods and approaches are listed in Table 35–2. It seems to be very difficult, however, to exclude all potential causes in the large group of heterogeneous disorders when investigating individual cases. Therefore, the following factors should be considered before the diagnostic technique is chosen: (1) invasive versus noninvasive approach (noninvasive tests like sonography and maternal blood sampling harbor no risks for the fetus and, therefore, should be applied first); (2) incidence of the potential disorders at the specific gestational age; and (3) necessity to promptly exclude fetal anemia causing nonimmune hydrops, which is life-threatening and can usually be successfully treated if diagnosis is achieved in time.

Noninvasive Procedures

Noninvasive examination by maternal blood sampling includes the antibody screening test for exclusion of alloimmune hemolytic anemia, the Kleihauer-Betke stain for HbF cells for diagnosis of fetomaternal hemorrhage, and a search for infectious diseases such as parvovirus B19; cytomegaly; syphilis; toxoplasmosis; and adeno-, coxsackie-, and herpes simplex virus infections. If family history or actual findings indicate a special etiology, more sophisticated investigations may be necessary: hemoglobin electrophoresis, determination of enzyme activity, or exclusion of autoimmune antibodies (anti-SSA, anti-SSB).

Sonography, echocardiography, and Doppler sonography as noninvasive and repeatable methods are the most important tools for the diagnosis and surveillance of cases with nonimmune fetal hydrops:

1. Distribution and extent of fluid accumulation, amount of amniotic fluid, and placental structure should be registered.
2. Sonographic detection of malformations and hygromata colli indicates specific chromosomal and nonchromosomal disorders; specific causes of hydrops may be detected in other pathologic conditions such as lung masses, tumors, heart defects, arteriovenous malformation, gastrointestinal and renal diseases, fetofetal transfusion, parasitic twin; sustained arrhythmia.
3. Echocardiography and Doppler sonography of arterial and venous vessels may demonstrate high cardiac output in cases of anemia and arteriovenous malformations.
4. Echocardiography and Doppler sonography of the venous system may indicate or exclude cardiac failure, which may be the primary or the secondary cause in the advanced stage of diseases other than anemia. Cardiac dilatation, AV valve incompetence, and increased pulsatility of venous blood flow velocity waveforms are signs of cardiac decompensation. Evaluation of the cardiothoracic ratio for detection of cardiomegaly as a noninvasive assessment of cardiac function in nonimmune hydrops is validated by the measurement of umbilical venous pressure.[431]
5. Fetal heart rate monitoring should repeatedly be performed for longer periods to exclude paroxysmal tachyarrhythmia over 24 hours.

Invasive Procedures

As fetal hydrops is an emergency situation, rapid karyotyping is indicated in most situations. The method of sampling depends on the gestational age and the necessity of other invasive procedures. These are chorionic

T A B L E 35–2. DIAGNOSTIC APPROACH IN CASES OF NONIMMUNE HYDROPS FETALIS*

Maternal history
  Ethnic background
  Diseases: anemia, infection, diabetes mellitus, connective tissue
    disease
  Consanguinity
  Family history
Past obstetric history
  Previous affected sibling
  Spontaneous abortions/stillbirths
Pregnancy history
  Gravida/para
  Gestational age
  Multiple gestations
  Infectious diseases
  Medication

Maternal studies
  Blood group typing
  Indirect Coombs testing
  Complete blood count with indices such as mean corpuscular
    volume
  Peripheral blood smear for erythrocyte morphology
  Kleihauer-Betke stain
  Syphilis, parvovirus B19, cytomegalovirus, toxoplasmosis, and
    other infections
  Additional examinations (as indicated):
    Hemoglobin electrophoresis
    Maternal blood chemistry
    G6PD, pyruvate kinase deficiency screening

Fetal studies
  Ultrasound
    Two- or three-dimensional ultrasound
  Fetal echocardiography
    Two-dimensional ultrasound (dimension, cardiac structures,
      rhythm)
    Pulsed and color flow Doppler (intracardiac and postcardiac for
      detection of flow abnormalities such as valve regurgitation,
      stenosis, ductus arteriosus constriction, shunts, high cardiac
      output)

M-mode (dimension, rhythm, contractility)
Venous Doppler studies (cardiac function, rhythm)
Arterial Doppler (high cardiac output, arteriovenous
  malformations)
Cardiotocography
  Fetal condition
  Arrhythmias, especially paroxysmal tachyarrhythmia
  Fetal anemia
Amniocentesis[†]
  Fetal karyotype
  α-Fetoprotein
  Antigen tests by PCR and amniotic fluid culture for syphilis,
    cytomegalovirus, toxoplasmosis, and other infections
  Metabolic testing of amniotic fluid
  Amniotic cell morphology and culture for metabolic disorders
Fetal blood sampling[†]
  Fetal karyotype
  Fetal complete blood count with indices
  Peripheral blood smear
  Reticulocyte count
  White blood cell differentiation
  Blood group typing
  Direct Coombs test
  Fetal albumin
  Fetal liver function tests
  Fetal antigen-specific IgM, IgA, and PCR for infectious causes
Additional examinations (as indicated)
  Hemoglobin electrophoresis
  Osmotic fragility
  Heinz body preparation
  Erythrocyte enzyme determination
  Special testing of erythrocyte membrane skeleton proteins
  Metabolic testing
Chorionic villus sampling[†]
  Fetal karyotype
Additional examinations (as indicated):
  Morphologic examination for storage diseases
  Metabolic testing

* This table is modified from corresponding tables in the following publications: Holzgreve et al., 1985[12]; Machin, 1989[15]; Norton, 1994[17]; Jones, 1995[18]; and Arcasoy & Gallagher, 1995.[200]
[†] If there is an index case or specific symptoms, *molecular genetic DNA-based analysis* can be performed from chorionic villus sampling, fetal blood, and amniotic cells (e.g., for diagnosing storage diseases, cystic fibrosis, skeletal dysplasia, or congenital myotonic dystrophy).

villus sampling or placentesis and fetal blood sampling, of which the latter has the advantage of an additional exclusion of many other potential disorders, especially anemia and infection. Amniocentesis allows the rapid exclusion of the most important chromosomal anomalies by fluorescent in situ hybridization (FISH) or PCR, but does not achieve a complete karyogram in contrast to the conventional karyogram rapidly achieved by sampling of fetal blood and chorionic villi. This is an important disadvantage especially in cases of detected fetal anomalies, where more subtle and less common chromosomal abnormalities are more frequent than in low-risk screening programs.[432] In a high-risk population, Evans and colleagues[433] could detect only 65% of chromosomal abnormalities by FISH using probe combinations (13, 18, 21, X, and Y), whereas other trisomies and chromosomal rearrangements such as mosaics, translocations, deletions, inversions, rings, and markers were missed within this combination of probes.[432, 433]

Therefore, fetal blood sampling is usually the preferential method for rapid karyotyping, except if the fetal phenotype strongly suggests an aneuploidy and an ob-

stetric decision is required immediately. In these situations, placental biopsy with direct preparation of the chromosomes can identify the karyotype on the same day. Moreover, its additional advantages are exclusion and differentiation of anemia (reticulocyte count, detection of hemoglobinopathies, signs of hemolytic anemia), thrombocytopenia, leukemia, detection of liver dysfunction, and infectious diseases. In special cases, some biochemical tests and DNA analysis are also possible from fetal blood for various diseases such as infectious diseases, metabolic disorders, and congenital myotonic dystrophy. Measurement of umbilical venous pressure during fetal blood sampling may assess cardiac function and differentiate between cardiac and noncardiac causes of hydrops[431, 434]; nevertheless, noninvasive measurement of cardiac size and/or venous blood flow pattern show a good correlation to cardiac function and systemic central venous pressure.[197, 431, 435, 436]

Amniocentesis offers karyotyping, but amniocytes may also be used for biochemical tests and DNA analysis of infectious diseases, metabolic disorders, congenital myotonic dystrophy, and cystic fibrosis.

Chorionic villus sampling allows rapid karyotyping, DNA analysis of various diseases, particularly congenital myotonic dystrophy, hemoglobinopathies, and special investigations for metabolic storage disease (DNA analysis, microscopy, biochemical testing).

Cystic hygroma paracentesis of a large nuchal cystic hygroma is seldom performed for karyotyping from lymphocytes, but may be an alternative to chorionic villus and fetal blood sampling in these special cases, which are often associated with severe oligohydramnios.[437]

The first diagnosis of hydrops fetalis is established sonographically. A rapid increase in the abdominal circumference of the pregnant woman, preterm labor, maternal preeclampsia, vaginal bleeding, or a suspicious family history may be an indication for the sonographic examination, if no screening is performed. Many causes of hydrops such as sustained arrhythmias, tumors of the fetus, lung masses, skeletal dysplasia, or TTTS can often be detected during this first scan. Other typical pathologic findings like cystic nuchal hygroma indicating chromosomal disorders or rare syndromes may lead to further diagnostic procedures such as rapid karyotyping. Especially in the first and early second trimesters, hydrops or generalized skin edema indicates a chromosomal aberration or a rare syndrome with poor prognosis. Fetal hydrops caused by anemia prior to 16 weeks' gestation is a rare finding. It may occur in cases of homozygous α-thalassemia, which should be considered in people from Southeast Asia and, according to a few case reports, in parvoviral infection also. Furthermore, primary ultrasound has to define the exact distribution of the fluid accumulation, such as skin edema, ascites, uni- or bilateral pleural effusion, pericardial effusion, hydrops placentae, and amount of amniotic fluid. Furthermore, a semiquantification of these fluid accumulations is the basis for further monitoring and sometimes for prognostic assessment. A graduated classification as mild, moderate, or severe is helpful and can additionally be specified by measurements (e.g., of the prehepatic ascites [diameter of fluid between the abdominal wall and liver], of the diameter between the lung and lateral thoracic wall, of the systolic and diastolic diameters of pericardial effusion, of the parietal or frontal and abdominal skin thickness, of the placental thickness, and of the amniotic fluid index or maximal vertical amniotic fluid pocket). Presence and extent of mediastinal shifting and biventricular heart diameter should always be documented. The distribution of fluid accumulations may be helpful for the diagnosis of the underlying cause. In hydropic fetuses with anemia, tachyarrhythmia, and complete heart block, signs like ascites, skin edema, hydrops placentae, and polyhydramnios are usually present, but pleural effusion can be noted only in more advanced stages of the disease.[7, 78, 438–440] In other underlying diseases like alteration of lymphatic drainage and chromosomal anomalies, pleural effusion is predominant and other fluid accumulations are less often seen.[7]

If the first sonographic examination does not reveal the etiology of hydrops, a high-level ultrasound examination should immediately be arranged, including fetal echocardiography and Doppler examination of the arterial and venous vessels. On the one hand, this leads to the detection of anomalies causing hydrops that are difficult to diagnose with a usual scan; and on the other hand, anomalies like associated cardiac defects can be detected that can again lead to the diagnosis of a chromosomal aberration or a rare syndrome. The peripheral arterial and venous Doppler examination may reveal a high cardiac output by demonstration of increased blood flow velocities and/or a cardiac dysfunction with increased pulsatility of the venous Doppler indicating the primary disease.

Hydrops is a fetal emergency condition that requires fast diagnosis and therapy. Therefore, some noninvasive diagnostic procedures should always be directly initiated, even if an adequate sonographic examination is not possible. This includes antibody screening, Kleihauer-Betke test for fetal hemoglobin, and an infectious serology from maternal blood. In cases of associated anomalies or hydrops prior to 16 weeks' gestation, rapid karyotyping should be performed. Chorionic villus or fetal blood sampling should be the preferable invasive technique, as they rapidly offer a complete karyogram, in contrast to amniocentesis with FISH and PCR.

In cases of hydrops after 16 weeks' gestation where sonography does not reveal a causative disease, fetal blood sampling should be performed to exclude fetal anemia (e.g., due to parvovirus B19 infection or fetomaternal transfusion), which would make an urgent blood transfusion necessary. Additionally, many diagnostic procedures can be performed on the basis of fetal blood sampling, such as complete blood count, red cell differentiation, liver enzymes, specific IgM, and PCR for infectious diseases. In cases with evidence for α-thalassemia or a lysosomal storage disease or for a rare cause of fetal anemia, special diagnostic steps should be initiated. Furthermore, amniocentesis may be useful to exclude an infectious etiology of hydrops, especially by PCR-based detection of viral DNA in the amniotic fluid. In many circumstances, especially for the exclusion of an infectious cause of hydrops, it is justified to combine examinations for maternal and fetal blood as well as amniotic fluid.

Hydrops without evidence for anemia or other causes can be due to a spontaneous remission of anemia subsequent to a parvoviral infection and more rarely to fetomaternal transfusion or to fetal bleeding. In these cases, mild cardiomegaly, polyhydramnios, thickened placenta, and an increased number of reticulocytes and normoblasts in fetal blood may be demonstrated. As negative specific IgM and also negative parviviral B19 DNA in maternal blood do not completely exclude parvovirus B19 infection, an examination should also be performed in amniotic fluid and fetal blood including PCR, as well as specific IgM and PCR, respectively. Again, this cannot completely exclude an infection that happened more than 6 to 8 weeks previously. Alternatively, paroxysmal supraventricular tachycardia should always be taken into consideration. Diagnosis of paroxysmal tachyarrhythmia is best established by repeated sonographic heart rate monitoring or easier by long-term cardiotocography several times per day. The definitive diagnosis is confirmed by fetal echocardiography, which also enables the identification of the specific type of arrhythmia. Also in these cases, cardiomegaly, polyhydramnios, and hydrops placentae may be present. In some cases, increased pulsatility of venous Doppler flow velocity waveforms during the periods of sinus rhythm can be seen, indicating cardiac dysfunction due to repeated tachycardia.

Prognostic Parameters

The prognosis in cases of NIHF is crucially dependent on the etiology of hydrops (i.e., it is extremely poor in fetuses with chromosomal anomalies, lysosomal storage diseases, homozygous α-thalassemia, and structural cardiac defects as cause of hydrops). The most favorable prognosis is given in fetuses with tachyarrhythmia and parvovirus B19 infection, which can usually be successfully treated in utero. Furthermore, there is a significantly lower survival rate in fetuses with the presence of hydrops before 24 weeks' gestation.[13] This is mainly caused by the high percentage of fetuses with more severe abnormalities, especially chromosomal aberrations, in this group. The high percentage of survivors in the group with later onset of hydrops, however, include fetuses with successfully treated tachyarrhythmias.[13] In some diseases, even if treated in utero, the gestational age at the onset of detectable fluid accumulation is an important prognostic factor (e.g., in fetuses with primary or secondary hydrothorax associated with lung masses, which may critically disturb the development of lungs during the second trimester). Although the etiology of hydrops remains the most important factor for the prognosis, and the pattern of fluid distribution does not predict subsequent outcome,[439] the extent of interstitial fluid accumulation may indicate the progression of the alteration and, thus, the individual prognosis in a special group of the same underlying disease.[441] Relatively independent from the etiology, cardiomegaly usually indicates a distinct compromise of cardiac function and is correlated with a more unfavorable prognosis.[442] The documented correlation of pulsatile umbilical venous blood flow with poorer outcome is caused by a similar pathomechanism,[196, 435] which indicates a large increase of fetal venous pressure following cardiac dysfunction.[431, 434] An important exception is tachyarrhythmia, where pulsation in the umbilical venous blood flow is usually present during tachycardia even in fetuses without hydrops and excellent prognosis.[94-96] Therefore, prognosis is crucially dependent on the etiology of hydrops, which has to be identified for the adequate perinatal management, assessment of prognosis, and counseling of the parents.

Conclusion

In summary, hydrops fetalis in its various manifestations is easily detected by ultrasound (screening), but the enormous spectrum of etiologies and associations requires highly specialized knowledge in order to apply the noninvasive and invasive diagnostic and sometimes therapeutic steps in a systematic and effective way. Due to the time pressure that is often present with progressing severity of hydrops, NIHF is a situation in prenatal medicine where a good cooperation between screening investigators and specialized centers not only allows for a realistic assessment of the prognosis and subsequent proper counseling about recurrence risks, but can also often mean the difference between life and death for an affected child in utero.

REFERENCES

1. Holzgreve W: The fetus with nonimmune hydrops. *In* Harrison MR, Golbus MS, Filly RA (eds): The Unborn Patient. Prenatal Diagnosis and Treatment, 2nd ed. Philadelphia: WB Saunders Company, 1990, pp 228–245.
2. Macafee CA, Fortune DW, Beischer NA: Non-immunological hydrops fetalis. J Obstet Gynaecol Br Commonw 77:226–237, 1970.
3. Maidman JE, Yeager C, Anderson V, et al: Prenatal diagnosis and management of nonimmunological hydrops fetalis. Obstet Gynecol 56:571–576, 1980.
4. Hutchinson AA, Drew JE, Yu VYH, et al: Nonimmunologic hydrops fetalis: A review of 61 cases. Obstet Gynecol 59:347–352, 1982.
5. Snijders RJM, Holzgreve W, Cuckle H, Nicolaides KH: Maternal age-specific risks for trisomies at 9-14 weeks' gestation. Prenat Diagn 14:543–552, 1994.
6. McCoy MC, Katz VL, Gould, Kuller JA: Non-immune hydrops after 20 weeks' gestation: Review of 10 years' experience with suggestions for management. Obstet Gynecol 85:578–582, 1995.
7. Anandakumar C, Biswas A, Wong YC, et al: Management of non-immune hydrops: 8 years' experience. Ultrasound Obstet Gynecol 8:196–200, 1996.
8. Iskaros J, Jauniaux E, Rodeck C: Outcome of nonimmune hydrops fetalis diagnosed during the first half of pregnancy. Obstet Gynecol 90:321–325, 1997.
9. Jauniaux E: Diagnosis and management of early non-immune hydrops fetalis. Prenat Diagn 17:1261–1268, 1997.
10. Im SS, Rizos N, Joutsi P, et al: Nonimmunologic hydrops fetalis. Am J Obstet Gynecol 148:566–569, 1984.
11. Holzgreve W, Curry CJR, Golbus MS, et al: Investigation of nonimmune hydrops fetalis. Am J Obstet Gynecol 148:805–812, 1984.
12. Holzgreve W, Holzgreve B, Curry CJR: Nonimmune hydrops fetalis: Diagnosis and management. Semin Perinatol 9:52–67, 1985.
13. Hansmann M, Gembruch U, Bald R: New therapeutic aspects in nonimmune hydrops fetalis based on four hundred and two prenatally diagnosed cases. Fetal Ther 4:29–36, 1989.
14. Hansmann M, Gembruch U, Bald, R: Management of the fetus with nonimmune hydrops. *In* Harrison MR, Golbus MS, Filly RA (eds): The Unborn Patient. Prenatal Diagnosis and Treatment, 2nd ed. Philadelphia: WB Saunders Company, 1990, pp 246–248.
15. Machin GA: Hydrops revisited: Literature review of 1,414 cases published in the 1980s. Am J Med Genet 34:366–390, 1989.
16. Wafelman LS, Pollock BH, Kreutzer J, et al: Nonimmune hydrops fetalis: Fetal and neonatal outcome during 1983–1992. Biol Neonate 75:73–81, 1999.
17. Norton ME: Nonimmune hydrops fetalis. Semin Perinatol 18:321–332, 1994.
18. Jones DC: Nonimmune fetal hydrops: Diagnosis and obstetrical management. Semin Perinatol 19:447–461, 1995.
19. Forouzan I: Hydrops fetalis: Recent advances. Obstet Gynecol Surv 52:130–138, 1997.
20. Apkon M: Pathophysiology of hydrops fetalis. Semin Perinatol 19:437–446, 1995.
21. Anderson PAW, Kleinman CS, Lister G, Talner NS: Cardiovascular function during normal fetal and neonatal development and with hypoxic stress. *In* Polin RA, Fox WW (eds): Fetal and Neonatal Physiology, 2nd ed. Philadelphia: WB Saunders Company, 1998, pp 837–890.
22. Wu PYK: Colloid osmotic pressure and osmoregulation in the pregnant woman, fetus, and neonate. *In* Polin RA, Fox WW (eds):

Fetal and Neonatal Physiology, 2nd ed. Philadelphia: WB Saunders Company, 1998, pp 1721–1726.

23. Brace RA: Fluid distribution in the fetus and newborn. *In* Polin RA, Fox WW (eds): Fetal and Neonatal Physiology, 2nd ed. Philadelphia: WB Saunders Company, 1998, pp 1703–1713.

24. Brace RA, Christian JL: Transcapillary Starling pressure in the fetus, newborn, and pregnant adult. Am J Physiol 240:H843–H847, 1981.

25. Adamson SL, Whiteley KJ, Langille BL: Pulsatile pressure-flow relation and pulse-wave propagation in the umbilical circulation of fetal sheep. Circ Res 70:761–772, 1992.

26. Faber JJ, Anderson DF: Angiotensin mediated interaction of fetal kidney and placenta in the control of fetal arterial pressure and its role in hydrops fetalis. Placenta 18:313–326, 1997.

27. Powell TL, Brace RA: Elevated fetal plasma lactate produces polyhydramnios in sheep. Am J Obstet Gynecol 165:1595–1607, 1991.

28. Gest AL, Hansen TN, Moise AA, Hartley CJ: Atrial tachycardia causes hydrops in fetal lambs. Am J Physiol 258:H1159–H1163, 1990.

29. Gold PS, Brace RA: Fetal whole-body permeability-surface area product and reflection coefficient for plasma protein. Microvasc Res 36:262–274, 1988.

30. Brace RA, Gold PS: Fetal whole-body interstitial compliance, vascular compliance, and capillary filtration coefficient. Am J Physiol 247:R800–R805, 1984.

31. Brace RA: Effect of outflow pressure on fetal lymph flow. Am J Obstet Gynecol 160:494–497, 1989.

32. Gest AL: The effect of outflow pressure upon thoracic duct lymph flow rate in fetal sheep. Pediatr Res 32:585–588, 1992.

33. Nimrod C, Keane P, Harder J, et al: Atrial natriuretic peptide production in association with nonimmune fetal hydrops. Am J Obstet Gynecol 159:625–628, 1989.

34. Nageotte MP, Hurwitz SR, Kaupke CJ, et al: Atriopeptin in the twin-to-twin transfusion syndrome. Obstet Gynecol 73:867–870, 1989.

35. Ville Y, Proudler A, Abbas A, Nicolaides K: Atrial natriuretic factor concentration in normal, growth retarded, anemic, and hydropic fetuses. Am J Obstet Gynecol 171:777–783, 1994.

36. Ville Y, Proudler A, Kuhn P, Nicolaides KH: Aldosterone concentration in normal, growth retarded, anemic, and hydropic fetuses. Obstet Gynecol 84:511–514, 1994.

37. Faber JJ, Anderson DF: Angiotensin mediated interaction of fetal kidney and placenta in the control of fetal arterial pressure and its role in hydrops fetalis. Placenta 18:313–326, 1997.

38. Kessel I, Makhoul IR, Sujov P: Congenital hypothyroidism and nonimmune hydrops fetalis: Associated? Pediatrics 103:E9, 1999.

39. Knilans TK: Cardiac abnormalities associated with hydrops fetalis. Semin Perinatol 19:483–492, 1995.

40. McFadden DE, Taylor GP: Cardiac abnormalities and nonimmune hydrops fetalis: A coincidental, not causal, relationship. Pediatr Pathol 9:11–17, 1989.

41. Gembruch U, Hansmann M, Redel DA, et al: Fetal complete heart block: Antenatal diagnosis, significance and management. Eur J Obstet Gynecol Reprod Biol 31:9–22, 1989.

42. Gembruch U, Knöpfle G, Chatterjee M, et al: First trimester diagnosis of congenital heart disease by transvaginal two-dimensional and Doppler echocardiography. Obstet Gynecol 75:496–498, 1990.

43. Gembruch U, Knöpfle G, Chatterjee M, et al: Prenatal diagnosis of atrioventricular canal malformation using up-to-date echocardiographic technology (a report of 14 cases). Am Heart J 121:1489–1497, 1991.

44. Hornberger LK, Sahn DJ, Kleinman CS, et al: Tricuspid valve disease with significant tricuspid insufficiency in the fetus: Diagnosis and outcome. J Am Coll Cardiol 17:167–173, 1991.

45. Lang D, Oberhoffer R, Cook A, et al: The pathological spectrum of malformations of the tricuspid valve in pre- and neonatal life. J Am Coll Cardiol 17:1161–1167, 1991.

46. Ettedgui JA, Sharland GK, Chita SK, et al: Absent pulmonary valve syndrome with ventricular septal defect: Role of the arterial duct. Am J Cardiol 66:233–234, 1990.

47. Persutte WH, Yeasting RA, Lenke RR, Levine MM: Prenatal ultrasonographic appearance of "agenesis" of the ductus arteriosus

and pulmonic valve hypoplasia. A case report and review of the embryogenesis. J Ultrasound Med 9:541–545, 1990.

48. Liang CC, Tsai CC, Hsieh CC, et al: Prenatal diagnosis of tetralogy of Fallot with absent pulmonary valve accompanied by hydrops fetalis. Gynecol Obstet Invest 44:61–63, 1997.

49. Huhta JC: The fetal ductus arteriosus. *In* Copel JA, Reed KL (eds): Doppler Ultrasound in Obstetrics and Gynecology. New York: Raven Press, 1994, pp 325–331.

50. Hofstadler G, Tulzer G, Altmann R, et al: Spontaneous closure of the human fetal ductus arteriosus—a cause of fetal congestive heart failure. Am J Obstet Gynecol 174:879–883, 1996.

51. Leal SD, Cavalle-Garrido T, Rynan G, et al: Isolated ductal closure in utero diagnosed by fetal echocardiography. Am J Perinatol 14:205–210, 1997.

52. Tulzer G, Gudmundsson S, Tewes G, et al: Incidence of indomethacin-induced human fetal ductal constriction. J Matern Fetal Invest 1:267–269, 1992.

53. Moise KJ: Effect of advancing gestational age on the frequency of fetal ductal constriction in association with maternal indomethacin use. Am J Obstet Gynecol 168:1350–1353, 1993.

54. Gembruch U, Chatterjee M, Bald R, et al: Prenatal diagnosis of aortic atresia by colour Doppler flow mapping. Prenat Diagn 10:211–217, 1990.

55. Bharati S, Patel AG, Varga P, et al: In utero echocardiographic diagnosis of premature closure of the foramen ovale with mitral regurgitation and large left atrium. Am Heart J 122:597–600, 1991.

56. Bitar F, Byrum CJ, Kveseli DA, et al: In utero management of hydrops fetalis caused by critical aortic stenosis. Am J Perinatol 14:389–391, 1997.

57. Redel DA, Hansmann M: Fetal obstruction of the foramen ovale detected by two-dimensional Doppler echocardiography. *In* Rijsterbourgh H (ed): Echocardiography. The Hague: Martinus Nijhoff Publishers 1981, pp 425–429.

58. Pesonen E, Haavisto H, Ammala P, Teramo K: Intrauterine hydrops caused by premature closure of the foramen ovale. Arch Dis Child 58:1015–1016, 1983.

59. Buis-Liem TN, Ottenkamp J, Meerman RH, Verwey R: The occurrence of fetal supraventricular tachycardia and obstruction of the foramen ovale. Prenat Diagn 7:425–431, 1987.

60. Phillipos EZ, Robertson MA, Still DK: Prenatal detection of foramen ovale obstruction without hydrops fetalis. J Am Coll Echocardiogr 3:342–344, 1990.

61. Benirschke K, Swartz WH, Leopold G, Sahn D: Hydrops due to myocarditis in a fetus. Am J Cardiovasc Pathol 1:131–133, 1987.

62. Atkin J, Snow JW, Zellweger H, Rhead WJ: Fatal infantile cardiac glycogenosis without acid maltase deficiency presenting as congenital hydrops [letter]. Eur J Pediatr 142:150, 1984.

63. Schmidt KG, Birk E, Silverman NH, Scagnelli SA: Echocardiographic evaluation of dilated cardiomyopathy in the human fetus. Am J Cardiol 63:599–605, 1989.

64. Steenhout P, Elmer C, Clercx A, et al: Carnitine deficiency with cardiomyopathy presenting as neonatal hydrops: Successful response to carnitine therapy. J Inherit Metab Dis 13:69–75, 1990.

65. Patel CR, Judge NE, Muise KL, Levine MM: Prenatal myocardial infarction suspected by fetal echocardiography. J Am Soc Echocardiogr 9:721–723, 1996.

66. Calhoun BC, Watson PT, Hegge F: Ultrasound diagnosis of an obstructive cardiac rhabdomyoma with severe hydrops fetalis and hypoplastic lungs. J Reprod Med 36:317–319, 1991.

67. Groves AM, Fagg NL, Cook AC, Allan LD: Cardiac tumours in intrauterine life. Arch Dis Child 67:1189–1192, 1992.

68. Holley DG, Martin GR, Brenner JI, et al: Diagnosis and management of fetal cardiac tumors: A multicenter experience and review of published reports. J Am Coll Cardiol 26:516–520, 1995.

69. Beghetti M, Gow RM, Haney I, et al: Pediatric primary benign cardiac tumors. A 15-year review. Am Heart J 134:1107–1114, 1997.

70. Sonigo P, Elmaleh A, Fermont L, et al: Prenatal MRI diagnosis of fetal cerebral tuberous sclerosis. Pediatr Radiol 26:1–4, 1996.

71. Platt LD, Geierman CA, Turkel SB, et al: Atrial hemangioma and hydrops fetalis. Am J Obstet Gynecol 141:107–109, 1981.

72. Wedemeyer AL, Breitfeld V: Cardiac neoplasm, tachyarrhythmia, and anasarca in an infant. Am J Dis Child 129:738–741, 1975.

73. Rheuban KS, McDaniel NL, Feldman PS, et al: Intrapericardial teratoma causing nonimmune hydrops fetalis and pericardial tamponade: A case report. Pediatr Cardiol 12:54–56, 1991.

74. Perez-Aytes A, Sanchis N, Barbal A, et al: Nonimmunological hydrops fetalis and intrapericardial teratoma: Case report and review. Prenat Diagn 15:859–863, 1995.
75. Bruch SW, Adzik NS, Reiss R, Harrison MR: Prenatal therapy of pericardial teratomas. J Pediatr Surg 32:1113–1115, 1997.
76. Riskin-Mashiah S, Moise KJ Jr, Wilkins I, et al: In utero diagnosis of intrapericardial teratoma: A case for in utero open fetal surgery. Prenat Diagn 18:1328–1330, 1998.
77. Gembruch U, Hansmann M, Bald R: Fetales Vorhofflattern bei komplettem atrioventrikulärem Kanal und Trisomie 18. Geburtsh Frauenheilk 48:445–447, 1988.
78. Gembruch U, Redel DA, Bald R, Hansmann M: Longitudinal study in 18 cases of fetal supraventricular tachycardia: Doppler-echocardiographic findings and pathophysiological implications. Am Heart J 125:1290–1301, 1993.
79. Naheed ZJ, Strasburger JF, Deal BJ, et al: Fetal tachycardia: Mechanisms and predictors of hydrops fetalis. J Am Coll Cardiol 27:1736–1740, 1996.
80. Crum AK, Lenington W, Jeanty P: Idiopathic infantile arterial calcification. Fetus 2:74781–74786, 1992.
81. Juul S, Ledbetter D, Wight TN, Woodrum D: New insights into idiopathic infantile arterial calcinosis. Am J Dis Child 144:229–233, 1990.
82. Lopes LM, Cha SC, Scanavacca MI, et al: Fetal idiopathic ventricular tachycardia with nonimmune hydrops: Benign course. Pediatr Cardiol 17:192–193, 1996.
83. Kleinman CS, Copel JA, Weinstein EM, et al: Treatment of fetal supraventricular tachyarrhythmias. J Clin Ultrasound 13:265–273, 1985.
84. Kleinman CS, Copel JA: Electrophysiological principles and fetal antiarrhythmic therapy. Ultrasound Obstet Gynecol 1:286–297, 1991.
85. Ko JK, Deal BJ, Strasburger JF, et al: Supraventricular tachycardia mechanisms and their age distribution in pediatric patients. Am J Cardiol 69:1028–1032, 1992.
86. Gest AL, Bair DK, Vander Straten MC: Thoracic duct lymph flow in fetal sheep with increased venous pressure from electrically induced tachycardia. Biol Neonate 64:325–330, 1993.
87. Nimrod C, Davies D, Harder J, et al: Ultrasound evaluation of tachycardia-induced hydrops in the fetal lamb. Am J Obstet Gynecol 157:655–659, 1987.
88. Stevens DC, Hilliard JK, Schreiner RL, et al: Supraventricular tachycardia with edema, ascites, and hydrops in fetal sheep. Am J Obstet Gynecol 142:316–322, 1982.
89. Gest AL, Martin CG, Moise AA, Hansen TN: Reversal of venous blood flow with atrial tachycardia and hydrops in fetal sheep. Pediatr Res 28:223–226, 1990.
90. Spinale FG, Holzgrefe HH, Mukherjee R, et al: LV and myocyte structure and function after early recovery from tachycardia-induced cardiomyopathy. Am J Physiol 268:H836–H847, 1995.
91. Packer DL, Bardy GH, Worley SJ, et al: Tachycardia-induced cardiomyopathy: A reversible form of left ventricular dysfunction. Am J Cardiol 57:563–570, 1986.
92. Spinale FG, Tanaka R, Crawford FA, Zile MR: Changes in myocardial blood flow during development of and recovery from tachycardia-induced cardiomyopathy. Circulation 85:717–729, 1992.
93. Tomita M, Spinale FG, Crawford FA, Zile MR: Changes in left ventricular volume, mass, and function during the development and regression of supraventricular tachycardia-induced cardiomyopathy: Disparity between recovery of systolic versus diastolic function. Circulation 83:635–642, 1991.
94. Gembruch U, Krapp M, Baumann P: Changes of venous blood flow velocity waveforms in fetuses with supraventricular tachycardia. Ultrasound Obstet Gynecol 5:394–399, 1995.
95. Krapp M, Gembruch U, Baumann P: Venous blood flow pattern suggesting tachycardia-induced "cardiomyopathy" in the fetus. Ultrasound Obstet Gynecol 10:32–40, 1997.
96. Gembruch U, Krapp M, Germer U, Baumann P: Venous Doppler in the sonographic surveillance of fetuses with supraventricular tachycardia. Eur J Obstet Gynecol Reprod Biol 84:187–192, 1999.
97. Schmidt KG, Ulmer HE, Silverman N, et al: Perinatal outcome of fetal complete atrioventricular block: A multicenter experience. J Am Coll Cardiol 17:1360–1366, 1991.
98. Baschat AA, Gembruch U, Knöpfle G, Hansmann M: First trimester fetal heart block: A marker for cardiac anomaly. Ultrasound Obstet Gynecol 14:311–314, 1999.
99. Groves AMM, Allan LD, Rosenthal E: Outcome of isolated congenital complete heart block diagnosed in utero. Heart 75:190–194, 1996.
100. Richards DS, Wagman AJ, Cabaniss ML: Ascites not due to congestive heart failure in a fetus with lupus-induced heart block. Obstet Gynecol 76:957–959, 1990.
101. Copel JA, Buyon JP, Kleinman CS: Successful in utero therapy of fetal heart block. Am J Obstet Gynecol 173:1384–1390, 1995.
102. Hansmann M, Gembruch U, Bald R, et al: Fetal tachyarrhythmias: Transplacental and direct treatment of the fetus—a report of sixty fetuses. Ultrasound Obstet Gynecol 1:162–170, 1991.
103. Van Engelen AD, Weijtens O, Brenner JI, et al: Management, outcome and follow-up of fetal tachycardia. J Am Coll Cardiol 24:1371–1375, 1994.
104. Simpson JM, Sharland GK: Fetal tachycardias: Management and outcome of 127 consecutive cases. Heart 79:576–581, 1998.
105. Jaeggi E, Fouron JC, Drblik SP: Fetal atrial flutter: Diagnosis, clinical features, treatment, and outcome. J Pediatr 132:336–339, 1998.
106. Gembruch U, Hansmann M, Redel DA, Bald R: Intrauterine therapy of fetal tachyarrhythmias: Intraperitoneal administration of antiarrhythmic drugs to the fetus in fetal tachyarrhythmias with severe hydrops fetalis. J Perinat Med 16:39–44, 1988.
107. Gembruch U, Manz M, Bald R, et al: Repeated intravascular treatment with amiodarone in a fetus with refractory supraventricular tachycardia and hydrops fetalis. Am Heart J 118:1335–1338, 1989.
108. Groves AM, Allan LD, Rosenthal E: Therapeutical trial of sympathomimetics in three cases of complete heart block in the fetus. Circulation 15:3394–3396, 1995.
109. Harris JP, Alexson CG, Manning JA, Thompson HO: Medical therapy for the hydropic fetus with congenital complete atrioventricular block. Am J Perinatol 10:217–219, 1993.
110. Anandakumar C, Biswas A, Chew SSL, et al: Direct fetal therapy for hydrops secondary to congenital atrioventricular heart block. Obstet Gynecol 87:835–837, 1996.
111. Carpenter RJ, Strasburger JF, Garson A, et al: Fetal ventricular pacing for hydrops secondary to complete heart block. J Am Coll Cardiol 8:1434–1436, 1986.
112. Walkinshaw SA, Welch CR, McCormack J, Walsh K: In utero pacing for fetal congenital heart block. Fetal Diagn Ther 9:183–185, 1994.
113. Aubard Y, Derouineau I, Aubard V, et al: Primary fetal hydrothorax: A literature review and proposed antenatal clinical strategy. Fetal Diagn Ther 13:325–333, 1998.
114. Rice HE, Estes JM, Hedrick NH, et al: Congenital adenomatoid malformation of the lung: A sheep model of fetal hydrops. J Pediatr Surg 29:692–696, 1994.
115. Barret J, Chitayat D, Sermer M, et al: The prognostic factors in the prenatal diagnosis of the echogenic fetal lung. Prenat Diagn 15:849–853, 1995.
116. Adzik NS, Harrison MR, Crombleholme TM, et al: Fetal lung lesions: Management and outcome. Am J Obstet Gynecol 179:884–889, 1998.
117. Silva da O, Ramanan R, Romano W, et al: Nonimmune hydrops fetalis, pulmonary sequestration, and favorable neonatal outcome. Obstet Gynecol 88:681–683, 1996.
118. Rosado-de-Christenson ML, Stocker JT: Congenital cystic adenomatoid malformation. Radiographics 11:865–886, 1991.
119. Thorpe-Beeston JG, Nicolaides KH: Cystic adenomatoid malformation of the lung: Prenatal diagnosis and outcome. Prenat Diagn 14:677–688, 1994.
120. Sullivan KM, Adzick NS: Fetal surgery. Clin Obstet Gynecol 37:355–371, 1994.
121. Dommergues M, Louis-Sylvestre C, Mandelbrot L, et al: Congenital adenomatoid malformation of the lung: When is active fetal therapy indicated. Am J Obstet Gynecol 177:953–958, 1997.
122. Morrow R, Macphail S, Johnson J, et al: Midtrimester thoracoamniotic shunting for the treatment of fetal hydrops. Fetal Diagn Ther 10:92–94, 1995.
123. Benacerraf BR, Frigoletto FD Jr: In utero treatment of a fetus with diaphragmatic hernia complicated by hydrops. Am J Obstet Gynecol 155:817–818, 1986.
124. Martinez Ferro M, Milner R, Voto L, et al: Intrathoracic alimentary tract duplication cysts treated in utero by thoracoamniotic shunting. Fetal Diagn Ther 13:343–347, 1998.

125. Liechty KW, Crombleholme TM, Quinn TM, et al: Elevated platelet-derived growth factor-B in congenital cystic adenomatoid malformations requiring fetal resection. J Pediatr Surg 34:805–809, 1999.

126. Valcamonico A, Goncalves LF, Jeanty P: Larynx, atresia. Fetus 2:7483–7489, 1992.

127. DeCou JM, Jones DC, Jacobs HD, Touloukian RJ: Successful ex utero intrapartum treatment (EXIT) procedure for congenital high airway obstruction syndrome (CHAOS) owing to laryngeal atresia. J Pediatr Surg 33:1563–1565, 1998.

128. Fryns JP, van Schoubroeck D, Vandenberghe K, et al: Diagnostic echographic findings in cryptophthalmos syndrome (Fraser syndrome). Prenat Diagn 17:582–584, 1997.

129. Blisard KS, Barlow SA: Neonatal hemochromatosis. Hum Pathol 17:646–648, 1986.

130. Wisser J, Schreiner M, Diem H, Roithmeier A: Neonatal hemochromatosis: A rare cause of nonimmune hydrops fetalis and fetal anemia. Fetal Diagn Ther 8:273–278, 1993.

131. Knisely AS: Neonatal hemochromatosis: A rare cause of nonimmune hydrops fetalis and fetal anemia [comment]. Fetal Diagn Ther 10:139–140, 1995.

132. Kassem E, Dolfin T, Litmanowitz I, et al: Familial perinatal hemochromatosis: A disease that causes recurrent non-immune hydrops. J Perinat Med 27:122–127, 1999.

133. Pletcher BA, Williams MK, Mulivor RA, et al: Intrauterine cytomegalovirus infection presenting as fetal meconium peritonitis. Obstet Gynecol 78:903–905, 1991.

134. Leikin E, Lysikiewicz A, Garry D, Tejani N: Intrauterine transmission of hepatitis A virus. Obstet Gynecol 88:690–691, 1996.

135. Schild RL, Plath H, Thomas P, et al: Fetal parvovirus B19 infection and meconium peritonitis. Fetal Diagn Ther 13:15–18, 1998.

136. McDuffie RS Jr, Bader T: Fetal meconium peritonitis after maternal hepatitis A. Am J Obstet Gynecol 180:1031–1032, 1999.

137. Seward JF, Zusman J: Hydrops fetalis associated with small-bowel volvulus [letter]. Lancet ii:52–53, 1978.

138. Witter FR, Molteni RA: Intrauterine intestinal volvulus with hemoperitoneum presenting as fetal distress at 34 weeks' gestation. Am J Obstet Gynecol 155:1080–1081, 1986.

139. Decoret E, Sibony O, Vuillard E, et al: Prenatal diagnosis of in utero fetal gastrointestinal bleeding. Fetal Diagn Ther 9:252–255, 1994.

140. Rijhsinghani A, Smith D: Self-limiting nonimmune hydrops and acute small bowel distention following maternal trauma. Obstet Gynecol 90:700–701, 1997.

141. Störmann J, Kuwertz-Bröking E, Fründ S, et al: Ergebnisse der pränatalen Diagnostik bei 62 Feten mit obstuktiver Uropathie. Eine retrospektive Analyse. Monatsschr Kinderheilk 144:204–230, 1996.

142. Suren A, Grone HJ, Kallerhoff M, et al: Prenatal diagnosis of congenital nephrosis of the Finnish type (CNF) in the second trimester. Int J Gynaecol Obstet 41:165–170, 1993.

143. Kim CK, Kim SK, Yang YH, et al: A case of recurrent infantile polycystic kidney associated with hydrops fetalis. Yonsei Med J 30:95–103, 1989.

144. Zerres K, Hansmann M, Mallmann R, Gembruch U: Autosomal recessive polycystic kidney disease. Problems of prenatal diagnosis. Prenat Diagn 8:215–229, 1988.

145. Geipel A, Germer U, Gortner L, et al: McKusick-Kaufman syndrome: Prenatal diagnosis and clinical management. Prenat Neonat Med 3:269–273, 1998.

146. Straub W, Zarabi M, Mazer J: Fetal ascites associated with Conradi's disease (chondrodysplasia punctata): Report of a case. J Clin Ultrasound 11:234–236, 1983.

147. Al-Tawil KI, Ahmed GS, Al-Hathal MM, Al-Zuwayed MA: Sporadic congenital infantile cortical hyperostosis (Caffey's disease). Am J Perinatol 15:629–633, 1998.

148. Perez del Rio MJ, Fernandez-Toral J, Madrigal B, et al: Two new cases of Cumming syndrome confirming autosomal recessive inheritance. Am J Med Genet 12:340–343, 1999.

149. Holzgreve W, Mahoney BS, Glick PL, et al: Sonographic demonstration of sacrococcygeal teratoma. Prenat Diagn 5:245–257, 1985.

150. Weinraub Z, Gembruch U, Födisch HJ, Hansmann M: Intrauterine mediastinal teratoma associated with non-immune hydrops fetalis. Prenat Diagn 9:368–372, 1989.

151. Sherer DM, Abramowicz JS, Eggers PC, et al: Prenatal ultrasonographic diagnosis of intracranial teratoma and massive craniomegaly with associated high-output cardiac failure. Am J Obstet Gynecol 168:97–99, 1993.

152. Sherer DM, Onyeije CI: Prenatal ultrasonographic diagnosis of fetal intracranial tumors: A review. Am J Perinat 15:319–328, 1998.

153. Kuller JA, Laifer SA, Martin JG, et al: Unusual presentation of fetal teratoma. J Perinatol 11:294–296, 1991.

154. Cyr DR, Guntheroth WG, Nyberg DA, et al: Prenatal diagnosis of an intrapericardial teratoma: A cause for nonimmune hydrops. J Ultrasound Med 7:87–90, 1988.

155. Holterman A-X, Filiatrault D, Lallier M, Youssef S: The natural history of sacrococcygeal teratomas diagnosed through routine obstetric sonogram: A single institution experience. J Pediatr Surg 33:899–903, 1998.

156. Graf JL, Housley T, Albanese CT, et al: A surprising histological evolution of preterm sacrococcygeal teratoma. J Pediatr Surg 33:177–179, 1998.

157. Navajas A, Astigarraga I, Fernandez-Teijeiro A, et al: Hydrops fetalis and fibrosarcoma: Case report of an uncommon association. Eur J Pediatr 156:62–64, 1997.

158. Van der Slikke JW, Balk AG: Hydramnios with hydrops fetalis and disseminated fetal neuroblastoma. Obstet Gynecol 55:250–253, 1980.

159. Jennings RW, LaQuaglia MP, Leong K, et al: Fetal neuroblastoma: Prenatal diagnosis and natural history. J Pediatr Surg 28:1168–1174, 1993.

160. Lynn AAA, Parry SI, Morgan MA, Mennuti MT: Disseminated congenital neuroblastoma involving the placenta. Arch Pathol Lab Med 121:741–744, 1997.

161. Bessho T, Kubota S, Ohtsuka Y, et al: Prenatally detected hepatic hamartoma: Another cause of non-immune hydrops. Prenat Diagn 16:337–341, 1996.

162. Dickinson JE, Knowles S, Phillips JM: Prenatal diagnosis of hepatic mesenchymal hamartoma. Prenat Diagn 19:81–84, 1999.

163. Kazzi NJ, Chang C, Roberts EC, Shankaran S: Fetal hepatoblastoma presenting as nonimmune hydrops. Am J Perinatol 6:278–280, 1989.

164. Liu Y, Mai Y, Chang C, et al: The presence of hydrops fetalis in a fetus with congenital mesoblastic nephroma. Prenat Diagn 16:363–365, 1996.

165. Wu TJ, Teng RJ: Diffuse neonatal haemangiomatosis with intrauterine haemorrhage and hydrops fetalis. A case report. Eur J Pediatr 153:759–761, 1994.

166. Drut R, Sapia S, Gril D, et al: Nonimmune hydrops fetalis, hydramnios, microcephaly, and intracranial meningeal hemangioepithelioma. Pediatr Pathol 13:9–13, 1993.

167. Seifer DB, Ferguson JE 2d, Behrens CM, et al: Nonimmune hydrops fetalis in association with hemangioma of the umbilical cord. Obstet Gynecol 66:283–286, 1985.

168. Carles D, Maugey-Laulom B, Roux D, et al: Lethal hydrops fetalis secondary to an umbilical cord hemangioma. Ann Pathol 14:244–247, 1994.

169. Jones CE, Rivers RP, Taghizadeh A: Disseminated intravascular coagulation and fetal hydrops in a newborn infant in association with a chorangioma of placenta. Pediatrics 50:901–907, 1972.

170. D'Ercole C, Cravello L, Boubli L, et al: Large chorioangioma associated with hydrops fetalis: Prenatal diagnosis and management. Fetal Diagn Ther 11:357–360, 1996.

171. Horigome H, Hamada H, Sohda S, et al: Large placental chorioangiomas as a cause of cardiac failure in two fetuses. Fetal Diagn Ther 12:241–243, 1997.

172. Anai T, Miyakawa I, Ohki H, Ogawa T: Hydrops fetalis caused by fetal Kasabach-Merritt syndrome. Acta Paediatr Jpn 34:324–327, 1992.

173. Gonen R, Fong K, Chiasson DA: Prenatal sonographic diagnosis of hepatic hemangioendothelioma with secondary nonimmune hydrops fetalis. Obstet Gynecol 73:485–487, 1989.

174. Skopec LL, Lakatua DJ: Non-immune fetal hydrops with hepatic hemangiothelioma and Kasabach-Merritt syndrome: A case report. Pediatr Pathol 9:87–93, 1989.

175. Albano G, Pugliese A, Stabile M, et al: Hydrops foetalis caused by hepatic haemangioma. Acta Paediatr 87:1307–1309, 1998.

176. Sharara FI, Khoury AN: Prenatal diagnosis of a giant cavernous hemangioma in association with nonimmune hydrops. A case report. J Reprod Med 39:547–549, 1994.

177. Nakamura Y, Komatsu Y, Yano H, et al: Nonimmunologic hydrops fetalis: A clinicopathological study of 50 autopsy cases. Pediatr Pathol 7:19–30, 1989.

178. Mor Z, Schreyer P, Weinraub Z, et al: Nonimmune hydrops fetalis associated with angioosteohypertrophy (Klippel-Trenaunay) syndrome. Am J Obstet Gynecol 159:1185–1186, 1988.

179. Sheu BC, Shyu MK, Lin YF, et al: Prenatal diagnosis and corticosteroid treatment of diffuse neonatal hemangiomatosis; case report. J Ultrasound Med 13:495–499, 1994.

180. Mejides AA, Adra AM, O'Sullivan MJ, Nicholas MC: Prenatal diagnosis and therapy for a fetal hepatic vascular malformation. Obstet Gynecol 85:850–853, 1995.

181. Ordorica SA, Marks F, Frieden FJ, et al: Aneurysm of the vein of Galen: A new cause for Ballantyne syndrome. Am J Obstet Gynecol 162:1166–1167, 1990.

182. Sepulveda W, Platt CC, Fisk NM: Prenatal diagnosis of cerebral arteriovenous malformation using color Doppler ultrasonography: Case report and review of the literature. Ultrasound Obstet Gynecol 6:282–286, 1995.

183. McElhinneey DB, Halbach VV, Silverman NH, et al: Congenital cardiac anomalies with vein of Galen malformations in infants. Arch Dis Child 78:548–551, 1998.

184. Moore L, Toi A, Chitayat D: Abnormalities of the intra-abdominal fetal umbilical vein: Reports of four cases and a review of the literature. Ultrasound Obstet Gynecol 7:21–25, 1996.

185. Jörgensen C, Andolf E: Four cases of absent ductus venosus: Three in combination with severe hydrops fetalis. Fetal Diagn Ther 9:395–397, 1994.

186. Sivén M, Ley D, Hägerstrand I, Svenningsen N: Agenesis of the ductus venosus and its correlation to hydrops fetalis and fetal hepatic circulation: Case reports and review of the literature. Pediatr Pathol Lab Med 15:39–50, 1995.

187. Gembruch U, Baschat AA, Caliebe A, Gortner L: Prenatal diagnosis of ductus venosus agenesis: A report of two cases and review of the literature. Ultrasound Obstet Gynecol 11:185–189, 1998.

188. Benatar A, Vaughan J, Nicolini U, et al: Prenatal pericardiocentesis: Its role in the management of intrapericardial teratoma. Obstet Gynecol 79:856–859, 1992.

189. Sklansky M, Greenberg M, Lucas V, Gruslin-Giroux A: Intrapericardial teratoma in a twin fetus: Diagnosis and management. Obstet Gynecol 89:807–809, 1997.

190. Suzuki N, Tsuchida Y, Takahashi A, et al: Prenatally diagnosed cystic lymphangioma in infants. J Pediatr Surg 33:1599–1604, 1998.

191. Gembruch U, Hansmann M, Bald R, et al: Prenatal diagnosis and management in fetuses with cystic hygromata colli. Eur J Obstet Gynecol Reprod Biol 29:241–255, 1988.

192. Fumia FD, Edelstone DI, Holzman IR: Blood flow and oxygen delivery to fetal organs as functions of fetal hematocrit. Am J Obstet Gynecol 150:274–282, 1984.

193. Blair DK, Vander Straten MC, Gest AL: Hydrops in fetal sheep from rapid induction of anemia. Pediatr Res 35:560–564, 1994.

194. Weiner CP, Pelzer GD, Heilskov J, et al: The effect of intravascular transfusion on umbilical venous pressure in anemic fetuses with and without hydrops. Am J Obstet Gynecol 161:1498–1501, 1989.

195. Hecher K, Snijders R, Campbell S, Nicolaides K: Fetal venous, arterial, and intracardiac blood flows in red blood cell isoimmunization. Obstet Gynecol 85:122–128, 1995.

196. Tulzer G, Gudmundsson S, Wood DC, et al: Doppler in nonimmune hydrops fetalis. Ultrasound Obstet Gynecol 4:279–283, 1994.

197. Hecher K, Campbell S: Characteristics of fetal venous blood flow under normal circumstances and during fetal disease. Ultrasound Obstet Gynecol 7:68–83, 1996.

198. Brace RA: Fetal blood volume responses to acute fetal hemorrhage. Circ Res 52:730–734, 1983.

199. Brace RA: Mechanisms of fetal blood volume restoration after slow fetal hemorrhage. Am J Physiol 256:R1040–R1043, 1989.

200. Arcasoy MO, Gallagher PG: Hematologic disorders and nonimmune hydrops fetalis. Semin Perinatol 19:502–515, 1995.

201. Old J: Hemoglobinopathies. Prenat Diagn 16:1181–1186, 1996.

202. Chan V, Chan WY, Tang M, et al: Molecular defects in Hb H hydrops fetalis. Br J Haematol 96:224–228, 1997.

203. Chui D, Waye S: Hydrops fetalis caused by α-thalassemia: An emerging health care problem. Blood 91:2213–2222, 1998.

204. Ko TM, Tseng LH, Hsu PM, et al: Ultrasonographic scanning of placental thickness and the prenatal diagnosis of homozygous alpha-thalassemia 1 in the second trimester. Prenat Diagn 15:7–10, 1995.

205. Tongsong T, Wanapirak C, Srisomboon J, et al: Antenatal sonographic features of 100 alpha-thalassemia hydrops fetalis fetuses. J Clin Ultrasound 24:73–77, 1996.

206. Lam YH, Ghosh A, Tang M, et al: Second trimester hydrops fetalis in pregnancies affected by homozygous α-thalassaemia-1. Prenat Diagn 17:267–269, 1997.

207. Lam YH, Tang M: Prenatal diagnosis of haemoglobin Bart's disease by cordocentesis at 12–14 weeks' gestation. Prenat Diagn 17:501–504, 1997.

208. Lam YH, Tang MHY, Lee CP, Tse HY: Prenatal ultrasonographic prediction of homozygous type 1 α-thalassemia at 12 to 13 weeks of gestation. Am J Obstet Gynecol 180:148–150, 1999.

209. Lam YH, Tang MH, Lee CP, Tse HY: Cardiac blood flow studies in fetuses with homozygous alpha-thalassemia-1 at 12–13 weeks of gestation. Ultrasound Obstet Gynecol 13:48–51, 1999.

210. Lam YH, Tang MH, Lee CP, Tse HY: Nuchal translucency in fetuses affected by homozygous alpha-thalassemia-1 at 12–13 weeks of gestation. Ultrasound Obstet Gynecol 13:238–240, 1999.

211. Yong KN, Wadsworth D, Langlois S, et al: Thalassemia carrier screening and prenatal diagnosis among the British Columbia (Canada) population of Chinese descent. Clin Genet 55:20–25, 1999.

212. Cheung MC, Goldberg JD, Kan YW: Prenatal diagnosis of sickle cell anemia and α-thalassemia by analysis of fetal cells in maternal blood. Nat Genet 14:264–268, 1996.

213. Carr S, Rubin L, Dixon D, et al: Intrauterine therapy for homozygous α-thalassemia. Obstet Gynecol 85:876–879, 1995.

214. Fung TY, Kin LT, Kong LC, Keung LC: Homozygous alpha-thalassemia associated with hypospadias in three survivors. Am J Med Genet 29:225–227, 1999.

215. Ng PC, Fok TF, Lee CH, et al: Is homozygous alpha-thalassaemia a lethal condition in the 1990s? Acta Paediatr 87:1197–1199, 1998.

216. Hayward A, Ambruso D, Battaglia F, et al: Microchimerism and tolerance following intrauterine transplantation and transfusion for α-thalassemia-1. Fetal Diagn Ther 13:8–14, 1998.

217. Hennekam RC, Beemer FA, Cats BP, et al: Hydrops fetalis associated with red cell pyruvate kinase deficiency. Genet Couns 1:75–79, 1990.

218. Gilsanz F, Vega MA, Gomez-Castillo E, et al: Fetal anaemia due to pyruvate kinase deficiency. Arch Dis Child 69:523–524, 1993.

219. Ravindranath Y, Paglia DE, Warrier I, et al: Glucose phosphate isomerase deficiency as a cause of hydrops fetalis. N Engl J Med 31:258–261, 1987.

220. Perkins RP: Hydrops fetalis and stillbirth in a male glucose-6-phosphate dehydrogenase-deficient fetus possibly due to maternal ingestion of sulfisoxazole; a case report. Am J Obstet Gynecol 111:379–381, 1971.

221. Mentzer WC, Collier E: Hydrops fetalis associated with erythrocyte G-6-PD deficiency and maternal ingestion of fava beans and ascorbic acid. J Pediatr 86:565–567, 1975.

222. Masson P, Rigot A, Cecile W: Hydrops fetalis and G-6-PD deficiency. Arch Pediatr 2:541–544, 1995.

223. Lienhardt A, Aubard Y, Laroche C, et al: A rare cause of fetal ascites: A case report of Günther's disease. Fetal Diagn Ther 14:257–261, 1999.

224. Özmen S, Seckin N, Turhan NÖ, et al: Fetal methemoglobinemia: A cause of nonimmune hydrops fetalis. Am J Obstet Gynecol 173:232–233, 1995.

225. Gallagher PG, Weed SA, Tse WT, et al: Recurrent fatal hydrops fetalis associated with a nucleotide substitution on the erythrocyte α-spectrin gene. J Clin Invest 95:1174–1182, 1995.

226. Whitfield CF, Follweiler JB, Lopresti-Morrow L, Miller BA: Deficiency of β-spectrin synthesis in burst-forming units-erythroid in lethal hereditary spherocytosis. Blood 78:3043–3051, 1991.

227. Giacoia GP: Severe fetomaternal hemorrhage: A review. Obstet Gynecol Surv 52:372–380, 1997.

228. Baschat AA, Harman CR, Alger LS, Weiner CP: Fetal coronary and cerebral blood flow in acute fetomaternal hemorrhage. Ultrasound Obstet Gynecol 12:128–131, 1998.

229. Hanigan WC, Ali MB, Cusack TL, et al: Diagnosis of subdural hemorrhage in utero. J Neurosurg 63:977–979, 1985.

230. Barozzino T, Sgro M, Toi A, et al: Fetal bilateral subdural haemorrhages. Prenatal diagnosis and spontaneous resolution by time of delivery. Prenat Diagn 18:496–503, 1998.

231. Buxton PJ, Maheswaran P, Dewbury KC, Moore IE: Neonatal hepatic calcification in subcapsular haematoma with hydrops fetalis. Br J Radiol 64:1058–1060, 1991.

232. Øie BK, Hertel J, Seip M, Früs-Hansen B: Hydrops foetalis in 3 infants of a mother with acquired chronic pure red cell aplasia: Transitory red cell aplasia in 1 of the infants. Scand J Haematol 33:466–470, 1984.

233. Bock JE, Bang J, Trolle D, Skaeraasen J: Successful ultrasound-guided intravascular transfusion in severe fetal anemia without blood group incompatibility. Acta Obstet Scand 64:681–682, 1985.

234. Carter C, Darbyshire PJ, Wickramasinghe SN: A congenital dyserythropoietic anaemia variant presenting as hydrops fetalis. Br J Haematol 72:289–290, 1989.

235. Williams G, Lorimer S, Merry CC, et al: A variant congenital dyserythropoietic anaemia presenting as a fetal hydrops foetalis [comment]. Br J Haematol 76:438–439, 1990.

236. Roberts DJ, Nadel A, Lage J, Rutherford CJ: An unusual variant of congenital dyserythropoietic anaemia with mild maternal and lethal fetal disease. Br J Haematol 84:549–551, 1993.

237. Jijina F, Ghosh K, Yavagal D, et al: A patient with congenital dyserythropoietic anaemia type III presenting with stillbirth. Acta Haematol 99:31–33, 1998.

238. Stone P, Zuccollo J: Lethal congenital dyserythropoietic anaemia type 1 in siblings presenting as pericardial effusion in the second trimester. Fetal Diagn Ther 14:11–14, 1999.

239. McLennan AC, Chitty LS, Rissek J, Maxwell DJ: Prenatal diagnosis of Blackfan-Diamond syndrome: Case report and review of the literature. Prenat Diagn 16:349–353, 1996.

240. Scimeca PG, Weinblatt ME, Slepowitz G, et al: Diamond-Blackfan syndrome: An unusual cause of hydrops fetalis. Am J Pediatr Hematol Oncol 10:241–243, 1988.

241. Rogers BB, Bloom SL, Buchanan GR: Autosomal dominantly inherited Diamond-Blackfan's anemia resulting in nonimmune hydrops. Obstet Gynecol 89:805–807, 1997.

242. Zwi LJ, Becroft DM: Intrauterine aplastic anemia and fetal hydrops: A case report. Pediatr Pathol 5:199–205, 1986.

243. Creutzig U, Baumann M: Spontaneous remission in neonates with Down's syndrome and acute myelogenous leukemia—transient myeloproliferative disease. Onkologie 21:184–188, 1998.

244. Gray ES, Balch NJ, Kohler H, et al: Congenital leukaemia: An unusual cause of stillbirth. Arch Dis Child 61:1001–1006, 1986.

245. Nunez E, Varela S, Cervilla K, Shalper J: Hydrops fetalis caused by congenital leukemia. Rev Child Pediatr 62:186–188, 1991.

246. Baschat AA, Wagner T, Malisius R, Gembruch U: Prenatal diagnosis of a transient myeloproliferative disorder in trisomy 21. Prenat Diagn 18:731–736, 1998.

247. Zerres K, Schwanitz G, Niesen M, et al: Prenatal diagnosis of acute non-lymphoblastic leukaemia in Down syndrome [letter]. Lancet 335:117, 1990.

248. Hendricks SK, Sorensen TK, Baker ER: Trisomy 21, fetal hydrops, and anemia: Prenatal diagnosis of transient myeloproliferative disorder. Obstet Gynecol 82:703–705, 1993.

249. Donnenfeld AE, Scott SC, Hensefelder-Kimmel M, Dampier D: Prenatally diagnosed non-immune hydrops caused by congenital transient leukaemia. Prenat Diagn 14:721–724, 1994.

250. Macones GA, Johnson A, Tilley D, et al: Foetal hepatosplenomegaly associated with transient myeloproliferative disorder in trisomy 21. Fetal Diagn Ther 10:131–133, 1995.

251. Gembruch U, Niesen M, Hansmann M, Knöpfle G: Listeriosis: A cause of non-immune hydrops fetalis. Prenat Diagn 7:277–282, 1987.

252. Pretorius DH, Hayward I, Jones KL, Stamm E: Sonographic evaluation of pregnancies with maternal varicella infection. J Ultrasound Med 11:459–463, 1992.

253. Barrow SD, Pass RF: Infectious causes of hydrops fetalis. Semin Perinatol 19:493–501, 1995.

254. Jordan J: Identification of human parvovirus B19 infection in idiopathic nonimmune hydrops fetalis. Am J Obstet Gynecol 174:37–42, 1996.

255. Yaegashi N, Okamura K, Yajima A, et al: The frequency of human parvovirus B19 infection in nonimmune hydrops fetalis. J Perinat Med 22:159–163, 1994.

256. Van den Veyver IB, Ni J, Bowles N, et al: Detection of intrauterine viral infection using the polymerase chain reaction. Mol Genet Metab 63:85–95, 1998.

257. Markenson GR, Yancey MK: Parvovirus B19 infections in pregnancy. Semin Perinatol 22:309–317, 1998.

258. Levy R, Weissman A, Blomberg G, Hagay ZJ: Infection by parvovirus B 19 during pregnancy: A review. Obstet Gynecol Surv 52:254–259, 1997.

259. Brown KE, Anderson SM, Young NS: Erythrocyte P antigen: Cellular receptor for B19 parvovirus. Science 262:114–117, 1993.

260. Brown KE, Hibbs JR, Gallinella G, et al: Resistance to parvovirus B19 infection due to lack of virus receptor (erythrocyte P antigen). N Engl J Med 330:1192–1196, 1994.

261. Porter HJ, Quantrill AM, Fleming KA: B19 parvovirus infection of myocardial cells. Lancet 5:535–536, 1988.

262. Naides SJ, Weiner CP: Antenatal diagnosis and palliative treatment of non-immune hydrops fetalis secondary to fetal parvovirus B19 infection. Prenat Diagn 9:105–114, 1989.

263. Petrokovsky B, Baker D, Schneider E: Fetal hydrops secondary to human parvovirus infection in early pregnancy. Prenat Diagn 16:342–344, 1996.

264. Smulian J, Egan J, Rodis F: Fetal hydrops in the first trimester associated with maternal parvovirus infection. J Clin Ultrasound 26:314–316, 1998.

265. Van Elsacker-Niele AM, Salimans MM, Weiland HT, et al: Fetal pathology in human parvovirus B19 infection. Br J Obstet Gynaecol 96:768–775, 1989.

266. Katz VL, Chescheir NC, Bethea M: Hydrops fetalis from B19 parvovirus infection. J Perinatol 10:366–369, 1990.

267. Morey AL, Keeling JW, Porter HJ, Fleming KA: Clinical and histopathological features of parvovirus B19 infection in the human fetus. Br J Obstet Gynaecol 99:566–574, 1992.

268. Brandenburg H, Los FJ, Cohen-Overbeek TE: A case of early intrauterine parvovirus B19 infection. Prenat Diagn 16:75–77, 1996.

269. Bhai PS, Davies NJ, Westmoreland D, Jones A: Spontaneous resolution of non-immune hydrops fetalis secondary to transplacental parvovirus B19 infection. Ultrasound Obstet Gynecol 7:55–57, 1996.

270. Parilla BV, Tamura RK, Ginsberg NA: Association of parvovirus infection with isolated fetal effusions. Am J Perinatol 14:357–358, 1997.

271. Rodis JF, Quinn DL, Gary GW Jr, et al: Management and outcome of pregnancies complicated by human B19 parvovirus infection: A prospective study. Am J Obstet Gynecol 163:1168–1171, 1990.

272. Searle K, Guillard C, Enders G: Parvovirus B19 diagnosis in pregnant women—quantification of IgG antibody levels (IU/ml) with reference to the international parvovirus B19 standard serum. Infection 25:32–34, 1997.

273. Bernstein IM, Capeless EL: Elevated maternal serum alpha-fetoprotein and hydrops fetalis in association with fetal parvovirus B-19 infection. Obstet Gynecol 74:456–457, 1989.

274. Komischke K, Searle K, Enders G: Maternal serum alpha-fetoprotein and human chorionic gonadotropin in pregnant women with acute parvovirus B19 infection with and without fetal complications. Prenat Diagn 13:1039–1046, 1997.

275. Johnson DR, Fisher RA, Helwik JJ, et al: Screening maternal serum alpha-fetoprotein levels and human parvovirus antibodies. Prenat Diagn 14:455–458, 1994.

276. Schwarz TF, Nerlich A, Hottenträger B, et al: Parvovirus B19 infection of the fetus. Histology and in situ hybridization. Am J Clin Pathol 96:121–126, 1991.

277. Torok TJ, Wang Q, Gary GW Jr, et al: Prenatal diagnosis of intrauterine infection with parvovirus B19 by the polymerase chain reaction technique. Clin Infect Dis 14:149–155, 1992.

278. Schwarz TF, Jäger G, Holzgreve W, Roggendorf M: Diagnosis of human parvovirus B19 infections by polymerase chain reaction. Scand J Infect Dis 24:691–696, 1992.

279. Gentilomi G, Zerbini M, Gallinella G, et al: B19 parvovirus induced fetal hydrops: Rapid and simple diagnosis by detection of B19 antigens in amniotic fluids. Prenat Diagn 18:363–368, 1998.

280. Schild RL, Bald R, Plath H, et al: Intrauterine management of fetal parvovirus B19 infection. Ultrasound Obstet Gynecol 13:161–166, 1999.

281. Essary LR, Vnencak-Jones CL, Manning SS, et al: Frequency of parvovirus B19 infection in nonimmune hydrops fetalis and utility of three diagnostic methods. Hum Pathol 29:696–701, 1998.

282. Wright C, Hinchliffe DA, Taylor C: Fetal pathology in intrauterine death due to parvovirus B19 infection. Br J Obstet Gynaecol 103:133–136, 1996.

283. Mielke G, Enders G: Late onset of hydrops fetalis following intrauterine parvovirus B19 infection. Fetal Diagn Ther 12:40–42, 1997.

284. Holzgreve W: Fetal anomalies. Curr Opin Obstet Gynecol 2:215–222, 1990.

285. Rodis JF, Borgida AF, Wilson M, et al: Management of parvovirus infection in pregnancy and outcomes of hydrops: A survey of members of the Society of Perinatal Obstetricians. Am J Obstet Gynecol 179:985–988, 1998.

286. Fairley C, Smoleniec J, Caul O, Miller E: Observational study of effect of intrauterine transfusion on outcome of fetal hydrops after parvovirus B 19 infection. Lancet 346:1335–1337, 1995.

287. Rodis JF, Rodner C, Hansen AA, et al: Long-term outcome of children following maternal human parvovirus B19 infection. Obstet Gynecol 91:125–128, 1998.

288. Miller E, Fairley CH, Cohen BJ, Seng C: Immediate and long term outcome of human parvovirus B19 infection in pregnancy. Br J Obstet Gynaecol 105:174–178, 1998.

289. Hudon L, Moise KJ Jr, Hegemier SE, et al: Long-term neurodevelopmental outcome after intrauterine transfusion for the treatment of fetal hemolytic disease. Am J Obstet Gynecol 179:858–863, 1998.

290. Brown HL, Abernathy MP: Cytomegalovirus infection. Semin Perinatol 22:260–266, 1998.

291. Ville Y: The megalovirus [editorial]. Ultrasound Obstet Gynecol 12:151–153, 1998.

292. Donner C, Liesnard C, Content J, et al: Prenatal diagnosis of 52 pregnancies at risk for congenital cytomegalovirus infection. Obstet Gynecol 82:481–486, 1993.

293. Peters MT, Lowe TW, Carpenter A, Kole S: Prenatal diagnosis of congenital cytomegalovirus infection with abnormal triple-screen results and hyperechogenic fetal bowel. Am J Obstet Gynecol 173:953–954, 1995.

294. Nelson CT, Demmler GJ: Cytomegalovirus infection in the pregnant mother, fetus, and newborn infant. Clin Perinatol 24:151–160, 1997.

295. Filloux F, Kerlsey DK, Bose CL, et al: Hydrops fetalis with supraventricular tachycardia and cytomegalovirus infection. Clin Pediatr 24:534–536, 1985.

296. Fadel HE, Ruedrich DA: Intrauterine resolution of nonimmune hydrops associated with cytomegalovirus infection. Obstet Gynecol 71:1003–1005, 1988.

297. Binder ND, Buckmaster JW, Benda GI: Outcome for fetuses with ascites and cytomegalovirus infection. Pediatrics 82:100–103, 1988.

298. Mazeron MC, Cordovi-Voulgaropoulos L, Perol Y: Transient hydrops fetalis associated with intrauterine cytomegalovirus infection: Prenatal diagnosis. Obstet Gynecol 84:692–694, 1994.

299. Hagay ZJ, Biran G, Ornoy A, Reece EA: Congenital cytomegalovirus infection: A long-standing problem still seeking a solution. Am J Obstet Gynecol 174:241–245, 1996.

300. Donner C, Liesnard C, Brancart F, Rodesch F: Accuracy of amniotic fluid testing before 21 weeks' gestation in prenatal diagnosis of congenital cytomegalovirus infection. Prenat Diagn 14:1055, 1999.

301. Nicolini U, Kustermann A, Tassis B, et al: Prenatal diagnosis of congenital human cytomegalovirus infection. Prenat Diagn 14:903–906, 1994.

302. Nigro G, La Torre R, Anceschi MM, et al: Hyperimmunoglobulin therapy for a twin fetus with cytomegalovirus infection and growth retardation. Am J Obstet Gynecol 180:1222–1226, 1999.

303. Hollier LM, Cox SM: Syphilis. Semin Perinatol 22:323–331, 1998.

304. Berkowitz K, Baxi L, Fox HE: False-negative syphilis screening: The prozone phenomenon, nonimmune hydrops, and diagnosis of syphilis during pregnancy. Am J Obstet Gynecol 163:975–977, 1990.

305. Levine Z, Sherer DM, Jacobs A, Rotenberg O: Nonimmune hydrops fetalis due to congenital syphilis associated with negative intrapartum maternal serology screening. Am J Perinatol 15:233–237, 1998.

306. Grimprel E, Sanchez PJ, Wendel GD, et al: Use of polymerase chain reaction and rabbit infectivity testing to detect Treponema pallidum in amniotic fluid, fetal and neonatal sera, and cerebrospinal fluid. J Clin Microbiol 29:1711–1718, 1991.

307. Nathan L, Twickler DM, Peters MT, et al: Fetal syphilis: Correlation of sonographic findings and rabbit infectivity testing of amniotic fluid. J Ultrasound Med 12:97–101, 1993.

308. Wendel GD Jr, Sanchez PJ, Peters MT, et al: Identification of Treponema pallidum in amniotic fluid and fetal blood complicated by congenital syphilis. Obstet Gynecol 78:890–895, 1991.

309. Barton JR, Thorpe EM Jr, Shaver DC, et al: Nonimmune hydrops fetalis associated with maternal infection with syphilis. Am J Obstet Gynecol 467:56–58, 1992.

310. Daffos F, Forestier F, Capella-Pavlovsky M, et al: Prenatal management of 746 pregnancies at risk for congenital toxoplasmosis. N Engl J Med 318:271–275, 1988.

311. Beazley DM, Egerman RS: Toxoplasmosis. Semin Perinatol 22:332–338, 1998.

312. Dunn D, Wallon M, Peyron F, et al: Mother-to-child transmission of toxoplasmosis: Risk estimates for clinical counselling. Lancet 353:1829–1833, 1999.

313. Zornes SL, Anderson PG, Lott RL: Congenital toxoplasmosis in an infant with hydrops fetalis. South Med J 81:391–393, 1988.

314. Berrebi A, Kobuch WE, Bessieres MH, et al: Termination of pregnancy for maternal toxoplasmosis. Lancet 344:36–39, 1994.

315. Pratlong F, Boulot P, Issert E, et al: Fetal diagnosis of toxoplasmosis in 190 women infected during pregnancy. Prenat Diagn 14:191–198, 1994.

316. Pratlong F, Boulot P, Villena I, et al: Antenatal diagnosis of congenital toxoplasmosis: Evaluation of the biological parameters in a cohort of 286 patients. Br J Obstet Gynaecol 103:552–557, 1996.

317. Hohlfeld P, Daffos F, Costa JM, et al: Prenatal diagnosis of congenital toxoplasmosis with a polymerase-chain-reaction test on amniotic fluid. N Engl J Med 331:695–699, 1994.

318. Desmonts GD, Couvreur J: Congenital toxoplasmosis: A prospective study of 378 pregnancies. N Engl J Med 29:1110–1116, 1974.

319. Hohlfeld P, Daffos F, Thulliez P, et al: Fetal toxoplasmosis: Outcome of pregnancy and infant follow-up after in utero treatment. J Pediatr 115:765–769, 1989.

320. Foulon W, Villena I, Stray-Pedersen B, et al: Treatment of toxoplasmosis during pregnancy: A multicenter study of impact on fetal transmission and children's sequelae at age 1 year. Am J Obstet Gynecol 180:410–415, 1999.

321. Couvreur J, Thulliez PH, Daffos F: In utero treatment to toxoplasmic fetopathy with the combination pyrimethamine-sulfadiazine. Fetal Diagn Ther 8:45–50, 1993.

322. McAuley J, Boyer KM, Patel D, et al: Early and longitudinal evaluation of treated infants and children of untreated historical patients with congenital toxoplasmosis: The Chicago Collaborative Treatment Trial. Clin Infect Dis 18:38–72, 1994.

323. Friedman S, Ford-Jones LE, Toi A, et al: Congenital toxoplasmosis: Prenatal diagnosis, treatment and postnatal outcome. Prenat Diagn 19:330–333, 1999.

324. Kohl S: Neonatal herpes simplex virus infection. Clin Perinatol 24:129–150, 1997.

325. Riley LE: Herpes simplex virus. Semin Perinatol 22:284–292, 1998.

326. Jacobs RF: Neonatal herpes simplex virus infections. Semin Perinatol 22:64–71, 1998.

327. Smith JR, Cowan FM, Munday P: The management of herpes simplex virus infection in pregnancy. Br J Obstet Gynaecol 105:255–260, 1998.

328. Greene D, Watson WJ, Wirtz PS: Non-immune hydrops fetalis with congenital herpes simplex infection. South Dakota J Med 46:219–220, 1993.

329. Lanouette JM, Duquette DA, Jacques SM, et al: Prenatal diagnosis of fetal herpes simplex infection. Fetal Diagn Ther 11:414–416, 1996.

330. Towbin JA, Griffin LD, Martin AB, et al: Intrauterine adenoviral myocarditis presenting as nonimmune hydrops fetalis: Diagnosis by polymerase chain reaction. Pediatr Infect Dis J 13:144–150, 1994.

331. Ranucci-Weiss D, Uerpairojkit B, Bowles N, et al: Intrauterine adenoviral infection associated with fetal non-immune hydrops. Prenat Diagn 18:182–185, 1998.

332. Forsnes EV, Eggleston MK, Wax JR: Differential transmission of adenovirus in a twin pregnancy. Obstet Gynecol 91:817–818, 1998.

333. Wenstrom KD, Andrews WW, Bowles NE, et al: Intrauterine viral infection at the time of second trimester genetic amniocentesis. Obstet Gynecol 92:420–424, 1998.

334. Jauniaux E, van Maldergem L, Munter CD, et al: Nonimmune hydrops fetalis associated with genetic abnormalities. Obstet Gynecol 75:568–572, 1990.

335. Hovav M, Nadjari M, Dagan J, et al: Nonimmune hydrops fetalis in a 49,XXXXY fetus at 16 menstrual weeks. Am J Med Genet 47:529–530, 1993.

336. Steiner RD: Hydrops fetalis: Role of the geneticist. Semin Perinatol 19:516–524, 1995.

337. Rotmensch S, Liberati M, Bronshtein M, et al: Prenatal sonographic findings in 187 fetuses with Down syndrome. Prenat Diagn 17:1001–1009, 1997.

338. Knoblauch H, Sommer D, Zimmer C, et al: Fetal trisomy 10 mosaicism: Ultrasound, cytogenetic and morphologic findings in early pregnancy. Prenat Diagn 19:379–382, 1999.

339. Snijders RJM, Noble P, Sebire N, et al: UK multicentre project on assessment of risk of trisomy 21 by maternal age and fetal nuchal-translucency thickness at 10-14 weeks of gestation. Lancet 352:343–346, 1998.

340. Azar G, Snijders RJM, Gosden CM, Nicolaides KH: Fetal nuchal cystic hygromata: Associated malformations and chromosomal defects. Fetal Diagn Ther 6:46–57, 1991.

341. Rejjal AL, Nazer H: Resolution of cystic hygroma, hydrops fetalis, and fetal anemia. Am J Perinatol 10:455–459, 1993.

342. Hyett JA, Moscoso G, Nicolaides KH: Abnormalities of the heart and great arteries in first trimester chromosomally abnormal fetuses. Am J Med Genet 69:207–216, 1997.

343. Gembruch U, Baschat AA, Knöpfle G, Hansmann M: Results of chromosomal analysis in fetuses with cardiac anomalies as diagnosed by first- and early second-trimester echocardiography. Ultrasound Obstet Gynecol 10:391–396, 1997.

344. Clark EB: Neck web and congenital heart defects: A pathogenic association in 45 X0 Turner syndrome? Teratology 29:355–361, 1984.

345. Hyett J, Perdu M, Sharland G, et al: Using fetal nuchal translucency to screen for major congenital cardiac defects at 10-14 weeks of gestation: Population based cohort study. BMJ 318:81–85, 1999.

346. Gembruch U, Knöpfle G, Bald R, Hansmann M: Early diagnosis of fetal congenital heart diseases by transvaginal echocardiography. Ultrasound Obstet Gynecol 3:310–317, 1993.

347. Huisman TWA, Bilardo CM: Transient increase in nuchal translucency thickness and reversed end-diastolic ductus venosus flow in a fetus with trisomy 18. Ultrasound Obstet Gynecol 10:397–399, 1997.

348. Matias A, Gomes C, Flack N, et al: Screening for chromosomal abnormalities at 10-14 weeks: The role of ductus venosus blood flow. Ultrasound Obstet Gynecol 12:380–384, 1998.

349. Bloomfield FH, Hadden W, Gunn TR: Lymphatic dysplasia in a neonate with Noonan's syndrome. Pediatr Radiol 27:321–323, 1997.

350. Fahnenstich H, Schmid G, Kowalewski S, et al: Familiärer nichtimmunologischer Hydrops fetalis. Klin Pädiatr 201:396–399, 1989.

351. Njolstad PR, Reigstad H, Westby J, Espeland A: Familial nonimmune hydrops fetalis and congenital pulmonary lymphangiectasia. Eur J Pediatr 157:498–501, 1998.

352. Williams MS, Josephson KD: Unusual autosomal recessive lymphatic anomalies in two unrelated Amish families. Am J Med Genet 73:286–289, 1997.

353. Bulas DI, Saal HM, Allen JF, et al: Cystic hygroma and congenital diaphragmatic hernia: Early prenatal sonographic evaluation of Fryns' syndrome. Prenat Diagn 12:867–875, 1992.

354. Hösli IM, Tercanli S, Rehder H, Holzgreve W: Cystic hygroma as an early first-trimester ultrasound marker for recurrent Fryns' syndrome. Ultrasound Obstet Gynecol 10:422–424, 1997.

355. Ptacek L, Johnson K, Griggs R: Genetics and physiology of the myotonic muscle disorders. N Engl J Med 328:482–489, 1993.

356. Geifman-Holtzman O, Fay K: Prenatal diagnosis of congenital myotonic dystrophy and counseling of the pregnant mother: Case report and literature review. Am J Med Genet 78:250–253, 1998.

357. Affi AM, Bhatia AR, Eyal F: Hydrops fetalis associated with congenital myotonic dystrophy. Am J Obstet Gynecol 166:929–930, 1992.

358. Dufour P, Berard J, Vinatier D, et al: Myotonic dystrophy and pregnancy. A report of two cases and a review of the literature. Eur J Obstet Gynecol Reprod Biol 72:159–164, 1997.

359. Stratto RF, Paterson RM: DNA confirmation of congenital myotonic dystrophy in non-immune hydrops fetalis. Prenat Diagn 13:1027–1030, 1993.

360. Igarashi H, Momoi MY, Yamagata T, et al: Hypertrophic cardiomyopathy in congenital myotonic dystrophy. Pediatr Neurol 18:366–369, 1998.

361. Joseph JT, Richards CS, Anthony DC, et al: Congenital myotonic dystrophy pathology and somatic mosaicism. Neurology 49:1457–1460, 1997.

362. Keller C, Reynolds A, Lee B, Garcia-Prats J: Congenital myotonic dystrophy requiring prolonged endotracheal and noninvasive assisted ventilation: Not a uniform fatal condition. Pediatrics 101:704–706, 1998.

363. Spearritt DJ, Tannenberg AE, Payton DJ: Lethal multiple pterygium syndrome: Report of a case with neurological anomalies. Am J Med Genet 47:45–49, 1993.

364. Kirkinen P, Herva R, Leisti F: Early prenatal diagnosis of a lethal syndrome of multiple congenital contractures. Prenat Diagn 7:189–196, 1987.

365. Vuopala K, Herva R: Lethal congenital contracture syndrome: Further delineation and genetic aspects. J Med Genet 31:521–527, 1994.

366. Vardon D, Chau C, Sigodi S, et al: Congenitally rapidly fatal form of nemaline myopathy with fetal hydrops and arthrogryposis. A case report and review. Fetal Diagn Ther 13:244–249, 1998.

367. Sepulveda W, Stagiannis KD, Cox PM, et al: Prenatal findings in generalized amyoplasia. Prenat Diagn 15:660–664, 1995.

368. Verloes A, Dodinval P, Retz MC, et al: A hydropic fetus with translucent ribs, arthrogryposis multiplex congenita and congenital myopathy: Etiological heterogeneity of A.M.C., Toriello-Bauserman type? Genet Couns 2:63–66, 1991.

369. Karimi-Nejad MH, Khajavi H, Gharavi MJ, Karimi-Nejad R: NeuLaxova syndrome: Report of a case and comments. Am J Med Genet 28:17–23, 1987.

370. Souka AP, Snijders RJM, Novakov A, et al: Defects and syndromes in chromosomally normal fetuses with increased nuchal translucency thickness at 10-14 weeks of gestation. Ultrasound Obstet Gynecol 11:391–400, 1998.

371. Lake BD, Young EP, Winchester BG: Prenatal diagnosis of lysosomal storage discases. Brain Pathol 8:133–149, 1998.

372. Dorpe van J, Moermann PH, Pecceu A, Steen van den P: Nonimmune hydrops fetalis caused by β-glucuronidase deficiency (mucopolysaccharidosis VII). Study of a family with 3 affected siblings. Genet Consel 7:105–112, 1996.

373. Vervoort R, Islam MR, Sly WS, et al: Molecular analysis of patients with β-glucuronidase deficiency presenting as hydrops fetalis or as early mucopolysaccharidosis VII. Am J Hum Genet 58:457–471, 1996.

374. Tasso MJ, Martinez-Gutierrez A, Carrascosa C, et al: GMI-Gangliosidosis presenting as nonimmune hydrops fetalis: A case report. J Perinat Med 24:445–449, 1996.

375. Tayebi N, Cushner SR, Kleijer W, Lau EK, et al: Prenatal lethality of a homozygous null mutation in the human glucocerebrosidase gene. Am J Med Genet 73:41–47, 1997.

376. Lemyre E, Russo P, Melancon SB, et al: Clinical spectrum of infantile free sialic acid storage disease. Am J Med Genet 19:385–391, 1999.

377. Patel MS, Callahan JW, Zhang S, et al: Early-infantile galactosialidosis: Prenatal presentation and postnatal follow-up. Am J Med Genet 85:38–47, 1999.

378. Dorland L, de Koning TJ, Toet M, et al: Poll-The BT: Recurrent non-immune hydrops fetalis associated with carbohydrate-deficient glycoprotein syndrome [abstract]. J Inherit Metab Dis 20(Suppl 1):88, 1997.

379. Handyside AH, Delhanty JDA: Preimplantation genetic diagnosis: Strategies and surprises. Trends Genet 13:270–275, 1997.

380. Hahn S, Sant R, Holzgreve W: Fetal cells in maternal blood: Current and future perspectives [editorial]. Mol Hum Reprod 4:515–521, 1998.

381. Hatjis CG: Diagnosis and successful treatment of fetal goitrous hyperthyroidism caused by maternal Graves disease. Obstet Gynecol 81:837–839, 1993.
382. Watson WJ, Fiegen MM: Fetal thyrotoxicosis associated with nonimmune hydrops. Am Obstet Gynecol 172:1039–1040, 1995.
383. Treadwell MC, Sherer DM, Sacks AJ, et al: Successful treatment of recurrent non-immune hydrops secondary to fetal hyperthyroidism. Obstet Gynecol 87:838–840, 1996.
384. Sebire NJ, Snijders RJM, Hughes K, et al: The hidden mortality of monochorionic twin pregnancies. Br J Obstet Gynaecol 104:1203–1207, 1997.
385. Bajoria R, Wigglesworth J, Fisk NM: Angioarchitecture of monochorionic placentas in relation to the twin-twin transfusion syndrome. Am J Obstet Gynecol 172:856–863, 1995.
386. Bajoria R, Kingdom J: The case of routine determination of chorionicity and zygosity in multiple pregnancy. Prenat Diagn 17:1207–1225, 1997.
387. Duncan KR, Denbow ML, Fisk NM: The aetiology and management of twin-twin transfusion syndrome. Prenat Diagn 17:1227–1236, 1997.
388. Machin GA, Still K: The twin-twin transfusion syndrome: Vascular anatomy of monochorionic placentas and their clinical outcomes. In Keith LG, Papiernik E, Keith DM, Luke B (eds): Multiple Pregnancy: Epidemiology, Gestation and Perinatal Outcome. New York - London: Parthenon Publishing Group, 1995, pp 367–394.
389. Fries MH, Goldstein RB, Kilpatrick SJ, et al: The role of velamentous cord insertion in the etiology of twin-twin transfusion syndrome. Obstet Gynecol 81:569–574, 1992.
390. Strong TH Jr: The umbilical pump: A contributor to twin-twin transfusion. Obstet Gynecol 89:812–813, 1997.
391. Fesslova V, Villa L, Nava S, et al: Fetal and neonatal echocardiographic findings in twin-twin transfusion syndrome. Am J Obstet Gynecol 179:1056–1062, 1998.
392. Hecher K, Ville Y, Snijders R, Nicolaides K: Doppler studies of the fetal circulation in twin-twin transfusion syndrome. Ultrasound Obstet Gynecol 5:318–324, 1995.
393. Zosmer N, Bajoria R, Weiner E, et al: Clinical and echographic features of in utero cardiac dysfunction in the recipient twin in twin-twin transfusion syndrome. Br Heart J 72:74–79, 1994.
394. Berry SM, Puder KS, Bottoms SF, et al: Comparison of intrauterine hematologic and biochemical values between twin pairs with and without stuck twin syndrome. Am J Obstet Gynecol 172:1403–1410, 1995.
395. Fusi L, McParland P, Fisk N, et al: Acute twin-twin transfusion: A possible mechanism for brain-damaged survivors after intrauterine death of a monochorionic twin. Obstet Gynecol 78:517–520, 1991.
396. Okamura K, Murotsuki J, Tanigawara S, et al: Funipuncture for evaluation of hematologic and coagulation indices in the surviving twin following co-twin's death. Obstet Gynecol 83:975–978, 1994.
397. Sebire NJ, D'Ercole C, Hugues K, et al: Increased nuchal translucency thickness at 10-14 weeks as a predictor of severe twin-to-twin transfusion syndrome. Ultrasound Obstet Gynecol 10:86–89, 1997.
398. Elliot JP, Urig MA, Clewell WH: Aggressive therapeutic amniocentesis for treatment of twin-twin transfusion syndrome. Obstet Gynecol 77:537–540, 1991.
399. Mahoney BS, Petty CN, Nyberg DA, et al: The "stuck twin" phenomenon: Ultrasonographic findings, pregnancy outcome, and management with serial amniocentesis. Am J Obstet Gynecol 163:1513–1522, 1990.
400. Pinette MG, Pan Y, Pinette SG, Stubblefield PG: Treatment of twin-twin transfusion syndrome. Obstet Gynecol 82:841–846, 1993.
401. De Lia JE, Kuhlmann RS, Harstadt TW, Cruikshank DP: Fetoscopilar ablation of placental vessels in severe previable twin-twin transfusion syndrome. Am J Obstet Gynecol 172:1202–1211, 1995.
402. Deprest JA, Lerut TE, Vandenberghe K: Operative fetoscopy: New perspective in fetal therapy? Prenat Diagn 17:1247–1260, 1997.
403. Ville Y, Hyett J, Hecher K, Nicolaides KH: Preliminary experience with endoscopic laser surgery for severe twin-twin transfusion syndrome. N Engl J Med 332:224–227, 1995.
404. Ville Y, Hecher K, Gagnon A, et al: Endoscopic laser coagulation in the management of severe twin-to-twin transfusion syndrome. Br J Obstet Gynaecol 105:446–453, 1998.
405. Hecher K, Plath H, Bregenzer T, et al: Endoscopic laser surgery versus serial amniocenteses in the treatment of severe twin-twin transfusion syndrome. Am J Obstet Gynecol 180:717–724, 1999.
406. Dommergues M, Mandelbrot L, Delezoide AL, et al: Twin-to-twin transfusion syndrome: Selective fetocide by embolization of the hydropic fetus. Fetal Diagn Ther 10:26–31, 1995.
407. Hecher K, Hackelöer BJ, Ville Y: Umbilical cord coagulation by operative microendoscopy at 16 weeks gestation in an acardiac twin. Ultrasound Obstet Gynecol 10:130–132, 1997.
408. Holzgreve W, Tercanli S, Krings W, Schuierer G: A simpler technique for umbilical-cord blockade of an acardic twin. N Engl J Med 331:56–57, 1994.
409. Sepulveda W, Bower S, Hassan J, Fisk NM: Ablation of acardiac twin by alcohol injection into the intra-abdominal umbilical artery. Obstet Gynecol 86:680–681, 1995.
410. Porreco RP, Barton SM, Haverkamp AD: Occlusion of umbilical artery in acardiac, acephalic twin. Lancet 337:326–327, 1991.
411. Quintero RA, Reich H, Puder KS, et al: Brief report: Umbilical-cord ligation of an acardiac twin by fetoscopy at 19 weeks of gestation. N Engl J Med 17:469–471, 1994.
412. Rodeck C, Deans A, Jauniaux E: Thermocoagulation for the early treatment of pregnancy with an acardiac twin. N Engl J Med 339:1293–1295, 1998.
413. Soma H, Watanabe Y, Hata T: Chorangiosis and chorangioma in three cohorts of placentas from Nepal, Tibet, and Japan. Reprod Fertil Dev 7:1533–1538, 1995.
414. Jauniaux E, Zucker M, Meuris S, et al: Chorangiosarcoma: An unusual tumour of the placenta. The missing link? Placenta 9:607–613, 1988.
415. Makino Y, Horiuchi S, Sonoda M, et al: A case of large placental chorioangioma with non-immunological hydrops. J Perinat Med 27:128–131, 1999.
416. Hirata GI, Masaki DI, O'Toole M, et al: Color flow mapping and Doppler velocimetry in the diagnosis and management of a placental chorangioma associated with nonimmune fetal hydrops. Obstet Gynecol 81:850–852, 1993.
417. Drut RM, Drut R: Nonimmune fetal hydrops and placentomegaly: Diagnosis of familial Wiedemann-Beckwith syndrome with trisomy 11p15 using FISH. Am J Med Genet 15:145–149, 1996.
418. Fritz MA, Christopher CR: Umbilical vein thrombosis and maternal diabetes mellitus. J Reprod Med 26:320–324, 1981.
419. Collins JH: Prenatal observation of umbilical cord torsion with subsequent premature labor and delivery of a 31-week infant with mild nonimmune hydrops. Am J Obstet Gynecol 172:1048–1049, 1995.
420. Sherer DM, Anyaegbunam A: Prenatal ultrasonographic morphologic assessment of the umbilical cord: A review. Part I. Obstet Gynecol Surv 52:506–514, 1997.
421. Sherer DM, Anyaegbunam A: Prenatal ultrasonographic morphologic assessment of the umbilical cord: A review. Part II. Obstet Gynecol Surv 52:515–523, 1997.
422. Novak PM, Sander CM, Yang SS, von Oeyen PT: Report of fourteen cases of nonimmune hydrops fetalis in association with hemorrhagic endovasculitis of the placenta. Am J Obstet Gynecol 165:945–950, 1991.
423. Knisely AS: The pathologist and the hydropic placenta, fetus, or infant. Semin Perinatol 19:525–531, 1995.
424. Uchide K, Suzuki N, Murakami K, et al: Subchorial hematoma: A probable cause of reversible nonimmune hydrops fetalis. Am J Perinatol 14:281–283, 1997.
425. Mallmann P, Gembruch U, Mallmann R, Hansmann M: Investigations into a possible immunological origin of idiopathic nonimmune hydrops fetalis and initial results of prophylactic immune treatment of subsequent pregnancies. Acta Obstet Gynecol Scand 70:35–40, 1991.
426. Van Selm M, Kanhai HH, Gravenhorst JB: Maternal hydrops syndrome: A review. Obstet Gynecol Surv 46:785–788, 1991.
427. Dorman SL, Cardwell MS: Ballantyne syndrome caused by a large placental chorangioma. Am J Obstet Gynecol 173:1632–1633, 1995.
428. Carbillon L, Oury JF, Guerin JM, et al: Clinical biological features of Ballantyne syndrome and the role of placental hydrops. Obstet Gynecol Surv 552:310–314, 1997.

429. Gherman RB, Incerpi MH, Wing DA, Goodwin TM: Ballantyne syndrome: Is placental ischemia the etiology? J Matern Fetal Invest 7:227–229, 1998.
430. Duthie SJ, Walkingshaw SA: Parvovirus associated fetal hydrops: Reversal of pregnancy induced proteinuric hypertension by in utero fetal transfusion. Br J Obstet Gynaecol 102:1011–1013, 1995.
431. Johnson P, Sharland G, Allan LD, et al: Umbilical venous pressure in nonimmune hydrops fetalis: Correlation with cardiac size. Am J Obstect Gynecol 167:1309–1313, 1992.
432. Evans MI, Henry GP, Miller WA, et al: International, collaborative assessment of 146000 prenatal karyotypes: Expected limitations if only chromosome-specific probes and fluorescent in-situ hybridization are used. Hum Reprod 14:1213–1216, 1999.
433. Evans MI, Ebrahim SA, Berry SM, et al: Fluorescent in situ hybridization utilization for high-risk prenatal diagnosis: A trade-off among speed, expense, and inherent limitations of chromosome-specific probes. Am J Obstet Gynecol 171:1055–1057, 1994.
434. Weiner CP: Umbilical pressure measurement in the evaluation of nonimmune hydrops fetalis. Am J Obstet Gynecol 168:817–823, 1993.
435. Gudmundsson S, Huhta JC, Wood DC, et al: Venous Doppler ultrasonography in the fetus with nonimmune hydrops. Am J Obstet Gynecol 164:33–37, 1991.
436. Reed KL, Chaffin DG, Anderson CF: Umbilical venous Doppler-velocity pulsations and inferior vena cava pressure elevation in fetal lambs. Obstet Gynecol 87:617–620, 1996.
437. Chen CP, Liu FF, Jan SW, et al: Cytogenetic evaluation of cystic hygroma associated with hydrops fetalis, oligohydramnios or intrauterine fetal death: The roles of amniocentesis, postmortem chorionic villus sampling and cystic hygroma paracentesis. Acta Obstet Gynecol Scand 75:454–458, 1996.
438. Saltzman DH, Frigoletto FD, Harlow BL, et al: Sonographic evaluation of hydrops fetalis. Obstet Gynecol 74:106–111, 1989.
439. Skoll MA, Sharland GK, Allan LD: Is the ultrasound definition of fluid collections in the non-immune hydrops fetalis helpful in defining the underlying cause or predicting outcome? Ultrasound Obstet Gynecol 1:309–312, 1991.
440. Smoleniec J, James D: Predictive value of pleural effusions in fetal hydrops. Fetal Diagn Ther 10:95–100, 1995.
441. Castillo RA, Devoe LD, Hai HA, et al: Nonimmune hydrops: Clinical experience and factors related to a poor outcome. Am J Obstet Gynecol 155:812–816, 1986.
442. Carlson DE, Platt LD, Medearis AL, Horenstein J: Prognostic indicators of the resolution of nonimmune hydrops fetalis and survival of the fetus. Am J Obstet Gynecol 163:1785–1787, 1990.

36

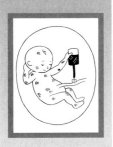

The Fetus at Risk
for Thrombocytopenia

RICHARD L. BERKOWITZ and JAMES B. BUSSEL

Thrombocytopenia

Normal Platelet Function

Platelets function in conjunction with factors present in the blood to produce hemostasis. Injury or damage to a blood vessel causes platelets to adhere to collagen microfibrils or other components that are part of the exposed subendothelium. This process is mediated in part by a fall in prostacyclin levels at the site of the injury. In addition, thrombin inhibition is reduced secondary to the decreased interaction of antithrombin III (AT-III) with cell surface glycosaminoglycans, and the interaction of von Willebrand factor with platelet glycoprotein IB-IX and the subendothelium. Once the platelets adhere to the underlying subendothelium, they then become activated and release the contents of their granules into the surrounding area. These granules contain, among other substances, strong procoagulants. These procoagulants not only stimulate coagulation but also attract other platelets to the site and induce aggregation, the irreversible process of binding platelets to each other via a fibrinogen bridge.

Platelet counts vary; however, the normal range is 150,000 to 400,000/μL. Therefore, thrombocytopenia is defined as any value less than 150,000/μL. Counts between 100,000 and 150,000/μL are considered mild thrombocytopenia, between 50,000 and 100,000/μL moderate thrombocytopenia, and less than 50,000/μL severe thrombocytopenia. Counts below 20,000/μL may be associated with significant spontaneous bleeding and will often require physician intervention.

Excessive bleeding may occur when the platelet count is sufficiently low. Unlike other bleeding disorders in which bruising is often the initial clinical manifestation, platelet disorders instead result in bleeding into mucous membranes. Petechiae, epistaxis, gingival and oral bleeding, and menometrorrhagia are commonly observed. Platelet disorders may be distinguished from disorders involving decreased concentrations of blood factors, such as hemophilia, by the fact that bleeding into joints does not occur in the case of platelet disorders.

Causes of Thrombocytopenia

Thrombocytopenia is a decrease in the number of platelets. Thrombocytopenia may be due either to decreased platelet production or increased platelet destruction. In pregnancy the latter is responsible for the vast majority of cases.[1] Platelet destruction can be caused by an immune response (e.g., isoimmune thrombocytopenic purpura [ITP] or autoimmune thrombocytopenia [AIT], abnormal platelet activation [e.g., gestational thrombocytopenia]), or platelet consumption in abnormal vessels (e.g., hemolysis, elevated liver enzymes, low platelets [HELLP] syndrome, thrombotic thrombocytopenic purpura–hemolytic-uremia syndrome [TTP-HUS]. Decreased platelet production is usually associated with either leukemia or aplastic anemia. It is important to remember that in certain cases, total platelet number may be sufficient, but bleeding can still occur due to a defect in platelet function.[2]

When a pregnant woman is discovered to be thrombocytopenic, it is important to make as accurate a diagnosis as possible. All preexistant diseases, especially human immunodeficiency virus (HIV) infection, should be considered, as well as any drugs that are being taken. The importance of a complete and accurate history cannot be overstated. This must include a family history of any bleeding disorders. Many causes of thrombocytopenia can be readily discovered by the physician who is thorough in his or her history-taking. A complete physical examination must also be performed, with special attention directed towards detecting hepatosplenomegaly, lymphadenopathy, and any signs of bleeding. Laboratory tests must be ordered as necessary. Abnormalities in the complete blood count (CBC), partial thromboplastin time (PTT), or prothrombin time (PT) must be investigated. Coombs testing or a search for antiplatelet antibodies must be performed if indicated. Some cases might require a peripheral smear to be performed early in the investigation.[3]

Immune reactions to drugs and systemic medical disorders are the primary causes of thrombocytopenia, in pregnancy. If drugs and other medical disorders are excluded, the primary differential diagnosis in the first and second trimesters includes gestational thrombocy-topenia (GTP)[4] and ITP.[5] It should be noted that while GTP can occur in the first trimester, it more typically becomes manifest later in pregnancy. In general, the milder the thrombocytopenia in a woman with no prior history of thrombocytopenia, the more likely she is to have GTP. If the platelet count is less than $70,000/\mu L$, and certainly less than $50,000/\mu L$, ITP is likely to be present. A complete family history may reveal evidence of a familial thrombocytopenia. Familial thrombocyto-penias are a poorly defined group of clinical entities. They can effectively be ruled out by a normal distribu-tion of platelet size on peripheral smear, and the absence of a history of other family members with thrombocyto-penia. During the third trimester or postpartum period the sudden onset of significant maternal thrombocyto-penia should lead to consideration of the HELLP syn-drome, TTP-HUS, or disseminated intravascular coagu-lation (DIC), although ITP can present in this fashion as well.[1]

Special Considerations During Pregnancy

During normal pregnancy numerous physical and bio-chemical changes occur in the pregnant woman. Some of these changes will affect hemostasis. Some clotting factors increase in quantity, some decrease, and others remain the same. In most cases the maternal platelet count does not change significantly, but as many as 5% of otherwise healthy women can develop mild gesta-tional thrombocytopenia when they are pregnant. Fur-thermore, the dilutional aspect of a pregnancy-induced increase in plasma volume can in and of itself cause platelet concentration to apparently decrease. During pregnancy, thrombocytopenia can occur in the fetus as well as in the mother. In the case wherein a mother is producing antiplatelet antibodies, in certain pathologic situations these IgG antibodies can actually pass through the placental barrier and cause a fetal thrombo-cytopenia.

In a study of more than 15,000 women and their neo-nates delivered at a single tertiary care hospital over a 7-year period, 6.6% had maternal platelet counts of $150,000/\mu L$ or less at the time of admission to the labor floor, and 1.2% had maternal counts of $100,000/\mu L$ or less. In this same series only 19 infants (0.12%) had birth platelet counts less than $50,000/\mu L$, and only six (0.04%) had birth counts less than $20,000/\mu L$.[6]

Almost 74% of the thrombocytopenic women in this series had gestational thrombocytopenia, and yet only one of these delivered a baby with a low platelet count. A significant number (21%) of the thrombocytopenic women had a hypertensive disorder. However, only four of these patients (1.8%) delivered babies with severe thrombocytopenia, and three of those four neonates were found to have independent causes for their low platelet counts. Slightly less than 4% of the thrombocyto-penic women had an immunologic disorder complicat-ing their pregnancy. It is interesting to note that al-though systemic lupus erythematosis (SLE) is a disease commonly associated with thrombocytopenia, in this study none of the eight patients with SLE delivered babies with platelet counts less than $50,000/\mu L$, but 4 of 46 women (8.7%) with ITP did. Importantly, two of the mothers with ITP whose neonates were thrombocy-topenic had normal platelet counts, while the other two were thrombocytopenic themselves. Finally, 9 of 19 women (47%) at risk for neonatal alloimmune thrombo-cytopenia (NAIT) delivered babies with cord platelet counts less than $50,000/\mu L$, and all six of the babies in the entire series with counts less than $20,000/\mu L$ were in this group.[6]

In this large series, only 3 of the 19 babies with birth platelet counts less than $50,000/\mu L$ were born to women with platelet counts less than $100,000/\mu L$. Therefore, it can be concluded from the results of this study that the overall incidence of severe fetal thrombocytopenia is very low and, when it is present, it has no correlation with the maternal platelet count.[7] Furthermore, in the clear majority of cases severe neonatal thrombocyto-penia is caused by either alloimmune (AIT) or, less com-monly, autoimmune (ITP) thrombocytopenia.[8]

Specific Disorders

Gestational Thrombocytopenia

GTP is by far the most common cause of mild thrombo-cytopenia during pregnancy. Gestational thrombocyto-penia is defined by the following five criteria: (1) platelet counts ranging from 70,000 to $150,000/\mu L$ without treat-ment of the low count, (2) no clinically evident bleeding attributable to the thrombocytopenia, (3) no history of thrombocytopenia prior to the pregnancy other than during prior pregnancies, (4) return of the platelet count to normal within 2 to 12 weeks following the delivery, and (5) no neonatal thrombocytopenia.[9]

Gestational thrombocytopenia may recur in subse-quent pregnancies. The exact cause of GTP is unknown; however, some investigators believe that the cause of this disorder is accelerated platelet consumption. This has not been confirmed, nor has the mechanism of the activation been identified. In GTP, antiplatelet antibod-ies may be detectable, but neither their presence nor their absence can be used to diagnose this disorder or differentiate it from ITP.[9] Unfortunately, there are no specific diagnostic tests to definitively distinguish GTP from mild ITP. This is a diagnosis that is established by fulfilling the five criteria described above. The primary means to differentiate this disorder from other similar conditions is to closely follow the platelet counts in order to look for levels that fall below 50,000 to $70,000/\mu L$, and also to document a normal neonatal platelet count and a restoration of maternal values to normal after completion of the pregnancy.

Immunologic Thrombocytopenia

Autoimmune (ITP) and alloimmune (AIT) thrombocyto-penia in pregnancy may have a significant impact on the mother and/or her fetus. However, it is important to note that although these diseases are pathophysiologically similar, they have important differences in their clinical manifestations.[10] This is especially true in the severity of the maternal, fetal, and neonatal outcome. ITP affects both mothers and fetuses, but with good management is usually fairly benign for both groups. In contrast, AIT has no impact whatsoever on the mother, but it is almost certainly responsible for more intracranial fetal and neonatal hemorrhage due to thrombocytopenia than all the other primary thrombocytopenic conditions combined.[11] Because of these important differences, one must consider these two entities separately in order to better understand their effects in pregnancy, and to counsel the mother on the most appropriate and optimal management strategies.

Immune Idiopathic Thrombocytopenia

ITP is the most common autoimmune disorder affecting pregnant women. Acute immune thrombocytopenic purpura is a self-limited disorder. It usually occurs in childhood, may follow a viral infection, and rarely enters a chronic stage.[2, 3] Chronic ITP, on the other hand, more typically presents in the second or third decade of life, rarely regresses spontaneously, and has a female/male ratio of 3:1. In this disorder the patient produces IgG antiplatelet antibodies that adhere to his or her own platelets. This leads to the sequestration and premature destruction of these platelets by the spleen. As IgG molecules are quite small and the placenta is of necessity rather permeable to small molecules, when a woman with ITP is pregnant these autoantibodies can physically cross the placenta, attach to fetal platelets, and cause fetal thrombocytopenia as well.

Estimates of the frequency of ITP during pregnancy vary widely and have not been well validated. These estimates have ranged from between 1 in 1,000 to 1 in 10,000 pregnancies.[1] Approximately 10% of these women will deliver infants with platelet counts less than 50,000/μL, but at most 1% of these women will have babies who develop an intracranial hemorrhage (ICH).[6, 12]

The classic diagnostic criteria for ITP include the following four findings:

1. Persistent thrombocytopenia less than 100,000/μL with or without accompanying megathrombocytes on the peripheral smear.
2. Bone marrow aspiration and biopsy, if performed, demonstrate normal or possibly increased numbers of megakaryocytes.
3. Other systemic disorders or drugs that are known to be associated with thrombocytopenia have been excluded.
4. Splenomegaly has been excluded.[3]

As is clear from the above discussion, ITP is basically a diagnosis of exclusion. Bone marrow aspiration is not required to establish the diagnosis in most cases. Antiplatelet antibodies are often detectable but, as they are present in several other disorders, they are not yet diagnostic.[3] Their quantitative titers have no correlation with the degree of thrombocytopenia in either the mother or her fetus.

Many women with ITP have a history of petechiae and easy bruisability. Some may also have a history of epistaxis and gingival bleeding that precedes their pregnancy. However, some patients with ITP are completely asymptomatic. Important hemorrhagic symptoms rarely occur unless the maternal platelet count is less than 20,000/μL.[13] It is believed that the course of ITP is usually not affected by pregnancy; however, the converse is not necessarily true. A pregnancy may certainly be adversely affected by ITP. The primary risk to the mother is significant hemorrhage during the peripartum period or at the time of the performance of invasive procedures such as amniocentesis or administration of an epidural anesthetic. Because, as discussed above, maternal IgG antiplatelet antibodies can cross the placenta and gain access to the fetal circulation, the fetus may also develop thrombocytopenia. This can result in bleeding at either the time of delivery or during the neonatal period. It is extremely difficult if not impossible to predict which patients are at greatest risk for hemorrhaging, as the fetal platelet count has no consistent relationship to the platelet count of the mother.[7]

Fortunately, the platelet function of these patients is usually excellent and thus it is not necessary to maintain their platelet counts within the normal range. A maternal platelet count of 30,000/μL is generally considered to be adequate for most circumstances. Higher counts are desirable for invasive procedures and delivery. A maternal platelet count of greater than 50,000/μL is considered to be sufficient for delivery in the great majority of patients, although greater than 80,000/μL may be ideal. Obstetric anesthesia textbooks suggest that 100,000/μL is needed in order to give epidural anesthesia. Bleeding times are not considered to be useful in assessing platelet function in ITP,[14] although newer methods of platelet function analysis may prove to be useful. To again emphasize the need for an excellent and detailed past medical history, it is important to note that a careful history relating episodes of bleeding to specific platelet counts will provide the most reliable estimation of the risk of hemorrhage in the peripartum period.

Treatment

Treatment of this disorder begins with steroid therapy. Generally, prednisone is the initial drug of choice. Depending on the past treatment history and urgency of increasing the platelet count, prednisone is used to treat this disorder at doses between 10 to 20 mg/d and 60 to 80 mg/d until a response is obtained. Clinical response is followed by a tapering off of the drug. Treatment with intravenous μ-globulin (IVIG) may also be considered, especially if a rapid increase in the platelet count is required or if the side effects of steroids would be unacceptable. IVIG at a total dose of 1,000 to 2,000 mg/kg over 1 to 3 days is generally effective in the treatment of ITP. These therapeutic regimens may be used alone or in combination and are successful in the treatment of virtually all cases of ITP. Splenectomy in the treatment of ITP should only be used as a last resort, and is almost never necessary during pregnancy. It should be noted that women who have undergone splenectomy prior to their pregnancy are at risk to have thrombocytopenic fetuses, even if their platelet counts remain within the normal range without additional therapy. Platelet transfusions are generally not necessary and should be reserved for women who are actively bleeding, or those with platelet counts less than 20,000/μL who have failed all other therapy and are about to undergo an invasive procedure.

The management of pregnant women with ITP at the time of delivery is controversial. Virtually all experts agree that maternal platelet counts must be raised to appropriate levels, but experts differ considerably as to how, or even whether, one should assess the fetus for thrombocytopenia. Some authors argue that because the incidence of fetal intracranial hemorrhage proven to be due to labor in thrombocytopenic fetuses of women with ITP is so low, there is no need to perform a cesarean section unless it is obstetrically indicated, nor is there a need to document fetal platelet counts prior to delivery. These authors do, however, caution against the use of both scalp electrodes and fetal scalp sampling. They also generally advocate that forceps and vacuum instrumentation be avoided.

Other authors make exactly the opposite argument. They feel that although the value of cesarean section has not been documented to prevent intracranial bleeding in fetuses with platelet counts of less than 50,000/μL, or even 20,000/μL, it makes sense to avoid a long and potentially traumatic labor in these cases. They, therefore, advocate determination of the fetal platelet count before the onset of labor, or minimally during early labor. They also advocate performing elective cesarean section where platelet counts of less than 50,000/μL are documented. The optimal method to determine the fetal platelet counts is controversial. Percutaneous umbilical cord blood sampling (PUBS) can be performed prior to the onset of labor. However, a review of 173 cases in which this was done revealed that the platelet count was successfully determined in 96% of the cases, and 6% of the fetuses were found to have counts less than 50,000/μL, but that 3% of the patients required emergency cesarean section for fetal distress caused by the PUBS procedure itself. This highlights the need to be circumspect about performing PUBS procedures in this clinical setting. An alternative approach is to perform a platelet count on a fetal scalp sample obtained in early labor after the patient is 2 to 3 cm dilated. One main objection to this approach is a technical one. Fetal platelets frequently clump when exposed to the heparin that is present in most collecting pipettes, resulting in falsely lowered platelet counts. This in turn may lead to unindicated cesarean section. If, however, a smear is made of the fetal scalp blood and examined, it has been demonstrated that detection of any aggregates of ten or more platelets in a high-power field correlates with a platelet count of 50,000/μL or greater.[15] This lends importance to the need to perform a blood smear in these patients. The controversy over these various approaches has not yet been resolved. It must be remembered that

the risk of fetal intracranial hemorrhage associated with labor in patients with ITP is very low, but not zero. Great care should therefore be taken to minimize any risk to the fetus caused by invasive testing. It goes without saying that it is also extremely important to avoid performing unnecessary cesarean sections. The difficulty lies in the fact that there is no conclusive evidence that fetuses with very low platelet counts would not benefit from a cesarean delivery performed early in the course of labor.[10]

Neonatal Alloimmune Thrombocytopenia

AIT is the platelet equivalent of hemolytic disease of the newborn (Rh factor incompatibility).[16] Like hemolytic disease of the newborn, AIT develops as a result of maternal sensitization to fetal antigens. Whereas in the former disorder, the antigens are present on red blood cells, in AIT, they are present on the surface of platelets. These women, who lack the specific antigen that the fetus has inherited from its father, produce IgG antibodies that cross the placenta and mediate the destruction of fetal platelets. Fetal platelets gain access to the maternal circulation and institute an immunologic reaction with the production of these IgG antibodies, which subsequently traverse the placenta to reach the fetal circulation, causing destruction of the fetus' platelets. Unlike Rh disease, however, prior sensitization is not necessary, as approximately half of the clinically evident cases of AIT are discovered in the first live-born infant. This finding suggests that one of three things is happening: either the fetal platelets gain access to the maternal circulation more easily than red blood cells; the platelet antigens are highly immunogenic and therefore stimulate production of high quantities of IgG during the first pregnancy; and/or the fetal reticuloendothelial system is particularly aggressive in destroying platelet antigen–antibody complexes. Furthermore, when one neonate has been affected, all subsequent siblings who carry the same platelet antigen will also be affected. There are currently no published reports of a P1A1-positive neonate who was unaffected by AIT after having a prior affected sibling. There are also no immunizations analogous to the RhoGAM injection given for Rh incompatibility that can prevent the sensitization which results in this subsequent platelet destruction.

Platelets possess specific alloantigen polymorphisms that are expressed on surface membrane glycoproteins. Although there are at least 14 officially recognized platelet-specific antigens at this time, more than 50% of the reported cases in Caucasians, and the majority of severe cases, have occurred as a result of P1A1 incompatibility.[11] The P1A system consists of two alleles, P1A1 and P1A2, which are inherited in a co-dominant fashion. Although prospective studies indicate that approximately 2% of Caucasian women are P1A1 negative, the incidence of NAIT is only 1 in 500 to 1,000 pregnancies. Clinical studies examining cases through affected neonates have reported an estimated frequency of only 1 in 5,000 neonates. These data indicate that only some women who are at risk to develop this disorder actually form antibodies that are capable of destroying their fetuses' platelets. Sensitization to the P1A1 antigen appears to require the presence of the HLA-Dw52A gene located in the major histocompatibility complex. The role of immune responsiveness is not well established for other platelet antigens.

The difficulty in predicting the occurrence of AIT lies in the fact that the affected mothers appear to be totally healthy. In typical cases of unanticipated AIT the mother is well and has a normal platelet count. Her pregnancy, labor, and delivery are indistinguishable from those of other low-risk obstetric patients. Rarely, a fetal ICH is detected in utero, which in turn leads to the diagnosis of AIT. The disorder in the neonate most often appears almost immediately after birth. The infants are either born with evidence of profound thrombocytopenia, or develop symptomatic thrombocytopenia within hours of birth. Affected neonates often manifest generalized petechiae and/or ecchymoses over the presenting fetal part, most often the scalp. Hemorrhage into viscera and bleeding following circumcision or venipuncture may also ensue. Of greatest concern, however, is the potential for intracranial hemorrhage in 10 to 20% of cases, as many as half of which occur in utero prior to the onset of labor. Fortunately, the neonatal thrombocytopenia is self-limited. It rarely lasts for more than a month, and can usually be treated with IVIG with or without steroids and transfusions of random or maternal platelets. In mild cases, simple observation is adequate. However, there are a significant number of infants affected with intracranial hemorrhage. The sequelae of an intracranial hemorrhage can be devastating and irreversible, although it can initially be clinically silent.[17] The discovery of an intracranial bleed would most certainly have implications for neonatal therapy. Furthermore, the occurrence of an intracranial hemorrhage places subsequent siblings at higher risk for a similar episode. Therefore, it is essential that ultrasound examinations be performed in all thrombocytopenic neonates in order to identify those with an ICH.

The laboratory diagnosis of AIT requires that three requirements be fulfilled. First, a platelet antigen incompatibility must be identified between the parents. This incompatibility is the pathophysiologic basis behind AIT. Second, a platelet antibody needs to be identified in the maternal sera that binds with paternal but not maternal platelets. Finally, and most importantly, the specificity of this antibody must be demonstrated to match the identified platelet antigen incompatibility. The laboratory testing for these antibodies is difficult and time consuming and requires a significant degree of experience in order to be properly performed. All testing for this disorder should be performed in regional laboratories with demonstrated competence in detecting multiple platelet antigens, and sufficient controls to distinguish antibodies directed at each of those antigens.

Subsequent fetuses who carry the same platelet antigen are generally affected to an even greater degree than was a prior sibling who had been affected with AIT.[11] We believe that if the father is unavailable for zygosity testing or known to be a heterozygote for the antigen in question, or there is a question of paternity, amniocentesis, or rarely chorionic villus sampling (CVS), should be performed to determine whether or not the fetus will be affected. In a review of 107 affected fetuses studied in utero prior to receiving any therapy, 50% were found to have initial platelet counts of less than $20,000/\mu L$. This was also true for 21 of 46 fetal platelet counts obtained prior to 24 weeks. Furthermore, this series documented that the fetal platelet count falls at a rate of greater than $15,000/\mu L$ per week if treatment is not administered. Neither the previous affected sibling's birth platelet count nor history of ICH predicted the initial platelet count in utero. In 42% of the cases the initial fetal platelet count was already less than the birth platelet count of the previous affected sibling. This strongly suggests that if treatment is going to be offered in an attempt to prevent intracranial bleeding in utero, it will have to be initiated fairly early in gestation, emphasizing the need for early diagnosis.

The hope that maternal antiplatelet antibody titers could be used to both identify affected fetuses and predict the severity of disease has unfortunately not been realized. While it is true that women with detectable antibodies are at risk of delivering an affected infant, changes in titer do not correlate with the severity of disease, nor does the absence of antibodies guarantee a normal fetal platelet count. At the present time, the only accurate means of estimating the fetal platelet count is to directly sample the fetal blood.

Once fetal thrombocytopenia has been documented, maternal platelets can be transfused into the fetal circulation. These platelets obviously will have different antigens upon their surfaces than those of the fetus, but they will not be destroyed by the maternal antibodies that are directed against paternally derived antigens. However, the transfusion will introduce additional maternal antibody into the fetal circulation and, theoretically, sensitize the fetus to other platelet antigens. This may turn out to be of significant clinical importance.[18] Of even greater importance, however, is the fact that platelets have a short half-life. The half-life of transfused platelets is less than 1 week, as compared to red blood cells, which survive in the fetal circulation for much longer periods of time.[19] Therefore, many weekly fetal platelet transfusions may be necessary if the objective of therapy is to correct the thrombocytopenia up until the time of delivery, resulting in an increased risk of fetal loss due to the multiple procedures. A less invasive approach is to minimize or avoid platelet transfusion altogether by medially treating the fetus through administering IVIG, with or without steroids, to the mother. This therapy is thought to be effective by either reducing maternal antibody production or decreasing its transport across the placenta.[20] A randomized, prospective study of 55 patients with documented AIT has been reported comparing the use of IVIG at a dose of 1 g/kg maternal weight per week, with or without low-dose dexamethasone therapy (1.5 mg/d). This study showed a significant fetal platelet response in approximately 70% of cases. The low-dose dexamethasone did not have any measurable effect on the fetal platelet count, but adding high-dose prednisone (60 mg/d) caused a significant increase in the fetal platelet count in 50% of those who failed treatment with the original regimen. Perhaps most importantly, there were no cases of ICH in the entire series,[21] or in a pilot series of 18 patients that proceeded it.[22, 23] This suggests that IVIG may have a beneficial effect in preventing ICH even if it fails to adequately correct the fetal thrombocytopenia. These results are exciting, as ICH is, as discussed above, the most severe consequence of thrombocytopenia. Other data from smaller studies have been mixed, with some reporting responses to IVIG, and others not.[24] The fetus of one woman being treated with IVIG had an ICH in utero, but that patient, and most other nonresponders, were simultaneously undergoing frequently repeated fetal platelet transfusions.[25]

The issue of performing a diagnostic PUBS procedure to determine the platelet count before initiating therapy is controversial. The risk of bleeding and serious potential sequelae must always be kept in mind. One report describes five fetuses with extremely low platelet counts who exsanguinated at the time of a fetal blood sampling procedure performed for this indication. All of them had platelet counts of less than $20,000/\mu L$, and four had counts less than $10,000/\mu L$. However, if transfusions of packed maternal platelets are administered at the time of the procedure to all fetuses who are found to have counts less than $50,000/\mu L$ this problem can likely be avoided.[26] Despite the controversy, two rationales have been proposed for performing fetal blood sampling in women with AIT.

The first is to determine the severity of the fetal thrombocytopenia before starting therapy, and the other is to determine the effectiveness of the therapy being administered. Simply stated, one is attempting to determine a baseline measurement and follow the progression of treatment. Since there are currently no noninvasively obtainable markers for differentiating severely thrombocytopenic fetuses from those with a higher platelet count, it is impossible to tailor the initial therapy for a particular patient without knowing the actual platelet count. Furthermore, once therapy has been started it is impossible to detect treatment failures or to empirically document treatment successes unless fetal blood sampling is performed.

In summary, AIT is a potentially devastating disease of the fetus that is silent in the mother. Fetal platelet counts are generally much lower in this disorder than in ITP, and the potential for intracranial bleeding is much higher. Effective medical therapy exists for most but not all fetuses with AIT. Optimal management for this disease requires close cooperation between specialists in maternal-fetal medicine and pediatric hematology working with a laboratory that has demonstrated its excellence in typing platelet antigens and detecting specific antiplatelet antibodies.

HELLP Syndrome

The HELLP syndrome is well known to be a serious complication of severe preeclampsia. Women with this condition are at increased risk to develop infection, DIC, renal failure, adult respiratory distress syndrome (ARDS), hepatic infarction and rupture, and congestive heart failure.[1] Reported mortality rates have ranged from 1 to 24%. Management requires expeditious delivery of the fetus and treatment of the associated hypertension and renal, cardiovascular, hematologic, and hepatic abnormalities when indicated.

Thrombocytopenia can most definitely occur in women with severe preeclampsia. The cause of this thrombocytopenia is not known. The underlying vascular disease is associated with activation of the platelets and nonspecific binding of immunoglobulins to their surface. This platelet activation may lead directly to platelet consumption. Alternatively, the bound immunoglobulin molecules may mediate immune platelet destruction, even though they are not specific antiplatelet antibodies.[27]

The thrombocytopenia in this disorder is usually moderate, and the platelet counts rarely fall below $20,000/\mu L$. Clinical hemorrhage is uncommon unless the patient develops DIC. However, a falling maternal platelet count is generally considered to be a sign of worsening disease and is an indication for delivery. Platelet counts usually improve within 24 to 48 hours of delivery, and platelet transfusions should be avoided unless a major hemorrhage occurs. Some evidence suggests that intravenous dexamethasone if given 10 mg at delivery and 12 hours later, followed by 5 mg given at 24 and 36 hours postpartum to women with platelet nadirs below $100,000/\mu L$, results in more rapid reductions in mean arterial pressure and abnormal liver enzymes and increases in urinary output and platelet counts than in those women who were not treated with this regimen.[28] This, however, should be substantiated by larger studies.

The neonates of mothers with the HELLP syndrome have been reported to have an increased incidence of transient leukopenia, but rarely have significant thrombocytopenia or significant bleeding.[29]

TTP-HUS

Thrombotic thrombocytopenic purpura (TTP) and hemolytic uremic syndrome (HUS) are vascular disorders with similar clinical manifestations. In both conditions moderate to severe thrombocytopenia is present. Hemolysis with schistocytes on a peripheral smear, elevated reticulocyte counts, and increased indirect bilirubin and lactate dehydrogenase (LDH) levels are also detected.[30] The differential diagnosis for both of these conditions includes the HELLP syndrome, systemic lupus erythematosis, disseminated intravascular coagulation, sepsis, chronic renal disease, Evans syndrome (autoimmune hemolytic anemia and thrombocytopenia), and HIV infection.

TTP is generally considered to be an acute disorder characterized by the pentad of hemolytic anemia, thrombocytopenia, neurologic symptoms, renal abnormalities, and fever. It can occur in either sex at any age, but is commonly seen in women in the reproductive years, and in pregnancy during the peripartum period. Presenting symptoms can include some or all of the following:

bleeding into mucous membranes, the skin, or per vagina, and jaundice. The patient may also present with a variety of neurologic abnormalities, some of which may be transient and fluctuate in severity. Fever may also be present. Laboratory analysis reveals evidence of a microangiopathic hemolytic anemia, and the blood urea nitrogen (BUN) and creatinine are usually elevated, but rarely go above 100 mg/dL and 3 mg/dL, respectively. Microscopic and, infrequently, macroscopic hematuria may also be present.

The cause of this disorder is unknown; however, it has been hypothesized that it is due to a preponderance of ultra-high-molecular-weight von Willebrand factor multimers released by inflamed vascular endothelium.[31] These multimers induce pathophysiologic platelet adherence and aggregation. This hypothesis, however, has not been proven. The management of TTP consists of plasma infusions (10 mL/kg every 6 hours) or, more definitively, plasma exchange. If the former is ineffective or cannot be tolerated because of problems with fluid overload and hypertension, plasmapheresis should be repeated daily until the LDH level is reduced to less than 300 IU/L. This is usually accomplished in three to five procedures and is associated with an 80 to 90% success rate. Delivery should be performed in patients who are not already postpartum. Plasmapheresis failures have been treated with a variety of modalities including splenectomy, IVIG, and vincristine.[32]

HUS rarely has associated neurologic abnormalities. It does, however, have a far greater degree of renal dysfunction than does TTP. The management of HUS is more difficult because plasma replacement or exchange appears to be less effective than in TTP. Supportive care is critical, and close attention must be paid to impending renal failure and control of hypertension. Peritoneal dialysis or hemofiltration may be required. IVIG has been reported to increase the platelet count in children with this disorder, but its efficacy during the peripartum period is unknown. Platelet transfusions are virtually contraindicated in both HUS and TTP because massive posttransfusion platelet consumption has been associated with fatal thromboembolic events.

In summary, TTP and HUS are rare causes of severe peripartum thrombocytopenia. The degree of maternal illness and hemolytic anemia should differentiate these disorders from more common causes of gestational thrombocytopenia, but DIC and the HELLP syndrome must be ruled out.

Summary

There are numerous causes of thrombocytopenia in pregnancy. These include reactions to drugs or medications, systemic disease, and immunologic phenomena. The presentation of these disorders may vary enormously, and this makes the determination of the cause of the thrombocytopenia particularly challenging. At this time, it is also difficult to predict which fetus will be affected without direct invasive testing, with its attendant risks. As our understanding of the pathophysiology of the various types of fetal thrombocytopenia grows, safer and more accurate means of detecting those who are affected must be developed. It is hoped that this will lead to both earlier diagnosis and more effective treatment of that condition. The dangers and difficulties of performing multiple fetal platelet transfusions have been demonstrated. Expansion of research in the areas of alternative treatments must be undertaken. It is also hoped that through the combined efforts of all involved, better methods of prevention, detection, and treatment of the various types of thrombocytopenia will be developed, leading to a reduction in the potential serious consequences of these disorders.

REFERENCES

1. McCrae KR, Samuels P, Schreiber AD: Pregnancy-associated thrombocytopenia: Pathogenesis and management. Blood 80:2697, 1992.
2. Bussel JB, Cines D: Immune thrombocytopenic purpura, neonatal alloimmune thrombocytopenia and post-transfusion purpura. In Hoffman R, Benz EJ, Shattil S, et al (eds): Hematology: Basic Principles and Practice, 3rd ed. New York: Churchill Livingstone, 1999.
3. George JN, Woolf SH, Gary MPH, et al: Idiopathic thrombocytopenic purpura: The recommendations of the American Society of Hematology. A practice guideline developed by explicit methods for the American Society of Hematology. Blood 88:1:3–40, 1996.
4. Burrows RF, Kelton JG: Incidentally detected thrombocytopenia in healthy mothers and their infants. N Engl J Med 319:142–145, 1988.
5. Samuels P, Bussel JB, Braitman L, et al: Estimation of the risk of thrombocytopenia in the offspring of pregnant women with presumed immune thrombocytopenic purpura. N Engl J Med 323:229–235, 1990.
6. Burrows RF, Kelton JG: Fetal thrombocytopenia and its relation to maternal thrombocytopenia. N Engl J Med 329:1463–1466, 1993.
7. Scott JR, Cruikshank DP, Kochenour NK, et al: Fetal platelet counts in the obstetric management of immunologic thrombocytopenic purpura. Am J Obstet Gynecol 136:495, 1980.
8. Bussel JB, Kramer K, McFarland JG, et al, and the Neonatal Alloimmune Thrombocytopenia Registry Group: The clinical features of neonatal alloimmune thrombocytopenia: A bedside diagnostic index. (Submitted.)
9. Lescale KB, Eddleman KA, Cines B, et al: Antiplatelet antibody testing in the thrombocytopenic pregnant women. Am J Obstet Gynecol 3:1014–1018, 1996.
10. Bussel JB: Immune thrombocytopenia in pregnancy: Autoimmune and alloimmune. J Reprod Immunol 37:35–61, 1997.
11. Bussel JB, Zabusky MR, Berkowitz RL, McFarland JG: Fetal alloimmune thrombocytopenia. N Engl J Med 337:22–26, 1997.
12. Bussel JB, Druzin ML, Cines DB, Samuels P: Thrombocytopenia in pregnancy. Lancet 337:251, 1991.
13. Medeiros D, Buchanan GR: Major hemorrhage in children with idiopathic thrombocytopenic purpura: Immediate response to therapy and long-term outcome. J Pediatr 133:334–339, 1998.
14. Ballem PJ, Buskard N, Wittman BK, et al: ITP in pregnancy: Use of the bleeding time as an indicator for treatment. Blut 59:132, 1989.
15. Adams DM, Bussel JB, Druzin ML: Accurate intrapartum estimation of fetal platelet count by fetal scalp sample smear. Am J Perinatol 11:42–45, 1994.
16. Schulman NR, Marder VJ, Heller MC, Collier EM: Platelet and leukocyte isoantigens and their antibodies: Serologic, physiologic and clinical studies. Prog Hematol 4:222–304, 1964.
17. Bussel JB, Tanli S, Peterson HC: Favorable neurological outcome in 7 cases of perinatal intracranial hemorrhage due to immune thrombocytopenia. Am J Pediatr 13:156–159, 1991.
18. Murphy MF, Waters AH, Doughty HA, et al: Antenatal management of fetomaternal alloimmune thrombocytopenia—report of 15 affected pregnancies. Transfus Med 4:281–292, 1994.
19. Kaplan C, Daffos F, Forestier F, et al: Management of alloimmune thrombocytopenia: Antenatal diagnosis and in utero transfusion of maternal platelets. Blood 72:340–343, 1988.

20. Bussel JB, Berkowitz RL, McFarland JG: Mechanisms of IVIG effect in fetal alloimmune thrombocytopenia [letter]. Br J Haematol 98:495–497, 1997.
21. Bussel JB, Berkowitz RL, Lynch L, et al: Antenatal management of alloimmune thrombocytopenia with intravenous gammaglobulin: A randomized trial of the addition of low dose steroids to IVIG in fifty-five maternal-fetal pairs. Am J Obstet Gynecol 174:1414–1423, 1996.
22. Bussel JB, Berkowitz RL, McFarland JG, et al: Antenatal treatment of neonatal alloimmune thrombocytopenia. N Engl J Med 319:1374–1378, 1998.
23. Lynch L, Bussel JB, McFarland JG, et al: Antenatal treatment of alloimmune thrombocytopenia. Obstet Gynecol 80:67–71, 1992.
24. Bussel JB, Skupski DW, McFarland J: Fetal alloimmune thrombocytopenia: Consensus and controversy. J Matern Fetal Med 5:281–292, 1996.
25. Kroll H, Kiefel V, Giers G, et al: Maternal intravenous immunoglobulin treatment to prevent intracranial haemorrhage in fetal alloimmune thrombocytopenia. Transfus Med 4:293–296, 1994.
26. Paidas MJ, Berkowitz RL, Lynch L, et al: Alloimmune thrombocytopenia: Fetal and neonatal losses related to cordocentesis. Am J Obstet Gynecol 172:475–479, 1995.
27. Saphier CJ, Repke JT: Hemolysis, elevated liver enzymes, and low platelets (HELLP) syndrome: A review of diagnosis and management. Semin Perinatol 22:118–133, 1988.
28. Vigil-De Gracia P, Garcia-Caceres E: Dexamethasone in the postpartum treatment of HELLP syndrome. Int J Gynaecol Obstet 59:217–221, 1997.
29. Koenig JM, Christensen RD: Incidence, neutrophil kinetics, and natural history of neonatal neutropenia associated with maternal hypertension. N Engl J Med 321:557–562, 1989.
30. Moschcowitz E: Hyaline thrombosis of the terminal arterioles and capillaries: A hitherto undescribed disease. Proc N Y Pathol Soc 24:21, 1924.
31. Moake JL, Rudy CK, Troll JH, et al: Usually large plasma factor VIII: von Willebrand factor multimers in chronic relapsing thrombotic thrombocytopenic purpura. N Engl J Med 23:1432–1435, 1982.
32. Moake JL: Thrombotic thrombocytopenic purpura and the hemolytic uremic syndrome. Hematology 127:1879–1889, 1995.

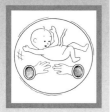

37

The Fetus with a Hematopoietic Stem Cell Defect

ALAN W. FLAKE

The engraftment and clonal proliferation of a relatively small number of normal hematopoietic stem cells (HSC) can sustain normal hematopoiesis for a lifetime. This observation provides the compelling rationale for bone marrow transplantation (BMT) and is now supported by thousands of long-term survivors of BMT who would otherwise have succumbed to lethal hematologic disease. However, realization of the full potential of BMT continues to be limited by a critical shortage of immunologically compatible donor cells, the inability to specifically control the recipient or donor immune response, and the requirement for recipient myeloablation to achieve engraftment. The price of HLA mismatch remains high: the greater the mismatch, the higher the incidence of graft failure, graft-versus-host disease (GVHD), and delayed immunologic reconstitution. Current methods of myeloablation cause high morbidity and mortality. In combination, these problems remain prohibitive for the majority of patients who might benefit from BMT. A theoretically attractive alternative, which can potentially address many of the limitations of BMT, is in utero HSC transplantation. This approach is potentially applicable to any congenital hematopoietic disease that can be diagnosed prenatally, and can be cured or improved by engraftment of normal HSCs.

With the application of biochemical and molecular approaches to prenatal diagnosis, there are an increasing number of congenital hematopoietic diseases that can now be prenatally diagnosed. Indeed, in the future, it is likely that all potential target diseases will be diagnosed at an early stage of gestation. In this circumstance, unique aspects of fetal development may allow treatment of the disease with reduced morbidity, mortality, and cost, relative to treatment after birth. It is the purpose of this chapter to review the theoretical, experimental and, at the present time, limited clinical support, for this approach.

An Experiment of Nature

Perhaps the most compelling argument for the potential of in utero HSC transplantation comes from an experiment of nature. Owen[1] in 1945 observed that dizygotic cattle twins with shared placental circulation were chimeric for their siblings' blood cells after birth. Subsequent investigators confirmed that chimeric animals were specifically tolerant for skin grafts[2] and organ grafts[3] from their sibling donor. Natural chimerism arising from shared placental circulation has also been observed in a number of other species, most notably primates,[4] and humans.[5] The cotton-top tamarin, a New World primate species, has a high incidence of natural chimerism with documentation of stable donor cell chimerism of greater than 80% in some animals. The incidence of human chimerism in monochorionic, dizygotic pregnancies is around 8% when sensitive detection methodology is used, and natural human chimeras with all levels of donor cell chimerism, including marked donor cell predominance, have been observed.[6] These observations are proof of principle for in utero stem cell transplantation. They confirm that under specific circumstances, circulating allogeneic stem cells can effectively compete, and stably engraft, and that normal host hematopoiesis is not prohibitive to the engraftment of donor cells.

Fetal Immunologic Tolerance

Owen's observations of natural chimerism led to the experimental work of Billingham, Brent, and Medawar[7] that promoted the concept of "acquired" immunologic tolerance. These studies suggested that early presentation of cellular antigen resulted in specific immunologic tolerance. Long-term tolerance could only be achieved during a period of immunologic immaturity and was best accomplished by transplantation of living cells. Evidence is now overwhelming that the fetal thymic microenvironment plays a primary role in determination of self-recognition and repertoire of response to foreign antigen. Pre–T cells undergo positive and negative selection during a series of maturational steps in the fetal thymus that are controlled by thymic stromal cells.[8, 9] The end result is deletion of T-cell clones with high affinity for self-antigen in association with self-MHC, and preservation of a T-cell repertoire against foreign

591

antigen. Single positive (post-thymic) lymphocytes are first seen in the peripheral circulation of the fetus at around 12 to 14 weeks' gestation.[10] Theoretically, introduction of foreign cells prior to completion of the thymic negative selection process would result in processing of foreign antigen as "self" with secondary specific tolerance on the basis of clonal deletion of alloreactive T-cells. It is important to note, however, that the mechanism of central thymic tolerance has been defined primarily in T-cell-receptor (TCR) transgenic mice. In these mice, thymic maturation of lymphocytes occurs in an environment of unregulated high levels of TCR with high affinity for a specific self-antigen, and which is expressed from the earliest to the latest stages of thymic development.[10–13] This is distinct from the clinical situation following in utero HSC transplantation in which there are a large number of circulating antigens interacting with recipient TCRs which vary in affinity for donor antigen. Differences in thymic maturation of lymphocytes in normal mice from the defined mechanisms in TCR transgenic mice have been recognized.[14, 15]

It is important to emphasize that the presence of phenotypically mature lymphocytes does not necessarily equate to their immunologic function and the capacity for rejection, and that the limit of tolerance in the human fetus has not been defined. Also, there are undoubtedly other mechanisms of tolerance that must occur to allow long-term engraftment.[16] Mechanisms of B-cell or peripheral tolerance exist but are less well understood. It is known that exposure of immature B cells to foreign antigen can result in clonal deletion or anergy depending upon the complexity and valency of the antigen presented. Thus, early gestational exposure, when the majority of B cells in the marrow and other sites are phenotypically immature,[17] should facilitate these mechanisms.

The Fetal Hematopoietic Environment

One of the biologically unique aspects of in utero HSC transplantation is the recipient microenvironment. Postnatal bone marrow transplantation generally requires ablative radiation or chemotherapy to achieve donor HSC engraftment, with a goal of replacement of all recipient-derived hematopoiesis. In contrast, engraftment following in utero transplantation is based on competitive population of available receptive sites (Fig. 37–1), with a goal of achieving an adequate level of mixed chimerism to ameliorate a disease. The receptive sites for homing and engraftment of transplanted cells are dynamic and dependent upon the gestational age of the recipient. Fetal hematopoiesis is characterized by an orderly series of migrational events proceeding from the yolk sac and/or periaortic splanchnopleure, to the fetal liver, and finally to the bone marrow (Fig. 37–2).[18, 19] Although regulation of these events is poorly understood, this process is presumably controlled by sequential expression and/or down-regulation of homing receptors and their corresponding ligands on the surface of microenvironmental cells and HSCs. Thus, the migration of fetal hematopoiesis is probably best viewed as

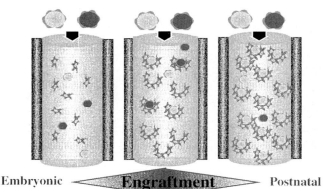

FIGURE 37–1. Schematic of the fetal hematopoietic microenvironment and the concept of "competitive population" of receptive sites. Donor and host HSC, depicted by pink and purple nuclei, respectively, circulate through the fetal microenvironment following transplantation. Prior to development of the fetal liver or bone marrow there are no receptive sites for engraftment of circulating cells (embryonic). As the microenvironment forms, stromal elements form into supportive "niches" which allow homing and engraftment of HSC. During this "window of opportunity" donor cells can compete for new receptive sites. Once the bone marrow is fully populated (postnatal), the receptive sites are occupied preventing engraftment of donor cells without a myeloablative preparative regimen. The critical independent role of immunologic ontogeny in the permissive fetal environment is discussed in the text. *See Color Plate.*

a sequential development of organ-specific microenvironmental "niches" of increasing HSC affinity. After in utero HSC transplantation, homing and engraftment of donor cells will depend upon the gestational age of the recipient and the availability of open niches. Studies of homing after in utero transplantation suggest that the pattern of engraftment recapitulates ontogeny.[20]

The human bone marrow begins as a cartilaginous matrix. Calcification and breakdown of the matrix accompany the arrival of osteoclasts at around 10 weeks' gestation. The marrow cavity becomes populated by macrophages and other stromal elements prior to the migration of hematopoietic elements and contains only stromal elements at 12 weeks' gestation. The first hematopoietic elements begin to appear around 15 weeks' gestation, and bone marrow hematopoiesis is not predominant until around 34 weeks' gestation.[21] During this period there is exponential expansion of the bone marrow compartment accompanied by expansion of the number and density of hematopoietic cells. This suggests that there is a period during gestation when the bone marrow is forming new "niches" and may be receptive to the engraftment of circulating HSC.

In the context of in utero transplantation, these concepts combined with the phenomenon of fetal tolerance suggest that there is a "window of opportunity" (Fig. 37–3) in the fetus during which donor cells could be engrafted without myeloablation or the risk of rejection. At the same time, the success of engraftment is clearly dependent upon the ability of donor cells to compete with recipient cells for available sites. The biology of specific disease states may influence this competitive balance favorably, or unfavorably. For the majority of

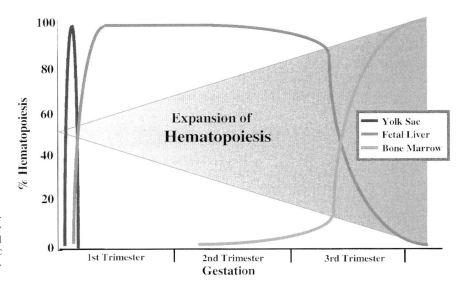

FIGURE 37–2. Normal hematopoietic ontogeny. Schematic depiction of normal migratory events during hematopoietic development and the exponential expansion in the hematopoietic compartment which occurs during this period. *See Color Plate.*

diseases, however, it is likely that strategies that improve the competitive advantage of donor cells will be required for success.

Animal Studies Supporting In Utero Transplantation

The first experimental studies supporting engraftment of donor cells after in utero transplantation were the classic studies of Billingham, Brent, and Medawar, who documented donor-specific tolerance for skin grafts after fetal or neonatal transplantation in mice.[7] Although chimerism was not analyzed, it can now be assumed that tolerant animals were chimeric for donor cells.[22, 23] Subsequent animal studies are best analyzed in the context of the model and whether or not a competitive advantage is present for donor cells.

Experimental Hematopoietic Chimerism After In Utero HSC Transplantation in Normal Animal Models

The most successful normal animal model is the sheep. Early gestational transplantation of allogeneic fetal liver-derived HSC into normal sheep fetuses results in a high rate of sustained multilineage hematopoietic chimerism that persists for many years[24] and is typically in the range of 10 to 15% BM and peripheral blood donor cell expression. The fetal sheep model is also permissive for widely disparate xenogeneic engraftment. Multilineage hematopoietic chimerism has been well documented after human fetal liver-derived HSC transplantation[25] and after transplantation of a variety of human cord blood and adult BM-derived populations.[26–30] In addition, we have shown that chimerism in the human sheep model is due to the engraftment of pluripotent HSC by documentation of long-term repopulation by donor cells

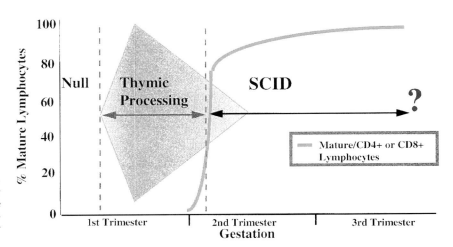

FIGURE 37–3. A schematic of normal immunologic ontogeny, depicting the concept of a "window of opportunity" for in utero transplantation. The late limit for successful engraftment in humans has not been defined, particularly for immunodeficiency disorders like SCID. *See Color Plate.*

on retransplantation into second-generation fetal lamb recipients.[31] In contrast to the sheep, however, other normal animal models have shown much greater resistance to engraftment after in utero transplantation. Although chimerism has been achieved in the normal primate,[32] goat,[33] rat,[34] and mouse,[34–39] the levels of engraftment are much lower and well below what might be expected to be therapeutic in most hematologic target diseases. Chimerism achieved in the normal mouse model following allogeneic or xenogeneic in utero HSC transplantation has generally been below the level of flow cytometric detection but has been detectable by the polymerase chain reaction (PCR).

Experimental Hematopoietic Chimerism after In Utero HSC Transplantation in Impaired Animal Models

In contrast to normal animal models, it is clear that under circumstances where there is a competitive advantage for normal cells, high levels of donor cell engraftment can be expected. This was first demonstrated by Fleischman and Mintz[40] in studies in W mutant anemic mouse strains which have a stem cell deficiency based on the absence of c-kit. In utero transplantation of normal allogeneic fetal liver cells by transplacental injection at 11 days' gestation resulted in rescue of severely anemic mice and complete replacement by donor hematopoiesis. The degree of erythroid replacement correlated with the degree of underlying anemia, with complete early replacement by donor erythroid cells in the lethally anemic W/W homozygotes, and partial but progressively increasing replacement by donor erythroid cells in the sublethally anemic W^v/W^v homozygotes. Donor white blood cell engraftment was also seen (in the W^v/W^v recipients) but was not as extensive as erythroid engraftment, mirroring the underlying severity of the lineage defect. Similarly, in the mouse severe combined immunodeficiency (SCID) model in which there is early arrest of T and B cell development, Blazar et al. have demonstrated lymphoid reconstitution following in utero HSC transplantation.[36] In successfully reconstituted animals, T and B lymphocytes were entirely of donor origin. Although donor myeloid and erythroid elements could not be consistently detected, the engraftment of donor HSC in the marrow was clearly documented by retransplantation experiments. Thus, in the presence of a lineage deficiency in utero HSC transplantation can selectively reconstitute the defective lineage, but it appears that competitive pressure from the normal nonaffected host lineages prevents high-level multilineage donor cell expression. Recent studies in the NOD/SCID mouse confirm and expand upon these observations.[41] In this model, the defect in T- and B-cell development is the same as the SCID mouse but in addition there are known defects in natural killer (NK) cells and antigen presentation.[42] In utero HSC transplantation in NOD/SCID recipients results in multilineage engraftment with increasing donor cell expression over time. The differences between donor cell engraftment in the SCID and NOD/SCID recipient include increased my-

eloid and B-cell expression with higher levels of BM hematopoiesis in NOD/SCID.

To summarize, experimental results in animal models support the feasibility of in utero HSC transplantation. Although limited studies have been performed in animal models that replicate the biology of human disease, there is evidence that if there is a selective advantage for normal cells, in utero transplantation can be curative. It is also clear that even in hematopoietically normal recipients, host cell competition is not prohibitive to limited donor HSC engraftment and that, in the sheep model, this engraftment can be substantial. Once engraftment occurs it appears to be stable with no evidence of immunologic rejection. Although engraftment can be achieved, the primary limitation to successful clinical application is the relatively low level of donor cell expression. The low levels of chimerism achieved in experimental studies, particularly in normal animal models other than the sheep, are inadequate to effectively treat the majority of potential target diseases. The future of in utero HSC transplantation depends upon developing successful strategies to provide a competitive advantage for donor cell engraftment with an ultimate increase in donor cell expression.

Considerations for Clinical Application

Consideration of the above supports the rationale for prenatal HSC transplantation. The potential clinical advantages of the prenatal approach over postnatal BMT are summarized in Table 37–1. These potential advantages must be weighed against the associated maternal and fetal risk. It should be emphasized that prenatal transplantation does not preclude conventional postnatal therapy. From an ethical perspective, it would be inappropriate to withhold beneficial postnatal therapy if prenatal transplantation fails or is only partially effective.

Maternal and Fetal Risk

Maternal and fetal risk can be divided into procedural and nonprocedural risk. The risk of fetal loss with chorionic villus sampling (CVS) has been well documented and is less than 1%.[43] The risk of procedure-related fetal loss with intraperitoneal or intravascular transplanta-

T A B L E 37–1. POTENTIAL ADVANTAGES OF IN UTERO HSC TX

ADVANTAGE	EFFECT
Immunologic tolerance	No HLA-restriction/immunosuppression
BM space available	No myeloablation
Sterile "isolation"	No posttransplant isolation
Proliferative environment	Potential competitive advantage—normal cells
Preempts clinical disease	Avoids morbidity/suffering

tion of HSC in the first to second trimester is unknown, but extrapolation from the extensive experience with intraperitoneal transfusion for fetal Rh disease is reasonable. There are differences, however, which need elaboration. There are a number of factors that increase the risk of fetal loss in treatment of Rh disease that are not present with in utero HSC transplantation. Intraperitoneal transfusion when used for treatment of Rh disease involves placement of a catheter into the fetal peritoneal cavity via the lumen of a 16-gauge needle with infusion of a relatively large volume of cells. In contrast, in utero HSC transplantation is usually carried out using no larger than a 22-gauge needle and involves less than 1 mL of injectate. The early gestational age and small size of the fetal recipient, on the other hand, may increase the relative risk of in utero stem cell transplantation. In balance, the increased risk of fetal loss following a single in utero transplant procedure is probably on the lower end of the risk for intraperitoneal transfusion, which has been estimated to be between 0.8 and 3.5% in various series,[44] and we currently estimate a risk of around 1% per transplant when counseling patients. It goes without saying that these risk assessments only apply to centers with extensive experience with these techniques.

Nonprocedural risks to the mother and fetus include the risk of transmissible infectious disease, and GVHD. The risk of transmissible infectious disease is dependent upon the donor source used and the donor cell screening process. This represents the primary obstacle to the use of fetal tissue,[45] as there currently exist no quality controls on procurement, preparation, or donor screening. With adult-derived tissues, standard protocols and procedures used to screen donors for bone marrow transplantation can be utilized. Clinical bone marrow transplant laboratories can be utilized and the high level of quality control established for cell processing for bone marrow transplantation maintained. The risk of fetal GVHD is also dependent upon the donor tissue used. Postnatal experience in immunocompromised bone marrow transplant recipients suggests that transplantation of more than 1×10^5 mature T lymphocytes per kilogram introduces the risk of GVHD.[46] Undoubtedly, fetuses with immunodeficiency disorders are at greater risk than other disease groups for this complication. It is well documented that newborns with severe combined immunodeficiency disease have a significant incidence of maternal versus fetal GVHD without transplantation.[47, 48] The two surviving recipients of CD34-enriched adult marrow with X-SCID received doses of 1.1×10^5 CD3+ cells/kg fetal weight, or less, per injection and neither had clinical evidence of GVHD.[49, 50] Thus, this appears to be a relatively safe minimal dose of T cells for clinical in utero transplantation.

Diseases Potentially Amenable to In Utero HSC Transplantation

Theoretically, any disease that can be diagnosed early in gestation and can be cured by postnatal BMT could potentially be treated by in utero stem cell transplantation. In reality, each disease is biologically unique and some diseases are clearly more favorable candidates than others. Diseases in which there is a selective advantage favoring normal cells, or diseases that can be corrected by expression of a small percentage of donor cells are the most favorable. Other diseases may have distinct biologic disadvantages. Table 37–2 is a partial list of candidate diseases arranged into groups, each of which are discussed below.

Immunodeficiency Disorders

The immunodeficiency disorders are a heterogeneous group of diseases that may or may not be biologically favorable for in utero transplantation. However, most of the highly favorable diseases are in this category. As already demonstrated in X-SCID,[49, 50] a survival advantage for a specific host lineage, particularly when manifest at the early stages of lineage commitment, can result in a powerful amplification of peripheral donor cell expression of the affected lineage. In one case,[49] although only 3% of bone marrow CD34+ cells and 20% of CD34 + CD38− cells were donor in origin, the patient had split chimerism with 100% of his peripheral T cells of donor origin. Most other known forms of SCID (i.e., ADA deficiency, Jak 3, ZAP-70) as well as some other

TABLE 37–2. CONGENITAL DISEASES POTENTIALLY AMENABLE TO IN UTERO STEM CELL TRANSPLANTATION (INCOMPLETE LIST)

Hemoglobinopathies
  β-Thalassemia major
  α-Thalassemia major
  Sickle cell disease

Immunodeficiency Diseases
  Severe combined immunodeficiency syndrome
  Bare lymphocyte syndrome
  Chronic granulomatous disease
  Wiskott-Aldrich syndrome
  Chediak-Higashi syndrome
  Infantile agranulocytosis (Kostman syndrome)
  Neutrophil membrane GP-180 deficiency
  X-linked lymphoproliferative syndrome
  X-linked hyper-IgM syndrome

Inborn Errors of Metabolism

Mucopolysaccharidoses
  Hurler disease (MPS-1) (α-iduronidase deficiency)
  Hurler-Scheie syndrome
  Hunter disease (MPS-II) (iduronate sulfatase deficiency)
  Sanfilippo B (MPS-IIIB) (α-glycosaminidase deficiency)
  Morquio (MPS-IV) (hexosamine-6-sulfatase deficiency)
  Maroteaux-Lamy syndrome (MPS-VI) (arylsulfatase B deficiency)
  Sly syndrome (MPS-VII) (β-glucuronidase deficiency)

Mucolipidoses
  Fabry disease (α-galactosidase A deficiency)
  Gaucher disease (glucocerebrosidase deficiency)
  Krabbe disease (galactosylceramidase deficiency)
  Metachromatic leukodystrophy (arylsulfatase A deficiency)
  Niemann-Pick disease (sphingomyelinase deficiency)
  Adrenal leukodystrophy
  I-cell mucolipidosis II

Other Hematopoietic Disease
  Osteopetrosis
  Diamond-Blackfan syndrome
  Fanconi anemia

diseases, such as X-linked (Bruton's) agammaglobulinemia,[51] could be expected to have similar amplification. In other immunodeficiency diseases, such as chronic granulomatous disease[52] or hyperimmunoglobulin M (IgM) syndrome,[53] even very low levels of donor cell engraftment may suffice to effect a cure. Each immunodeficiency disorder has its own biologic considerations and they must be considered on an individual basis. A unique aspect of the immunodeficiency disorders, particularly those with defective cellular immune response, is the potential for extension of the immunologic "window of opportunity." It may be possible to transplant these diseases much later than those with intact immune systems because of their inherent defect in cellular rejection.

Hemoglobinopathies

Hemoglobinopathies are another biologically attractive target for in utero HSC therapy. Although clinical efforts to treat β–thalassemia by in utero transplantation have thus far failed, there is reason to be optimistic. The Italian experience with postnatal bone marrow transplantation for β–thalassemia has been informative. Lucarreli and his group have reported that stable mixed chimerism of 20% donor cell engraftment is adequate to clinically ameliorate the disease.[54] Similarly, in sickle cell anemia, a patient has been reported after postnatal transplantation with mixed chimerism with 10 to 20% donor cell engraftment in the bone marrow but greater than 70% normal hemoglobin (Hb) in peripheral blood and clinical cure of the disease.[55] There is clearly a profound survival advantage of normal red cells (half-life, 120 days) compared to thalassemia or sickle red cells (half-life, <10 days) after release from the bone marrow compartment. Thus, with levels of engraftment comparable to those achieved in the allogeneic sheep model, clinical cure might be achieved. Even with low-level engraftment, a strategy of prenatal transplantation with induction of low-level chimerism and specific hematopoietic tolerance, followed by postnatal "booster" transplants from the same donor, may be feasible. In our opinion, an exception to the favorable status of the hemoglobinopathies is homozygous α-thalassemia. Since synthesis of hemoglobin F is α-globin dependent and Hb F is the major Hb of the fetus after 8 weeks' gestation,[56] ineffective erythropoiesis and fetal anemia are present by 10 weeks' gestation.[57] This leads to hypercellularity of hematopoietic sites in the fetus and abnormal extramedullary hematopoiesis that, at least theoretically, would make it even more difficult for donor cells to effectively compete for engraftment sites.

Inborn Errors of Metabolism

A final group of diseases are the inborn errors of metabolism. These are a heterogeneous group of diseases that are caused by a deficiency of a specific lysosomal hydrolase, which results in the accumulation of substrates such as mucopolysaccharide, glycogen, or sphingolipid.[58] Depending upon the specific enzyme abnormality and the compound(s) that accumulates, specific patterns of tissue damage and organ failure occur. The purpose of BMT in these diseases is to provide HSC-derived mononuclear cells that can repopulate various organs in the body including the liver (Kupffer cells), skin (Langerhans cells), lung (alveolar macrophages), spleen (macrophages), lymph nodes, tonsils, and the brain (microglia). Those that have been corrected by postnatal BMT such as Gaucher disease[59] or Maroteaux-Lamy syndrome[60] (minimal central nervous system [CNS] involvement) may be reasonable candidates for prenatal transplantation. In some diseases postnatal BMT has corrected the peripheral manifestations of the disease and has arrested the neurologic deterioration, but not reversed preexisting neurologic injury (i.e., metachromatic leukodystrophy and Hurler disease).[61] In these diseases the neurologic injury may begin before birth. This provides a compelling rationale for prenatal treatment. The primary question is whether donor HSC-derived microglial elements would populate the CNS providing the necessary metabolic correction within the blood-brain barrier. In a sheep model, ceroid-lipofuscinosis prenatal transplantation, with average levels of donor cell chimerism in the bone marrow, failed to affect the clinical course of the disease.[62] Maturation of the blood-brain barrier restricts access to the CNS of transplanted cells or the deficient enzyme. Although there is good evidence for origin of CNS glial cells from HSC, the timing of their differentiation and migration to the CNS is unclear and probably quite early.[63] Thus, even with relatively high levels of systemic engraftment, there may be inadequate enzyme production within the CNS to effect a cure. At the present time, this group of diseases is the least biologically attractive group for in utero HSC transplantation, although a number of prenatal gene therapy strategies appear promising.

Source of Donor Cells

Early experimental and clinical efforts at in utero hematopoietic stem cell transplantation utilized fetal liver- or fetal liver- and thymus-derived cells because of the fear of GVHD, and the potential proliferative and engraftment advantages of fetal donor cells placed into a fetal environment. However, there are significant practical, safety, and ethical issues associated with fetal tissue. Using standard techniques for abortion, there is a very high rate of fetal abdominal disruption and bacterial or fungal contamination of the liver.[45] The risk of transmissible viral disease is difficult to eliminate. In addition, the cell yields may be low, requiring the use of multiple fetal specimens. Because fetal tissue is not always electively available, the cells may have to be frozen or cultured ex vivo with a resultant potential loss of hematopoietic stem cells. A reported experience with in utero transplantation of three fetuses with hemoglobinopathies using cryopreserved fetal liver-derived cells failed to document engraftment.[64] In the absence of freezing or ex vivo culture and expansion, fetal cells are not renewable, making postnatal transplants in the prenatally tolerized recipient impossible. Finally, there are ethical issues intrinsic to the use of tissue from abortuses that are difficult to resolve.[65]

Because of the problems with fetal cells, postnatal donor sources have been investigated. Studies have confirmed that the fetus is exquisitely susceptible to GVHD. Experiments in which unprocessed adult bone marrow has been transplanted into fetal lambs have uniformly resulted in fatal GVHD.[66] Early experimental efforts at fetal transplantation of T-cell–depleted bone marrow had high rates of failure of engraftment or much lower levels of engraftment than similar studies using fetal cells. The rate of GVHD was found to be directly related to the number of T cells transplanted.[67] Clinical attempts at fetal transplantation using T-cell–depleted marrow, which were followed to term, failed to engraft, although donor cells were found in extramedullary sites of one fetus with α–thalassemia aborted at 24 weeks, after transplantation at 18 weeks, because a fetal blood sampling revealed no donor cell expression.[68] Thus, it would appear that T-cell–depleted bone marrow, using current techniques, is probably not an optimal source of donor cells.

Recently, methods have been developed to enrich hematopoietic cell populations for stem cells based on surface differentiation markers specific for early hematopoietic progenitors. These methods simultaneously deplete mature T cells to varying degrees, reducing the likelihood of GVHD. A number of highly enriched human BM-derived cell populations have been transplanted in the fetal lamb model with successful creation of sustained multilineage xenogeneic chimerism without GVHD.[26–28, 30, 69] The level of chimerism, however, is very low in the xenogeneic human/sheep model, making quantitative comparisons of levels of chimerism between donor sources difficult. The extent of stem cell enrichment and accompanying depletion of accessory bone marrow cells that is optimal for successful engraftment without GVHD has not been clearly defined. What is clear is that the number of T cells transplanted must be minimized. The recent clinical successes of two different methods of CD34 enrichment of adult marrow-derived donor cells is encouraging and, at the present time, CD34-enriched donor cells with an adequate degree of T-cell depletion may be the safest and most practical source of donor cells for clinical transplantation.

Other possible sources worthy of consideration include cord blood and peripheral blood-derived stem cells. Stem cells derived from cord blood may have proliferative and engraftment advantages over postnatal cells,[70] similar to fetal-derived cells, but do not have the associated risk of contamination. Cord blood does contain mature T lymphocytes and has induced GVHD after in utero transplantation in the fetal lamb model.[71] Peripheral stem cell harvest may provide an excellent, renewable source of donor HSC, but unanswered questions exist regarding a possible increased risk of GVHD as well as the durability of reconstitution after transplantation.

In summary, the predominant concerns in the consideration of potential donor sources remain fetal and maternal safety. Thus, emphasis should be placed on sterility, absence of transmissible viral infection, and absolute T-cell depletion. In addition, the practical concern of renewability of specific donor cells, at the present time, favors adult sources. In the future, progress in ex vivo culture, expansion, and preservation of fetal- or cord blood-derived HSC may favor the use of these potentially valuable and currently wasted resources.

Dose of Donor Cells and Number of Transplants

There is little evidence supporting the concept that donor cell engraftment can be dramatically increased by increasing the dose of donor cells in a single administration. In the fetal lamb model, log-fold increases in either allogeneic or xenogeneic cells between 10^4 and 10^{11} cells/kg fetal weight results in a dose-engraftment curve consistent with saturation kinetics.[72] This would make sense if the number of available receptive sites limited engraftment. The fetal environment can be viewed as a competitive environment where host and donor cells are competing for a fixed number of receptive sites. Although these "niches" are presumably expanding in number during development, they are probably limited at any particular time. Clinical transplantation of a very large number of cells in a single dose is therefore unlikely to increase engraftment, but may increase the absolute number of T cells transplanted above the threshold for GVHD. This probably occurred in a reported case of in utero transplantation for globoid leukodystrophy in which an effort to transplant a large number of cells resulted in transplantation of in excess of 10^7 CD3+ cells/kg fetal weight into a 13-week-gestation fetus. The fetus died at 20 weeks' gestation, with autopsy findings in an autolyzed fetus of massive "extramedullary hematopoiesis."[73] The authors of this report have not convincingly excluded GVHD as the cause of fetal demise. Thus at the current time it seems that cell doses in the range of 10^6 to 10^8 cells/kg fetal weight are probably adequate to achieve engraftment and log-fold higher doses may have deleterious effects unless concomitant T-cell depletion can be achieved.

The relative benefit versus risk of transplanting donor cells in one versus divided doses has not been fully resolved. Theoretically, based on the argument above, repeated injections spaced far enough apart to allow generation of new niches in the recipient should result in increased numbers of engrafted donor HSC. There is experimental evidence in the fetal lamb model that supports the efficacy of dividing a dose of cells into three transplants versus a single transplant (E. Zanjani and A. Flake, unpublished data). Further experimental work needs to be done before absolute recommendations can be made.

Clinical Experience with In Utero HSC Transplantation

At the present time there has been limited clinical success with in utero HSC transplantation. We are aware of a total of 24 in utero HSC transplants reported or discussed in the literature including the initial report by Linch[74] in 1986. They have been performed for a variety of diseases, at various gestational ages, using different donor cell preparations. We will discuss transplants performed for each disease category separately.

Immunodeficiency Disorders

Clinical success with in utero HSC transplantation has thus far been limited to the immunodeficiency diseases. There have been eight reported attempts to treat fetuses with immunodeficiency disorders by in utero transplantation (Table 37–3). Four of these have been reported successful, one was terminated prior to adequate analysis, two did not engraft, and one had a procedure-related death. Touraine has reported three immunodeficiency cases; one patient with "bare lymphocyte syndrome"[75] one patient a female with presumed autosomal SCID,[76] and one fetus with chronic granulomatous disease (CGD) who died following the transplant.[77] In both survivors, fetal engraftment was achieved by transplantation of fetal liver- and thymus-derived donor cells with the initial transplant at 28 and 26 weeks. Multiple transplants from different donors, including postnatal transplants in the SCID patient, complicate analysis. There has been minimal engraftment data published on these patients, particularly beyond 1 year of age, but they are reported to be healthy. There have been two cases of X-linked SCID treated using a similar approach. We recently reported an unequivocally successful case of treatment of X-linked SCID by the in utero transplantation of CD34-enriched paternal bone marrow.[49] This patient received a series of three intraperitoneal transplants at 16, 17.5, and 18.5 weeks' gestation. He is now 40 months old with split chimerism (Fig. 37–4) and full T-lymphocyte reconstitution. He has had no significant infections or hospitalizations. He has evidence of donor-derived stem cells in the marrow and has increasing evidence of donor NK-cell and B-cell expression and humoral response. He has required four doses of intravenous immunoglobulin (IVIG) during his life for low IgG levels but currently maintains low normal IgG levels and has normal titers of specific antibodies to tetanus, diphtheria, haemophilus, and polio 1 and 2 vaccines.

Using a similar protocol, Wengler[50] reported a second case of X-SCID transplanted with CD34-enriched paternal marrow at 21 and 22 weeks' gestation. Donor T cells were present in cord blood; however, the child was only 4 months old at the time of this report.

The failures in this category include an autosomal SCID fetus transplanted by combined intraperitoneal and intravenous injection with T-cell–depleted maternal marrow at 20 weeks' gestation.[78] Analysis of umbilical blood at 24 weeks revealed no donor cells, and the fetus was aborted. No autopsy was performed. Possible explanations for failure in this patient include premature analysis and the use of T-cell–depleted marrow. We have shown in the sheep that there is no peripheral donor cell expression even in successful transplants until near term.[20] Hence, strategies of fetal blood sampling to determine engraftment are likely to be misleading. We have also been unable to engraft adult BM that has been T-cell depleted without enrichment in the sheep model, providing another possible explanation for failure. The Chediak-Higashi fetus was transplanted with T-cell–depleted maternal marrow by intraperitoneal injection at 19 weeks' gestation.[78] There was no evidence of engraftment or tolerance after birth and the child underwent conventional BMT. Possible explanations for failure in this case are late transplantation (there is no T-cell dysfunction in this disease) and once again the use of T-cell–depleted marrow. We attempted to treat a fetus with chronic granulomatous disease by a series of three transplants of CD34-enriched paternal marrow by intraperitoneal injection at 13, 14, and 15 weeks' gestation. The father's cells clumped in the presence of bovine serum albumin, which was used in the enrichment protocol. The child is healthy on γ-interferon therapy at 1 year of age without evidence of engraftment or tolerance for donor cells (A.W. Flake and E.D. Zanjani, unpublished material, 1995). Subsequent experimental work in the sheep model suggests that no engraftment is achieved if donor cells are intentionally allowed to clump, which provides one explanation for failure.

From this combined experience it appears that in utero HSC transplantation can successfully treat X-linked SCID and perhaps autosomal SCID and bare lymphocyte syndrome. The failures were flawed transplants either in the methodology used or their execution and

T A B L E 37–3. CLINICAL EXPERIENCE WITH IN UTERO HSC TRANSPLANTATION FOR IMMUNODEFICIENCY DISEASES

GESTATIONAL AGE (WK)	DONOR CELL SOURCE	DISEASE TREATED	NO. OF CASES	POSTNATAL OUTCOME	REFERENCE NO.
28	Fetal liver and fetal thymus	Bare lymphocyte syndrome	1	Clinically normal, 26% donor HLA expression at 1 yr	75
26		SCID	1	Alive, engrafted by PCR for Y	76
18	Fetal liver	CGD	1	Procedure-related death	77
19		SCID	1	Terminated at 24 wk, no autopsy performed	78
26	Maternal TCD BM	Chediak-Higashi	1	No engraftment at birth	
15	Paternal CD34 enriched	CGD	1	Alive, no detectable engraftment	See text
16	Paternal CD34 enriched	X-linked SCID	1	Alive at 40 mo, normal immune function, split chimerism	49
20	Paternal CD34 enriched	X-linked SCID	1	Alive at 3.5 mo, split chimerism	50

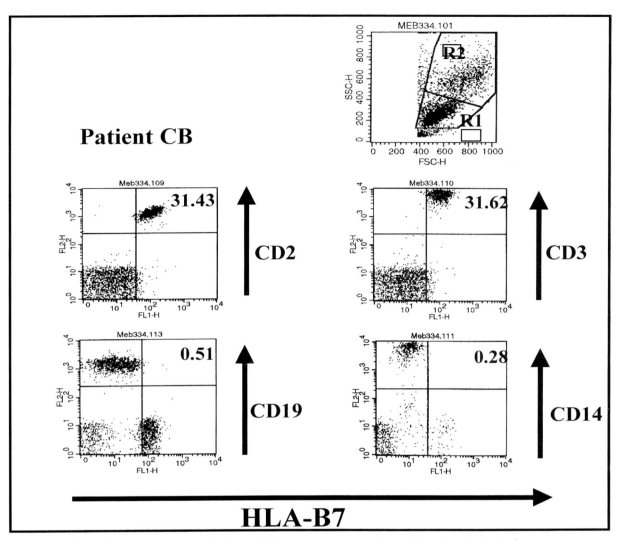

FIGURE 37–4. HLA-B7 and phenotypic analysis of an X-SCID patient's cord blood by dual color flow cytometry after in utero transplantation. Embedded numbers on the scans represent percentage of gated events that are lineage positive (R2 gated). Essentially all of the CD2 and CD3+ cells (T-cells) are HLA-B7+ (donor in origin), whereas CD19+ (B-cells) and CD14+ (monocytes) cells are all HLA-B7– (recipient origin). (CB = cord blood).

therefore did not adequately test the approach. We would currently recommend treatment of this category of disease by a series of two or three transplants of CD34-enriched adult bone marrow that has been thoroughly T-cell depleted to prevent transplantation of greater than 1×10^5 CD3+ cells/kg fetal weight. This degree of T-cell depletion is particularly important in SCID patients. With the exception of SCID, the first transplant would ideally be performed prior to 14 weeks' gestation.

Hemoglobinopathies

We are aware of nine attempts to treat fetuses with hemoglobinopathy, none of which have been clinically successful (Table 37–4). Of these nine, four were performed at 18 weeks' gestation or later, one of which was an intrauterine fetal demise. We feel that it is likely that these patients were transplanted too late to expect

engraftment in the absence of underlying immunodeficiency. Nevertheless, a patient with α-thalassemia transplanted at 18 weeks was aborted at 24 weeks, after donor cells were not detected by fetal blood sampling.[78] Analysis at autopsy revealed marked extramedullary hematopoiesis with donor cells identified in extramedullary sites. This case is important in that it confirms the sheep data in which donor cells are not peripherally expressed until later in gestation. We feel strongly that peripheral blood sampling should not be used as an indicator of engraftment. There was one additional intrauterine death from septic abortion after the transplantation of fetal tissue.[78] Of the remaining four cases that were transplanted prior to 15 weeks, there was one fetus with β-thalassemia major, two fetuses with homozygous α-thalassemia, and one fetus with sickle cell disease. The patient with β-thalassemia was initially reported as engrafted by Touraine with PCR evidence of Y chromosome at birth and an HbA of 0.9% at birth rising to 30%

T A B L E 37-4. CLINICAL EXPERIENCE WITH IN UTERO HSC TRANSPLANTATION FOR HEMOGLOBINOPATHIES

GESTATIONAL AGE (WK)	DONOR CELL SOURCE	DISEASE TREATED	NO. OF CASES	POSTNATAL OUTCOME	REFERENCE NO.
12	Fetal liver	β-Thalassemia major	1	Alive, not engrafted	77, 79
19	Fetal liver	β-Thalassemia major	1	Intrauterine death	
25	Sibling TCD BM	β-Thalassemia	1	No engraftment, clinical status c/w primary disease	83
18	Maternal TCD BM	α-Thalassemia-1	1	Terminated at 24 wk, + donor cells in extramedullary hematopoiesis	78
14	Fetal liver	β-Thalassemia major	1	Septic abortion	78
15		α-Thalassemia-1	1		
18	Cryopreserved fetal liver	β-Thalassemia major	1	No detectable engraftment	64
13		Sickle cell disease	1		
13	Paternal CD34 enriched	α-Thalassemia-1	1	PCR detectable α-gene, ?tolerance	82

at 1 year of life.[77, 79] This patient has since been stated to have lost the engraftment and remains transfusion dependent. It is, in our opinion, somewhat doubtful that this patient was ever engrafted by donor HSCs because of the transient presence of PCR-detectable donor cells, and the normal variability of HbA levels in β-thalassemia patients. Two cases, one of homozygous α-thalassemia, and one of sickle cell disease, were transplanted at 15 and 13 weeks, respectively, with a single injection of cryopreserved fetal liver-derived cells.[64] There are data to suggest that cryopreservation may damage the ability of fetal liver HSC to engraft in the human. Postnatal treatment of SCID patients failed when cryopreserved fetal liver was used but was successful when similar doses of fresh fetal liver cells were used.[80, 81] In addition, as discussed above, there may be biologic disadvantages in α-thalassemia for donor cell competition and engraftment. The final case of α-thalassemia was transplanted by a series of three transplants of CD34-enriched paternal marrow, at 13, 18, and 23 weeks' gestation. The fetus required repeated intrauterine transfusions to survive to term and by report has a trace-positive PCR signal for α-globin gene in cord blood and bone marrow and evidence of donor-specific tolerance by mixed lymphocyte reaction. The child remains healthy but transfusion dependent at 1 year of age.[82]

In summary, there is not yet convincing evidence for the efficacy of in utero transplantation for hemoglobinopathies, but once again it does not appear to have been adequately tested. There have been very few cases attempted and with the exception of the final case of α-thalassemia, none of the transplants were performed in what we would consider an optimal manner. Our current strategy for the treatment of hemoglobinopathies would be to transplant fetuses with β-thalassemia major or sickle cell disease by a series of at least three transplants using CD34-enriched adult BM beginning prior to 14 weeks' gestation. We would hope that this would provide at least low-level engraftment and tolerance so that engraftment could be boosted after birth if necessary by further transplants from the same donor.

Inborn Errors of Metabolism

There have been five attempts to treat fetuses with inborn errors of metabolism by in utero HSC trans-

plantation (Table 37-5). Two have been performed for metachromatic leukodystrophy, one for globoid leukodystrophy, one for Hurler disease, and one for Niemann-Pick disease. Two attempts for metachromatic leukodystrophy were at 23 and 34 weeks using TCD adult BM with, as could be predicted, no evidence of engraftment.[83] One patient with Hurler disease was transplanted with fetal liver-derived cells at 14 weeks' gestation. Low-level engraftment was observed at birth (1% donor cells in cord blood) with slowly increasing engraftment (5 to 10% at 1 year) and α-L-iduronidase activity (<10 pmol/mg tissue per minute at birth, 98.3 pmol/mg tissue per minute at 22 months of age) after birth. The child died at 2 years of age from complications of his disease (E.D. Zanjani, unpublished material). The patient with Niemann-Pick disease was transplanted with fetal liver at 14 weeks and was still in utero at the time of the report,[77] with no subsequent report published. The third patient with metachromatic leukodystrophy was transplanted at 13 weeks' gestation with a massive dose of CD34-enriched paternal marrow that also contained 5% CD3+ cells for a total dose of over 1×10^8 T cells/kg fetal weight.[73] The fetus died at 20 weeks' gestation with autopsy findings of massive infiltration of all tissues with donor cells that stained positive for myeloperoxidase. DNA-restriction fragment length polymorphism (RFLP) analysis of liver, spleen, and skin revealed 95%, 50%, and 9% of DNA, respectively, to be of donor origin. It is important to note that the fetus was severely autolyzed preventing morphologic characterization of the infiltrating cells. The authors of this report have interpreted this as massive extramedullary donor myelopoiesis but have not convincingly excluded GVHD as the cause of fetal demise.

In summary, there is to date little clinical or experimental evidence that in utero HSC transplantation can successfully achieve adequate levels and distribution of engraftment to treat the inborn errors of metabolism. Nevertheless, in the two cases in which transplantation was performed at an early gestational age some evidence of donor cell expression was present at the time of death. However, the rationale for prenatal treatment of diseases in this category in which the neurologic damage may begin before birth, or for diseases in which fetal demise or compromise may occur in utero (fetal hydrops and hepatic dysfunction in sialidosis and Wolman disease, respectively) remains compelling. In order to effec-

TABLE 37–5. CLINICAL EXPERIENCE WITH IN UTERO HSC TRANSPLANTATION FOR THE INBORN ERRORS OF METABOLISM

GESTATIONAL AGE (WK)	DONOR CELL SOURCE	DISEASE TREATED	NO. OF CASES	POSTNATAL OUTCOME	REFERENCE NO.
34, 23	Paternal TCD BM	MCLD	2	No evidence of engraftment, clinical status c/w primary disease	83
14	Fetal liver	Hurler disease	1	Low level engraftment, death at age 2 from complications of the disease	See text
13	Paternal CD34 enriched	MCLD	1	Intrauterine death at 20 wk, extensive donor cell infiltration	73
14	Fetal liver	Niemann-Pick disease	1	Alive in utero—no subsequent report	77
		Other hematologic diseases			
12	Maternal TCD BM	Rh-disease	1	No detectable engraftment + tolerance	85
17	Maternal TCD BM	Rh-disease	1	Survived with no engraftment	74

tively treat these diseases, however, strategies to increase donor cell engraftment and increase early donor cell expression are needed. In addition, CNS-directed prenatal gene therapy strategies may be promising.[84] Thsese are all active areas of investigation and may lead to future success in the prenatal treatment of the inborn errors of metabolism.

Other Hematologic Disorders

In addition to the above, two attempts to treat fetuses with erythroblastosis fetalis by in utero HSC transplantation have been made (Table 37–5). In each case, TCD maternal BM was transplanted. A 17-week fetus received the transplant intravenously,[74] and a 12-week fetus received the transplant by intraperitoneal injection.[85] In neither case was the prenatal course of the disease influenced (both required multiple intrauterine transfusions), and in both cases there was no detectable engraftment after birth. The patient transplanted at 17 weeks had no evidence of tolerance by mixed lymphocyte reaction (MLR), whereas the patient transplanted at 12 weeks had a decreased frequency of maternal antigen-directed cytotoxic T lymphocytes relative to predicted and controls, suggesting the presence of donor-specific tolerance. The rationale for treatment of Rh disease by in utero transplantation must be questioned, since it can be treated by in utero transfusion, and the recipient does not need engraftment of HSC for long-term cure.

Conclusions

In utero hematopoietic stem cell transplantation is currently in its embryonic stage of development, but holds considerable developmental promise as a therapeutic approach for the treatment of a large number of congenital hematologic diseases. Despite, until recently, limited evidence of clinical efficacy, interest in the field has been gaining momentum, and clinical application is likely to increase. Parallel advances in prenatal diagnosis, fetal intervention, and hematopoietic stem cell technology have removed many of the practical, technical, and ethical obstacles to clinical application. With this progress, there has been a significant increase in the number of centers around the world with both the stated interest and perceived expertise to develop clinical programs. At this point in the evolution of in utero hematopoietic stem cell transplantation there are more questions than answers. Widespread clinical application is premature based on the extremely limited clinical success that has been achieved. The biology of each disease is unique, and expectations of success or failure can only be based upon sound clinical investigation guided by an understanding of the relevant issues and careful selection and evaluation of patients. Clinical centers should be associated with an active research effort to solve the remaining problems with this potentially valuable therapeutic approach. In the near future, advances in our understanding of stem cell biology, developmental ontogeny, and gene therapy may allow prenatal stem cell and gene therapy to achieve their full potential.

REFERENCES

1. Owen RD: Immunogenetic consequences of vascular anastomoses between bovine cattle twins. Science 102:400–401, 1945.
2. Anderson D, Billingham R, Lampkin G, Medawar P: The use of skin grafting to distinguish between monozygotic and dizygotic twins in cattle. Heredity 5:379–397, 1951.
3. Simonsen M: The acquired immunity concept in kidney homotransplantation. Ann N Y Acad Sci 59:448–452, 1955.
4. Picus J, Aldrich W, Letvin N: A naturally occurring bone-marrow chimeric primate. Transplantation 39:297–303, 1985.
5. van Dijk B, Bommsma D, de Man A: Blood group chimerism in human multiple births is not rare. Am J Med Genet 61:264–268, 1996.
6. Gill T: Chimerism in humans. Transplant Proc 9:1423–1431, 1977.
7. Billingham R, Brent L, Medawar PB: Actively acquired tolerance of foreign cells. Nature 172:603–607, 1953.
8. Sprent J: Central tolerance of T cells. Int Rev Immunol 13:95–105, 1995.

9. Goodnow C: Balancing immunity and tolerance: Deleting and tuning lymphocyte repertoires. Proc Natl Acad Sci U S A 93:2264–2271, 1996.

10. Strominger JL: Developmental biology of T cell receptors. Science 244:943–949, 1989.

11. Sha WC, Nelson CA, et al: Positive and negative selection of an antigen receptor on T-cells in transgenic mice. Nature 336:73–76, 1988.

12. Schwartz R: Acquisition of immunologic self tolerance. Cell 57:1073–1081, 1989.

13. Blackman M, Kappler J, Marrack P: The role of the T-cell receptor in positive and negative selection of developing T-cells. Science 248:1335–1342, 1990.

14. Guidos CJ, Danska JS, Fathman CG, Weissman IL: T cell receptor-mediated negative selection of autoreactive T lymphocyte precursors occurs after commitment to the CD4 or CD8 lineages. J Exp Med 172:835–845, 1990.

15. Weissman IL: Developmental switches in the immune system. Cell 76:207–218, 1994.

16. Goodnow C, Adelstein S, Basten A: The need for central and peripheral tolerance in the B cell repertoire. Science 248:1373–1379, 1990.

17. LeBien T, Wormann B, Villablanca J, et al: Multiparameter flow cytometric analysis of human fetal bone marrow B-cells. Leukemia 4:354–358, 1990.

18. Metcalf D, Moore MAS: Embryonic aspects of haemopoiesis. In Neuberger A, Tatum EL (eds): Haemopoietic Cells, vol 24, Frontiers in Biology. Amsterdam, London: North-Holland Publishing Co, 1971, pp 471–497.

19. Tavian M, Coulombel L, Luton D, et al: Aorta-associated CD34+ hematopoietic cells in the early human embryo. Blood 87:67–72, 1996.

20. Zanjani ED, Ascensao JL, Tavassoli M: Liver-derived fetal hematopoietic stem cells selectively and preferentially home to the fetal bone marrow. Blood 81:399–404, 1993.

21. Hunn I, Bodger M, Hoffbrand A: Development of pluripotent hematopoietic progenitor cells in the human fetus. Blood 62:118–123, 1983.

22. Kaufman CL, Ildstad ST: Induction of donor-specific tolerance by transplantation of bone marrow. Ther Immunol 1:101–111, 1994.

23. Sykes M: Immunobiology of transplantation [review]. FASEB J 10:721–730, 1996.

24. Flake AW, Harrison MR, Adzick NS, Zanjani ED: Transplantation of fetal hematopoietic stem cells in utero: The creation of hematopoietic chimeras. Science 233:776–778, 1986.

25. Zanjani ED, Pallavicini MG, Ascensao JL, et al: Engraftment and long-term expression of human fetal hemopoietic stem cells in sheep following transplantation in utero. J Clin Invest 89:1178–1188, 1992.

26. Srour EF, Zanjani ED, Brandt JE, et al: Sustained human hematopoiesis in sheep transplanted in utero during early gestation with fractionated adult human bone marrow cells. Blood 79:1404–1412, 1992.

27. Srour EF, Zanjani ED, Cornetta K, et al: Persistence of human multilineage, self-renewing lymphohematopoietic stem cells in chimeric sheep. Blood 82:3333–3342, 1993.

28. Civin CJ, Lee MJ, Hedrick M, et al: Purified CD34+/lineage-/38- cells contain hematopoietic stem cells [abstract 707]. Blood 82 (Suppl 1):180a, 1993.

29. Kawashima I, Zanjani E, Almaida-Porada G, et al: CD34+ human marrow cells that express low levels of Kit protein are enriched for long-term marrow-engrafting cells. Blood 87:4136–4142, 1996.

30. Zanjani ED, Almeida-Porada G, Livingston AG, et al: Human bone marrow CD34- cells engraft in vivo and undergo multilineage expression that includes giving rise to CD34+ cells. Exp Hematol 26:353–360, 1998.

31. Zanjani ED, Flake AW, Rice H, et al: Long-term repopulating ability of xenogeneic transplanted human fetal liver hematopoietic stem cells in sheep. J Clin Invest 93:1051–1055, 1994.

32. Harrison MR, Slotnick RN, Crombleholme TM, et al: In-utero transplantation of fetal liver haemopoietic stem cells in monkeys. Lancet 2:1425–1427, 1989.

33. Pearce R, Kiehm D, Armstrong D, et al: Induction of hematopoietic chimerism in the caprine fetus by intraperitoneal injection of fetal liver cells. Experientia 45:307–308, 1989.

34. Rice HE, Hedrick MH, Flake AW: In utero transplantation of rat hematopoietic stem cells induces xenogeneic chimerism in mice. Transplant Proc 26:126–128, 1994.

35. Pallavicini MG, Flake AW, Madden D, et al: Hemopoietic chimerism in rodents transplanted in utero with fetal human hemopoietic cells. Transplant Proc 24:542–543, 1992.

36. Blazar BR, Taylor PA, Vallera DA: In utero transfer of adult bone marrow cells into recipients with severe combined immunodeficiency disorder yields lymphoid progeny with T- and B-cell functional capabilities. Blood 86:4353–4366, 1995.

37. Blazar BR, Taylor PA, Vallera DA: Adult bone marrow-derived pluripotent hematopoietic stem cells are engraftable when transferred in utero into moderately anemic fetal recipients. Blood 85:833–841, 1995.

38. Carrier E, Lee T, Busch M, Cowan M: Induction of tolerance in nondefective mice after in utero transplantation of major histocompatibility complex-mismatched fetal hematopoietic stem cells. Blood 86:4681–4690, 1995.

39. Carrier E, Lee TH, Busch MP, Cowan MJ: Recruitment of engrafted donor cells postnatally into the blood with cytokines after in utero transplantation in mice. Transplantation 64:627–633, 1997.

40. Fleischman R, Mintz B: Prevention of genetic anemias in mice by microinjection of normal hematopoietic cells into the fetal placenta. Proc Natl Acad Sci U S A 76:5736–5740, 1979.

41. Archer DR, Turner CW, Yeager AM, Fleming WH: Sustained multilineage engraftment of allogeneic hematopoietic stem cells in NOD/SCID mice after in utero transplantation. Blood 90:3222–3229, 1997.

42. Shultz LD, Schweitzer PA, Christianson SW, et al: Multiple defects in innate and adaptive immunologic function in NOD/LtSz-scid mice. J Immunol 154:180–191, 1995.

43. Rhoads G, Jackson L, Schlesselman S, et al: The safety and efficacy of chorionic villus sampling for early prenatal diagnosis of cytogenetic abnormalities. N Engl J Med 320:609–617, 1989.

44. Bowman J: Hemolytic disease (erythroblastosis fetalis). In Creasy R, Resnick R (eds): Maternal-Fetal Medicine. Principles and Practice, 3rd ed. Philadelphia: WB Saunders Company, 1994, pp 730–733.

45. Rice HE, Hedrick MH, Flake AW, et al: Bacterial and fungal contamination of human fetal liver collected transvaginally for hematopoietic stem cell transplantation. Fetal Diagn Ther 8:74–78, 1993.

46. McKinnon S, Papadopoulos E, Carabasi M, et al: Adoptive immunotherapy. Evaluating escalating doses of donor leukocytes for relapse of CML after BMT: Separation of GvL responses from GvHD. Blood 86:1261–1268, 1995.

47. Alain G, Carrier C, Beaumier L, et al: In utero acute graft-versus-host disease in a neonate with severe combined immunodeficiency. J Am Acad Dermatol 29:862–865, 1993.

48. Sottini A, Quiros-Roldan E, Notarangelo LD, et al: Engrafted maternal T cells in a severe combined immunodeficiency patient express T-cell receptor variable beta segments characterized by a restricted V-D-J junctional diversity. Blood 85:2105–2113, 1995.

49. Flake A, Roncarolo M-G, Puck J, et al: Treatment of X-linked severe combined immunodeficiency by in utero transplantation of paternal bone marrow. N Engl J Med 335:1806–1810, 1996.

50. Wengler G, Lanfranchi A, Frusca T, et al: In-utero transplantation of parental CD34 haematopoietic progenitor cells in a patient with X-linked severe combined immunodeficiency (SCIDX1). Lancet 348:1484–1487, 1996.

51. Manis J: Agammaglobulinemia and insights into B-cell differentiation. N Engl J Med 335:1523–1525, 1996.

52. Bjorgvinsdottir H, Ding C, Pech N, et al: Retroviral-mediated gene transfer of gp91phox into bone marrow cells rescues defect in host defense against Aspergillus fumigatus in murine X-linked chronic granulomatous disease. Blood 89:41–48, 1997.

53. Hollenbaugh D, Wu LH, Ochs HD, et al: The random inactivation of the X chromosome carrying the defective gene responsible for X-linked hyper IgM syndrome (X-HIM) in female carriers of HIGM1. J Clin Invest 94:616–622, 1994.

54. Andreani M, Manna M, Lucarelli G, et al: Persistence of mixed chimerism in patients transplanted for the treatment of thalassemia. Blood 87:3494–3499, 1996.

55. Walters MC, Patience M, Leisenring W, et al: Bone marrow transplantation for sickle cell disease. N Engl J Med 335:369–376, 1996.

56. Bunn H, Forget B: Hemoglobin structure. *In* Hemoglobin: Molecular, Genetic, and Clinical Aspects. Philadelphia: WB Saunders Company, 1986, pp 13–35.
57. Lam Y, Ghosh A, Tang M, et al: Second-trimester hydrops fetalis in pregnancies affected by homozygous alpha thalassemia-1. Prenat Diagn 17:267–269, 1997.
58. Moses S: Pathophysiology and dietary treatment of the glycogen storage diseases. J Pediatr Gastroenterol Nutr 11:155–174, 1990.
59. Kaye E: Therapeutic approaches to lysosomal storage diseases. Curr Opin Pediatr 7:650–654, 1995.
60. Imaizumi M, Gushi K, Kurobane I, et al: Long-term effects of bone marrow transplantation for inborn errors of metabolism: A study of four patients with lysosomal storage diseases. Acta Paediatr Jpn 36:30–36, 1994.
61. Krivit W, Lockman L, Watkins P, et al: The future for treatment by bone marrow transplantation for adrenoleukodystrophy, metachromatic leukodystrophy, globoid cell leukodystrophy and Hurler syndrome. J Inherit Metab Dis 18:398–412, 1995.
62. Westlake V, Jolly R, Jones B, et al: Hematopoietic cell transplantation in fetal lambs with ceroid-lipofuscinosis. Am J Med Genet 57:365–368, 1995.
63. Barron K: The microglial cell. A historical review. J Neurol Sci 134 (Suppl):57–68, 1995.
64. Westgren M, Ringden O, Sturla E-N, et al: Lack of evidence of permanent engraftment after in utero fetal stem cell transplantation in congenital hemoglobinopathies. Transplantation 61:1176–1179, 1996.
65. Cefalo RC, Berghmans RL, Hall SP: The bioethics of human fetal tissue research and therapy: Moral decision making of professionals. Am J Obstet Gynecol 170:12–19, 1994.
66. Zanjani ED, Lim G, McGlave PB, et al: Adult haematopoietic cells transplanted to sheep fetuses continue to produce adult globins. Nature 295:244–246, 1982.
67. Crombleholme TM, Harrison MR, Zanjani ED: In utero transplantation of hematopoietic stem cells in sheep: The role of T cells in engraftment and graft-versus-host disease. J Pediatr Surg 25:885–892, 1990.
68. Diukman R, Golbus MS: In utero stem cell therapy. J Reprod Med 37:515–520, 1992.
69. Kawashima I, Zanjani ED, Almaida-Porada G, et al: CD34+ human marrow cells that express low levels of Kit protein are enriched for long-term marrow-engrafting cells. Blood 87:4136–4142, 1996.
70. Lansdorp P, Dragowska W, Mayani H: Ontogeny-related changes in proliferative potential of human hematopoietic cells. J Exp Med 178:787–791, 1993.
71. Zanjani E, Flake A, Rice H, et al: An in-vivo comparison of potential human donor hematopoietic stem cell (HSC) sources for bone marrow transplantation using the human/sheep xenograft model. Blood 82 (Suppl 1):655A, 1993.
72. Flake A, Zanjani E: Cellular therapy. New trends and controversies in fetal diagnosis and therapy. Obstet Gynecol Clin North Am 24:159–177, 1997.
73. Bambach BJ, Moser HW, Blakemore K, et al: Engraftment following in utero bone marrow transplantation for globoid cell leukodystrophy. Bone Marrow Transplant 19:399–402, 1997.
74. Linch D, Rodeck C, Nicolaides K, et al: Attempted bone marrow transplantation in a 17 week fetus [letter]. Lancet 1:1382, 1986.
75. Touraine JL, Raudrant D, Royo C, et al: In-utero transplantation of stem cells in bare lymphocyte syndrome [letter]. Lancet 1:1382, 1989.
76. Touraine JL: Stem cell transplantation in primary immunodeficiency, with special reference to the first prenatal, in utero, transplants. Allergol Immunopathol (Madr) 19:49–51, 1991.
77. Touraine J: Treatment of human fetuses and induction of immunological tolerance in humans by in utero transplantation of stem cells into fetal recipients. Acta Haematol 96:115–119, 1996.
78. Cowan M, Golbus M: In utero hematopoietic stem cell transplants for inherited disease. Am J Pediatr Hematol Oncol 16:35–42, 1994.
79. Touraine JL, Raudrant D, Rebaud A, et al: In utero transplantation of stem cells in humans: Immunological aspects and clinical follow-up of patients. Bone Marrow Transplant 1:121–126, 1992.
80. Gupta S, Pahwa R, O'Reilly R, et al: Ontogeny of lymphocyte subpopulations in human fetal liver. Proc Natl Acad Sci U S A 73:919–922, 1976.
81. Pahwa R, Pahwa S, Good R, et al: Rationale for combined use of fetal liver and thymic for immunological reconstitution in patients with severe combined immunodeficiency. Proc Natl Acad Sci U S A 74:3002–3005, 1977.
82. Hayward A, Ambruso D, Battaglia F, et al: Microchimerism and tolerance following intrauterine transplantation and transfusion for α-thalassemia-1. Fetal Diagn Ther 13:8–14, 1998.
83. Slavin S, Naparstek E, Ziegler M, et al: Clinical application of intrauterine bone marrow transplantation for treatment of genetic disease—feasibility studies. Bone Marrow Transplant 1:189–190, 1992.
84. Snyder E, Wolfe J: Central nervous system cell transplantation: A novel therapy for storage diseases? Curr Opin Neurol 9:126–136, 1996.
85. Thilaganthan B, Nicolaides K: Intrauterine bone-marrow transplantation at 12 week's gestation. Lancet 342:243, 1993.

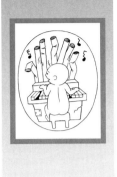

CHAPTER 38

Ontogeny of the Fetal Immune System: Implications for Fetal Tolerance Induction and Postnatal Transplantation

CRAIG T. ALBANESE and ALICIA BÁRCENA

History of Chimerism and Tolerance

Successful prenatal and postnatal cellular transplantation is dependent on the establishment of chimerism. In Greek mythology, a chimera was depicted as a fire-breathing monster resembling a lion in the forepart, with additional components of goat and dragon combined. It was invoked to explain the magical and often capricious forces of nature. The "immunologic" chimera is also a hybrid individual, formed after engraftment of hematopoietic tissue between two immunologically disparate individuals, and represents the only true state of donor-specific transplantation tolerance. This is a state in which the recipient is specifically hyporeactive to the donor yet fully reactive to third-party antigens both in vivo and in vitro.

To understand the relationship between chimerism and tolerance, one needs to examine its relatively short history, starting from an experiment of nature in the late 1940s. Two nearly simultaneous observations established that engraftment of bone marrow stem cells in a genetically different recipient renders the recipient tolerant to tissue, solid organ, and cellular grafts specifically from that same donor. Owen[1] made the seminal observation that freemartin cattle (genetically different dizygotic cattle twins that share a common placental circulation) were red blood cell chimeras. Several years later, Billingham, Brent, and Medawar[2] were commissioned by the British government to develop and apply a skin grafting technique for histocompatibility typing in order to distinguish between the potentially sterile (thus less economically useful) freemartin cattle and identical cattle twins (Fig. 38–1). To their surprise, when reciprocal skin grafts were exchanged between the adult cattle twin pairs, they were accepted by the genetically disparate freemartin twins. Based on Owen's observations, the group reasoned that perhaps red blood cell chimerism was present in freemartin cattle and was as-sociated with "actively acquired immunological tolerance" to subsequent donor-specific grafts. These observations were further supported by the permanent acceptance of kidney allografts by the chimeric cattle.[3] In 1953, Billingham applied these observations in a rodent model of bone marrow transplantation.[4] Chimerism was not achieved using adult recipients, but was successful when neonatal mice were transplanted. The neonates accepted donor-specific skin grafts while MHC-disparate third-party grafts were rejected. Newborn (and presumably, fetal) mice are distinct from adult recipients in that no conditioning (i.e., cytoreduction and/or cytoablation) is required to achieve engraftment of transplanted bone marrow cells. This immunologically "privileged" state exists until 72 hours after birth in mice. Since Billingham's mouse studies, numerous allogeneic and xenogeneic transplantation studies have been published demonstrating that the establishment of stable hematopoietic chimerism, in both adults and fetuses, induces tolerance to donor-matched organs.[5–14] Natural chimerism from shared placental circulation has also been observed in primates and humans,[15, 16] and the incidence of human chimerism in monochorionic dizygotic pregnancies is approximately 8%.[17, 18]

In 1984, Ildstad and Sachs[19] reported that mixed allogeneic and xenogeneic chimerism could lead to specific acceptance of donor strain-matched grafts in adult mice without the need for long-term immunosuppression. Subsequently, donor-specific transplantation tolerance across major histocompatibility barriers has been achieved through chimerism in other species of adult animals including rats,[7, 8] dogs,[9] pigs,[10] and monkeys.[11] Unfortunately, the incidence of toxicity in adults is high due to the conditioning regimens necessary to achieve adequate bone marrow engraftment.

The demonstration of acquired immunologic tolerance to donor antigens in neonatal mice has opened the door to a potentially new recipient of cellular transplan-

PLACENTAL CROSS CIRCULATION

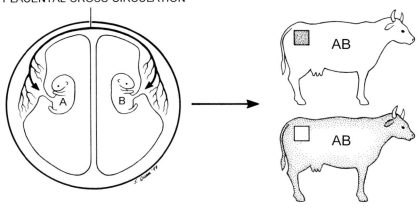

FIGURE 38–1. An experiment of nature. Genetically different dizygotic cattle that shared a common placental circulation were immunologic chimeras and accepted reciprocal skin grafts. Thus emerged the concept of actively acquired donor-specific immunologic tolerance.

tation—the human fetus. The development of durable chimerism may prove to be the most physiologic way to achieve replacement of abnormal hemoglobin, immune cells, or enzyme defects diagnosed prenatally. Moreover, prenatal tolerance can be achieved, allowing postnatal solid organ transplantation without immunosuppression. Based on the presumptive ontogeny of immunologic development, the early gestation fetus (<14 weeks' gestation) has been proposed as a recipient of a cellular transplant that will allow engraftment without conditioning. It is believed that the early human fetus, much like the fetal/early neonatal rodent, is immunologically immature and naive, especially with respect to T-cell development. Furthermore, the early human fetus' bone marrow is believed to be relatively devoid of cellular elements, thus there may be ample "space" into which donor cells may home to, reside, and divide.

This chapter highlights the current knowledge of the development and function of the fetal imune system, focusing on those elements critical in the establishment of cellular immunity. It is the interaction (or lack thereof) of fetal cells and the donor inoculum that will establish whether chimerism and tolerance can be achieved prenatally. We will discuss in detail recent data that may partially challenge the current notion of the fetus as an immunologically immature and nonfunctional recipient for cellular transplantation.

Ontogeny of the Fetal Immune System

General Considerations

Understanding the development of the fetal immune system is required in order to improve our ability to treat a fetus affected with a hematopoietic cellular disorder or a newborn that requires organ transplantation soon after birth. Certainly, within the first trimester of pregnancy, few elements of the fetal immune system have developed, thus severely hampering the ability of the fetus to respond to infection, although this might offer the theoretical opportunity window to introduce hematopoietic stem cells into the affected fetus. Beginning early

in the second trimester, most of the cellular elements of the immune system can be found circulating in the human fetus, although the functional status of these cells is not yet known (see below). Studies on the immune systems of newborns have shown that all elements of the adult immune system are present, but deficiencies in their functional status have been reported. It follows that deficiencies in the functioning of the fetal immune system may also exist.

The following section will review the current data on the development of the hematopoietic system in the human embryonic and fetal periods. In addition, we will summarize the developmental and functional status of the key elements of the fetal hematopoietic system responsible for cellular immunity—T lymphocytes and natural killer (NK) cells. These cellular subpopulations, when functionally mature and competent, are responsible for the establishment of a state of tolerance or, conversely, for the rejection of a hematopoietic stem cell allograft.

Development of the Human Embryonic and Fetal Hematopoietic System

The hematopoietic system is one of the most dynamic and complex systems of the human body. Hematopoietic stem cells (HSCs) that are generated in the hematopoietic environment (yolk-sac, aorta-gonad-mesonephros [AGM], liver, or bone marrow) undergo a series of divisions and maturational steps that are required to generate all the cellular lineages found in the blood and the immunologic organs (e.g., spleen, lymph nodes, and mucosa-associated lymphoid tissues). HSCs are functionally defined as those hematopoietic progenitor cells that have self-renewing capabilities, long-term repopulating activity, and multilineage potential. They are poorly studied and defined in humans, since there are no good in vivo assays to determine whether the functional behavior of several cellular subsets observed in vitro correlates with long-term repopulating ability. It is generally accepted that stem cells express the cell-surface glycoprotein "cluster of differentiation" 34 (CD34). During embryonic (from conception to 7 weeks' gestation) and fetal (from 8 weeks' gestation to term) development, the anatomic sites of hematopoiesis switch from extraembryonic tissue to a variety of intraembryonic and fetal sites. Historically, it has been believed that hematopoiesis first begins at 3 to 5 weeks' gestation in the extraembryonic yolk sac (Fig. 38–2). It is also believed that yolk sac–derived HSCs migrate inside the embryo around 5 to 6 weeks' gestation and seed the liver. Recently, two independent groups have shown that at least some HSCs identified by their ability to long-term repopulate all the lymphoid and myeloid lineages of blood cells in mice, are generated in an intraembryonic hematopoietic site defined as the para-aortic splanchnopleure or AGM region.[20, 21] In humans, a similar AGM region (ventral to the aorta) has been found to generate CD34+ hematopoietic progenitor cells (Fig. 38–2) between 3 and 7 weeks' gestation.[22]

Several groups have reported the presence of hematopoietic islets in the embryonic liver around the fifth week of gestation. During the second half of the embryonic period, three hematopoietic tissues coexist: yolk sac, AGM, and liver. The differences and the relationship between these different hematopoietic sites has not been yet determined. The liver, which is mainly erythropoietic,[23] constitutes the major site of hematopoiesis throughout the end of the embryonic period and through a good portion of the fetal period.[24] The bone marrow (BM) becomes the predominant hematopoietic organ at around 34 weeks' gestation.

The development of the human long BM has been extensively studied by Charbord et al.[25] They reported that between 8 and 10.5 weeks' gestation, the bone is entirely cartilaginous and that around 11 to 12.5 weeks' gestation, vascularization of the developing BM cavity (without detectable hematopoiesis) takes place. Intramedullary hematopoiesis begins between 12.5 and 17 weeks' gestation. Therefore, around the end of the first trimester of pregnancy and the beginning of the second trimester, hematopoiesis overlaps between two hematopoietic organs, the liver and the BM. The fetal BM is less erythropoietic and more myelopoietic than the fetal liver, but a fine characterization of the different hematopoietic environments and the hematopoietic potential of HSCs generated in these two sites has not yet been studied.

A model of fetal liver and BM hematopoiesis is presented in Figure 38–3. This model presents the current knowledge of the phenotypical profile that defines HSCs, B-lymphoid progenitors, and myeloid progenitors. Figure 38–3 illustrates that HSCs can be defined as CD34^{bright} CD33^{dull}CD7$^{+/-}$CD38$^-$ cells, and lack the expression of markers specific for erythrocytes (glycophorin A), mature T cells (CD3), NK cells (CD16, CD56), monocytes (CD14), pre-B cells (CD10), and B cells (CD19, CD20). This stem cell population also expresses CD13, Thy-1, and c-kit.[26] As the stem cells differentiate during hematopoietic development, the expression of CD38 is up-regulated while CD34 expression is decreased.[27] Further differentiation is characterized by the acquisition of CD10 followed by a loss of Thy-1, CD13, and CD33 expression when generating B-cell committed progenitors, or up-regulation of CD33 expression when generating myeloid-committed progenitors, that are CD13$^+$ Thy-1$^-$CD10$^-$.

T-Cell Development in the Human Fetus

Understanding T-cell development and function in the human fetus is very relevant for in utero cellular transplantation (IUT), since T cells are the major mediators of postnatal graft rejection, and thus could play an adverse role prenatally. It is largely unknown which events drive a pluripotent hematopoietic stem cell to generate lymphoid-committed progenitors capable of differentiation into T, B, and NK cells. Therefore, the paucity of these cells in the early fetal circulation and hematopoietic tissues has been used to define the optimal timing of IUT. Based on the low frequency of mature T cells (CD3$^+$CD4$^+$ helper and CD3$^+$CD8$^+$ cytotoxic cells, respectively) in the peripheral fetal blood, most recent attempts at IUT have been made before 14 weeks' gestation. However, as we will discuss below, the accumulation of T cells in the periphery begins before 14 weeks' gestation and, in light of the poor results of cellular transplants made before this time period, the function of the fetal immune system before 14 weeks' gestation deserves further analysis.

The thymus is the organ responsible for the generation of T cells. The thymic rudiment formation is very well characterized and it is detectable around 4 to 5 weeks'

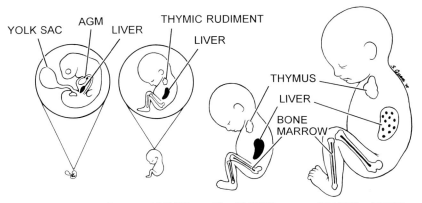

FIGURE 38–2. Ontogeny of the human hematopoietic system. The development of the embryonic and fetal hematopoietic organs are depicted. (AGM = aorta-gonad-mesonephros.)

YOLK SAC   AGM   LIVER   THYMIC RUDIMENT   LIVER   THYMUS   LIVER   BONE MARROW

BEFORE 5 WKS. → 5 - 12 WKS. → 12 - 22 WKS. ⟶ 22 WKS. - TERM

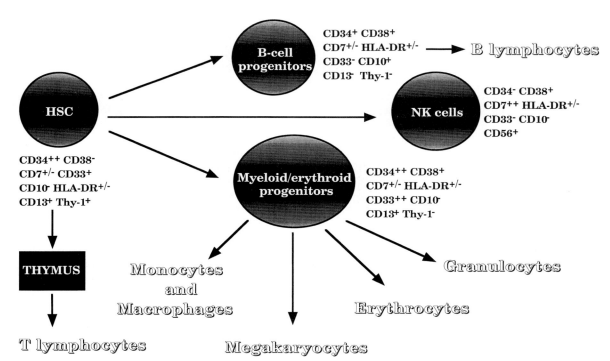

FIGURE 38–3. Model for fetal hematopoiesis in the fetal liver and bone marrow. Hematopoietic stem cells (HSCs), characterized by the high cell surface expression of CD34 and lack of CD38 expression, are generated in the fetal liver and bone marrow. They differentiate into B-cell progenitors, myeloid progenitors, and NK cells in situ. T-cell generation will take place in the thymus.

gestation (Fig. 38–4). Between 8 and 9 weeks' gestation, hematopoietic progenitors presumably generated in the fetal liver migrate to and colonize the thymus.[28] The presence of few but detectable CD3[+] T cells in the thymic rudiment has been reported at 9 to 10 weeks' gestation.[29] The detailed scheme of fetal T-cell development will be discussed below. The thymus is anatomically mature, with differentiated cortex and medulla, at 14 weeks' gestation, although it will continue to grow in size well into the postnatal period.

Pre–T-cell progenitors are believed to reside in the fetal liver and BM. This has been demonstrated by isolating fetal hematopoietic progenitors (CD34[++]) by cell sorting and phenotypically and functionally analyzing the resulting population for T-cell progenitor potential. The cell surface antigen CD7, as proposed by Haynes, may be the first marker expressed on the surface of cells committed to the T-cell lineage,[30] although not exclusively, since it has been found on mature NK cells and normal myeloid- and lymphoid-progenitor populations in the BM.[31, 32] Immunohistochemical studies performed on sections of embryonic and fetal hematopoietic tissues such as yolk sac and fetal liver have demonstrated the presence of CD45[+]CD7[+] cytoplasmic (cy) CD3[+] cells.[28, 33] This population lacked surface expression of CD3–T-cell receptor (TCR), CD4, or CD8 markers, and it was detected as early as 7 weeks' gestation. Similar analyses performed in the fetal upper thorax, where the thymic rudiment is located, indicated that there is a lymphoid population in the perithymic mesenchyme between 7 and 9.5 weeks' gestation that displays a comparable phenotypic profile of that observed in the fetal

liver.[28] Taken together, these results led to the hypothesis that the CD45[+]CD7[+]cyCD3[+]CD4[-]CD8[-] fetal liver cells constitute the prethymic T-cell committed progenitor that migrates to the fetal thymus early in ontogeny. This conclusion was founded on the premise that CD3 expression is solely restricted to cells belonging to the T-cell lineage. Recent data show, however, that this is not the case, since fetal liver CD7[+]CD56[+] NK cells express cyCD3.[34] Moreover, functionally mature NK cells comprised 35 to 70% of the CD45[+] leukocytes in embryonic and fetal liver of 6 to 24 weeks' gestation[34] (and our own unpublished observations). These data suggest that most of the CD45[+]CD7[+]cCD3[+] cells previously assumed to be fetal liver T-cell precursors contain a significant proportion of NK cells. Nevertheless, these findings do not preclude the possibility that CD7 is expressed very early in T and NK development. Some investigators have used additional markers such as CD2 and CD5 to define prethymic T-cell precursors. Multiparametric immunofluorescence analyses in fetal BM have indicated the presence of a very minor population of cells characterized by the expression of CD34, CD7, CD2, and CD5.[35] The existence of a prethymic T-cell committed population in the fetal BM is exclusively supported by phenotypic data, and definitive evidence of the lineage commitment of such a population requires its isolation and functional characterization in comparison with the counterpart CD34[+]CD7[-] population. Figure 38–3 depicts a model of intrathymic fetal T-cell development. Commitment to the T-cell lineage takes place in the thymus, to where CD34[bright] CD33[dull]CD38[-] would migrate and acquire CD2, CD5, CD7, and CD28. The acqui-

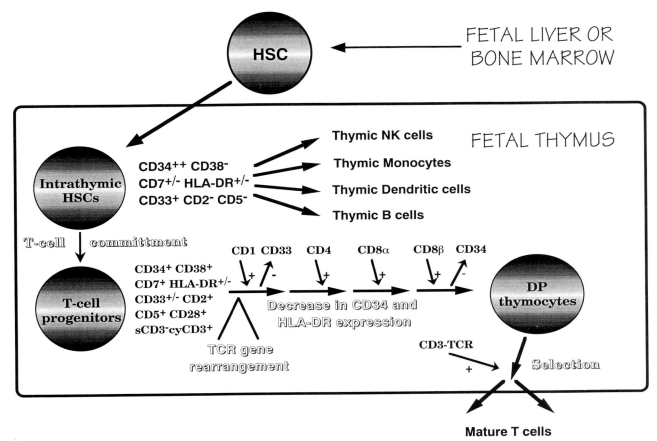

FIGURE 38-4. Intrathymic differentiation of HSCs into T cells. HSCs generated in the fetal liver and bone marrow home to the thymus and differentiate into a multipotent HSC, mainly committed to lymphoid lineages (T, B, and NK cells). This intrathymic progenitor is still able to differentiate into cells of the myeloid lineage. The sequence of acquisition and loss of characteristic cell surface markers of thymocytes is indicated.

sition of these markers is accompanied by an increase in CD38 expression, that correlates with a down-regulation in CD34, CD33, and HLA-DR. The T-cell committed progenitors, which express cytoplasmic CD3-γ and -δ, and rearrange the TCR genes, will sequentially acquire CD1, CD4, CD8α, CD8β, and CD3-TCR to ultimately generate double-positive cells, which co-express CD4 and CD8. The double-positive thymocytes then undergo positive and negative selection to give rise to a MHC-restricted mature repertoire of CD3$^+$CD4$^+$ or CD3$^+$CD8$^+$ single-positive thymocytes. Around this same time, single-positive T cells begin to rapidly accumulate in the peripheral immune system, hence the desire to transplant by 14 weeks' gestation. However, recent analyses have indicated that T-cell numbers in the fetal liver increase tenfold, from 2.3 × 10^3 to 2.4 × 10^4, between 12 and 13 weeks' gestation.[36] Haynes et al. also observed a low number of T cells in the liver at 12 weeks' gestation.[28] These findings indicate that before 14 weeks' gestation the numbers of T cells in the periphery are low, but they are clearly detectable and their numbers are rapidly increasing from 12 weeks onward. Another possible concern with transplanting cells just prior to the complete maturation of the thymus is the time required for donor cells to take part in the selection process

of T cells in the thymus. It may take up to several weeks for cells derived from donor stem cells to colonize the thymus and contribute to the selection of developing T cells.[37] Meanwhile, T cells are generated which may not be tolerant towards donor human leukocyte antigens (HLA). The critical question that remains to be answered before the validity of these concerns can be addressed is whether the relatively few T cells present before 14 weeks' gestation are capable of mediating rejection of donor stem cells.

The functional capacity of T cells present at different stages of fetal development is currently unknown. Studies of umbilical cord blood (UCB) T cells have suggested that fetal T cells may not be functionally similar to their adult counterparts.[38, 39] In comparison to adult peripheral-blood leukocytes (aPBLs), UCB T cells were normal in their proliferative responses to alloantigens in primary mixed leukocyte reactions.[40, 41] The phenotypic profile of activation or co-stimulatory molecules on activated UCB T cells was also similar to that of aPBL T cells.[41–42] Purified CD5$^+$ UCB T cells were also tested for their cytotoxic capabilities. Cytotoxic UCB and aPBL CD5$^+$ T cells were stimulated with allogeneic aPBLs in primary mixed leukocyte cultures and tested for cytotoxicity after 7 days of culture. The cytotoxic activity of the UCB T cells was comparable or even exceeded that of aPBL T cells.[42] However, UCB T cells did differ from adult T cells in their secondary proliferative response after a primary alloantigen stimulation.[38] Secondary stimulation of UCB T cells failed to induce a proliferative response of a similar magnitude to that of adult T cells. This unresponsiveness is likely to be due to defective signaling by Ras, a molecule active in signal transduction in the T-cell receptor signaling pathway.[39] It is hypothesized that a defect in the functioning of UCB T cells is responsible for the low incidence of graft-versus-host disease (GVHD) associated with UCB transplants. Whether such a defect exists, and to what degree, in preterm fetal T cells is not known.

The capacity of fetal T cells to mediate graft rejection needs to be determined before any final conclusions can be drawn. If fetal T cells are found to be functional, then the in utero transplantation of stem cells may have to occur even earlier than the currently accepted limit of 14 weeks' gestation. However, if the cytotoxic capacity of fetal T cells is reduced or absent from fetal T cells, then the window of opportunity for the introduction of foreign cells into the fetus may be longer than expected.

Natural Killer Cell Development in the Human Fetus

NK cells are another type of lymphocyte capable of mediating the killing of foreign cells and, like T cells, have been implicated in postnatal bone marrow rejection.[21] The role (if any) of fetal NK cells in the outcome of IUT has, however, received little attention. In contrast to T cells, NK cells appear in the liver as early as 6 weeks' gestation and NK cells have been found to comprise 35 to 70% of the CD45[+] leukocytes in embryonic and fetal livers of 6 to 24 weeks' gestation.[34] It is hypothesized that these NK cells are generated in the fetal liver, although this has not been demonstrated by the isolation of NK-committed progenitors early in gestation. We have hypothesized that the fetal NK population might be derived directly from HSC, but the existence of an NK-committed progenitor in the fetal liver cannot be ruled out.[43] NK cells are known to be capable of killing virally infected cells and tumor cells and, if found to be active early in fetal development, may provide the fetus' first and only defense against such threats. Indeed, analysis of NK cell frequencies in fetal blood at different gestational ages has suggested that NK cells are most frequent early in gestation (29% at 13 weeks) and decrease exponentially until term (6% at 38 weeks).[44]

NK cells are also generated in the fetal thymus. Hematopoietic stem cells residing in the liver are believed to be a source of the stem cells/progenitors which colonize the fetal thymus,[37, 45–47] since NK cells and their progenitors have also been detected in the fetal thymus.[48–50] A close developmental relationship between T and NK cells has been hypothesized based on a number of antigenic similarities between these two lineages,[34, 47] and there is evidence of an intrathymic common progenitor for fetal T and NK cells.[49] As mentioned above, there are several reports demonstrating evidence for a very early development of NK cells in the perithymic mes-

enchyma between 7 and 9.5 weeks' gestation. This lymphoid population was characterized as CD45[+]CD7[+] cyCD3[+] and lacked surface expression of CD3, TCR, CD4, or CD8 markers.[28, 33, 51] Furthermore, fetal NK cells are defined by a high expression of CD7, suggesting that the thymic CD45[+]CD7[+]cyCD3[+] cells are NK cells.[45] Flow cytometric analyses of fetal thymi at later time points in gestation have unequivocally demonstrated the presence of CD56[+]CD3[−] NK cells.[48–50] The finding that NK cells are generated in at least two fetal hematopoietic organs, starting most likely at the time when the liver and thymus first begin to become hematopoietic, suggests an important role for these cells in fetal immunity. CD56[+]CD3[−] NK cells are in fact plentiful in the fetal liver and blood weeks before T cells begin to be found outside of the thymus.[34, 44]

A better understanding of the functional capacities of these embryonic and fetal NK cells is, however, required before determining the threat that these cells pose to donor cells. In Figure 38–5, we show our data indicating the presence of NK cells in fetal liver CD45[+] cells as early as 8 weeks' gestation. Preliminary studies on older fetal tissues suggest that fetal NK cells are functionally active and, thus, may interfere with donor cell engraftment in utero. The cytolytic activity of purified fetal CD56[+]CD3[−] NK cells was examined by Phillips et al.[34] NK cells from liver specimens, of gestational ages ranging from 15 to 24 weeks, were demonstrated to kill tumor cell lines. Although not tested directly in parallel with NK cells isolated from adult peripheral blood leukocytes, the cytotoxic activity of the fetal NK cells appeared to be somewhat less than that historically observed with adult PBLs. Brief interleukin-2 (IL-2) exposure also appeared to induce lymphokine-activated killer (LAK) cell activity in cultures of fetal NK cells. LAK cells are capable of killing NK tumors and cell lines resistant to killing by freshly isolated NK cells. Together, these observations demonstrated that fetal NK cells older than 15 weeks' gestation are functional. These investigators also reported that there may be a link between the gestation age of the NK cells and their functional activity, with younger NK cells appearing to exhibit less cytotoxic activity than older cells.

Studies on UCB NK cells offer indirect data on the functional capacity of fetal NK cells. NK cells present in UCB have been shown to be deficient in lytic activity. However, the defect in UCB NKC is readily restored to levels comparable to those of adult PBLs by a brief exposure of less than or equal to 24 hours to either of the cytokines IL-2 or IL-12.[52–59] Interestingly, one report showed that the functional capacity of purified CD56[+]CD3[−] UCB NK cells was indistinguishable from that of the same cell population isolated from adult PBLs.[34] These results suggest that the decreased NKC activity of UCB may be in part mediated by the accessory cells found in the UCB leukocyte preparations tested by most investigators. UCB NK cells were also found to generate LAK cells in a manner similar to adult NK cells when stimulated by IL-2 and/or IL-12.[54, 57–60] These data demonstrate that any functional deficiencies of UCB NK cells are readily reversed in vitro by exposure to known NK cell stimulators. However, one study found that

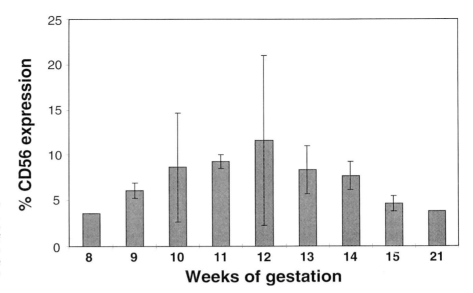

FIGURE 38–5. NK cells are present in the fetal immune system from the 8th week onward. Fetal livers (n = 3 to 5) from the indicated gestational ages were analyzed for the presence of CD56 among CD45$^+$ glycophorin A$^-$ light density cells. Percentages of CD56$^+$ cells among live cells (propidium iodide negative) are represented ± S.E.

unlike adult NK cells, UCB NK cells did not generate LAK cells in response to IL-7, TNF-α, or IFN-γ.[57] The lack of response to TNF-α and IFN-γ is apparently not due, however, to a lack of receptors for these cytokines, since over 90% of UCB NK cells have been found to express these receptors.[61]

In conclusion, the functional status of the cellular arm of the immune system in the early human fetus needs to be characterized further. Studies on the functional capacity of embryonic and fetal lymphocytes may prove these cells to be capable of rejecting donor stem cells. Presently, we hypothesize that host T and NK cells might be critical in the rejection of the donor HSCs (Fig. 38–6). Notwithstanding, in utero transplants performed as early as technically feasible may have the greatest chance of evading the developing fetal immune system.

Prenatal Tolerance Induction for Postnatal Organ Transplantation

The studies by Medawar suggested that early presentation of cellular antigen resulted in specific immunologic

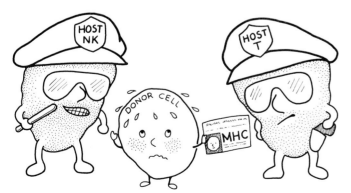

FIGURE 38–6. The fate of a donor cell transplanted into the fetus is largely determined via recognition (or lack of recognition) by host T and NK cells. Depending on a variety of factors, donor MHCs may play an important role in its survival.

tolerance. Theoretically, introduction of foreign cells prior to completion of fetal thymic T-cell maturation would result in processing of foreign antigen as "self." Diseases producing organ failure such as obstructive uropathy and hypoplastic left heart syndrome can be diagnosed prenatally and potentially treated by organ replacement postnatally (Fig. 38–7). However, the morbidity and mortality of lifelong immunosuppression coupled with the extreme shortage of size-appropriate organs has greatly limited the field of neonatal solid organ transplantation. Bone marrow is the only graft that, once accepted, does not require immunosuppression agents to prevent rejection.[62, 63] Moreover, bone marrow chimerism is associated with systemic donor-specific transplantation tolerance for solid organ and cellular grafts. The acquisition of prenatal chimerism can circumvent the three most significant limitations to conventional postnatal bone marrow transplantation: (1) the requirement for lethal conditioning of the recipient with its attendant morbidity and mortality, (2) GVHD, and (3) lack of suitable HLA-matched donors. Approximately 50% of BMT recipients who develop GVHD die as a result of complications associated with it.[64] It is well established that the incidence and severity of GVHD are directly correlated with the degree of genetic disparity.[64] In HLA-identical related donor and recipient combinations, the incidence of GVHD is 30 to 50%. In the event of one class I or class II HLA antigen disparity, the incidence increases to 65%. If greater than two antigen disparities exist between donor and recipient, 100% develop GVHD and 80% die. The chance of finding an HLA-identical or a one-antigen disparate donor is only 30%. GVHD is believed to be mediated primarily by T cells. However, B cells and NK cells have also been implicated as the effector cells in GVHD.[65] Removal of T cells from the allogeneic BM inoculum has been shown to prevent GVHD.[66] However, up to 70% of patients fail to engraft, suggesting that T cells are critical for engraftment of the BM stem cell. In order to extend the applicability of BMT to MHC-

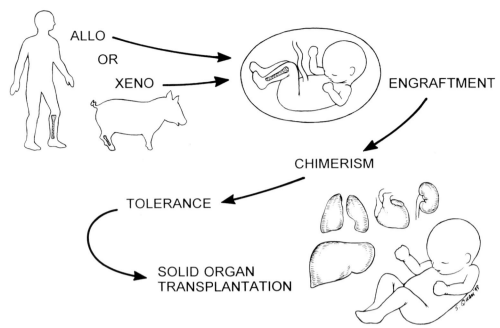

FIGURE 38–7. Simplified paradigm for fetal tolerance induction. Early presentation of cellular antigen results in specific immunologic tolerance. Theoretically, introduction of foreign cells prior to completion of fetal thymic T cell maturation would result in processing of foreign antigen as "self" and engraftment of allogeneic or xenogeneic cells. Diseases producing organ failure such as obstructive uropathy and hypoplastic left heart syndrome can be diagnosed prenatally and potentially treated by organ replacement postnatally.

mismatched donor/recipient pairs, transplantation of a highly enriched or purified stem cell population rather than unmodified BM has been attempted. However, although purified stem cell transplants reliably engraft in MHC-matched combinations, they do not engraft in genetically disparate recipients.

Ideally, predicted neonatal organ failure could be treated by establishing donor-specific tolerance to either living-related allogeneic or xenogeneic organs prenatally by establishing hematopoietic chimerism before birth. This would theoretically allow postnatal solid organ transplantation without the need for immunosuppression and also potentially solve the organ shortage problem. Studies in mice,[67] sheep,[68] monkeys,[12] and humans[69] suggest that the early gestation fetus is susceptible to tolerance induction by the transplantation of allogeneic cells.

Mechanisms of Chimerism-Induced Transplantation Tolerance

The way in which hematopoietic chimerism induces transplantation tolerance is not known. It is believed that persistence of donor-derived cells is crucial to the stability of allograft tolerance. In support of this notion, Sharabi et al.[70] demonstrated that in stable, allogeneic, irradiated chimeras, elimination of donor cells abrogated tolerance to subsequent skin grafts. Conversely, Starzl[71, 72] suggested that successful long-term solid organ transplants are a result of the transplanted organ carrying a small population of hematopoietic stem cells that establish microchimerism (<1% demonstrable chimerism) in the recipients' bone marrow. Microchime-

rism contributes to the induction and maintenance of tolerance, allowing some solid organ allografts to survive without immunosuppression. Starzl's observations on microchimerism are supported by the work of Liegeois[73] that showed that mice given antilymphocyte serum and bone marrow but not skin grafts had much less microchimerism than similarly treated mice given skin grafts. This suggests that the presence of the graft is an added stimulus for proliferation of donor bone marrow cells. Other explanations are that the persistent donor-specific bone marrow cells, after proliferating in response to the graft, exert a suppressor or veto effect on recipient antidonor alloreactivity; or that persistent donor bone marrow cells might act as surrogate targets for donor alloreactive cells. Kim et al.[74] and Alard et al.[67] demonstrated that microchimerism in a rodent model fails to predict tolerance, but microchimerism is necessary for tolerance to skin grafts. Carrier et al.[75] demonstrated tolerance to skin grafts from in utero fully allogeneic fetal liver stem cell transplants in a nondefective mouse model with levels of engraftment of less than 0.1%. Although Hedrick et al.[76] were unable to induce tolerance to a renal allograft by in utero stem cell injection that resulted in a 3 to 5% level of engraftment in a sheep model, Mychaliska et al.[77] reported that in utero transplantation of T-cell–depleted paternal bone marrow can increase the survival of a kidney allograft in the rhesus monkey. Microchimerism resulted as well as donor-specific tolerance by mixed lymphocyte reaction. There was, however, delayed (after approximately 1 month) mild rejection of the renal allografts. Yuh et al.[78] used an in utero rat model that resulted in approximately 1% chimerism. Some chimeric animals accepted skin grafts and 100% of those went on to accept lung or heart allografts.

T lymphocytes are thought to be the mediators of rejection during classic organ transplantation.[79] There are currently three proposed mechanisms for the maintenance of T-cell tolerance[80]: (1) central or clonal deletion in which potentially self-reactive T cells are negatively selected (deleted) during development in the thymus; (2) clonal anergy, or the inability of a T cell to respond and be activated by its cognate antigen; and (3) active suppression by other circulating cells (clonal suppression). These various mechanisms are needed to downregulate the reactive T-cell clones that escape into the periphery. In addition, there may be mechanisms of tolerance that involve the B-cell repertoire. Exposure of early-gestation B cells to foreign antigen may result in clonal deletion or anergy.

An alternate theory on the development of tolerance has been proposed in a study by Ridge et al.[81] They suggested that the immune system does not discriminate between self- and non-self but between dangerous and harmless entities, and that the primary distinction is made by antigen-presenting cells (APCs), which are activated to up-regulate co-stimulatory molecules (i.e., fetal T and B cells) only when induced by alarm signals from their environment. They proposed that Medawar's classic experiments in neonatal tolerance resulted from the mixture (and dose) of cells in the donor inocula, which contained very few professional APCs (e.g., dendritic cells) and a large percentage of T and B cells, which cannot co-stimulate virgin T cells. Thus the tiny number of virgin T cells in newborn mice might easily be overwhelmed by the tolerogenic cells in the donor inoculum before ever having an opportunity to meet an activating APC such as a dendritic cell.

Summary

The data presented in this chapter, although promising, demonstrate that the field of in utero cellular transplantation and induction of prenatal tolerance is still in its infancy. The observation that T and NK cells might be present in the fetal immune system earlier than initially recognized suggests that we need to expand our knowledge of the ontogeny and function of the fetal immune system. The early-gestation fetus may not be the "ideal" recipient of a cellular graft—its "primitive" immune system may, in part, be a deterrent to successful prenatal chimerism. Figure 38–8 summarizes the potential pitfalls that might prevent the successful transfer of HSCs in utero.

Regarding the transfer of HSCs in utero, there are several basic questions that need to be addressed in future research in the field. In one hand, we need to determine what is the ideal source of HSCs for in utero transplantation. Are fetal cells better suited to engraft in the fetal environment than neonatal or postnatal HSCs? The recent findings indicating that the most primitive and quiescent HSCs reside in the CD34⁻ subpopulation of hematopoietic progenitors challenges the well-accepted concept of HSCs expressing high levels of

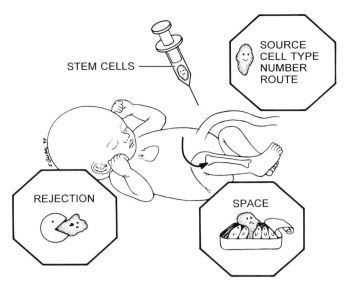

FIGURE 38–8. Potential obstacles and unanswered questions that may influence the ability to achieve successful cellular transplantation in utero.

CD34.[82] In addition, how many cells should be transferred into a human fetus to ensure long-term engraftment? Which route of cellular injection is the most efficient and practical: intraperitoneal, intraplacental, intrahepatic, or intravenous? The presence of functional NK cells in the immature immune system of the early-gestation fetus suggests that this cellular compartment might play a crucial role in the rejection of the graft. And finally, is the fetal immune system really "empty," as it has been theorized for decades? Or, on the contrary, are we dealing with space issues in the fetal hematopoietic environment that are similar to the considerations made for postnatal transplantation?

REFERENCES

1. Owen RD: Immunologic consequences of vascular anastomoses between bovine twins. Science 102:400–401, 1945.
2. Anderson D, Billingham R, Lampkin G, et al: The use of skin grafting to distinguish between monozygotic and dizygotic twins in cattle. Heredity 5:379–397, 1951.
3. Simonsen M: The acquired immunity concept in kidney homotransplantation. Ann N Y Acad Sci 59:448–452, 1955.
4. Billingham R, Brent L, Medawar P: Actively acquired tolerance of foreign cells. Nature 172:603, 1953.
5. Ildstad ST, Sachs DH: Reconstitution with syngeneic plus allogeneic or xenogeneic bone marrow leads to specific acceptance of allografts or xeno-grafts. Nature 307:168–170, 1984.
6. Ildstad ST, Wren SM, Boggs SS, et al: Cross-species bone marrow transplantation: Evidence for tolerance induction, stem cell engraftment, and maturation of T lymphocytes in a xenogeneic stromal environment (rat—mouse). J Exp Med 174:467–478, 1991.
7. Chabot JA, Pepino P, Wasfie T, et al: UVB pretreatment of rat bone marrow allografts. Prevention of GVHD and induction of allochimerism and donor-specific unresponsiveness. Transplantation 49:886–889, 1990.
8. Orloff MS, Fallon MA, DeMara E, et al: Induction of specific tolerance to small-bowel allografts. Surgery 116:222–228, 1994.
9. Caridis DT, Liegeois A, Barrett I, et al: Enhanced survival of canine renal allografts of ALS-treated dogs given bone marrow. Transplant Proc 5:671–674, 1973.
10. Smith CV, Suzuki T, Guzzetta PC, et al: Bone marrow transplantation in miniature swine: IV. Development of myeloablative regi-

mens that allow engraftment across major histocompatibility barriers. Transplantation 56:541–549, 1993.

11. Thomas F, Carver F, Foil M: Long-term incompatible kidney survival in outbred higher primates without chronic immunosuppression. Ann Surg 198:370, 1993.

12. Harrison MR, Slotnick RN, Crombleholme TM, et al: In-utero transplantation of fetal liver haemopoietic stem cells in monkeys. Lancet 2:1425–1427, 1989.

13. Srour EF, Zanjani ED, Cornetta K, et al: Persistence of human multilineage, self-renewing lymphohematopoietic stem cells in chimeric sheep. Blood 82:3333–3342, 1993.

14. Zanjani ED, Flake AW, Rice H, et al: Long-term repopulating ability of xenogeneic transplanted human fetal liver hematopoietic stem cells in sheep [see comments]. J Clin Invest 93:1051–1055, 1994.

15. Picus J, Aldrich WR, Letvin NL: A naturally occurring bone-marrow-chimeric primate. I. Integrity of its immune system. Transplantation 39:297–303, 1985.

16. van Dijk P, Narins PM, Wang J: Spontaneous otoacoustic emissions in seven frog species. Hear Res 101:102–112, 1996.

17. Gill TJD: Chimerism in humans. Transplant Proc 9:1423–1431, 1977.

18. Thomas JM, Carver FM, Kasten-Jolly J: Further studies of veto activity in rhesus monkey bone marrow in relation to allograft tolerance and chimerism. Transplantation 57:101, 1994.

19. Ildstad ST, Sachs DH: Reconstitution with syngeneic plus allogeneic or xenogeneic bone marrow leads to specific acceptance of allografts or xenografts. Nature 307:168–170, 1984.

20. Godin I, Dieterlen-Lièvre F, Cumano A: Emergence of multipotent hemopoietic cells in the yolk sac and paraaortic splanchnopleura in mouse embryos, beginning at 8.5 days postcoitus. Proc Natl Acad Sci U S A 92:773–777, 1995.

21. Medvinski A, Samoylina L, Muller A, et al: An early pre-liver intraembryonic source of CFU-S in the developing mouse. Nature 364:64–66, 1993.

22. Tavian M, Coulombel L, Luton D, et al: Aorta-associated CD34+ hematopoietic cells in the early human embryo. Blood 87:67–72, 1996.

23. Rowley PT, Ohlsson-Wilhelm BM, Farley BA: Erythroid colony formation from human fetal liver. Proc Natl Acad Sci U S A 75:984–988, 1978.

24. Migliaccio G, Migliaccio AR, Petti S, et al: Human embryonic hemopoiesis. Kinetics of progenitors and precursors underlying the yolk sac/liver transition. J Clin Invest 78:51–60, 1986.

25. Charbord P, Tavian M, Humeau L, et al: Early ontogeny of the human marrow from long bones: An immunohistochemical study of hematopoiesis and its microenvironment [see comments]. Blood 87:4109–4119, 1996.

26. Muench MO, Cupp J, Polakoff J, et al: Expression of CD33, CD38 and HLA-DR on CD34+ human fetal liver progenitors with a high proliferative potential. Blood 83:3170–3181, 1994.

27. Terstappen LWMM, Huang S, Safford M, et al: Sequential generation of hematopoietic colonies derived from single nonlineage-committed CD34+CD38− progenitor cells. Blood 77:1218–1227, 1991.

28. Haynes BF, Martin ME, Kay HH, et al: Early events in human T cell ontogeny: Phenotypic characterization and immunohistological localization of T-cell precursors in early human fetal tissues. J Exp Med 168:1061–1080, 1988.

29. Haynes BF, Heinly CS: Early human T cell development: Analysis of the human thymus at the time of initial entry of hematopoietic stem cells into the fetal thymic microenvironment. J Exp Med 181:1445–1458, 1995.

30. Lobach DF, Haynes BF: Ontogeny of the human thymus during fetal development. J Clin Immunol 7:81–97, 1987.

31. Grümayer ER, Griesinger F, Hummell DS, et al: Identification of novel B-lineage cells in human fetal bone marrow that coexpress CD7. Blood 77:64–68, 1991.

32. Chabannon C, Wood P, Torok-Storb B: Expression of CD7 on normal human myeloid progenitors. J Immunol 149:2110–2113, 1992.

33. Lobach DF, Hensley LL, Ho W, et al: Human T-cell antigen expression during early stages of fetal thymic maturation. J Immunol 1351:1752–1759, 1985.

34. Phillips JH, Hori T, Nagler A, et al: Ontogeny of human natural killer (NK) cells: Fetal NK cells mediate cytolytic function and express cytoplasmic CD3 epsilon, delta proteins. J Exp Med 175:1055–1066, 1992.

35. Terstappen LW, Huang S, Picker LJ: Flow cytometric assessment of human T-cell differentiation in thymus and bone marrow. Blood 79:666–677, 1992.

36. Mychaliska GB, Muench MO, Rice HE, et al: The biology and ethics of banking fetal liver hematopoietic stem cells for in utero transplantation. J Pediatr Surg 33:394–399, 1998.

37. Bárcena A, Galy AHM, Punnonen J, et al: Lymphoid and myeloid differentiation of fetal liver CD34+ lineage-cells in human thymic organ culture. J Exp Med 180:123–132, 1994.

38. Risdon G, Gaddy J, Horie M, et al: Alloantigen priming induces a state of unresponsiveness in human umbilical cord blood T cells. Proc Natl Acad Sci U S A 92:2413–2417, 1995.

39. Porcu P, Gaddy J, Broxmeyer HE: Alloantigen-induced unresponsiveness in cord blood T lymphocytes is associated with defective activation of Ras. Proc Natl Acad Sci U S A 95:4538–4543, 1998.

40. Roncarolo MG, Bigler M, Ciuti E, et al: Immune responses by cord blood cells. Blood Cells 20:573–586, 1994.

41. Risdon G, Gaddy J, Stehman FB, et al: Proliferative and cytotoxic responses of human cord blood T lymphocytes following allogeneic stimulation. Cell Immunol 154:14–24, 1994.

42. Roncarolo MG, Bigler M, Martino S, et al: Immune functions of cord blood cells before and after transplantation. J Hematother 5:157–160, 1996.

43. Bárcena A, Muench MO, Roncarolo MG, et al: Tracing the expression of CD7 and other antigens during T- and myeloid-cell differentiation in the human fetal liver and thymus. Leuk Lymphoma 17:1–11, 1995.

44. Thilaganathan B, Abbas A, Nicolaides KH: Fetal blood natural killer cells in human pregnancy. Fetal Diagn Ther 8:149–153, 1993.

45. Bárcena A, Muench MO, Galy AHM, et al: Phenotypic and functional analysis of T-cell precursors in the human fetal liver and thymus: CD7 expression in the early stages of T- and myeloid-cell development. Blood 82:3401–3414, 1993.

46. Bárcena A, Muench MO, Roncarolo MG, et al: In search of T-cell progenitors in the human fetal liver. Res Immunol 145:120–123, 1994.

47. Spits H, Lanier LL, Phillips JH: Development of human T and natural killer cells. Blood 85:2654–2670, 1995.

48. Sánchez MJ, Spits H, Lanier LL, et al: Human natural killer cell committed thymocytes and their relation to the T cell lineage. J Exp Med 178:1857–1866, 1993.

49. Sánchez MJ, Muench MO, Roncarolo MG, et al: Identification of a common T/NK cell progenitor in the human fetal thymus. J Exp Med 180:569–576, 1994.

50. Beecher MS, Baiocchi RA, Linett ML, et al: Expression of the zeta protein subunit in CD3− NK effectors derived from human thymus. Cell Immunol 155:508–516, 1994.

51. Campana D, Janossy G, Coustan-Smith E, et al: The expression of T cell receptor-associated proteins during T cell ontogeny in man. J Immunol 142:57–66, 1989.

52. Merrill JD, Sigaroudinia M, Kohl S: Characterization of natural killer and antibody-dependent cellular cytotoxicity of preterm infants against human immunodeficiency virus-infected cells. Pediatr Res 40:498–503, 1996.

53. Lau AS, Sigaroudinia M, Yeung MC, et al: Interleukin-12 induces interferon-gamma expression and natural killer cytotoxicity in cord blood mononuclear cells. Pediatr Res 39:150–155, 1996.

54. Gaddy J, Risdon G, Broxmeyer HE: Cord blood natural killer cells are functionally and phenotypically immature but readily respond to interleukin-2 and interleukin-12. J Interferon Cytokine Res 15:527–536, 1995.

55. Bradstock KF, Luxford C, Grimsley PG: Functional and phenotypic assessment of neonatal human leucocytes expressing natural killer cell-associated antigens. Immunol Cell Biol 71:535–542, 1993.

56. Malygin AM, Timonen T: Non-major histocompatibility complex-restricted killer cells in human cord blood: Generation and cytotoxic activity in recombinant interleukin-2-supplemented cultures. Immunology 79:506–508, 1993.

57. Webb BJ, Bochan MR, Montel A, et al: The lack of NK cytotoxicity associated with fresh HUCB may be due to the presence of soluble HLA in the serum. Cell Immunol 159:246–261, 1994.

58. Keever CA, Abu-Hajir M, Graf W, et al: Characterization of the alloreactivity and anti-leukemia reactivity of cord blood mononuclear cells. Bone Marrow Transplant 15:407–419, 1995.
59. Harris DT: In vitro and in vivo assessment of the graft-versus-leukemia activity of cord blood. Bone Marrow Transplant 15:17–23, 1995.
60. Harris DT, LoCascio J, Besencon FJ: Analysis of the alloreactive capacity of human umbilical cord blood: Implications for graft-versus-host disease. Bone Marrow Transplant 14:545–553, 1994.
61. Han P, Hodge G, Story C, et al: Phenotypic analysis of functional T-lymphocyte subtypes and natural killer cells in human cord blood: Relevance to umbilical cord blood transplantation. Br J Haematol 89:733–740, 1995.
62. Slavin S, Morecki S, Weigensberg M, et al: Functional clonal deletion versus suppressor cell-induced transplantation tolerance in chimeras prepared with a short course of total-lymphoid irradiation. Transplantation 41:680–687, 1986.
63. Ildstad ST, Wren SM, Bluestone JA, et al: Characterization of mixed allogeneic chimeras. Immunocompetence, in vitro reactivity, and genetic specificity of tolerance. J Exp Med 162:231–244, 1985.
64. Ferrara J, Deeg H: Graft-versus-host disease. Review article. N Engl J Med 324:667–674, 1991.
65. Onoe K, Fernandes G, Good R: Humoral and cell-mediated immune responses in fully allogeneic bone marrow chimeras in mice. J Exp Med 151:115–132, 1980.
66. Korngold R, Sprent J: Lethal GVHD after bone marrow transplantation across minor histocompatibility barriers in mice: Prevention by removing mature T-cells from marrow. J Exp Med 148:1687–1698, 1978.
67. Alard P, Matriano J, Socarras S, et al: Detection of donor-derived cells by polymerase chain reaction in neonatally tolerant mice. Microchimerism fails to predict tolerance. Transplantation 60:1125–1128, 1995.
68. Flake AW, Harrison MR, Adzick NS, et al: Transplantation of fetal hematopoietic stem cells in utero: The creation of hematopoietic chimeras. Science 233:776–778, 1986.
69. Rolles K, Burroughs AK, Davidson BR: Donor specific bone marrow infusion after orthotopic liver transplantation. Lancet 343:263–265, 1994.
70. Sharabi Y, Sachs DH: Mixed chimerism and permanent specific transplantation tolerance induced by a nonlethal preparative regimen. J Exp Med 169:493, 1989.
71. Starzl TE, Demetris AJ, Murase N, et al: Cell migration, chimerism and graft acceptance. Lancet 339:1579–1582, 1992.
72. Starzl TE, Demetris AJ, Murase N: Donor cell chimerism permitted by immunosuppressive drugs: A new view of organ transplantation. Immunol Today 14:326–332, 1993.
73. Liegeois A, Gaillard MC, Ouvre E, et al: Microchimerism in pregnant mice. Transplant Proc 13:1250–1252, 1981.
74. Kim H, Shaaban A, Yang E, et al: Microchimerism and tolerance after in utero bone marrow transplantation in mice. J Surg Res 77:1–5, 1998.
75. Carrier E, Lee TH, Busch MP, et al: Induction of tolerance in nondefective mice after in utero transplantation of major histocompatibility complex-mismatched fetal hematopoietic stem cells. Blood 86:4681–4690, 1995.
76. Hedrick MH, Rice HE, MacGillivray TE, et al: Hematopoietic chimerism achieved by in utero hematopoietic stem cell injection does not induce donor-specific tolerance for renal allografts in sheep. Transplantation 58:110–111, 1994.
77. Mychaliska GB, Rice HE, Tarantal AF, et al: In utero hematopoietic stem cell transplants prolong survival of postnatal kidney transplantation in monkeys. J Pediatr Surg 32:976–981, 1997.
78. Yuh DD, Gandy KL, Reitz BA, et al: Perinatal induction of immunotolerance to cardiac and pulmonary allografts. J Thorac Cardiovasc Surg 114:64–75, 1997.
79. Sharabi Y, Abraham V, Sykes M, et al: Mixed allogeneic chimeras prepared by a non-myeloablative regimen: Requirement for chimerism to maintain tolerance. Bone Marrow Transplant 9:191–198, 1992.
80. Streilin JW: Neonatal tolerance of H-2 antigens: Procuring graft acceptance the old fashioned way. Transplantation 52:1–10, 1991.
81. Ridge J, Fuchs E, Matzinger P: Neonatal tolerance revisited: Turning on newborn T cells with dendritic cells. Science 271:1723–1730, 1996.
82. Zanjani ED, Almeida-Porada G, Livingston AG, et al: Human bone marrow CD34⁻ cells engraft in vivo and undergo multilineage expression that includes giving rise to CD34⁺ cells. Exp Hematol 26:353–360, 1998.

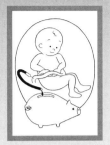

CHAPTER 39

Fetal Hematopoietic Stem Cell Transplantation

MARCUS O. MUENCH and FRANÇOIS GOLFIER

Fetal cellular therapy has the potential of providing a cure or ameliorating an array of inherited diseases. There are a number of tissues that can be transplanted in the form of a cellular suspension which then have the ability to integrate, in a normal fashion, into the host's own tissues. Hematopoietic stem cells (HSCs) represent one such cell type. There is extensive experience with the postnatal transplantation of HSCs and a rapidly growing experience with this form of cellular therapy in utero. Fetal cellular therapy is very attractive because it builds on a well-established foundation of diagnostic and therapeutic techniques in prenatal care. Genetic tests can be performed early in gestation to identify fetuses with a particular inheritable disease. The transplantation procedure itself can be as simple as a percutaneous injection of cells into the fetus' peritoneum performed under ultrasonic guidance.

Nonetheless, there are many hurdles that must be overcome before cellular therapy becomes a reliable form of treatment for the fetus with an inherited disease. One of the challenges that remain in making fetal cellular therapy a reality is choosing the best cells to transplant. Since there are many developmental changes that occur to tissues between fetal and adult life, it is reasonable to assume that the best tissues to transplant into a fetus are those of fetal origin. However, there is little experience with fetal tissue transplantation relative to the extensive experience with postnatal transplantation of adult cells and organs. Methods of tissue processing, quality control measures, and cryopreservation need to be adapted from the experience with postnatal tissues to use with fetal tissues. This chapter reviews recent breakthroughs in the field of fetal HSC transplantation and delves into some of the many outstanding issues and future possibilities surrounding the transplantation of fetal HSCs both in utero and after birth.

Availability of Fetal Tissues

The large number of pregnancies terminated each year worldwide represents a vast, largely untapped reservoir of transplantable tissue. In the United States alone, a total of 1,210,883 legal abortions were reported to the Centers for Disease Control in 1995.[1] Approximately 34% of the abortions were performed between 9 and 13 weeks' gestation. Abortions between 16 and 20 weeks' gestation accounted for approximately 4% of the total abortions representing over 45,000 abortions. Abortions at 21 weeks' gestation or older represented 1.4%, or over 15,000 abortions. It is important to note, however, that not all fetal specimens are suitable for the harvest of tissues for transplantation, since some mothers will be at high risk for communicable disease or the pregnancies will be terminated due to fetal abnormality. Nonetheless, an effective program to procure, process, and bank fetal tissues could result in a sizable tissue bank within a short period of time.

Advantages of Fetal Tissues

Human fetal tissue is a rich source of HSCs that has been proven to be suitable for in utero hematopoietic stem cell transplantation (IUT) and may also be suitable for postnatal transplantation. Although both animal experiments and experience with human IUT have shown that adult HSCs will engraft a fetus,[2, 3] it remains to be determined if fetal HSCs have an engraftment advantage in the fetal environment. There are, however, a number of advantages that may favor the use of fetal tissue for transplantation.

First, fetal liver (FL) and fetal bone marrow (FBM) contain low numbers of T lymphocytes, the major mediators of graft-versus-host disease (GVHD).[4–6] Indeed, GVHD was not found to be a major problem in the limited experience with postnatal and in utero transplantation of FL cells harvested from fetuses at an early gestational age.[4, 7] In fact, there is no other source of HSCs that has as few mature lymphocytes as that of fetal tissues. This is not to say that there are no mature lymphocytes present in fetal tissues capable of causing GVHD. Midtrimester fetal tissues contain significant numbers of T, B, and natural killer (NK) cells, and their numbers increase with the gestational age of the tissue. The presence of at least the T lymphocytes, the major cells responsible for GVHD, must be taken into consideration when processing these tissues for transplantation.

Nonetheless, the ultimate number of T cells present in a graft that has been prepared for transplantation by some method of HSC enrichment is dependent on the number of T cells in the starting tissues, since no purification procedure used in the clinical setting is yet capable of removing all contaminating T cells. The low numbers of T cells present in fetal tissues to begin with helps to ensure that processed grafts are virtually free of T cells.

Second, concerns about the durability of a graft are warranted when considering HSC transplantation as a lifelong cure of hematopoietic diseases, especially those afflicting a fetus. The findings that the levels of HSC engraftment following IUT are low underscore this concern. In a healthy person the longevity of the hematopoietic system may make it appear that the pool of HSCs, the precursors of a lifetime of blood cell production, is immortal. Indeed, HSC transplantation in adults relies on the capacity of a fraction of one person's HSCs to reconstitute the entire hematopoietic system of another individual. Although HSC transplantation does result in durable engraftment, it is exactly under the stressful conditions of a transplant that HSCs begin to reveal their mortality. Serial transplantation of HSCs from one mouse to another results in the eventual death of recipients due to a decline in HSC function.[8–12] The conclusion from a number of different studies performed in the mouse is that HSCs have a limited capacity to proliferate. These findings also predicted that fetal HSCs should have a more extensive proliferative capacity than those of adult HSCs because of the short proliferative history of fetal cells (Fig. 39–1). Indeed, recent studies in the mouse comparing fetal and adult HSCs demonstrated that fetal HSCs could outgrow their adult counterparts.[13, 14] Another way in which these findings can be viewed is that the transplantation of FL and FBM results in nearly the entire HSC pool of one young individual being transplanted as opposed to the small fraction of the HSC pool that can be obtained from umbilical cord blood (UCB), adult BM, or mobilized peripheral blood stem cells (PBSCs). It is important to note that the capacity of a human HSC to proliferate is unknown; consequently, the longevity of a graft cannot be calculated. Thus, it is imposible at this time to quantify the advantage that fetal HSCs have over their adult counterparts. Nonetheless, the most cautious approach to IUT would be to opt for transplanting the highest number of HSCs with the shortest proliferative history possible.

Third, the propensity of fetal progenitors and HSCs to grow in vitro suggests that the number of progenitors in a fetal graft could be expanded in vitro before transplantation to aid engraftment.[15] Ex vivo expansion of fetal progenitors is likely to be most useful in the postnatal transplantation setting, where the size of the recipient requires that a larger number of progenitors be transplanted if rapid engraftment is to be achieved. Although murine studies have demonstrated the advantages of ex vivo progenitor expansion by demonstrating accelerated peripheral blood cell reconstitution in mice receiving expanded bone marrow, human studies have not yet demonstrated a clear benefit of progenitor expansion.[15–17] Culture conditions have not yet been found to induce the expansion of progenitors derived from human adult bone marrow or PBSCs to the degree observed with murine bone marrow cells. Consequently, in humans ex vivo culture does not generate a large enough expansion of progenitors to significantly shorten the period of time required for leukocyte engraftment. However, fetal progenitors and UCB-derived progenitors have been shown to be much more responsive to cytokines than adult progenitors.[18] Not only do a higher frequency of fetal progenitors grow in response to cytokine stimulation but, on average, each fetal progenitor generates a larger number of cells than its adult counterpart. Since FL, FBM, and UCB have a high frequency of early progenitors and HSCs but lack the overall progenitor content found in an adult graft, the engraftment potential of these tissues is likely to be improved by increasing the progenitor content before transplantation. Our own studies have demonstrated that over 100-fold increases in FL progenitors can be generated ex vivo, suggesting that the size of fetal grafts can be significantly

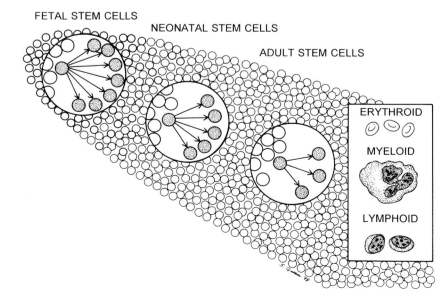

F I G U R E   39–1. Hierarchy of hematopoietic stem cells in human ontogeny. A pool of hematopoietic stem cells provides for a lifetime of hematopoiesis, generating a vast number of erythroid, myeloid, and lymphoid cells on a daily basis. The proliferative capacity of stem cells is great, but there is evidence that stem cells are not immortal. This figure illustrates the decline in proliferative capacity that occurs to the stem cell compartment over the course of human development.

increased to promote a rapid engraftment.[19, 20] However, HSCs are likely to be differentiated into committed progenitors during culture. Thus, until conditions are identified that maintain HSC activity, only a portion of a fetal graft is likely to be used for progenitor expansion and the remainder left unmanipulated as the main source of HSCs.

A fourth benefit to the use of fetal tissue again relates to the in vitro proliferative advantage fetal cells have over adult cells. Many vectors used for the transduction of genes into cells require that the target cells are actively growing. For instance, the resistance of adult HSCs to proliferate in vitro has made them difficult targets of retroviral transduction, thus stymieing many efforts at hematopoietic gene therapy in the adult. In contrast, the relative ease of stimulating fetal cells to proliferate in vitro makes these cells more prone to transduction by retroviral vectors. Indeed, FL HSCs were shown to be susceptible to retroviral transduction using an animal model of human bone marrow reconstitution. Candidate FL HSCs were isolated and transduced in culture. (We use the term "candidate HSC" because the exact phenotypic characteristics of HSCs are not known and, therefore, caution must be expressed in discussing the results of experiments that have not conclusively proven that the cells being studied are a homogeneous population of HSCs.) Afterwards, these cells were injected into human fetal bone fragments transplanted in severe-combined immunodeficiency (SCID) mice. Multilineage engraftment by transduced HSCs was documented after several months in vivo, suggesting that true HSCs were transduced. Interestingly, similar experiments performed using adult PBSCs failed to achieve bone marrow reconstitution.[21, 22] Thus, genetic modification of HSCs appears more likely in the near future using fetal cells rather than adult cells. This technology may prove useful in a number of ways. Genes may be introduced into fetal HSCs that aid in engraftment of these cells in the IUT setting. Such genes have not yet been identified, but studies are underway to identify gene products that play a role in HSC homing and proliferation. Genetic modification of HSCs to provide a greater resistance to chemotherapeutic drugs is being tested as novel treatment for cancer.[23] Allogeneic transplantation of modified fetal HSCs could contribute to such a therapy. The delivery of therapeutic gene products by genetic modification of fetal HSCs may also be possible. HSCs may be engineered to overexpress particular enzymes that are deficient in lysosomal and peroxisomal storage diseases. Furthermore, the enhanced susceptibility of fetal HSCs to genetic modification may also be used to modify a fetus' own stem cells. Future fetal therapies may be designed based on the harvest, ex vivo modification, and return of modified HSCs back to a fetus. Autologous IUT goes beyond the current practice of allogeneic IUT, but offers the advantages of treatment later in gestation and avoids any risk of graft rejection.

Sources of Fetal and Neonatal Hematopoietic Stem Cells

There are several different tissues that are sources of fetal HSCs (Fig. 39–2). The availability and suitability

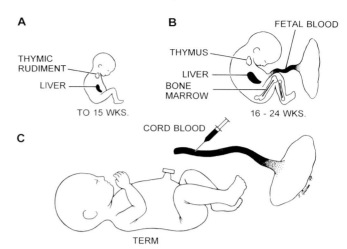

F I G U R E 39–2. Different sources of fetal hematopoietic stem cells. Fetal stem cells can be harvested from a number of different tissues depending on the gestational age of the fetus. Before 15 weeks' gestation the liver is the primary site of hematopoiesis in the human fetus. Fetal livers harvested before 15 weeks' gestation are small but have the advantage over other fetal tissues in that the number of T cells present in the liver at this developmental stage are few because the thymus is not fully developed until the end of the first trimester (A). In the second trimester, hematopoiesis begins to develop in the bone marrow but also continues in the liver. Both these tissues can be harvested and used as a source of stem cells. These tissues require processing because the thymus is actively producing large numbers of T cells, which can be found throughout the fetal circulation. Fetal blood also contains large numbers of progenitors, which are difficult to harvest from aborted specimens but may be used as a source of stem cells in ex utero gene therapy protocols. Fetuses identified with a genetic disease may have blood drawn and the stem cells genetically modified before return into the fetal circulation (B). The most widely available source of fetal hematopoietic stem cells available for autologous or allogeneic transplantation come from the umbilical cord blood. Umbilical cord blood can be harvested at the time of birth without harm to either the mother or newborn (C).

of these tissues for transplantation depends upon the legal restrictions on abortion faced in different countries and the method of abortion used. From biologic and technical perspectives, we have chosen to separate fetal tissues available in the United States into four categories: Before 15 weeks' gestation the liver is the primary hematopoietic organ and represents the major source of HSCs available from first-trimester abortions. Mid-trimester fetuses offer two sources of HSCs: the liver and the bone marrow. UCB is a fourth source of fetal tissue that can be easily obtained and used for transplantation.

First-Trimester Fetal Liver

FLs younger than 15 weeks' gestation are advantageous as a source of HSCs because the number of mature T cells in these tissues is very small. The mean number of CD3$^+$ T cells was found to be 2.3 × 10^3 at 12 weeks' gestation, 2.4 × 10^4 at 13 weeks' gestation, and 2.2 × 10^4 at 14 weeks' gestation.[24] Thus, these tissues require little if any processing to remove T cells in order to make them suitable for IUT. The drawback of using first-trimester FLs is that these tissues are very small in size and contain a modest number of progenitors and HSCs. In our experience, total viable cell counts averaged from 4.36×10^7 cells at 12 weeks' gestation to 2.0×10^8 cells at 14 weeks' gestation.[24] The numbers of HSCs present in these tissues has been shown to be sufficient for IUT[25] but are likely to be too few for postnatal transplantation unless methods can be developed to expand HSC and progenitor numbers in vitro.

Mid-Trimester Fetal Liver

We have studied FLs older than 16 weeks' gestation as a potential source of HSCs instead of following the approach of most past studies, which focused on younger, first-trimester FLs. These older FL tissues are much larger and contain greater numbers of progenitors and HSCs than first-trimester FLs. We analyzed 80 livers between 16 and 24 weeks' amenorrhea for the number of viable cells that can be obtained. The median number of cells was 1.9×10^9 (range, 3.9×10^8 to 1.1×10^{10}, $n = 80$) compared to the average 2.0×10^8 cells harvested from livers of 14 weeks' gestation. Figure 39–3 indicates the variations in cell counts we obtained at different gestational ages. These results do not necessarily reflect a biologic phenomena but, rather, reveal the practical yield of cells that can be expected from frequently fragmented livers obtained after abortion. Wide cellularity ranges can be explained by the variation in the size of the livers after procurement.

The large size of mid-trimester FLs correlates with an increase in progenitor content over that observed with first-trimester FLs. Using CD34 as a marker for progenitors and HSCs, the content of CD34+ cells was estimated by flow cytometric analyses. The CD34+ population represented a mean 2.9% of all FL cells, resulting in a mean 1.3×10^8 CD34+ cells per liver. However, cells expressing the CD34 antigen represent a heterogeneous cell population of which most are already committed progenitors.

Only a small minority of the CD34+ cells are thought to be HSCs responsible for durable engraftment. These HSCs have been tentatively defined as CD34+CD4+, CD34+CD90+, or CD34+CD38−.[26–33] The average content of CD34+CD4+ cells was 3.5×10^6 per liver, whereas an average of 8.9×10^6 CD34+CD90+ cells were detected per liver. The mean number of CD34+CD38− cells per liver was 2.6×10^6, representing a mean 0.06% of total FL cells. These findings suggest that the HSC content of a single FL is comparable to that of an adult bone marrow graft. This number of HSCs is certainly sufficient for IUT and is likely to even be sufficient for postnatal transplantation.

Unlike first-trimester FLs, mid-trimester FLs contain significant numbers of mature lymphocytes. T-cell (CD3+) numbers have been shown to increase progressively during ontogeny, as well as NK cell numbers (CD56+CD3−).[34] We observed that a mean of 1.7×10^7 liver cells expressed CD3. NK cell numbers were found to represent a mean of 4.7×10^7 per liver. These numbers of lymphocytes require that the FLs undergo processing to decrease the burden of lymphocytes if the tissue is to be safe for IUT.

Mid-Trimester Fetal Bone Marrow

The FBM begins to develop late in the first trimester, and by the second trimester sufficient numbers of cells can be found in the long bones to consider the bone marrow as a source of transplantable HSCs.[35] We observed a median number of 1.8×10^9 (range, 4×10^7 to 5×10^9) cells in the long bones of fetuses between 16 and 24 weeks' gestation. The best yields were from bones obtained from fetuses older than 19 weeks' gestation. At these gestational ages the total number of bone marrow cells that can be obtained is similar to that of the liver. The median number of cells in the bone marrow expressing CD34 was 1.5×10^8, which was again similar to the content of progenitors in the FL at the same gestational ages. The frequency of CD34+ cells was higher in the bone marrow than in the liver, an average 5.1% of all cells. The candidate HSC populations were present at 1.0×10^6 CD34+CD38− cells, 1.5×10^6 CD34+CD4+ cells, and 2.1×10^6 CD34+CD90+ cells per average bone marrow harvest.

Phenotypic analyses showed that a mean of 2.5×10^7 bone marrow cells expressed CD3. NK cell numbers were assessed using a CD56+CD3− staining and were found to represent a mean of 2.2×10^7 cells per bone marrow harvest. The presence of high numbers of mature lymphocytes in mid-trimester FBM requires that this tissue undergo processing in order to remove the lymphocytes that may cause GVHD when transplanted.

Umbilical Cord Blood

UCB has received a great deal of recent attention as a source of HSCs for transplantation.[36] The advantages of using UCB as a source of HSCs include its wide availability, low rate of infectious agents, and ethnic

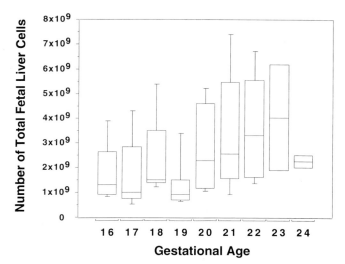

FIGURE 39–3. Box plot of the total number of cells available from mid-trimester fetal livers. This plot shows the 10th, 25th, 50th (median), 75th, and 90th percentiles of the number of cells harvested from fetal livers between 16 and 24 weeks' gestation. The median number of total fetal liver cells for all gestational ages shown was 1.9×10^9 (range, 3.9×10^8 to 1.1×10^{10}, $n = 80$).

diversity. There is no harm to either mother or infant by the harvest of UCB. UCB shares many of the proliferative advantages fetal cells have over adult cells as discussed above. The transplantation of UCB cells into fetuses may, however, be currently ill advised. The greatest limitation to the use of UCB for IUT is the presence of T cells in the graft. Although the use of rigorous methods of HSC purification may make UCB suitable in the IUT setting, most common methods of HSC purification cannot remove T cells from UCB with an efficiency needed for IUT. Consequently, other sources of fetal tissues may be better for IUT than UCB. Nonetheless, with the encouraging results achieved with UCB transplantation in children and adults, the use of this source of HSCs is likely to grow in the future.[37, 38]

The Need for Fetal Tissue Banking

The establishment of a fetal tissue bank is essential for the safe transplantation of fetal tissue. The risks of fetal tissue contamination preclude the immediate transplantation of fetal tissue, since appropriate screening and culture results require at least 2 weeks to complete. Therefore, the fetal tissues need to be cryopreserved before use unless culture methods can be found that maintain fetal HSCs during the time in which they are evaluated for viral and microbial contaminants.[39] Even the remote possibility of a very low level of microbial contamination must be taken seriously when considering the use of fetal tissue for IUT. A recipient fetus is very vulnerable to microbial infection, especially a fetus with an inherited deficiency in immune function. Any degree of bacterial, fungal, or viral contamination could be catastrophic in the IUT setting.

The possibility of microbial contamination of fetal tissues depends on the manner in which the abortion was performed and the fetal organ being harvested. The vast majority of available fetal tissue in the United States comes from elective abortions using suction curettage or forceps delivery. These methods result in varying degrees of fetal disruption and subject the fetal tissues to vaginal contaminants. An analysis performed at our center of unprocessed FL specimens found an 85% rate of bacterial or fungal contamination when the fetal specimens were disrupted during the abortion procedure.[40] However, this rate of contamination was found to be reduced to 14% by minimal processing of the fetal tissues.[24] In contrast, abortions performed using the RU486 technique in the United Kingdom, which allows for the retrieval of FL from intact fetuses, significantly reduces the risk of tissue contamination.[41] Ek and colleagues in Sweden reported a similarly low contamination rate of 5.7%.[42] We have also observed that FBM can be collected without contamination if the bones are intact. Nonetheless, the threat of contamination remains and there are legal and ethical mandates not to alter the abortion method to benefit the collection of fetal tissues.

The cryopreservation and banking of UCB specimens has also been adopted as the best method to utilize this HSC resource.[36, 43–46] Although UCB can be collected in a sterile fashion, testing for viral contaminants still re-

mains prudent. A bank of either fetal or UCB tissues has a number of other advantages. These tissues are available on demand and eliminate the need to search for and harvest a suitable donor. Frozen tissues can be shipped anywhere and thawed just prior to transplantation. Cryopreservation of UCB cells results in a minimal loss of primitive progenitor activity.[43, 45, 47, 48] Likewise, a high frequency of FL progenitors can be recovered after cryopreservation with a tendency for the more primitive progenitors to be most resistant to the effects of cryopreservation.[24, 49, 50] There are, therefore, no major technical limitations to the freezing and long-term storage of fetal and neonatal HSCs.

Procurement of Fetal Tissues

In the United States, fetal tissue from legal elective abortions is available up to 24 weeks' gestation. These tissues can be used for transplantation following national guidelines that have been enacted to protect donor confidentiality and to eliminate financial incentives for tissue donation. To ensure strict adherence to these legal mandates, we have developed a system for collecting fetal tissue that separates a woman's decision to have an abortion from her decision to donate fetal tissue. This system also maintains donor and recipient confidentiality (Fig. 39–4).

Our method of tissue collection employs a third-party agent, Advanced Biosciences Resources (ABR). This nonprofit agency is not affiliated with UCSF. ABR is regulated by the Internal Revenue Service, because of its nonprofit status, and by the Uniform Anatomical Gift Act (UAGA) and the National Organ Transplant Act (NOTA). These statutes regulate the use of human organs and tissues for medical transplantation and research. The use of ABR for the procurement of fetal tissue separates those involved in the enterprise of fetal tissue banking from the fetal-tissue donor as well as the donor's obstetrician. In our method of tissue collection, a pregnant women first decides to terminate her pregnancy, after which she is approached by the abortion providers as to her desire to donate her fetus as a potential source of tissue for transplantation. She is also asked to complete a consent form and a questionnaire and to donate a small amount of peripheral blood. The consent and questionnaire for donating fetal tissue are presented by the physician performing the abortion or by an assistant who otherwise has no involvement in this study. Likewise, the blood is drawn by the staff of the abortion clinic, and ABR has no direct contact with women who have chosen to donate fetal tissue and is not aware of their identity. The signed consent form remains on file at the medical facility as a part of the donor's medical records. Neither ABR nor persons involved in the use of the fetal tissue have access to the consent forms to ensure confidentiality of the donor. The questionnaire was designed to exclude donors at high risk for human immunodeficiency virus (HIV) and other acute and chronic viral diseases. The questionnaire and blood are identified by a unique number assigned by the staff of

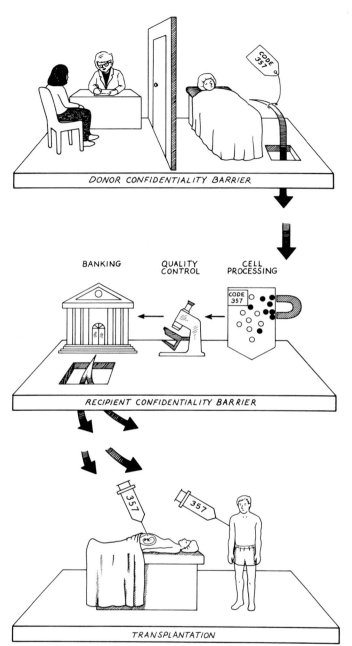

FIGURE 39–4. Schematic representation of the process for procuring, processing, banking, and transplanting fetal tissue. Investigator conflict of interest is avoided and donor confidentiality is ensured by using an independent third party to procure fetal tissue. Consent to donate fetal tissue is sought after a patient has independently decided to have an abortion. Furthermore, the identity of the donor remains unknown to the third party responsible for tissue procurement, the investigators involved in the banking of the tissue, and the transplant recipient. Quality control measures are implemented to ensure the safety of the processed fetal tissue. Recipient confidentiality is maintained by not disclosing recipient identity to the donor or third-party procurement team.

ABR. ABR is responsible for delivery of the questionnaire, blood, and fetal tissues to our center.

The questionnaire is evaluated for any indication of risk factors and only tissues obtained from women who appear to be at low risk for communicable disease are processed. The blood sample of the woman donating fetal tissue is used to determine the health status of the donor with regard to specific viral pathogens. The maternal serum is screened for HIV, human T-cell lymphotropic virus types I and II (HTLV I/II), hepatitis B surface antigen (HBsAg), hepatitis B core antibody (HBcAb), hepatitis C virus antibody (HCVAb), rapid plasma reagin (RPR), and toxoplasmosis immunoglobulin M (IgM) using standard laboratory procedures. Other pathogens are tested for by direct measurement of the fetal tissues themselves. A small piece of unprocessed fetal tissue is removed before processing and is tested for active cytomegalovirus (CMV) infection using the CMV Shell-vial test, parvovirus infection using a polymerase chain reaction (PCR) assay for parvovirus B-19 DNA, and *Chlamydia* organisms tested by culture. The processed tissues are screened for microbial contaminants using the U.S. Pharmacopoeia Assay and definitive negative results are made on the 14th day of culture. It is important to note that the confidentiality barrier that has been established between the fetal tissue donor and clinical staff involved in the use of the fetal tissues prevents the notification of the donor in the case that she has been found to suffer from an infection. Although this practice may at first appear to be unethical, it is nevertheless necessary to maintaining donor confidentiality. In consenting to donate fetal tissues, the donors are aware that they will not benefit from the act of donation, which includes remaining blind to the results of the pathogen screenings performed on their blood and the fetal tissue.

Processing of Fetal Tissues

The size of the fetus at the time of transplant limits the volume that the donor cells can be suspended in for injection. The average weight of a fetus between 12 and 14 weeks' gestation ranges from approximately 25 to 50 g.[51] Cells should be injected in no more than a 1-mL volume. This small volume necessitates the enrichment of HSCs from whole FL and/or FBM. There are a number of devices currently available or being tested for the enrichment of HSCs based on their expression of the cell surface antigen CD34. Enrichment of CD34+ cells serves both to remove the bulk of the cells present as well as to deplete the number of T cells, which do not express CD34. Some contamination by T cells is likely to occur in any purification procedure and may limit the number of processed cells that can be injected. The dose of T cells that can be tolerated by a fetus is unknown. Studies in sheep have demonstrated that the in utero administration of high numbers of T cells can result in GVHD. However, no GVHD was detected in animals given less than or equal to 2×10^7 T cells/kg fetal weight.[52] Such a cell dose is considerably higher than the 1×10^5 T cells/kg threshold suggested for human postnatal transplants.[53] Until further studies are conducted, a conservative approach should be taken, with the dose of T cells injected being limited to that acceptable for postnatal transplants.

Techniques for the enrichment of stem cells typically rely on immunomagnetic bead technology to select cells sensitized with an anti-CD34 monoclonal antibody (Fig. 39–5). Such devices positively select a spectrum of hematopoietic progenitors resulting in an enriched population of CD34[+] cells. However, because T-cell depletion is not complete, other methods of purifying stem cells have been considered for IUT. Fluorescence-activated cell sorting (FACS) can be used to achieve the highest possible cell purity. Although the preparation of cells for transplantation with FACS is not yet common, successful autologous reconstitution with HSCs purified on the basis of the CD34[+]CD90[+] phenotype has been reported in patients with multiple myeloma.[54] IUT using HSCs enriched by FACS has the advantages that T cells are very few in the graft and only a small number of cells may need to be transplanted, reducing the volume of cells infused. There are some outstanding questions, however, concerning the optimal makeup of HSC grafts for IUT. Further research is required to determine the positive roles that cell populations other than HSCs, such as T cells,[52] may play in promoting hematopoietic engraftment in utero before the best method of HSC purification can be determined. Recent findings that some HSCs do not express the CD34 antigen also caution us to consider carefully the method of HSC purification.[55, 56]

Our approach to processing FL and FBM tissues for transplantation into fetuses has differed depending on the gestation age of the fetal tissue. FLs less than 15 weeks' gestation undergo limited processing, since there is no need to remove the few T cells present in these tissues.[24] Alternatively, we have used positive selection procedures to enrich CD34[+] cells from mid-trimester FL and FBM specimens.[57] Both methods begin with the arrival of the fetal tissues to our institute after procurement by the staff of our third-party provider, ABR. The tissues are shipped on ice in a transportation medium consisting of phosphate-buffered saline supplemented with 0.5% human serum albumin and an antibiotic solution consisting of erythromycin lactobionate, gentamicin sulfate, vancomycin hydrochloride, and amphoteri-

cin B. The processing of the tissues usually begins within 2 to 4 hours after abortion.

First-Trimester Fetal Livers

The major objectives of performing any processing procedure on these tissues, other than the preparation of a single-cell suspension, are to reduce the size of the graft and to reduce the rate of microbial contamination.[24] A single-cell suspension can be easily created by passing these small FLs through a 70-μm nylon mesh. The cells are washed once, followed by isolation of the light-density ($\leq$1.077 g/mL) cells by centrifugation using a standard high-density cell-isolation medium such as Lymphoprep (Nycomed Pharma AS, Oslo, Norway). The pellet from the density-gradient is subjected to a second density gradient to increase the cell yield. In our experience the FL cells are very prone to clumping, resulting in variable recoveries of light-density cells. Addition of a second round of density-step centrifugation was found to result in more consistent yields. The light-density cells are washed twice to remove any of the cell separation medium and to help eliminate microbial contamination. The final cell suspension is cryopreserved after the removal of a small aliquot of cells for quality control analyses. This technique was found to result in a low frequency of tissues with microbial contamination and satisfied the requirements for a reduced cell volume. However, as discussed above the overall number of progenitors that can be obtained from first-trimester FLs is much less than what can be harvested from mid-trimester FLs and FBM. Thus, our more recent efforts have focused on processing these older fetal tissues to make them safe for transplantation.

Mid-Trimester Fetal Liver and Bone Marrow

The size of mid-trimester fetal tissues requires that these tissues undergo some degree of processing to reduce the size of the graft if their intended use is for IUT. The

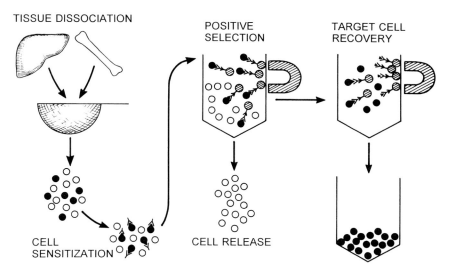

FIGURE 39–5. Overview of the isolation of CD34[+] cells from fetal tissues. The fetal livers and bone marrow are dissociated to produce a single-cell suspension. Target cells are sensitized using an anti-CD34 monoclonal antibody. The target cells are magnetically selected using magnet beads coated with an antibody recognizing the anti-CD34 monoclonal antibody bound to the target cells. The unbound cells are purged from the chamber after which the target cells are released from the magnetic beads using a peptide that competes for the binding of the anti-CD34 monoclonal antibody. The target cells are recovered free of any magnetic beads and without enzymatic or physical disruption.

TISSUE DISSOCIATION

POSITIVE SELECTION

TARGET CELL RECOVERY

CELL SENSITIZATION

CELL RELEASE

T-cell content of both mid-trimester FL and FBM also necessitates the removal of these cells if GVHD is to be avoided. Processing also serves to remove microbial contaminants that are likely to be present in liver specimens and to a lesser degree in the FBM. We have evaluated a number of different methods for the purification of these fetal tissues and have had the greatest success using a positive selection system based on the isolation of CD34$^+$ cells (Isolex 50 magnetic cell separation system; Baxter Healthcare Immunotherapy Division, Irvine, CA).[57] The procedure for isolating CD34$^+$ cells using this system is similar to the one described by the manufacturer for the isolation of adult bone marrow progenitors. However, fetal hematopoietic tissues have unique properties that require modifications to the standard protocol to obtain the best results. We describe here briefly our procedure for the isolation of fetal CD34$^+$ cells with an emphasis on the modifications that we have made to the standard protocol.

The selection procedure begins with the delivery of the FL and FBM samples, which have been kept on ice and in the transport medium described above (Fig. 39–5). The tissues are bathed in an antibiotic solution and disrupted to produce a single-cell suspension. The liver is disrupted by grinding the tissue through a series of progressively smaller pore-size sieves, ending with a sieve with a 105-μm pore size. A working buffer consisting of phosphate-buffered saline with 1% human serum albumin and the four antibiotics is used throughout the isolation procedure until the final wash of rosetted cells, before the use of the releasing agent, at which time antibiotics are withheld from the working medium. To harvest the FBM, first the long bones are isolated by peeling the soft tissues, including the periost, from the bones. Attention is paid to not break the bones or detach the cartilage, so as not to expose the medulla. These precautions are the likely reason that we have had great success in isolating FBM in a sterile fashion. To remove the bone marrow, each bone is cut in half lengthwise. The FBM is scraped from the bone with a scalpel blade and then ground through a wire mesh with a glass pestle. The FBM is then filtered through a 70-μm mesh to remove bone fragments and any large clumps of cells. We have found that the purity and efficiency of the isolation procedure is largely dependent on removal of any cell aggregates, since these clumps, which often are comprised of dead cells, block the binding of the target cells to the immunomagnetic beads.

The single-cell suspensions from the liver and bone marrow are processed separately. All work is done at room temperature except for the sensitization procedure with the anti-CD34 monoclonal antibody, which is done at 4°C. The cell suspensions are first mixed with a solution containing human immunoglobulin to prevent nonspecific binding of the CD34 monoclonal antibody. The target cells are then sensitized using the anti-CD34 monoclonal antibody. After incubation with the monoclonal antibody the cell suspensions are washed twice. After these washes, which are done to remove any unbound monoclonal antibody, cell clumps usually arise, in the liver samples in particular. This is because of cell death that occurs due to the centrifugation procedure.

It is important to remove any clumps at this step in the procedure. Thus, the cell suspensions are gently filtered through a 70-μm mesh, with care taken not to force the cell clumps through the sieve. The sensitized cells are then mixed with human IgG immunoglobulin and immunomagnetic beads. The cells are then exposed to a magnetic field and unrosetted, nontarget cells are drained from the chamber. The remaining target cells are released from the beads by incubation with PR34$^+$ stem cell releasing agent. The releasing agent competes for the binding of the anti-CD34 monoclonal antibody with the CD34 expressed on the target cells. Thus, no enzymatic cleavage of cell surface proteins on the target cells occurs. Target cells are then drained from the chamber and concentrated by centrifugation. The final cell preparations are cryopreserved after removal of a small sample for quality control analyses.

The purity and yield of progenitors as well as the levels of T-cell contamination are analyzed by flow cytometric analyses. The results of one such analysis, before and after purification, on a 24-week's-gestation FL are shown in Figure 39–6. Using the procedure described, an average purity of 74% and recovery of 29% of CD34$^+$ cells was achieved from FL tissues. The yield averaged 8.2 × 10^6 CD34$^+$ cells. From FBM samples, an average purity of 87% and recovery of 19% of CD34$^+$ cells was achieved, representing a final number of 1.9 × 10^7 cells expressing CD34. The recovery of cells that express the highest levels of CD34 is more efficient than the recovery of those that express only low levels of CD34. Fortunately, HSCs are thought to be among the fraction of hematopoietic cells expressing high levels of CD34.[58] The average recoveries of candidate HSCs (CD34$^+$CD38$^-$ and CD34$^+$CD4$^+$ cells) was higher than the overall yield of cells expressing CD34. The recoveries of CD34$^+$CD38$^-$ cells was 30% from the FL and 40% from the FBM. CD34$^+$CD4$^+$ cell recovery was 52% from the FL and 63% from the FBM.

Colony assays were also performed to measure the recovery of functional progenitors. We measure progenitor numbers using serum-deprived conditions, since these conditions support the growth of fetal progenitors better than traditional culture media containing fetal bovine serum.[57] The serum-deprived culture medium consists of a base of Iscove's modified Dulbecco's medium supplemented with 7.5 × 10^{-5} M α-thioglycerol, 50 μg/mL gentamicin, 2% bovine serum albumin, 200 μg/mL human iron-saturated transferrin, 10 μg/mL insulin, and 20 μg-protein/mL human low-density lipoprotein. Use of this serum-deprived culture medium eliminates the variability introduced by the use of different lots of fetal bovine serum. The same culture medium can be used in different laboratories, helping to standardize the method for measuring fetal colony-forming cells. The growth of primitive progenitors and candidate HSCs is supported by a combination of the cytokines c-kit ligand and granulocyte-macrophage colony-stimulating factor.[19, 26] Two types of progenitors are detected based on colony size: low-proliferative potential colony-forming cells (LPP-CFCs) are defined as progenitors giving rise to colonies of 50 or more cells but smaller than colonies derived from high-proliferative

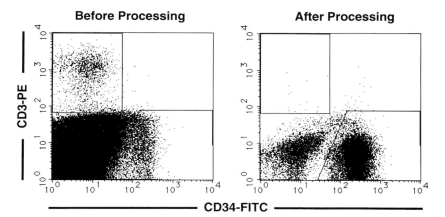

FIGURE 39-6. Phenotypic analyses of CD34⁺ fetal liver cells selected using the Baxter Isolex 50 system. The frequencies of T cells (CD3⁺CD34⁻) and total progenitor/stem cells (CD34⁺CD3⁻) are calculated based on the number of cells found in the two boxed regions shown in the figure. The dot plot on the right was obtained from total fetal liver cells before processing. The dot plot on the left represents cells after positive selection. Note the preferential selection of cells expressing high levels of CD34.

potential colony-forming cells (HPP-CFCs). HPP-CFCs are defined as progenitors giving rise to colonies that are approximated to consist of 1×10^4 to 1×10^6 cells. On average, HPP-CFCs are more primitive than LPP-CFCs.[26] After the processing of FLs, a 38% recovery of HPP-CFCs was achieved compared to only 15% of LPP-CFCs. The recovery of HPP-CFCs from processed FBM samples was 49% compared to the recovery of only 21% of LPP-CFCs. Thus, the colony assay data demonstrated a preferential enrichment of early progenitors versus more mature progenitors.

Processing of fetal tissues using the Isolex system was also found to be very effective at depleting T cells (Fig. 39-6). Phenotypic analyses of CD3⁺ cells before and after processing FL tissues showed a mean 99.96% depletion of T cells, with a mean 6.6×10^3 CD3⁺ cells remaining. In the FBM samples, a mean 99.92% depletion of T cells was achieved with a mean 4.8×10^3 CD3⁺ cells remaining. Indeed, in some samples the number of T cells remaining after processing was below the level of detection using flow cytometry.

All processed tissues are also analyzed for the presence of microbial contamination and the presence of *Chlamydia* organisms. Microbial contamination of FLs has been a major problem limiting the use of these tissues for transplantation. After abortion through the vaginal tractus, rates of contamination as high as 85% have been reported for FL cells.[40] This rate of contamination decreased to 9 to 14% with the use of antibiotics in the transport medium.[24, 39] The problem of microbial contamination is not limited to fetal tissues. Reported rates of bacterial contamination in bone marrow and peripheral blood collections have ranged from 0 to 17%.[59–65] We showed in our study that the purification of FL CD34⁺ progenitors in the presence of antimicrobial agents could provide grafts free of contamination.[57] Both unprocessed and processed FBM specimens were also free of microbial contamination. The lack of contamination in processed FL tissues can be explained by the large reduction in tissue size, effects of repeated washes during the selection procedure, and the effect of the antibiotic solution used through most of the processing procedure. Our experience has demonstrated that the majority of processed fetal tissues are free of microbial contaminants

and free of specific viral contaminants and are, thus, safe for transplantation.

Experience with Fetal Hematopoietic Stem Cell Transplantation

Although several hundred people have been the recipients of FL transplants, currently UCB transplantation is the premier form of fetal cellular transplantation.[6, 38, 66–68] Success with FL transplantation has been greatest in instances were the recipients were suffering from immunodeficiences. Both postnatal and IUT transplants of FL cells have successfully reconstituted the immune system in these patients.[69–76] FL transplantation has also been attempted for aplastic anemia, leukemia, and various other inherited disorders.[77–82] Although the transplantation of fetal tissue for these diseases demonstrated some degree of improvement in some patients, engraftment of donor-derived cells was not confirmed. It should be noted that the levels of immunosuppressive and cytoablative therapy given before these transplants was minimal and was likely to be a major cause of the lack of engraftment in these patients. It has been hypothesized that factors other than cellular reconstitution are responsible for the transient improvements observed in host hematopoiesis in some patients.[66] However, controlled studies have not been performed to test this hypothesis. First-trimester FLs have also been transplanted in utero as a treatment for α-thalassemia, sickle cell anemia, and β-thalassemia but no engraftment was reported.[83] The lack of engraftment in these transplants was likely due to competition with the fetus' own hematopoietic cells or rejection by the fetus' immune system rather than a deficiency in the fetal cells transplanted. Thus, to date little success has been achieved with FL transplantation with the exception of the prenatal and postnatal transplants for immunodeficiency. However, the recent success with unrelated transplants using UCB cells to treat a number of malignant and nonmalignant diseases suggests that, with the improvements that have been made in HSC transplantation, it is likely that FL and FBM cells can also be used as a source of HSC for postnatal transplantation.

The Future of Fetal Tissue Transplantation

HSC transplantation is a critical component of medical therapy for congenital immunodeficiences, inborn errors of metabolism, and various malignant and nonmalignant hematologic diseases. Shortages in human leukocyte antigen (HLA)-identical bone marrow will undoubtedly press the search for alternative sources of HSCs. UCB offers an excellent alternative source of transplantable HSCs which has been proven capable of reconstituting an adult recipient. Mid-trimester FL and FBM may further supplement the supply of tissues for postnatal transplantation. We have shown that the numbers of early progenitors and candidate HSCs present in these tissues is comparable to those present in a graft of adult origin.

The greatest challenge to the use of FL and FBM for postnatal transplantation is the establishment of a bank of these tissues that is large enough to contain a useful portion of the spectrum of HLA types. Large-scale programs in UCB banking have begun and have contributed to the available supply of transplantable HSCs. The financial burden of banking UCB cells is minimal because these tissues do not require extensive processing before cryopreservation. The high incidence of sterility among FBM samples suggests that these tissues may also be cryopreserved without undergoing extensive processing first. Those FBM samples that have passed quality control analysis and are deemed to have the correct HLA type for a particular transplant could then be thawed and the progenitors and HSCs selected before transplantation. This protocol would minimize the up-front cost of banking FBM, but the same protocol is likely not to be practical in the case of banking FL cells. The high incidence of contamination in FL specimens before processing would result in most FL samples being discarded because of microbial contamination. Cost-effective methods of decontaminating FL samples need to be identified before large-scale banking of these tissues is financially feasible.

In the case of IUT, HLA disparity need not be considered because this form of HSC transplantation seeks to establish a state of hematopoietic chimerism before the full establishment of the fetal immune system. Only a minimal number of FL and FBM samples need be processed and stored for near-term use. The greater numbers of progenitors that can be harvested from mid-trimester tissues versus first-trimester FLs would suggest that the older tissues are the preferable choice for IUT. However, mid-trimester tissues are not available in all countries due to restrictions on late-term abortions. The large numbers of HSCs available from a combination of mid-trimester FL and FBM also suggests that these tissues may be used for a two-step therapy involving IUT and a subsequent postnatal boost to increase the levels of engraftment. Such a strategy relies on the primary in utero transplant to induce a state of immune tolerance to the donor tissues, thus preventing the rejection of the secondary transplant. The subject of in utero tolerance induction is taken up more extensively in another chapter.

This chapter has focused on fetal sources of HSCs. However, there are a number of other cell types that could be harvested from aborted fetuses and used for cellular therapy in utero or in the postnatal patient. Other cell types that deserve consideration for transplantation include hepatocytes, fibroblasts, and mesenchymal stem cells. There are a large number of diseases that could be cured by hepatocyte transplantation if this form of treatment can be perfected. FBM-derived fibroblasts and mesenchymal stem cells may also be transplanted and contribute to the cure of various lysosomal and peroxisomal storage diseases. Gene transfer into these cell types may be used to further increase the production of particular enzymes by these cells, thus making them efficient vehicles for the delivery of therapeutic gene products. Little is known about the biology of these different cell types found in the fetus. In vitro and animal studies are required, however, to test the potential of these different therapies before they can be seriously considered for human use. To be certain, there are no limitations to the clinical use of various fetal tissues should they be deemed useful in the treatment of human disease. Experience with fetal HSCs has shown that fetal tissue should be seriously considered as a source of tissues for human transplantation.

REFERENCES

1. Koonin LM, Smith JC, Ramick M, Strauss LT: Abortion surveillance—United States, 1995. MMWR Morb Mortal Wkly Rep 47:31, 1998.
2. Fleischman RA, Mintz B: Development of adult bone marrow stem cells in H-2 compatible and noncompatible mouse fetuses. J Exp Med 159:731, 1984.
3. Flake AW, Roncarolo MG, Puck JM, et al: Treatment of X-linked severe combined immunodeficiency by in utero transplantation of paternal bone marrow. N Engl J Med 335:1806, 1996.
4. Royo C, Touraine JL, Veyron P, Aitouche A: Survey of experimental data on fetal liver transplantation. Thymus 10:5, 1987.
5. Gale RP: Development of the immune system in human fetal liver. Thymus 10:45, 1987.
6. O'Reilly RJ, Pollack MS, Kapoor N, et al: Fetal liver transplantation in man and animals. In Recent Advances in Bone Marrow Transplantation. New York: Alan R Liss, Inc, 1983, p 799.
7. Touraine JL, Roncarolo MG, Bacchetta R, et al: Fetal liver transplantation: Biology and clinical results. Bone Marrow Transplant 11:119, 1993.
8. Harrison DE: Normal function of transplanted mouse erythrocyte precursors for 21 months beyond donor life spans. Nature 237:220, 1972.
9. Ogden DA, Micklem HS: The fate of serially transplanted bone marrow cell populations from young and old donors. Transplantation 22:287, 1976.
10. Botnick LE, Hannon EC, Obbagy J, Hellman S: The variation of hematopoietic stem cell self-renewal capacity as a function of age: Further evidence for heterogenicity of the stem cell compartment. Blood 60:268, 1982.
11. Harrison DE, Stone M, Astle CM: Effects of transplantation on the primitive immunohematopoietic stem cell. J Exp Med 172:431, 1990.
12. Harrison DE, Astle CM, Delaittre JA: Loss of proliferative capacity in immunohemopoietic stem cells caused by serial transplantation rather than aging. J Exp Med 147:1526, 1978.
13. Rebel VI, Miller CL, Eaves CJ, Lansdorp PM: The repopulation potential of fetal liver hematopoietic stem cells in mice exceeds that of their liver adult bone marrow counterparts. Blood 87:3500, 1996.
14. Harrison DE, Zhong RK, Jordan CT, et al: Relative to adult marrow, fetal liver repopulates nearly five times more effectively long-term than short-term. Exp Hematol 25:293, 1997.

15. Muench MO, Roncarolo M-G, Namikawa R, et al: Progress in the ex vivo expansion of hematopoietic progenitors. Leuk Lymphoma 16:1, 1994.

16. Muench MO, Moore MAS: Accelerated recovery of peripheral blood cell counts in mice transplanted with in vitro cytokine-expanded hematopoietic progenitors. Exp Hematol 20:611, 1992.

17. Muench MO, Firpo MT, Moore MAS: Bone marrow transplantation with interleukin-1 plus kit-ligand ex vivo expanded bone marrow accelerates hematopoietic reconstitution in mice without the loss of stem cell lineage and proliferative potential. Blood 81:3463, 1993.

18. Lansdorp PM, Dragowska W, Mayani H: Ontogeny-related changes in proliferative potential of human hematopoietic cells. J Exp Med 178:787, 1993.

19. Muench MO, Roncarolo MG, Menon S, et al: FLK-2/FLT-3 ligand (FL) regulates the growth of early myeloid progenitors isolated from human fetal liver. Blood 85:963, 1995.

20. Muench MO, Roncarolo M-G, Rosnet O, et al: Colony-forming cells expressing high levels of CD34 are the main targets for granulocyte colony-stimulating factor and macrophage colony-stimulating factor in the human fetal liver. Exp Hematol 25:277, 1997.

21. Humeau L, Chabannon C, Firpo MT, et al: Successful reconstitution of human hematopoiesis in the SCID-hu mouse by genetically modified, highly enriched progenitors isolated from fetal liver. Blood 90:3496, 1997.

22. Humeau L, Namikawa R, Bardin F, et al: Ex vivo manipulations alter the reconstitution potential of mobilized human CD34$^+$ peripheral blood progenitors. Leukemia 13:348, 1999.

23. Brenner MK: Gene transfer into human hematopoietic progenitor cells: A review of current clinical protocols. J Hematother 2:7, 1993.

24. Mychaliska GB, Muench MO, Rice HE, et al: The biology and ethics of banking fetal liver hematopoietic stem cells for *in utero* transplantation. J Pediatr Surg 33:394, 1998.

25. Touraine JL: In utero transplantation of fetal liver stem cells in humans. Blood Cells 17:379, 1991.

26. Muench MO, Cupp J, Polakoff J, Roncarolo MG: Expression of CD33, CD38 and HLA-DR on CD34+ human fetal liver progenitors with a high proliferative potential. Blood 83:3170, 1994.

27. Zauli G, Furlini G, Vitale M, et al: A subset of human CD34$^+$ hematopoietic progenitors express low levels of CD4, the high-affinity receptor for human immunodeficiency virus-type 1. Blood 84:1896, 1994.

28. Louache F, Debili N, Marandin A, et al: Expression of CD4 by human hematopoietic progenitors. Blood 84:3344, 1994.

29. Muench MO, Roncarolo MG, Namikawa R: Phenotypic and functional evidence for the expression of CD4 by hematopoietic stem cells isolated from human fetal liver. Blood 89:1364, 1997.

30. Baum CM, Weissman IL, Tsukamoto AS, et al: Isolation of a candidate human hematopoietic stem-cell population. Proc Natl Acad Sci U S A 89:2804, 1992.

31. Craig W, Kay R, Cutler RL, Lansdorp PM: Expression of Thy-1 on human hematopoietic progenitor cells. J Exp Med 177:1331, 1993.

32. Issaad C, Croisille L, Katz A, et al: A murine stromal cell line allows the proliferation of very primitive human CD34++/CD38- progenitor cells in long-term cultures and semisolid assays. Blood 81:2916, 1993.

33. Terstappen LWMM, Huang S, Safford M, et al: Sequential generation of hematopoietic colonies derived from single nonlineage-committed CD34+CD38- progenitor cells. Blood 77:1218, 1991.

34. Phillips JH, Hori T, Nagler A, et al: Ontogeny of human natural killer (NK) cells: Fetal NK cells mediate cytolytic function and express cytoplasmic CD3 epsilon, delta proteins. J Exp Med 175:1055, 1992.

35. Charbord P, Tavian M, Humeau L, Peault B: Early ontogeny of the human marrow from long bones: An immunohistochemical study of hematopoiesis and its microenvironment. Blood 87:4109, 1996.

36. Rubinstein P, Rosenfield RE, Adamson JW, Stevens CE: Stored placental blood for unrelated bone marrow reconstitution. Blood 81:1679, 1993.

37. Kernan NA, Schroeder ML, Ciavarella D, et al: Umbilical cord blood infusion in a patient for correction of Wiskott-Aldrich syndrome. Blood Cells 20:245, 1994.

38. Kurtzberg J, Laughlin M, Graham ML, et al: Placental blood as a source of hematopoietic stem cells for transplantation into unrelated recipients. N Engl J Med 335:157, 1996.

39. Rice HE, Skarsgard ED, Emani VR, et al: An effective strategy for decontamination, ex vivo expansion, and storage of human fetal liver hematopoietic stem cells. Transplant Proc 26:3352, 1994.

40. Rice HE, Hedrick MH, Flake AW, et al: Bacterial and fungal contamination of human fetal liver collected transvaginally for hematopoietic stem cell transplantation. Fetal Diagn Ther 8:74, 1993.

41. Anderson EM, Jones DR, Liu DT, Evans AA: Gestational age and cell viability determine the effect of frozen storage on human fetal hematopoietic progenitor cell preparations. Fetal Diagn Ther 11:427, 1996.

42. Ek S, Westgren M, Pschera H, et al: Screening of fetal stem cells for infection and cytogenetic abnormalities. Fetal Diagn Ther 9:357, 1994.

43. Rubinstein P, Dobrila L, Rosenfield RE, et al: Processing and cryopreservation of placental/umbilical cord blood for unrelated bone marrow reconstitution. Proc Natl Acad Sci U S A 92:10119, 1995.

44. Newton I, Charbord P, Schaal JP, Herve P: Toward cord blood banking: Density-separation and cryopreservation of cord blood progenitors. Exp Hematol 21:671, 1993.

45. Almici C, Carlo-Stella C, Wagner JE, Rizzoli V: Density separation and cryopreservation of umbilical cord blood cells: Evaluation of recovery in short- and long-term cultures. Acta Haematol 95:171, 1996.

46. Denning-Kendall P, Donaldson C, Nicol A, et al: Optimal processing of human umbilical cord blood for clinical banking. Exp Hematol 24:1394, 1996.

47. Harris DT, Schumacher MJ, Rychlik S, et al: Collection, separation and cryopreservation of umbilical cord blood for use in transplantation. Bone Marrow Transplant 13:135, 1994.

48. Nicol A, Nieda M, Donaldson C, et al: Analysis of cord blood CD34+ cells purified after cryopreservation. Exp Hematol 23:1589, 1995.

49. Ek S, Ringden O, Markling L, et al: Effects of cryopreservation on subsets of fetal liver cells. Bone Marrow Transplant 11:395, 1993.

50. Jones DR, Anderson EM, Evans AA, Liu DT: Long-term storage of human fetal haematopoietic progenitor cells and their subsequent reconstitution. Implications for in utero transplantation. Bone Marrow Transplant 16:297, 1995.

51. Guihard-Costa AM, Larroche JC, Droulle P, Narcy F: Fetal biometry. Growth charts for practical use in fetopathology and antenatal ultrasonography. Introduction. Fetal Diagn Ther 10:215, 1995.

52. Crombleholme TM, Harrison MR, Zanjani ED: In utero transplantation of hematopoietic stem cells in sheep: The role of T cells in engraftment and graft-versus-host disease. J Pediatr Surg 25:885, 1990.

53. Kernan NA, Collins NH, Juliano L, et al: Clonable T lymphocytes in T cell-depleted bone marrow transplants correlate with development of graft-v-host disease. Blood 68:770, 1986.

54. Tricot G, Gazitt Y, Leemhuis T, et al: Collection, tumor contamination, and engraftment kinetics of highly purified hematopoietic progenitor cells to support high dose therapy in multiple myeloma. Blood 91:4489, 1998.

55. Goodell MA, Rosenzweig M, Kim H, et al: Dye efflux studies suggest that hematopoietic stem cells expressing low or undetectable levels of CD34 antigen exist in multiple species. Nat Med 3:1337, 1997.

56. Zanjani ED, Almeida-Porada G, Livingston AG, et al: Human bone marrow CD34$^-$ cells engraft in vivo and undergo multilineage expression that includes giving rise to CD34$^+$ cells. Exp Hematol 26:353, 1998.

57. Golfier F, Bárcena A, Cruz J, et al: Mid-trimester fetal livers are a rich source of CD34$^{+/++}$ cells for transplantation. Bone Marrow Transplant 24:451, 1999.

58. Di Giusto D, Chen S, Combs J, et al: Human fetal bone marrow early progenitors for T, B, and myeloid cells are found exclusively in the population expressing high levels of CD34. Blood 84:421, 1994.

59. Rowley SD, Davis J, Dick J, et al: Bacterial contamination of bone marrow grafts intended for autologous and allogeneic bone marrow transplantation. Incidence and clinical significance. Transfusion 28:109, 1988.

60. D'Antonio D, Iacone A, Fioritoni G, et al: Detection of bacterial contamination in bone marrow graft. Haematologica 76(Suppl): 44, 1991.

61. Lazarus HM, Magalhaes-Silverman M, Fox RM, et al: Contamination during in vitro processing of bone marrow for transplantation: Clinical significance. Bone Marrow Transplant 7:241, 1991.

62. Stroncek DF, Fautsch SK, Lasky LC, et al: Adverse reactions in patients transfused with cryopreserved marrow. Transfusion 31:521, 1991.

63. Schwella N, Zimmermann R, Heuft HG, et al: Microbiologic contamination of peripheral blood stem cell autografts. Vox Sang 67:32, 1994.

64. Prince HM, Page SR, Keating A, et al: Microbial contamination of harvested bone marrow and peripheral blood. Bone Marrow Transplant 15:87, 1995.

65. Webb IJ, Coral FS, Andersen JW, et al: Sources and sequelae of bacterial contamination of hematopoietic stem cell components: Implications for the safety of hematotherapy and graft engineering. Transfusion 36:782, 1996.

66. Gale RP, Touraine JL, Kochupillai V: Synopsis and prospectives on fetal liver transplantation. Thymus 10:1, 1987.

67. Broxmeyer HE: Cord blood as an alternative source for stem and progenitor cell transplantation. Curr Opin Pediatr 7:47, 1995.

68. Kögler G, Callejas J, Hakenberg P, et al: Hematopoietic transplant potential of unrelated cord blood: Critical issues. J Hematother 5:105, 1996.

69. Keightley RG, Lawton AR, Cooper MD, Yunis EJ: Successful fetal liver transplantation in a child with severe combined immunodeficiency. Lancet 2:850, 1975.

70. Buckley RH, Whisnant KJ, Schiff RI, et al: Correction of severe combined immunodeficiency by fetal liver cells. N Engl J Med 294:1076, 1976.

71. Ackeret C, Lluss HJ, Hitzig WH: Hereditary severe combined immunodeficiency and adenosine deaminase deficiency. Pediatr Res 10:67, 1976.

72. Aiuti F, Businco L, Fiorilli M, et al: Fetal liver transplantation in two infants with severe combined immunodeficiency. Transplant Proc 11:230, 1979.

73. Betend B, Touraine JL, Hermier M, Francois R: [Restoration of mixed and severe immunologic deficiency, by fetal liver and thymus graft]. Arch Fr Pediatr 36:995, 1979.

74. Seto S, Miyake T, Hirao T: Reconstitution of cell-mediated immunity in severe combined immunodeficiency following fetal liver transplantation. Tokai J Exp Clin Med 10:233, 1985.

75. O'Reilly RJ, Kirkpatrick D, Kapoor N, et al: A comparative review of the results of transplants of fully allogeneic fetal liver and HLA-haplotype mismatched, T-cell depleted marrow in the treatment of severe combined immunodeficiency. Prog Clin Biol Res 193:327, 1985.

76. Touraine JL: In-utero transplantation of fetal liver stem cells into human fetuses. Hum Reprod 7:44, 1992.

77. Kansal V, Sood SK, Batra AK, et al: Fetal liver transplantation in aplastic anemia. Acta Haematol 62:128, 1979.

78. Lucarelli G, Izzi T, Procellini A, et al: Fetal liver transplantation in 2 patients with acute leukaemia after total body irradiation. Scand J Haematol 28:65, 1982.

79. Izzi T, Polchi P, Galimberti M, et al: Fetal liver transplant in aplastic anemia and acute leukemia. Prog Clin Biol Res 193:237, 1985.

80. Kochupillai V, Sharma S, Francis S, et al: Fetal liver infusion in acute myelogenous leukaemia. Thymus 10:117, 1987.

81. Kochupillai V, Sharma S, Francis S, et al: Fetal liver infusion in aplastic anaemia. Thymus 10:95, 1987.

82. Pajor A, Janossa M, Kelemen E: Pregnancy in aplastic anemia treated with fetal liver and bone marrow hemopoietic cells and antithymocyte globulin. Arch Gynecol Obstet 251:207, 1992.

83. Westgren M, Ringden O, Eik-Nes S, et al: Lack of evidence of permanent engraftment after in utero fetal stem cell transplantation in congenital hemoglobinopathies. Transplantation 61:1176, 1996.

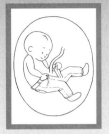

CHAPTER 40

The Fetus with a Genetic Defect Correctable by Gene Therapy

ESMAIL D. ZANJANI and W. FRENCH ANDERSON

Gene therapy for the treatment of disease in children and adults is being actively pursued by many medical centers. However, there are genetic disorders that result in irreversible damage to the fetus before birth. Success with in utero gene transfer in animals supports the suggestion that it may now be appropriate to design clinical protocols to evaluate in utero gene therapy in human patients.

Gene therapy, the treatment of disease by the transfer and appropriate expression of an exogenous normal gene into somatic cells of an organism, is the subject of intensive experimental and clinical investigation.[1] All of the currently active clinical gene therapy protocols concern the treatment of postnatal (i.e., pediatric and adult) patients, and many employ a form of ex vivo retroviral vector transduction of hematopoietic stem/progenitor cells (HSCs) followed by transplantation of the gene-engineered cells back into the patient.[2] This approach relies on the high proliferative and multilineage differentiation potential of HSCs for delivering the corrective gene to the patient, and many protocols use ex vivo transduction of the patient's bone marrow or mobilized peripheral blood HSCs. For a few diseases, such as severe combined immunodeficiency (SCID) caused by adenosine deaminase (ADA) deficiency, there is a positive pressure for the engraftment and growth of treated blood cells.[3] For most other diseases, however, the reengraftment of the transduced HSCs is facilitated by some form of marrow ablation therapy. Although difficulties with the ex vivo transduction of human HSCs and the poor expression of the transgenes in vivo have limited the wide application of this procedure, results from these studies have been very informative and progress in improving the delivery and expression of genes is rapid. As more efficient transduction strategies become available, HSC gene therapy promises to serve as a highly desirable therapeutic measure for the treatment of a variety of genetic and acquired disorders in man.

Although most genetic diseases would be treated after birth, there are some disorders that produce irreversible damage to the fetus during gestation. Examples are listed in Table 40–1. For these diseases, an in utero ap-proach would be optimal. The success of recent animal studies evaluating gene transfer in utero raise the possibility that somatic cell gene therapy may be effective in human prenatal patients. In this review, we will examine the rationale and experimental evidence that form the basis for suggesting that clinical trials of somatic cell gene therapy in unborn patients may now be appropriate.

In Utero Gene Transfer: Animal Studies

The persistence and expression of vector-encoded genes following transfer in utero have been evaluated in rodents, sheep, and monkeys. The majority of studies have been with the hematopoietic system.

Studies in Rodents

In a series of experiments, Jaenisch et al.,[4] employing retroviruses to map the murine genome, demonstrated that wild-type Moloney murine leukemia virus could be used to permanently transfer exogenous genes into the genome of mice at very early points in development, and that these genes were expressed in a wide variety of tissues following the birth of the animal. These studies showed that it was possible to insert exogenous genes into a developing organism, and suggested that many of the tissues in the developing fetus might be amenable targets for in utero gene transfer.

Clapp et al.,[5] using a direct injection approach into the fetal liver, demonstrated that fetal liver HSCs are a suitable target for in utero gene transfer, and these in situ transduced HSCs ultimately homed to the nascent fetal marrow and persisted for long periods within the animal, producing gene-marked progeny of multiple hematopoietic lineages. Although the direct injection into the fetal liver led to a high rate of mortality, the long-term persistence of the transgene indicated that this in utero approach had resulted in the transduction of the long-term engrafting HSCs. In shorter term stud-

T A B L E 40–1. CANDIDATE DISEASES FOR IN UTERO
GENE THERAPY

1. Neurologic/metabolic
   Lesch-Nyhan syndrome
   Tay-Sachs
   Sandhoff disease
   Niemann-Pick disease
   Leukodystrophy
     Canavan
     Krabbe
     Metachromatic
   Generalized gangliosidosis
   Leigh disease
2. Metabolic
   Wolman disease
   Type II Gaucher disease
   Pompe disease
   Osteopetrosis
3. Immunologic
   SCID
   Wiscott-Aldrich syndrome
4. Hematologic
   α-Thalassemia
   Fanconi anemia
   Chronic granulomatous disease

ies, similar fetal gene transfer strategies have been employed to achieve the transfer of exogenous genes into skin,[6] pulmonary epithelium,[7] hepatocytes,[8] and heart,[9] among others.[10]

Studies in Sheep

Long-term persistence and expression of a marker gene, the bacterial neomycin resistance gene (Neo[R]), following transfer in utero was demonstrated in sheep using two different approaches.

Ex Vivo HSC Gene Transfer

In the first approach, an autologous retroviral/HSC transplantation protocol, but without myeloablation, was used to introduce the bacterial Neo[R] gene into sheep fetuses. Circulating mononuclear cells obtained from sheep fetuses by exchange transfusion at about 100 days' gestation (term: 145 days) were incubated in medium containing retroviral particles for about 18 hours and reinfused into respective donor fetuses intravenously.[11] Examination of the lambs after birth revealed the presence of a functioning Neo[R] gene in a significant number of these animals. The results, reported in detail previously,[11] revealed that of the ten recipients that could be evaluated, six were positive for G418-resistant progenitor cells colony-forming unit–Mix ([CFU-Mix], colony-forming unit–granulocyte-macrophage [CFU-GM], blast-forming unit–erythroid [BFU-E], and colony-forming unit–erythroid [CFU-E]). Vector DNA sequences were present in both the blood and the bone marrow of two animals. In addition, the presence of the gene product, neomycin phosphotransferase (NPT) activity, was documented in bone marrow of another animal. These findings established that the in utero gene-engineered HSC transplantation protocol resulted in the transfer and expression of the Neo[R] gene in these large animals.

That the protocol resulted in the transfer of the Neo[R] gene into the pluripotent HSCs was demonstrated by the results from two of the animals that were studied for extended periods of time: 43 and 59 months after birth. Both animals continued to exhibit significant numbers of G418-resistant progenitors (CFU-Mix, CFU-GM, BFU-E) throughout the study period.[11] Although these early studies were carried out with retroviral supernatant that was contaminated with amphotropic helper virus, no viral toxicity was noted in any of the animals. Moreover, lambs born to in utero–treated ewes expressing the Neo[R] gene did not exhibit any drug-resistant hematopoietic progenitors.[11] Overall, the gene-engineered HSC transplantation protocol in sheep resulted in long-term expression of the Neo[R] gene at a low but significant efficiency. The fetal HSCs appear to be transduced in vitro much more efficiently than adult HSCs and the developmental potential of the hematopoietic system in the fetus promotes the proliferation/expansion of engrafted HSCs in the bone marrow (see discussion below).

*Direct Intraperitoneal Injection **In Utero** of Retroviral Vector*

The need for a significant volume of blood to serve as the source of HSCs limits the applicability of autologous gene-engineered HSC transplantation to older fetuses. However, most genetic disorders in humans can now be diagnosed very early in gestation. It is thus possible to treat these patients very early during intrauterine life. While the size of the fetus at these early gestational ages readily permits the injection of materials (cells, reagents, etc.), it is not possible to obtain sufficient amounts of blood or other HSC-containing tissues from very young fetuses for gene transfer purposes. In a second approach, therefore, the efficacy and safety of the direct injection of vectors into preimmune sheep fetuses was evaluated.[13]

Twenty-nine preimmune sheep fetuses (57 to 67 days old; term: 145 days) were injected with helper-free retroviral preparations (supernatant [at a titer of 5×10^4 CFU/mL], producer cells, or irradiated producer cells) intraperitoneally. Twenty-two fetuses survived to term, four of which were sacrificed at birth for analysis. Of the remaining 18 animals, three were controls and 15 had received vector preparations. Twelve of these 15 exhibited transduction of hematopoietic cells when blood and marrow were analyzed by Neo[R]-specific polymerase chain reaction (PCR). Expression of the Neo[R] gene was demonstrated by G418-resistant hematopoietic colony growth. In eight of the animals that were followed for over 5 years; the presence/expression of the transgene was consistently observed by PCR and G418-resistance assays. The expression of the Neo[R] gene was confirmed by functional NPT activity assay, and by immunofluorescence, enzyme-linked immunosorbent assay (ELISA), and fluorescence-activated cell sorter (FACS) analyses. The long-term presence and expression of the transgene in hematopoietic cells/progenitors of the primary animals suggested that the pluripotent HSCs were transduced. This conclusion was confirmed when secondary lambs transplanted with HSCs obtained from the primary transduced sheep exhibited Neo[R] activity in both their bone marrow and blood.

PCR analysis of tissues from sacrificed primary animals revealed that vector sequences were present in almost all tissues analyzed, including the reproductive organs. However, no pathology was noted in any of the organs, and breeding experiments and extensive analysis of purified sperm from the three semen-positive rams indicated that no vector sequences were present in the sperm. The positive semen samples were due to vector integration into nongermline cells.[12]

Exogenous genes were detected in the brain of several animals that were sacrificed at various time points throughout the studies. It is not known whether the presence of proviral DNA in the brain was the result of entry of the vector into the central nervous system (CNS) with subsequent transduction of the nervous tissue, since it is also possible that the presence of the vector may reflect the migration of transduced hematopoietic microglial precursors into the brain during development. Regardless of the mechanism, however, the ability to deliver exogenous genes to the brain in utero offers the possibility of treating a number of patients with storage diseases that affect the CNS.

In recent follow-up studies,[13] a much higher titer retroviral vector was used that resulted in more efficient transduction and expression of the transgenes in the hematopoietic cells of the animals injected in utero. Sixteen preimmune sheep fetuses were injected intraperitoneally with the G1nBgSvNa8.1, a helper-free retroviral vector supernatant encoding both the bacterial Neo[R] and the β-galactosidase genes. This vector was concentrated to a titer of 1×10^8 CFU/mL. All recipients survived to term and were born alive and healthy. However, two animals died within a few days after birth due to causes unrelated to these studies. Bone marrow and blood samples from the remaining 14 experimental sheep were collected soon after birth and at intervals thereafter for Neo[R] and β-galactosidase–specific PCR analysis. Over the 2-year time course of these studies, proviral DNA and high levels of G418-resistant hematopoietic progenitors were consistently observed in 12 of the 14 experimental sheep that were evaluated. The presence and expression of the Neo[R] and β-galactosidase genes were demonstrated in 12 of 14 evaluable animals by several immunologic and biochemical methods, including (1) immunofluorescence, (2) ELISA, (3) flow cytometric analysis, and (4) x-gal staining. Seven of the 12 sheep examined by flow cytometric analysis exhibited greater than or equal to 6% transduced peripheral blood lymphocytes. Once again, extensive analyses of offspring and of the purified sperm separated from other semen components demonstrated that the germline cells were not transduced in these animals.

Thus the direct injection of a retroviral vector into the peritoneal cavity of preimmune fetal recipients appears to represent a relatively efficient way of delivering a foreign gene to the developing fetus. It is possible to obtain long-term expression of the transgene in hematopoietic cells without apparent serious risk to the fetus or its germline.

Studies in Monkeys

The effectiveness of the in utero gene-engineered HSC transplantation protocol was evaluated in monkeys. Helper virus–contaminated (N2) and helper virus–free (LNL6) retroviral supernatant were used in an in utero gene-engineered HSC transplantation protocol to transfer the bacterial Neo[R] gene into two cynomolgus and five rhesus monkeys.[14] An autologous protocol similar to that used in sheep fetuses was used in six of the recipients at a gestational age between 113 and 144 days (term: 165 days). In addition, an allogeneic gene-engineered HSC transplantation protocol without cytoablation was used to treat the one remaining rhesus fetus at about 60 days' gestation.

In the autologous in utero gene-engineered HSC transplantation protocol carried out in the six animals, blood (1.3 to 3.0 mL) was obtained from each fetus at 113 to 144 days' gestation. Low-density mononuclear cells from four samples were incubated with N2 retroviral supernatant overnight, washed, and reinfused into respective donor fetuses intraperitoneally. Whole blood from the remaining two rhesus monkey fetuses was incubated with helper virus–free LNL6 retroviral supernatant overnight, pelleted by centrifugation, and reinfused into each fetus intraperitoneally. All bleedings and injections were carried out under ultrasound guidance. One cynomolgus fetus was delivered prematurely and was not evaluated. Bone marrow samples obtained from the remaining five newborn monkeys soon after birth and at intervals thereafter were cultured in methylcellulose in the presence or absence of lethal doses of G418, and the total numbers and relative percentages of resistant colonies (CFU-Mix, CFU-GM, BFU-E, CFU-E) were determined and compared to untreated controls. Three animals, including one animal treated with the LNL6 vector, exhibited significant numbers of G418-resistant progenitors on several occasions after birth, signifying the successful transfer/expression of the exogenous genes in these monkeys.[14]

These results demonstrate the successful transfer and long-term expression of the bacterial Neo[R] gene in the primate using the in utero gene-engineered HSC transplantation approach without cytoablation of the host. However, although the transfer appears to have occurred at a greater efficiency than postnatal gene transfer in dogs and monkeys, the expression levels are still low.

Finally, in the allogeneic study,[14] a mixture of male and female cells obtained from livers of 62-day-old rhesus monkey fetuses were incubated with helper virus–contaminated N2 retroviral supernatant overnight, washed and injected (3×10^8 cells/kg estimated fetal body weight) intraperitoneally into an unrelated female rhesus fetus. Bone marrow and blood samples were obtained from the newborn monkey at 1 month of age, and at intervals thereafter, for the determination of donor cell engraftment and transgene expression. Engraftment of significant numbers of donor-derived cells accompanied by low levels of G418-resistant hematopoietic progenitors of donor origin were documented at 1 month of age and for more than 1 year thereafter. Even though this was only a single animal study, the persistence of donor cell/exogenous gene activity was encouraging.

Preimmune Status of Recipients

The successful long-term gene transfer and expression in these large animals (sheep, monkeys) is likely to be the result of the preimmune status of the early-gestational-age fetuses studied. There is a period in early immunologic development, prior to thymic processing of mature lymphocytes, during which the fetus is tolerant of foreign antigens. Exposure to foreign antigens during this period results in sustained tolerance that can be permanent if the presence of the antigen is maintained.[15] Cellular tolerance appears to be secondary to clonal deletion of reactive lymphocytes in the thymus, whereas the mechanism of B-lymphocyte tolerance (peripheral tolerance) appears to involve both clonal deletion and clonal suppression.[16] The end result is an immune system that is specifically tolerant of foreign antigenic sources. The use of preimmune fetuses and the intraperitoneal route of administration may have also circumvented the rapid inactivation of murine retroviral vectors that has been reported to occur in vivo.[17]

In Utero Hematopoietic Stem Cell Transplantation

Convincing experimental and clinical support for the efficacy of an in utero approach for the treatment of genetic diseases comes from prenatal HSC transplantation studies. Permanent hematopoietic chimerism with specific transplantation tolerance to skin and organ transplants from their siblings has been observed in normal dizygotic cattle twins with shared placental circulation.[18] In cattle with mannosidosis, hematopoietic chimerism resulted in the cross-correction of the genetic defect.[19] Experiments of nature resulting in hematopoietic chimerism have also been observed in multiple gestations in a number of species including primates[20] and humans.[21] Experiments designed to reproduce this phenomenon by the early gestational transplantation of allogeneic cells in mice, goats, sheep, and monkeys[22] have shown that long-term multilineage chimerism can be achieved across major histocompatibility, barriers without evidence of rejection or the need for immunosuppression. The anemia in W/W^v mice and the immunodeficiency in SCID mice can be successfully treated by in utero HSC transplantation.[23]

Clinical application of in utero HSC transplantation is in its early stages of development. To date, success has been limited to fetal patients with immunodeficiency disorders.[24] However, with advances in prenatal diagnosis, fetal intervention, and HSC technologies, most of the practical, technical, and ethical obstacles to the use of this procedure are increasingly being resolved and clinical application of in utero HSC transplantation is increasing. These improvements are likely to also facilitate the development of approaches for in utero gene therapy.

Rationale for In Utero Human Gene Therapy

There are a number of reasons for treating patients with certain specific diseases before birth. An in utero approach to gene therapy would benefit from the advantages that the developing fetal hematopoietic system provides, which can help circumvent some of the major difficulties encountered with postnatal treatments.[25] These include, among others:

1. The naturally occurring transition in the primary sites of hematopoiesis from yolk sac to liver/spleen and finally bone marrow during ontogeny is accomplished by the migration of HSCs from one site (e.g., liver) to another site (e.g., bone marrow) via the circulation.[26] This process results in the presence of considerable numbers of transient (migratory) HSCs in the fetal circulation during much of gestation, a process also demonstrable at birth and thereafter.

2. Since this mechanism was developed to provide for a hematopoietic bone marrow after birth, it is possible that both the circulating HSCs and the developing hematopoietic sites within the fetus are "primed" for the homing and engraftment of HSCs. Thus, fetal circulation is likely to contain relatively large numbers of "primed" HSCs destined to populate the developing bone marrow system of the fetus. In this regard, it has been established that the efficiency of retroviral-mediated gene transfer in HSCs is significantly influenced by the cell cycle status of HSCs. Primitive adult HSCs are rarely in an active phase of the cell cycle, and require activation (e.g., by cytokines) for transduction in vitro,[27] a process that may result in the relative loss of long-term repopulating ability of the HSCs.[28] By contrast, HSCs in the circulation in the fetus are probably actively dividing and can serve as a more ready target for gene transfer than adult progenitors.[11,14]

3. The availability of bone marrow spaces (possibly also already "primed") for "homing" and engraftment of HSCs in the fetus allows for the engraftment of transduced HSCs without the need for cytoablation of the patient's own marrow, thus avoiding the risks associated with this procedure.[25] That significant HSC engraftment can occur in unprepared fetuses was demonstrated in large animal species[30] and humans[31] by the long-term engraftment and expression of HSCs from allogeneic donors.

4. Another possible handicap in postnatal gene therapy is the large number of cells that are needed to reconstitute the patient. The procedure requires a large volume of retroviral supernatant. Performing

this procedure before birth when only a small volume is needed circumvents this problem. The relatively small size of most mammalian fetuses, combined with the cellular expansion that occurs in association with fetal growth and development, permit the application of in utero gene therapy with relatively few gene-engineered HSCs.

5. Although most infants born with genetic disorders are essentially unaffected by the disease at birth, there are a number of inherited metabolic diseases that cause irreversible damage to the fetus before birth (see Table 40–1). Performing gene therapy in utero may prevent the disease or its therapeutic modalities from clinically compromising the patient.

6. Evidence is now accumulating that in postnatal gene transfer employing adenoviral vectors, host immune responses result in almost complete cessation of transgene expression together with immune-mediated tissue damage to the recipient.[32] Immunologic responses to E1-deleted recombinant adenoviruses also limited the duration of transgene expression soon after the direct introduction into the trachea of immunocompetent fetal lambs relatively late in gestation.[33] Although a number of different strategies involving vector modification and immune suppression of the host currently under development[34] may allow the transgene to evade the host immune defenses, recent observations in mice[35] and sheep[36] suggest that the humoral and/or cellular immune responses to these vectors may be avoided or significantly dampened in young, preimmune fetuses. Thus, as was previously shown with the Moloney murine leukemia retrovirus-based vectors in young sheep fetuses,[37] no evidence of tissue inflammation or neutralizing antibodies was observed at any time after the injection of recombinant adenovirus into preimmune fetal sheep.[36] This observation may be explained by the fact that normal immunologic ontogeny includes a period of immunologic immaturity during which foreign antigens can be tolerated.[15] During this period, transplantation of allogeneic or xenogeneic HSCs results in the creation of permanent chimeras.[38] Even highly immunogenic vectors and/or gene products could be introduced into the fetus during this period of immunologic naivete without eliciting an immune response. The possible development of tolerance to the vector/gene product[39] may permit postnatal treatment of the patient, if required, with relative safety.

Safety and Ethical Considerations

In addition to the risks associated with early prenatal diagnosis using chorionic villus sampling, which appears to be less than 1%,[40] the incidence of significant fetal and maternal complications with removal of blood from older fetuses and injections of vectors into very young fetuses is not known. Even though the injection-related risk is likely to be small, since it would involve needles no larger than 22 gauge and relatively small volumes of cells or vectors, experience with in utero treatment for Rh disease would indicate a 1 to 3.5% risk factor.[41] The risk of transfer of the exogenous genetic material to the mother also has to be considered. Three of the ewes in the direct vector injection studies whose fetuses were given producer cells were found to transiently contain trace quantities of vector sequences in their peripheral blood. By contrast, none of the ewes whose fetuses received retroviral supernatant were found to be positive for vector sequences.[12] There is evidence that placental tissue is readily infected with a variety of retroviruses[42] and that the placenta allows the transfer of retroviral-like particles from mother to the fetus.[43] However, in the sheep studies, the transfer of genetic material that occurred was short-lived, since it was detected only at one time point soon after the fetal treatment, with all subsequent samplings being devoid of vector sequences.[12]

Transduction of the germline with the potential of transmission of the transgene to future generations is another risk with significant societal implications. The possibility exists that future studies may demonstrate germline transmission of the transgene with direct intraperitoneal injection of retroviral supernatant or producer cells. The risk of germline transmission is considerably reduced with the in utero gene-engineered HSC transplantation protocol, since only transduced cells, and no retroviral vector, are given to the fetus. The experimental nature of in utero gene therapy dictates that an ethical framework, from which patients can be counseled and clinical decisions made, be established. There are well-established criteria involving fetal therapy that can also serve to facilitate the process for in utero gene therapy.[44] The ethical considerations unique for in utero gene therapy have been well-discussed by Fletcher.[45]

REFERENCES

1. Anderson WF: Human gene therapy. Nature 392 (Suppl 6679): 25–30, 1998.
2. Malech HL, Maples PB, Whiting-Theobald N, et al: Prolonged production of NADPH oxidase-corrected granulocytes after gene therapy of chronic granulomatous disease. Proc Natl Acad Sci U S A 94:12133–12138, 1997.
3. Anderson WF: Human gene therapy. Science 256:808–813, 1992.
4. Jaenisch R: Retroviruses and embryogenesis: Microinjection of Moloney leukemia virus into midgestation mouse embryos. Cell 19:181–188, 1980.
5. Clapp DW, Freie B, Lee WH, Zhang YY: Molecular evidence that in situ-transduced fetal liver hematopoietic stem/progenitor cells give rise to medullary hematopoiesis in adult rats. Blood 86:2113–2122, 1995.
6. Hayashi SI, Morishita R, Aoki M, et al: In vivo transfer of gene and oligodeoxynucleotides into skin of fetal rats by incubation in amniotic fluid. Gene Therapy 3:878–885, 1996.
7. Sekhon HS, Larson JE: In utero gene transfer into the pulmonary epithelium. Nat Med 1:1201–1203, 1995.
8. Koch KS, Brownlee GG, Goss SJ, et al: Retroviral vector infection and transplantation in rats of primary fetal rat hepatocytes. J Cell Sci 99(Pt 1):121–130, 1991.
9. Woo YJ, Raju GP, Swain JL, et al: In utero cardiac gene transfer via intraplacental delivery of recombinant adenovirus. Circulation 96:3561–3569, 1997.

10. Holzinger A, Trapnell BC, Weaver TE, et al: Intraamniotic administration of an adenoviral vector for gene transfer to fetal sheep and mouse tissues. Pediatr Res 38:844–850, 1995.
11. Kantoff PW, Flake AW, Eglitis MA, et al: In utero gene transfer and expression: A sheep transplantation model. Blood 73:1066–1073, 1989.
12. Porada CD, Tran N, Eglitis M, et al: In utero gene therapy: Transfer and long-term expression of the bacterial neo(r) gene in sheep after direct injection of retroviral vectors into preimmune fetuses. Hum Gene Ther 9:1571–1585, 1998
13. Zanjani ED, Flake AW, Almeida-Porada G, et al: Homing of human cells in the fetal sheep model: Modulation by antibodies activating or inhibiting very late activation antigen-4-dependent function. Blood 94:2515–2522, 1999.
14. Ekhterae D, Crombleholme T, Karson E, et al: Retroviral vector-mediated transfer of the bacterial neomycin resistance gene into fetal and adult sheep and human hematopoietic progenitors in vitro. Blood 75:365–369, 1990.
15. Binns RM: Bone marrow and lymphoid cell injection of the pig foetus resulting in transplantation tolerance or immunity, and immunoglobulin production. Nature 214:179–180, 1967.
16. Marrack P, Lo D, Brinster R, et al: The effect of thymus environment on T cell development and tolerance. Cell 53:627–634, 1988.
17. Takeuchi Y, Cosset FL, Lachmann PJ, et al: Type C retrovirus inactivation by human complement is determined by both the viral genome and the producer cell. J Virol 68:8001–8007, 1994.
18. Rother RP, Squinto SP, Mason JM, Rollins SA: Protection of retroviral vector particles in human blood through complement inhibition. Hum Gene Ther 6:429–435, 1995.
19. Jolly RD, Thompson KG, Murphy CE, et al: Enzyme replacement therapy—an experiment of nature in a chimeric mannosidosis calf. Pediatr Res 10:219–224, 1976.
20. Picus J, Aldrich WR, Letvin NL: A naturally occurring bone-marrow-chimeric primate. I. Integrity of its immune system. Transplantation 39:297–303, 1985.
21. Zanjani ED, Mackintosh FR, Harrison MR: Hematopoietic chimerism in sheep and nonhuman primates by in utero transplantation of fetal hematopoietic stem cells. Blood Cells 17:349–363, 1991.
22. Blazar BR, Taylor PA, Vallera DA: In utero transfer of adult bone marrow cells into recipients with severe combined immunodeficiency disorder yields lymphoid progeny with T- and B-cell functional capabilities. Blood 86:4353–4366, 1995.
23. Fleischman RA, Mintz B: Prevention of genetic anemias in mice by microinjection of normal hematopoietic stem cells into the fetal placenta. Proc Natl Acad Sci U S A 76:5736–5740, 1979.
24. Wengler GS, Lanfranchi A, Frusca T, et al: In-utero transplantation of parental CD34 haematopoietic progenitor cells in a patient with X-linked severe combined immunodeficiency (SCIDXI). Lancet 348:1484–1487, 1996.
25. Flake AW, Harrison MR, Zanjani ED: In utero stem cell transplantation. Exp Hematol 19:1061–1064, 1991.
26. Zanjani ED, Ascensao JL, Tavassoli M: Liver-derived fetal hematopoietic stem cells selectively and preferentially home to the fetal bone marrow. Blood 81:399–404, 1993.
27. Moore KA, Deisseroth AB, Reading CL, et al: Stromal support enhances cell-free retroviral vector transduction of human bone marrow long-term culture-initiating cells. Blood 79:1393–1399, 1992.
28. Kittler EL, Peters SO, Crittenden RB, et al: Cytokine-facilitated transduction leads to low-level engraftment in nonablated hosts. Blood 90:865–872, 1997.
29. Wells S, Malik P, Pensiero M, et al: The presence of an autologous marrow stromal cell layer increases glucocerebrosidase gene transduction of long-term culture initiating cells (LTCICs) from the bone marrow of a patient with Gaucher disease. Gene Ther 2:512–520, 1995.
30. Harrison MR, Slotnick RN, Crombleholme TM, et al: In-utero transplantation of fetal liver haematopoietic stem cells in monkeys. Lancet 2:1425–1427, 1989.
31. Flake AW, Roncarolo MG, Puck JM, et al: Treatment of X-linked combined immunodeficiency by in utero transplantation of paternal bone marrow. N Engl J Med 335:1806–1810, 1996.
32. Vincent MC, Trapnell BC, Baughman RP, et al: Adenovirus-mediated gene transfer to the respiratory tract of fetal sheep in utero. Hum Gene Ther 6:1019–1028, 1995.
33. McCray PB Jr, Armstrong K, Zabner J, et al: Adenoviral-mediated gene transfer to fetal pulmonary epithelia in vitro and in vivo. J Clin Invest 95:2620–2632, 1995.
34. Yap J, O'Brien T, Tazelaar HD, McGregor CG: Immunosuppression prolongs adenoviral mediated transgene expression in cardiac allograft transplantation. Cardiovasc Res 35:529–535, 1997.
35. Larson JE, Morrow SL, Happel L, et al: Reversal of cystic fibrosis phenotype in mice by gene therapy in utero. Lancet 349:619–620, 1997.
36. Yang EY, Flake AW, Adzick NS: Prospects for fetal gene therapy. Semin Perinatol 23:524–534, 1999.
37. Pitt BR, Schwarz MA, Pilewski JM, et al: Retrovirus-mediated gene transfer in lungs of living fetal sheep. Gene Ther 2:344–350, 1995.
38. Zanjani ED, Flake AW, Rice HE, et al: Long-term repopulating ability of xenogeneic transplanted human fetal liver hematopoietic stem cells in sheep. J Clin Invest 93:1051–1055, 1994.
39. Mychaliska GB, Rice HE, Tarantal AF, et al: In utero hematopoietic stem cell transplants prolong survival of postnatal kidney transplantation in monkeys. J Pediatr Surg 32:976–981, 1997.
40. Rhoads GG, Jackson LG, Schlesselman SE, et al: The safety and efficacy of chorionic villus sampling for early prenatal diagnosis of cytogenetic abnormalities. N Engl J Med 320:609–617, 1989.
41. Bowman J: In Creasy R, Resnick R (eds): Maternal-Fetal Medicine: Principles and Practice, 3rd ed. Philadelphia: WB Saunders Company, 1994, pp 730–733.
42. Bui T, Watanabe R, Kennedy B, et al: Simian immunodeficiency virus infection of macaque primary placental cells. AIDS Res Hum Retrovir 11:955–961, 1995.
43. Tsukamoto M, Ochiya T, Yoshida S, et al: Gene transfer and expression in progeny after intravenous DNA injection into pregnant mice. Nat Genet 9:243–248, 1995.
44. Fletcher JC: Fetal therapy, ethics, and public policies. Fetal Diagn Ther 7:158–168, 1992.
45. Fletcher JC, Richter G: Human fetal gene therapy: Moral and ethical questions. Hum Gene Ther 7:1605–1614, 1996.

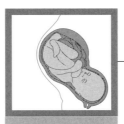

P A R T V

Postnatal Management: Social Security for the Fetus

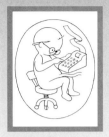

CHAPTER 41

Postnatal Follow-up and Outcomes

ROBERT PIECUCH and JODY A. FARRELL

Since the early 1980s, fetal surgery has been selectively offered as a treatment option to mothers carrying fetuses with specific life-threatening anomalies. Risks of the procedure to the fetus are weighed against the benefit of correction of a lethal or debilitating anomaly. But, for the mother, maternal safety is paramount as most fetal malformations do not directly threaten her health. Postnatal maternal and infant follow-up and outcome data are extremely important in counseling families considering fetal intervention. They often have many questions concerning maternal safety, maternal long-term morbidity, infant risk, and infant long-term follow-up. Centers that perform these procedures have a responsibility to provide data on past patients, make recommendations for maternal and infant postnatal follow-up, and ensure that the necessary support services for the child and mother are available after discharge.

Maternal Outcome After Fetal Surgery

Short-term maternal morbidity from open fetal surgery and postoperative tocolytic therapy is significant. All patients develop preterm labor, suffer the adverse reactions of tocolytic therapy, and deliver their infants preterm. Equally important, however, is the possibility of significant long-term maternal morbidity. Two potentially serious sequelae from fetal surgery are effects on future fertility and uterine rupture in subsequent pregnancies. A mother must be able to conceive again (if she desires) and to deliver her infant without significant obstetric morbidity that can be attributed to the prior fetal surgical procedure.

The vast majority of fetal surgical procedures have been performed using a non–lower uterine segment open hysterotomy. Due to the constraints placed upon the fetal surgeon by placental and fetal location, most hysterotomies used for fetal exposure cannot be placed in the lower uterine segment. The incisions may be transverse, vertical, or oblique, on either the anterior, fundal, or posterior uterine walls, depending on placental and fetal location. Because of the unique and variable hysterotomy incision, long-term uterine function could be

compromised. Two studies have looked at the impact of fetal surgery on maternal fertility.[1] A study published in 1991 looking at 17 open hysterotomy fetal surgeries concluded that a midgestation hysterotomy, closed with absorbable sutures, had no detrimental effect on the mother's future fertility.[1] A recent survey of over 60 women who had undergone fetal surgery—the largest fetal surgery experience at a single institution—clearly demonstrated that maternal fertility is not adversely affected by fetal surgery.[2] Every woman without a prior history of infertility who wanted to become pregnant after fetal surgery has been successful. Table 41–1 summarizes maternal postnatal outcome.

Fetal surgery may bring an increased risk of uterine rupture or a greater incidence of preterm labor in future pregnancies. Due to these unique incisions, it has been recommended that all subsequent pregnancies be delivered by cesarean section. Classic cesarean section has a reported incidence of uterine rupture of 12%,[3] abnormal scarring of 13%, and dehiscence of 6%.[4] Our most recent follow-up of 64 women who have undergone fetal surgery reports a 10% incidence of uterine scar dehiscence, which is consistent with maternal outcomes of subsequent pregnancies after cesarean section,[2] and an 11% incidence of preterm labor that is not greater than that found in the general population.[5, 6] Furthermore, preterm labor was well controlled in these women because the average gestational age of their infants at birth was 36 weeks.[2]

The development of less invasive percutaneous techniques to correct specific fetal problems (e.g., endoscopic tracheal clip placement for congenital diaphragmatic hernia, radiofrequency ablation for sacrococcygeal teratoma, or umbilical cord divison by harmonic scalpel) may alter obstetric management in fetal surgery patients. There is not enough experience with the newer, less invasive technique of fetoscopic surgery to determine how future pregnancies should be managed. Because of the lack of a large hysterotomy, the benefits of this technique should include a decreased risk of uterine dehiscence and/or rupture and enable women to labor with future pregnancies. To date only two mothers have labored using this new technique. One was able to de-

T A B L E 41–1. MATERNAL POSTNATAL OUTCOME FOLLOWING FETAL SURGERY

NAME	YEAR OF SURGERY	PREGNANCY ATTEMPT	SUCCESS	SAB/# TAB/#	LIVE BIRTH	GESTATIONAL AGE AT BIRTH	OB COMPLICATION	NEONATAL COMPLICATION
KA	1996	Y	Y	S/1				
TA	1990	Y	Y		1	36	PTL (26 wk)	Jaundiced
CA	1991	Y	N				Hx of infertility	
JB	1992	Y	Y		1	38		
KB	1995	Y	Y		1	38		Irregular HR
LB	1988	Y	Y	S/1	1	40		
LC	1990	Y	Y		1	36		
LC	1985	Y	Y		2	38		
						39	Uterine dehiscence	
JC	1995	Y	Y		1	37		
SC	1992	Y	Y		1	38		
JC	1994	Y	Y		1	37	Preeclampic	Jaundiced
AC	1993	Y	Y	S/1	1	37		
LD	1989	Y	Y	S/1	2	37	Uterine dehiscence	RDS
						34	Uterine dehiscence	RDS
SF	1993	Y	Y	T/1				
AF	1995	Y	Y		1	38		
DH	1993	Y	Y		1	37	PTL (29 wk)	
	1986	Y	Y		1	37		
TK	1994	Y	N				Hx of infertility	
DK	1993	Y	Y		1	39		
JK	1996	Y	N		1	38		
PL	1993	Y	Y	S/1			Hx of infertility	
CL	1987	Y	Y	S/2	1	37		
SM	1994	Y	Y		2	35		
DM	1989	Y	Y		2	36.5		
						37		
SN	1997	Y	Y	S/1	1	38		
KN	1993	Y	Y		1	38		
JO	1994	Y	Y	S/1	2	38		
						38		
JP	1991	Y	Y		2	34		Craniosyn
KR	1995	Y	Y			38.5		
						37		
CR	1995	Y	Y	S/1	1			
KR	1991	Y	Y		1	39		
MS	1991	Y	Y		1	32	Ruptured uterus	RDS
DS	1990	Y	Y		1	36		
FS	1990	Y	Y			40		
	TOTALS			S/7 T/1	33	m = 37.2		

SAB, spontaneous abortion; TAB, therapeutic abortion; PTL, preterm labor; RDS, respiratory distress syndrome.

liver vaginally without complications, and the other underwent a low-transverse cesarean section for failure to progress. Current recommendation in this select group is to allow the mother to labor and attempt a vaginal delivery.

Outcome for Survivors of Fetal Surgery

Improved techniques in prenatal diagnosis and perinatal treatment have dramatically altered the approach to some fetuses with certain congenital anomalies. Although the survival of these fetuses has been reviewed extensively, their clinical courses can still be complicated. There have been ongoing concerns that the fetal procedure itself may have significant impact on the hemodynamics of the fetus, affecting brain blood flow that might have implications for the long-term neurologic and developmental outcomes of children who have un-

dergone fetal surgery. Despite fetal intervention, the clinical course especially for infants with pulmonary hypoplasia may be long and complicated, and chronic illness itself may result in developmental delays. Postnatal assessment and long-term follow-up are integral aspects of the fetal intervention program. Outcome data can assist in the development of patient management plans and early intervention when indicated.

Neurodevelopmental Outcome

To date the only information available on the neurodevelopmental outcome of survivors of fetal surgery is our experience with a small group of original survivors of the technique. In the 6-year period between 1989 and 1994, 36 fetuses underwent open surgical intervention for congenital diaphragmatic hernia (CDH) and congenital cystic adenomatoid malformations (CCAM) at the Fetal Treatment Center at the University of California at San Francisco.[7] Sixteen of the nonsurvivors died in utero. Twelve patients survived to discharge. Four of these 12 survivors were prenatally diagnosed with CCAM, had hydrops, and underwent fetal resection of the masses. Eight were diagnosed with left-sided CDH. Seven of these fetuses had complete repairs performed, utilizing various techniques, while the last fetus was the first at our institution to undergo tracheal occlusion. Currently, there are eight survivors of a tracheal clip procedure, all of which are less than 2 years of age and are too young to report any reliable outcome data.

Medical records of the older children were reviewed retrospectively for diagnosis, gestational age at fetal surgery and at birth, central nervous system imaging abnormalities evaluated by ultrasound both before and after birth, per protocol, and postnatal clinical course including days on ventilator support and days in supplemental oxygen. One child who had open fetal surgery for a congenital diaphragmatic hernia was excluded from the analysis because he was a victim of abuse at 6 months of age and suffered severe brain injury with significant neurodevelopmental deficits. He had been reported previously to be developing normally.

Fetal surgery survivors underwent complete physical, neurologic, and age-appropriate developmental examinations. These tests were performed on the children at follow-up at 1, 1.5, and 2.5 years with age adjusted for prematurity and at 4.5 years' chronologic age. Children were seen in our follow-up program where possible, on our assessment schedule (see Table 41–3), but as the candidates for open fetal surgery are referred from across the United States, reports were obtained from community caregivers where families could not travel back for assessment.

Suspect neurologic findings included clumsiness, tremors, or mild tone and reflex changes without fixed impairment. Abnormal findings included cerebral palsy, defined as moderate to severe abnormalities associated with fixed impairment such as diplegias and hemiplegias.

Developmental assessments performed by us included the Bayley Scales of Infant Development II at 1 and 1.5 years adjusted age, the Stanford Binet Intelligence Scale at adjusted age 2.5 years, and the McCarthy Scales of Children's Abilities at 4.5 years (Table 41–2). Adjusted age, or conceptional age, was defined as the age at which the child would have been had birth occurred at term. Cognitive developmental abnormalities were defined as mild if scores on the age-appropriate scale were between 1 and 2 standard deviations (SD) below the mean (70 to 85) and as severe if scores were 2 SD or more below the mean ($\leq$69). Results of tests given by community caregivers were categorized similarly, based on the criteria for tests given for normal, borderline, or abnormal results.

The clinical course of these children is shown in Table 41–3. The four infants with CCAM resections had fairly uncomplicated clinical courses after birth. One infant born at 25 weeks' gestation had a prolonged need for ventilator support related to prematurity, but did not go on to develop chronic lung disease. Infants with CDH had more complicated courses. Three infants were repeatedly hospitalized in the first year for respiratory disease. Two infants were identified with central nervous system (CNS) lesions, one with periventricular leukomalacia and one with grade III intracranial hemorrhage (ICH), both recognized after fetal intervention and before birth.

Neurologic and developmental outcomes are shown in Table 41–4. Both children with CNS abnormalities demonstrated abnormal neurologic outcomes. Two other children with CDH have mild cognitive delays.

In sick premature neonates who have not undergone fetal surgery, both intracranial hemorrhage and periventricular leukomalacia are associated with subsequent neurologic problems such as cerebral palsy.[8-11] Intracranial hemorrhage is a known risk of fetal surgery as well, occurring in as many as 21% of fetuses, and is likely related to a combination of medical risk factors including fetal stress, transient maternal and fetal hemo-

TABLE 41–2. SCHEDULE OF ASSESSMENTS

This protocol is followed for children who are developing normally and have adequate family support. Infants with atypical development are seen as needed during the diagnostic phase and referred to appropriate community agencies. We will continue to follow them on our regular schedule. For premature infants, ages are adjusted until their third birthday.
Within the first month after discharge, children have a neurodevelopmental exam either at clinic or on a home visit.

3 months	Neurodevelopmental exam	Bayley Infant Neurodevelopmental Screener (BINS)
5 months	Neurodevelopmental exam	Bayley Infant Neurodevelopmental Screener (BINS)
8 months*	Neurodevelopmental exam	Bayley Infant Neurodevelopmental Screener (BINS)
12 months	Neurodevelopmental exam	Bayley Scales of Infant Development II
18–24 months[†]	Neurodevelopmental exam	Bayley Scales of Infant Development II
2½ years	Neurodevelopmental exam	Bayley Scales of Infant Development II
4½ years	Neurodevelopmental exam	Wechsler Preschool and Primary Scale of Intelligence—Revised (WPPSI-R)
		Conners' Parent Reading Scale—Revised
8 years	Neurodevelopmental exam	Wechsler Intelligence Scale for Children III
		Wide Range Achievement Test–3
		Conners' Parent Rating Scale—Revised
12 years	Neurodevelopmental exam	Wechsler Intelligence Scale for Children III
		Wide Range Achievement Test–3
		Conners' Parent Rating Scale—Revised

* Physical therapy consultation if needed.
[†] All infants meeting criteria followed to this age; all infants <1,250 g and ECMO infants followed to age 8; all infants <800 g followed to age 12; infants in research studies followed per protocol.

TABLE 41–3. CLINICAL COURSE AFTER OPEN FETAL SURGERY

PT. #	DIAGNOSIS	GA AT FETAL SURGERY (WK)	GA AT BIRTH (WK)	BIRTH WEIGHT (G)	CNS IMAGING PATHOLOGY	DAYS ON VENTILATOR	DAYS ON OXYGEN
1	CCAM	24	34	2,420	None	5	15
2	CCAM	25	33	2,000	None	3	9
3	CCAM	25	30	1,500	None	14	20
4	CCAM	22	25	1,050	None	48	60
5	CDH	25	32	1,749	None	2	8
6	CDH	24	28	1,378	None	65	90
7	CDH	25	32	1,640	Grade 1 ICH	7	14
8	CDH	24	32	2,205	None	1	180
9	CDH	24	32	1,820	Unknown	37	—
10	CDH	23	30	1,680	Right PVL	84	85
11	CDH	24	33	2,100	Grade III ICH	22	30

GA, gestational age; CNS, central nervous system; CCAM, congenital cystic adenomatoid malformations; CDH, congenital diaphragmatic hernia; ICH, intracranial hemorrhage; PVL, periventricular leukomalacia.

dynamic instability, and the anatomy of the premature brain.[12] In our small group, specific etiologies for fetal compromise could not be associated with operative or tocolytic regimens.

These were the earliest experiences with fetal open surgical intervention, and variable approaches to care were utilized. Subsequently, more standardized and less invasive approaches have been adopted. The most significant advance in fetal intervention has been the movement away from open fetal surgery to minimally invasive fetoscopic surgery, or FETENDO. The new generation of survivors will presumably reflect the outcome of the newer advances for CDH, including less invasive FETENDO clip procedures, eliminating, it is hoped, many of the current complications from hysterotomy and open fetal surgery. Decreased uterine manipulation may have a positive impact on preterm labor, thereby decreasing the incidence and sequelae of premature delivery.

In sick premature infants who have not undergone fetal surgery, pulmonary disease resulting in chronic lung disease and bronchopulmonary dysplasia is a risk factor for subsequent developmental delays. In our group of fetal surgery patients, all eight fetuses with congenital diaphragmatic hernia delivered prematurely and had significant degrees of pulmonary hypoplasia and immaturity, despite their fetal intervention. Some of these infants had significant ventilator and oxygen requirements, resulting in elements of chronic lung disease and bronchopulmonary dysplasia, similar to that seen in infants with CDH who are repaired postnatally.

In this small group of infants, fetal surgery does not appear to put these survivors at a greater risk of poor neurologic and developmental outcome beyond already identified medical risk factors related to prematurity and lung disease that contribute to poor neurodevelopmental outcome.

Unfavorable outcomes appear to be related to intracranial hemorrhage and requirement of prolonged respiratory support. Follow-up of children who have undergone fetal surgery should include a careful search for intracranial hemorrhage. Less invasive fetoscopic therapies, reduction of fetal stress, improved maternal and fetal hemodynamic stability, and improved tocolysis allowing delivery later in gestation may decrease the incidence of intracranial hemorrhage and prolonged respiratory support and lead to less intensive postnatal courses. These improvements should lead to continued improvement in the neurologic and developmental outcomes for fetuses undergoing surgery. We look forward to long-term follow-up of these children as they progress through school to examine for the possibility of more

TABLE 41–4. NEURODEVELOPMENTAL OUTCOME AFTER OPEN FETAL SURGERY

PT. #	DIAGNOSIS	NEUROLOGIC OUTCOME	COGNITIVE OUTCOME	AGE AT FOLLOW-UP (MO)
1	CCAM	Normal	Normal	47
2	CCAM	Normal	Normal	11
3	CCAM	Normal	Normal	25
4	CCAM	Normal	Normal	38
5	CDH	Normal	Normal	25
6	CDH	Normal	Normal	56
7	CDH	Normal	Normal	16
8	CDH	Normal	Mild delay	18
9	CDH	Normal	Mild delay	69
10	CDH	Abnormal	Normal	25
11	CDH	Suspect	Normal	15

CCAM, congenital cystic adenomatoid malformations; CDH, congenital diaphragmatic hernia.

subtle developmental abnormalities, and likewise will follow the next generation of survivors of more advanced techniques of fetal intervention.

Medical Outcome

As already mentioned, the medical outcome of fetal surgery survivors may be fairly complex despite fetal intervention. Although pulmonary hypoplasia and chronic lung disease will significantly affect the survivor's immediate hospital course, medical needs within the first year of life may be complex. Outcomes may be affected by failure to thrive, gastroesophageal reflux, and bony deformities related to CDH, conditions not necessarily unique to fetal surgery patients. Nobuhara et al.[13] reported significant long-term morbidities in these patients, including developmental delay, poor growth, gastroesophageal reflux, hearing loss, and musculoskeletal abnormalities.

Failure to thrive in infants with CDH may be due to a number of causes, including increased work of breathing both from pulmonary hypoplasia and from chronic lung disease, requiring increased calories for growth, or gastroesophageal motility abnormalities resulting in reflux. Van Meurs[14] has shown that even at 2 years of age, half of her CDH survivors were measured at less than the fifth percentile for weight. Almost 90% of this group had evidence of gastroesophageal reflux (GER). Our experience has been similar, and has alerted us to early identification and medical treatment of GER, with decision for surgical intervention made if necessary before discharge. If medical management is successful, a regimen of chronic treatment and increased caloric supply maintained into the second year of life may be warranted.

Thoracic growth in infants recovering from CDH may be abnormal. In our own population, approximately 10% of CDH survivors have developed some element of pectus and/or scoliosis. This may be from underlying pathophysiology as a result of pulmonary hypoplasia, but may also be a complication of surgical repair, especially in infants with little remnant diaphragm, requiring patch repair. Lund[15] has reported that as many as one third of CDH survivors seen in their follow-up clinic had evidence of pectus deformities, with a much smaller number requiring intervention for scoliosis. We have outlined a schedule of physical therapy evaluations as part of our follow-up of these infants.

Recent advances in fetal intervention for congenital diaphragmatic hernia have led to the fetal endoscopic tracheal clip procedure (FETENDO clip). This procedure has evolved from placing an internal plug into the fetal trachea to placing multiple stainless steel clips transversely across the trachea. In the survivors of this procedure, the external clips produced little tracheal damage.[16] At the time of birth, these infants' tracheas opened to normal caliber and had little visible mucosal damage. Long-term follow-up in this subset of patients has been significant for vocal cord paresis in two patients who required tracheostomy placement.[17] We remain committed to performing long-term examination and assessment of patients who undergo this innovative treatment.

REFERENCES

1. Longaker MT, Golbus MS, Filly RA, et al: Maternal outcome after open fetal surgery: A review of the first 17 human cases. JAMA 265:737–741, 1991.
2. Farrell JA, Albanese CT, Jennings RW, et al: Maternal fertility is not affected by fetal surgery. Fetal Ther Diagn (in press).
3. Carroll SG, Turner MJ, Stronge JM, O'Herlhy C: Management of antepartum spontaneous membrane rupture after one previous caesarean section. Eur J Obstet Gynecol Reprod Biol 173:618–628, 1995.
4. Halperin MD, Moore DC, Hannah WJ: Classical versus low-segment transverse incision for preterm caesarean section: Maternal complications and outcome of subsequent pregnancies. Br J Obstet Gynecol 95:990–996, 1988.
5. Creasy RK: Preterm birth prevention: Where are we? Am J Obstet Gynecol 168:1223–1230, 1993.
6. Keirse MJNC: New perspectives for the effective treatment of preterm labor. Am J Obstet Gynecol 173:618–628, 1995.
7. Gibbs DL, Piecuch R, Graf J, et al: Neurodevelopmental outcome after open fetal surgery. J Pediatr Surg 33:1254–1256, 1998.
8. Papile L, Munsick-Bruno G, Schaefer A: Relationship of cerebral intraventricular hemorrhage and early childhood neurologic handicaps. J Pediatr 103:273–277, 1983.
9. Guzzetta F, Shackleford G, Volpe S, et al: Periventricular intra-parenchymal echodensities in the premature newborn: Critical determinant of neurologic outcome. Pediatrics 78:995–1006, 1986.
10. Graziani L, Pasto, Stanley C, et al: Neonatal neurosonographic correlates of cerebral palsy in preterm infants. Pediatrics 78:88–95, 1986.
11. Piecuch R, Leonard C, Cooper B, Sehring S: Outcome of extremely low birth weight infants (500 to 999 grams) over a twelve-year period. Pediatrics 100:633–639, 1997.
12. Bealer JF, Raisanen J, Skarsgard ED, et al: The incidence and spectrum of neurological injury after open fetal surgery. J Pediatr Surg 30:1150–1154, 1995.
13. Nobuhara K, Lund D, Mitchell J, et al: Long-term outlook for survivors of congenital diaphragmatic hernia. Clin Perinatol 23:873–886, 1996.
14. Van Meurs K, Robbins S, Reed V, et al: Congenital diaphragmatic hernia: Long term outcome in neonates treated with extracorporeal membrane oxygenation. J Pediatr 1222:893–899, 1993.
15. Lund D, Mitchell J, Kharasch V, et al: Congenital diaphragmatic hernia: The hidden morbidity. J Pediatr Surg 29:258–264, 1994.
16. Harrison MR, Adzick NS, Flake AW, et al: Correction of congenital diaphragmatic hernia in utero, VIII. The response of the hypoplastic lung to temporary tracheal occlusion. J Pediatr Surg 31:1339–1348, 1996.
17. Harrison MR, Mychaliska GB, Albanese CT, et al: Correction of congenital diaphragmatic hernia in utero IX. Fetuses with poor prognosis (liver herniation and low lung-to-head ratio) can be saved by fetoscopic temporary tracheal occlusion. J Pediatr Surg 33:1017–1023, 1998.

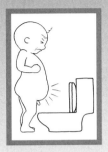

The Fetus with Complex Genitourinary Anomalies

RICHARD W. GRADY and MICHAEL E. MITCHELL

The Developing Bladder

Normal bladder development results in an organ that functions to store and evacuate urine. This process, known as bladder cycling, requires the bladder to store urine at low intravesical pressures during filling while maintaining continence at the level of the bladder neck. Subsequent evacuation of urine from the bladder requires a coordinated contraction of the detrusor in conjunction with relaxation of the bladder outlet. Both normal storage and emptying require intact sensation.[1]

During embryogenesis, components of the urologic system such as the ureteral buds first appear during the fourth week of gestation. At this time the bladder has not completely formed from the anterior urogenital sinus (Fig. 42–1). The urinary bladder subsequently arises during the eighth week of fetal development when the ventral portion of the urogenital sinus begins to expand.[1] With bladder filling, the mesenchymal tissue surrounding this structure differentiates into smooth muscle, which will eventually become the detrusor muscle. Ingrowth of neuronal tissue into this smooth muscle to form motor units is also critical to the development of a functional bladder.[2] Embryogenesis of the pelvic floor is also important in normal fetal bladder development and function; the pelvic floor acts as a dynamic support for the bladder, which aids in both continence and volitional voiding.[3]

Factors Involved in Bladder Development

Recent work by investigators in basic science and clinical research demonstrates the complex and interdependent interaction of a variety of factors in bladder development. Mechanical processes such as cell stretch and pressure are intimately involved in the expression of growth factors, which act to influence cell growth and cell signal transduction.[4] Park and co-workers have demonstrated in vitro and in vivo that mechanical stretch of urothelium results in the production of keratinocyte growth factor (KGF) and vascular epidermal growth factor (VEGF), which act as potent mitogens.[5] These factors in turn influence and are influenced by neural develop-

ment in utero and in the newborn period. The interplay between these processes affects cellular and extracellular matrix development of the bladder as well (Fig. 42–2).

Role of Neuronal Development

During fetal development, innervation of the pelvic floor and bladder occurs as the nerve cell bodies of the neuroectoderm (precursor to the spinal cord) grow motor nerve axons that eventually reach and innervate the developing muscle in the mesoderm. Ingrowth of neural tissue occurs between 8 weeks and 3 months of gestation. In conjunction the muscle fibers of the developing bladder mature by 19 weeks of gestation.[2] However, bladder cycling does not begin until the formation of neuromuscular junctions in the fifth month of development.[1, 6] These nerves and accompanying nerve growth factors are critical to the normal growth and development of the fetus. With normal development, these motor nerve axons provide a wide range of possible function including fine motor regulation of the muscular diaphragm of the pelvis and bladder. Aberrations in this neural developmental process are apparent in conditions such as spina bifida, where they result in pelvic floor and bladder dysfunction.[7] Neural development is also likely affected in other congenital defects such as bladder exstrophy and cloacal anomalies as well and may be one component of bladder dysfunction in these patients.

Experiments by Steers and co-workers support the concept that neuronal development is critical to normal bladder development. In the fetal and neonatal periods, neurons, which fail to access end-organs, undergo programmed cell death. Various growth factors appear critical to neuronal development. In particular, nerve growth factor (NGF) is required for adrenergic and sensory neurons to survive and mature. NGF levels increase in the rat bladder during embryogenesis simultaneously with closure of the urachus and the onset of bladder cycling. In vitro experiments also reveal increased production of protein kinase C–dependent NGF production with cyclic stretching of bladder smooth muscle. These findings lend support to and highlight the role of mechanical factors in bladder development as well. Immu-

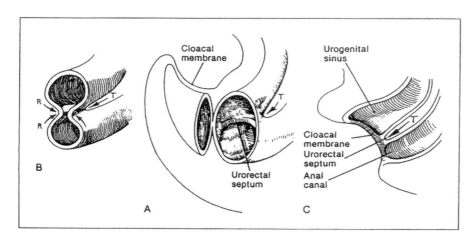

F I G U R E 42–1. Bladder embryology: Process of cloacal division into urogenital sinus and rectum. (From Hinman F Jr: Atlas of UroSurgical Anatomy. Philadelphia: WB Saunders Company, 1993, p 314, with permission.)

nization to NGF in utero causes newborn rats to perish secondary to urinary retention.[8] Studies by Keating and others also support the concept of neuronal change during development. They demonstrated marked changes in cholinergic and purinergic response between day 1 and week 4 of bladder development in a rabbit model.[9]

Postnatally, bladder function continues to develop; this has been well documented in animal models; evidence suggests that this is also true in the human.[1] Children do not achieve volitional voiding and continence until several years after birth. These developmental milestones require: (1) adequate bladder capacity, (2) volitional control of the bladder neck and striated external urethra sphincter muscle, and (3) the initiation of detrusor contraction inhibition via control of the spinal reflex. Progression from the spontaneous voiding of infancy triggered by intravesical pressure via the spinal reflex to volitional control of the storage and emptying of urine occurs as a gradual transition. Detrusor instability, high-pressure voiding, and incomplete emptying are common and well-documented phenomena in healthy infants. Detrusor instability can be found to varying degrees in as many as 57% of children between 3 and 14 years old.[10]

Because maturation of the developing nervous system relies on continuous restructuring and growth of both the end-organs and involved nerves, the immature nervous system possesses incredible reserve inherent in its plasticity during development. Neuronal proliferation and death in conjunction with neuronal migration and targeting allow neural networks to be refashioned in response to environmental stimuli.[11] Evidence of this remodeling is apparent in the development of speech, vision, hearing, language, etc. Because maturation of the nervous system eventually results in limited plasticity, the developing nervous system also represents a window of opportunity. Evidence suggests that bladder development is subject to similar plasticity in development and that early intervention in the abnormal bladder may permit the achievement of developmental milestones in bladder function.[12]

Role of Mesenchymal-Epithelial Interaction

Normal bladder development also relies on the interplay between urothelium and mesenchyme; this results in induction of smooth muscle function and differentiation by urothelium and vice versa. The role of mesenchymal-epithelial interactions is not unique to bladder development. The gastrointestinal tract, skeletal system, and integument also rely on this interaction during organogenesis.[13, 14] In a series of elegant experiments, Baskin et al. separated bladder mesenchyme from urothelium in an embryonic rat model before smooth muscle differentiation had begun to occur. Through tissue recombination experiments, they showed mesenchymal to smooth muscle differentiation in the bladder required the presence of epithelium.[14] Urothelial development is similarly influenced by the mesenchyme associated with it. Tissue recombination experiments using urogenital sinus

F I G U R E 42–2. Complex patterns of interaction between factors affecting bladder development.

mesenchyme and urothelium demonstrate prostatic ductal morphogenesis, epithelial androgen receptor expression, prostatic functional cytodifferentiation, and prostate-specific secretory protein expression from normally planar bladder epithelium.[13]

Growth and Mechanical Factors

Growth factors such as KGF, transforming growth factor-α or -β (TGF-α or TGF-β), and epidermal growth factor (EGF) are likely the principal mediators of differentiation during development, although the specific factors underlying this complex cell–cell signaling in bladder development remain to be elucidated. Investigators have shown in vitro and in vivo that cell stretch and pressure influence the production of these factors by urothelium and smooth muscle.[4, 5, 15] In vitro studies of urothelium exposed to mechanical stretch demonstrate expression of potent growth factors by these cells. Urothelial stretch rather than intravesical pressure is important to elicit these factors; the specific mechanical influences that affect mesenchymal and smooth muscle growth factor expression have been less well defined.[5] Researchers have shown, however, that phasic pressure exerted on smooth muscle cells in vitro also elicits growth factor expression.[4]

Furthermore, mechanical forces exerted on bladder smooth muscle and urothelium result in changes in collagen types I and III synthesis in vitro.[16] In utero, these mechanical forces occur with bladder cycling, which begins as early as the fifth month of gestation in human embryogenesis. Antenatal ultrasonography has demonstrated voiding cycles every 50 to 150 minutes in the fetus after the fifth month of gestation.[1]

From a structural standpoint, Levin and co-workers have demonstrated that during development, the normal bladder (1) increases proportionately in weight and capacity in early and midgestation and that the rate accelerates in the last trimester, (2) becomes significantly more compliant during gestation, (3) has low intravesical pressure during early gestation that appears to be calcium-mediated tonic tension, and (4) has poor contractile response to field stimulation in the early gestational period that appears to be a nitric oxide–mediated phenomenon[17] (Fig. 42–3).

These studies highlight our increasing understanding that multiple factors acting interdependently including neuronal development, mechanical forces, cell signal transduction factors, growth factors, and other forces that remain to be identified significantly impact bladder development during embryogenesis.

Genitourinary Anomalies— Clinical Correlations

Complex genitourinary anomalies influence bladder development principally by producing urinary outlet obstruction or by creating urinary diversion. In humans, congenital anomalies such as posterior urethral valves cause antenatal urinary outlet obstruction, whereas other conditions such as bladder exstrophy result in antenatal urinary diversion. Study of these congenital anomalies and their equivalent animal models helps us to understand the consequences of these conditions on bladder development and function.

Urinary Tract Outlet Obstruction

Experimental Models

Effects on Muscle and Extracellular Matrix Development

Animal models of urinary outflow obstruction show marked increases in bladder mass (four to eight times) secondary to proportional increases in smooth muscle via hyperplasia and hypertrophy and connective tissue volume via increased volume content. These bladders demonstrate acceleration in the maturation pattern of myosin and actin development. Up-regulation of neurotransmitter receptor (i.e., muscarinic cholinergic receptors) expression also occurs with obstruction. Urinary outlet obstruction causes changes in the extracellular matrix as well. Collagen concentration increases in parallel with smooth muscle hyperplasia and hypertrophy. This phenomenon appears due to increased gene and protein expression along with increased activity of tissue inhibitors of metalloproteinases (TIMPS), which prevent enzymes that normally degrade connective tissue (matrix metalloproteinases) from functioning.[18]

Obstruction also alters collagen subtype expression in a fetal rabbit model (Fig. 42–4). Collagen type I and III predominate in the bladder extracellular matrix (ECM). As the bladder develops, these collagen types change in spatial distribution. Experiments by Yao and co-workers in the developing rabbit bladder demonstrate collagen αI (I) mRNA expression peaking at 2 weeks of development in the lamina propria, whereas collagen αI (III) peaks at 3 to 4 weeks in the lamina propria and urothelium. Partial obstruction up-regulates mRNA of both collagen subtypes and ultimately results in protein deposition in the lamina propria and muscularis mucosa.[16, 19] With chronic obstruction, these changes likely produce fibrosis and poor bladder compliance and function. We recognize this entity clinically in several disease states such as the valve bladder secondary to posterior urethral valves.

Animal studies also show that as the bladder develops the amount and composition of ECM and smooth muscle in the bladder changes. Collagen production and smooth muscle development in the ECM is likely mediated by cell signal transduction, perhaps in response to urothelial cell–cell signals. Interestingly, the fetal bladder appears to respond differently to partial outlet obstruction than the adult bladder.[17] Histologic comparison between the two shows increased bladder mass for both adults and fetal rabbits after outlet obstruction. This increase is due to ECM deposition in the adults versus smooth muscle hypertrophy in the fetal rabbits. Furthermore, the ECM in the fetal rabbits is largely type III collagen in the muscularis compared to type I collagen outside the serosal layer in adults.[16]

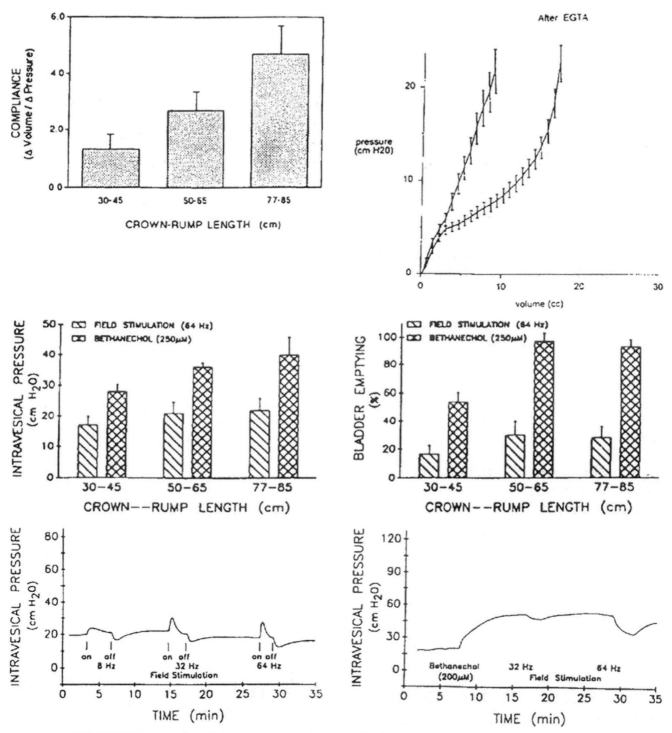

FIGURE 42–3. Summary for the developmental aspects of both passive and active properties of the fetal bovine bladder. (From Levin R: Developmental aspects of urinary bladder physiology and pharmacology. Dialogues in Pediatric Urology 19:3, 1996, with permission.)

In vivo experiments in fetal rodents have implicated the growth factors TGF-β2, TGF-β3, and TGF-α in the changes that occur in the obstructed fetal bladder. TGF-β is a known mitogen for mesenchymal cells such as fibroblasts and smooth muscle cells. In partial outlet obstruction, mesenchyma located next to the serosa of the bladder differentiates into myofibroblasts and smooth muscle. Alteration in the production of these growth factors in bladder obstruction suggests that mechanical processes such as obstruction or diversion of the urinary tract can have profound effects on the developing bladder.[14]

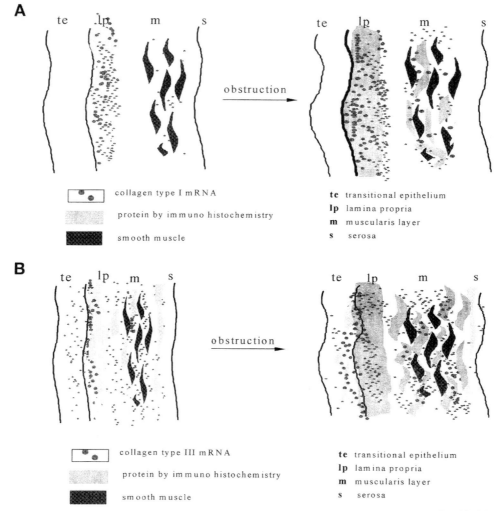

FIGURE 42–4. Changes in collagen types I (A) and III (B) gene and protein distribution after bladder outlet obstruction. (From Tekgul S: Collagen types I and III localization by in situ hybridization and immunohistochemistry in the partially obstructed young rabbit bladder. J Urol 156:585, 1996, with permission.)

Ultimately, these changes produce effects on the storage and voiding characteristics of the obstructed bladder largely due to impaired compliance; poor compliance accelerates the bladder's compensatory changes by producing further smooth muscle hypertrophy and collagen deposition. Therapeutic intervention largely resides in arresting this cycle and reversing the changes that the bladder has undergone to compensate for outlet obstruction.[18]

Effects on Neuromotor Function

Studies in adult animal models demonstrate neuropathic changes in the obstructed bladder. These changes are most dramatic in the cholinergic and adrenergic neurotransmitter systems and correlate with smooth muscle hypertrophy and high-pressure voiding. Lin and co-workers found mild urinary outlet obstruction produced diminished emptying ability in conjunction with decreased compliance and capacity using an adult animal model.[20] In a fetal rabbit model, partial bladder outlet obstruction produces denervation supersensitivity—the bladder strips from these animals decreased responsiveness to field stimulation but significantly increased responsiveness to bethanechol and potassium chloride[21] (Fig. 42–5).

Clinical Studies

Posterior Urethral Valves

Posterior urethral valves (PUVs) have been recognized as a disease state for about 100 years. Since that time, advances in imaging technology have allowed the diagnosis of this entity in utero, and clinical observations by Hendren and others have more fully elucidated the spectrum of this disease.[22] The underlying cause of valve formation in the posterior urethra remains unclear. Stephens and co-workers believe PUVs represent abnormal placement and reabsorption of the wolffian duct orifices; this creates a valve-like malformation in the posterior urethra at the level of the verumontanum.[23]

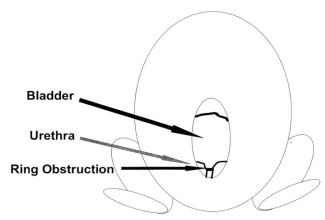

FIGURE 42–5. Creation of partial bladder outlet obstruction by incomplete ligation of the urethra with a suture ligature or jeweler's ring in a rabbit model.

Clinically, PUVs can have a wide spectrum of effects on bladder function; this likely results from the timing at which obstruction develops during embryogenesis, the severity of obstruction, and the anatomic configuration of the upper genitourinary system. The term "valve bladder syndrome" has been coined to describe the poorly compliant, dysfunctional bladders that are produced by obstruction by PUV (Fig. 42–6). These bladders demonstrate not only high urine storage pressure but also decreased sensation. The syndrome also includes poor ureteral function and a renal concentrating defect.[24] Bladder function in these patients can adversely impact renal function both in utero and after birth. Consequently, treatment of PUVs has been driven by efforts to protect kidney function, with preservation of bladder function only recently receiving clinical attention.[12]

The investigator who first described PUVs, H. H. Young, also proposed early primary valve ablation in

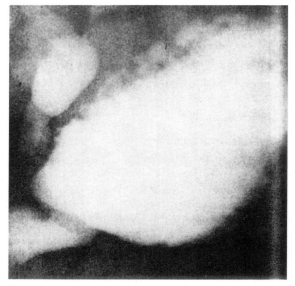

FIGURE 42–6. Cystogram of valve bladder in a newborn male infant prior to posterior urethral valve ablation.

these patients in 1929.[25] However, the predominant management strategy at that time remained suprapubic urinary diversion. Later, other investigators favored upper urinary tract diversion via high cutaneous ureterostomy or pyelostomy. The effects of urinary diversion soon became obvious. Unlike otherwise normal bladders, these bladders did not demonstrate a return to normal function after urinary undiversion.[12] Hendren subsequently championed the return to early valve ablation in the 1970s with reconstruction of the urinary tract.[26] Other surgeons at this time, however, argued that lower urinary tract diversion via cutaneous ureterostomy or vesicostomy had a beneficial effect on renal function and preservation.[27] Currently, the early treatment of PUVs remains a topic of debate because of the concern that "valve bladders" may have a detrimental effect on renal function. However, clinical studies suggest that urinary diversion does *not* have a beneficial effect on renal function compared to early valve ablation. Furthermore, recent studies suggest that early valve ablation may restore bladder function.[28]

Close and Mitchell have demonstrated that early ablation of PUVs (within the first 8 months of life) permits nonobstructive bladder storage and filling and subsequent development of normal bladder function as the bladder develops (Fig. 42–7). In their series, patients who underwent delayed treatment for posterior urethral valves (after the first year of life) never regained normal bladder function, suggesting that they had missed a critical developmental milestone.[28] Using the same logic, it is the authors' opinion that early treatment of the exstrophic bladder represents a similar opportunity to salvage normal bladder function, which may be lost with delayed or staged treatment. In contrast, urinary diversion of otherwise normal bladders produces decreased compliance and capacity, but these effects are reversible if the bladder is refunctionalized. This suggests that important developmental events occur in utero and that aberrations in these developmental sequences by diseases such as bladder exstrophy or posterior urethral valves may be reversible early in postnatal life.

Urinary Diversion

Experimental Model

Animal models to study the effect of urinary diversion have proven more difficult to create. Levin studied ureteral diversion in adult canines and found that intravesical capacity, compliance, and bladder weight decreased significantly compared to control values. These changes proved reversible after ureteral undiversion in this model. However, the results have questionable application to a developing bladder model. Slaughenhoupt and colleagues have created an exstrophy model using sheep but have not published any data regarding its effects on bladder development.[29] Atala has created a vesicostomy in utero lamb model to demonstrate the feasibility of closing the defect after delivery with urothelium grown in vitro on a substrate. This research represents

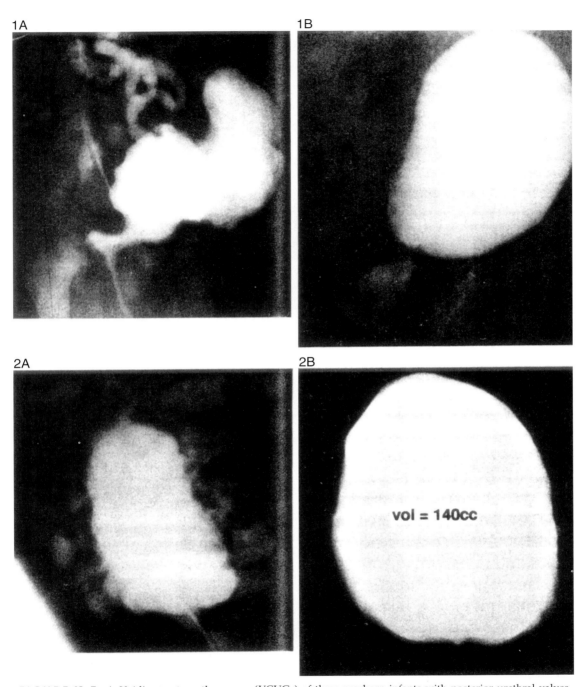

FIGURE 42–7. *A,* Voiding cystourethrograms (VCUGs) of three newborn infants with posterior urethral valves demonstrating trabeculated bladders and upper tract dilation. *B,* VCUGs of same infants at 1 year of age after early valve ablation. The bladders demonstrate smooth walls and normal capacities. Patient 1 also completely resolved bilateral high-grade vesicoureteral reflux. (From Mitchell M: Early primary valve ablation for posterior urethral valves. Semin Pediatr Surg 5:69, 1996, with permission.)

Illustration continued on following page

3A

3B

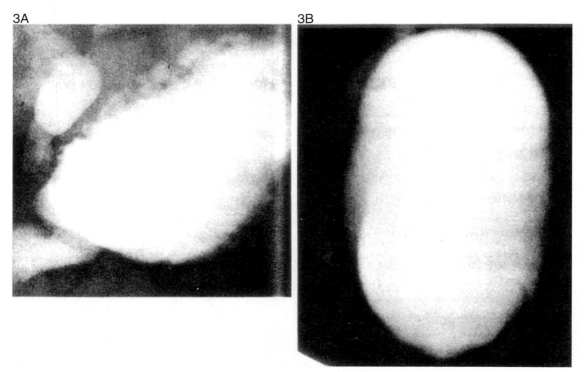

F I G U R E 42–7 *Continued*

state-of-the-art technology in tissue engineering but has not been used to study the effect of urinary diversion on bladder development.[30]

Lipski and co-workers have developed a unique rabbit urinary diversion model in 3-week-old New Zealand white rabbits by defunctionalizing one half of the bladder and isolating it from urine flow. The other half was left to serve as an internal control. Early results from this model demonstrated increased connective tissue in the diverted bladder halves compared to controls.[31] However, most of our knowledge regarding urinary diversion arises from observations of clinical conditions, most notably bladder exstrophy (Figs. 42–8 and 42–9).

Clinical Studies

Bladder Exstrophy

Exstrophia vesicae, or bladder exstrophy, has long been considered one of the scourges of genitourinary anomalies. Samuel Gross referred to it as "the most distressing malformation of the bladder" in 1876. Since that time little has changed in the perception that most people have of this anomaly. It is perhaps best considered as a complex, encompassing cloacal exstrophy and epispadias as well as classic bladder exstrophy.[32]

Exstrophy occurs in 1 in 20,000 to 1 in 50,000 live births. Interestingly, bladder exstrophy has been re-

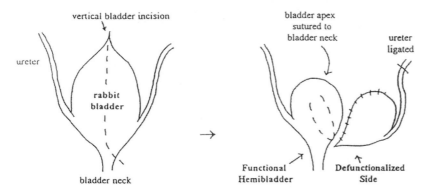

F I G U R E 42–8. Bladder diversion model. The rabbit bladder is incised vertically. Half is refunctionalized and formed into a reservoir. The other half is defunctionalized due to ureteral ligation. (From Lipski B, Yoshino K, Yao LY, et al: A unique new model to study the effects of urinary diversion in the developing rabbit bladder. J Urol 160[4]:154–158, 1998, with permission.)

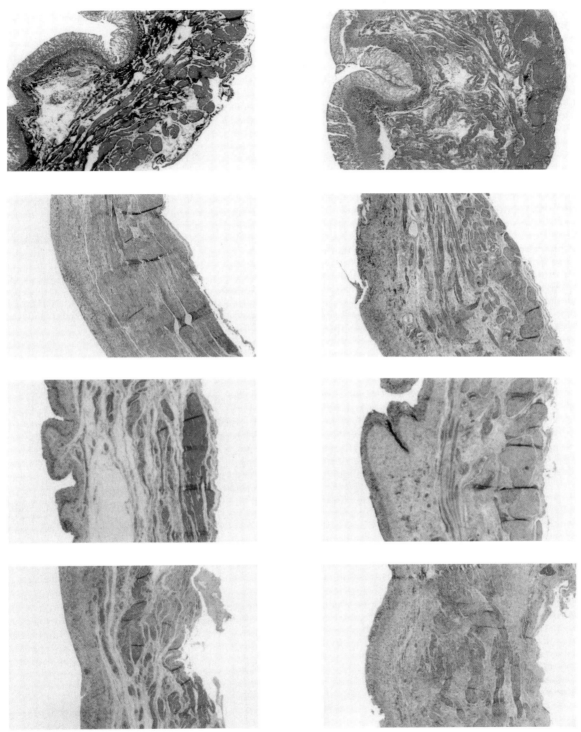

FIGURE 42–9. Histologic comparison of full-thickness bladder wall sections of defunctionalized and functional bladders 3, 7, 14, and 28 days after urinary diversion. Epithelium appears at left and serosa appears at right of sections. Connective tissue is more prevalent in bladder wall between muscle bundles in defunctionalized specimens. Blue areas represent connective tissue, including collagen. Red areas represent muscle and cytoplasm. (Masson's trichrome stain, reduced from × 5.) (From Lipski B, Yoshino K, Yao LY, et al: A unique new model to study the effects of urinary diversion in the developing rabbit bladder. J Urol 160:154–158, 1998, with permission.)

ported at a higher incidence (1 in 1,002) in an autopsy series of 19,000 children; no direct role of exstrophy has been implicated in the deaths of these fetuses.[33]

Inheritance patterns of exstrophy have also been studied. Until recently, fertility rates of patients with bladder exstrophy have been compromised by their primary disease state. Messelink and co-workers, in a review of published studies, found 18 patients with a probable heritable pattern of exstrophy.[34] However, most do not consider exstrophy to be a primarily genetic event. Estimates of risk vary from 1 in 70 to 1 in 100 for offspring of parents with exstrophy.[35]

Other anomalies associated with exstrophy include omphalocele and neurologic abnormalities. Gearhart et al. found a 10% incidence of neurologic abnormalities based on a retrospective review of radiographs of exstrophy patients.[36] The most common anomolies include sacral agenesis and spina bifida occulta. Overt neurologic sequelae such as myelomeningocele occur rarely. Renal development anomalies such as fusion and migration defects are also unusual. This relative lack of associated abnormalities suggests a mechanical process in the development of exstrophy.

Theories to explain the cause of exstrophy in the prescientific era focused mainly on trauma during pregnancy to the unborn child. Berstungs hypothesized that abnormal retention of fluid in the bladder resulted in its rupture during embryogenesis. Others have suggested that bladder exstrophy occurs secondary to a closed membrane defect or developmental arrest. Certainly, developmental arrest is an unlikely cause of exstrophy, since the embryo does not normally pass through a stage of development corresponding to exstrophy.

In brief review, the cloacal membrane forms between the second and third weeks after fertilization as a consequence of ectodermal and endodermal apposition in the midline without mesodermal ingrowth. By the fourth week of embryogenesis, the cloacal membrane forms the ventral wall of the urogenital sinus with the paired primordia of the genital tubercle lateral to its upper borders. Rapid enlargement of the primordia and growth of the mesoderm toward the midline then replace the cloacal membrane during the fifth week of development.[37]

In our modern era, Muecke and Marshall hypothesized that persistence of the cloacal membrane during embryogenesis would result in this anomaly. Using a chick embryo model, Muecke demonstrated that placement of a plastic segment into the cloacal membrane would produce exstrophy. This represented the first animal model of exstrophy.[38] However, Thomalla and co-workers[39] found that selective ablation of the cloacal membrane in the chick embryo below the level of the omphalomesenteric vessels using a CO_2 laser also produced bladder or cloacal exstrophy in a timing dependent fashion (Fig. 42–10). Their observations led them to conclude that ablation and not persistence of the cloacal membrane during embryogenesis is the critical factor in the development of exstrophy.[39] Timing of this "single-hit" phenomenon can explain cloacal exstrophy if it occurs early in development, classic exstrophy if it occurs later (approximately the seventh week of devel-

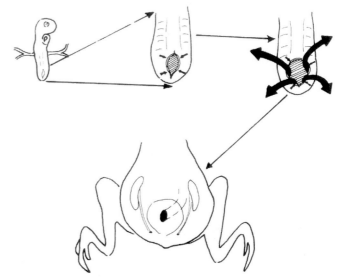

F I G U R E 42–10. Diagrammatic representation of cloacal exstrophy chick model induced by CO_2 laser. (From Thomalla V: Induction of cloacal exstrophy in the chick embryo using the CO_2 laser. J Urol 134:991, 1987, with permission.)

opment), or epispadias if it occurs even later (eighth to tenth week of development).

ANTENATAL DETECTION

Mirk published the first report of prenatally detected bladder exstrophy by ultrasonography in 1986. The ultrasonographic features of this anomaly include (1) persistent nonvisualization of the urinary bladder in association with normal amniotic fluid levels, (2) caudal insertion of the fetal umbilical cord, and (3) a ventral solid mass protruding from the fetal abdomen (representing the exstrophic bladder)[40] (Fig. 42–11). The fetal kidneys and bladder can usually be identified at 15 weeks of gestation; by 20 weeks, most kidneys are visualized by ultrasonography. Fetal bladder cycling occurs at a rate of every 50 to 155 minutes. Therefore, prolonged or serial observation should identify the urinary bladder in most normal fetuses. In practice, many babies with exstrophy are not diagnosed until after delivery.

Prenatal diagnosis allows for coordinated care of these patients at institutions experienced in the treatment of bladder exstrophy and early treatment of this birth defect. Early surgical management of bladder exstrophy is an important component in the successful treatment of exstrophy. It is also important that health care providers experienced in the treatment of these patients counsel the parents of fetuses with antenatally diagnosed exstrophic anomalies because significant improvement in the treatment of bladder exstrophy has occurred in the last 20 years.

SURGICAL MANAGEMENT OF BLADDER EXSTROPHY

Clinicians involved in the treatment of bladder exstrophy have made significant progress since the first attempts were made to repair this defect. Ureterosigmoidostomy emerged as the procedure of choice for

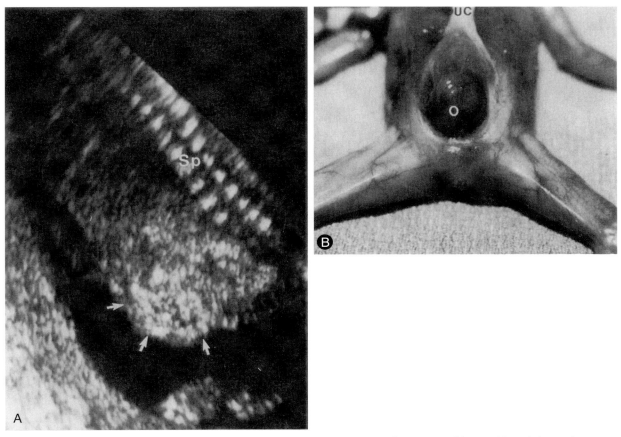

FIGURE 42-11. Antenatal ultrasonographic examination. *A*, Transvaginal sonogram of fetus at 16 weeks' gestation demonstrates a small soft tissue mass (*arrows*) protruding from the anterior abdominal wall. The urinary bladder is not visualized. This finding is consistent with the diagnosis of bladder or cloacal exstrophy. (Sp = spine.) *B*, Postmortem photograph confirms bladder exstrophy with an associated infraumbilical omphalocele, O. Anorectal atresia is also present. (UC = umbilical cord.) (From Cullinan J, Nyberg D: Fetal abdominal wall defects. *In* Rumack C, Wilson S, Charboneau J [eds]: Diagnostic Ultrasound, 2nd ed. St. Louis: Mosby-Yearbook, Inc, 1998, p 1171, with permission.)

bladder exstrophy in the early part of the 20th century. Urinary diversion became the accepted treatment for exstrophy because of the poor results reported by surgeons who attempted primary bladder closure for bladder exstrophy. As the complications of metabolic acidosis, chronic pyelonephritis, and increased risk of adenocarcinoma of the colon were recognized other forms of urinary diversion such as ileal conduits, colon conduits, and modified rectal reservoirs eventually replaced ureterosigmoidostomy. During this time, various surgeons attempted functional reconstruction of the exstrophic bladder—usually in a single stage—with inconsistent but occasionally successful results. Staged reconstructive approaches pioneered by Robert Jeffs and others in the 1970s demonstrated improved continence rates and less risk of renal damage. Series using this operative technique note continence rates ranging from 30 to 88%.[41-43] Staged reconstruction has subsequently been accepted as the standard form of surgical management for bladder reconstruction in the exstrophic patient. Our recent efforts, however, suggest that improvements in single-stage reconstruction may be feasible, successful, and reproducible.

COMPLETE PRIMARY REPAIR OF BLADDER EXSTROPHY

Our interest in complete primary closure of the exstrophic bladder arose as an extension of the complete penile disassembly technique developed by Mitchell for the surgical correction of epispadias.[44] This technique applied to exstrophy repair facilitated the complete anatomic reconstruction of the exstrophic bladder at one setting. Previous success by other surgeons noted above suggested that successful primary repair was possible. However, no consistent, reliable operation to achieve this result existed. We have subsequently attempted primary closure of the exstrophic bladder in all newborns with this anomaly to evaluate the results of this procedure.

Primary closure of the exstrophic bladder offers several advantages. From a practical standpoint, complete repair would decrease the number of subsequent surgical procedures required to repair this defect. Early complete repair also would take advantage of the plasticity inherent in the developing bladder by allowing the bladder to cycle. This would also allow any benefits from mechanical forces acting on the bladder at an early stage

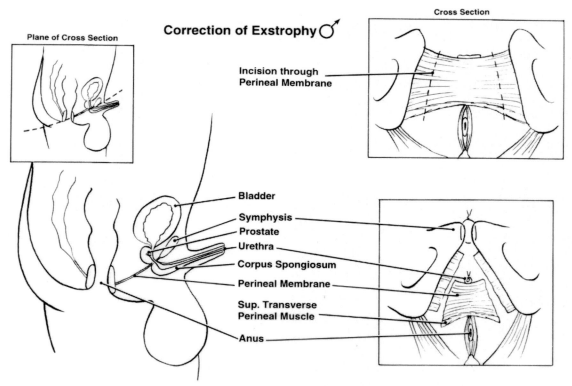

FIGURE 42–12. Schematic diagram of male exstrophy anatomy and application of complete primary repair of exstrophy to the correction of exstrophy in boys.

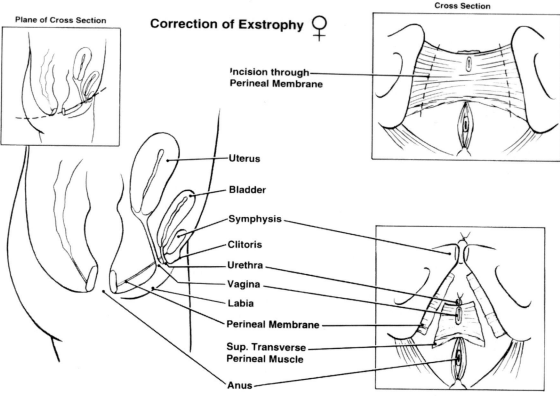

FIGURE 42–13. Schematic diagram of female exstrophy anatomy and application of complete primary repair of exstrophy to the correction of exstrophy in girls.

of development to accrue as well. We feel primary closure of bladder exstrophy in the neonatal period provides the best opportunity to optimize bladder development in this patient population. The principles of bladder exstrophy repair that we employ are similar in males and females (Figs. 42–12 and 42–13). A complete description of the surgical technique we employ can be reviewed in the literature.[45]

Conclusions

The bladder undergoes marked changes in utero and in the postnatal period. Evidence from clinical and laboratory research studies suggest that these changes result from the interaction of a variety of paracrine, autocrine, neural, and mechanical influences that act in a pleiomorphic fashion to produce an organ that stores and empties urine safely and efficiently. Aberrations in normal bladder development due to obstruction or urinary diversion directly impact bladder development. Abnormal bladder development due to obstruction in utero, in particular, has far-reaching consequences on pulmonary and renal development as well.

In clinical situations such as posterior urethral valves, we have observed that early intervention can restore normal bladder function to abnormal bladders. Our clinical data suggest that the postnatal period provides an opportunity to take advantage of the transient plasticity of the bladder to restore normal bladder function. Progress in our understanding of bladder development at a molecular biologic level also holds the promise of gene therapy intervention that would allow us to exploit the plasticity of early bladder development to restore function to abnormal bladders in a variety of situations.

REFERENCES

1. Klimberg I: The Development of Voiding Control. AUA Update Series 7:162–167, 1988.
2. Hoyes A, Ramus NI, Martin BGH: Ultrastructural aspects of the development of the innervation of the vesical musculature in the early human fetus. Invest Urol 10:307–311, 1973.
3. Galloway N: The biology of continence. In Department of Urology. Seattle, WA: University of Washington Medical Center Grand Rounds, 1997, p 4.
4. Park J, Freeman M, Peters C, et al: Stretch-induced cyclooxygenase-2 expression in bladder smooth muscle cells. San Francisco, CA: International Bladder Research Congress, 1998.
5. Park J, Freeman M, Peters C: Mechanical stretch mediates heparin-binding EGF-like growth factor expression in bladder smooth muscle cells by autocrine release of angiotensin II. San Francisco, CA: International Bladder Research Congress, 1998.
6. Wadhwa S, Bijlani V: Ultrastructural and histochemical observations of innervation of developing human urinary bladder. Acta Histochem Cytochem 17:93–99, 1984.
7. Shapiro E, Seller MJ, Lepor H, et al: Altered smooth muscle development and innervation in the lower genitourinary and gastrointestinal tract of the male human fetus with myelomeningocele. J Urol 160(3 Pt 2):1047–1053, 1998.
8. Steers W: Role of NGF in bladder innervation during development. In The Developing Bladder: It's Impact on Practice. Dialogues in Pediatric Urology, 1996.
9. Keating M, Duckett JW, Snyder HM, et al: Ontogeny of bladder function in the rabbit. J Urol 144:766–769, 1990.
10. Koff S: Non-neuropathic vesicourethral dysfunction in children. In O'Donnel B (ed): Pediatric Urology. Oxford: Reed Elsevier, 1996, pp 217–228.
11. Diamond J: Modeling and competition in the nervous system. Curr Top Dev Biol 17:147, 1982.
12. Close C: Urethral valves and the potential for healing in very young patients. AUA Update Series: pp 1–20, 1999.
13. Hayashi N, Cunha GR, Parker M: Permissive and instructive induction of adult rodent prostatic epithelium by heterotypic urogenital sinus mesenchyme. Epithel Cell Biol 2:66–78, 1993.
14. Baskin L, Sutherland R, Thomson A, et al: Growth factors and receptors in bladder development and obstruction. Lab Invest 75:157–166, 1996.
15. Baskin L: The effect of physical forces on the bladder. In The Developing Bladder: Its Impact on Practice. Dialogues in Pediatric Urology, 1996.
16. Yao L, Tekgul S, Kim KK, et al: Developmental regulation of collagen differential expression in the rabbit bladder. J Urol 156 (2 Pt 2):565–570, 1996.
17. Levin R: Developmental aspects of urinary bladder physiology and pharmacology. In The Developing Bladder: Its Impact on Practice. Dialogues in Pediatric Urology, 1996.
18. Peters C: The impact of obstruction on bladder development. In The Developing Bladder: Its Impact on Practice. Dialogues in Pediatric Urology, 1996.
19. Tekgul S, Yoshino K, Bagli D, et al: Collagen types I and III localization by in situ hybridization and immunohistochemistry in the partially obstructed young rabbit bladder. J Urol 156(2 Pt 2):582–586, 1996.
20. Lin V, McConnell JD: Molecular aspects of bladder outlet obstruction. Adv Exp Med Biol 385:65–74, 1995.
21. Rohrmann D, Monson FC, Damaser MS, et al: Partial bladder outlet obstruction in the fetal rabbit. J Urol 158:1071–1074, 1997.
22. Hendren H: Posterior urethral valves in boys: A wide clinical spectrum. J Urol 106:298–307, 1971.
23. Stephens F, Smith ED, Hutson JM: Congenital Anomalies of the Urinary and Genital Tracts. Oxford: Isis Medical Media, 1996, pp 93–94.
24. Mitchell M: Persistent ureteral dilation following valve resection. Dialogues Pediatr Urol 5:8–9, 1982.
25. Young H, McKay RW: Congenital valvular obstruction of the prostatic urethra. Surg Gynecol Obstet 48:509–535, 1929.
26. Hendren W: A new approach to infants with severe obstructive uropathy: Early complete reconstruction. J Pediatr Surg 5:184–199, 1970.
27. Johnson J: Temporary cutaneous ureterostomy in the management of advanced congenital urinary obstruction. Arch Dis Child 38:161–166, 1963.
28. Close C, Carr MC, Burns MW, Mitchell ME: Lower urinary tract changes after early valve ablation: Is early diversion warranted? J Urol 157:984–988, 1997.
29. Slaughenhoupt B, Chen CJ, Gearhart JP: Creation of a model of bladder exstrophy in the fetal lamb. J Urol 156(2 Pt 2):816–818, 1996.
30. Fauza D, Fishman SJ, Mehegan K, Atala A: Videofetoscopically assisted fetal tissue engineering: Bladder augmentation. J Pediatr Surg 33:7–12, 1998.
31. Lipski B, Yoshino K, Yao LY, et al: A unique new model to study the effects of urinary diversion in the developing rabbit bladder. J Urol 160:154–158, 1998.
32. Gross S: A Practical Treatise on the Diseases, Injuries, and Malformations of the Urinary Bladder, the Prostate Gland, and the Urethra, 3rd ed. Philadelphia: Henry C Lea, 1876.
33. Campbell M, Harrison JH: Urology, 3rd ed. Philadelphia: WB Saunders Company, 1970.
34. Messelink E, Aronson D, Knuist M, et al: Four cases of bladder exstrophy in two families. J Med Genet 31:490–492, 1994.
35. Shapiro E, Lepor H, Jeffs R: The inheritance of classical bladder exstrophy. J Urol 308:132–135, 1984.
36. Cadeddu J, Benson JE, Silver RI, et al: Spinal abnormalities in classic bladder exstrophy. J Urol 79:975–978, 1997.
37. Maizels M: Normal development of the urinary tract. In Walsh P, Retik AB, Stamey T, Vaughan D (eds): Campbell's Urology. Philadelphia: WB Saunders Company, 1996, pp 1315–1320.

38. Muecke E: The role of the cloacal membrane in exstrophy: The first successful experimental study. J Urol 92:659–667, 1964.

39. Thomalla V, Rudolph R, Rink R, Mitchell M: Induction of cloacal exstrophy in the chick embryo using the CO_2 laser. J Urol 134:991–995, 1984.

40. Mirk P, Calisti A, Fileni A: Prenatal sonographic diagnosis of bladder exstrophy. J Ultrasound Med 5:291–294, 1986.

41. Megalli M, Lattimer J: Review of the management of 140 cases of exstrophy of the bladder. J Urol 109:243–248, 1973.

42. Lepor HAJ, Jeffs R: Primary bladder closure and bladder neck reconstruction in classical bladder exstrophy. J Urol 130:1142–1145, 1983.

43. Kramer S, Kelalis PP: Assessment of urinary continence in epispadias: A review of 94 patients. J Urol 128:290–293, 1982.

44. Mitchell M, Bagli D: Complete penile disassembly for epispadias repair: The Mitchell technique. J Urol 155:300–304, 1996.

45. Grady RW, Carr MC, Mitchell ME: Complete primary repair of bladder exstrophy. Urol Clin North Am 26:95–108, 1999.

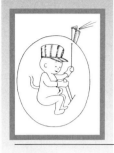

Fetal Tissue Engineering

DARIO O. FAUZA and JOSEPH P. VACANTI

Major congenital anomalies are present in approximately 3% of all newborns.[1] These diseases are responsible for nearly 20% of deaths occurring in the neonatal period and even higher morbidity rates during childhood.[2] By definition, birth defects entail loss and/or malformation of tissues or organs. Treatment of many of these congenital anomalies is often hindered by the scarce availability of normal tissues or organs, either in autologous or allologous fashion, mainly at birth. Autologous grafting is frequently not an option in newborns due to donor site, size limitations, and the well-known severe donor shortage observed in practically all areas of transplantation is even more critical during the neonatal period.

Recently, a novel concept in perinatal surgery has been introduced, involving minimally invasive harvest of fetal tissue, which is then engineered in vitro in parallel to the remainder of gestation, so that an infant with a prenatally diagnosed birth defect can benefit from having autologous, expanded tissue readily available for surgical implantation in the neonatal period (Fig. 43–1).[3, 4] The engineered fetal tissue can also be implanted in utero, genetically or otherwise manipulated in vitro, or frozen and stored for further applications including implantation later in life.[5]

Tissue engineering is an interdisciplinary field in which the principles and methods of engineering merge with those of biologic sciences for the fundamental understanding of structure/function relationships in normal and pathologic tissues and organs, as well as for the development of biologic substitutes that can restore, maintain, or improve tissue or organ function.[6] In that context, new tissues or organs can be created through three general strategies, or a combination of them, as follows[7]:

1. *Isolated cells or cell substitutes.* In this approach, cells are manipulated in vitro and then infused or implanted to supply a specific function.
2. *Tissue-inducing substances.* In this process, appropriate signal molecules, such as growth factors, are delivered to specific targets by different methods for the stimulation or control of tissue growth and/or maturation.
3. *Cells placed on or within matrices.* This methodology can be further subdivided in two systems: In closed systems, the cells are isolated from the host's body by a membrane that allows permeation of nutrients and wastes, but prevents large structures, such as antibodies or immune cells, from destroying the transplant. These systems can be either implanted or used as extracorporeal devices. In open systems, the cells are attached to matrices, bioabsorbable or not, and become incorporated into the body after implantation. The matrices can be fashioned from natural polymers or from artificial substances, including synthetic polymers and ceramics.

All of these strategies can be applied in autologous, heterologous, or xenologous fashion. They all may carry problems, including immunologic rejection, growth limitations, differentiation and function restraints, incorporation barriers and cell/tissue delivery difficulties. Many of those problems can be better managed, if not totally prevented, when fetal tissue is used. Compared with mature cells, fetal cells usually proliferate much more rapidly, are significantly more plastic in their differentiation potential, frequently produce more angiogenic and trophic factors, express histocompatibility antigens at lower levels, can survive at lower oxygen tensions, commonly lack strong intercellular adhesions, and display better survival after refrigeration and cryopreservation protocols.[8–16]

Attempts at engineering virtually every mammalian tissue have already taken place.[7] Surprisingly, however, although a relatively large body of data has come out of research involving fetal tissue, most fetal cell lines are yet to be explored for tissue engineering purposes. The first reported transplantation of human fetal tissue took place in 1922, when fetal adrenal tissue was transplanted into a patient with Addison disease.[17] This experiment, as well as others involving fetal tissue from different sources that followed, failed.[18, 19] It was only in the last three decades that successful outcomes after fetal tissue transplantation in humans started to be consistently observed.

A number of properties and therapeutic applications of fetal tissue have already been explored. However, to

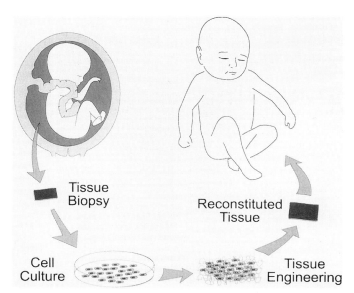

F I G U R E 43–1. Diagram representing the concept of fetal tissue engineering for surgical treatment of birth defects. A fetus with a prenatally diagnosed congenital anomaly undergoes tissue harvest, preferably through minimally invasive technique. The tissue is then processed and engineered in vitro while pregnancy continues, so that the newborn can benefit from having autologous, expanded tissue promptly available for reconstruction at birth.

date, the vast majority of the studies have involved just fetal cell, tissue, or organ transplantation, without any tissue engineering per se. Other chapters are devoted to discussing these subjects in detail.

The true engineering of fetal tissue, through culture and placement of fetal cells into matrices or membranes, or other in vitro manipulations, has barely begun to be investigated, with very few studies reported so far.[3–5, 20, 21] This chapter offers an overview of the general principles of tissue engineering and of how they can be applied in fetal medicine.

Methods of Tissue Engineering

In tissue engineering, living cells are not only cultured in vitro but can also be genetically, chemically, mechanically, electrically, or otherwise manipulated prior to implantation. Cell organization and delivery methods can vary, depending on the kind of tissue or organ replacement considered. Summarized discussions and examples of postnatal applications of such methods follow, as well as observations on other topics of general interest in tissue engineering.

Cell Transfer

In this process, after manipulation in vitro, isolated cells are infused into the bloodstream or implanted into specific sites of the recipient for the performance of a particular function. When implanted, the cells attach to the host tissue stroma, reorganize, and use its native blood supply.[22]

For example, normal myoblasts from unaffected relatives have been transplanted into patients with Duchenne muscular dystrophy and have been shown to produce dystrophin for 1 to 6 months after transplant, although the efficiency of myoblast transfer was low.[23–25] Preliminary results in a canine model showed short-term muscle formation after autotransplanted skeletal muscle satellite cells multiplied in vitro were implanted into the heart.[26] Intraportal injection of gene-transfected hepatocytes previously isolated from the recipient's own liver has been shown to reduce cholesterol levels in a patient with homozygous familial hypercholesterolemia.[27] Bone marrow transplantation can also be considered another example of this methodology.

Usually, this method can be successfully applied for the replacement of metabolic and certain cellular functions. On the other hand, its usefulness in replacing structural functions, such as heart valves, bone, or cartilage, is unlikely. In addition, without a template to guide new tissue development, even the fulfillment of a metabolic function is frequently unsatisfactory for lack of sufficient cell mass, due to growth and structure limitations of the neotissue within the host.

Tissue-Inducing Substances

In this case, injected substances or implanted constructs can induce, modulate, or guide the formation of new tissue.

For instance, implantable synthetic polymers can be designed so that they slowly release growth factors, which may allow regeneration of a damaged nerve over a greater distance.[28, 29] Patients with skin loss have undergone implantation of a composite material whose upper layer consists of silicone (to prevent fluid loss) and whose lower layer consists of chondroitin sulfate and collagen (which induces new blood vessels and connective tissue ingrowth). Three weeks later, the upper layer is replaced by a thin epidermal graft. This has been followed by good graft acceptance and minimal scarring.[30–33] In a further refinement of this procedure, the skin graft was eliminated and substituted by epidermal cells seeded onto the lower layer of the composite prior to implantation.[34] Partial esophageal substitution has been achieved experimentally through the interposition of copolymer tubes made of lactic and glycolic acid. Over time, connective tissue and epithelium covered the polymer graft, which slowly degraded, and the animals were able to drink and eat semisolid food.[35] Implantation of demineralized bone powder (which stimulates bone growth) in association with bone morphogenic proteins (which induce formation of cartilage and bone, including marrow) or growth factors such as transforming growth factor-β (TGF-β; which augments bone growth) have been shown to be promising strategies in bone and cartilage replacement.[36–38]

Closed Systems

In closed systems, the transplanted cells are isolated from the host by a semipermeable membrane that allows transport of nutrients and wastes, but prevents large structures such as antibodies or immune cells from destroying the transplant. This selective separation may also protect the recipient in case the implanted cells can be potentially harmful in any way.

For example, in the treatment of certain brain conditions where there is loss of dopamine production, such as Parkinson's disease, immortalized cells derived from rat pheochromocytoma (PC12 cells) have been encapsulated in polymer membranes and implanted in the striatum of guinea pigs. Dopamine release from the capsules was detected for up to 6 months following implantation.[39] In a similar manner, encapsulated bovine adrenal chromaffin cells have been implanted into the subarachnoid space in rats and, through continuous release of enkephalins and catecholamines, appeared to relieve chronic pain.[40]

Similar approaches, but with special variations, have been experimentally explored as a means to transplant islets of Langerhans for the treatment of *diabetes mellitus.* A tubular membrane (ID ≅ 1 mm) was coiled in a housing containing islets and connected to a polymer graft which, in turn, connected the whole device to blood vessels. The membrane had a 50-kDa molecular mass cutoff that allowed diffusion of glucose and insulin, but no passage of antibodies and lymphocytes. Pancreatectomized dogs treated with this device maintained long-term normoglycemia.[41] Hollow fibers containing rat islets were immobilized in polysaccharide alginate forming macrocapsules (diameter between 0.5 and 1.0 mm) and implanted intraperitoneally in diabetic mice. Normoglycemia was sustained for more than 2 months without relevant complications.[42] Islets have also been placed into microcapsules composed of alginate or polyacrylates (diameter <0.5 mm) and shown to control glycemia for years in rodents.[43–47]

Major limitations of these systems include biocompatibility problems, leading to tissue reaction and overgrowth, reducing diffusion of nutrients and waste products, as well as foreign body reaction with macrophage-generated nitric oxide, which is cytotoxic and may reach and destroy the transplanted cells.[48] Microcapsules offer better flow of nutrients and wastes than macrocapsules and can be administered by injection. Macrocapsules, on the other hand, are physically more stable and easier to retrieve should complications develop.

Closed systems can also be used as extracorporeal devices. The patient's blood or plasma can be pumped extracorporeally through systems housing cells separated from the bloodstream/plasma by a semipermeable membrane. An example is the extracorporeal liver support system with xenogeneic hepatocytes used until the patient's own liver function recovers or as a bridge to transplantation.[49]

Open Systems

In open systems, the transplanted cells are attached to scaffolds made of either naturally occurring substances such as collagen, laminin, and chondroitin sulfate, or from synthetic polymers or ceramics, such as polylactic and polyglycolic acids, polyvinyl alcohol hydrogels, and porous calcium phosphates. The cells are in direct contact with the host's body and become fully incorporated into the recipient after implantation, permanently replacing living tissue.

A number of facts support both the rationale and the viability of this concept: tissue renewal and remodeling are continuous processes universally observed; detached cells in culture tend to structurally reorganize themselves when exposed to appropriate substrata (e.g., endothelial cells form tubular structures spontaneously when properly cultivated in vitro[50]); such capacity for reorganization, however, is limited in vitro as well as in vivo, unless a template (scaffold) is present to guide restructuring[20]; anchorage-dependent cell shape is a determining factor in cell division and differentiation[51, 52]; and a scaffold is also necessary for the maximization of nutrient and waste diffusion, as well as gas exchange.[20]

In an open system implant, the polymer scaffold guides cell organization and growth and maximizes diffusion of nutrients and waste products.[20] Preferably, the scaffold is made of either a degradable material or a naturally occurring one, minimizing biocompatibility limitations. The cell/polymer matrix construct can be prevascularized and/or become vascularized after implantation. The vascularization of the implant is usually a natural response from the host, but can also be accelerated by the sustained release of angiogenic factors previously embedded in the scaffold.[53]

Efforts aimed at engineering virtually all mammalian tissues through this technique have already taken place. Some examples follow.

Human neonatal dermal fibroblasts have been cryopreserved, grown on a degradable polyglycolic acid mesh, and placed onto the wound bed in deep injuries affecting all skin layers, with an epidermal skin graft placed on top. The engineered graft vascularizes and evolves into an organized tissue resembling dermis, with good graft acceptance.[54] In engineered skin replacement, the scaffold can also be an important component of the final graft. For instance, fibroblasts have been placed on a hydrated collagen gel which, after implantation, is enzymatically digested by the fibroblasts themselves, resulting in reorganization of the collagen fibrils.[55]

Neocartilage has been engineered based on collagen-glycosaminoglycan templates, isolated chondrocytes, and chondrocytes attached to natural or synthetic polymers.[56–63] The chondrocytes secrete their own supporting matrix onto the engineered scaffold. The final construct's three-dimensional (3-D) shape and size are the same as that of the scaffold, whose conformation is designed in accordance with the structure to be replaced.[62, 63] Chondrocytes cultivated in agarose gel have been shown to produce tissue with physical characteristics similar to that of articular cartilage.[64] Nasoseptal implants, cartilage discs for joint resurfacing, and cartilage in the shape of a human ear have already been successfully engineered.[65]

Valve leaflets of the heart and major vessels have been created through open systems in animal models.[66]

Autologous myofibroblasts and endothelial cells harvested from a femoral artery were expanded in culture and then separately seeded in layers onto a polymer scaffold made of polyglactin woven mesh sandwiched between two nonwoven polyglycolic acid sheets. The construct was then trimmed to the size of the valve leaflet to be replaced and implanted. The polymer scaffold was completely degraded with time. Thereafter, the histologic, histochemical and mechanical properties of the engineered leaflet resembled those of normal leaflets.[66]

Hepatocytes have been cultivated in vitro, seeded onto polylactic or polyglycolic acid polymer scaffolds, and implanted heterotopically onto the omentum or mesentery.[67] Soon after implantation, before vascular ingrowth takes place, hepatocyte survival is limited by hypoxia. Their survival can be enhanced by the following adjunctive measures. A portacaval shunt performed prior to implantation distributes systemically growth factors and other mitogens normally present only in the portal circulation.[68] Epidermal growth factor, which is mitogenic to hepatocytes, can be locally released from embedded polymer microspheres seeded onto the scaffold.[69] The hepatocytes can be co-transplanted with other cell types known to secrete hepatotrophic growth factors, such as islet of Langerhans cells and nonparenchymal liver cells.[70] By controlling the density of extracellular matrix substrate used to coat the polymer, the extent of differentiated function and cell proliferation of the hepatocytes can be controlled.[71] Transplanted liver cells placed on appropriate polymers have formed tissue structures resembling those found in a normal liver (including bile ducts), have produced albumin and other liver function markers, and have removed bilirubin and urea metabolism products.[68]

Attempts at engineering small intestine have also begun to yield results. Intestinal crypt cells were heterotopically transplanted as epithelial organoid units seeded on polyglycolic/polylactic tubular scaffolds. They survived following implantation, reorganized, and produced brush-border enzymes and basement membrane, regenerating complex composite tissue resembling small intestine.[72]

While promising, a number of limiting factors related to the open system concept remain to be overcome. Depending on the cell line considered, proliferation in vitro may be significantly limited. The blood supply of the implant is still dependent, almost exclusively, on microvascular ingrowth from the host. A reliable method of engineering a major vascular circuitry integrated within parenchymal constructs, which could then be anastomosed to the host's vascular bed during implantation, is yet to be determined. The same applies to other complex "accessory" circuitries, such as the urinary and biliary tracts, as well as major neural networks.

Scaffold Engineering

Along with cell manipulation in vitro, tissue engineering is intimately dependent on scaffold composition and design. In open systems, the scaffold should be biocompatible, resorbable, amenable to different shape configurations, and able to promote cell adhesion. It should also maximize diffusion of nutrients and waste products, as well as gas exchange, after implantation. A scaffold's composition can influence the extent of differentiated function and proliferation of the cells.[71] Its cell adhesion properties can also be made selective for specific cell types, for instance, through chemical surface modification (e.g., by plasma discharge), allowing for particular arrangements in complex, multicellular constructs.[73, 74] In addition, polymers can be used for controlled local release of substances such as growth and angiogenic factors.[69]

Synthetic polymers usually carry many advantages over natural ones regarding degradation control, manufacturing, processing, spatial design, homogeneity, and even biocompatibility. A good example is one class of biodegradable polymers, namely, polyesters of the family of polylactic and polyglycolic acids and their copolymers. They degrade by hydrolysis, with minimal tissue reaction, yielding naturally occurring metabolites. Their resorption rates and spatial layout can be easily controlled. Clinically, these polymers have been used extensively as suture materials, support fabrics, and controlled-release devices.[75] Recently, these substances have been fashioned into 3-D scaffolds with different compartments, analog to vascular/ductal networks, along with a platform for parenchymatous cells, for liver engineering.[76] This technique involves computer-guided 3-D-polymer printing and allows for the construction of polymer scaffolds in any desired shape, size, or microconfiguration, including the possibility of automatically linking the 3-D-printing process to magnetic resonance imaging (MRI) or computer-assisted tomography. This automatic link between 3-D-polymer construction and high-resolution imaging techniques renders possible the reproduction of normal 3-D organ architecture in scaffold manufacture.

On the other hand, natural materials may contain information, such as special amino acid sequences, that may promote cell adhesion or maintenance of differentiated cell function. Disadvantages of natural scaffolds include possible antigenicity, heterogeneity, and manufacturing difficulties. The advantages of both natural and synthetic matrices can be combined, for instance, through grafting of critical amino acid sequences onto synthetic polymers.[77, 78]

A special application of either synthetic or natural polymers is their use to improve normal tissue regeneration. It has been shown in animal models that synthetic guides or conduits composed of natural polymers (such as laminin, collagen, and chondroitin sulfate), or synthetic ones, can enhance nerve regeneration. The conduits protect the regenerating nerve from infiltrating scar tissue and/or better direct the new axons toward their target.[79–81]

In closed systems, because the implanted cells have to be separated from the host by nonresorbable membranes, biocompatibility is critical. Otherwise, tissue reaction would hamper gas exchange, the flow of nutrients and waste and, possibly, lead to local release of cytotoxic agents, such as macrophage-generated nitric oxide.[48] Microcapsules are commonly made of hydrogels, particularly polysaccharide alginate, because of the extremely mild conditions required for gel formation.[7] Further coatings of the alginate with polyanions, such as polylysine, and again with alginate, if necessary, can affect the flow of nutrients and waste, mechanical strength, and biocompatibility.[7] Macrocapsules and vascular devices are usually made of acrylonitrile-vinyl chloride copolymers.[82, 83]

Bioreactors

After seeding expanded cells onto a scaffold and until implantation, the resulting construct can be either maintained in culture without any further manipulation (static culture), or submitted to a so-called bioreactor. The latter provides special, controlled conditions or stimuli in vitro, aimed at improving cell organization, differentiation, and growth, hence bettering final construct composition and architecture.

A bioreactor can assume different formats and provide different conditions. For instance, vascular or heart valve leaflet constructs exposed to pulsatile flow evolve into more organized structures, when compared with static culture, with better performance after implantation.[84] Well-stirred bioreactors enable nutrients to better penetrate the center of cartilaginous constructs, leading to stronger, thicker implants.[85] Flow bioreactors enhance albumin synthesis in 3-D hepatocyte constructs.[76] Mechanical stretch of the scaffold leads to myocyte orientation in the same direction of the stretch forces in skeletal muscle composites.[86] Low-frequency electric fields can induce reorganization of cellular microfilaments and cytoskeletal structures.[87]

Depending on the cell line(s) considered, the effectiveness of a bioreactor is a major limiting factor for successful engineering. This concept is relatively new and several in vitro conditions and stimuli to numerous different cell lines still remain to be explored.

Fetal Tissue Engineering

Given the relatively large body of data involving fetal cell and tissue transplantation, it is somewhat surprising that so little has been done in fetal tissue engineering *sensu strictu* so far. Fetal cells were first used experimentally in engineered constructs by Vacanti et al. in 1987.[20] The experiment, in rats, used fetal cells from the liver, intestine, and pancreas, which were cultured, seeded on bioabsorbable matrices, and later implanted. This investigation was part of the introductory study on selective cell transplantation using bioabsorbable, synthetic polymers as matrices, which also included adult cell lines. The fetal constructs were implanted in heterologous fashion and heterotopically, namely, in the interscapular fat, omentum, and mesentery, with no structural replacement, and were removed for histologic analysis no later than 2 weeks after implantation. Successful engraftment was observed in some animals that received hepatic and intestinal constructs, but in none that received pancreatic ones.

A related study was performed by the same group in 1995, involving only liver constructs, also implanted in heterologous and heterotopic fashion in rats.[21] Then, fetal hepatocytes were shown to proliferate to a greater extent than adult ones in culture and to yield higher cross-sectional cell area at the implant. As in the first experiment, no structural replacement or functional studies were included.

Fetal constructs as a means of structural replacement, in autologous fashion, in large animal models, were first reported experimentally in 1997.[3, 4] The studies involved videofetoscopic harvest of fetal tissue, which was then

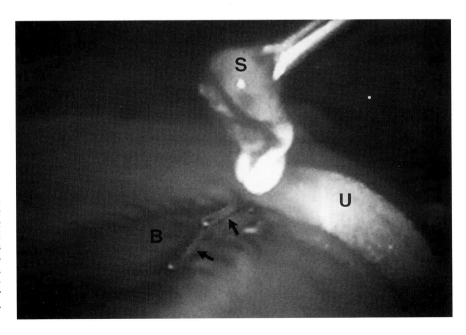

FIGURE 43–2. Videofetoscopic view of the harvest of a fetal lamb's bladder specimen for tissue engineering purposes. (B = exstrophic bladder; S = bladder specimen; U = umbilical cord.) The *arrows* point toward titanium clips placed on the harvested bed of the bladder to prevent fetal evisceration. (From Fauza DO, Fishman S, Mehegan K, et al: Videofetoscopically assisted fetal tissue engineering: Bladder augmentation. J Pediatr Surg 33:7–12, 1998, with permission.)

engineered in vitro while pregnancy was allowed to continue, so that a newborn with a prenatally diagnosed anomaly could benefit from having autologous, expanded tissue readily available for surgical reconstruction at birth (Fig. 43–1). This concept was first applied for the treatment of experimental bladder exstrophy and skin defects.[3, 4] Videofetoscopic harvest was through three ports with balloon-tipped cannulas and either saline or medical air as intra-amniotic working media (Fig. 43–2).

In the bladder reconstruction study, one group of animals had their experimental bladder exstrophy primarily closed and another group underwent bladder augmentation with engineered, autologous fetal bladder tissue at birth. Fetal detrusor cells proliferated in culture significantly faster than adult ones (up to fourfold; Fig. 43–3). Fetal urothelial cells proliferated at expected postnatal rates. The engineered bladders were radiologically normal at 3 weeks following implantation (Fig. 43–4). At 2 months, after the synthetic matrix had already been reabsorbed, the engineered bladders were more compliant than those primarily closed (Fig. 43–5). Histologically, engineered bladders resembled normal ones, with a multilayered, pseudostratified urothelial lining overlying layers of smooth muscle (Fig. 43–6). The muscular layer was hypertrophied in the exstrophic bladders primarily closed, as expected, but normal in the engineered bladders (Fig. 43–7).

In the skin replacement study, animals were their own controls, each with two experimental skin defects treated either with an engineered, autologous fetal skin tissue, or with an acellular biodegradable scaffold equal to the one used for the engineered skin. Fetal dermal fibroblasts multiplied significantly faster in vitro (approximately fivefold) than the same cells harvested postnatally. Fetal keratinocytes multiplied at expected postnatal rates. The engineered skin grafts induced faster epithelization of the wound (partial at 1 week and complete between 2 and 3 weeks postoperatively) compared with the acellular ones (partial at 3 weeks and complete

between 3 and 4 weeks postoperatively) (Fig. 43–8). Time-matched histologic analysis of skin architecture showed a higher level of epidermal/dermal organization, richer vascularization, and less dermal scarring in the wounds that received the engineered skin, compared with those that received the acellular matrices (Fig. 43–8). Normal skin annexes were not observed in any grafted area up to 2 months postoperatively, although some areas that received engineered skin showed an architectural pattern compatible with ongoing adnexal development at 8 weeks following implantation (Fig. 43–8).

Given the limitations of autologous grafting and transplantation during the neonatal period, autologous fetal tissue engineering may well become the only alternative for the treatment of a number of life-threatening congenital anomalies in which new tissue is needed to repair a defect at birth. In many severe but non–life-threatening conditions, this therapeutic concept may also become the first choice, as suggested by the functional results of the bladder augmentation study.[3] This concept can be applied to any cell line and include in utero implantation of the engineered construct, as well as different forms of cell manipulation in vitro, prior to implantation.[5, 86] Fetal cells can also be frozen, stored, and implanted later in life, either in autologous or allologous fashion.[86]

Further advantages of the use of fetal cells for tissue engineering are likely to be demonstrated in the near future, due to their proliferation and differentiation potential, enhanced production of angiogenic and trophic factors, low histocompatibility antigen expression, higher tolerance to lower concentrations of oxygen, lack of strong intercellular adhesions, and cryopreservation endurance.[8-16]

Ethical Considerations

The National Institutes of Health, the American Obstetrical and Gynecological Society, and the American Fer-

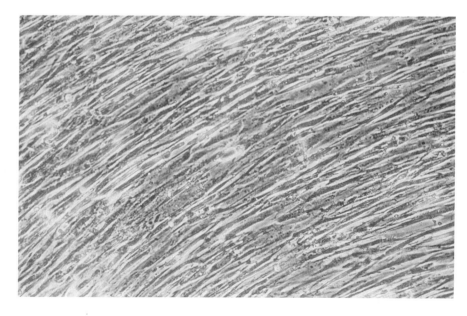

F I G U R E 43–3. Phase microscopy view of fetal detrusor cells completely filling the culture plate only 3 days after harvest. (Original magnification × 100.)

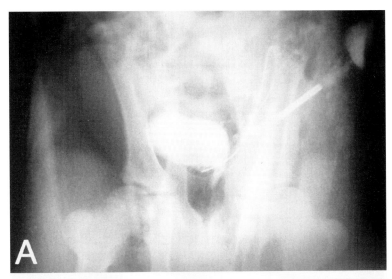
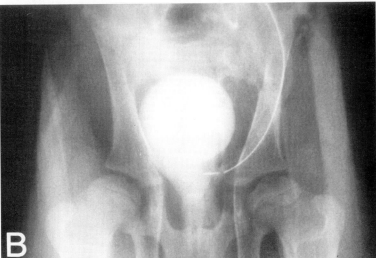

FIGURE 43–4. Contrast cystograms performed 3 weeks postoperatively after primary closure of an exstrophic bladder (*A*) and after augmentation of an exstrophic bladder with autologous engineered fetal tissue (*B*). (From Fauza DO, Fishman S, Mehegan K, et al: Videofetoscopically assisted fetal tissue engineering: Bladder augmentation. J Pediatr Surg 33:7–12, 1998, with permission.)

FIGURE 43–5. Bladder compliance curves obtained 60 days after either engineered bladder augmentation or primary closure of experimental exstrophic bladders. (From Fauza DO, Fishman S, Mehegan K, et al: Videofetoscopically assisted fetal tissue engineering: Bladder augmentation. J Pediatr Surg 33:7–12, 1998, with permission.)

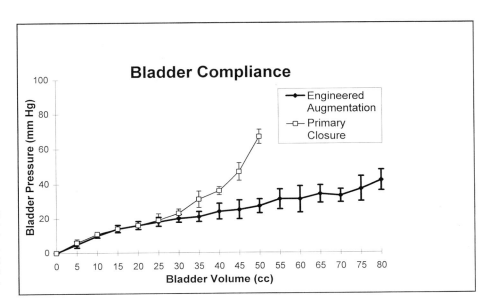

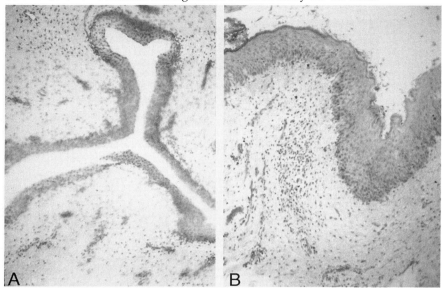

FIGURE 43–6. Microscopic view of mucosa from an exstrophic bladder primarily closed (*A*) and from an engineered fetal bladder tissue (*B*), 60 days postoperatively. (H&E, original magnification × 100.) (From Fauza DO, Fishman S, Mehegan K, et al: Videofetoscopically assisted fetal tissue engineering: Bladder augmentation. J Pediatr Surg 33:7–12, 1998, with permission.)

tility Society have all proposed ethical guidelines for the use of fetal tissue.[88–90] Centers involved with fetal medicine and research have also established principles related to this matter.[91]

However, tissue engineering, as a novel development in fetal tissue processing, adds a new dimension to the discussion concerning the use of fetal tissue for therapeutic or research purposes. If fetal specimens are to be used for the engineering of tissue, which in turn is to be implanted in autologous fashion, no ethical objections should be anticipated, as long as the procedure is a valid therapeutic choice for a given perinatal condition. In that case scenario, ethical considerations are the very same that apply to any fetal intervention. On the other hand, if fetal engineered tissue is to be implanted in heterologous fashion, ethical issues are analogous to the ones involving fetal tissue/organ transplantation, independent of whether the original specimen comes from a live or deceased fetus.

The distinction between autologous and heterologous implantation of engineered fetal tissue is a critical one in that, again, no condemnation of autologous use could be ethically justified.

Future Perspectives

Fetal tissue engineering is one of the newest developments of the still infantile fields of tissue engineering

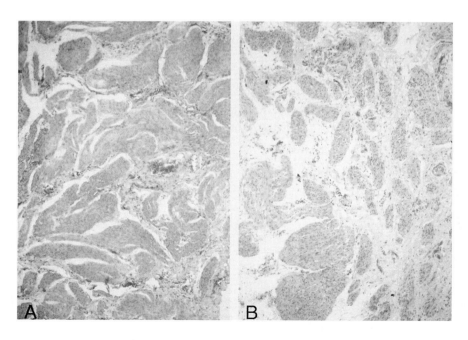

FIGURE 43–7. Microscopic view of muscular layer from an exstrophic bladder primarily closed (*A*) and from an engineered fetal bladder tissue (*B*), 60 days postoperatively. Notice evident hypertrophy of the muscular bundles in the exstrophic bladder closed primarily, as expected. Muscular hypertrophy was not observed in the engineered bladders. (H&E, original magnification × 100.) (From Fauza DO, Fishman S, Mehegan K, et al: Videofetoscopically assisted fetal tissue engineering: Bladder augmentation. J Pediatr Surg 33:7–12, 1998, with permission.)

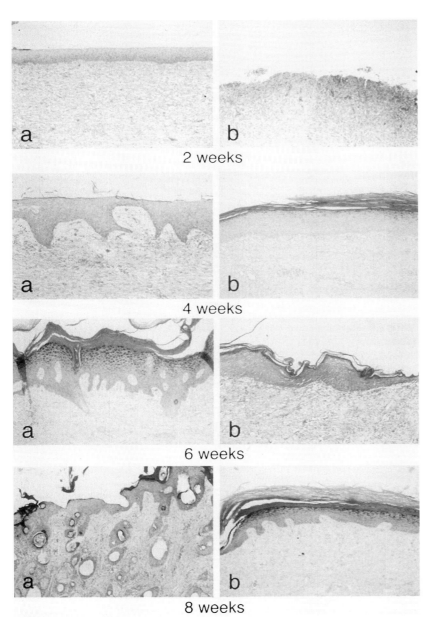

2 weeks

4 weeks

6 weeks

8 weeks

FIGURE 43–8. Comparative neoskin histologies from engineered (*A*) and acellular (*B*) sites at different times following implantation, in weeks. Notice the faster epithelization time and higher level of organization of the engineered specimens. (H&E, original magnification × 100.) (From Fauza DO, Fishman S, Mehegan K, et al: Videofetoscopically assisted fetal tissue engineering: Skin replacement. J Pediatr Surg 33:357–361, 1998, with permission.) *See Color Plate 6*

and fetal surgery. It is a very promising concept that has barely started to be explored, with many questions yet to be answered and numerous evolutionary paths, including unsuspected ones, yet to be pursued.

Unlike postnatal cells, most fetal cell lines are yet to be studied for tissue engineering purposes. The optimal timing for harvest of each kind of fetal cell remains to be determined, along with their growth, differentiation, preservation, and antigenic properties. Different timings for in utero implantation are also yet to be established, as is the feasibility of instituting banks of diverse fetal cells, either for autologous implantation later in life, or for allologous, or maybe even xenologous applications.[92–95]

As a new dimension of it, fetal tissue engineering shall benefit from the progress expected for tissue engineering in general, which should include several aspects of this multidisciplinary field. For instance, genetic manipulation could maximize certain specialized cell functions, such as insulin synthesis in islet cells, which could be intentionally overproduced for therapeutic purposes.[7] Genetic engineering could also provide missing genes to replace proteins (e.g., LDL receptor or factor IX).[96–99] Cell surface modulation techniques, including but not restricted to gene manipulation, currently under investigation, could delete immunogenic sites and prevent immunorecognition, raising the possibility of unrestricted allologous and possibly xenologous implantation of different cryopreserved cells.[65] Polymer and bioreactor development and manufacturing, along with large-scale cell culture systems, should broaden the range and facilitate dissemination of tissue engineering applications.[7, 53, 100, 101] Optimizing vascularization of engineered constructs will be essential for generating larger tissues/

organs, as will be a deeper understanding, at the molecular level, of the phenomena that govern cell growth, differentiation, and intercellular interaction and organization. Methods for studying interfaces between cell and different materials, along with mathematical models and in vitro systems that can predict in vivo events, will be useful as well.[102–107] Finally, cell and construct manipulation at zero gravity will be examined, as tissue engineering in space starts to be explored.[108]

As a component of the general promise of tissue engineering, fetal tissue engineering may well become the only perinatal alternative for treatment of a number of life-threatening birth defects in the future. Its reach, nonetheless, will likely go beyond the perinatal period, offering unique novel perspectives to various aspects of surgery in the 21st century.

REFERENCES

1. McKusick VA (ed): Mendelian Inheritance in Man: Catalogs of Autosomal Dominant, Autosomal Recessive, and X-linked Phenotypes. Baltimore: Johns Hopkins University Press, 1990.
2. Contribution of birth defects to infant mortality—United States, 1986. MMWR Morb Mortal Wkly Rep 38:633–635, 1989.
3. Fauza DO, Fishman S, Mehegan K, et al: Videofetoscopically assisted fetal tissue engineering: Bladder augmentation. J Pediatr Surg 33:7–12, 1998.
4. Fauza DO, Fishman S, Mehegan K, et al: Videofetoscopically assisted fetal tissue engineering: Skin replacement. J Pediatr Surg 33:357–361, 1998.
5. Fauza DO, Marler J, Koka R, et al: Fetal tissue engineering: Diaphragmatic replacement. J Pediatr Surg (in press).
6. Skalak R, Fox CF (eds): Tissue engineering: Proceedings of a workshop held at Granlibakken, Lake Tahoe, CA, February 26–29, 1988. New York: Alan R. Liss, Inc, 1988.
7. Langer R, Vacanti JP: Tissue engineering. Science 260:920–926, 1993.
8. Kirkwood KJ, Billington WD: Expression of serologically detectable H-2 antigens on mid-gestation mouse embryonic tissues. J Embryol Exp Morphol 61:207–219, 1981.
9. Foglia RP, Dipreta J, Statter MB, et al: Fetal allograft survival in immunocompetent recipients is age dependent and organ specific. Ann Surg 204:402–410, 1986.
10. Foglia RP, LaQuaglia M, DiPreta J, et al: Can fetal and newborn allografts survive in an immunocompetent host? J Pediatr Surg 21:608–612, 1986.
11. Groscurth P, Erni M, Balzer M, et al: Cryopreservation of human fetal organs. Anat Embryol 174:105–113, 1986.
12. Bjorklund A, Lindvall O, Isacson O, et al: Mechanisms of action of intracerebral neural implants: Studies on nigral and striatal grafts to the lesioned striatum. Trends Neurosci 10:509–516, 1987.
13. Wong L: Medical Research Council Tissue Bank (presentations at Sept. 1988 panel meeting). In Report of the Human Fetal Tissue Transplantation Research Panel, Vol 2, Consultants to the Advisory Committee to the Director, National Institutes of Health, Dec: D267-D282, 1988.
14. Crombleholme TM, Langer JC, Harrison MR, et al: Transplantation of fetal cells. Am J Obstet Gynecol 164:218–230, 1991.
15. Edwards RG (ed): Fetal Tissue Transplants in Medicine. Cambridge, England: Cambridge University Press, 1992.
16. Fine A: Transplantation of fetal cells and tissue: An overview. Can Med Assoc J 151:1261–1268, 1994.
17. Hurst AF, Tanner WE, Osman AA: Addison's disease with severe anemia treated by suprarenal grafting. Proc R Soc Med 15:19, 1922.
18. Fichera G: Implanti omoplastici feto-umani nei cancro e nel diabete. Tumori 14:434, 1928.
19. Thomas ED, Lochte HL, Lu WC, et al: Intravenous infusion of bone marrow in patients receiving radiation and chemotherapy. N Engl J Med 247:491, 1957.
20. Vacanti JP, Morse MA, Saltzman WM, et al: Selective cell transplantation using bioabsorbable artificial polymers as matrices. J Pediatr Surg 23:3–9, 1988.
21. Cusick RA, Sano K, Lee H, et al: Heterotopic fetal rat hepatocyte transplantation on biodegradable polymers. Surg Forum XLVI: 658–661, 1995.
22. Matas AJ, Sutherland DER, Steffes MW, et al: Hepatocellular transplantation for metabolic deficiencies: Decrease of plasma bilirubin in Gunn rats. Science 192:892–894, 1976.
23. Partridge TA, Morgan JE, Coulton GR, et al: Conversion of mdx myofibres from dystrophin-negative to -positive by infection of normal fibroblasts. Nature 337:176–179, 1989.
24. Webster C, Blau HM: Accelerated age-related decline in replicative life-span of Duchenne muscular dystrophy myoblasts: Implications for cell and gene therapy. Somatic Cell Mol Genet 16:557–565, 1990.
25. Karpati E, Acsadi G: The principles of gene therapy in Duchenne muscular dystrophy. Clin Invest Med 17:499–509, 1994.
26. Marelli D, Desrosiers C, el-Alfy M, et al: Cell transplantation for myocardial repair: An experimental approach. Cell Transplant 1:383–390, 1992.
27. Grossman M, Raper SE, Kozarsky K, et al: Successful ex vivo gene therapy directed to liver in a patient with familial hypercholesterolaemia. Nat Genet 6:335–341, 1994.
28. Aebischer P, Salessiotis AN, Winn SR: Basic fibroblast growth factor released from synthetic guidance channels facilitates peripheral nerve regeneration across long nerve gaps. J Neurosci Res 23:282–289, 1989.
29. Krewson CE, Saltzman WM: Transport and elimination of recombinant human NGF during long-term delivery to the brain. Brain Res 727:169–181, 1996.
30. Yannas IV, Burke JF, Orgill DP, et al: Wound tissue can utilize a polymeric template to synthesize a functional extension of skin. Science 215:174–176, 1982.
31. Heimbach D, Luterman A, Burke J, et al: Artificial dermis for major burns. A multicenter randomized clinical trial. Ann Surg 208:313–320, 1988.
32. Michaeli D, McPherson M: Immunologic study of artificial skin used in the treatment of thermal injuries. J Burn Care Rehabil 11:21–26, 1990.
33. Stern R, McPherson M, Longaker MT: Histologic study of artificial skin used in the treatment of full-thickness thermal injury. J Burn Care Rehabil 11:7–13, 1990.
34. Murphy GF, Orgill DP, Yannas IV: Partial dermal regeneration is induced by biodegradable collagen-glycosaminoglycan grafts. Lab Invest 62:305–313, 1990.
35. Grower MF, Russell EA Jr, Cutright DE: Segmental neogenesis of the dog esophagus utilizing a biodegradable polymer framework. Biomater Artif Cells Artif Organs 17:291–314, 1989.
36. Toriumi DM, Kotler HS, Luxenberg DP, et al: Mandibular reconstruction with a recombinant bone-inducing factor. Functional, histologic, and biomechanical evaluation. Arch Otolaryngol Head Neck Surg 117:1101–1112, 1991.
37. Yasko AW, Lane JM, Fellinger EJ, et al: The healing of segmental bone defects, induced by recombinant human bone morphogenetic protein (rh BMP-2). A radiographic, histological, and biomechanical study in rats [published erratum appears in J Bone Joint Surg 74:1111, 1992]. J Bone Joint Surg 74A:659–670, 1992.
38. Noda M, Camilliere JJ: In vivo stimulation of bone formation by transforming growth factor-beta. Endocrinology 124:2991–2994, 1989.
39. Aebischer P, Tresco PA, Winn SR, et al: Long-term cross-species brain transplantation of a polymer-encapsulated dopamine-secreting cell line. Exp Neurol 111:269–275, 1991.
40. Sagen J: Chromaffin cell transplants for alleviation of chronic pain. ASAIO J 38:24–28, 1992.
41. Sullivan SJ, Maki T, Borland KM, et al: Biohybrid artificial pancreas: Long-term implantation studies in diabetic, pancreatectomized dogs. Science 252:718–721, 1991.
42. Lacy PE, Hegre OD, Gerasimidi-Vazeou A, et al: Maintenance of normoglycemia in diabetic mice by subcutaneous xenografts of encapsulated islets. Science 254:1782–1784, 1991.
43. Lim F, Sun AM: Microencapsulated islets as bioartificial endocrine pancreas. Science 210:908–910, 1980.

44. O'Shea GM, Goosen MF, Sun AM: Prolonged survival of transplanted islets of Langerhans encapsulated in a biocompatible membrane. Biochim Biophys Acta 804:133–136, 1984.

45. Sugamori ME, Sefton MV: Microencapsulation of pancreatic islets in a water insoluble polyacrylate. Trans Am Soc Artif Intern Organs 35:791–799, 1989.

46. Levesque L, Brubaker PL, Sun AM: Maintenance of long-term secretory function by microencapsulated islets of Langerhans. Endocrinology 130:644–650, 1992.

47. Lum ZP, Krestow M, Tai IT, et al: Xenografts of rat islets into diabetic mice. An evaluation of new smaller capsules. Transplantation 53:1180–1183, 1992.

48. Wiegand F, Kröncke KD, Kolb-Bachofen V: Macrophage-generated nitric oxide as cytotoxic factor in destruction of alginate-encapsulated islets. Transplantation 56:1206–1212, 1993.

49. Rozga J, Podesta L, LePage E, et al: A bioartificial liver to treat severe acute liver failure. Ann Surg 219:538–546, 1994.

50. Folkman J, Haudenschild C: Angiogenesis in vitro. Nature 288:551–556, 1980.

51. Folkman J, Moscona A: Role of cell shape in growth control. Nature 273:345–349, 1978.

52. Ben-Ze'ev A, Farmer A, Penman S: Protein synthesis requires cell-surface contact while nuclear events respond to cell shape in anchorage-dependent fibroblasts. Cell 2:365–372, 1980.

53. Langer R: New methods of drug delivery. Science 249:1527–1533, 1990.

54. Hansbrough JF, Cooper ML, Cohen R, et al: Evaluation of a biodegradable matrix containing cultured human fibroblasts as a dermal replacement beneath meshed skin grafts on athymic mice. Surgery 111:438–446, 1992.

55. Bell E, Ivarsson B, Merrill C: Production of a tissue-like structure by contraction of collagen lattices by human fibroblasts of different proliferative potential in vitro. Proc Natl Acad Sci U S A 76:1274–1278, 1979.

56. Takigawa M, Shirai E, Fukuo K, et al: Chondrocytes dedifferentiated by serial monolayer culture form cartilage nodules in nude mice. Bone Miner 2:449–462, 1987.

57. Grande DA, Pitman MI, Peterson L, et al: The repair of experimentally produced defects in rabbit articular cartilage by autologous chondrocyte transplantation. J Orthop Res 7:208–218, 1989.

58. Wakitani S, Kimura T, Hirooka A, et al: Repair of rabbit articular surfaces with allograft chondrocytes embedded in collagen gel. J Bone Joint Surg 71B:74–80, 1989.

59. Stone KR, Rodkey WG, Webber RJ, et al: Future directions. Collagen-based prostheses for meniscal regeneration. Clin Orthop 252:129–135, 1990.

60. Vacanti CA, Langer R, Schloo B, et al: Synthetic polymers seeded with chondrocytes provide a template for new cartilage formation. Plast Reconstr Surg 88:753–759, 1991.

61. von Schroeder HP, Kwan M, Amiel D, et al: The use of polylactic acid matrix and periosteal grafts for the reconstruction of rabbit knee articular defects [published erratum appears in J Biomed Mater Res 26: following 553, 1992]. J Biomed Mater Res 25:329–339, 1991.

62. Freed LE, Marquis JC, Nohria A, et al: Neocartilage formation in vitro and in vivo using cells cultured on synthetic biodegradable polymers. J Biomed Mater Res 27:11–23, 1993.

63. Kim WS, Vacanti JP, Cima L, et al: Cartilage engineering in predetermined shapes employing cell transplantation on synthetic biodegradable polymers. Plast Reconstr Surg 94:233–237, 1994.

64. Buschmann MD, Gluzband YA, Grodzinsky AJ, et al: Chondrocytes in agarose culture synthesize a mechanically functional extracellular matrix. J Orthop Res 10:745–758, 1992.

65. Pollok J-M, Vacanti JP: Tissue engineering. Semin Pediatr Surg 5:191–196, 1996.

66. Shinoka T, Ma PX, Shum-Tim D, et al: Tissue engineering heart valves: Autologous valve leaflet replacement study in a lamb model. Circulation 94(9 Suppl):II-164–II-168, 1996.

67. Johnson LB, Aiken J, Mooney D, et al: The mesentery as a laminated vascular bed for hepatocyte transplantation. Cell Transplant 3:273–281, 1994.

68. Uyama S, Kaufmann PM, Takeda T, et al: Delivery of whole liver-equivalent hepatocyte mass using polymer devices and hepatotrophic stimulation. Transplantation 55:932–935, 1993.

69. Mooney D, Sano K, Kaufmann PM, et al: Long-term engraftment of hepatocytes transplanted on biodegradable polymer sponges. J Biomed Mater Res 37:413–420, 1997.

70. Kaufmann PM, Sano K, Uyama S, et al: Heterotopic hepatocyte transplantation using three-dimensional polymers: Evaluation of the stimulatory effects by portocaval shunt or islet cell transplantation. Transplant Proc 26:3343–3345, 1994.

71. Mooney D, Hansen L, Vacanti J, et al: Switching from differentiation to growth in hepatocytes: Control by extracellular matrix. J Cell Physiol 151:497, 1992.

72. Choi RS, Riegler M, Pothoulakis C, et al: Studies of brush border enzymes, basement membrane components, and electrophysiology of tissue-engineered neointestine. J Pediatr Surg 33:991–997, 1998.

73. Lopina ST, Wu G, Merrill EW, et al: Hepatocyte culture on carbohydrate modified star polyethylene oxide hydrogels. Biomaterials 17:559–569, 1996.

74. Hubbell JA, Massia SP, Desai NP, et al: Endothelial cell-selective materials for tissue engineering in the vascular graft via a new receptor. Biotechnology 9:586–572, 1991.

75. Cima LG, Vacanti JP, Vacanti C, et al: Tissue engineering by cell transplantation using degradable polymer substrates. J Biomech Eng 113:143–151, 1991.

76. Utsunomiya H, Kim SS, Koski JA, et al: The fabrication and function of a novel three dimensional hepatocyte device allowing flow for mass transfer of oxygen and nutrients. J Pediatr Surg (in press).

77. Hubbell JA, Massia SP, Drumheller PP: Surface-grafted cell-binding peptides in tissue engineering of the vascular graft. Ann N Y Acad Sci 665:253–258, 1992.

78. Lin HB, Garcia-Echeverria C, Asakura S, et al: Endothelial cell adhesion on polyurethanes containing covalently attached RGD-peptides. Biomaterials 13:905–914, 1992.

79. Madison R, da Silva CF, Dikkes P, et al: Increased rate of peripheral nerve regeneration using bioresorbable nerve guides and a laminin-containing gel. Exp Neurol 88:767–772, 1985.

80. Valentini RF, Vargo TG, Gardella JA, et al: Electrically charged polymeric substrates enhance nerve fibre outgrowth in vitro. Biomaterials 13:183–190, 1992.

81. Chang AS, Yannas IV: In Smith B, Adelman G (eds): Neuroscience Year. Boston: Birkhauser, 1992, pp 125–126.

82. Christenson L, Dionne KE, Lysaght MJ: In Goosen MFA (ed): Fundamentals of Animal Cell Encapsulation and Immobilization. Boca Raton, FL: CRC Press, 1993, pp 7–41.

83. Lanza RP, Sullivan SJ, Chick WL: Perspectives in diabetes islet transplantation with immunoisolation. Diabetes 41:1503–1510, 1992.

84. L'Heureux, Paquet S, Labbe R, et al: A completely biological tissue-engineered human blood vessel. FASEB J 12:47–56, 1998.

85. Freed LE, Vunjak-Novakovic G, Langer R: Cultivation of cell-polymer cartilage implants in bioreactors. J Cell Biochem 51:257–264, 1993.

86. Fauza DO, Marler J, Vacanti JP: Unpublished data.

87. Cho MR, Thatte HS, Lee RC, et al: Reorganization of microfilament structure induced by ac electric fields. FASEB J 10:1552–1558, 1996.

88. Consultants of the Advisory Committee to the Director of the National Institutes of Health. Report of the Human Fetal Tissue Transplantation Panel. Bethesda, MD: National Institutes of Health, Vol I, 1988.

89. Greeley HT, Hamm T, Johnson R, et al: The ethical use of human fetal tissue in medicine. N Engl J Med 320:1093–1096, 1989.

90. Gershon D: Fetal tissue research. New panel for ethical issues (news). Nature 349:184, 1991.

91. Annas GJ, Elias S: The politics of transplantation of human fetal tissue. N Engl J Med 320:1079–1082, 1989.

92. Gluckman E, Devergie A, Thierry D, et al: Clinical applications of stem cell transfusion from cord blood and rationale for cord blood banking. Bone Marrow Transplant 9:114–117, 1992.

93. Gluckman E, Wagner J, Hows J, et al: Cord blood banking for hematopoietic stem cell transplantation: An international cord blood transplant registry. Bone Marrow Transplant 11:199–200, 1993.

94. Rubinstein P: Placental blood-derived hematopoietic stem cells for unrelated bone marrow reconstitution. J Hematother 2:207–210, 1993.

95. Borel Rinkes IH, Toner M, Sheeha SJ, et al: Long-term functional recovery of hepatocytes after cryopreservation in a three-dimensional culture configuration. Cell Transplant 1:281–292, 1992.

96. Armentano D, Thompson AR, Darlington G, et al: Expression of human factor IX in rabbit hepatocytes by retrovirus-mediated gene transfer: Potential for gene therapy of hemophilia B. Proc Natl Acad Sci U S A 87:6141–6145, 1990.

97. Chowdhury JR, Grossman M, Gupta S, et al: Long-term improvement of hypercholesterolemia after ex vivo gene therapy in LDLR-deficient rabbits. Science 254:1802–1805, 1991.

98. Raper SE, Wilson JM: Cell transplantation in liver-directed gene therapy. Cell Transplant 2:381–400, 1993.

99. Grossman M, Raper SE, Kozarsky K, et al: Successful ex vivo gene therapy directed to liver in a patient with familial hyper-cholesterolaemia. Nat Genet 6:335–341, 1994.

100. Hu WS, Anning JG: Large-scale mammalian cell culture. Curr Opin Biotech 8:148–153, 1997.

101. Mikos AG, Bao Y, Cima LG, et al: Preparation of poly (glycolic acid) bonded fiber structures for cell attachment and transplantation. J Biomed Mater Res 27:183–189, 1993.

102. Ratner BD: Surface modification of polymers: Chemical, biological and surface analytical challenges. Biosens Bioelectron 10:797–804, 1995.

103. Lauffenberger DA: Models for receptor-mediated cell phenomena: Adhesion and migration. Annu Rev Biophys Chem 20:387–414, 1991.

104. Hsieh HJ, Li NQ, Frangos JA: Pulsatile and steady flow induces c-fos expression in human endothelial cells. J Cell Physiol 154:143–151, 1993.

105. Nerem RM, Girard PR: Hemodynamic influences on vascular endothelial biology. Toxicol Pathol 18:572–582, 1990.

106. Parkhurst MR, Saltzman WM: Quantification of human neutrophil motility in three-dimensional collagen gels. Effect of collagen concentration. Biophys J 61:306–315, 1992.

107. Guido S, Tranquillo RT: A methodology for the systematic and quantitative study of cell contact guidance in oriented collagen gels. Correlation of fibroblast orientation and gel birefringence. J Cell Sci 105:317–331, 1993.

108. Saltzman WM: Weaving cartilage at zero g: The reality of tissue engineering in space. Proc Natl Acad Sci U S A 94:13380–13382, 1997.

CHAPTER *44*

Fetal Wound Healing: The Role of Homeobox Genes

ERIC J. STELNICKI and COREY LARGMAN

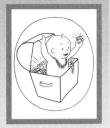

Most of the previous chapters in this book have dealt with the general topic of how we, as physicians, can intervene on behalf of an abnormally developing fetus. This chapter will turn this topic on its head, and instead explore some ways that human fetal biology may potentially benefit those of us who have already wandered outside the womb.

The mammalian fetus is unique in many ways, but perhaps one of its most exciting attributes is its ability to heal cutaneous wounds without scar in a manner more akin to tissue regeneration than classic wound repair. This phenomenon is a complex process that results in the scarless repair of fetal skin if the injury occurs within the first two trimesters of development. After this developmental stage the fetus begins to show increasing signs of adult-like wound healing, so that by birth all wounds are repaired by generating a large amount of scar[1] (Fig. 44–1). Scarless wound healing is seen frequently in lower organisms like the newt, but is without precedent in mammalian tissues. How this process of tissue regeneration occurs is poorly understood, but we hypothesize that developmentally restricted genes that regulate normal skin formation also orchestrate this regenerative repair.

Comparison of this process to adult wound healing has revealed several important differences, summarized in Table 44–1, including changes in connective tissue matrix deposition[2]; alterations in the type of cellular migration into the wound site[3]; and the differential expression of growth factors such as transforming growth factor-1 (TGF-1), whose expression is up-regulated in adult wound healing but remains low during the process of scarless tissue repair.[4–6] Tenascin, an extracellular matrix molecule, has been shown to be deposited more expeditiously in fetal compared to adult wounds. This molecule, which is also spatially restricted during placode formation in early skin development, is regulated in vitro by homeodomain proteins.[3, 7]

The process of wound healing is also dramatically different between fetal and adult wounds. In the adult, dermal wound healing is initiated via an inflammatory response mediated by macrophages, which in turn at-

tract fibroblasts into the wound. These adult fibroblasts then lay down an extracellular matrix, consisting mostly of type I collagen, in an irregular pattern that results in scar formation over a period of weeks to months. In contrast, fetal dermal wound healing is mediated by local fibroblasts, which are rapidly activated in response to cutaneous injury.[8] These fibroblasts lay down an extracellular matrix and then deposit predominantly type III collagen, resulting in the restoration of normal dermal architecture within 3 to 7 days.[9] This enhanced process carries over to reepithelialization, which also occurs at an accelerated rate in the fetal wound.

In general, however, little is understood about how the mammalian process of tissue regeneration is regulated at the level of gene transcription, as most of the above findings likely represent changes that are occurring at the end of a complex regulatory cascade. Understanding how this process is initiated would have implications not only for adult wound healing but also for the treatment of other diseases characterized by scar formation.

Since fetal wound healing appears to be a tissue regenerative process rather than a repair mechanism, we and others have tried to better understand it by studying the model of newt and frog limb regeneration.[10, 11] Like fetal wound healing, the processes involved in regrowing an amputated part are complex. What is clear is that in both the newt and frog, the regeneration of limbs is marked by the induction of homeobox gene expression.[12] Thus the process of dedifferentiation of tissues appears to be correlated with reexpression of homeobox genes whose original function was to regulate proper limb development. It is also striking that mesodermal signals associated with the zone of polarizing activity, which regulates limb development, can be mimicked by either exogenous retinoic acid or sonic hedgehog protein, both of which appear to activate homeobox gene expression.[13, 14] Building on these data, it has been suggested that a similar set of homeobox genes may also be important for the process of tissue regeneration in the mammalian fetus.[15, 16] Our work has been centered on defining (1) which homeobox genes are expressed throughout human skin development, (2) what are the temporal

669

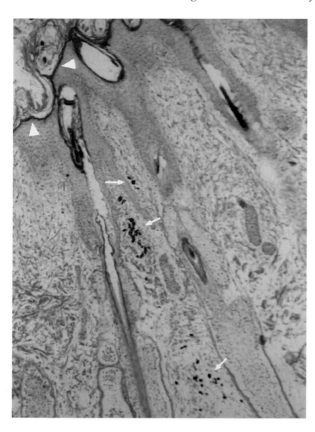

FIGURE 44–1. Adult versus fetal wound healing. The figure is a Mason's trichrome stained full-thickness incisional fetal wound, 5 days after wounding. Here the normal skin architecture is restored and there is no scar. *Arrows* mark the India ink showing the wound site, and *arrowheads* denote the dermal/epidermal junction.

and spatial expression patterns of these genes that may coordinate tissue skin generation, and (3) which homeobox genes are directly involved in the process of scarless cutaneous wound repair.

What Are Homeobox Genes?

Homeobox genes were initially described as a set of developmental genes in *Drosophila* that delineate body pattern.[17, 18] These genes share a highly conserved 183 nucleotide sequence (the homeobox), which encodes a 61-amino-acid DNA-binding motif (the homeodomain).[19] The protein products of these genes are thought to function as transcription factors. In early studies, the *Antennapedia* gene was used to isolate a large number of related mammalian homeobox genes. These so-called *Antennapedia*-like or class I homeobox genes are referred to as the *HOX* genes and are found in four genomic clusters (A, B, C, and D)[20] (Fig. 44–2). Individual genes can be aligned in paralog groups on the basis of sequence homology, such that *HOXA13* and *HOXB13* share extremely conserved homeoproteins and would be expected to bind to the same gene regulatory targets. In addition to the *HOX* homeobox genes, a large number of divergent non-*HOX* homeobox genes have now been described, including the *Pbx, Meis,* and *Prx* subclasses.[21] The non-*HOX* genes are also expressed in specific spatial and temporal patterns during fetal development. One example is the mouse *Prx-2* gene, which is expressed in the developing skin, heart, and forebrain, as well as in diverse mesenchymal tissues during murine development.[22] These non-HOX proteins may bind to DNA in isolation or form cooperative DNA-binding complexes with homeobox gene products.[23, 24]

Homeobox genes are thought to be master developmental regulators on the basis of their specific temporal and spatial expression patterns in the developing mouse embryo.[25, 26] Perhaps the best evidence for the importance of *HOX* gene expression in control of developmental processes are studies that show that mice with homeobox gene deletions produced by homologous recombi-

TABLE 44–1. COMPARISON OF ADULT AND FETAL WOUND HEALING

WOUND HEALING CHARACTERISTICS	ADULT	FETAL
Scar	Present	Absent
Effector cell	Macrophage	Fibroblast
Cell proliferation	Slower	Faster
Speed of closure	Slower (14 days)	Faster (2–3 d)
Acute inflammation	Greater	Lesser
Matrix deposition		
Tenascin	Slow deposition	Rapid deposition
Laminin	Slow deposition	Rapid deposition
Collagen type I	Increased	Decreased
Collagen type III	Decreased	Increased
Hyaluronic acid	Decreased	Increased 3 X over adult
Angiogenesis	Greater	Lesser
	Slow	Rapid
Epithelialization		
Growth Factors		
TGF-β_1	High within 6 hours	Low at all times
bFGF	Present	Absent

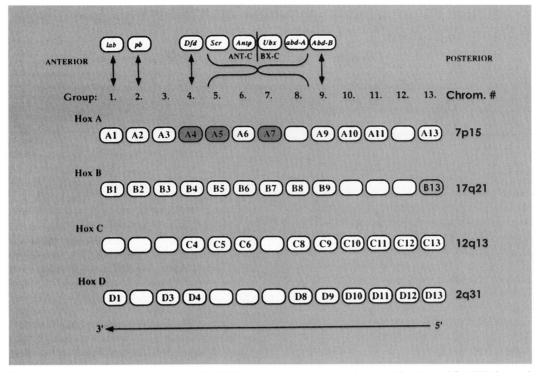

FIGURE 44-2. Mammalian and *Drosophila HOX* genes are arrayed in clusters. The *Drosophila HOX* homeobox genes are aligned along a chromosomal locus that corresponds to their regional expression across the body. The mammalian *HOX* genes can be aligned with the *Drosophila* genes according to the degree of homology within the homeobox. For instance, *HOXA4, HOXB4, HOXC4,* and *HOXD4* are so-called paralog genes and are most closely related to the *Dfd* gene. Thus the human or murine *HOX* genes can be aligned into four clusters (A through D) that parallel the *Drosophila* genes. The three *HOXA* genes most clearly identified with fetal skin development (see Fig. 44-3) are highlighted in red, while the *HOXB13* gene, which is associated with fetal wound healing, is highlighted in yellow.

nation exhibit severe disruption of specific morphologic structures.[27] In most cases, the phenotypic changes occur in tissues derived from the section of underlying mesoderm that represents the anterior expression limit of the deleted gene. Defects in homeobox genes have also been linked to human developmental defects. A mutation in *HOXD13* has been shown to cause an autosomal dominant inherited congenital hand anomaly called synpolydactyly.[28] The overexpression of the *MSX1* homeobox gene results in a skull malformation called Boston type craniosynostosis.[29, 30]

Epidermal Growth and Differentiation

The process of epidermal differentiation is organized by the underlying dermis which, in turn, arises from mesodermal tissues.[31] Experimental ablation of portions of the early chicken notochord result in specific patterned defects in skin formation.[32] The role of the dermis in skin development involves not only furnishing the supporting structures, but also in supplying a variety of inductive signals that orchestrate the differentiation process in the overlying ectoderm. These inducers are incompletely understood but probably include epidermal growth factors, retinoids, *sonic hedgehog* (*shh*), and bone morphogenetic protein (BMP)-type molecules.[33–36]

In *Drosophila Hox* homeobox genes expressed in mesodermal cells regulate the production of diffusable signals which, in turn, regulate expression of other homeobox genes in the overlying epidermal cells. Thus certain genes, such as *decapentaplegic* (*dpp*) and *wingless genes* (*wg*), both homologs of mammalian growth factors, appear to be downstream targets of homeobox proteins.[37] In the developing vertebrate blastula as well as in the limb bud there are close spatial and temporal expression relationships between BMPs, fibroblast growth factors (FGFs), and homeodomain transcription factors that are thought to regulate the expression of these putative morphogens.

Which Homeobox Genes are Expressed in the Developing Human Skin?

To date, there have been few studies that have examined the role of homeobox genes in skin development.[38] Scott and Goldsmith proposed on theoretical grounds that the *HOX* homeobox genes play a major regulatory role in human skin formation.[39] Early studies revealed that *Hoxc6* and *Hoxc8* were expressed in the developing mouse ectoderm.[40, 41] In terms of human skin development, screening for expression of individual *HOX* genes has shown that *HOXC4* was localized to the upper epidermis, and mRNA for *HOXA7* and *HOXB3* expression has been detected in developing skin.[42] *HOXB7* mRNA was noted in 7- to 10-week human fetal whole skin and evidence was obtained suggesting that *HOXB4* is expressed in hair follicles as well as the placode bodies that form between the mesoderm and the initial developing epidermal layer in areas destined to become hair follicles.[43, 44] In addition, *Hoxc6* and *Hoxd4* are expressed in chicken feathers, which is an epidermal appendage equivalent to hair.[45]

In order to begin to assess the role of homeobox genes in scarless regeneration we recently categorized the expression of both *HOX* and non-*HOX* homeobox genes throughout human skin development.[46] We utilized a reverse transcriptase polymerase chain reaction (RT-PCR) technique with a set of degenerate PCR primers designed to detect homeobox-containing transcripts in fetal, neonatal, and adult human skin. The majority of the *HOX* gene transcripts detected in fetal skin belonged to the *HOXA* and *HOXB* clusters (Table 44–2). Of these, *HOXA4*, *HOXA5*, *HOXA7*, and *HOXB13* appeared to be predominant. Transcripts for *HOXA6*, *HOXA10*, *HOXA11*, and *HOXB7* were also detected with lower frequency in whole fetal skin. Like the fetal tissue, the majority of *HOX* gene transcripts detected in the human neonatal scalp were *HOXA4*, *HOXA5*, and *HOXA7*. This same trend continued in the adult tissue, with the additional detection of several members of the *HOXB* cluster (*HOXB1*, *HOXB3*, and *HOXB6*) and one member of the *HOXC* locus (*HOXC4*).

In order to obtain spatial localization of *HOX* gene transcripts, in situ hybridization was used to determine where these genes were expressed during skin development. *HOX* gene expression in the mid second-trimester fetal scalp was detected throughout the epidermis, except in the stratum corneum (Fig. 44–3). *HOX* expression was down-regulated in the basal and stratum spinosum layers of the newborn and adult skin, where expression appeared to be localized to the upper granular layers of the epidermis. Essentially identical results were obtained using skin from the back and arm. Moreover, with the exception of *HOXB7*, which was only weakly expressed in the basal and suprabasal layers of the epidermis, most of the *HOX* gene expression patterns were similar.

Non-*HOX* Homeobox Genes Are Expressed in Developing Skin

In addition to these *HOX* mRNAs, sequences corresponding to several non-*HOX* homeobox-containing gene transcripts were also detected in human fetal or adult skin (Table 44–2). *MSX-1* and *MSX-2* transcripts were detected in both fetal and adult cutaneous tissues throughout the body.[47] In contrast, *MOX-1*, *Caudal*, and *PRX-2* expression were detected only in the fetal samples. The largest number of transcripts for *MOX-1* were detected during weeks 11 to 18 of development, while no *MOX-1* transcripts were detected in adult skin.

In the early and mid second-trimester of gestation (15 to 18 weeks), *MSX-1* and *MSX-2* were both clearly expressed in the cells of the dermal stroma (Fig. 44–4). At this stage both the reticular and papillary dermis are developing and the dermal signals for both *MSX-1* and *MSX-2* appeared to be localized to fibroblasts. Both *MSX-1* and *MSX-2* were detected in the hair follicles that were beginning to grow downward from the overlying epithelium. Within each follicle the expression of both genes seemed to be in the dermal papilla, the collar epithelium that lines the inner root sheath, and in the

T A B L E 44–2. EXPRESSION OF HOMEOBOX GENES DURING SKIN DEVELOPMENT AND IN SCARLESS WOUNDS*

HOMEOBOX GENE	FETAL SKIN ($N = 167$)	NEONATAL SKIN ($N = 30$)	ADULT SKIN ($N = 90$)	FETAL FIBROBLASTS ($N = 20$)	WOUNDED SKIN ($N = 40$)
HOX Genes					
A4	17	13	22	—	—
A5	5	10	19	—	—
A6	1	—	—	—	—
A7	25	26	43	—	3
A10	1	—	—	—	—
A11	1	—	—	—	—
B1	—	—	1	—	—
B3	—	—	1	—	—
B6	—	—	1	—	—
B7	2	—	—	—	—
B13	35	7	—	40	40
Non-*HOX* Genes					
Msx-1	2	17	8	—	—
Msx-2	3	7	5	—	—
MOX-1	5	17	—	—	—
Caudal	1	3	—	—	—
Prx-2	2	—	—	60	57

* Data represent the percentage of each DNA sequence found following RT-PCR amplification and cloning of mRNA from skin samples, cultured fetal fibroblasts, or wounded fetal human skin in a SCID mouse transplantation model. N = number of gene sequences examined for each sample.

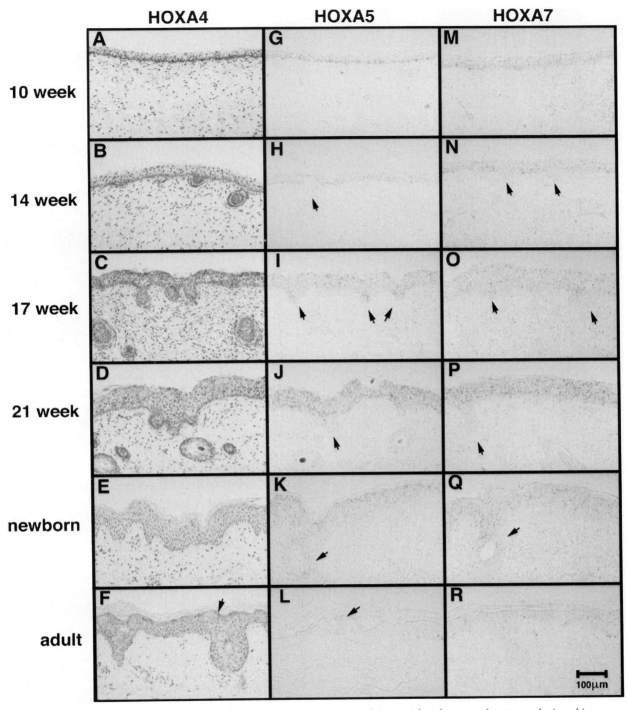

FIGURE 44–3. *HOXA4, HOXA5,* and *HOXA7* genes are expressed in spatial and temporal patterns during skin development. In situ hybridization analysis was used to detect expression of *HOXA4, HOXA5,* and *HOXA7* in serial sections from 10- through 21-week fetal, newborn, and adult skin. Panels *A* through *F* were counterstained with hematoxylin to visualize tissue morphology. Digoxigenin-labled RNA probes were hybridized with tissue sections, and a tyramide amplification and peroxidase detection was used to visualize *HOX* gene expression. All the *arrows* point to developing hair follicles except the *arrow* in panel *L*, which denotes the weak expression of *HOXA5* in the granular layer of the adult skin. Peak *HOXA* gene expression appears at week 17 of fetal development. These signals are absent in the adult dermis. The expression of each of these genes in also seen in the epidermis, but the regions of protein expression vary with each gene at each chronologic stage of development.

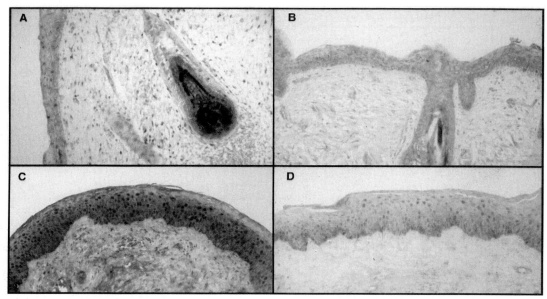

FIGURE 44–4. Msx-1 and Msx-2 proteins are differentially localized in developing fetal and adult skin. Msx-1 or Msx-2 proteins were detected using specific antisera which were affinity purified against the respective proteins. *A* and *C*, Blue staining shows Msx-1 protein expression in 17-week fetal scalp and adult scalp, respectively. *B* and *D*, Blue staining shows Msx-2 protein expression in 17-week fetal scalp and adult scalp, respectively.

papillary ectoderm. This expression pattern coincides with the findings of Noveen et al., who showed that *Msx-1* and *Msx-2* were expressed in similar regions in the feather.[48]

However, unlike the expression of *Msx* genes in chicken skin, human *MSX-1* and *MSX-2* were also strongly expressed in the developing overlying epithelium. *MSX-1* was expressed most strongly in the basal epithelial cells that line the basement membrane. *MSX-2*, although also expressed in this region, showed its greatest level of expression in the suprabasal epithelium. In early to mid second-trimester fetal skin (15 to 18 weeks), the expression of the *MOX-1* homeobox gene was similar to that observed for the *MSX* genes. *MOX-1* was expressed in the dermal fibroblasts, the epithelial and mesenchymal cells of the developing hair follicles, and in the overlying epithelium. One noticeable difference, however, was that several pericytes in the overlying periderm stained strongly for *MOX-1* transcripts. These expression patterns changed markedly in late second-trimester human fetal skin (22 to 24 weeks). As initially suggested by the RT-PCR analysis, *MOX-1* expression was dramatically down-regulated, and was detected only in a few specific epithelial cells located at the innermost layer of the outer root sheath, and expression of *MOX-1* was lost in adult skin.

PRX-2, however, showed a more distinct pattern.[49] It was barely detected in normal fetal skin as a weak signal concentrated over the papilla of the developing hair shaft, with no signal detected in the epidermis, and little signal above background in the dermal tissue (Fig. 44–5*A* to *C*). Thus at least a portion of the signal detected by PCR amplification in the dermis may be due to actual ectodermally derived cells within the hair bulb. However, *PRX-2* expression was detected in cultured fibro-

blasts, suggesting that a portion of the *PRX-2* signal is also mesodermal. Figure 44–6 shows a schematic summary of the major homeobox genes detected in developing skin.

How Homeobox Proteins Might Influence Skin Growth and Regeneration

Although how these various homeobox genes affect skin generation and regeneration is currently unknown, Figure 44–7 shows a summary of proposed regulators of homeobox gene expression and some of the downstream targets of the homeodomain proteins. There is growing evidence from work on both reepithelializing keratinocytes and fibroblasts migrating into the wound site that surface integrins modulate cellular migration during wound repair. Among the few gene targets identified for homeobox proteins, cell surface adhesion molecules predominate. Several CAM genomic regulatory regions are activated in vitro by HOX proteins, including N-CAM by Hoxb8, Hoxb9, and Hoxc6, and L-CAM by Hoxd9.[50–52] The promoter region of the α_2-integrin gene contains both activator and repressor regions with putative homeodomain-binding sites.[53] Gould et al. obtained data that the connectin gene, which encodes a novel cell adhesion molecule, is regulated by the Ubx homeodomain protein.[54, 55] These data support the concept that homeodomain proteins regulate tissue patterning by controlling cell–cell and cell–matrix interactions. There is growing evidence from work on keratinocytes that cell surface integrins modulate cellular proliferation and differentiation.[56] It is intriguing that many cell surface

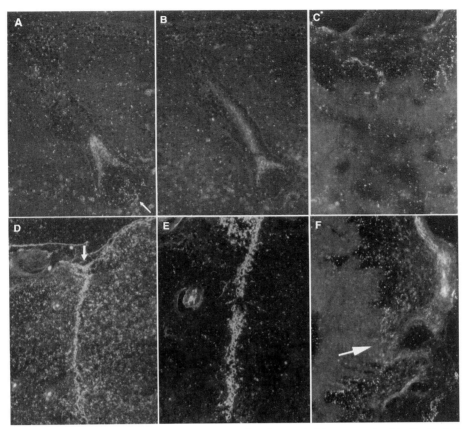

FIGURE 44–5. Localization of *PRX-2* expression in normal and wounded human scalp skin. In situ hybridization was used to localize *PRX-2* expression. *A,* Antisense *PRX-2* probe on second-trimester fetal skin showing expression localized to the dermal papillae (*small arrow*). *B,* Control sense *PRX-2* probe on second-trimester fetal skin. *C,* Antisense *PRX-2* probe on normal adult skin. *D,* Antisense *PRX-2* probe on wounded second-trimester fetal skin, showing up-regulation of the signal for *PRX-2.* The *thick arrow* represents birefringence from the India ink used to mark the wound site. The majority of *PRX-2* expression is in the dermis. *E,* Control sense *PRX-2* probe on wounded second-trimester fetal skin. The strong signal seen in the middle of the section represents birefringence from the India ink used to mark the wound site. There is no signal in the dermis surrounding the wound site as seen in panel *D.* *F,* Antisense *PRX-2* probe on wounded adult skin. In contrast to the fetal skin, there is moderate up-regulation of *PRX-2* that is localized to the epidermis, with essentially no signal in the dermis surrounding the wound site (*arrow*). The strong signal in the stratum corneum is nonspecific birefringence.

adhesion molecules appear to be regulated by homeodomain proteins.

Are Homeobox Genes Expressed in Wound Healing Effector Cells?

We conducted a set of experiments to determine which homeobox genes expressed in fetal skin might be involved in fetal wound repair. We had three criteria for candidate wound healing regulatory proteins: (1) they would be expressed in developing fetal dermis, but not in adult dermis; (2) they would be differentially expressed in regenerating fetal skin compared to healing adult skin; and (3) they would not be expressed in adult wounded dermis. An RT-PCR–based survey of homeobox gene expression was performed on cultured fetal and adult dermal fibroblasts, which are thought to be the effector cells during fetal tissue regeneration. In second-trimester fetal fibroblasts, only two homeobox gene transcripts were detected (*PRX-2* and *HOXB13*).[49] The expression of only these two homeobox gene transcripts in cultured fetal fibroblasts was in contrast to the broad array of homeobox mRNAs detected using the same RT-PCR protocol in fetal or adult skin (Table 44–2). Substantial expression of *HOXB13* but very low levels of *PRX-2* were detected in skin samples from second-trimester scalp, back, or leg. Consistent with their detection in proliferating fibroblasts, both *PRX-2* and *HOXB13* were detected in the dermis of second-trimester fetal skin and were not detected in adult skin. Weak *PRX-2* expression was detected in adult skin within the basal layers of the epidermis, with no signal detected in the dermis.

Does Homeobox Gene Expression Change During Fetal Wound Healing?

In order to access changes in homeobox gene expression during fetal wound healing, we employed a fetal wound

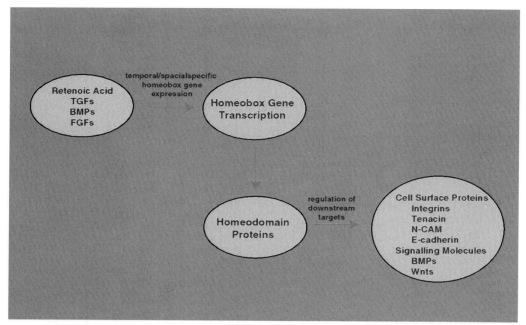

FIGURE 44–6. Summary of homeobox genes expressed in developing skin. A complication of RT-PCR, RNAse protection, and in situ hybridization data for RNA levels and immunohistochemical localization of proteins is summarized. Although most of the same genes are detected in dermis and epidermis, their relative expression levels are different, with *HOXB13* and *PRX-2* being most strongly expressed in developing and wounded fetal skin.

regeneration model, in which second-trimester fetal or adult human scalp skin was transplanted into severe combined immunodeficiency (SCID) mice. In this model, full-thickness wounds made in transplanted second-trimester fetal skin heal without scar formation, while wounded adult skin heals with scarring. At both 4 and 12 hours after wounding, over 80% of homeobox gene sequences detected in three separate samples of wounded fetal skin consisted of human *PRX-2* and *HOXB13* (Table 44–2). Thus the same homeobox genes expressed in cultured fetal fibroblasts were also detected in fetal skin immediately after wounding. These data provided the impetus to further characterize and quanti-

tatively assay these genes during fetal and adult wound repair.

RNase protection analysis was used to quantitate *PRX-2* gene expression in total RNA isolated from (1) wounded versus control transplanted fetal skin, (2) wounded versus control transplanted adult skin, and (3) untreated fetal and adult skin (Fig. 44–8). It is important to recognize that the model employed entails two wounds: (1) the initial placement of a piece of fetal or adult human skin into the SCID mice, and (2) the subsequent wounding of the human tissues. Therefore, an important control was considered to be unwounded transplanted human skin tissue. RNase protection analysis of three independent graft transplantation and wounding experiments revealed a statistically significant fourfold increase in *PRX-2* expression in fetal wounds compared to adult wounded skin transplants, as well as a significant 2.5-fold increase compared to transplanted fetal tissue. Neither wounded adult skin nor transplanted adult skin showed an increase in expression of *PRX-2*. In situ hybridization confirmed that *PRX-2* expression is dramatically up-regulated in the entire dermis surrounding the wound site in the scarless fetal wound model (Fig. 44–5*D* and *E*). In contrast, wounded adult skin failed to show increased expression of *PRX-2* by RNase protection, and expression was still localized to the epidermis at levels similar to those observed in the unwounded adult skin. Most importantly, no *PRX-2* expression was detected in the dermis of the scarred adult wound.

We used a semiquantitative PCR approach to estimate the relative expression levels of *HOXB13* in fetal and

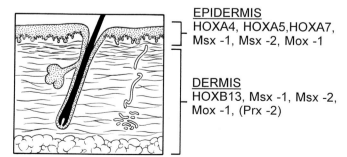

FIGURE 44–7. Proposed regulators and targets of homeobox genes in skin. Retenoic acid has been shown to up-regulate *HOX* gene expression in vitro and in vivo, while several growth factors are expressed in spacial and temporal patterns consistent with *HOX* gene regulation. Among the few downstream targets identified for *HOX* gene regulation are a series of cell surface proteins and a few growth factor genes.

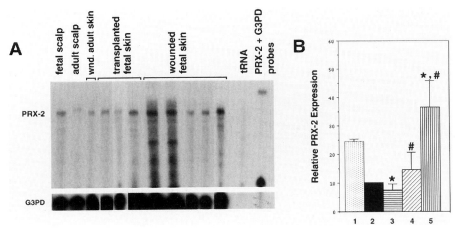

FIGURE 44–8. *PRX-2* expression in normal and wounded fetal and adult human skin. *A, PRX-2* expression in unwounded skin was compared to that in transplanted but not wounded fetal skin and in wound skin using RNase protection analysis. Expression in wounded and unwounded adult skin is shown for comparison. G3PD was used as a control for RNA loading. *B,* Quantitation of the *PRX-2* expression shown in panel *A.* (⬚ = fetal skin; ■ = adult skin; ▤ = adult wound; ▨ = fetal transplanted skin; ▥ = fetal wound; *, $p < 0.01$; #, $p < 0.04$.)

adult skin. *HOXB13* signal appeared to be similar in total fetal and adult skin (Fig. 44–9). However, there was a statistically significant decrease in *HOXB13* expression in wounded second-trimester fetal skin compared to unwounded fetal skin and adult tissue. Taken together, these data suggest that *HOX* genes, such as *HOXB13,* may play a role in controlling the fetal wound.

What's Next?

In order to effect wound regeneration rather than wound scar formation, the migration, proliferation, and differentiation of fetal fibroblasts must predominate over infiltration, proliferation, and activation of wound macrophages, the principal early component of adult wound healing. We hypothesize that the function of homeodomain proteins in the fetal fibroblast is to activate or repress diffusible signals that control the process of tissue growth and development (see Fig. 44–7). Moreover, the changes observed in expression of the homeobox genes during fetal but not adult wound healing suggest a possible role for the protein products in mechanisms that control mammalian dermal regeneration and prevent the formation of scar response to wounding. Understanding this process would provide the first step in controlling not only scar formation, but also in treating fibroproliferative diseases such as cirrhosis, as well as in the eventual realization of the long sought goal of possible induction of mammalian tissue regeneration.

Acknowledgments

The authors wish to thank the Research Service of the Department of Veterans Affairs (CL) and the the American Plastic Surgery Education Foundation/Ethicon Research Fellowship (EJS) for support, and members of

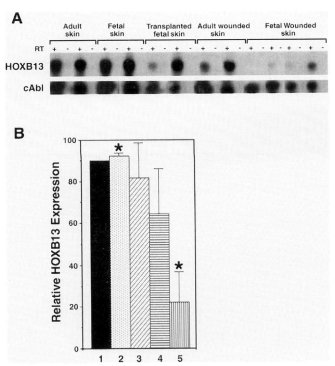

FIGURE 44–9. *HOXB13* is down-regulated in scarless wound healing. *A,* RT-PCR was used to compare *HOXB13* message levels in normal skin, transplanted but not wounded skin, and wounded second-trimester fetal or adult skin. A radiolabeled internal primer was used to detect *HOXB13* expression by Southern blotting of the PCR products. *B,* Quantitation of *HOXB13* expression in the various wounded and control skin tissues. (■ = adult skin; ⬚ = fetal skin; ▤ = fetal transplanted skin; ▨ = adult wounded skin; ▥ = fetal wounded skin.) Gels from the Southern analysis of the PCR reactions were scanned and quantitated. *HOXB13* values were normalized to the cAbl levels. Means and standard deviations are reported. (*, $p < 0.01$.)

the Largman and Harrison Laboratories for continuing technical assistance.

REFERENCES

1. Adzick NS, Longaker MT: Scarless fetal healing. Therapeutic implications [see comments]. Ann Surg 215:3–7, 1992.
2. Longaker MT, Chiu ES, Adzick NS, et al: Studies in fetal wound healing. V. A prolonged presence of hyaluronic acid characterizes fetal wound fluid. Ann Surg 213:292–296, 1991.
3. Adzick NS, Lorenz HP: Cells, matrix, growth factors, and the surgeon. The biology of scarless fetal wound repair. Ann Surg 220:10–18, 1994.
4. Whitby DJ, Ferguson MW: Immunohistochemical localization of growth factors in fetal wound healing. Dev Biol 147:207–215, 1991.
5. Nath RK, LaRegina M, Markham H, et al: The expression of transforming growth factor type beta in fetal and adult rabbit skin wounds. J Pediatr Surg 29:416–421, 1994.
6. Shah M, Foreman DM, Ferguson MW: Control of scarring in adult wounds by neutralising antibody to transforming growth factor beta. Lancet 339:213–214, 1992.
7. Whitby DJ, Longaker MT, Harrison MR, et al: Rapid epithelialisation of fetal wounds is associated with the early deposition of tenascin. J Cell Sci 99(Pt 3):583–586, 1991.
8. Lorenz HP, Lin RY, Longaker MT, et al: The fetal fibroblast: The effector cell of scarless fetal skin repair. Plast Reconstr Surg 96:1251–1261, 1995.
9. Nath RK, Parks WC, Mackinnon SE, et al: The regulation of collagen in fetal skin wounds: mRNA localization and analysis. J Pediatr Surg 29:855–862, 1994.
10. Crews L, Gates PB, Brown R, et al: Expression and activity of the newt Msx-1 gene in relation to limb regeneration. Proc R Soc Lond B Biol Sci 259:161–171, 1995.
11. Brockes JP: New approaches to amphibian limb regeneration. Trends Genet 10:169–173, 1994.
12. Gardiner DM, Blumberg B, Komine Y, et al: Regulation of HoxA expression in developing and regenerating axolotl limbs. Development 121:1731–1741, 1995.
13. Niswander L, Jeffrey GR, Martin GR, Tickle C: A positive feedback loop coordinates growth and patterning of the vertebrate limb. Nature 371:609–612, 1994.
14. Brickell P, Tickle C: Morphogens in chick limb development. Bioessays 11:145–149, 1989.
15. Weeks PM, Nath RK: Fetal wound repair: A new direction [editorial] [see comments]. Plast Reconstr Surg 91:922–924, 1993.
16. Brockes JP: Amphibian limb regeneration: Rebuilding a complex structure. Science 276:81–87, 1997.
17. Gehring WJ: The homeobox: A key to the understanding of development. Cell 40:3–5, 1985.
18. Scott MP, Weiner AJ: Structural relationships among genes that control development: Sequence homology between the Antennapedia, Ultrabithorax, and fushi tarazu loci of Drosophila. Proc Natl Acad Sci U S A 81:4115–4119, 1984.
19. Desplan C, Theis J, O'Farrell PH: The sequence specificity of homeodomain-DNA interaction. Cell 54:1081–1090, 1988.
20. Scott MP, Tamkun JW, Hartzel GW: The structure and function of the homeodomain. Biochim Biophys Acta 989:25–48, 1989.
21. Burglin T: A comprehensive classification of homeobox genes. In Duboule D (ed): Guidebook to the homeobox gene. Oxford, England: Oxford University Press, 1994, pp 25–71.
22. de Jong R, Meijlink F: The homeobox gene S8: Mesoderm-specific expression in presomite embryos and in cells cultured in vitro and modulation in differentiating pluripotent cells. Dev Biol 157:133–146, 1993.
23. Chang C-P, Shen W-F, Rozenfeld S, et al: Pbx proteins display hexapeptide-dependent cooperative DNA binding with a subset of Hox proteins. Genes Dev 9:663–674, 1995.
24. Shen W-F, Chang C-P, Rozenfeld S, et al: HOX homeodomain proteins exhibit selective complex stabilities with Pbx and DNA. Nucl Acids Res 24:898–906, 1996.

25. Dolle P, Izpisua-Belmonte J-C, Falkenstein H, et al: Coordinate expression of the murine Hox-5 complex homeobox-containing genes during limb pattern formation. Nature 342:767–772, 1989.
26. Krumlauf R, Holland PW, McVey JH, et al: Developmental and spatial patterns of expression of the mouse homeobox gene, Hox 2.1. Development 99:603–617, 1987.
27. Capecchi MR: Targeted gene replacement. Sci Am 270:54–61, 1994.
28. Muragaki Y, Mundlos S, Upton J, et al: Altered growth and branching patterns in synpolydactyly caused by mutations in HOXD13. Science 272:548–551, 1996.
29. Lewanda AF, Jabs EW: Genetics of craniofacial disorders. Curr Opin Pediatr 6:690–697, 1994.
30. Jabs EW, Muller U, Li X, et al: A mutation in the homeodomain of the human MSX2 gene in a family affected with autosomal dominant craniosynostosis. Cell 75:443–450, 1993.
31. Dhouailly D: La peau: un autre modele pour etudier la formation des profiles morphogenetiques chez les vertebres. Lexique Embryologie 8:858–862, 1992.
32. Sengel P: Pattern formation in skin development. Int J Dev Biol 34:33–50, 1990.
33. Carpenter G, Cohen S: Epidermal growth factor. J Biol Chem 265:7709–7712, 1990.
34. Asselineau D, Bernard BA, Bailly C, et al: Retinoic acid improves epidermal morphogenesis. Dev Biol 133:322–335, 1989.
35. Francis-West PH, Robertson KE, Ede DA, et al: Expression of genes encoding bone morphogenetic proteins and sonic hedgehog in talpid (ta3) limb buds: Their relationships in the signalling cascade involved in limb patterning. Dev Dyn 203:187–197, 1995.
36. Lyons KM, Hogan BL, Robertson EJ: Colocalization of BMP 7 and BMP 2 RNAs suggests that these factors cooperatively mediate tissue interactions during murine development. Mech Dev 50:71–83, 1995.
37. Immergluck K, Lawrence PA, Bienz M: Induction across germ layers in Drosophila mediated by a genetic cascade. Cell 62:261–268, 1990.
38. Detmer K, Lawrence HJ, Largman C: Expression of class I homeobox genes in fetal murine skin. J Invest Dermatol 101:517–522, 1993.
39. Scott GA, Goldsmith LA: Homeobox genes and skin development: A review. J Invest Dermatol 101:3–8, 1993.
40. Oliver G, Wright CVE, Hardwicke J, et al: A gradient of homeodomain protein in developing forelimbs of Xenopus and mouse embryos. Cell 55:1017–1024, 1988.
41. Bieberich CJ, Ruddle FH, Stenn KS: Differential expression of the Hox 3.1 gene in adult mouse skin. Ann N Y Acad Sci 642:346–354, 1991.
42. Reiger E, Bijl JJ, van Oostveen JW, et al: Expression of the homeobox gene HOXC4 in keratinocytes of normal skin and epithelial tumors correlate with differentiation. J Invest Dermatol 103:341–346, 1994.
43. Simeone A, Mavilio F, Acampora D, et al: Two human homeobox genes, C1 and C8: Structure analysis and expression in embryonic development. Proc Natl Acad Sci U S A 84:4914–4918, 1987.
44. Whiting J, Marshall H, Cook M, et al: Multiple spatially specific enhancers are required to reconstruct the pattern of Hox 2.6 gene expression. Genes Develop 5:2048–2059, 1991.
45. Chuong CM: The making of a feather: Homeoproteins, retinoids and adhesion molecules. Bioessays 15:513–521, 1993.
46. Stelnicki EJ, Homes D, Largman C, et al: HOX homeobox genes exhibit spatial and temporal changes in expression during human skin development. J Invest Dermatol 110:115–115, 1997.
47. Stelnicki EJ, Holmes D, Largman C, et al: The human homeobox genes MSX-1, MSX-2, and MOX-1 are differentially expressed in the dermis and epidermis of fetal and adult skin. Differentiation 62:33–41, 1997.
48. Noveen A, Jiang TX, Ting-Berreth SA, et al: Homeobox genes Msx-1 and Msx-2 are associated with induction and growth of skin appendages. J Invest Dermatol 104:711–719, 1995.
49. Stelnicki EJ, Arbeit J, Cass DL, et al: Changes in expression of human homeobox genes PRX-2 and HOX B-13 are associated with scarless fetal wound healing. J Invest Dermatol 111:57–63, 1998.

50. Jones FS, Holst BD, Minowa O, et al: Binding and transcriptional activation of the promoter for the neural cell adhesion molecule gene by HOXC6 (HOX-3.3). Proc Natl Acad Sci U S A 90:6557–6561, 1993.
51. Jones FS, Prediger EA, Bittner DA, et al: Cell adhesion molecules as targets for Hox genes: Neural cell adhesion molecule promoter activity is modulated by cotransfection with Hox-2.5 and -2.4. Proc Natl Acad Sci U S A 89:2086–2090, 1992.
52. Goomer RS, Holst BD, Wood IC, et al: Regulation in vitro of an L-CAM enhancer by homeobox genes HOXD9 and HNF-1. Proc Natl Acad Sci U S A 91:7985–7989, 1994.
53. Zutter MM, Santoro SA, Painter AS, et al: The human a2 integrin gene promoter. Identification of positive and negative regulatory elements important for cell type and developmentally restricted gene expression. J Biol Chem 269:463–469, 1994.
54. Gould AP, Brookman JJ, Strutt DI, et al: Targets of homeotic gene control in Drosophila. Nature 348:308–312, 1990.
55. Gould AP, White RA: Connectin, a target of homeotic gene control in Drosophila. Development 116:1163–1174, 1992.
56. Watt FM, Hodivala KJ: Cell adhesion. Fibronectin and integrin knockouts come unstuck. Current Biol 4:270–272, 1994.

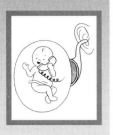

Advanced Technologies for Future Fetal Treatment: Surgical Robotics

OMAR S. BHOLAT and THOMAS M. KRUMMEL

In his satirical drama *Rossum's Universal Robots*,[1] Karel Capek, a Czech playwright of the 1920s, coined the term "robot," a word derived from the Czech "robota" meaning slave labor. Originally machines created to do mundane work, freeing people to pursue more creative interests, Capek's robots develop an increasing amount of artificial intelligence as robotic technology improves and eventually, in his portrayal, become more capable than their human masters. Ultimately, they view mankind's presence as a nuisance rather than a collaborative coexistence that must, therefore, be exterminated as a population. Even in the 1920s, the play caused an uproar; people were fearful that robots would replace human laborers on the assembly line. Some interpreted Capek's play as a forwarning that the robotic solution to repetitive, grinding work might be worse than the original problem.

The actual development of robotics is a recent phenomenon, as the first programmable industrial manipulators were developed in the 1940s. George Devol, credited as the father of the robot, developed a magnetic process controller that could be used to control these machines.[2] As computer technology developed, so did the field of robotics and, in 1954, Devol patented the first manipulator with playback memory. His device was capable of point-to-point motion and was the forerunner of devices used by industry today. This development marks the beginning of modern robotics.

In 1961, Joseph F. Engelberger formed a company called Unimation, and the commercial production of industrial robots was initiated. Since then, robots have been used in industry for everything from arc welding to complex electronic device assembly. Applications for these devices have reached beyond the industrial area, into areas such as agriculture, oceanographic and space exploration, education, and now, into surgery.[2]

With the development of minimally invasive surgical techniques in the late 1980s, surgeons no longer needed to physically place their hands within the body to perform certain operations. Thus, minimally invasive surgery (MIS) has revolutionized our concept of a surgical procedure. In MIS, instruments and viewing equipment are inserted into the body through small incisions; long manipulators are used to perform operations under manual guidance. As imaging and manipulating systems become more enabling, and surgeons become more facile and ingenious, MIS will continue to become more evolved in scope. It has been projected that MIS may eventually be used in as many as 75% of abdominal and thoracic operations, with conventional open surgery relegated to a secondary role.[3]

It was in the field of neurosurgery that the potential for increased precision and safety by using robotic technology during surgical procedures was first recognized. In 1989, a robot was used in the resection of a thalamic astrocytoma[4] and, since that time, robotic technology has been used by surgeons as an assistant in MIS procedures, by gynecologists to increase precision in tubal anastomoses, and by cardiothoracic surgeons in the performance of coronary artery bypass grafting.

Development of Robotics

According to Eiji Nakano, there have been three generations of robots.[2] First-generation robots, created before 1980, consisted of stationary mechanical arms and lacked artificial intelligence (AI) which, by definition, is the ability of a machine to learn through real-life experiences. These robots, which had the ability to perform precise tasks rapidly and repeatedly, were first used in automating factories and continue to be widely used in industry. This technology served as the basis for the development of the Aesop robot, the first robot to receive Food and Drug Administration (FDA) approval for surgical procedures.

Second-generation robots were developed between 1980 and 1990, and differed from first-generation robots in their degree of artificial intelligence and equipment with sensors providing sensory input about the robot's environment. Processing of such sensory data by a microcomputer allows for adjustment of the robot based on collected data, and these robots had the ability to stay synchronized with each other without having to be overseen by a human operator. The Robodoc system, a robot that is used in hip replacement surgery, functions in this fashion. It uses a microprocessor to analyze information from computed tomography (CT) scans and position registration input to plan the procedure. Milling of the femur is performed by the robot in a semiautonomous fashion and is more precise than the conventional method of performing this procedure.[5]

A third-generation of robots have evolved since 1990, and are characterized as mobile, autonomous creatures that make extensive use of AI. They contain a controller and can perform tasks without either human or computer supervision. Current medical applications of these robots include the development of microrobots that can travel autonomously within the human body to make exploration of body cavities even less invasive. In this direction, researchers at the California Institute of Technology and Massachusetts Institute of Technology are developing microrobots that could be used to perform colonoscopy. These devices are between 2 and 4 cm in length and propel themselves through the colon.[6]

Rationale for Using Robotics

In industry, robots allow increased productivity in a cost-effective fashion; robots are relatively inexpensive and hard working, and perform tasks precisely and repetitively without fatigue. Robots can be employed for tasks too dangerous or impossible for a human and, at their current state, require relatively little maintenance to function properly. Robotic technology has the potential for markedly increasing control of human factors, and therein lies the reason the medical profession would seek to harness this technology.

However, the potential problems created by the introduction of robots into the operating room are real, and mirror those that arose when robots were introduced into industry in the 1960s. As in Capek's play, workers feared that robots would displace them. In the United States, organized labor lobbied extensively to delay the introduction of robots into industry. However, while the goal of these efforts was to maintain jobs, it had the opposite effect: the United States lost its competitive edge and countries such as Japan that embraced this new technology thrived.[7] Presently, in a similar, double-edged fashion, while operating room personnel may fear displacement, the introduction of a device that could increase precision and decrease error may result in an economic advantage for facilities using these devices. Just as in industry, hospitals that implement such technology may have an advantage; as elsewhere, automation and related high technology may be the keys to economic survival for some institutions.[7]

The use of robotics for retinal surgery readily illustrates these points. Retinal surgery requires precise positioning of a laser, within 25 μm of a target, in order to avoid damaging retinal blood vessels. If a retinal vessel is damaged, a retinal hematoma and subsequent blindness may occur. The unaided human hand cannot reliably direct a surgical instrument to within less than 100 μm of its target,[8] and as surgeons become fatigued they develop an intention tremor that further decreases their accuracy. Finally, the eye itself has a natural motion of 200 Hz and acts as a moving target.[8] The combination of these factors creates a situation that lacks the precision that both the surgeon and the patient demand, but is well within the capabilities of current robotic technology.

Robotic systems have been developed that overcome human limitations for this application. Using computer integration, the motion of the eye can be tracked and the eye made to appear stationary; similarly, the surgeon's tremor can be electronically filtered out. The end result is a system that can position a laser to within 10 μm of a target, making it ten times more accurate than an unaided human hand.[8] The major benefit of using a robotic system with this level of precision is improved task performance, with subsequent improvement in patient outcome. Other perceived benefits include diminished use of medical personnel and decreased operative expense.

Ethical Considerations

One of the fundamental principles of medicine is "first, do no harm." Thus, the safety of any new device is critical. Although there are some standards for devices that rely on computer software for significant aspects of their function, the use of computer and robotic system in surgery is still novel.[9] Isaac Asimov first dealt with such ethical issues regarding the use of robotic technology in 1942. His short story, *Runaround*, describes "The Three Rules of Robotics":

1. A robot may not injure a human being or, through inaction, allow one to come to harm.
2. A robot must obey all orders given to it from humans, except where such orders would contradict the First Law.
3. A robot must protect its own existence, except when to do so would contradict the First Law or the Second Laws.

Most ethicists agree that this is a good basic outline for governing robots that act autonomously. For the moment, most robots currently in FDA trials lack autonomy; they either mimic the motions made by a surgeon or perform a task under the direct supervision of a surgeon. Thus, they are as safe as the surgeon using this new technology. As medical robots are refined and robots are allowed to function more autonomously, these three rules will become more germane. Engineers designing these systems will need to incorporate redundant safety systems, preventing robots from causing harm.

Current Clinical Applications

Research in the use of robotic technology to perform surgical procedures has reached a critical stage; multiple laboratories around the world have developed robotics systems currently undergoing clinical trials or are being implemented into clinical practice. The use of robots to perform surgical procedures has three main advantages over humans: they have greater three-dimensional (3-D) spatial accuracy, are more reliable, and can achieve much greater precision.[11]

The robots currently in use for automated surgical operations are modified industrial robots. At their current state of development, these industrial robots are readily applied to surgical tasks. As their applications continue to expand and as they prove themselves, specific surgical robots may follow.

General Surgery

In recent years, MIS has replaced many conventional open surgical procedures. The application of MIS to more complex procedures has been slow because many surgeons find the current equipment awkward and cumbersome. Robotics systems have been developed to aid in the performance of MIS so as to overcome this limitation. The first robot to receive FDA approval and enter into routine clinical use was the Aesop robotic arm (Computer Motion Inc., Santa Barbara, CA) (Fig. 45–1).

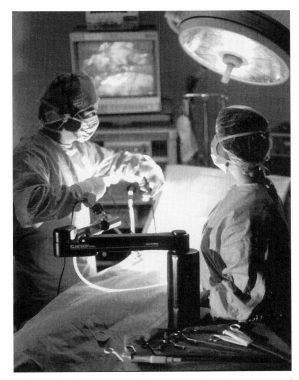

FIGURE 45–1. The Aesop robotic arm can serve as an assistant during laparoscopic surgery and eliminates the need for a human assistant. (Photograph by Bobbi Bennett for Computer Motion Inc., Santa Barbara, CA, copyright 1999.) *See Color Plate 6*

This multiaxis robotic arm is capable of movement along the x- and y-axes in addition to rotational motion, allowing it to maneuver with 6 degrees of freedom. Its primary function is to control the endoscopic camera during minimally invasive surgery. While camera control is a critical component of the successful performance of laparoscopic procedures, it is usually relegated to the least experienced member of the operating team. An unskilled assistant can impair the successful performance of the procedure and increase the stress associated with the performance of the procedure. With the Aesop robotic system, the surgeon controls the position of the endoscope, through either voice or foot control of the robotic arm. Unlike human assistants, robotic arms are able to hold instruments perfectly still, providing a more efficient operating environment.[12]

The Aesop system has, in some situations, been used to replace surgical assistants. Complete robotic-assisted, single-surgeon surgery has been successfully performed with no perioperative complications.[13] Studies have demonstrated that this technology is safe and can significantly decrease operative time while decreasing the use of operating room personnel.[12] This robot has been used successfully during various procedures, including cholecystectomy, herniorrhaphy, appendectomy, nephrectomy, pyeloplasty and, most recently, complex cardiovascular bypass surgery.

Another limitation of MIS is caused by the placement of instruments into the body through small incisions. These incisions serve as fulcrums and cause the surgeon's hand to move in an unnatural fashion. Adding to this is a sense of disconnection, caused by the lack of alignment of the video axis with the hand axis. The surgeon looks up at the instrument tips on a video screen across the operating room table instead of down at the operative field. This arrangement makes hand-eye coordination very difficult, and engenders a feeling of disconnectedness.[14] Consequently, every motion is deliberate rather than natural, with relatively simple maneuvers becoming difficult and time consuming. SRI International has developed a telepresence system to overcome these limitations.

The Telepresence Minimally Invasive Surgery (TMIS) system is a prototype robotic system that was developed to overcome the loss of hand-eye coordination and touch sensitivity that occurs with conventional MIS technology (Fig. 45–2).[15] It served as the forerunner of the Intuitive Computer-Enhanced Minimally Invasive Surgery System, which is currently being used for microsurgical applications. The TMIS system employs a pair of force-reflecting manipulators with 4 degrees of freedom that maintain a remote center of rotation aligned with the surgical incision. Through the use of a computer workstation remote from the patient, the hand-eye axis is restored and the surgeon's hands are placed on the correct side of the fulcrum. This permits the performance of complex tasks in an environment that feels more natural to the surgeon. Procedures including suturing, hemorrhage control, enterotomy closure, cholecystectomy, nephrectomy, ureteral anastomoses, and intestinal anastomosis were successfully performed in animal models with this system.[16–18]

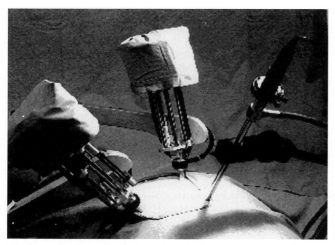

FIGURE 45–2. An example of the Telepresence Minimally Invasive Surgery (TMIS) system performing a laparoscopic procedure. (Courtesy of SRI International, Stanford, CA.)

Orthopedic Surgery

One of the most critical steps in performing total hip replacement surgery is creating a cavity in the femur to accept the prosthetic component. This procedure is performed manually by pounding a broach into the femur using a mallet, and if not performed precisely, multiple complications including hip dislocation may occur. The application of robotics to orthopedics is a natural one, as bones are rigid and can be fixed in known positions. A robotic system called the Robodoc Surgical Assistant System (Fig. 45–3) has been developed to permit precise milling of the femoral canal,[5] and create a cavity that accepts a prosthesis so precisely that it produces total contact between the stem of the prosthesis and the femoral medullary canal. Current methods of femur preparation allow the prosthesis to make contact with the bone over only 18 to 20% of its surface; use of the Robodoc Surgical Assistant System results in as much as 90% contact between bone and the prosthesis.[11]

Before performing the procedure, three titanium locator pins are implanted into the greater trochanter and condyles of the patient's femur, and a CT scan of the femur and locator pins is obtained. Computer software is used to render a 3-D image of the femur, plan the milling of the femoral canal, and select the most appropriate prosthesis for the patient. The patient is then taken to the operating room, where the robot performs the procedure in a semiautonomous fashion.[19] The previously placed titanium pins serve as reference points and the CT scan serves as a road map. Once the reference points have been used to register the location of the femur, the robot drills a cavity in the end of the femur that will accept the prosthesis precisely. The robot can create a cavity to house any make of prosthesis and is accurate to within 0.4 mm, ten times more accurate than the conventional method.[11] Additional benefits from using robotics include a significant reduction in femoral fractures, improved implant fit, decreased prosthetic loosening, fewer surgical revisions, and improved long-

term fixation of implant to bone in young patients.[20] The end result is a major cost savings for the health care system and less time lost for the patient.

Robodoc could also reduce the cost of prostheses, which currently account for almost half the cost of this procedure.[6] Presently, surgeons take measurements during the procedure and select the prosthetic component just prior to placing it into the patient. A representative of the prosthesis company is usually present in the operating room with a selection of devices. This practice is much more expensive than just ordering a single prosthetic device. The Robodoc system can select the prosthesis well before an operation with 100% accuracy, which is 22% better than its human counterparts.[6] Other applications of this technology include revision of total hip replacement, tunnel placement for anterior cruciate ligament surgery, and total knee replacement surgery. This robot is currently in clinical use in Europe, with FDA approval pending in the United States.

Microsurgery

Although the human hand is amazing in its capabilities, there are procedures in microsurgery at or beyond the limits of the position resolution of the hand. This is especially important when tremor becomes more accentuated because of fatigue, stress, or the use of caffeine.[21] Perhaps nowhere else in surgery is precision as important as it is when one is working on structures that are on the order of 1 mm in diameter. The improvements in precision that robots can provide have already been discussed; thus consideration of robotics in this field is logical.[8]

In 1994, the National Aeronautics and Space Administration's (NASA) Jet Propulsion Laboratory began development of a Robot Assisted MicroSurgery (RAMS) workstation, a 6-degrees-of-freedom, "slave"-type robot with programmable controls (Fig. 45–4). This system provides haptic feedback and permits the surgeon to interactively designate automated control of robot trajectories. It can scale hand motions down to 10 μm, filter tremor, and magnify tool forces as displayed to the surgeon.[22] The result is a system that allows for the control of mechanical input and allows for better control of instruments in the operative field. Microsurgical applications for this robot include procedures on the retina, middle ear, brain, spinal cord, nerves, and blood vessels.[21]

One of the more recent advances in robotic-assisted microsurgery is the application of these techniques to coronary artery bypass surgery. Robotic systems have been developed that provide the potential for increased precision and the application of minimally invasive techniques. They permit endoscopic coronary artery anastomoses to be performed without the need for large incisions and hold the potential for significantly reducing surgical trauma. To date, two robotic systems have been developed and used successfully to perform coronary artery anastomoses.

The Zeus™ Robotic Surgical System (Computer Motion Inc., Santa Barbara, CA) is comprised of three slave-

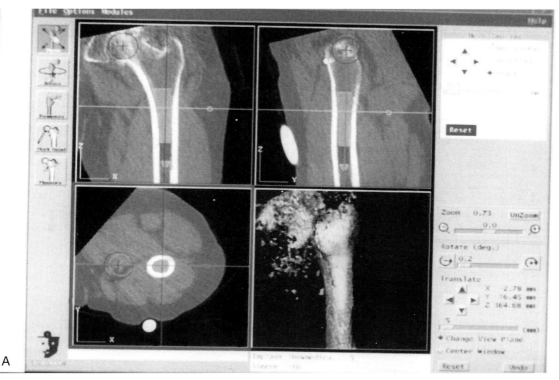

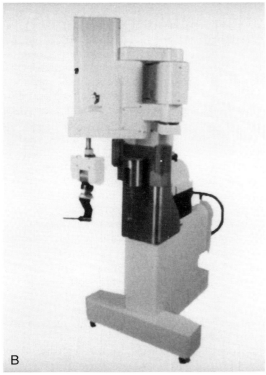

F I G U R E 45–3. Using the Orthodoc workstation (*A*), total hip replacement surgery can be planned, with the prosthesis chosen preoperatively. The Robodoc Surgical Assistant System (*B*) is then used to mill the femoral canal to precisely accept the preselected prosthesis. (Courtesy of Integrated Surgical Systems, Davis, CA.)

type robotic arms, a dedicated computer controller, and an operating console (Fig. 45–5). One robotic arm is used to control the endoscope, while the other two robotic arms manipulate surgical instruments with 6 degrees of freedom.[23] While seated at the console, the surgeon views the operative site with a high-resolution monitor and operates with handles that simulate conventional surgical instruments. The surgeon controls movement of the endoscope with voice commands, just as with an Aesop robotic arm. The surgeon's hand movements are scaled and any tremor is filtered out through the use of computer technology.[23] The end result is pre-

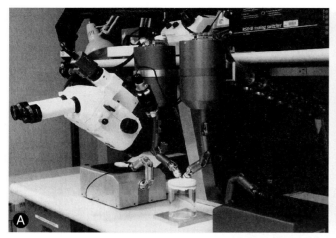
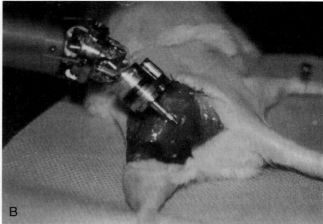

FIGURE 45–4. The Robot Assisted MicroSurgery workstation (*A*) is comprised of two robotic arms and a standard operative microscope. An example (*B*) of a microvascular anastomosis in a rat is shown. (Courtesy of NASA's Jet Propulsion Laboratory.)

cise micromovements of the robotic arms, enabling the surgeon to perform complex, minimally invasive microsurgical procedures with great precision. This device was used to perform the first robotic assisted coronary artery anastomosis in the United States and is currently in phase III FDA trials comparing outcomes to conventional surgery.

The Intuitive Computer-Enhanced da Vinci Surgery System (Intuitive Surgical, Mountain View, CA) is a robotic system that has been used in Europe to perform a variety of MIS procedures (Fig. 45–6), and specifically used in France to perform the first robotic-assisted coronary artery anastomoses. Like the Zeus robotic system, it is a slave-type robot and is composed of three robotic arms that permit a minimally invasive approach to cardiac surgery. Computer integration is once again used to permit scaling of motion and the elimination of tremor. A benefit of this robotic system is that it provides the surgeon with a seventh degree of freedom.[24] This is accomplished by placing a wrist joint at the effector end of its instruments and results in an instrument that behaves more like a human hand.[25] This permits the surgeon to perform procedures in the same fashion as they would for conventional procedures, and provides surgeons with a high degree of dexterity while minimizing the amount of training required to use the equipment.

By applying the benefits of computer processing and the optics of minimally invasive surgery to robotics, these three systems permit complex surgical procedures to be performed with exacting precision. Just as with the conventional method of performing an operation, the key to technical success is exposure; the use of computers, optics, and robotics optimizes this exposure. While the level of precision that has been achieved is impressive, it will be improved over time. Just as computers have been used to remove the tremor of the surgeon, they will be used to subtract the motion of the patient. For example, a beating heart could be electronically tracked and be made apparently still, perhaps obvi-

ating the need for an arrested heart for direct coronary revascularization.

Neurosurgery

Precision is critical to the successful performance of neurosurgical procedures. Minor errors in positioning can result in injury to critical structures and cause permanent disability. Unlike most of the surgical subspecialties, visual landmarks are rare and previous methods of tumor localization were relatively imprecise.[26] For this reason, craniotomies for biopsy or resection of intra-axial brain tumors were performed through large skin flaps and cranial openings. With the advent of CT scanning and magnetic resonance imaging (MRI), computer-based imaging modalities that provided precise information on the anatomic localization and extent of intracranial tumors became available. These imaging modalities revolutionized neurosurgery and continue to allow for the evolution of more precise techniques.

Stereotactic biopsy of subcortical lesions, performed through a burr hole, was certainly less invasive than a classic craniotomy. In the latter method, a metallic frame was firmly fixed to the patient's head and then a CT scan was performed. Reference points on the head frame permitted the physician to calculate a trajectory to any intracranial target visible on the CT scan, and in the operating room the surgeon used an adjustable arc to manually approach these intracranial lesions. This method did not permit direct visualization of the lesion or the instruments that the surgeon uses. Additionally, the transfer of this 3-D information to the surgical field was imprecise, as it relied on a surgeon's hand-eye coordination and knowledge of neuroanatomy for lesion localization. The end result was a procedure that continued to lack precision.

It is easy to see the potential that robotics offers to this type of a procedure. The movements of the robot are more precise and regular. It can work faster and in

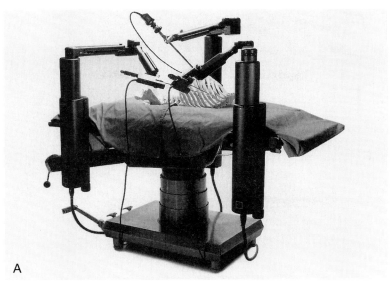

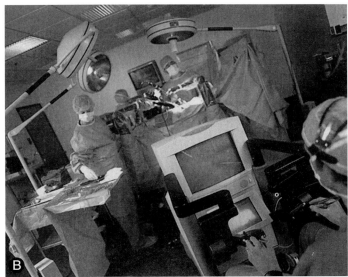

FIGURE 45-5. The Zeus™ Robotic Surgical System (*A*) is comprised of three slave-type robotic arms. During surgery (*B*), the surgeon sits at the workstation and performs delicate procedures using familiar instrumentation. (Photograph by Bobbi Bennett for Computer Motion Inc., Santa Barbara, CA, copyright 1999.) *See Color Plate 6*

a much reduced working space, and can be used to operate directly inside the CT scanner, permitting the acquisition of new images at any stage of the procedure. In essence, the CT scanner acts as virtual eyes for both the robot and the surgeon. In addition, CT and MRI provide precise 3-D anatomic information that can be transported to a stereotactically defined surgical field. The incorporation of imaging-based stereotaxis into tumor neurosurgery not only improved the accuracy with which CT and MRI information could be used in surgical planning but also made minimally invasive techniques possible.

Minimally invasive techniques are attractive because they have the potential for making operations more accurate, with less damage to normal tissues and fewer complications. When combined with some of the newer imaging modalities, such as functional MRI, positron

emission tomography, and magnetoencephalography, it should be possible to reduce inadvertent operative injury to eloquent brain areas.[27] While the use of robotics have been limited to improving the precision of stereotactic biopsy, their application to the resection of tumors continues to be explored. The advantage of using robotic technology in combination with these imaging modalities provides the surgeon with information on the location of the lesion, the location of the instruments, and the location of the eloquent areas of the brain.

Telepresence Surgery

The concept of telepresence surgery was first proposed by NASA in 1972 as a method for providing remote surgical care to orbiting astronauts.[28] At that time, the

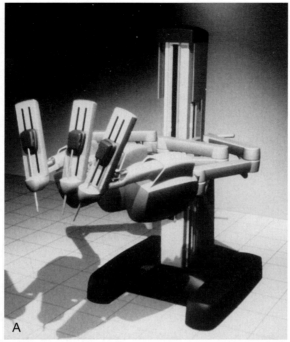

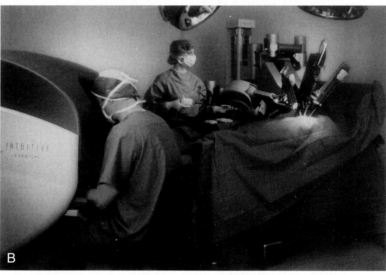

F I G U R E 45–6. The Intuitive Computer-Enhanced da Vinci™ Surgery System (*A*) is a slave-type robotic system that has been used in Europe to perform a variety of minimally invasive procedures. Surgical procedures (*B*) are performed at a workstation, with the surgeon using specially designed instruments that enhance dexterity. (Courtesy of Intuitive Surgical, Mountain View, CA.)

limitations of robotic and computer systems made the development of such a system impossible. However, rapid advances in computing power and component miniaturization, coupled with the emergence of minimally invasive surgical techniques for the performance of complex operative procedures, have lead to renewed interest in the application of telepresence surgery, driven by the needs of the military and space programs.

Telepresence surgery refers to the remote operation of robots to perform surgery and was an inadvertent outcome of attempting to use computer systems to enhance the surgeon's dexterity.[8] This occurred when com-

puters and electrical systems were placed between the surgeon and the patient and physical motion was converted into electrical signals by the computer. This signal was sent between robots on an operating table and a surgeon at a computer console in the operating room. It was rapidly discovered that the proximity of the surgeon to the patient was not a factor in performing the procedure. A signal could be transmitted from remote sites to a surgeon performing tasks at a computer console and, thus, telepresence surgery was born.

Telepresence employs an immersive user interface, permitting the user to work with high effectiveness in inaccessible or remote environments.[14] Surgical procedures are performed through the use of a workstation that uses familiar instruments (Fig. 45–7). Surgeons are given a stereoscopic view of the operative field, with the usual proprioceptive, haptic, and auditory cues. The goal of telesurgery is to create a system that permits a surgeon to remotely perform complex surgical tasks without the need of specialized training. This technology has the potential for providing surgeons and patients with many benefits. Lifesaving surgical care can be rapidly delivered to patients in isolated environments (e.g., rural areas, a battlefield, or aboard a ship). It provides an environment where a surgeon can telementor multiple students without displacing the very person they are trying to teach.[29] Finally, an environment that improves the surgeon's ergonomics can be created.

While the technology for telepresence exists right now, there are some problems that prevent it from being widely implemented. For example, when an operation is performed from a distant location, a signal must be sent and received. If the time involved to send a signal back and forth is more than 0.1 second, it is detectable by the human eye.[2] As the delay becomes longer, it becomes more and more difficult to accurately perform tasks, and when the delay is greater than 0.2 second, tasks can no longer be performed.[8] Thus, the current limiting distance for remote operation is about 200 miles.[8] When one considers that satellites in geosynchronous orbits are 22,300 miles above the earth, it becomes clear that the current delay is prohibitive.

Despite these limitations, surgery has been successfully performed using telepresence technology. At first, these procedures were performed in animal models us-

ing a workstation located 5 miles away from the animals and without any operative complications.[17] Subsequently, in 1997, the first cholecystectomy was performed clinically using this technology.[8] In addition, in the clinical setting, telepresence surgery has been used to assist surgeons during conventional surgical procedures and teach minimally invasive techniques.[30] Open surgical procedures have been performed on abdominal and vascular structures, with results equal to conventional methods, and advanced laparoscopic procedures have been successfully performed using this technique.[14] The benefit of having surgical specialists no farther away than a phone call is readily apparent.

Role in Pediatric Surgery

All of the robotically assisted procedures presented in the previous section have been successfully performed in children.[17, 20, 22, 31, 32] When the size of anatomic structures in children is taken into consideration, the benefits of magnification and the precision introduced by a stable operative platform cannot be overstated. For the neonate or pediatric patient, any modifications made to anatomic structures must be durable; they must be able to last well into and beyond adulthood. The application of robotics to total hip replacement in children serves as a good example of their utility. It is clear that, as children grow, they frequently require revision of their prior procedure, and the number of revisions that can be performed is affected by the precision with which the prior procedure was performed. The precision of robotics pro-

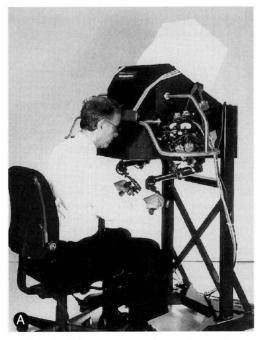
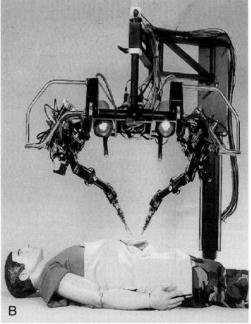

FIGURE 45–7. Telepresence employs an immersive user interface, permitting the user to work with high effectiveness in inaccessible or remote environments. Surgical procedures are performed through the use of a workstation (A) that uses familiar instruments. Robotic manipulators (B) interface with the patient and permit procedures to be performed. (Courtesy of SRI International, Stanford, CA.)

vides these patients with the best chance for an acceptable outcome.

Fetal surgery is another area where the application of robotics is particularly attractive. The rationale for fetal surgery is that the prenatal treatment of certain disorders can prevent permanent damage or death. In the past, open fetal surgery has been used to treat a variety of congenital disorders including congenital diaphragmatic hernia, congenital cystic adenomatoid malformation, and obstructive uropathy. However, the Achilles' heel of fetal surgery has been preterm labor, triggered by large uterine incisions. More recently, a minimally invasive approach, termed operative fetoscopy, has been applied to fetal surgery to overcome or minimize this limitation. Operative fetoscopy has previously been explored in animal models and is now applied in humans for certain fetal anomalies.[33] Unlike typical MIS techniques, CO_2 cannot be used because it causes fetal hypothermia, dehydration, and acidosis. Instead, a small working space is created with Hartmann solution. In general, as anatomic structures become smaller, robotic technology confers an advantage over conventional methods of performing surgery, and in theory the application of robotics to fetal surgery should enable surgeons to perform more complex procedures while further decreasing trauma.[34] While the application of robotics to fetal surgery remains in its infancy, it gives fetal surgical therapy a new stimulus and inspires alternative approaches to treatment of prenatal disease.

Future Directions

As the role of surgical robotics expands, advances in technology will increase their utility. Flexible instruments with versatile end effectors will be developed in order to increase versatility of robots; smart materials may change our notion of how a surgical instrument should be designed; and advanced robotic systems such as microelectrical mechanical systems and artificial intelligence will further expand our capabilities.

Microelectrical Mechanical Systems

Imagine a machine so small that it cannot be seen by the naked eye. Microelectromechanical systems (MEMS) are integrated microdevices that combine electrical and mechanical components.[8] These working machines have gears no bigger than a grain of pollen (Fig. 45–8), and current technology permits these machines to be batch fabricated, tens of thousand at a time, at a cost of only a few pennies for each device.[35] They are fabricated using integrated circuit batch processing techniques and they range from micrometers to millimeters in size. These systems can sense, control, and actuate on the micro scale, and function individually or in arrays to generate effects on the macro scale.[36]

In the most general form, MEMSs consist of mechanical microstructures, microsensors, microactuators, and electronics integrated onto a silicon chip. Miniaturization of mechanical systems promises unique opportuni-

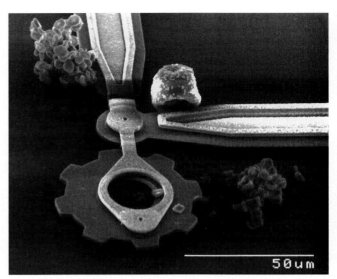

FIGURE 45–8. An example of a microengine with two clots of blood and a grain of pollen providing a reference scale. (Courtesy of Sandia National Laboratories' Intelligent Micromachine Initiative.)

ties for new directions of scientific and technological progress. Importantly, the role of MEMS is not limited to miniaturization of mechanical systems—it opens a new paradigm for designing mechanical devices and systems. The microfabrication technology enables fabrication of large arrays of devices, which individually perform simple tasks but in combination can accomplish complicated functions. This technology has been used to build devices such as microengines, microtransmissions, microlocks, and micromirrors. These devices have also been combined to yield intricate mechanical systems on a chip. Current applications in industry include accelerometers; pressure, chemical, and flow sensors; microoptics, optical scanners; and fluid pumps.[36]

The medical application of this technology remains in its infancy. MEMS will be used on both the micro and macro scales to provide new methods of patient care. Imagine robots so small that they could actually fit inside a single living cell, or travel around the body in the bloodstream, using on-board computers for navigation. At its most microscopic level, robots could be designed to repair damaged DNA. Some researchers have even suggested that robots could be designed specifically to act as antibodies against viruses and resistant strains of bacteria that defy biologists' attempts to find cures.[2] Systems for precise delivery of medication could also be developed. At a slightly larger level, an implantable device, capable of functioning as a miniature lab, could be placed into diabetics to measure glucose levels continuously and deliver insulin as needed. At the macroscopic level, MEMS could develop "smart" instruments for endoscopic procedures—perhaps a laparoscopic instrument that can navigate around corners, allowing greater access for the performance of more complex procedures. Microscopic pressure sensors and actuators will provide realistic haptic feedback. The solid state construction of these devices eliminates moving parts so that there is nothing to disassemble, clean, and reassemble. The result is a device that is easier to use and provides more realistic information about the operating environment.

Artificial Intelligence

Human beings learn through their experiences and, most importantly, by making mistakes. Each year, physicians and surgeons learn by repeating the mistakes of preceding generations. Yet there is no other profession less tolerant of mistakes than medicine. One of the primary motivations for developing AI applications for medicine is to prevent clinicians from learning by making mistakes while performing critical tasks. Heuristic knowledge, or the ability of a machine to learn based on real-life experiences, is the basis of AI. For a machine to behave in an intelligent fashion, it needs to respond to situations very flexibly, take advantage of opportunities, make sense of contradictory information, identify and sort important factors of a situation, synthesize new concepts, and come up with ideas that are novel.[37] The rigid design of computer logic makes this very difficult to achieve.

Although this research effort began in the late 1950s, the first large-scale success was not until the mid 1970s with a program developed at Stanford and used to help physicians diagnose and treat bacterial infections.[38] These expert systems were designed based on the knowledge of an expert in a particular field and, while this program could be used to perform diagnostic tasks, it did not make mistakes or have the opportunity to learn through making mistakes. In essence, all of its choices were preselected.

That biologic organisms outperform any computational system yet developed was the impetus to develop a different approach to problem solving. Thus, in the 1980s came the development of neural networks, computational systems that use organizational principles of biologic nervous systems.[38] Insects are a good example of a simple life form that is capable of a large range of sophisticated adaptive behaviors involving complex sensorimotor coordination. These behaviors are generated by remarkably few nerve cells, which might suggest that they are based on simple mechanisms.[39] They are not. Biologic organisms make use of parallel processing to perform as many as 10^{16} operations per second while using very little energy.[40] Neural networks consist of several simple, highly interconnected data processing units and approximate the complexity used by the human brain to process information.[38] Just as a neuron represents a tiny computer and a system of interconnected neurons forms an intelligent organism, neural networks create intelligent computers. These computers have the ability to "learn" from experience by adjusting the strength of their connections, much like networks of organic neurons. A limitation of this technology is that neural nets are not physical devices. They are simulated devices running as software on conventional digital computers and, as such, have all the limitations of these rigid systems.

Future directions for AI include neuromorphic engineering, genetic algorithms, and artificial evolution. The goal of neuromorphic engineering is to transform microcircuitry into an analog computing medium that resembles neural tissue.[40] The resulting structure captures the essence of neurons in hardware (i.e., transistors, capacitors, and resistors of a silicon chip), generating hardware that can reliably store analog information as an electrical charge. Current research is working to mimic the dense interconnections of the human brain.

Genetic algorithms and artificial evolution attempt to apply Darwin's theory of evolution to AI. That is, the artificial evolution approach maintains a population of viable genotypes (chromosomes), coding for control architectures.[39] The genotypes are interbred according to a selection pressure, much as in standard genetics, with a gradual emergence of the more evolutionarily favored control architecture. The combination of these three techniques holds promise for developing robots that learn, remember, and even evolve.

Cybersurgery

Technological advances have occurred over the last three decades that have changed our lives. Not a day goes by without using integrated circuitry technology in both our personal and professional lives. The integration of high-performance computers, artificial intelligence, and robotics into surgery remains in its infancy. Technology aspect experts agree that these advances in technology will be an integral part of our future operating rooms, and integrated man–machine environments will be introduced into the daily practice of medicine. Highly interactive information networks will be developed and will use human interface technology to permit surgeons to acquire sophisticated medical information. Smart materials and robotic technology will be used to increase both the precision and quality of care. As Dr. Richard Satava has said, "The future of surgery—and of medicine in general—is no longer in blood and guts, but in bits and bytes."[8]

REFERENCES

1. Capek K: Rossum's Universal Robot, English version by P. Selver and N. Playfair. New York: Doubleday, Page & Company, 1923.
2. Gibilisco S: The McGraw-Hill Illustrated Encyclopedia of Robotics & Artificial Intelligence. New York: McGraw-Hill, 1994.
3. Freudenheim M: Surgery: The kindest cut of all is no cut at all. The New York Times, D1, 1991.
4. Drake JM, Joy M, Goldenberg A, Kreindler D: Computer- and robot-assisted resection of thalamic astrocytomas in children. Neurosurgery 29:27–33, 1991.
5. Cain P, Kazanzides P, Zuhars J, et al: Safety considerations in a surgical robot. Biomed Sci Instrum 29:291–294, 1993.
6. Hatlestad L: Biotech: The next great entrepreneurial wave. The Red Herring, May 1998.
7. Klafter RD, Chmielewski TA, Negin M: Robotic engineering an integrated approach. Englewood Cliffs, NJ: Prentice-Hall, Inc, 1989.
8. Satava RM: Cybersurgery: Advanced technologies for surgical practice. New York: Wiley-Liss, Inc, 1998.
9. Taylor RH, Lavallee S, Burdea GC, Mosges R: Computer-Integrated Surgery: Technology and Clinical Applications. Cambridge, MA: MIT Press, 1996.

10. Asimov I: The Complete Robot. Garden City, NY: Doubleday & Company, 1982.
11. Buckingham RA, Buckingham RO: Robots in operating theatres. BMJ 311:1479–1482, 1995.
12. Geis WP, Kim HC, McAfee PC, et al: Synergistic benefits of combined technologies in complex, minimally invasive surgical procedures. Surg Endosc 10:1025–1028, 1996.
13. Cadeddu JA, Stoianovici D, Kavoussi LR: Robotics in urologic surgery. Urology 49:501–507, 1997.
14. Hill JW, Jensen JF: Telepresence technology in medicine: Principles and applications. Proc IEEE 86:569–580, 1998.
15. Bowersox JC: Telepresence surgery. Br J Surg 83(4):433–434, 1996.
16. Bowersox JC, LaPorta AJ, Cordts PR, et al: Complex task performance in Cyberspace. Surgical procedures in a telepresence environment. Stud Health Technol Inform 29:320–326, 1996.
17. Bowersox JC, Cornum RL: Remote operative urology using a surgical telemanipulator system: Preliminary observations. Urology 52:17–22, 1998.
18. Bowersox JC, Cordts PR, LaPorta AJ: Use of an intuitive telemanipulator system for remote trauma surgery: An experimental study. J Am Coll Surg 186:615–621, 1998.
19. Taylor RH, Mittelstadt BD, Paul HA, et al: An image-directed robotic system for precise orthopaedic surgery. IEEE Trans Robotics, Automat 10:261–275, 1994.
20. Spencer EH: The ROBODOC clinical trial: A robotic assistant for total hip arthroplasty. Orthop Nurs 15:9–14, 1996.
21. Tendick F, Sastry SS, Fearing RS, Cohn M: Applications of micromechatronics in minimally invasive surgery. IEEE–ASME Trans Mechatron 3:34–42, 1998.
22. Schenker PS, Das H, Ohm T: A New Robot for High Dexterity Microsurgery. Proceedings of Technology 2004, 1994, pp 115–122.
23. Stephenson ER, Sankholkar S, Ducko CT, Damiano RJ: Robotically assisted microsurgery for endoscopic coronary artery bypass grafting. Ann Thorac Surg 66:1064–1067, 1998.
24. Shennib H, Bastawisy A, Mack MJ, Moll FH: Computer-assisted telemanipulation: An enabling technology for endoscopic coronary artery bypass. Ann Thorac Surg 66:1060–1063, 1998.
25. Skari T: The cutting edge: Heart surgery enters the age of robotics. Life Special Issue. Fall, 1998, pp 14–23.
26. Spetzger U, Gilsbach JM, Mosges R, et al: The computer-assisted localizer, a navigational help in microneurosurgery. Eur Surg Res 29:481–487, 1997.
27. Wilkins RH: Neurological surgery. JAMA 275:1825–1826, 1996.
28. Alexander AD: Impacts of telemation on modern society. Proceedings of the First CISM-ITOMM Symposium, 1972, pp 121–136.
29. Fenton C: Bionic surgery: Advanced technology training telepresence surgery system. USU 1998, pp 3–7.
30. Kavoussi LR, Moore RG, Partin AW, et al: Telerobotic assisted laparoscopic surgery: Initial laboratory and clinical experience. Urology 44:15–19, 1994.
31. Drake J: Computer- and robot-assisted resection of thalamic astrocytomas in children. Neurosurgery 29:27–31, 1991.
32. Deprest JA, Lerut TE, Vandenberghe K: Operative fetoscopy: New perspective in fetal therapy. Prenat Diagn 17:1247–1260, 1997.
33. Garcia-Ruiz A, Gagner M, Miller JH, et al: Manual vs robotically assisted laparoscopic surgery in performance of basic manipulation and suturing tasks. Arch Surg 133:957–961, 1998.
34. Sniegowski J, Miller S, LaVigne G, et al: Monolithic geared-mechanisms driven by a polysilicon surface-micromachined on-chip electrostatic microengine. Proceedings of the Solid-State Sensor and Actuator Workshop, 1996, pp 178–182.
35. Howe R: Polysilicon integrated microsystems: Technologies and applications. Proceedings of Transducers '95, 1995, pp 43–46.
36. McKerrow PJ: Introduction to Robotics. Singapore: Addison-Wesley Publishers Ltd, 1991.
37. Wildman D, Zagorski E, Ekmann J: Enhancing process control through artificial intelligence. Dynam Systems Control 55:460–469, 1994.
38. Husbands P, Harvey I, Cliff D, Miller G: Artificial evolution; a new path for artificial intelligence? Brain Cogn 34(1):130–159, 1997.
39. Watson A: Why can't a computer be more like a brain? Science 277(5334):1934–1936, 1997.

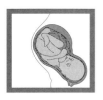

Index

Note: Page numbers in *italics* refer to illustrations; page numbers followed by t refer to tables.

DATE DUE

DEMCO 13829810

ISBN 0-7216-8446-7